AF479052

Medicine in the Tropics

Medicine in the Tropics

Edited by

A. W. WOODRUFF, MD PhD FRCP FRCPE DTM&H

Director, Department of Clinical Tropical Medicine,
London School of Hygiene and Tropical Medicine;
Physician, Hospital for Tropical Diseases, London

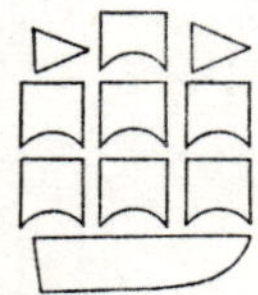

CHURCHILL LIVINGSTONE
Edinburgh and London 1974

CHURCHILL LIVINGSTONE

Medical Division of Longman Group Limited

Represented in the United States of America by Longman Inc., New York, and by associated companies, branches and representatives throughout the world.

© **Longman Group Limited 1974**

All rights reserved. No part of this publication may be reproduced, stored in a retrieval system, or transmitted in any form or by any means, electronic, mechanical, photocopying, recording or otherwise, without the prior permission of the publishers (Churchill Livingstone, 23 Ravelston Terrace, Edinburgh EH4 3TL).

First published 1974

ISBN 0 443 00956 2

Library of Congress Catalog Card Number 73-92051

Printed in Great Britain

Preface

Medicine of the tropics is of great and increasing importance to
all practitioners be they working in temperate or tropical regions.
Much of this importance derives from the enormous increase in
world travel which has taken place in recent years and which has
brought persons from all countries into close contact with one
another and exposed many persons of particular regions to
diseases of other regions. Even in temperate regions a significant
proportion of the community has now been exposed to disease in
tropical and subtropical regions within the recent past. This
increasing importance of tropical medicine to the medical
profession comes at a time when the subject has expanded
enormously and has become too large for any one person, or small
group of persons, to write authoritatively on the range of subjects
it comprises. Moreover there are now experts in many countries
who over many years have made exhaustive studies of particular
diseases encountered by them locally. The book that aims at
authoritative treatment of medicine in the tropics must call on
these experts and for this reason a team of internationally
recognised authorities have been invited to write in this book on
their particular subject. The result, it is hoped, is a volume in which
may be found an authoritative account of current medicine in the
tropics. The approach is clinical and is aimed at physicians
dealing with patients in or from tropical and subtropical regions.
The subject matter comprises not only those diseases which are
peculiar to the tropics or encountered there more commonly than
in temperate regions but also many which, though cosmopolitan,
present in the tropics in a way different from that in which they
are seen in non-tropical regions.

It is hoped that practitioners both in the tropics and in
temperate regions and undergraduates as well as postgraduate
students will find in this volume a working manual for study and
practice, a reference text, and a comprehensive and authoritative
account of clinical medicine of the tropics.

I should like to thank Miss L. Chapman for secretarial assistance
in the compilation of this book. Great appreciation is also expressed
to the publishers for all their help and cooperation.

A. W. WOODRUFF

List of Contributors

1 A. C. Allison MSc MA DPhil BM BCh
Head, Cell Pathology Division, Clinical Research Centre, Harrow;
Consultant Pathologist, Northwick Park Hospital, Harrow, Middlesex

2 B. G. Maegraith CMG DPhil MB BS FRCP FRCPE
Dean and Emeritus Professor of Tropical Medicine, Liverpool School of
Tropical Medicine

3 K. C. Willett MB BS MRCS LRCP
Former Director of the West African Institute of Trypanosomiasis Research

4 P. D. Marsden MD FRCPE MRCP DTM&H DAP&E
Senior Lecturer, London School of Hygiene and Tropical Medicine;
Physician, Hospital for Tropical Diseases, London; Visiting Research
Worker, Fundacao Goncalo Moniz, Brazil; Visiting Professor of Public
Health, Cornell Medical Center, New York, USA

5 Sir James Baird KBE MD FRCP FRCPE
Lieutenant-General, Director-General Army Medical Services; Formerly
Director of Medicine and Consulting Physician to the Army

6 A. J. Wilmot (deceased)
Late Associate Professor of Medicine, Department of Medicine, University
of Natal, Durban, South Africa

7 P. C. C. Garnham CMG MD DSc FRCP FRCPE FRS
Emeritus Professor of Medical Protozoology, University of London;
Senior Research Fellow, Imperial College of Science and Technology, London

8, 9 R. Knight MB BChir MRCP MRCS LRCP DTM&H
Lecturer, Medical Unit, Hospital for Tropical Diseases, London

10 L. Brumpt MD
Professeur de Pathologie Exotique, Faculté de Médecine, Paris; Institut de
Médecine Tropicale, Rue de l'Ecole de Médecine
Paris, France

11 A. Z. Shafei MD PhD MRCP
Senior Consultant Physician, General Hospital, Ilorin, Kwara State, Nigeria

12, 14 A. W. Woodruff MD PhD FRCP FRCPE DTM&H
Director, Department of Clinical Tropical Medicine, London School of
Hygiene and Tropical Medicine; Physician, Hospital for Tropical
Diseases, London

12, 25 W. H. Hargreaves CB OBE FRCP FRCPE
Major-General, late RAMC (retd). Formerly Professor of Medicine,
University of Baghdad; Lecturer in Tropical Medicine to the Middlesex
and London Hospital Medical Schools; Consulting Physician to the
Royal Hospital, Chelsea, London

12, 25 R. J. G. Morrison CB CBE MD FRCP
Major-General, late RAMC (retd). Physician, Royal Hospital, Chelsea,
London; Lecturer in Tropical Medicine, Middlesex Hospital Medical
School, London; Examiner in Tropical Medicine, University of London
and Royal College of Physicians, London

13 A. Abdallah MD
Director-General, Institute of Research for Tropical Medicine, Cairo;
Under-Secretary of State for the Ministry of Health, Egypt

13 A. H. Mousa MD FRCP DTM&H
Professor of Endemic Medicine, Cairo University; Supervisor, Theodor
Bilharz Institute, Academy of Science and Technology, Egypt

14 P. G. Janssens MD
Director, Prince Leopold Institut de Médecine Tropicale, Antwerp, Belgium

15, 16 B. H. Kean MD FACP
Clinical Professor of Medicine (Tropical Medicine), Cornell University
Medical College; Director, Parasitology Laboratory, The New York
Hospital; Attending Physician, The New York Hospital, New York,
USA

15 D. T. Dennis MD
Formerly Fellow in Tropical Medicine and Assistant Physician, The New
York Hospital–Cornell Medical Center; Presently attached to US Naval
Medical Research Unit no. 3, Ethiopia

17 R. N. Chaudhuri MB FRCPE TDD(Wales) FNA
Emeritus Medical Scientist, Indian Council of Medical Research;
Formerly Director and Professor of Tropical Medicine, Calcutta School of
Tropical Medicine, and Superintendent and Senior Physician, Carmichael
Hospital for Tropical Diseases, Calcutta, India

18 R. L. Huckstep CMG MD BChir FRCSE FRCS
Professor of Orthopaedic Surgery, University of New South Wales;
Chairman, Departments of Orthopaedic Surgery, Prince of Wales and
Prince Henry's Hospitals, Sydney, Australia; Hunt Professor, Royal
College of Surgeons

19 U E (deceased)
Late Rector, Institute of Medicine, Rangoon, Burma

20 F. J. Wright MD FRCP FRCPE DTM&H
Physician, Kilimanjaro Christian Medical Centre, Moshi, Tanzania;
Recently Senior Lecturer, Diseases of Tropical Climates, University of
Edinburgh; Formerly Medical Specialist, Kenya

21 W. H. Jopling FRCP FRCPE DTM&H
Consultant Leprologist, Hospital for Tropical Diseases, London;
Consultant in Tropical Dermatology, St John's Hospital for Diseases of
the Skin, London

22 C. E. Gordon Smith CB MD FRCP FRCPath
Dean, London School of Hygiene and Tropical Medicine

23 C. J. Hackett MD PhD FRCP DTM&H
Honorary Research Fellow, Institute of Orthopaedics, Royal National
Orthopaedic Hospital, London

24 L. H. Turner MBE MD MRCS LRCP DTM&H
Director, Leptospirosis Reference Laboratory (Public Health Laboratory
Service, WHO/FAO), London School of Hygiene and Tropical Medicine

26 P. E. C. Manson-Bahr MD FRCP DTM&H
Senior Lecturer, Department of Clinical Tropical Medicine, London School
of Hygiene and Tropical Medicine; Consultant Physician, Seamen's
Hospital, Greenwich, London

27 D. B. Jelliffe MD FRCP FAAP FAPHA DCH DTM&H
Head, Population, Family and International Health Division, University
of California, Los Angeles; Visiting Professor of Tropical Medicine,
Tulane School of Public Health, New Orleans, Louisiana, USA; Formerly
Director, Caribbean Food and Nutrition Institute, Kingston, Jamaica;
Formerly Professor of Paediatrics and Child Health, Makerere Medical
School, Kampala, Uganda

28 C. Gopalan MD(Madras) PhD DSc FRCPE
Director, National Institute of Nutrition, Indian Council of Medical
Research, Hyderabad, India

28 K. Krishnaswamy MD
Senior Research Officer, National Institute of Nutrition, Indian Council of
Medical Research, Hyderabad, India

29 R. H. Girdwood MD PhD FRCP FRCPE FRCPath
Professor of Therapeutics, University of Edinburgh

30 H. Lehmann PhD ScD MD(Basle) FRCP FRCPath FRS
Professor of Clinical Biochemistry, University of Cambridge; Honorary
Director, MRC Abnormal Haemoglobin Unit

31 J. S. Weiner PhD DSc LRCP MRCS FInstBiol FSA
Director, MRC Environmental Physiology Unit, London School of
Hygiene and Tropical Medicine; Professor of Environmental Physiology,
University of London

32 S. A. Hall (deceased)
Late Senior Lecturer in Occupational Hygiene, TUC Centenary Institute
of Occupational Health, London School of Hygiene and Tropical Medicine

32 R. S. F. Schilling MD DSc FRCP DPH DIH
Professor of Occupational Health, University of London; Director, TUC
Centenary Institute of Occupational Health, London School of Hygiene
and Tropical Medicine

33 H. A. Reid OBE MD FRCPE FRACP DTM&H
Honorary Consultant Physician, Liverpool Hospital Region; Senior
Lecturer, Liverpool School of Tropical Medicine

35 A. G. Shaper MB ChB(Cape Town) FRCP MRCPath DTM&H
Member of the Scientific Staff, MRC Social Medicine Unit, London
School of Hygiene and Tropical Medicine; Honorary Consultant
Physician, University College Hospital, London; Formerly WHO
Research Professor in Cardiovascular Diseases, Makerere University,
Kampala, Uganda

36 C. R. M. Wilson MB BS DPM MRCPsy
Research Assistant, University College Hospital and Hospital for Tropical
Diseases, London; Registrar (Psychiatry), University College Hospital,
London

Contents

CONTENTS

1

Immunity and Immunopathology

Immunity can be defined as the capacity to resist a noxious agent, such as an infection, a toxin or a venom. There are two main types of immunity, *innate* and *acquired*. Innate immunity is independent of prior infection and specific responses of immunocompetent cells. It is mainly due to the genetic constitution of the host, but can be modified by environmental factors such as nutritional status, and often acts synergistically with acquired immunity. There are several different types of acquired immune responses, involving synthesis of distinct classes of immunoglobulins and also cell-mediated immunity and non-specific cellular resistance. These can interact in a complex way to protect hosts against infection. In the case of chronic infections, such as those produced by many tropical parasites, immune responses make prominent and characteristic contributions to the observed pathological reactions of tissues. Since the number of different types of immune response is limited, these recur again and again in different combinations. Thus the immune responses to chronic bacterial, viral or fungal infections, and to tumours, have much in common.

In this chapter an attempt will be made to assess the relative importance of different types of immune response in some diseases of the tropics. The coverage is not intended to be comprehensive or systematic, but to illustrate general principles as they are at present understood. Frequent reference is made to animal experiments where these throw light on the situation in man. Sometimes immune responses are themselves injurious, and many immunopathological reactions have been described. These are again relevant to the pathogenesis of certain conditions observed in tropical countries.

INNATE IMMUNITY

Considering resistance against infection from the genetic standpoint, two aspects must be borne in mind: genetically controlled variation in invading organisms giving rise to differences in pathogenicity, and genetically controlled variation in the resistance of hosts. The outcome of an infection depends on the interaction of these two components with one another and with environmental influences. Several genetic factors are known to affect host susceptibility or resistance to particular infections in lower animals and man. Analysing the host response further, a distinction must be made between resistance under control of single major genetic factors (single cistrons or closely linked gene complexes) and resistance determined by many genes. When single factors are important, susceptibility in populations shows a bimodal or trimodal distribution, some hosts being much more resistant than others; and the resistance shows segregation among the progeny of matings between susceptible and resistant hosts. Where many genes are involved, susceptibility shows a continuous distribution and there is no clear-cut segregation among progeny.

Malaria

The influence of genetic constitution is shown by the well known species specificity of plasmodia, which can be manifested by different degrees of immunity. Thus, most monkeys (with the exception of *Aotus trivirgatus*) are completely insusceptible to all forms of human malaria. In chimpanzees, pre-erythrocytic forms of *Plasmodium ovale* and *P. falciparum* will develop in the liver, but blood infection does not occur. *P. vivax* goes a little further, develops in the liver of chimpanzees but only invades the blood in occult form. The simian *P. cynomolgi bastianelli* apparently develops normally in the liver of man and establishes itself in a low degree of blood parasitaemia.

Certain individuals within a species are resistant. Thus West Africans, and their descendants, show marked resistance against infection by *P. vivax* not shown by white Americans. This has been observed shortly after inoculation of American Negroes, who had no prior exposure to the parasite for generations, and so is evidently not due to an acquired immune response. African children with the sickle cell trait are relatively resistant to infections with *P. falciparum* and less frequently die of severe complications of malaria than children with normal adult haemoglobin. Hence through natural selection the sickle cell

1

trait, a relatively rare mutation, has become common in several areas where falciparum malaria was, until eradication, hyperendemic in Africa, Mediterranean countries, the Near East and India. The difference between sickling and non-sickling children is most marked in the age group 1–4 years, when the protective effect due to the abnormal haemoglobin is potentiated by acquired immunity. In older children and adults living in hyperendemic areas the effects of the sickle cell trait are overshadowed by acquired immunity. The distribution of or other haemoglobinopathies, e.g. β-thalassaemia and haemoglobin E, and also of glucose-6-phosphate dehydrogenase deficiency, suggests that these conditions also protect against malaria, but direct evidence for this is not yet compelling.

Viruses

Several examples of genetically controlled resistance against viruses have been studied in experimental animals (see Allison, 1965). One is the resistance of certain strains of mice against yellow fever virus and other arboviruses of the B group. The resistance is under the control of a single major dominant genetic factor. Cultured macrophages from susceptible animals support multiplication of the virus, whereas macrophages from resistant animals do so to a much lesser extent. Thus the innate resistance is manifested in individual cells and is not due to an immune response in the host. Similar observations have been made with hepatitis virus in mice, and one strain of mice (A2G) is resistant to infection with influenza and parainfluenza viruses. Again a single dominant genetic factor controls resistance.

Some genetic factors are known to affect susceptibility to virus infections in man. Thus individuals of blood group O are more susceptible to infection by influenza A2 than those with blood group A. Claims that blood groups influence susceptibility to smallpox have not been substantiated. Although certain virus infections are more serious in some populations than others (e.g. the severity of measles in Africans), it is not yet clear how far this is due to genetic factors.

The spread of myxomatosis illustrates the effects of inherited resistance and the potency of disease as a selective agent. When the virus was first introduced into the Australian rabbit population it was highly virulent and killed more than 95 per cent of infected animals. The small proportion of survivors multiplied and some of their progeny were susceptible, so there was a series of epidemics. However, when the animals were trapped year by year and tested under conditions which precluded the effects of antibody, the wild populations were found to have markedly increased resistance to a standard challenge of virus. The virus itself changed, isolates from wild animals became less virulent than the parent virus, but virulent enough to attain high concentrations in skins of infected animals, thereby ensuring continued transmission under natural conditions. This is a nice example of evolution of host and parasite so as to ensure survival of both.

Chediak-Higashi syndrome

This is an example of a genetic defect which increases susceptibility to infection without directly affecting the systems involved in immune responses. The condition is found in children homozygous for an autosomal recessive gene and is characterised by the presence of unusually large specific granules in leucocytes. This is accompanied by a fair or blotchy skin coloration, because pigment granules in the skin are also large. Affected children show increased susceptibility to infections such as pneumonia, oral ulceration or pyoderma. Many of the surviving children later show an accelerated phase of the disease which resembles a lymphoma.

Chronic granulomatous disease

This condition is inherited as a sex-linked recessive, or sometimes as an autosomal recessive. It is characterised by severe recurrent bacterial infections. Leucocytes do not destroy ingested bacteria or viruses normally, and show deficient NADH oxidase activity.

ACQUIRED IMMUNITY

Origin and maturation of immunocompetent cells

Cells are described as immunocompetent when they can respond to contact with an antigen by manifesting specific immunity. Many lymphoid cells in embryonic organs, or produced by the bone marrow in the adult, mature following interaction with lymphoepithelial tissue of the thymus. These are known as 'thymus-derived' lymphocytes, which are required for cell-mediated immunity. They also participate in formation of certain types of antibody, although antibody-producing plasma cells appear to be derived from bone marrow stem cells without passage through the thymus. The effects of the thymus are evident after neonatal thymectomy or adult thymectomy followed by radiation; the latter inactivates the thymus-dependent cells already circulating or seeded out to lymph nodes and spleen. All cell-mediated immune responses are markedly depressed, and so is antibody formation against certain antigens.

Lymphocytes from the thoracic duct can perform all immunological functions, including transformation in the presence of antigen. Experiments with labelled cells show that most of the macrophages in peritoneal exudates (and presumably in tissues) are derived from the bone marrow by way of the blood. Very few, if any, appear to be derived from lymphocytes.

Immunoglobulins

Serum antibodies belong to a complex family of related proteins which are known collectively as immunoglobulins. All have the same basic

IgM. Characteristically, this is the first antibody to appear after an antigenic stimulus. Later the level of IgM antibody falls as that of IgG rises. Only one molecule of IgM in the presence of complement is required to lyse a cell. Under mild reducing conditions, disulphide links in IgM molecules are broken. Certain blood group antibodies and those directed against pneumococcal polysaccharide are of IgM type.

IgA. Immunoglobulins of this class have variable sedimentation coefficients: 7S, 9S and 11S. These values suggest that IgA molecules include dimers (11S), and even higher polymers, of units the size of IgG. Like IgM, the IgA immunoglobulins have relatively high carbohydrate contents (about 12 per cent). Neither IgM nor IgA passes across the placenta from the maternal to the fetal circulation, whereas IgG molecules are readily transmitted. However, IgA molecules have the capacity to acquire a 'transport piece'

TABLE 1. *Properties of human immunoglobulin classes*

Property	Immunoglobulin class			
	IgG	*IgA*	*IgM*	*IgE*
Sedimentation coefficient (S)	7	7, 9, 11, 13	18–32	7
Molecular weight	150 000	150 000–600 000	900 000	150 000
Heavy chains	γ	α	μ	ε
Light chains	χ, λ	χ, λ	χ, λ	/ χ, λ
Carbohydrate %	3	12	12	?
Transmitted across placenta	+	−	−	−
Sensitisation for passive cutaneous anaphylaxis	−	−	−	+
Reaction with rheumatoid factor	+	−	−	−

structure, being made up of two heavy polypeptide chains (molecular weight 50 000) and two light chains (molecular weight 20 000) covalently linked by disulphide bonds. Five major classes of immunoglobulins have been recognised, all having common light chains but distinct heavy chains. Their molecular weights and biological properties are also different, as shown in Table 1.

IgG. Most of the antibody in serum is of this type, formerly known as 7S globulin. It is normally resistant to mercaptoethanol. Apart from variation in light chain structure (κ or λ), genetically controlled variation is known in both light and heavy chains (allotype specificity). IgG molecules have a complement-binding site, but two molecules of IgG in close apposition are required for complement-mediated lysis of cells (and presumably organisms).

which potentiates their passage into bodily secretions, e.g. saliva and nasal secretion.

Antibody formation

Experiments with labelled antigens have shown that these are very largely taken up by macrophages. The anatomical localisation depends on the site of injection of antigen: if this is into tissue spaces, there is appreciable uptake in lymph nodes, whereas after intravenous injection uptake occurs mainly in the liver, spleen and bone marrow. The majority of macromolecular material ingested by macrophages is broken down in the lysosomal system to low molecular weight, non-immunogenic material, but some persists for a relatively long time. Some antigens, such as pneumococcus capsular polysaccharide, are not readily degraded and can persist in macrophages for months. Antigen injected into mice after ingestion in syngenetic macrophages often elicits more antibody than if injected alone. Such experiments have suggested that macrophage 'processing' before passing antigen on to lymphocytes and plasma cells may facilitate production of antibody by these cells.

Immunofluorescence and electron microscopic observations on single cells releasing antibody have shown that these are usually plasma cells, although some cells morphologically indistinguishable from lymphocytes can do so. Selective ablation and immunofluorescence studies have shown that after intravenous injection of antigen most antibody is formed in the spleen, lung and bone marrow. When antigens are distributed by lymphatics from a local infection or site of injected antigen, antibody is made predominantly in the group of regional draining lymph nodes. When there is local granuloma formation, antibody synthesis takes place in the granuloma itself. How antibody formation is elicited by antigen, and whether this is due to selection of clones of cells genetically predisposed to form a particular antibody, is still a matter of speculation. The light and heavy immunoglobulin chains are synthesised independently on polyribosomes and join up afterwards to form antibody. After other additions, e.g. carbohydrate to heavy chains, the antibody is released.

CONGENITAL AND ACQUIRED IMMUNE
DEFICIENCY SYNDROMES

Many congenital defects of immune responses have been described (see *W.H.O. Technical Report Series*, No. 402, 1968). Some are inherited as sex-linked recessive or autosomal recessive conditions, while others have no obvious genetic basis. Some deficiencies are nearly complete, and affect either the capacity to produce all classes of antibodies (e.g. infantile sex-linked recessive agammaglobulinaemia) or all manifestations of cell-mediated immunity. Children with severe hypogammaglobulinaemia are highly susceptible to infections with pyogenic bacteria, *Candida albicans* and *Pneumocystis carinii*, and are able to survive only because of chemotherapy and immunoglobulin infusions.

Other defects are restricted to certain classes of immune responses, e.g. selective IgA deficiency, which has been associated in several cases with bronchitis, sinusitis and exudative enteropathy.

Sometimes there are deficient humoral and cell-mediated immune responses to some antigens but not to others, e.g. in patients with hereditary lymphopenic immunological deficiency; affected children often die in childhood of fungal or viral infections. Such defects can sometimes be highly selective: thus, patients with vaccinia gangrenosa do not have circulating antibody against vaccinia virus, though their immunoglobulin levels and responses to other antigens are usually normal. Children suffering from recurrent staphylococcal infections lack antibodies which inhibit the Müller reaction, although other immunological responses tested have been normal. Minor specific immunological defects of this kind may well play a part in the pathogenesis of infections by organisms which are normally well controlled by immune reactions (e.g. certain fungi, *P. carinii* and possibly leishmaniasis and leprosy).

Non-genetic processes can also influence the development of immunological function. Infants with congenital rubella infection have during the period of virus excretion markedly deficient levels of IgG and increased levels of IgM. The circulating lymphocytes of these patients do not respond with proliferation to phytohaemagglutinin, allogeneic lymphocytes or foreign antigens. Similar interference with the responses of lymphocytes to stimulation with these agents can be produced by infection of lymphocytes *in vitro* with measles, rubella or Newcastle disease virus or with mycoplasma. This has an *in vivo* counterpart in the depression of cell-mediated immune responses (e.g. the tuberculin reaction) observed during and shortly after measles infection. Depression of cell-mediated immunity occurs also in lymphoproliferative disorders such as Hodgkin's disease, chronic lymphocytic leukaemia, myeloma and Waldenström's macroglobulinaemia, and in lepromatous leprosy.

These immunosuppressive effects are general, and affect immune responses to a wide group of unrelated antigens. This is quite distinct from specific unresponsiveness or tolerance to particular antigens in the presence of normal responses to other antigens. Specific unresponsiveness can be induced readily in adult animals with some antigens, e.g. pneumococcus capsular polysaccharide. With most antigens, specific unresponsiveness is more readily induced in the neonatal period than later. This is not true for all antigens, and antibodies to some can be made even in the fetus. Some immunisation procedures favour the production of antibody but not cell-mediated immunity, as discussed below, and this is another type of specific induced unresponsiveness.

ANTIBODY-MEDIATED HYPERSENSITIVITY
REACTIONS

Immune reactions not only protect: under certain circumstances second access of antigen to immunised subjects can produce severe reactions or even death. Individuals who show immune reactivity to antigens are termed hypersensitive. The main distinction usually made is between reactions of immediate-type and those of delayed-type hypersensitivity. This reflects not only the classical time scale of visible reactions after challenge of sensitised animals with antigen, but also the type of immune response involved (antibody- and cell-mediated immunity respectively). Immediate-type reactions begin a few seconds or minutes after the contact of antigen with antibody, although visible effects may not be evident for many minutes or hours and may not disappear for days. Hence timing of reactions is insufficient to distinguish between immediate and delayed reactions, and other factors, such as the histology of the lesions and ability to transfer the reaction with antibody or with cells, must be taken into account. There are two main types of antibody-mediated hypersensitivity: anaphylactic reactions due to attachment of antibody to cells before contact with antigen, and a series of reactions following formation of antigen-antibody complexes.

Anaphylactic reactions

These are responsible for local manifestations such as asthma, hay fever or urticaria, as well as for generalised anaphylaxis occasionally observed in patients, e.g. those sensitised to animal serum and given a second injection. As shown by well known variants of the Schultz-Dale test, tissues such as strips of ileum or bronchial smooth muscle can take up antibody from the medium in which they are suspended; when washed and subsequently challenged with antigen the strips contract. In hypersensitivity reactions of this type at least four pharmacologically active mediators are released: histamine, slow-reacting substance of anaphylaxis (SRS–A), serotonin and bradykinin. Antibody must first become adsorbed on to the tissues. Such adsorption is shown by some subclasses of IgG, in which case the reaction usually crosses species barriers and is reversible, depending on the concentration of antibody used. It is also shown by antibodies of reaginic or IgE type, which have a higher affinity for tissues, so that adsorption is less readily reversible than with IgG. Antibodies of reaginic type were first demonstrated

by the test of Prausnitz and Küstner. Serum from a sensitised person is injected subcutaneously into an unsensitised person, and 1–2 days later the allergen is pricked into the skin at the same site and at another site. If reaginic antibodies are present a typical wheal and flare are produced at the prepared site. In experimental animals, tests for passive cutaneous anaphylaxis are usually carried out by injecting antibody into the skin, and 1–2 days later injecting antigen and a dye intravenously. Where the skin is sensitised by firmly adsorbed antibody, contact with antigen results in increased vascular permeability so that the skin is coloured by the dye. Two properties distinguish reaginic from other antibodies: reaginic antibodies are thermolabile and passive sensitisation is successful only in the homologous (or sometimes closely related) species.

Reaginic antibodies are not the only ones involved in anaphylactic reactions. The complexity of the subject can be illustrated by extrinsic asthma, in which some specific causative factor is identifiable as the exciting agent, e.g. pollen. Lungs of allergic subjects challenged *in vitro* with specific pollen antigen release histamine and SRS–A. However, it is not yet established that reaginic antibody (IgE) is responsible for the release. In the guinea pig and rat, antigen-induced release of SRS–A is not mediated by a heat-labile homologous antibody but by heat-stable antibodies of the γ-1 class in the guinea pig and the IgGa class in the rat. Thus even if (as seems likely) extrinsic asthma is due to an immunological reaction, the responsible immunoglobulins, participating cells and active chemical mediators are not certainly defined.

Two recent pharmacological developments may come to have relevance in tropical medicine. The only specific antagonists of chemical mediators widely used are antihistamines, which do not control all asthmatic and other acute allergic reactions. Mallén (1965) was impressed with the efficacy of diethylcarbamazine (Hetrazan) in relieving the intractable bronchospasm of tropical eosinophilia and reported a successful trial of this drug in patients with severe asthma without tropical eosinophilia. Altounyan (1967) reported that disodium cromoglycate (Intal) inhibits experimentally induced asthma in man. With experimental animal models, these drugs show remarkable properties: they act after antigen-antibody interaction to inhibit selectively the release of a chemical mediator; histamine release is inhibited by disodium cromoglycate and SRS–A release by diethylcarbamazine. Their action at this stage allows tissues to become

B

desensitised in the absence of inflammation because antigen-antibody interaction does not lead to the release of chemical mediators. However, further controlled trials are required to establish that these drugs, alone or in combination, are effective in the treatment of intractable asthma or other acute allergic reactions.

Immunopathological changes produced by antigen-antibody complexes

The second variant of antibody-mediated hypersensitivity is associated with the name of Maurice Arthus. If antigen is injected subcutaneously into an immunised animal, there is an inflammatory reaction with oedema followed, in severe cases, by haemorrhage and necrosis. The sequence of changes develops more slowly than that seen in acute anaphylaxis, and is characterised by marked infiltration of inflammatory cells, especially polymorphs. Sometimes acute anaphylaxis is succeeded by an Arthus reaction. Evidence has accumulated that the Arthus reaction is a severe inflammatory response following the formation of antigen-antibody complexes, especially within blood vessel walls. It is supposed that locally introduced antigen reacts with blood-borne antibody. Some complexes also form around the blood vessels, and ingestion of the complexes by polymorphs within and outside the vessel walls also brings about degranulation and release of hydrolytic enzymes and of permeability-producing factors from these cells. The importance of polymorphs is shown by the marked reduction in inflammation in Arthus reaction sites if circulating polymorphs are depleted, e.g. by specific antiserum. It seems likely that the local inflammatory reactions sometimes seen after treatment of helminth infections, syphilis or lepromatous leprosy are analogous to Arthus reactions: in this case release of antigen from dying infective agents corresponds to subcutaneous injection of antigen.

The third type of antibody-mediated hypersensitivity, serum sickness, also follows the formation of antigen-antibody complexes. It occurs when an excess of antigen in the circulation forms soluble antigen-antibody complexes, which are taken up by certain endothelial cells. Large complexes of antigen and antibody, especially when insoluble, are rapidly removed from the circulation by the reticuloendothelial system. The endothelial cells most affected by soluble complexes are those of the renal glomeruli. One type of experimental nephritis can be reproduced in animals by injection of soluble complexes of antigen and antibody, or by immunisation procedures that result in the formation of these complexes in the circulation. The complexes of antigen, antibody, and usually also of complement components, accumulate as granular deposits between the basement membranes and epithelial cells of the glomeruli, which are damaged as a consequence. The immunoglobulin and complement are demonstrable by specific immunofluorescence as granular deposits along the glomerular capillary walls, and the complexes are also visible in the characteristic subepithelial position by electron microscopy. Usually the damage is increased by local adhesion and degranulation of polymorphs. Human patients with post-streptococcal nephritis and lupus erythematosus have been shown to have such deposits of antigen and antibody (the antigen being of streptococcal origin and containing DNA, respectively). Similar deposits of immunoglobulin and complement, and presumably of *P. malariae* antigen, occur in African children with the nephrotic syndrome (see section on malaria). It should be recognised that this type of immunopathological reaction occurs independently of the nature of the antigen forming the soluble complexes: there need be no antigenic relationship to renal antigens. However, the second type of experimentally induced nephritis is produced by antibodies against renal glomerular basement membrane. In the latter, immunoglobulin and complement are visible as a smooth continuous immunofluorescent image along the glomerular capillary walls. Some cases of human autoimmune nephritis appear to be of this type.

Soluble antigen-antibody complexes can also localise in arterial walls, producing a widespread arteritis of varying severity, sometimes resembling that in polyarteritis nodosa. Since circulating antigen, and probably immune complexes, are often found in tropical parasitic infections, e.g. malaria and trypanosomiasis, the possible role of these complexes in other immunopathological manifestations deserves further investigation.

CELL-MEDIATED IMMUNITY

In many microbial and helminth infections the immunological responses of the host include not only the synthesis of antibodies against a variety of components of the invading organism but also the development of cell-mediated immunity to some of these components. The term cell-mediated immunity is a generic designation for immune responses that can be transferred to non-immunised recipients by lymphoid cells but not by antibody. The specific antigen-recognising mechanism on sensitised cells may, however, be a type of antibody firmly bound to the cells and not readily released. The main manifestations of cell-mediated immunity are delayed hypersensitivity, including contact hypersensitivity, and the destruction of cells antigenically distinct from host cells, including homografts and cells that have acquired new antigenic characteristics during the course of infection, neoplastic transformation or interaction with chemical sensitising agents. Such interactions are essentially destructive.

Delayed hypersensitivity

In a sensitised host intracutaneous antigen produces after several hours, redness and induration. This increases gradually up to 24–48 hours and then slowly subsides. Histological examination of delayed reaction sites reveals perivascular masses consisting mainly of mononuclear cells (lymphocytes and macrophages), although there may be an early, transient contribution by polymorphs. In contrast, immediate reactions (e.g. produced by injection of pollen extract into an asthmatic or hay fever subject) consist mainly of oedema fluid with few cells. Arthus reactions, due to formation of antigen-antibody complexes, may show a time course similar to delayed hypersensitivity; a distinguishing feature is that the cell infiltrate in Arthus reactions consists mainly of polymorphs, even in the later stages. Several delayed reactions in human subjects, including the tuberculin reaction, are often of mixed type, having both delayed hypersensitivity and Arthus components. This may well be true of some delayed reactions to tropical parasites described in this chapter, in which there has seldom been adequate histological control of reaction sites or confirmation of the nature of reactions by transfer to non-sensitised subjects. Transfer of delayed hypersensitivity can be achieved by mononuclear cells of peripheral blood, or of similar cells in exudates, bone marrow, spleen or lymph nodes. The duration of hypersensitivity transferred in this way depends on the length of time the transferred cells can survive in the recipient, and is short unless the transfer is into syngenetic recipients. In some species, such as the guinea pig and man, interpretation of skin transfer tests is complicated by a normal lymphocyte transfer reaction unless syngenetic recipients are used.

When the transferred cells are labelled, some are found to accumulate at the site of locally injected antigen, but the great majority (more than 90 per cent) of cells in reaction sites are of host origin. It is supposed that a small number of sensitised lymphocytes reacting with antigen can bring about accumulation of non-sensitised cells, especially macrophages. The combination of sensitised lymphocytes with antigen leads to release of a factor that immobilises macrophages. This has been used as an *in vitro* test for cell-mediated immunity in guinea pigs; in the presence of a minority of sensitised lymphocytes and specific antigen, macrophages are prevented from migrating out of a capillary tube.

Contact hypersensitivity

Sensitisation can result from contact with certain plants, drugs and simple chemicals (e.g. oxazalone, a strong sensitiser, picryl chloride or 2,4-dinitrochlorobenzene). The induction of sensitivity follows application to the skin or mucous membranes, and subsequent contact of the skin with the agent is followed by local dermatitis. This may begin within a day, and passes through the stages of red papules, serum-filled vesicles, oozing crusts and hyperkeratotic desquamation. The underlying histology in this situation and in homografts that are undergoing rejection is similar to that in delayed hypersensitivity. In all of these manifestations of cell-mediated immunity allergic hyper-reactivity to repeated contact with the relevant antigens can be built up, so that tissue damage becomes progressively greater. The tissue destruction that follows from this hyper-reactivity in chronic diseases, such as tuberculosis, leprosy or syphilis, is regarded as making a major contribution to the observed pathology.

Histology of lymph nodes

The histological changes associated with the development of cell-mediated immunity can be seen in the lymph nodes draining an area of application of a chemical sensitising agent or the site of application of a skin homograft. There is proliferation of lymphocytes in the paracortical areas, which rapidly enlarge and become packed by the fourth day after sensitisation with immunoblasts (large pyroninophilic cells) which divide and differentiate into small lymphocytes. Sensitised cells belong to the population of long-lived lymphocytes and are concentrated in the 'thymus-dependent' areas of lymphoid tissues, but they also circulate in blood and lymph. In contrast, when the only response is antibody synthesis, there is formation of localised germinal centres in the cortex and plasma cell production at the cortico-medullary junction and in the medullary cords. With many antigens both reactions occur side by side.

Lymphocyte transformation

Human peripheral blood lymphocytes survive in culture for several days without undergoing any marked morphological change unless they are stimulated by some agent that brings about 'transformation'. This process is characterised by increased RNA and protein synthesis, beginning within a few hours, and an increase in the number of lysosomes; after about 24 hours the cells

antibody formation often occur. Inclusion of the antigen in an incomplete adjuvant (mineral oil) favours antibody formation, whereas inclusion in a complete adjuvant (mineral oil with killed tubercle bacilli or certain other organisms) increases both antibody formation and delayed hypersensitivity. If, on first exposure to an antigen, conditions are chosen so that only antibody is formed, and the animal is then given the antigen in complete adjuvant, delayed hypersensitivity fails to develop. This phenomenon is known as immune deviation, and is one form of suppression of cell-mediated immunity. Under certain condi-

TABLE 2. *Some skin tests for delayed hypersensitivity*

Type of agent	Disease	Test material
Virus	Smallpox	Live virus from calf lymph
	Mumps	Killed virus from chick embryo allantoic fluid
	Herpes simplex	Killed purified virus from tissue culture
?virus	Cat-scratch fever	Heated extract from excised lymph node from the disease
Bacterium	Tuberculosis	Tuberculoprotein (purified protein derivative): from heated culture filtrate
	Leprosy	Lepromin: extract of infected skin
	Brucellosis	Brucellin: culture filtrate of *Br. melitensis* and *Br. abortus*
	Johne's disease (cattle)	Johnin: culture filtrate
	Psittacosis	Group (heated) and specific antigens
	Lymphogranuloma venereum	Heated pus from a bubo
Fungus	Dermatomycosis	Trichophytin: culture filtrate
	Coccidiomycosis	Coccidioidin: culture filtrate
	Histoplasmosis	Histoplasmin: culture filtrate
Protozoon	Leishmaniasis	Leishmanin: extract of cultured leishmania
Helminth	Hydatid disease	Casoni antigen: hydatid cyst fluid

synthesise DNA and divide. Transformation can be brought about in non-sensitised cells by agents such as phytohaemagglutinin, streptolysin S or a factor from pokeweed. If lymphocytes are taken from a sensitised subject, transformation of a proportion of cells can be achieved by exposure to specific antigen, e.g. tuberculin or a drug. This test has already proved useful in contact hypersensitivity and drug allergies, and could provide further information about the presence or absence of cell-mediated immunity in tropical parasitic infections.

Relationship of cell-mediated immunity to antibody formation

If an animal such as a guinea pig is immunised with a protein, both delayed hypersensitivity and

tions specific antibody can also prevent rejection of a homograft of tumour: this is known as enhancement.

Cell-mediated immunity in infectious disease

There is good evidence that cell-mediated immunity is mainly responsible for elimination of tumours antigenically different from host cells (see below). Delayed hypersensitivity is also demonstrable with a variety of viral, bacterial, protozoal, fungal and helminth infections (Table 2). Often antibody-mediated hypersensitivity is observed as well: thus, in patients recovering from lobar pneumonia it is usually possible to provoke an immediate wheal-and-flare reaction by injection of type-specific capsular polysaccharide and a delayed-type reaction by nucleoprotein antigen from *Streptococcus pneumoniae*. It is widely agreed that cell-mediated immune reactions, slowly increasing in intensity, play a part in the pathogenesis of chronic infections such as tuberculosis, leprosy, brucellosis and syphilis. However, even in the classical case of tuberculosis, it is far from clear as to what extent cell-mediated immunity is responsible for the observed resistance to reinfection with virulent organisms. Detailed discussion of tuberculosis is beyond the scope of this chapter, but the problem recurs in relation to tropical parasitic infections and will be considered in the appropriate sections.

Effects of drugs

Cortisone and related corticosteroids markedly inhibit the manifestations of cell-mediated immunity, perhaps because of a specific effect on lymphocytes, perhaps because of non-specific anti-inflammatory properties (e.g. prevention of lysosomal damage).

body weight. The capacity of macrophages to digest phagocytosed macromolecules can also be measured by using labelled materials, and the initial rate, at least, is found to follow the general time-course of enzyme-mediated reactions, from which a maximum rate of digestion for an excess of substrate, and a Michaelis-Menten constant, can be obtained.

The rate of phagocytosis of bacteria injected intravenously depends on amounts of natural or immune opsonins, so that serum opsonin levels can be measured from the kinetics of phagocytosis of microorganisms *in vivo*. Thus the non-specific role of the RES is potentiated by specific immune responses leading to antibody production, and the opsoninisation so produced is reinforced by the complement system. The role of macrophages in the initiation of immune responses has been considered above. This can be exerted by macrophages of the spleen and lymph nodes, but presumably not by Kupffer cells. The relative importance of liver or spleen in the phagocytosis

TABLE 3. *Classification of reticuloendothelial cells*

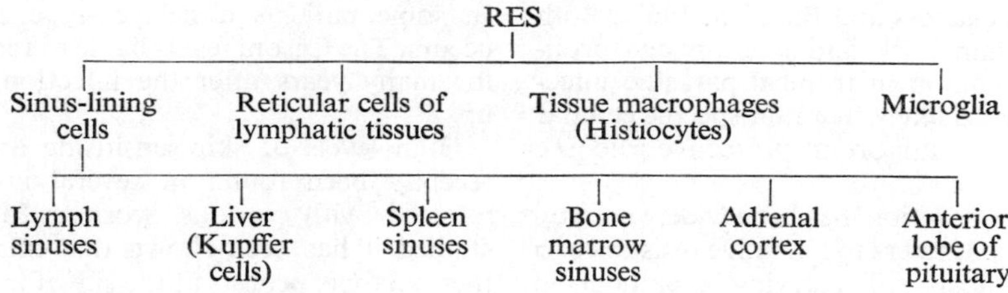

RETICULOENDOTHELIAL SYSTEM (RES)

The reticuloendothelial or macrophage system consists of cells with potent phagocytic ability widely distributed in the body, as shown in the accompanying diagram (Table 3). Depending on their situation, the cells of the RES exert their phagocytic action on materials in tissues (tissue macrophages or histiocytes); in the circulating lymph (sinus-lining cells of lymph nodes) or in the blood (peripheral blood macrophages and cells lining blood sinuses). The phagocytic activity of macrophages lining the blood stream can be quantitated by measuring the clearance from blood of colloidal particles. From the exponential function obtained a phagocytic index (K) is calculated. In normal animals most phagocytic uptake is in the liver (85 per cent) and spleen (10 per cent), and a corrected phagocytic index (α) expresses the activity of macrophages in relation to the weight of these organs as a fraction of total

of red cells depends largely on the nature of the opsonising antibody. The importance of the RES in defence against bacterial infections is well documented, but there has been surprisingly little systematic work on its importance in relation to tropical parasitic infections. However, it is obviously involved in the ingestion of several different types of parasites and parasitised red cells, as shown by histopathological examination. Further quantitative studies of the activity of the RES in parasitic infections are needed.

NON-SPECIFIC ACQUIRED CELLULAR RESISTANCE

Certain infections, such as tuberculosis, are associated with a proliferation and 'activation' of macrophages. The activated macrophages are larger than normal and have an increased content of lysosomes and lysosomal enzymes. They show also increased capacity for digestion and for intracellular inactivation of many different organisms. This is reflected in increased resistance of animals with activated macrophages against infection with organisms that can multiply intracellularly, such as some species of *Mycobacterium*, *Brucella*, *Listeria*, *Salmonella* and *Pasteurella*. This type of resistance is distinct from specific immunity because it is manifested against organisms antigenically different from those by which it is induced, so that it can be termed 'non-specific acquired cellular resistance'.

Proliferation and activation of macrophages is, however, related to cell-mediated immunity. After first exposure to an organism, non-specific acquired cellular resistance builds up slowly, over a period of several weeks, and may then subside; however, after challenge with a small dose of the original organism or antigen from it (e.g. tuberculin) non-specific cellular resistance builds up quickly. The capacity to develop such resistance can be transferred by lymphoid cells but not by serum antibody. This suggests that development of a cell-mediated immune response to one organism is associated with proliferation and activation of macrophages, and this in turn provides non-specific cellular resistance against other organisms (Mackaness and Blanden, 1967). Both cell-mediated immunity and macrophage proliferation are common in tropical parasitic infections, and it seems likely that non-specific cellular resistance plays an important protective role (see sections on protozoa).

The term 'premunition' has been widely used by protozoologists. It refers to a relative resistance to reinfection of hosts still carrying a pathogenic organism; it disappears with cure, is conferred by live but not killed vaccines, and is not transferable with antibodies. The conditions under which premunition is described suggest that it may be related to non-specific acquired cellular resistance.

The importance of macrophages in resistance against intracellular organisms such as *Mycobacterium tuberculosis* is illustrated by the effects of agents toxic for macrophages. One of the most striking is that of silica particles, which are taken up by macrophages and, in sufficient concentration, kill them. Sublethal concentrations of silica potentiate growth of *Myco. tuberculosis* in macrophages in culture, and silicosis in humans as well as experimental animals aggravates tuberculous infections.

HELMINTHIC INFECTIONS

Helminth infections can provide a large mass of foreign antigenic material in the host, and it is not surprising that they can elicit a variety of immune responses. A few examples will serve to illustrate the role of these responses in immunopathological reactions and the possibility that immunisation might be used to protect against infection. Conditions in which blood eosinophilia is common include intestinal infections with hookworms, roundworms or whipworms; various forms of filariasis; guinea-worm infection (dracontiasis); mite infection of the lungs (including some cases of 'tropical eosinophilia'); and hydatid disease due to *Taenia echinococcus*. In all such conditions there is opportunity for absorption of antigenic materials from the parasites, which can give rise to hypersensitivity reactions. Thus hydatid cysts contain excretory and breakdown products of the worms. The cysts are surrounded by inflammatory cells, with many eosinophils and some plasma cells. If cysts rupture and their contents are absorbed into the circulation, the patient is liable to undergo an acute anaphylactic attack. Furthermore, hydatid cyst fluid will often give precipitates with serum from infected subjects, and if such subjects are injected intracutaneously with hydatid cyst fluid (Casoni test) they produce a local wheal-and-flare and/or Arthus reaction. In some patients a delayed-type skin reaction occurs. The Casoni test is liable to remain positive for many years after the infection has cleared up.

High levels of skin-sensitising antibody have recently been found in several animal species infected with various worms. In all species studied it has been shown that this antibody is thermolabile, persists at the site of injection in the skin for long periods, and gives homologous but not heterologous passive cutaneous anaphylactic reactions after challenge with antigen (Ogilvie and Jones, 1969). The reactions are similar to those produced by reagenic antibody (IgE) in man. It seems likely that these and other allergic responses make an important contribution to the severe reactions produced in tissues by worm infections, e.g. lungworms (*Dictyocaulus vivaparus*) in cattle. In sheep and cattle infected with *Ostertagia* spp. and pigs infected with *Hyostrongylus* there is marked hyperplasia of the gastric gland area and loss of cellular differentiation, congestion, oedema and excess mucous secretion. These changes are extreme, but some of the lesser changes seen in human worm infections may well have an allergic basis. Acute allergic reactions are almost certainly responsible for the local inflammation following chemotherapy of patients with onchocerciasis.

Skin tests have shown delayed hypersensitivity reactions to a number of worm infections, and some of these have been transferred in experimental animals with lymphoid cells but not with serum, showing that they conform to the definition of cell-mediated immunity. Warren and his co-workers (1968) have provided evidence that a cell-mediated immune response to schistosome eggs plays an important part in the granulomatous reaction and consequent fibrosis which is characteristic of chronic schistosomiasis. Little reaction is produced by the adult worms. An accelerated reaction is seen in mice on second exposure to schistosome eggs, and this can be transferred by cells but not by serum.

One important question is how effective these various immune responses are in protecting the host against worm infection, and to what extent this can be exploited for vaccination. Vaccination with dead worms or extracted antigen has been unsuccessful, but in a few cases vaccination with attenuated living organisms has been found to confer protection against infection by worm larvae. Dineen and Wagland (1966) have shown that the fourth larval stage of *Trichostrongylus colubriformis* in the guinea pig is markedly affected by prior immunisation of the host. Immunity has been transferred by cells but not by serum, and many of the transferred immune cells have been found to migrate to the intestine, where the worms are situated, and undergo cytolysis there. Vaccination against larvae of the cattle lungworm (*D. viviparus*), using irradiated organisms, has proved commercially successful, and a similar vaccine against the dog hookworm (*Ancylostoma caninum*) has been effective in preliminary trials. The mechanism of protection is not fully understood, but in some cases immunity can be transferred with serum. It seems possible that in certain situations antibody is more important, in others cell-mediated immunity.

In contrast, many adult worms can persist in their hosts for long periods, which suggests that they are relatively resistant to immunological attack, and this resistance of adult worms has been confirmed by suitable animal experiments. The mechanisms underlying the resistance of adult worms are not fully understood: among the contributory factors may be release of large amounts of antigen (which might paralyse or neutralise immunological responses), the presence in many worms of a resistant cuticle, and antigenic variation. An interesting example of the latter is the acquisition by schistosomes of a coating of host antigen which allows them to masquerade as host tissue. Smithers and his colleagues (1969) found that portal inoculation of adult *S. mansoni* from donor hosts into monkeys is ineffective if the monkeys are previously immunised with donor tissue. The host antigens are confined to the surface of the worm, and antibodies against them damage the tegument. The antigens are rapidly lost or exchanged if the worm is transferred to another host species.

Innate immunity to leprosy is demonstrable by some degree of host specificity. Furthermore, non-specific factors such as temperature affect growth of the organisms, and the lower temperature of the skin and nasal passages in contrast to that of internal organs probably contributes to the predilection of the *Myco. leprae* for these sites.

Patients with leprosy present a wide range of symptoms, depending on their proximity to either of the two polar forms of the disease, *tuberculoid* or *lepromatous*. In the lepromatous form the number of bacilli in the tissues is enormous. The organisms multiply in macrophages, which on ageing appear either vacuolated (Virchow or foamy cells), or distended by parasites (lepra cells). Initially the infiltrated macrophages lie around blood vessels, nerves and dermal glands; later the infiltrate largely replaces the dermis, but is separated by a clear zone of stroma from the epidermis. Many bacteria invade nerves of the skin, where they are phagocytosed by Schwann cells or macrophages. In advanced cases skin lesions are widely distributed, and bacteria spread to other organs including the reticuloendothelial system. In lepromatous patients there is often a high titre of circulating antibody, in particular IgA and IgM, and lymph nodes show many plasma cells together with replacement of the paracortical cells by reticulo-histiocytes (see Turk and Walters, 1968). The paucity of immunoblasts in the paracortical areas of the nodes, and the absence of a lymphoid cell infiltration in the infected tissues, suggest that there is a deficient cell-mediated immune response. Unfortunately, the impaired cell-mediated immunity applies not only to *Myco. leprae* antigens (e.g. Mitsuda reaction). Lepromatous patients also have a deficiency in development of contact hypersensitivity, for example to picryl chloride and dinitrochlorobenzene. Moreover, their peripheral blood lymphocytes show impaired transformation to blast cells after exposure *in vitro* to phytohaemagglutinin, tuberculin or *C. albicans* extract (see Shepard, 1968). This impairment of cell-mediated immune responses is the most distinctive feature of lepromatous leprosy, and the question arises as to whether it is a primary abnormality (a small minority of subjects with deficient cell-mediated immunity tending to develop lepromatous leprosy when exposed to the organism) or follows secondarily as a result of the massive infection. When mice are heavily infected with *Myco. lepraemurium* (murine 'leprosy' bacillus) their contact hypersensitivity to chemical antigens is similarly depressed although their capacity to produce circulating antibodies is not, which suggests that the impairment of cell-mediated immunity can be secondary. However, this does not exclude the possibility that a minor constitutional impairment of cell-mediated immunity in human subjects may increase the initial likelihood that the lepromatous form of the disease, rather than the tuberculoid, will follow infection.

Skin lesions in tuberculoid leprosy are macular, and there is an early localised loss of sensation due to inflammation in nerves. Despite the fact that bacilli are scanty, infected tissues show massive infiltration of large and small mononuclear cells (epithelioid cells and lymphocytes, with some giant cells). In the skin there is no 'clear zone' between the cell infiltrate and the overlying epidermis. Lymph nodes have few plasma cells and a predominance of lymphocytes and blast cells. These induced changes are characteristic of a well developed cell-mediated immune reaction. In contrast to the lepromatous form, there is only a slight rise in total serum immunoglobulin levels or specific antibody to *Myco. leprae*. This polar form of leprosy is generally a self-limiting disease that requires medical attention only if signs arise of transformation to the lepromatous condition. Dimorphous or borderline leprosy includes features of both extreme forms of the disease; occasionally different skin areas of the body show a preponderance of one form or the other.

There are two acute exacerbations of the disease which probably have a complex immunopathological basis. The milder is known as the 'lepra' reaction, while erythema nodosum leprosum (ENL) is a more acute reaction which can endanger the life of the patient. It is seen only in the lepromatous or near-lepromatous forms of the disease. Symptoms include rapid onset of oedema, pain and fever, and there is an acute inflammatory reaction with polymorph infiltration around the lesions. This may be an acute hypersensitivity reaction, e.g. due to deposition of antigen-antibody-complement complexes. Moreover, autoimmunity may be somehow involved. Lupus erythematosus cells and antinuclear factors have been found in about one third of leprosy patients; rheumatoid factor, cryoglobulins, positive Coombs' tests and antitissue antibodies have also been demonstrated in the sera of some patients. It is unlikely that these originate as a result of cross-immunity between *Myco. leprae* and host tissues; more probably they are aberrant responses of hyper-reactive lymphoid tissues exposed to a large quantity of bacterial material, which may also act as an adjuvant, favouring immune reactions against antigenically modified host tissue constituents. Lepromatous leprosy, in which there is a large mass of antigen and at least some specific antibody, might be a situation in which circulation of antigen-antibody complexes in antigen excess could occur, with resulting damage to the renal glomeruli. It is of interest that glomerulonephritis has been recorded more often than expected by chance in lepromatous leprosy. Further observations on the localisation of complexes would be desirable.

The decisive role of immune responses in determining the clinical course of leprosy in man is confirmed by the results of experimental infection with *Myco. leprae* in mice (see Rees and Weddell, 1968). Injection of bacilli into mouse foot pads results in strictly limited local multiplication, whereas after injection into mice made immunologically deficient by thymectomy and irradiation there is widespread growth of organisms, with histological changes like those of lepromatous leprosy in man. Restoration of immunological capacity in these immunologically deficient lepromatous mice by injections of syngenetic lymphocytes results in rapid killing of the bacilli, and the transient histological changes often resemble those in intermediate or borderline leprosy in man; ultimately they simulate 'burnt out' leprosy. Nerve damage is permanent.

In conclusion, it seems that the wide spectrum of clinical and pathological features in human leprosy is determined by the effectiveness of the cell-mediated immune response. In the lepromatous form this response is depressed, and damage to nerves and other tissues coincides with massive multiplication of invading bacilli. In contrast there is in the tuberculoid form a powerful cell-mediated immune response, so that few bacilli survive; damage to nerves and other tissues follows a sustained inflammatory reaction of immunopathological nature. The factors initially responsible for either the presence or absence of a cell-mediated immune response are unknown. Only a minority of exposed subjects develop leprosy (less than 5 per cent), presumably because most humans (like most mice) can rapidly acquire effective immunity. Constitutional factors are likely to be involved in the defence mechanism in some way, as reflected in the preponderance of lepromatous leprosy both in males and in certain races. Once the infection is contracted and a good antibody response is evoked, specific cell-mediated immunity against *Myco. leprae* may be depressed by a mechanism akin to immune deviation, the Jancovic phenomenon, or enhancement of tumour growth (see appropriate sections). Later the massive infection has an immunosuppressive effect, of varying degree among individuals, so that cell-mediated immune responses to unrelated antigens are impaired. The opportunity for spontaneous regression of the leprosy infection itself is then drastically reduced, and there is increased susceptibility to secondary pathogens such as tuberculosis organisms.

RELAPSING FEVER

This disease is characterised by repeated pyrexias of sudden onset and rapid subsidence which, in the absence of chemotherapy, may recur almost indefinitely. Coincident with the fever is the appearance of *Borrelia* spp. in peripheral blood; the spirochaetes disappear about 4 hours before a crisis of dyspnoea and other symptoms suffered by the patient. This disease presents two interesting immunological features. One is the antigenic variation of the spirochaete, which accounts for their ability to produce relapsing infections. If infection with a particular variant is produced, antibodies (mainly IgM) rapidly appear which can agglutinate the organisms and presumably opsonise them for destruction by the RES. These antibodies are variant-specific, and the relapsing spirochaetes are found to be of a new antigenic variant not agglutinated by antisera already present. *Borrelia recurrentis* organisms are much less efficiently cleared from the blood in splenectomised rats than in intact controls, suggesting that the RES, especially in the spleen, plays an important part in clearing the peripheral blood of the organisms. The second phenomenon seen in splenectomised rats with late infections (after peak bacteraemia) is congestion of the lungs and eosinophilia, suggesting that an acute allergic reaction is taking place; many of the splenectomised rats die, whereas few intact controls are killed with the laboratory strain used. An immediate-type of wheal-and-flare reaction is seen in the skin of sensitised animals after injection of bacterial antigen. This laboratory model of the development of acute hypersensitivity in relapsing fever may have a human counterpart in the dyspnoea, arthralgia and skin rashes often seen in human *Borrelia* infections. Occasionally these complications are severe or even lethal.

MALARIA

Innate immunity to infection with malaria parasites has already been discussed. In regions where *P. falciparum* is holoendemic or hyperendemic, malaria parasites provide intense and prolonged antigenic stimulation. As is well known, after the neonatal period—when there is protection through passive immunity and possibly other ways—there is a period of about 3–5 years with a high parasite rate and splenomegaly; later parasite rates and counts and spleen rates fall as acquired immunity is built up. The immunological and immunopathological responses to malaria are complex and still incompletely understood (*W.H.O. Technical Report Series*, No. 396, 1968).

Antigenic structure of parasites

Immunodiffusion tests with isolated parasites show the presence of numerous antigens, some common to many different species of *Plasmodium*, others species-specific. Some antigens appear to be present only at certain phases in the life cycle. Of possible immunopathological importance are antigens appearing in the circulation concomitantly with, and shortly after, parasitaemia; these antigens are precipitated by immune sera. Immunofluorescence and agglutination tests have shown the presence of parasite-specific antigens on the surface of parasitised cells. An important factor in the repeated reinfection observed in children is likely to be antigenic variation in the parasite. This has been shown to occur in experimental animal infections, notably with *P. knowlesi* in monkeys. A series of peaks of parasitaemia is observed, the parasites in each relapse having a new major antigenic type, to which agglutinating antibodies are rapidly formed. These are involved in protection of animals against the earlier variants, but not the variants newly emerging.

Antibodies

One of the most striking results of malarial infection, in experimental animals as well as in man, is increase in the levels of circulating IgG and IgM, but not usually of IgA or IgD. Some of the IgG and IgM is specific antibody, directed against parasite antigens, and some is not. A substantial contribution to the high IgG levels found in Africans is made by malarial infection, as evidenced by the consequences of specific chemoprophylaxis. Antibodies measured in different ways appear at different times. Thus antibodies giving immunofluorescence reactions with *P. falciparum* parasites develop in young children, whereas in older children and adults additional antibodies develop giving precipitates in immunodiffusion tests.

Mechanism of immunity

Sometimes a true sterilising immunity develops in malaria, and the host is resistant to reinfection. This happens most readily in abnormal hosts, e.g. with *P. knowlesi* infections in man. It has also been reported with *P. malariae* and occasionally with strains of *P. vivax* in man. Immunity is manifested first against the parasites in the blood, but all stages are eventually affected. It is well established that in experimental animals and man antibodies against a particular strain of malaria parasite can confer a considerable measure of protection against the infection. Intravenous injections of immunoglobulins from pooled African sera have been shown to decrease the counts of *P. falciparum* trophozoites, but not gametocytes, in peripheral blood of children. The pooled globulins are supposed to have antibodies directed against many strains of *P. falciparum*, common to East and West Africa at least. Whether such antibodies neutralise the parasites, or merely opsonise parasites and infected cells for phagocytosis, is unknown.

It seems unlikely that antibody is the only factor involved in immunity against malaria. The older observations on 'premunition'—protection against the superinfection while malaria parasites are still present—raised the possibility that cell-mediated immunity and non-specific cellular resistance might be important. Some recent observations are consistent with this interpretation. Monkeys immunised with *P. knowlesi* parasite antigen in complete Freund's adjuvant and challenged with the same variant of *P. knowlesi* show parasitaemia followed by complete clearance (sterile immunity), whereas fatal infections were observed in monkeys immunised with parasite antigen in incomplete adjuvant. Antibody levels after the two immunisation procedures were about the same, but the complete adjuvant favours development of cell-mediated immunity. Neonatal thymectomy increases the mortality after *P. berghei* infections in rats, suggesting that some thymus-dependent function is required for normal recovery from infection. The reaction most consistently depressed by thymectomy is

cell-mediated immunity. Cell-mediated immune reactions are known to result in macrophage hyperplasia and non-specific acquired cellular resistance. The importance of the reticuloendothelial system in recovery from malarial infection is shown by the severity of infections, and their tendency to recrudesce, after splenectomy or blockade of the RES.

These reactions are seen in *P. falciparum* infections of the placenta, which acts almost as a culture medium for the parasite in infected pregnant women. Lymphocytes accumulate in large numbers in the blood spaces, and undergo transformation there, with increase in the size of cytoplasm and nucleus. Numerous macrophages are seen in the more advanced stages, deeply stained by vital dyes such as neutral red (showing that they have many lysosomes). The macrophages ingest parasites and pigment with great avidity. Many protozoologists regard the macrophages as derived from the transformed lymphocytes, but in the absence of specific labelling it seems possible that they have been recruited from monocytes and activated by the cell-mediated immune response. Whatever the origin of the macrophages, their reactions are similar to those in other types of non-specific cellular resistance. The increased susceptibility to malarial infection of Africans who return to a malarious region after living for some time in a malaria-free environment is well documented, and would be consistent with a loss of non-specific cellular resistance in the absence of continued antigenic stimulation.

Immunopathological complications

Nephrotic syndrome. Epidemiological evidence has suggested that the high incidence of the nephrotic syndrome observed in children living in tropical countries (e.g. Africa and South America) is related to *P. malariae* infection. The clinical syndrome is described in chapter 2; there is a proliferative glomerulonephritis, poorly selective proteinuria and lack of response to corticosteroids and other immunosuppressive drugs. Experimentally induced and naturally occurring nephritides fall into two groups: those due to antibodies against kidney constituents, especially glomerular basement membrane, and those due to deposition of antigen-antibody complexes. The latter arise from soluble complexes in antigen excess in the circulation. Either of these mechanisms concentrates an antigen-antibody reaction in a vulnerable site, the glomerular capillary walls; in the presence of an amplifying mechanism, often involving complement and polymorphs, there is tissue damage and proliferation. In the glomeruli of children with the nephrotic syndrome, granular deposits of immunoglobulin (IgG and IgM) and of complement (β_1C) have been shown along the capillary walls by immunofluorescence. In electron micrographs the deposits are seen on the epithelial side of the basement membrane. Both these are characteristic of the immune complex type of nephritis. Studies with specific fluorescein-labelled antibodies, and with eluates of antigen and antibody from nephrotic kidney, have provided no evidence that the antigen in the deposits is related to streptococci or to *P. falciparum*, but they are consistent with a relationship to *P. malariae*. Thus it seems that a minority of children infected with *P. malariae* respond in such a way that antigen-antibody-complement complexes circulate and are deposited in the renal glomeruli, causing the changes characteristic of the nephrotic syndrome. There is no evidence for the presence of antibody against renal glomerular basement membrane in these patients, or of a cross-reacting antigen common to *P. malariae* and a kidney constituent.

The possibility that immune complexes could cause other immunopathological complications in malaria deserves further consideration.

Autoimmunity. Various autoimmune processes have been described in malaria in humans as well as in experimental animals. Some of these will be discussed in other sections, e.g. rheumatoid factor, antibodies reacting with the Wassermann antigen, and the presence of circulating organ-specific antibodies. One manifestation attributed by some investigators to autoimmunity is malarial anaemia, particularly the haemolytic manifestations seen, for instance, in pregnant women with *P. falciparum* in peripheral blood. It seems in these cases (and in certain experimental animal infections) that the anaemia is disproportionate to the parasitaemia, so that it cannot be explained merely by destruction of parasitised cells; phagocytosis of apparently normal cells in the spleen has also been observed. It is thought that antibodies play a role in this process, either those directed against parasite antigens on non-parasitised cells (which are sometimes demonstrable by immunofluorescence), or autoantibodies against erythrocyte antigens.

TRYPANOSOMIASIS

The importance of genetic factors can be illustrated by the insusceptibility of West African Muturu and N'Dama cattle to trypanosomiasis, in contrast to the susceptibility of Zebu cattle. There are marked species differences in response to infections. Many monkeys are highly susceptible to blood-induced infection with *Trypanosoma rhodesiense* and *T. gambiense*, but baboons are not; nevertheless, the resistance of baboons can be overcome by inoculation of parasites into the cerebrospinal fluid. Humans are resistant to *T. brucei*, *T. congolense* and *T. vivax*, but are susceptible to *T. rhodesiense* and *T. gambiense* in Africa and *T. cruzi* in South America. Although the parasites provide intense and prolonged antigenic stimulation, and elicit a variety of immune responses, these usually fail to protect human subjects from progressive infections. This is not always true, however, and cases have been described with symptomless *T. gambiense* infections for as long as 8 years.

Antigenic structure

Many antigens have been demonstrated in trypanosomes, some group-specific, some species-specific and still others variant-specific. Some antigens are liberated from the parasites and found free in the plasma of infected animals. Trypanosomes have the capacity to undergo rapid antigenic changes. This is shown in animals by sequential changes in major protein antigens against which agglutinating and lytic antibodies are formed; these changes of the outer coat of the trypanosomes allow relapse of new variants (Brown, 1963). The wide range of antigenic variants in naturally occurring trypanosomes is one of the factors which makes immunisation difficult.

Antibodies

The most remarkable response to trypanosome infections, in experimental animals as well as humans, is the rapid increase in total IgM levels, which may be anything from twice to about six times normal. The high levels of IgM are detectable in field tests with fingerprick samples of blood dried on to filter paper, and provide a useful screening test for trypanosomiasis in the field. There may also be some elevation of IgG levels. Antibodies have been found which agglutinate parasites or lyse them in the presence of complement; these develop rapidly after infection and are initially of IgM type. Antibodies are also recognisable by immunofluorescent staining of parasites, complement fixation and immunodiffusion. Antibodies termed 'ablastins' which prevent multiplication of trypanosomes have also been described.

Heterophile antibodies. Patients with trypanosomiasis may have relatively high titres of antibodies that agglutinate sheep red blood cells. The titres have been higher in East Africans with *T. rhodesiense* infections than in West Africans with *T. gambiense* infections. In monkeys infected with either *T. rhodesiense* or *T. gambiense*, high titres of IgM heterophile antibodies agglutinating sheep red blood cells rapidly appeared. These are similar to antibodies against Forssmann antigen, but not identical. The possibility that heterophile antibodies could help in screening for trypanosomiasis deserves further consideration.

Mechanism of immunity

The effects of humoral immunity are shown in infections by pathogenic trypanosomes in laboratory animals. There is a build-up of trypanosomes in the blood followed by a massive destruction of the organisms by lysis. Presumably the organisms are also opsonised for phagocytosis by the RES. Usually a low-grade infection of peripheral blood remains until the organisms are cleared by antibodies against variants or by other immune responses. Goats and sheep acquire immunity to trypanosomes following recovery from patent infections; this is said to be mediated by a humoral mechanism. The role of cell-mediated immunity has not been carefully analysed, although it has been suggested that cellular responses may be important with *T. cruzi* infections. The infections are associated with lymphocytic infiltrations, many resembling transformed lymphocytes. The acquisition of immunity is reported to cause macrophages which normally support multiplication of the trypanosomes to change their characteristics and to destroy the parasites by phagocytosis. This is certainly reminiscent of the role of non-specific cellular resistance in other facultative intracellular organisms (*Mycobacteria*, *Listeria*, etc.). Practically useful immunisation of cattle has been achieved by allowing a low-grade infection to develop and then treating the infection periodically; perhaps this allows a build-up and maintenance of non-specific cellular resistance (see Manson-Bahr, 1963).

Immunopathology

Very little is known about immunopathological complications of trypanosomiasis, although the presence of antigen in plasma suggests that circulating antigen-antibody complexes could produce vascular abnormalities which might contribute to pathogenesis in chronic infections.

There is no good evidence for innate immunity against *Leishmania* infections. Their distribution appears to be determined by epidemiological and not immunological factors. Acquired immunity can be highly efficient and has already been quite widely used for immunoprophylaxis. It is most readily seen in single sores, the self-curing leishmanial infections like oriental sore and Chiclero's ulcer. These confer strong immunity to reinfection.

Antigens

Immunodiffusion studies have shown that the antigenic structure of *Leishmania* organisms is complex. Immunodiffusion, Noguchi-Adler and passive haemagglutination tests are now being used to compare strains of *Leishmania* from different parts of the world, and several antigenic variants have been found. However, the presence of common antigens in immunodiffusion tests, and cross-protection after infection, suggest that at least the major antigens involved in immunity may be shared by many different strains of *Leishmania* organisms.

Antibodies

In visceral leishmaniasis, due to *L. donovani*, and the widespread South American infection espundia due to *L. braziliensis*, serum antibodies against the organisms are demonstrable by complement-fixation, immunodiffusion and other tests. Serum IgG levels are usually high, sometimes very high. No serum antibody is demonstrable in self-curing leishmanial cutaneous ulcers. Attempts to transfer immunity against *Leishmania* with serum antibody have been unsuccessful, and there is no evidence that humoral antibody contributes to recovery from human infections. It may, in fact, have the opposite effect.

Delayed hypersensitivity

This is manifested by 48–72 hour reactions after skin testing with leishmanin (Montenegro reaction). The antigen is prepared from whole flagellates or an extract of flagellates (10^8 per mm^3 in visceral or new world cutaneous leishmaniasis or less in old world cutaneous leishmaniasis). The test is specific for leishmaniasis, but does not distinguish between different forms of human infections. Delayed hypersensitivity develops early in *L. mexicana* but later in *L. tropica*, and is found only after recovery in *L. donovani* infections. The presence of delayed hypersensitivity is said to imply immunity to infection in all forms of leishmaniasis. In areas endemic for any form of leishmaniasis positive leishmanin reactors are found who give no evidence of previous infection. It is thought that these individuals are immune to infection with the form of leishmaniasis prevalent in that area (Manson-Bahr, 1963).

Acquired immunity: underlying mechanisms

In oriental sore due to *L. tropica*, lifelong immunity is acquired when the lesions are allowed to run their natural course (4–6 months). Active immunisation is an established method of control. Following the ancient practice of inoculating children with material from sores on a covered part of the body to prevent unsightly scars, artificial lesions have been produced using material from sores or cultures of *L. tropica*. The immunity is sterilising, and organisms can only very rarely be isolated from recovered lesions. The immunity is supposed to be a local cellular reaction activated by parasites which grow in macrophages in the skin. Histological examination shows the presence of numerous lymphocytes, some large and resembling transformed lymphocytes. It seems likely that a cell-mediated immune response (demonstrated by the presence of delayed hypersensitivity) and related non-specific acquired cellular resistance is the main mechanism of immunity.

Bray and Bryceson (1968) have studied the recovery of guinea pigs from infection with *L. enrietti*, after which they are immune to reinfection. The guinea pigs show delayed hypersensitivity, which is transferable by cells but not by serum. They show no antibody detectable serologically and no cytophilic antibody. Peritoneal macrophages from recovered animals were cultured and found to take up more organisms than did macrophages from normal animals, but the growth of the organisms within the macrophages was not impaired. However, lymphocytes from immune animals (but not from normal animals) rapidly destroyed infected macrophages and the *Leishmania* were killed in the process. These results strongly support the view that cell-mediated immunity is of crucial importance in protection against *Leishmania* infections.

The finding of Bray and Bryceson that there was no increased ability of macrophages from convalescent guinea pigs to destroy *Leishmania* or impair their growth was taken as evidence against the presence of non-specific cellular resistance. However, the experiments do not provide a critical test, and evidence that the resistance is non-specific comes from observations of Adler (1963) on the mildness of *P. berghei*

infections, and increased phagocytosis of malaria parasites, in hamsters infected with *L. tropica* or *L. infantum*. In Sicily infants infected with *L. infantum* seldom contracted malaria when the disease was common on the island. Adler concludes that there is a definite antagonism between visceral leishmaniasis and malaria both in man and the hamster, and this non-specific protection may be due to the relatively enormous increase in immunologically competent cells. In bay sore due to *L. mexicana*, delayed hypersensitivity develops but the infection may persist for many years, so clearance of parasites by immune mechanisms is relatively inefficient; possibly the situation may be complicated by antigenic variation.

In visceral leishmaniasis due to *L. donovani* there is a delicate balance between proliferation of organisms in the reticuloendothelial cells and development of cell-mediated immunity. In most parts of the world 98 per cent of cases with kala-azar will die if they are not treated. In some cases resistant to treatment with drugs, splenectomy cures the disease (Manson-Bahr, 1963), suggesting that removal of the large mass of parasitised cells allows immunity to develop. In kala-azar, leishmanin skin tests are negative until after recovery, when they become positive. This suggests that in the active disease cell-mediated immunity does not develop. Whether this is a specific failure to respond to *Leishmania* antigen, or immunosuppression which would be manifested against other antigens, is unknown. The possibility that serum antibody might inhibit the action of the cell-mediated immune response, by a mechanism analogous to tumour enhancement, should also be considered. Emergence of immunity may account for the development of a post kala-azar dermal leishmanoid nodular rash, which may disappear with relapses, only to reappear again with final recovery. Antigen already present in the skin could account for a hypersensitivity reaction. Once cases have recovered completely, immunity prevents the appearance of a new primary skin lesion and thus the development of a visceral infection. In *L. braziliensis* infections an attack also confers lifelong immunity.

Two conditions in which the cell-mediated immune response is ineffective in clearing cutaneous parasites are leishmaniasis recidiva and leishmaniasis diffusa. In the former the parasites are walled-off in epithelioid cells surrounded by lymphocytes, forming typical delayed hypersensitivity granulomas. The parasites are inaccessible in such granulomatous lesions, which provoke a strong cell-mediated immune response, as shown by a high level of delayed hypersensitivity in skin tests. In contrast, diffuse cutaneous leishmaniasis is characterised by the absence of a cell-mediated immune response. The lesions show no lymphocytic invasion, parasites are not destroyed and there is no delayed hypersensitivity. For some unknown reason the lymph nodes fail to produce specifically sensitised lymphocytes.

Bryceson (1970) has examined this condition in Ethiopia. The disease occurs in a region where simple oriental sore is common. It begins as a small nodule which spreads to give nodular lesions on the face, arms and legs reminiscent of lepromatous leprosy. Histological examination of lesions shows only macrophages full of Leishman-Donovan bodies and a few plasma cells. The leishmanin skin test is negative, but delayed hypersensitivity to lepromin and tuberculin are unimpaired, and sensitivity to dinitrochlorobenzene can be induced. Thus there is no general immunosuppression and intercurrent diseases are handled normally. Patients relapse even after prolonged treatment, suggesting that the condition may be due to a specific immunological defect on the part of the patient. Whether this is a primary failure to respond in congenitally predisposed subjects, or whether it follows secondarily from antigen overloading, is still unknown. However, evidence already available suggests that in leishmaniasis, as in leprosy, the presence or absence of a cell-mediated immune response is a crucial factor determining the course of the disease produced by the infecting agent.

FUNGAL AND MISCELLANEOUS INFECTIONS

Increasing use is being made of immunological methods for diagnosis and treatment of fungal and other infections. Immunofluorescence, immunodiffusion, latex particle agglutination and other tests are already widely used, and this will be extended as other specific reagents are developed. Thus immunodiffusion can already be applied with sera from patients with mycetoma to determine whether infections are due to *Madurella*, *Allescheria*, *Streptomyces* or *Nocardia* spp.

An example of acute hypersensitivity is provided by farmer's lung, bagassosis and sisal disease. Diseases in this group are characterised by increasing respiratory distress, accompanied by fever and general malaise, brought on by inhalation of dust from mouldy hay, bagasse (sugar cane waste), sisal grass, etc. The symptoms are not typical of asthma—although asthma can be present—and they can occur in subjects without demonstrable skin-sensitising antibodies. The blood does, however, contain antibodies which give precipitates with aqueous extracts of the inciting agents, often thermophilic actinomycetes growing on hay or other plant fibres. The pathological changes are probably due to Arthus-type reactions occurring in bronchioles and alveoli, and are as a rule quite rapidly reversed when exposure to the antigen ceases.

Delayed hypersensitivity is widely used for testing for previous infection with *Histoplasma capsulatum* and *Coccidioides immitis*. Epidemics account for only a tiny fraction of the many human infections, and skin test surveys have contributed most of our current information on the geographical distribution and prevalence of infection with these organisms in man. Acute allergy may play a role in the erythema nodosum and multiforme observed in some histoplasmosis cases. Cell-mediated immunity may contribute to the chronic inflammatory process and tissue damage in mycetoma and blastomycosis. An important pathological feature is said to be a sort of arteritis obliterans, with proliferation of arterial endothelium. This could possibly represent a chronic immunopathological response of mild Arthus type.

VIRUS INFECTIONS

Innate immunity plays an important part in virus infections, as illustrated by the host specificity of many and strain differences in susceptibility within a single species, discussed in the section on innate immunity. An acquired response to virus infection is the production of interferon, which is host-specific but not virus-specific, which distinguishes it from an immune response. Nevertheless, interferon may act synergistically with acquired immunity in the resolution of virus infections. The antigenic structures of viruses, and the immune responses to them, are complex, but some broad generalisations can be made.

Antigenic structure

Large viruses, such as poxviruses and herpesviruses, have many antigens, as shown by immunodiffusion tests. Viruses of intermediate size, such as adenoviruses, have three major antigens, the disposition of which in the viruses is known. Lipid-containing viruses of intermediate size, such as myxoviruses, have three major antigens, two associated with the surface agglutinin complex and an interior ribonucleoprotein antigen. The structures of some arboviruses seem to be rather similar to those of myxoviruses. Small viruses such as poliovirus and encephalomyocarditis virus have a single major coat antigen. An important aspect of viral immunology is the number of antigenic types that can be exhibited by a virus. With some this is restricted, e.g. poliovirus has three. With others the number may be large, e.g. adenovirus and influenza virus. This allows repeated infection with different virus strains. Sometimes there are group-specific antigens, as well as type-specific antigens (e.g. influenza virus or arboviruses of group B); infection with one member of a group may confer some measure of protection against other members of the group. Although there may be a multiplicity of antigenic types, change from one to another only takes place occasionally. Viruses are not known to undergo the rapid, sequential major antigenic changes shown, for instance, by plasmodia, trypanosomes or *Borrelia* organisms as individual infections relapse.

Antibodies

As a rule, the sequence of immune responses to viruses follows the same pattern as with other antigens. IgM antibodies appear in the blood early, followed by IgG antibodies. With many viruses, serum antibodies passively transferred to recipients protect recipients against serious effects of virus infections (e.g. measles convalescent serum in man). This applies particularly to those viruses in which there is a viraemic stage between multiplication at the primary site of infection and that in a second, vulnerable organ (e.g. poliovirus in the gut and the central nervous system). However, this is not always true. High levels of IgG and IgM antibodies in serum (actively induced by systemic inoculation of killed vaccines or passively transferred) do not confer protection against upper respiratory tract infection with influenza or other myxoviruses. In this case protection is achieved by locally produced IgA antibody in the nasal secretions, stimulated by a natural infection or locally administered vaccine.

The recovery from virus infections of agammaglobulinaemic children (who have very low levels of immunoglobulins but essentially normal cell-mediated immune responses) is usually normal, and this has been taken as evidence that antibody is not involved in the recovery. However, generalised vaccinial infection sometimes occurs in agammaglobulinaemic children, and in adults who show no detectable antibody against the virus. Moreover, in animals treated with immunosuppressants, recovery from some virus infections

is abnormal. Hence it seems likely that recovery from virus infections is due to several factors, of which antibody is one and interferon may be another.

Cell-mediated immunity

Delayed hypersensitivity is manifested after intradermal injection of live viruses and virus antigens, e.g. vaccinia, herpes simplex and mumps. It can provide useful epidemiological evidence of past infections, sometimes being more reliable than antibody levels. Cell-mediated immunity makes an important contribution to the primary response following vaccination against smallpox and is mainly responsible for the 'accelerated' response seen in previously vaccinated subjects. (This is sometimes incorrectly termed an 'immediate' or 'immune' response.) Cell-mediated immunity appears to be important also in the pathogenesis of rashes characteristic of several virus infections. During the second viraemic phase virus lodges in the skin, where it grows focally. Enough antigen is produced to elicit local delayed hypersensitivity reactions, which histologically show cuffing of blood vessels with mononuclear cells. In experimental animals on immunosuppressants focal growth of viruses in the skin occurs, but the redness and induration characteristic of rashes do not develop.

Immunopathology

Antibody-mediated hypersensitivity can be demonstrated in virus infections, but little is known of its immunopathological significance. Children immunised with killed vaccine against respiratory syncytial virus have been found to suffer from more severe infections than unvaccinated children. It is thought that the absence of IgA antibodies in the upper respiratory tract accounts for the lack of protection, and the severity of the infection may have been increased by antibody-mediated hypersensitivity. Halstead has suggested that an immunopathological reaction may account for dengue haemorrhagic fever. Immune complexes, presumably formed during the initial phase of a dengue infection in persons with heterologous dengue antibody, are thought to give rise to abnormalities in haemostasis and shock. Immune complexes are certainly deposited in the renal glomeruli of experimental animals with some virus infections, and may produce nephritis.

Cell-mediated immune reactions play a part in pathogenesis in lymphocytic choriomeningitis infections of laboratory animals. Mice acquiring the virus from mothers or infected during the newborn period carry large amounts of virus throughout their lifespan. There is no cell-mediated immune response. However, when older mice are infected they show ill effects, including runting and lymphocytic infiltration of the meninges. Neonatal thymectomy or immuno-suppressant treatments ameliorate the effects of infection in older animals. Whether any comparable situation exists in man is at present unknown.

TUMOURS

Many experimentally induced tumours have been shown to carry antigens different from those present in normal cells of the original host. It is found, for example, that previous injections of irradiated tumour cells increase the number of live tumour cells required to establish a transplant. Usually tumours induced by chemical carcinogens have individual specificities, so that an animal immunised against one is not protected against others. In contrast, all tumours induced by a particular virus (e.g. polyoma, SV40, Rous sarcoma virus or murine sarcoma virus) have a common antigen shared by other tumours induced by the same virus, but not by other viruses.

Immunity against tumours can always be transferred by cells, so that it is cell-mediated. Serum antibodies against tumour antigens are often present as well, and can be demonstrated by *in vitro* tests, e.g. immunofluorescence or cytoxicity in the presence of complement. Usually, serum containing antibodies passively transferred has no detectable effect on tumour growth in recipients, but in some cases (especially where histocompatibility differences are involved) it can either enhance or retard tumour growth.

There is little doubt that cell-mediated immune responses represent an important 'policing system' protecting animals against the growth of tumour cells that arise from time to time. This can be shown, for instance, by the increased incidence of tumours observed in animals whose cell-mediated immune responses have been depressed, e.g. by neonatal thymectomy or treatment with anti-lymphocytic serum. There is a greatly increased risk of malignancy of the lymphoreticular system in patients with congenital immunological defects (e.g. primary immuno-globulin aberrations, ataxia-telangiectasia and Aldrich's syndrome) and in patients receiving immunosuppressive therapy after kidney grafts. The tendency to develop malignancy in these patients may be due to failure of normal resistance against oncogenic agents or failure to react to tumour-specific antigens. Secondary suppression of cell-mediated immune responses in Hodgkin's disease and some other lymphoreticular neoplasms has been mentioned above.

Recently there has been interest in the possibility that one factor in the aetiology of Burkitt's lymphoma may be some immunosuppressive event, such as intense malarial infection. The prolonged remissions sometimes observed after chemotherapy of this tumour may be due, at least in part, to acquired immunity. It is of interest that the other tumour responding well to chemotherapy, choriocarcinoma, is in fact a homograft against which a particularly strong immunological reaction would be expected.

AUTOIMMUNITY

Autoimmunity can be broadly defined as the situation in which an antibody or sensitised cells can react with some constituent of host tissues. Autoimmunity is found in association with a number of diseases, although it is usually unknown whether the antibodies or sensitised cells play any part in the causation of the disease, are a consequence of it or merely a concomitant. However, there is good evidence that autoimmune mechanisms can be causative factors in diseases of laboratory animals, e.g. experimental allergic encephalomyelitis and experimental thyroiditis. It seems likely that autoimmune mechanisms can also play a pathogenetic role in some human diseases, including antibody-related haemolytic anaemia, lupus erythematosus, certain renal disorders (e.g. chronic membranous nephritis) and certain endocrine disorders (e.g. Hashimoto's thyroiditis). Thus, antibodies against glomerular basement membrane eluted from kidneys of subjects with autoimmune glomerulonephritis injected into monkeys were fixed to their glomerular basement membranes (as shown by immuno-fluorescence) and caused a severe, progressive glomerulonephritis. Moreover, kidneys grafted into such patients rapidly fixed the antibody and developed glomerulonephritis (Dixon, 1968). The cytotoxicity of sensitised human lymphocytes on the appropriate target organs *in vitro* has also been demonstrated. However, it is still a matter of speculation to what extent most autoimmune manifestations are pathogenetic. During the past few years it has become clear that several reactions that can be termed autoimmune are even commoner in populations living in the tropics than they are in temperate climates. Some of these will be discussed briefly.

Rheumatoid-factor-like globulins

A group of proteins which can be regarded as autoantibodies circulate in the blood of most patients with rheumatoid arthritis. These rheumatoid factors (RF) are IgM molecules that have the capacity to combine with IgG. The reaction has provided the basis of tests for RF by agglutination of particles which have a layer of IgG at their surface, e.g. sheep erythrocytes coated with rabbit anti-sheep cell serum or treated with tannic acid and exposed to human IgG, or particles of polystyrene latex or the volcanic clay bentonite which have adsorbed human IgG. All these reactions test for antibody to IgG, but they are not identical. Sometimes human and sometimes animal IgG is used, and different tests do not always give the same results, so it seems that a number of RF-like globulins are involved. In the serum these usually circulate as a complex with IgG with a sedimentation coefficient of 22S. Apart from rheumatoid arthritis, reactions for RF have been reported in a number of infections, including leprosy, syphilis, trypanosomiasis, malaria, subacute bacterial endocarditis, tuberculosis, infectious mononucleosis and infective hepatitis. Usually positive reactions are transient and they may be atypical, showing no sharp endpoint. A relatively high incidence of RF-like globulins has been described in East and West Africans, especially those living in malarious regions or suffering from leishmaniasis. A particularly high incidence of RF has been described in Rwanda Africans from a non-malarious region who have emigrated to Buganda, which is malarious. RF reactions become positive in rabbits infected with trypanosomes and monkeys infected with malaria.

These anti-IgG antibodies may arise through several mechanisms including stimulation of the host by its own immunoglobulin altered by combination with antigen. An experimental model of this is provided by the production of RF following the injection of antigen-antibody complexes. Host immunoglobulin might be made antigenic by partial enzymatic breakdown; this can be achieved experimentally. In either of these situations the adjuvant activity of microorganisms might favour autoantibody formation.

Immunoconglutinins

Some of the components of complement are modified by combination with antigen-antibody complexes, and antibodies can be formed against the altered complement components. These are termed immunoconglutinins and have been observed in human and bovine trypanosomiasis.

Wassermann antibodies

Antibody against the Wassermann antigen can be regarded as an autoantibody because it will react with alcoholic extracts of normal human heart and to a lower titre with saline extracts. A positive reaction is seen in nearly all cases of untreated syphilis, pinta, yaws and bejel, at least during the first few years after infection. Positive Wassermann reactions have been reported in about 20 per cent of leprosy cases, 25 per cent of subjects after smallpox vaccination, 26 per cent of patients with ornithosis pneumonia and some patients with primary atypical pneumonia or infective hepatitis. Although positive reactions are seen in animals infected with trypanosomes, they do not appear to occur in human trypanosomiasis. Positive Wassermann reactions have also been reported in artificially induced human malaria and in chronic relapsing vivax malaria. The Wassermann reaction obtained with normal rabbit serum appears to be a consequence of coccidial infection.

Antinuclear factors

These are frequently seen in systemic lupus erythematosus, in which there is multiple autoantibody formation. Antinuclear factors have been reported in about 30 per cent of patients with leprosy, about one third of those with antibodies giving positive LE cell tests. Many of the patients with antinuclear factors also had rheumatoid factor and antibodies to thyroglobulin and the Wassermann antigen. Antinuclear factors have also been described in tuberculosis, but may have been due to treatment with isoniazid. This is related to hydralazine which is known to cause the formation of antinuclear antibodies in humans. Preliminary surveys suggest that antinuclear factors are uncommon in Africans living in areas where malaria is holoendemic.

Antibodies against red cells

In both human and laboratory animal infections with malaria, antibodies against erythrocyte stroma have been described. A raised incidence of cold agglutinins has been reported in trypanosomiasis, relapsing fever and malaria. There is a high incidence in Melanesian populations, reacting with a variant of the I blood group antigen, which may be a consequence of malarial infection. Cold agglutinins directed against the I antigen are common after *Mycoplasma pneumoniae* infections, and cold autoantibodies occur transiently in about 8 per cent of cases of infectious mononucleosis; these are distinct from the heterophile antibody to sheep red cells. The Donath-Landsteiner antibody is a cold agglutinin directed against P_1 and P_2 but not p^k antigen; about half the cases with this antibody are syphilitic.

Predisposition to autoimmune manifestations

A genetic predisposition to autoimmune disease has been clearly demonstrated in experimental animals, e.g. autoimmune haemolytic anaemia and glomerulonephritis in mice and experimental allergic encephalomyelitis and experimental thyroiditis in guinea pigs. Susceptibility to autoimmune phenomena differs in different strains. Mating of a highly susceptible inbred mouse strain with a low incidence strain (e.g. NZB × NZW) produces an FI with a high incidence of autoimmune syndromes with a different pattern from that found in the affected parental strain. The genetic differences are manifested both in the ease with which autoimmune antibodies are produced and in the susceptibility of target tissues. Although the human data are difficult to analyse because of the impossibility of obtaining adequately matched control families, certain families show remarkable clustering of autoimmune serological manifestations, with and without clinical disease.

Certain groups of humans are also especially prone to autoimmune manifestations. In Western Europe and America the incidence of auto-antibodies against tissues such as thyroid and gastric parietal cells rises with advancing age, even in subjects without any disease referable to autoimmunity. If the cells involved in immune responses are not functioning normally, the chance of developing autoimmune manifestations is greatly increased. Autoimmunity occurs with high frequency in several forms of immunological deficiencies, e.g. infantile sex-linked agammaglobulinaemia, primary immunoglobulin aberrations or agammaglobulinaemia and thymoma. The incidence of rheumatoid arthritis, dermatomysotis, diffuse vasculitis and antibody-related haemolytic anaemias in these patients is about thirty times that in the general population. An unusually high incidence of serological and clinical manifestations of autoimmunity is seen in first and second degree relatives of patients with primary immunoglobulin aberrations. Patients with neoplasms of the lymphoreticular system have an unusually high incidence of cold agglutinins and autoimmune haemolytic anaemias.

Predisposition to serological manifestations of autoimmunity may exist also in some populations exposed to tropical parasitic infections. In New Guinea, sera from subjects with high levels of gamma globulin living in a hyperendemic malarial area had significantly greater complement-fixing capacity against saline extracts of human liver and kidney than sera with lower gamma globulin levels from subjects not injected. Shaper (1968) has found that Africans with high titres of malarial antibodies, as shown by immunofluorescence, often have splenomegaly, very high levels of IgM, and a high incidence of rheumatoid factor and of antibodies against heart, thyroid and parietal cells. Most subjects with this combination were immigrants from a non-malarial region, but it was sometimes seen also in indigenous Africans living in the malarious Kampala region. Shaper suggests that hyper-responsiveness to malaria, and associated immunological changes, result in the production of autoantibodies to various tissues. These antibodies are not thought to produce tissue damage, but if damage does occur it might be aggravated by deposition of antibodies and complement. Shaper considers that this background may predispose subjects to endomyocardial fibrosis, rheumatic heart disease, 'big spleen disease' and possibly some other conditions (see chapter on heart disease).

REFERENCES

ADLER, S. (1963) In *Immunity to Protozoa*, ed Garnham, P. C. C., Pierce, A. E. and Roitt I., pp. 235–245, Oxford: Blackwell.

ALLISON, A. C. (1965) *Arch. ges. Virusforsch.*, **17**, 280.

ALTOUNYAN, R. E. C. (1967) *Acta Allergol.*, **22**, 487.

BRAY, R. S. and BRYCESON, A. D. M. (1968) *Trans. roy. Soc. trop. Med. Hyg.*, **44**, 493.

BROWN, K. N. (1963) In *Immunity to Protozoa*, ed. Garnham, P. C. C., Pierce, A. E. and Roitt, I., pp. 204–212, Oxford: Blackwell.

BRYCESON, A. D. M. (1970) *Trans. roy. Soc. trop. Med. Hyg.*, **64,** 380.
DINEEN, J. K. and WAGLAND, B. M. (1966) *Immunology*, **11,** 47.
DIXON, F. J. (1968) *Amer. J. Med.*, **44,** 493.
MACKANESS, G. B. and BLANDEN, R. V. (1967) *Progr. Allergy*, **11,** 89.
MALLEN, M. S. (1965) *Ann. Allergy*, **23,** 534.
MANSON-BAHR, P. E. C. (1963) In *Immunity to Protozoa*, ed. Garnham, P. C. C., Pierce, A. E. and Roitt, I.,
    pp. 246–252, Oxford: Blackwell.
REES, R. J. W. and WEDDELL, A. G. M. (1968) *Ann. N.Y. Acad. Sci.*, **154,** 214.
SHAPER, A. G., KAPLAN, M. H., MODY, N. J. and MCINTYRE, P. A. (1968) *Lancet*, **1,** 1342.
SHEPARD, C. C. (1968) *Int. J. Leprosy*, **36,** 87.
SMITHERS, S. R., TERRY, R. J. and HOCKLEY, D. J. (1969) *Proc. roy. Soc. (Biol.)*, **171,** 483.
TURK, J. L. and WALTERS, M. F. (1968) *Lancet*, **2,** 436.
WARREN K. S. (1968) *Bull. N.Y. Acad. Med.* **44,** 280.

Protozoal Diseases

Malaria

African Human Trypanosomiasis

South American Trypanosomiasis

Leishmaniases

Amoebiasis

Toxoplasmosis

Intestinal Protozoa Other Than
Entamoeba histolytica

Primary Amoebic Meningoencephalitis

2
Malaria

Human malaria is caused by infection with sporozoa of the genus *Plasmodium*, transmitted in nature by the bite of female *Anopheles* mosquitoes. Four subgenera and species are involved:

> *Plasmodium* (subgenus *Plasmodium*): *P. malariae, P. vivax, P. ovale*. These parasites have large erythrocytic schizonts and round gametocytes.

> *Plasmodium* (subgenus *Laverania*): *P. falciparum*. These parasites have large erythrocytic and elongated crescentic gametocytes.

Certain parasites of monkeys may also infect man including *P. knowlesi, P. cynomolgi bastianelli* and *P. simium*, and a few natural and several laboratory infections have been recorded. The significance of malaria as a zoonosis is at present uncertain.

Nomenclature. The English term for malaria caused by *P. falciparum* is malignant tertian or subtertian malaria. The specific name, falciparum malaria, is now commonly used internationally, as it avoids language confusion. This principle of nomenclature is also often adopted for *P. vivax* infection, which is called vivax malaria, and for *P. ovale* infection which is called ovale (tertian) malaria. *P. malariae* infection is still referred to most commonly as quartan malaria.

EPIDEMIOLOGY

All forms of human malaria are transmitted in nature by the bite of the female *Anopheles* mosquito.

Artificial infection may result from passage of infected blood containing the erythrocytic phase of the parasite. Such infection may follow transfusion of blood containing the parasites or injection of infected blood samples accidentally, e.g. in drug addicts, experimentally or for therapeutic purposes. It may also be achieved experimentally by injection of blood containing sporozoites (within 30–60 minutes of the infective mosquito bite). Malaria is occasionally transmitted to the child across the placenta; the exact mode of transmission in this case is not known.

The epidemiological picture in a given geographical area depends largely on the species of parasite and the habits and characteristics of the vector. Climatic and geographical factors of great importance in the vector are breeding places, host preferences, biting habits and length of life. The most active vectors are anthropophilic, others are zoophilic; some bite indoors, some out of doors.

The mosquito becomes infected by ingesting human blood containing male and female gametocytes. The life cycle of the parasite in the vector is usually completed in about 12 days depending on the ambient temperature (optimum lies between 17°C and 29°C; maximum 32°C; minimum 15°C). The interval of time elapsing from the ingestion of infective blood to the appearance of sporozoites in the saliva of the mosquito is known as the *extrinsic incubation period*.

Malaria is regarded as endemic in an area when there is measurable incidence and natural transmission over the years. Endemicity is commonly described in terms of the rate of enlarged spleens and the incidence of parasites (parasite rates) found in the community. The definitions of the various degrees of endemicity approved by the World Health Organization are:

1. *Holoendemic:* spleen rate in children of 2–9 years of age constantly over 75 per cent, adult spleen rate low, tolerance high.
2. *Hyperendemic:* spleen rate in children constantly over 50 per cent, high rate in adults.
3. *Mesoendemic:* spleen rate in children between 11 and 50 per cent.
4. *Hypoendemic:* spleen rate in children not exceeding 10 per cent.

The density of parasitic infection is low in all age groups at low levels of endemicity. As endemicity rises, the rates in young children increase in relation to those of adults; this disparity results largely from immunity acquired by older children and adults.

In a given area, endemicity is determined both by the factors affecting the vector mentioned above and by the host reaction.

Where there is constantly repeated infection from vectors with frequent man-biting habits (holoendemicity), the surviving population achieves a progressive and notable degree of resistance to infection and concurrent immunity to the clinical effects of infection. Malaria consequently appears in children but relatively rarely in adults, in whom the splenomegaly also disappears. In these circumstances and where the endemic level is unaffected by environmental changes, such as temperature and humidity and density of vectors, the malaria in the community is referred to as *stable*. The level of incidence tends to be constant and epidemics do not occur.

Where transmission is less intense and not continuous, or is interrupted or seasonal, stable immunity is not established and both adults and children are affected, with parasites present and with splenomegaly at all ages. In these circumstances the malaria in the community is regarded as *unstable* and considerable fluctuations in incidence tend to occur. Epidemics may develop, especially in populations inadequately or irregularly protected by entomological control measures or by antimalarial drugs. Epidemics may also occur after long periods of lowered transmission due to climatic interference with vector breeding, as occurred in Ceylon before the epidemic of 1934–35, following successive failure of the monsoons. An epidemic indicates a sharp decline or absence of communal immunity, so that most individuals in all age groups are highly susceptible; the parasite rates are approximately the same in all groups.

GEOGRAPHICAL DISTRIBUTION

The *Plasmodia* infecting man are distributed over a wide area stretching roughly from latitudes 60°N to 40°S. The distribution and local incidence have been considerably reduced by eradication campaigns.

Transmission occurs in suitable environmental conditions of warm ambient temperature and humidity, where vector mosquitoes are breeding, where there exists a human reservoir of infection, and where susceptible persons are available.

Height above sea level is an important factor in the transmission of malaria parasites, probably because of the effect which relatively low temperatures at high altitudes have on the breeding of the vector mosquitoes. The height at which transmission ceases depends in part on the local temperature: thus, in the African coastal belt there is little malaria above 1000 metres; in the

hotter interior it is present to 2000 metres and even higher. Outbreaks have occurred in Ethiopia at over 2200 metres.

Eradication programmes

The geographical distribution and importance of malaria in the world have been considerably modified and reduced by the global campaign for eradication sponsored by the World Health Organization.

Malaria eradication means the ending of transmission and the elimination of the reservoir of infective human cases. It does not necessarily imply eradication of the vector mosquitoes.

The standard eradication campaign consists of four self-explanatory phases: preparation, attack, consolidation and maintenance. To this, in certain difficult areas, particularly Africa, may be added a pre-eradication programme which is concerned with the initial development and training of adequate staff and health services.

The basic methods of attack are mosquito control (usually by spraying with residual insecticides) and chemotherapeutic cure of human infection. Progress has been brilliant in some areas, negligible in others. The most important technical difficulties have been insecticide resistance in the vectors and drug resistance in the parasites. Discussion of the former is outside the scope of this chapter. Parasite drug resistance is reviewed on page 68 et seq.

Imported malaria

In regions of the world in which malaria is not endemic the disease appears in immigrants and travellers who have been exposed in endemic areas. Many cases are recrudescences or relapses. Primary attacks are usually seen in travellers who, because of the speed of modern air transport, may enter a non-endemic area during the incubation period of an infection.

Malaria has become an important possibility in the differential diagnosis of the cause of a febrile illness. When considering this possibility, essential factors are clearly the geographical history of the individual patient and some knowledge of the global distribution of the disease.

Imported malaria seldom gives rise to public health problems. Transmission is rare, except in special circumstances, for instance the introduction of infection into areas in which the disease was previously endemic and in which adequate numbers of vectors still exist.

Falciparum malaria

Malaria caused by *P. falciparum* (falciparum malaria) was present in southern and eastern Europe until recently, when the disease was claimed to be eradicated.

In tropical Africa the most highly endemic areas are found on the coastal belts of West Africa from Senegal to Angola and South-west Africa, and in East Africa from Somaliland to Mozambique and parts of South Africa; it is common in large regions of Central Africa and in some of the adjacent islands including Madagascar.

Eradication programmes have been partly successful in French Somali, but the disease is still hyperendemic in areas of Ethiopia, the Somali Republic and in many parts of the Sudan, especially in the south. It occurs in scattered foci in Egypt, Libya, Algeria, Tunisia, Morocco and Spanish Sahara. In southern Africa it is hyperendemic in Botswana, Lesotho and Swaziland. In some of these areas the consolidation phase of eradication has been reached.

In the eastern Mediterranean and the Middle East falciparum malaria occurs in southern and western Turkey, in Muscat, Oman, Qatar, coastal districts of Saudi Arabia, eastern Iraq and southern, western and eastern Iran. It has been eradicated from Cyprus and Sardinia and eradication programmes are advanced in Israel, Jordan, Lebanon, Syria, parts of Turkey, Iraq and northern Iran.

In the East, eradication programmes are well advanced particularly in India and Ceylon; a severe epidemic has recently been reported in the latter. The disease is still highly endemic in Bangladesh and many areas of Pakistan, Nepal and Afghanistan.

In the Far East, falciparum malaria is dominant in large regions of Burma, Laos, Thailand, Cambodia, West and East Malaysia, Indonesia and in Portuguese Timor.

Eradication programmes have been successful in Singapore (complete eradication), Hong Kong (except in Sai Kiang peninsula), the Ryukyu Islands and southern Japan. The consolidation phase has been reached in Taiwan, parts of the Philippines, Sarawak and North Borneo. The situation in south-western and southern China is not certainly known; falciparum malaria exists in these areas but an active eradication programme is believed to be in operation.

In the Pacific it is endemic in New Guinea, Papua and many islands in Melanesia. It is absent from Polynesia and Micronesia. It occurs occasionally in northern Australia and in varying endemicity in the Admiralty Islands, Bismarck Archipelago, the Solomon Islands, some islands in the Torres Strait and the New Hebrides. It is absent from New Caledonia and certain island groups, including Loyalty, Futuna, Bellona and some islands in Torres Strait.

In Central and South America falciparum malaria is endemic in large areas, especially in El Salvador, Mexico, Nicaragua, Peru, Ecuador, Colombia, Venezuela and the Argentine. Considerable progress in eradication programmes has been made in some regions, notably in coastal Guyana (eradicated), Surinam, British Honduras, Bolivia, Costa Rica, Guatemala, the Panama Canal Zone, and large areas of Venezuela and Brazil.

Until recently it was highly endemic in many islands in the Caribbean region. The disease has now been eradicated from Barbados, Grenada, Carriacou, Martinique, Puerto Rico and St Lucia. The consolidation phase has been reached in Dominica, Guadeloupe, Jamaica, Trinidad and Tobago. Campaigns are in the early stages in the Dominican Republic and Cuba.

Malaria has been eradicated from the United States of America and does not exist naturally in Canada.

Vivax malaria

Infection caused by *P. vivax* has a very wide but patchy distribution, stretching from Europe (until recently) and Siberia in the north to the Argentine and South Africa in the south. It is common in parts of North and North-east Africa, including Ethiopia and Egypt and in Mauritius and Madagascar. It is present in relatively low distribution in East Africa and Central Africa.

It does not occur amongst the Negroes of West Africa, whether living in Africa or the Americas or Caribbean, although it apparently exists in West Africa, since occasional visitors to this region are infected.

Vivax malaria occurs in the Middle East in wide areas of Iran, in Bangladesh and Pakistan, many parts of India, Burma, Laos, Thailand, Malaysia, Indonesia, Vietnam, the Philippines and New Guinea. It is also present in Central and South America, including Mexico, Venezuela, Colombia and Brazil.

Ovale malaria

P. ovale infection is the rarest form of human malaria and the most geographically restricted.

It is found mainly in localised foci in tropical Africa in Nigeria, Ghana, Liberia, Sierra Leone, the Gambia and the Congo. Less frequently it is found in Central Africa. Isolated cases have been reported in Mauritius, Israel, India, Thailand, Malaysia, the Philippines and New Guinea and in northern South America, including Venezuela.

Quartan malaria

This infection has a very wide but patchy distribution. It was formerly common in Europe. It occurs in many parts of tropical West, Central and East Africa. It is present in foci in North Africa, North-east Africa, parts of southern India and Ceylon, the Andaman and Maldive Islands, Pakistan and Burma. In some areas of Malaysia it is the most prominent form of malaria. It occurs in many other parts of the Far East, including Indonesia and New Guinea, and is scattered through the Caribbean (Guadeloupe and Jamaica) and Central and South America, including Panama, Guyana and Brazil.

PARASITE LIFE CYCLES

Sporogony: life cycle in the mosquito

As pointed out above, apart from congenital malaria, natural transmission occurs through the mosquito. There is some argument about whether the insect should be regarded as the definitive host and man as the intermediate, or *vice versa*. The issue is best avoided by referring to invertebrate and mammalian hosts.

Host specificity is strict in that the sexual cycle normally takes place in *Anopheles* mosquitoes only. Experimentally, most species of anopheline mosquitoes prove to have some degree of susceptibility to human malaria parasites. However, in addition to susceptibility, a potent vector in an endemic area must feed frequently on man and must be reasonably long-lived in order to secure the production and transmission of sporozoites. In regard to longevity, it has been suggested that the reason why some species of *Anopheles* are successful in transmitting *P. falciparum* and *P. vivax* but not *P. malariae*, may be that they do not live long enough to allow the full development of *P. malariae*.

Which vectors are active in an endemic area is determined to some extent by local conditions. In nature the proportion of captured mosquitoes found infected is usually small, seldom exceeding 3 or 4 per cent, although it may reach 10 per cent of more in holoendemic areas such as those in West Africa, whereas 90 per cent or more of susceptible vectors such as *A. gambiae*, *A. maculipennis*, *A. stephensi* and *A. culicifacies* experimentally fed on gametocytes will become infected.

The life cycle in the insect is conveniently considered to begin when human blood containing gametocytes, the sexual forms of the parasites, is ingested by the appropriate female mosquito during the act of biting. Ingested asexual parasites are destroyed in the insect stomach but the gametocytes escape from the containing erythrocytes and mature into male and female gametes. The male cells exflagellate, producing eight long thin mobile flagellae (or *microgametes*) which break away from the parent body. One microgamete penetrates a female cell and fertilises it. The male and female nuclei fuse and the *ookinete* so formed grows larger and becomes very active, eventually piercing an epithelial cell in the gut wall by lysis. It rounds up on the inner side of the epithelial wall below the lining membrane and secretes a cyst wall around itself. The nucleus undergoes mitotic division around which cytoplasm condenses to produce large numbers of the infective parasitic forms, or *sporozoites*.

After about a week to a fortnight the cyst ruptures and the sporozoites are discharged into the haemocoele and invade all parts of the insect, some eventually reaching the acinal cells of the salivary glands. When the insect bites, the sporozoites penetrate the cell membrane and are injected with the acinal fluid (saliva) into the human host.

During the bite of the infective mosquito sporozoites are injected either directly into small blood vessels or into the tissue spaces and thence into blood vessels. They remain in the systemic blood stream for a surprisingly short period, usually less than an hour.

From the initial bite to the infection of the salivary glands the process takes 5–15 days, the period depending on the environmental circumstances. The insect usually remains infective for the rest of its life.

LIFE CYCLES IN MAN

Exoerythrocytic schizogony

The next stage of the life cycle, the *primary exoerythrocytic schizogony*, begins in the tissues of the host. This phase, which is also called the pre-erythrocytic (PE) phase, takes place in the ectodermal parenchymatous cells of the liver. On entering the cell the sporozoite rounds up and the nucleus undergoes repeated division. In the course of 6–16 days, the exoerythrocytic schizont matures and divides to produce small single-nucleated *merozoites*. The liver cell ruptures and the merozoites escape either into the blood stream or into contiguous liver cells where they may initiate a *secondary exoerythrocytic (EE) phase*.

In falciparum infection no secondary infection of the liver cells occurs, but in the other infections secondary exoerythrocytic schizogony takes place following invasion of the liver cells by the merozoites released by the primary exoerythrocytic phase. The secondary phase is involved in the continuation of the blood phase through the release of exoerythrocytic merozoites and eventually provides the mechanism for relapses (see later).

In human malaria only a single generation of primary exoerythrocytic schizogony is required before the merozoites entering the blood stream are capable of invading the erythrocytes and initiating the asexual blood cycle of the parasites, the *erythrocytic* or *E phase*.

There is no evidence that the merozoites formed during the erythrocytic phase can infect the tissue cells.

Erythrocytic (E) asexual phase

As explained above, the erythrocytic asexual cycle is started by the penetration into erythrocytes of merozoites arising from the exoerythrocytic schizonts in the liver cells. In falciparum malaria, this phase is initiated by merozoites coming from the primary exoerythrocytic phase only; in the other forms of infection it arises from merozoites issuing from both primary and secondary exoerythrocytic schizonts.

Once the merozoites enter the erythrocytes the asexual cycle proceeds. The parasites grow rapidly and a large central vacuole forms in the cytoplasm, leading to the so-called ring form. The cytoplasm then becomes amoeboid to form the single-nucleated *trophozoite*. At this stage it feeds on the host cell by the process of phagotrophy, during which the erythrocytic substance is incorporated into the parasite cytoplasm inside food vacuoles lined by a double membrane visible under the electron microscope and presumably derived from the plasma membrane lining the parasite. Several such vacuoles may be found in a single parasite at this stage. As the haemoglobin of the erythrocytic substance is metabolised, the contents of the vacuoles and the erythrocyte itself become paler, and insoluble malaria pigment (haemozoin) is formed as granules of variable size in which the iron remains in the haem molecule attached to denatured protein similar in

amino acid make-up to the globin of the original haemoglobin. The pigment granules are contained within the double membrane of the vacuole and thus, like the ingested erythrocyte substance, are not in direct contact with the cytoplasm of the parasite. There is some discussion about whether the parasite feeds solely by phagotraphy or also ingests the erythrocyte material via a cytostome, a structure resembling the micropyle of the merozoite; it is thought by some authorities that at any rate the first centrally placed vacuole which creates the signet ring appearance of the young parasite arises in this second manner.

The trophozoite grows rapidly and becomes less amoeboid. New vacuoles are no longer formed, and those already existing become irregular in size and shape. The nucleus divides by mitosis (chromosomes have not been observed) until the *mature schizont* is formed as a solid body containing variable numbers of nuclei, the number depending to some extent on the species. As in the exoerythrocytic schizont discrete merozoites now form, as individual small oval or round bodies each containing a nucleus of chromatin material. The erythrocyte ruptures and the merozoites escape into the blood stream. Some are destroyed in the plasma, others invade further erythrocytes and repeat the cycle.

At some stage of the infection merozoites entering erythrocytes form sexual parasites, the male and female *gametocytes*, instead of repeating the erythrocytic cycle. The production of gametocytes is primarily inherent in the life history of the parasites and is not directly influenced by the appropriate host, although in the *Plasmodia* invading man, several generations of schizogony in the blood usually take place before they are produced. The schizont of the E phase thus has the capacity of producing both asexual and sexual parasites.

The asexual erythrocytic (E) cycle is completed in 2 or 3 days, depending on the species of parasite concerned and ends with the discharge of merozoites and the destruction of the erythrocyte. The process is called *schizogony*.

Gametocytes take some days longer to mature. They then dwell in the individual erythrocyte for the remainder of its existence, which may be over 100 days.

Changes occur in the erythrocytes containing the asexual parasites, depending on the relevant infecting organism. As the haemoglobin is metabolised by the latter, the colour of the erythrocyte fades; as little as 4 per cent of the haemoglobin of the infected cell remains unchanged by the time the schizont reaches maturity. The host cell may remain normal, or become enlarged or reduced in size.

The disc shape is usually lost as the parasite grows and the cell becomes more spheroidal. Changes occur in the envelope in the form of various kinds of stippling (Schüffner's, Maurer's and Ziemann's dots) which apparently arise as a result of local concentrations of antigen derived directly from the growing parasite.

Summary

The life cycles of the malaria parasites naturally infecting man may be summarised as follows.

In all four parasites, sporozoites invade the liver parenchymal cells to form the primary exoerythrocytic phase; merozoites from this invade the blood stream at the end of the prepatent period and start up the erythrocytic (E) phase, which is responsible for the clinical response.

This may be written:

SP ⎯⎯⎯⟶ PE ⎯⎯⎯⟶ E

Sporozoites   Primary exo-   Erythrocytic
*   erythrocytic   phase*
*   or pre-*
*   erythrocytic*
*   phase*

For *P. falciparum* infection, this is the only pattern.

In *P. vivax*, *P. ovale* and *P. malariae*, the primary exoerythrocytic phase produces in addition to the blood-invading merozoites, others which invade contiguous liver cells, thus inducing a secondary exoerythrocytic cycle (the EE or persistent liver phase) which injects merozoites into the blood stream and at a later stage may initiate a relapse. For these parasites, therefore, the pattern is:

SP ⎯⎯⎯⟶ PE ⎯⎯⎯⟶ E
                ↓
                EE ⎯⎯⎯⟶ E (relapse)

Secondary
exoerythrocytic
phase

It will be noted that the patterns of parasites in patients with overt malaria are:

Falciparum malaria : E phase *only*.
Other malarias : E phase plus persistent
                  EE phase.

These patterns determine the relevant chemotherapy (see page 65 et seq.).

RELAPSES AND RECRUDESCENCES

A relapse is a renewed manifestation of malaria due to parasites in the blood which derive from a secondary exoerythrocytic source. This can occur only in a sporozoite-induced infection and in infection by a *Plasmodium* species in which secondary exoerythrocytic schizogony occurs. A true relapse may therefore occur in sporozoite-induced *P. vivax*, *P. ovale* and *P. malariae* infection. It does not occur in blood transmitted infections.

In *P. falciparum* infection, renewed manifestations of the malaria subsequent to the primary attack, if not resulting from fresh infection, are due to multiplication in the blood of an existing population of parasites surviving from the original infection. This is a recrudescence, not a relapse. It may occur also in a blood-induced infection.

Relapses are explained on the grounds that after replacing the primary exoerythrocytic schizonts some merozoites enter further parenchymatous cells; this process is repeated indefinitely, so that merozoites are discharged at regular intervals into the blood stream to initiate afresh the erythrocytic phase. As the infection progresses, some immunity becomes established and the merozoites are destroyed as they reach the blood. The immunity, however, has no effect on the tissue parasites, the merozoites from which continue to infect liver cells. In time the immunity declines and the merozoites thrown into the blood initiate a new erythrocytic phase and relapse occurs.

This theory of the origin of relapses is generally accepted but does not fit certain aspects of the life cycle in some parasites.

For instance, the prepatent period in certain strains of *P. vivax* parasites may be prolonged beyond the usual 8 days for periods as long as 6 months, over a time in which, because of the absence of the erythrocytic parasite, no immunity could develop. Prolongation of the incubation period can be induced artificially in laboratory strains of *P. vivax*, for instance, by administration of antimalarial drugs for the first few days after infection with sporozoites. The same effect can be produced in patients bitten by mosquitoes infected with both *P. vivax* and *P. falciparum*, in which case the appearance of the former parasites in the blood is delayed for many weeks; the patients are susceptible to superinfection with blood parasites during this period, indicating absence of immunity, presumably because no extraerythrocytic merozoites from the original infection are being discharged into the blood, and consequently immunity-engendering E parasites are not being produced.

Similar difficulties are found in explaining relapses of *P. vivax* and *P. malariae* occurring at intervals much longer than would be needed for the disappearance of acquired immunity. No single explanation fits the facts. There are arguments against the assumptions that the sporozoites lie dormant in such latency, that they begin to grow but growth becomes arrested at some point or that during latency the exoerythrocytic schizonts produce only histotropic merozoites.

PERIODICITY AND LENGTH OF VARIOUS STAGES OF LIFE CYCLE

The length of the life cycle in the mosquito (sporogony) is influenced by the ambient temperature. The time is shortened at high temperatures and lengthened at low temperatures. Above the maximum temperature, which is well below that tolerated by the parasite in the mammalian host, the parasite is killed. For a given temperature the time needed for sporogony depends on the species of parasite. It is usually about 1–2 weeks.

In man, the length of the tissue and blood cycles is nearly constant for a given parasite and little affected by the presence of even high fever.

In *P. falciparum*, primary exoerythrocytic schizogony takes about 6 days from the time of infection with sporozoites, 8 days in *P. vivax* and 9 days in *P. ovale* infections. The length of the cycle in *P. malariae* has not been measured in man but in the chimpanzee which is a natural host, it is estimated at between 13 and 16 days.

The asexual cycle in the erythrocyte takes 48 hours in *P. vivax*, 49–50 hours in *P. ovale*, 72 hours in *P. malariae*. In *P. falciparum* the cycle usually takes 48 hours but the completion of schizogony in the vessels of the deep tissues makes exact timing of the process difficult. Certain strains in India were at one time thought to take rather less than 48 hours for schizogony, producing subtertian rather than tertian fever (see later).

The length of the asexual schizogony cycle determines the periodicity of the fever once a rhythm has been established, in that the maturation and rupture of the schizonts corresponds closely in time to the early stages of the febrile paroxysms.

It will be noted that the duration of the three developmental phases of a given species, i.e. sporogony, exoerythrocytic and erythrocytic schizogony, are roughly proportional. Thus *P. malariae* requires 15–20 days at 25°C in the mosquito, 13–16 days in the liver cell and 3 days in the blood, and *P. falciparum* 9 days at 25°C in the insect, 5½–6 days in the liver cell and 2 days in the blood.

P. falciparum

Merozoites escaping from the mature exoerythrocytic schizonts in the liver cells between the fifth and sixth day invade erythrocytes in all stages of maturity and undergo rapid multiplication.

The young ring forms are very small, with thin cytoplasm around a large vacuole and with prominent single or double nucleus. The vacuole may be the same colour as the erythrocyte substance or it may be colourless. As in other parasites, it is thought to be a nutrient vacuole. The parasites are often applied along the edge of the erythrocyte (accolé or appliqué rings). Multiple infection of a single erythrocyte is common. The young rings grow rapidly in size, but do not show very active amoeboid movement. At 24 hours the parasite appears as thick rings with a relatively small vacuole in which the nucleus may be visible, giving a bird's eye appearance.

The vacuole now goes and the nucleus elongates and becomes bar-shaped. Black pigment granules appear in the cytoplasm.

At this stage in a synchronous infection the parasite numbers in the peripheral blood decline sharply due to their retreat to the blood vessels of the deep tissues to continue the schizogony cycle. The location of the parasites at this stage has not been fully established. The mature schizont is irregular in shape and in the distribution of its merozoites. It occupies about two thirds of the erythrocyte. The number of merozoites formed varies from strain to strain, but averages sixteen.

Following schizogony, a new generation of minute rings appears in the peripheral blood.

The erythrocyte does not change in size when infected with *P. falciparum* although it becomes more spheroid as the infection develops. With special staining techniques characteristic Maurer's clefts can be demonstrated in the infected erythrocyte, first appearing when the parasite is in the late ring stage, becoming most distinct in cells containing large rings and disintegrating at the schizont stage. The clefts are large, blurred and blotchy; they number up to twelve.

The crescentic shape of the mature gametocytes of *P. falciparum* gives the parasite its name. The sexual forms appear first in the blood about 10 days after the beginning of parasitaemia. The numbers rise to a peak and subside in the course of the next few weeks, often reaching a point where they are difficult to find after the fifth week of patency. A few are produced intermittently thereafter. Their appearance in the peripheral blood may be delayed by administration of non-curative doses of quinine and stimulated by other drugs, including sulphonamides. The gametocyte remains in the infected erythrocyte for the duration of its existence, a mean of about 50 days, with a maximum of about 120. In some highly endemic areas the maximum production of gametocytes occurs in children up to the fifth year. They are often hard to find in blood films from older children and adults; this is thought to result from the development of immunity or premunition.

The mature male gametocyte is sausage-shaped with blunt ends and a large diffuse nucleus made up in stained films of dark red dots partly covered by coarse dark-brown pigment granules which are always clustered in the nuclear region. The cytoplasm stains blue-mauve. The female gametocyte (macrogametocyte) is more crescentic-shaped and somewhat longer. The nucleus is compact and partly obscured by pigment granules; the cytoplasm is blue. Remnants of the host erythrocyte are stretched across the concavity of the crescent.

Because of the deep tissue schizogony, the peripheral blood picture in the infected patient normally contains only rings and gametocytes. Schizonts are rare, except in severe and heavy infections.

The overall number of parasites in the blood mounts rapidly with each schizogony, and 15–25 per cent of the surviving erythrocytes may be infected.

Man is the natural host of *P. falciparum*. The infection has been experimentally passed into young and splenectomised gibbons and into the splenectomised chimpanzee. It has recently been transmitted to the owl monkey *Aotus trivirgatus* in which a severe and fatal infection results. The latter infection may prove a useful tool for chemotherapeutic studies.

Plasmodium vivax

Merozoites differentially invade young red cells, particularly reticulocytes although older cells are not invulnerable. Multiple infection of an erythrocyte occurs, but less frequently than in *P. falciparum* infection. The invasion is rapid, and free merozoites are seldom seen in the blood. The parasite quickly develops a central vacuole, to form the ring stage. A few hours later the cytoplasm becomes actively amoeboid, rapidly projecting and withdrawing pseudopodia. The volume of cytoplasm increases rapidly, and about 8 hours after infection small granules of light brown haemozoin pigment appear in it. By 24 hours the parasite occupies about two thirds of the erythrocyte; it is now sluggish, the central vacuole disappears and the nucleus becomes large and oval or horseshoe shaped. Pigment granules increase in the cytoplasm. The trophozoite enlarges and the cytoplasm becomes denser. At about 36 hours the schizont is formed as the nucleus divides and redivides into 12 to 16 (occasionally up to 24) daughter nuclei.

Cytoplasm condenses around each nucleus of the maturing schizont and in this way individual merozoites are formed, leaving a residual mass of excess cytoplasm and pigment granules agglomerated into a few dense masses.

The mature schizont appears as a rosette occupying the bulk of the enlarged erythrocyte. The latter ruptures and releases the merozoites which immediately invade new erythrocytes. The pigment, the residual body and the debris of the disrupted erythrocyte are removed by phagocytosis.

The erythrocyte cycle occurs at regular intervals of about 48 hours. A single brood gives rise eventually to tertian fever. Two broods, developing on alternate days, are associated with quotidian fever. In the first few days of a primary attack the cycles are not fully synchronised and the fever is irregular.

The infected erythrocyte enlarges and becomes paler as the parasite develops. Stippling, known as Schüffner's dots, appears in stained preparations at the early ring stage. The pink-staining uniform small dots increase in number rapidly and cover the whole erythrocyte, obscuring details of the growing parasite.

At some stage in the erythrocytic cycle certain merozoites infecting erythrocytes do not reproduce the E phase but are converted into large non-vacuolated non-amoeboid male and female gametocytes, which become fully grown in about 4 days. These begin to appear about the fifth day of patency, but have been reported as early as the third day. In the latter case they may have originated from merozoites discharged from the liver exoerythrocytic parasites; this probably also occurs in relapses in which gametocytes may be present in the first batch of blood parasites.

The natural mammalian host of *P. vivax* is man. Racial immunity exists in the West African Negro who is remarkably insusceptible to infection, whether in Africa or after generations elsewhere. Other African races, including the Bantu, are fully susceptible. The chimpanzee is partially susceptible and more vulnerable after splenectomy, when mature gametocytes are produced. The owl monkey, *A. trivirgatus*, has recently been found to take the infection well and is proving a valuable animal for research. Rhesus monkeys are completely insusceptible.

The relapse pattern in *P. vivax* infections varies with the strain but is remarkably constant for the relevant parasite. Thus the Chesson strain, originally from New Guinea and widely used in human experiments, has a short period of 13 days; some strains from Rumania have intervals of as long as 260 days and from Siberia even longer. In an infected person removed from the endemic area relapses may occur for up to 3 years, but seldom later.

The diagnosis of *P. vivax* infection is made by the examination of parasites in thin blood smears stained by Giemsa's or Leishman's methods, in which the cytoplasm stains blue and the chromatin of the nucleus red or purple. The appearances of the various stages of the parasite are usually diagnostic, but abnormal forms may occur which may be mistaken for *P. ovale*. Small schizonts with relatively few merozoites may occur in partly immune hosts, and Schüffner's dots may be absent. The parasites are also distorted by antimalarial drugs and in severely anaemic patients. In doubtful cases, the probability of infection with simian malaria must be considered. The commonest source of error is probably bad film-making or staining techniques.

Plasmodium ovale

After a precise pre-patent period of 9 days, merozoites from the exoerythrocytic parasites in the liver invade reticulocytes, and in 49–50 hours develop into mature schizonts.

The ring form is relatively large with a rounded nucleus and a small central vacuole, in which the nucleus sometimes appears inserted. Growth is slow and amoeboid activity restricted. The vacuole disappears early and the solid-looking spherical parasite comes to half fill the erythrocyte. Pigment appears as fine brown granules, which tend to condense into dark brown lumps. The large nucleus divides into large daughter nuclei and 8 merozoites (range of 4 to 16) are formed and arranged irregularly in the mature schizont. The number of merozoites doubles in relapses.

The changes in the containing erythrocyte are characteristic. The cell enlarges, becomes spheroidal and is easily distorted during the making of a thin blood film in which the infected erythrocytes appear oval and may be fimbriated at one or both extremities. The characteristic features in the film are thus essentially artefacts.

The infected erythrocytes become stippled in a particular way, which is diagnostic. The cell soon becomes covered with Schüffner's dots, in the form of large violet spots which are larger and fewer than those in *P. vivax* and may partly obscure the parasite.

The density of parasites in the blood in *P. ovale* infection is low, probably because of the predilection for infection of reticulocytes; small numbers of parasites may persist for months.

Prolonged latency has been reported in *P. ovale* infections. Relapses are common in some strains and rare in others. They follow a frequency pattern for individual strains, as in *P. vivax* infections.

Gametocytes first appear about the fifth day of patency, and the numbers build up slowly so that it may be weeks before mosquitoes can be infected. The gametocyte completely fills the erythrocyte; the pigment is coarse and dark and may collect near the surface of the gametocyte. (Distinguishing features are listed in Table 1.)

Man is the natural host of *P. ovale*. As with *P. vivax* malaria, the parasite is liable to be suppressed by concurrent *P. falciparum* infection. The chimpanzee can be infected artificially, and is fully susceptible after splenectomy.

Plasmodium malariae

P. malariae invades mature erythrocytes; there is little evidence of reticulocyte invasion. The ring forms resemble those of *P. vivax* except that the cytoplasm is denser. In stained thin films made within the first 24 hours the growing parasite stretches across the erythrocyte to form a characteristic 'band' form, which is regarded by some as an artefact. The pigment is dark brown or black and may be concentrated along one edge of the band, with the elongated nucleus along the other. The ring form may persist until the parasite occupies most of the erythrocyte. Division of the nucleus begins after some 60 hours when the vacuole finally disappears. Six to 12 deeply staining daughter nuclei are formed and surrounded by dense cytoplasm to become merozoites. The pigment conglomerates and occupies the central region of the parasite. The mature schizont thus has a characteristic rosette appearance.

The erythrocyte remains unchanged in size and shape. Freshly stained films may disclose stippling, best seen at the ring and trophozoite stage. The dots are fine and regularly distributed. Stippling is not always visible in Romanowsky stained

TABLE 1. *Differentiation of human malaria parasites in thin blood films*

Parasite	Erythrocyte infection rate	Stages of asexual parasites in peripheral blood	Ring forms	Trophozoites	Schizonts	Gametocytes	Changes in erythrocyte
P. falciparum	Scanty, to 15% or more	Usually only rings. Late trophozoites and schizonts in heavy infection or complications	Small fine rings at first. Cytoplasm becoming thicker 1–2 chromatin dots. Thin cytoplasm. Appliqué forms. Multiple infection of erythrocytes common	Uncommon in peripheral blood. Solid, irregularly rounded; chromatin indistinct; pigment concentrated	Rare. 8–36 merozoites. Heavily pigmented. Occupies $\frac{2}{3}$ of normal-sized cell	Crescentic or bean-shaped	Not enlarged. Maurer's dots
P. vivax	Usually scanty, rarely greater than 2%	All stages	Small and large rings. Single chromatin dot, occasionally two	Large, amoeboid, of yellow-brown pigment	Common, especially in late stages of cycle, just before and early in the paroxysm. Rounded, occupying most of erythrocyte. 12–14 merozoites	Round. Occupy most of enlarged erythrocyte. Scattered pigment	Enlarged. Pale Schüffner's dots
P. ovale	As in *P. vivax*	All stages	As in *P. vivax*	As in *P. vivax* but less amoeboid	Rounded occupies $\frac{3}{4}$ of erythrocyte. 6–12 merozoites. Central mass of pigment	As in *P. vivax*	Enlarged. Pale. Oval with fimbriated ends in stained films. Schüffner's dots
P. malariae	Low, usually not more than 1%	All stages	Small or fat. Single chromatin dot	Narrow band forms	Round. Often rosette with central pigment mass. 6–12 merozoites. Fills erythrocyte	Round. Fills erythrocyte	Not enlarged. Ziemann's stippling

slides, but can usually be demonstrated by fluorescent tagged antibody techniques.

The density of infection is low. It is highest in children. Parasitaemia may persist at very low levels for long periods.

Gametocytes usually appear late in sporozoite-induced infections. They have been recorded for the first time after infection as early as the fifth day and as late as the twenty-third. In blood-induced infections they are commonly present by the sixth day. In endemic areas gametocytes are seen only in young children. The male gametocyte occupies the whole erythrocyte; it has a large nucleus and greyish-green cytoplasm dotted with fine black pigment granules. The female gameto-cytes are spherical with a large central nucleus and pigment granules finely dispersed in the cyto-plasm, which takes on a deep blue colour with Romanowsky stain. They closely resemble, and are difficult to distinguish morphologically, from the late single-nucleated asexual parasites.

Clinical recurrences of the disease may occur 5–10 years or even longer after the original infection. Periods of more than 30 years' latency have been recorded. The infection has been trans-mitted by blood transfusion over 20 years after a known attack of quartan malaria. The erythro-cytic infection may thus persist in the peripheral blood for long periods, or be initiated from time to time by merozoites from the long-persisting secondary exoerythrocytic phase in the liver.

P. malariae occurs naturally in animals other than man. The parasite of chimpanzees formerly called *P. rhodaini* is identical with *P. malariae*, and is therefore a potential zoonosis. Strains of *P. malariae* from man will produce heavy infec-tions in splenectomised chimpanzees in which may develop mature gametocytes infective to mosquitoes.

IMMUNITY AND ACQUIRED RESISTANCE

Some evidence of acquired immunity and resist-ance to homologous infection appears within a few days of the establishment of the erythrocytic parasites in all forms of human malaria. The pro-cesses involved are both cellular and humoral. Cellular immunity is manifested by hyperplasia and hyperactivity of the lymphoid macrophages, which specifically engulf the relevant parasites but show no abnormal reaction to other parasites. The avid phagocytosis is associated in these cells by excessive mitochondrial activity. In this way most of the erythrocytic parasites may be destroyed, although in some forms of malaria, notably avian

infections, some parasites survive and maintain the specific macrophage activity and other im-mune responses in the host. Such a situation is referred to as 'premunition'; it is believed to con-tinue only so long as the erythrocytic parasites survive. If the parasites are totally destroyed, immunity is rapidly lost. In mammalian infections, including those in man, the immune responses are also stimulated only by the asexual erythrocytic parasites and the other parasitic phases, including the exoerythrocytic and the sexual forms, are not involved.

In infections which have continued over a long period or in circumstances in which reinfection is frequent, acquired resistance develops to super-infection (infection with the same strain of the same species of parasite). Such resistance does not completely prevent reinfection as such but limits it and considerably modifies the clinical effects. Individuals who have acquired such resistance are commonly referred to as 'immunes' or 'semi-immunes'. In such persons the immunity is not absolute as usually indicated by the develop-ment of occasional attacks of clinically modified malaria. The significance of this in regard to chemotherapy is discussed elsewhere. Immunity in man is usually lost in a matter of months following eradication of the E parasites by treat-ment or by long absence from the endemic area. The continuance of resistance in man for this period indicates that the effect is partly humoral (as demonstrated in the gamma globulin) and not wholly dependent on premunition (persistence of E forms) as in avian malaria.

The acquisition of adequate immunity takes time, and those who eventually acquire it usually suffer from severe malaria in the early years of exposure.

In highly endemic areas infection is uncommon in infants below the age of 4–6 months. There-after malaria becomes increasingly common and more severe as the child gets older. After the third to fifth year attacks become fewer and less violent and survivors beyond this period show steadily increasing resistance to infection and to its clinical effects, so long as they remain in the endemic region.

The relative absence of infection or of the severe effects of infection in the first 6 months of life in holo- or hyperendemic areas has not yet been explained. Evidence of transmission of immune bodies to the fetus from the infected mother has been obtained in *P. falciparum* infections in which protective gamma globulins have been identified in the cord blood. There is also some evidence of inhibition of erythrocytic parasitic development

D

in *P. falciparum* infections in infants fed exclusively on breast milk or milk products. Such inhibition has been repeatedly demonstrated in rodent and simian malaria.

Acquired resistance may be easily lost. In communities normally subjected to continual reinfection and consequently highly resistant, long periods of interruption of transmission may lead to considerable loss of immunity, rendering the community open to epidemics. In areas where transmission is low, or seasonal, resistance may not fully develop.

Some individuals appear to be naturally more resistant than others on exposure to infection with human malaria parasites. Whether this is due to natural immunity or to other factors has not been determined. However, natural immunity undoubtedly occurs in man in relation to many species of malaria parasites of other mammals. It usually involves most stages of the parasite, including the E forms (especially the merozoites), the gametocytes and the sporozoites. The resistance of the Negro to infection with *P. vivax* is an example.

The nature of acquired immunity in human malaria is not fully understood, but there is no doubt that active humoral antibodies are formed which are capable of destroying the E parasites. In *P. falciparum* infection some of these protective antibodies have been demonstrated in the gamma globulin complex.

In unprotected indigenous children in holo-endemic falciparum areas, the serum gamma globulin concentrations are sometimes high at birth, then fall and begin to rise steadily. Beyond the age of 2 years they exceed those reached in children of the same age living in the same area but protected from birth from malaria by anti-malarial drugs. These differences persist up to the sixth year of life, after which the concentrations in the two groups are of the same order.

The significance of these changes in gamma globulin, which so closely follow the pattern of immune response in an area of stable malaria, has recently been disclosed by the discovery that the 7S fraction of the globulin extracted from immune adults has a powerful antiparasitic effect on the homologous parasite in indigenous children.

Immune individuals who have been protected against infection by chemotherapy and suppression or have been absent from the endemic area for long enough again become susceptible to the homologous strain. This is probably because of loss of protective gamma globulin, since it has recently been shown that a significant fall in serum concentration of this globulin occurs in immune subjects protected for 2 years by anti-malarial drugs.

In addition to the protective gamma globulins, antibodies capable of fixing complement, agglutinins, precipitins and fluorescent antibodies appear in the serum of infected individuals.

The development of fluorescent antibodies in children and adults exposed to *P. falciparum* infection closely mirrors that of gamma globulins and may thus be correlated with the specific protective antibody. This applies also to *P. malariae* and *P. ovale* infections.

Antibody titres increase rapidly after infection and reach maximal levels which fall very gradually after cure. Fluorescent antibody has been detected in the serum 12 months after infection with *P. vivax*.

P. falciparum infection is said to provoke effective 'premunition' in the indigenous host, in the sense that children in highly endemic areas may carry a continuous high parasitaemia while adults have a low parasitaemia. It is difficult to accept this interpretation in areas in which transmission is frequent and, indeed, practically continuous, since some of the parasites observed at any one time may well derive from a fresh primary exoerythrocytic phase. Immunity lasts for the homologous strain for 3–4 months or longer after eradication of the primary infection. It is strain specific. Individuals from a highly endemic area may develop severe infections of other strains of the same species on exposure in another area.

The declining parasitaemia in the untreated case of vivax malaria is clear evidence of the development of some form of resistance to the parasite which is probably humoral rather than premunitive, since recovery from infection is followed by a slowly declining residual immunity (in the absence of parasites, and therefore not premunity), which is strain rather than species specific and which may last as long as 3 years. A long period of infection, 6 months or more, is needed to evoke functional immunity. Humoral antibodies, including complement fixing factors and fluorescent antibodies have been demonstrated within a week of the first appearance of parasitaemia in sporozoite induced infections; they may persist for long periods, but it is uncertain how they relate to resistance to infection or to the associated clinical modification of attacks.

The immunity acquired against the erythrocytic parasites does not affect the exoerythrocytic phases in the liver. When it declines, merozoites from the latter will eventually initiate a new erythrocytic infection and a relapse will occur.

This applies also to *P. ovale* and *P. malariae* infections (see pages 35 and 37).

Infection with *P. ovale* produces active resistance to reinfection with the homologous strain and some resistance to heterologous strains of the same species.

P. malariae induces powerful immunity in the host. In hyperendemic areas it develops rapidly, so that the highest incidence of the infection occurs in childhood, after which it declines steadily. Unlike other species of man-infecting *Plasmodium* the parasites may not completely disappear from the blood, even over very long periods. Some authorities consider this evidence in favour of premunition rather than humoral immunity, but it is possible that the explanation lies in the very long-persisting exoerythrocytic phase, which may from time to time continue to top up the erythrocytic infection. The nephrotic syndrome (see below) commonly seen in children in endemic areas is believed to result from auto-antibody-antigen reactions in the kidney initiated by the *P. malariae* infection; the antibody-antigen complex has been demonstrated on the glomerular basement membrane.

HUMAN POPULATION GENETICS AND MALARIA

Four abnormal haemoglobins which are transmitted by autosomal genes transferred by mendelian inheritance occur in high frequencies in man, namely haemoglobins S (sickle), C and E, and thalassaemia. These represent states of balanced polymorphism. The high frequencies of heterozygotes could be explained by high rates of gene mutation, by differentially increased female fecundity or by some form of biological advantage operating in favour of the heterozygotes.

The first two factors are insignificant in any human situation so far examined, and it is generally accepted that the impressive polymorphic balance which exists must have developed through the operation of advantageous selection.

The selecting agent for the sickle cell gene (haemoglobin S) is *P. falciparum* malaria. This has not yet been proved for thalassaemia, although there is evidence in favour so far as β thalassaemia is concerned. It is not the case for haemoglobins C and E.

The serious nature of homozygous SS disease (sickle cell disease) and the high rate of mortality of homozygote infants and young children indicate that severe selection is operating against the sickle cell gene despite its persistence at high frequencies.

The possibility that heterozygotes of haemoglobin S are resistant to the fatal effects of *P. falciparum* infection is indicated by the parallel geographical distributions of present and former endemic areas of this species of malaria and of the sickle cell gene. Thus, in areas of Africa in which the frequency of the gene is high, *P. falciparum* malaria is either holoendemic or hyperendemic. This applies to other areas in which the gene is found, but of course there are some regions in the world where malaria is highly endemic but the gene does not exist.

Lower parasite rates and counts in young heterozygotes than in non-sicklers have been reported in endemic areas by many workers. There is considerable controversy, however, about whether there are valid differences of incidence of infection in the two groups, but the occurrence of densities of parasites greater than 100 000 per mm^3 blood (regarded as the potentially lethal level of infection) is significantly much lower in S heterozygotes than in normals. Moreover, fatal malaria infections rarely occur in heterozygotes.

The pattern is most obvious in young children in whom it has been suggested that the relative resistance to *P. falciparum* provided by haemoglobin S may be adequate to help the heterozygotes 'through the dangerous years of early childhood during which an active immunity to the disease is developed' (Allison). This seems to be the case.

Although the heterozygote does not often develop the severest manifestations of malaria, the parasites do infect him, and immunity is developed as in a normal individual. Indeed, there is evidence that, possibly because of increased phagocytosis, the immune response to invasion of the erythrocyte by the parasite is stimulated in the heterozygote. This is supported by evidence that heterozygous children develop higher gamma globulin plasma levels than do corresponding normal children. In holoendemic areas, therefore, the differences between heterozygotes and normals is evident mostly in the children in whom immunity is being developed, i.e. between 1 and 4 years. Beyond this age, the total surviving population has developed a high degree of immunity which overshadows the protection afforded by the gene, so that no differences between the malaria situation in the heterozygote and in normals are apparent, except perhaps during pregnancy.

It can be said, therefore, that the presence of the S gene in a heterozygote substantially protects the child from malignant malaria in a holoendemic area over the dangerous period of acquiring immunity, when the normal child may die from the infection. This amounts to human selection.

It is believed that *P. falciparum* infection may also be acting selectively in erythrocyte glucose-6-phosphate dehydrogenase (G-6-PD) deficiency. This deficiency is a sex-linked genetic phenomenon, more easily demonstrated in the male hemizygote than in the female heterozygote.

Again the distribution of the trait and that of *P. falciparum* malaria closely tally, and evidence is accumulating that the density of infection (not the incidence) rarely reaches the potential fatal level (100 000 parasites per mm³) in enzyme-deficient children, and that consequently fatal malaria is much less common in the carrier of the trait than in normals. Thus he survives where a normal child may die when exposed to the same epidemiological conditions during the period of 1–4 years when immunity is being built up.

PATHOLOGY AND PATHOGENESIS
OF ACUTE MALARIA

In the host no pathological changes are caused by the sporozoites beyond the invasion of the liver parenchymal cells and the initiation in them of the exoerythrocytic phase.

The development of exoerythrocytic parasites and the bursting of the liver cells containing the schizonts cause some ephemeral local cellular reaction. The area concerned is immediately invested by polymorphonuclear leucocytes and lymphoid macrophages which phagocytose the remains of the damaged cells. These changes occur after development of both primary and secondary exoerythrocytic schizonts. The destroyed cells are replaced, and there is no evidence of permanent damage or fibroblastic reaction.

This process has no general pathological effects beyond initiating in turn the asexual E phase in the erythrocytes via the merozoites ejected into the blood. Gametocytes are likewise pathologically inert. It is the E phase alone which is responsible for the clinical and pathological disturbances in the host which constitute malaria. The mechanisms by which the pathological changes are initiated and maintained in the host by this parasitic phase are discussed below. As in many acute medical conditions, the progress of the disease and its effects on the host depend on the balance struck between the pathological activity of the parasite and the development of immune responses in the host.

In human malaria most observations have been made in fatal *P. falciparum* infections. The other infections are largely self-limited and seldom cause death. The pathological processes involved have been examined mainly in falciparum malaria in man and in acute infections in animals, particularly *P. knowlesi* and *P. coatneyi* in monkeys, and *P. berghei* in rodents.

The importance of the individual phases of asexual schizogony in the pathogenesis of the disease has not yet been clearly determined. There is some evidence that circulating physiologically active factors may be involved in tissue dysfunction which block the basic metabolic activity of tissue cells. It is not known whether these substances are developed during the intracellular life of the parasite or at the time of the rupture of the mature schizont, when, in addition to the merozoites, granules of malaria pigment, the residual body and fragments of the cell substance, are thrown into the blood stream.

Malaria pigment is formed by the parasite from haemoglobin, which it converts into an insoluble combination of haem and denatured protein derived from globin. Although the pigment is thrown into the circulation when the schizont ruptures and is subsequently widely dispersed in tissue spaces and macrophages, it appears to be physiologically inert and is thought to take no part in the pathogenesis of malaria.

Over the course of the infection there is considerably greater loss of the circulating erythrocyte mass than can be accounted for by the parasitaemia. There is direct evidence in human falciparum infection that this depends in part on concurrent lysis of uninfected erythrocytes. In the later stages of the infection specific phagocytosis of both invaded and non-invaded erythrocytes may also be involved.

Anaemia results, but is seldom sufficient in itself to affect the host tissues.

The uptake, carriage and discharge of oxygen by haemoglobin in invaded and uninvaded cells is not grossly affected, so that it can be presumed that the oxygen supply at the tissue face is adequate for basic metabolic processes in all but the most severely haemolytic infections, for example in complicated falciparum malaria in which blackwater fever has appeared.

Nevertheless, profound disturbances of function and structure occur in the tissues of the non-immune host if an acute infection is allowed to run unchecked.

A feature of great importance in *P. falciparum* infections which distinguishes its pathological effects from those of other human malarias is the recession of the asexual parasites from the peripheral circulation to the blood vessels of the internal organs for the later stages of schizogony. In some undetermined way, the late trophozoites and early and mature schizonts remain in the deep tissues until the rupture of the schizonts and the liberation of merozoites. This leads to interference of local blood flow which must be at any rate a supporting factor in subsequent pathological events.

Notable circulatory changes occur during the characteristic febrile paroxysms, which include generalised peripheral vasoconstriction (in the cold stage) followed in a few hours by vasodilatation and increase in cardiac output. These events are probably of little significance unless the febrile stage persists, as it does in aperiodic falciparum malaria.

As the infection progresses, damage to cardiac muscle also exerts its effects on the output and blood flow and, although heart failure as such is unusual, generalised cardiovascular failure leading to the development of medical shock is common. The overall depression of the circulation is associated with specific circulatory disturbances in the organs and tissues arising from readjustment of internal blood flow which may occur independently of shock. It has been shown experimentally that the reduction of blood flow in the organs arises from intense vasoconstriction, itself due to hyperactivity of the sympathetic nervous system similar to that demonstrable in medical shock. The effect is to diminish local blood flow and disturb or heighten the activity of other factors which may be influencing tissue function, for example, the metabolic inhibitors mentioned above. Changes in local circulation may also upset the balance and production of the hormones of the adrenal and other endocrine glands, and lead to further vasomotor effects.

These physiological dynamic circulatory changes may be exacerbated by the production or uncovering of pharmacologically active substances such as kinins. They are also to some extent affected by mechanical interference with local blood flow. Functional damage to vascular endothelium leads to escape of protein and water and local increase in blood viscosity and finally stasis. This occurs in greatest degree in vessels lined with relatively impermeable endothelium, as in the brain. Stickiness of infected erythrocytes in relation to vascular endothelium may also impede the already slowing circulation. Swelling of the hyperactive Kupffer cells in the liver may provide some mechanical obstruction to the sinusoidal flow, and in the general circulation in the terminal stages of an infection clumping (so-called 'sludging') of the erythrocytes may occur and further impede the flow exacerbating the prevailing anoxaemia by interference with haemoglobin oxygenation in the alveoli of the lungs. The latter is disturbed to some degree in any case by the vascular changes occurring in the lungs.

Changes in organs

The pathological patterns seen in the tissues in acute falciparum malaria, *P. knowlesi* infection in monkeys and *P. berghei* infections in mice are essentially similar. They arise from the interaction of the three basic pathogenic factors; the disturbance of cellular function and structure; the dynamic and physiological changes in the vascular tree, and the background of anoxaemia and/or tissue anoxia.

A few changes are noted below. Details may be had from larger texts.

The spleen enlarges in all infections. The increase in size is at first due to dynamic vascular engorgement, but in long-continued or repeated infections hyperplasia of the reticuloendothelium and of the lymphoid tissue occurs, followed later by interstitial fibrosis, especially about the corpuscular blood vessels.

Malaria pigment is deposited in the tissue spaces and picked up by the macrophages, colouring the organ slaty-grey or black. In the acute stages of falciparum malaria the lymphoid cells of the splenic corpuscles are greatly reduced in numbers, and mitotic figures are sometimes seen. Some authors hold that the lymphoid macrophages appearing in the blood at this stage are derived from these cells. The Malpighian corpuscles are free from pigment except for occasional macrophages which may contain haemosiderin in excess of malaria pigment. The pulp macrophages are laden with granules and clumps of malaria pigment and some haemosiderin, and with infected and non-infected erythrocytes and free parasites. The sinuses are engorged with erythrocytes, many infected and containing pigmented stages of the parasites.

In spontaneously recovered cases of *P. falciparum* malaria or in cases after treatment, regeneration of the follicles gradually takes place. Eventually the only indication of past infection may be the malarial pigment still present in the macrophages and tissue spaces.

Localised infarcts and subperitoneal haemorrhage followed by fibrosis may occur; occasionally the organ may be completely infarcted by twisting on its pedicle or may be ruptured. In long-standing cases with good development of immunity, the spleen becomes small and fibrosed with practically no pulp left.

In repeated infection in children it grows very large, with gross congestion and with hyperplasia of the reticuloendothelial tissue.

The liver is enlarged early, following vascular engorgement which is prominent in the central lobular regions. The pronounced change in intrahepatic flow results from active constriction of the portal venous system. Flow through the liver is slowed and there is delay in passage of blood through the sinusoids, especially in the centrilobular area. The vasoconstriction and the reduction in flow can be reversed by adrenergic blockade and thus appear to arise from hyperactivity of the sympathetic nervous system.

The organ is slaty-grey or black owing to its content of malaria pigment. This colour change is most notable in *P. falciparum* infections.

Cloudy swelling of the parenchymal cells has been reported in acute *P. vivax* infection, but is not common in *P. falciparum* malaria in which there is degeneration and ultimately necrosis of the cells of the central zone and sometimes fatty degeneration of the cells of the lobular periphery. These lesions have been observed at biopsy and necropsy. The sinusoids in the mid and central zones are widely dilated, as are the central and sublobular veins. The Kupffer cells actively take up malaria pigment and haemosiderin and parasitised and unparasitised erythrocytes. They become swollen and may detach and enter the blood stream. The degenerative and necrotic lesions in the parenchymal cells extend peripherally, and in very severe cases may involve almost the whole lobule, short of the cells immediately contiguous to the portal tract. The cells involved in this reaction are devoid of glycogen which often disappears from the cells in the central zone before necrosis develops. This is concerned with altered adrenal activity since the glycogen can be restored in animal malaria by administration of cortisone and sugar.

The central lobular necrosis is essentially nonspecific, and arises from the dynamic local vascular changes in the portal venous tree. Very similar lesions occur in many other acute medical states. In infections in which immunity has been built up, lymphocytic infiltration of Glisson's capsule in the portal tracts is common.

Treatment of the malaria is followed by rapid restoration of the liver picture to normal. In the absence of complicating factors such as malnutrition or excessive alcoholism it is doubtful whether any permanent fibrosis or cirrhosis is produced.

Deviations of liver 'function' tests are the rule in acute infections. There is an appreciable rise in total bilirubin concentration and there may be overt jaundice. The plasma albumin concentration falls in the course of an acute infection and may reach low levels after repeated attacks. As the infection proceeds, the plasma globulins rise, mainly because of the production of gamma globulin containing antibodies.

Changes in the brain are common in falciparum malaria. At autopsy in so-called 'cerebral' malaria the capillaries are seen to be loaded with erythrocytes, many infected with schizonts and lying along the endothelial membrane. The vessels in a specimen of cortex pressed between two microscope slides are often outlined by the pigment contained in these infected cells. Small thrombi may be present but seldom in large numbers; they are probably formed in the very late stages of the disease.

There are sometimes small ring haemorrhages about the vessels and occasional larger discrete haemorrhages into the brain substance. In these lesions the extravascular erythrocytes are commonly uninfected. Where treatment has been given before death the erythrocytes within the vessels may be free from parasites, whereas a few of the erythrocytes in the surrounding haemorrhages may be parasitised. Granulomas may occur in such circumstances, consisting of a central vessel free of parasites, a clear zone of brain substance, a ring of erythrocytes and an enveloping collection of lymphocytes and glial cells.

Renal lesions develop in acute falciparum infections and in blackwater fever. The most serious arise as the renal anoxia syndrome with oliguria, sometimes proceeding to anuria and acute uraemia. This syndrome is common to many other acute medical states including shock, and is also known as the 'tubular-vascular syndrome' or 'lower nephron nephrosis'. The basic pathogenic process is an ischaemia of the kidney tissue, involving especially the cortex and arising from overall reduction in renal blood flow occurring independently or associated with shock. There is degeneration and necrosis of the tubular epithelium, with desquamation of cells and debris shed into the lumen, especially in the proximal and distal convoluted tubules and the ascending loop of Henle. The collecting tubules are irregularly filled with epithelial debris and sometimes blood from haemorrhages from the associated congested intertubular medullary capillaries. Many of the tubules are widely dilated. The glomerular capillary tufts are retracted. They are ischaemic in some areas, congested in others. The lesions in blackwater fever are similar except for dense eosinophilic granules containing iron found in the degenerate tubular epithelium and in the material filling the tubular lumen. This material is derived from haemoglobin.

The renal vessels usually contain many fewer parasites than those of other organs, particularly the brain. The kidneys are rarely pigmented heavily, but malaria pigment is present in interstitial tissues and in the parasitised cells containing late trophozoites and schizonts. There is usually some haemosiderin in the epithelial cells.

Protein is commonly found in the urine in acute malaria and epithelial casts and some erythrocytes are not unusual. In severe cases of *P. falciparum* infection there may develop a picture resembling acute nephritis with oliguria and rising blood urea, heavy proteinuria and hyaline and epithelial casts. This may be associated with frank haematuria and may proceed to anuria and uraemia as above.

In long-continued and repeated infections with *P. malariae* in children the so-called 'nephrotic syndrome' may develop, with salt and water retention and generalised oedema, but no increase in blood urea nitrogen concentration.

Recent studies of renal biopsies in this condition have shown thickening of the walls of the glomerular tuft capillaries with some endocapillary cell proliferation and hyaline deposits. Fluorescent studies have shown an antibody-antigen precipitation on the basement membrane. In advanced cases the glomerular tuft is retracted and Bowman's space exaggerated. The tubular epithelium is damaged in varying degree. The lesions are most pronounced in the proximal convoluted tubules, with vacuolar and fatty degeneration and desquamation of the epithelium into the lumen. Erythrocytes containing parasites and pigment may be present in small numbers, but there may be no local evidence of malarial infection. The interstitial tissue is infiltrated with lymphocytes. The kidneys are usually enlarged, pale, grey and tense. Both cortex and medulla are pale and swollen and demarcation is indistinct. Occasionally the kidneys are contracted, with irregular interstitial fibrosis, adherent capsules and cellular proliferation in the glomeruli.

The bone marrow in acute falciparum malaria is hyperplastic, representing compensatory normoblastic activity, but there is usually no increase in reticulocytes in the peripheral blood until some days after treatment has removed the parasites. It has been suggested that some inhibitory mechanism exists during parasitaemia which, while not restricting the production of young erythrocytes, obstructs their entrance into the peripheral blood, thus exacerbating the prevailing anaemia. In very severe infections there may be no erythropoietic response. Myeloblastic activity is usually depressed, as indicated by a granulocytic leucopenia. In repeated infection, there may be some general depression of both erythropoiesis and leucopoiesis.

Coagulation mechanisms and endothelial permeability

In some cases plasma fibrinogen concentration increases, in others there may be a dramatic decrease. Traces of clotting can be found in vessels, particularly those in the brain substance, but there is little evidence of intravascular coagulation in the so-called 'plugged' vessels in the brain which, in the untreated fatal case, are often filled with erythrocytes containing mature schizonts. It is possible that fresh clotting may be balanced by active fibrinolysis. The role of accelerated intravascular clotting with associated embolus and thrombosis as pathogenic mechanisms in falciparum malaria has still to be determined. In some acute cases the blood platelet count may be low and abnormal serial thrombin times and prolonged one-stage prothrombin times have been recorded. The development of physiological 'stasis' within the capillaries, arising from loss of protein and fluid from the local blood stream via damaged endothelial membrane is probably a more important factor in the pathological picture. Increases in permeability have been demonstrated in the small brain vessels and the blood brain barriers in simian and rodent malaria. In the former infections, a factor is present capable of increasing permeability of normal endothelium. Where stasis is allowed to continue, coagulation may occur as a terminal event.

Haemolysis

Recent work has shown that intravascular haemolysis occurs throughout the course of an acute *P. falciparum* infection. The mechanisms involved are not understood, although it is possible that lipids such as lysolecithin and unsaturated long-chain fatty acids (possibly cis-vaccinic acid, which accumulates in the infected erythrocytes) may be involved. The latter have been found to accumulate in the infected erythrocytes as the parasites mature. There is some evidence that an autoantigen-antibody reaction may be initiated as a result of the infection of the erythrocytes. The lysis involves both infected and non-infected cells.

Some loss of circulating erythrocytes probably results from specific phagocytosis by macrophage tissue cells. This factor is manifest at about the time humoral antibodies are first detectable in the blood. Erythrocytes are also lost to the general circulation as the result of pooling of blood in the subcutaneous tissues, the liver, spleen and skeletal muscles caused by the development of shock and fall of plasma volume. Corresponding changes occur in the haematocrit.

Pathogenesis of acute malaria

The synthesis of the clinical state of malaria involves the interaction of parasite on host and of host on parasite. Little is known about the latter, but information is accumulating about the overall responses of the host to the invader.

Many of the processes involved are essentially non-specific and occur in the evolution of other acute medical states. These include various physiological and pathophysiological phenomena which are mentioned above and are mainly concerned with tissue metabolism and blood circulation. These are modified and adjusted by the overall response of the host to the parasite and its products, including immunosensitivity reactions.

Although many processes are non-specific, it is clear that they must somehow be initiated by the parasite during its life cycle in the erythrocyte. The initiating factors are not yet determined, but a direct link between the parasite in the erythrocyte and the body tissues of the host has been found in the discovery of a soluble factor of low molecular weight and probably allied to lactic acid which can be detected in the serum of infected animals during the later stages of an acute attack of malaria.

This factor which arises from somewhere in the parasite-host complex causes inhibition of the respiratory activity and oxidative phosphorylation of host cell mitochondria and so grossly disturbs the function and ultimately destroys the cell.

This is probably one of several agents working and interacting at various points in the host bodily economy and influencing its physiological and biochemical balance. Others may include pharmacologically active substances such as kinins or histamine. A chain of pathogenic activities is set off, with interrelated processes involving membrane permeability, interference with hormone production and balance, hyperactivity of the sympathetic nervous system leading to changes in local blood circulation (as in the liver and kidneys) with or without total vascular collapse.

What is happening in one organ may affect the function of others, and the physiology of the body as a whole in this way becomes more and more involved. The effects vary from host to host, leading to local or general disturbances most of which are at first reversible but as time goes on become irreversible and lead to local tissue death. If unchecked, the chain reaction expands, more and more processes pass the irreversible stage and eventually the host is destroyed.

This concept of early factors initiating an expanding chain reaction of interrelated physiological phenomena governed by host : parasite responses makes the pattern of the development of the disease more understandable and offers a useful research hypothesis, but it has yet to be fully substantiated.

Biochemical changes

The chemical anatomy of the blood in malaria depends on the functional integrity of the tissues (for example the state of the liver, the kidney and the water : electrolyte balance) and is largely non-specific to the infection.

Where there is hepatic dysfunction there is increase in plasma bilirubin and deviation of the usual battery of liver 'function' tests.

Involvement of the kidneys is indicated in the acute attack by increasing blood urea nitrogen concentration and disturbances of the plasma sodium : potassium ratio.

In severe lysis there is haemoglobinaemia which may be accompanied by haemoglobinuria. In blackwater fever haematinalbumin may be present in the serum.

Total plasma protein is unaltered, or may be lowered in the early stages of an acute infection. As the disease proceeds, the protein content may increase as a result of increase in gamma globulin despite a fall in albumin, and the albumin/globulin ratio is correspondingly reversed.

The urine usually contains some protein. It contains bilirubin when the plasma concentration is high (over 3 mg per cent). The electrolyte concentration is low where the renal tubules have been functionally or structurally damaged, as in blackwater fever. When there is severe dehydration from sweating, diarrhoea and vomiting there may be no measurable sodium chloride in the urine. The unconcentrated urine has a low specific gravity, which may be masked by the presence of protein or haemoglobin.

The urine may be acid, neutral or alkaline in both malaria and blackwater fever. Hyaline and granular casts are usual in the acute attack and there may be erythrocytes.

In the late stages of severe falciparum malaria the blood sugar may be very low. As little as 4.0 mg per cent has been recorded.

CLINICAL PATTERNS IN MALARIA

The clinical manifestations of malaria arise from the invasion of the erythrocytes and the progress of the asexual erythrocytic E parasites.

In non-immunes, *P. falciparum* differs from other species in that it causes an acute and rapidly progressive disease in which serious and diverse complications may occur; it is often fatal if unchecked. Recrudescences occur in incompletely treated infections.

The other species of parasite give rise to serious and unpleasant but more benign illnesses in which complications are unusual, Fatality is rare, and the diseases are self-limited and relapses common.

Pre-patent period

This is the time which elapses between the infection by sporozoites and the first appearance of E parasites in the blood. The period is usually 6 to 9 days, except in *P. malariae*, depending on the species of infections, in which it ranges from 13 to 16 days. It ends with the discharge of merozoites from the primary exoerythrocytic liver phase into the blood, but these are seldom seen. Details for each parasite are given elsewhere (page 33).

In the pre-patent period the infected individual seldom notices any clinical effects, but thereafter as the parasitaemia builds up there may be prodromal signs, including vague malaise, headache and backache, sometimes short episodes of feeling cold and shivering.

Incubation period

This is the time lapsing between infection and the first appearance of fever with E parasites in the blood. In non-immune hosts the incubation period for all species is usually 10 to 15 days. There are exceptions to this, for example, in certain strains of *P. vivax* and *P. malariae* the period may be much longer. The incubation period may also be prolonged by the administration of antimalarial drugs at doses less than those needed for eradication of the parasites.

Periodicity of fever and febrile paroxysms

The completion of schizogony with the rupture of the schizonts and the liberation of merozoites, pigment and debris into the blood stream corresponds roughly in time to the development of a febrile reaction in the host. If the schizogony of broods of parasites is more or less contemporaneous, a febrile paroxysm occurs at this time, and the patient suffers from periodic fever. In *P. falciparum*, *P. vivax* and *P. ovale* in which schizogony takes about 48 hours, the febrile paroxysms occur every third day under these circumstances. This is called *tertian* periodicity. Where the parasites occur as two broods maturing on alternate days, the paroxysms appear each day during the attack and the periodicity is called *quotidian*. In *P. malariae* schizogony takes 72 hours, so that the febrile periodicity when all parasites mature simultaneously is once every fourth day (*quartan*).

In primary attacks of malaria some days are normally required before the rhythm of parasitic schizogony is determined. Hence for the first few days the fever is usually irregularly remittent or intermittent. After 5 to 7 days, however, periodicity is established and the fever becomes tertian, quotidian, etc. Once determined in a given infected individual, the periodicity tends to remain unchanged until the parasites are destroyed by chemotherapy or the infection subsides. On occasion, established periodicity may change, a tertian fever becoming quotidian, and *vice versa*. This usually occurs as a result of some change in circumstances, such as a superimposed viral or bacterial infection. Periodicity may also be changed experimentally, for example, by administration by typhoid vaccine, or by disturbing the normal rhythm of patients by reversing their periods of activity and rest.

In *P. vivax*, *P. malariae* and *P. ovale* infections the development of periodic fever, usually with paroxysms, is the rule. In many *P. falciparum* infections periodic fever may never develop, and whether or not the fever becomes periodic depends to some extent on the strain of infecting parasite.

Synchronicity of schizogony and related febrile paroxysms is most evident in *P. vivax* infections, least in *P. falciparum*.

In recrudescences and relapses of infections in which periodic fever was established, the attack usually presents with the same periodicity as the primary attack, or previous recurrence. Thus a relapse of a *P. vivax* infection with established tertian fever will develop tertian periodicity immediately, and there will be no preliminary interlude of irregular fever as in the primary attack.

Duration. The duration of an attack of malaria depends on both the species (and strain) of the parasite and on the immune status of the host. In a primary infection in a non-immune *P. falciparum* usually causes a short and savage attack which seldom lasts more than a few weeks and usually ends fatally without treatment.

Primary attacks caused by the other species of parasites may last for weeks or even months (over 300 days in one recorded case of *P. malariae* infection) The attacks are self-limited and commonly followed by relapses.

Relapses and recrudescences

The parasitological background to recurrence of malaria after an interval following a primary attack or a subsequent recurrence is discussed on page 32.

In *P. falciparum* infection, recurrence of a malarial attack results from multiplication in the blood of E parasites already present and representing the original asexual infection of the primary attack. In the other infections, although recrudescences of existing blood infections may theoretically occur, the reappearance of malaria is a true relapse in that the recurrence follows the establishment in the blood of new broods of E parasites following discharge of merozoites from secondary exoerythrocytic schizonts in the liver.

It is therefore better to talk of *recrudescences* of *P. falciparum* and *relapses* of the other infections.

On the whole, secondary attacks tend to be less severe and of shorter duration in *P. vivax*, *P. malariae* and *P. ovale* infections. This is probably dependent on the more rapid acquisition of functional immunity than in the primary attack. This may not be the case in *P. falciparum* infections, since many of the serious complications may arise as a result of incomplete removal of the parasites from the blood.

Reinfection occurs in endemic areas in individuals who are currently infected or have been infected. The clinical picture depends on the strain of parasite and the prevailing state of acquired resistance to infection.

Malaria in non-immunes and semi-immunes

The response of an individual to infection is largely determined by his immune status. The development of immunity in the sense of modifying the clinical and pathological effects of an infection and of resistance to reinfection is determined by the presence of the asexual erythrocytic (E) parasite. After long periods of infection and reinfection the immunity acquired minimises the response of the host, leading to a milder clinical reaction than that seen in the non-immune.

For this reason the clinical features of malaria in non-immunes and in semi-immunes will be discussed separately.

NON-IMMUNE PATIENTS

Vivax malaria (benign tertian malaria; infection with *P. vivax*).

During the last few days of the incubation period prodromal symptoms are common. The patient may feel irregular headache, backache and limb pains. He is sometimes anorexic, may be nauseated and even vomit. Transient feelings of cold associated with shivering are common. In relapses these may have the periodicity of the subsequent febrile paroxysms of the attack. Otherwise prodromata are uncommon in relapses.

The *onset* of the primary attack begins with a rapid rise of body temperature to 38–39°C or higher, accompanied by the usual febrile response of feeling cold and having short bursts of shivering. At this stage rigor does not occur. Asexual erythrocytic E parasites are present in the blood, usually in small numbers.

An irregularly remittent or intermittent fever continues for several days, with peaks of up to 40°C but seldom higher.

The patient feels ill. The pulse is rapid, breathing fast, the skin flushed and moist. Sweating is free and irregular.

Towards the end of the first week in the majority of cases periodic fever becomes established and febrile paroxysms begin. In relapses periodic fever is usually evident from the onset.

The *febrile paroxysms* are composed of short bursts of fever succeeded by heavy sweating. They are physiologically similar to other febile paroxysms such as those following injection of typhoid vaccine. They are more common in the day than in the night and usually develop in the *post meridian* hours. They exhibit three well-defined stages: the cold stage or chill, the hot or fever stage and the sweating stage. These are followed by the interval, after which the succeeding paroxysm occurs, and so on.

The *cold stage* begins abruptly with a sharp rise of body temperature, and is characterised by subjective feelings of intense cold accompanied by shivering and then rigor, which may be very severe, involving most of the muscles of the body. The temperature continues to rise rapidly but the skin remains pale and may feel cold. There is sometimes cyanosis of the visible mucous membranes. The blood pressure rises and the pulse is small and fast. There is often some epigastric discomfort and the patient is anorexic and nauseated. Vomiting may occur, particularly towards the end of the cold stage. The patient demands external warmth and, if he has his way, will continue to shake, shudder and chatter under blankets.

The chills of the cold stage are violent and unpleasant. They accompany the febrile episodes from the establishment of periodicity, but vary in intensity from one paroxysm to the next. In quotidian fever severe rigors may appear only in association with every other febrile attack, as though the reaction were related to the activity of one brood of parasites rather than the other.

At the beginning of the primary attack the cold stage lasts about an hour and the maximum temperature reached is seldom over 40°C. Within a week or two its duration commonly increases by about a third and the temperature reached may be as high as 41°C.

The *hot stage* abruptly replaces the cold. The situation now resembles that in any other pyrexia of the same degree. The patient loses his subjective feelings of cold. Rigors and shivering cease. He feels hot and kicks away his blankets. The temperature remains at about the level reached at the end of the cold stage, but may rise slightly; very occasionally, hyperpyrexia may develop. The skin flushes and is hot and dry. Blood pressures fall and the pulse becomes full and bounding. Respiration is rapid and there is often some unproductive coughing. The patient complains of throbbing headache and often intense thirst. He is restless, excited and euphoric; as the stage progresses he may become disorientated and incoherent or pass into delirium or light coma. The hot stage lasts 2–6 hours and is succeeded by the *sweating stage*. Sweating first appears on the temples and becomes generalised in a few minutes. Sweat pours off all parts of the body and the patient very rapidly feels better. The temperature usually begins to fall before the sweating starts and once the latter has begun drops within an hour or two to normal or below. Concurrently the pulse slows, the signs and symptoms of the hot stage disappear and the patient feels increasingly relieved, but exhausted. He commonly falls into deep sleep and wakes considerably refreshed and subjectively much better.

The *interval* follows. The temperature remains within normal limits in most cases, but may sometimes rise to a low peak before settling again. The patient feels well during the interval, but deteriorates rapidly once the next paroxysm begins.

Paroxysms of this nature repeat at regular intervals throughout the clinical activity of the infection. In the first weeks of an untreated case they tend to become more severe. Towards the end of the self-limited attack which may last 6–8 weeks or more, they tend to become less intense, the peak temperatures reached become lower, rigor becomes less vigorous and occasional episodes of short peaks of fever with few accompanying symptoms occur. Finally, paroxysms cease and the untreated disease enters a quiescent stage of weeks or months until a relapse develops.

Other signs and symptoms of importance occur during the attack:

Parasites are present in the peripheral blood during the attack. All stages of the asexual E phase may be seen from one paroxysm to the next but one tends to predominate at a given time. Just before the paroxysm commences, schizonts predominate. A few hours later, most parasites are in the ring stage and over the next 24 hours trophozoites and early schizonts are the commonest forms (for details, see page 34).

Anaemia develops as the disease progresses. In the early stages it is not pronounced, but it may become notable in a long-sustained attack. The erythrocyte count in an established infection varies from 4.9 to about 3.0 million cells per mm³ with a mean of about 4.0 million. The mean cell diameter may be greater than normal during parasitaemia, probably because of the increase in size of the infected cells. The bone marrow response is normoblastic and sometimes hyperplastic. Reticulocyte numbers are not increased during the attack but rise within a week of successful treatment.

The *spleen* invariably increases in size during the attack and is commonly palpable in the costal angle by the end of the second week. Thereafter it enlarges slowly, It is usually tender and there may be some local pain in the splenic area.

The *liver* is sometimes tender and palpable. Transient biochemical evidence of hepatic dysfunction has been reported in some cases but no evidence of pronounced structural damage. The serum total bilirubin may be slightly raised, but clinical jaundice is rare.

As in many febrile conditions, *herpes labialis* may appear once the disease is established. It is usually confined to the mouth and lips but may spread laterally to the nose and even the ears. It subsides with the treatment of the malaria.

Course and prognosis. *P. vivax* infections rarely cause death, although a few fatal cases have been reported in young children, in whom anaemia may become very severe; figures of as low as 0.4 million cells per mm³ have been recorded. The usual course in untreated cases is one of chronic ill health developing after successive relapses. In areas where reinfection occurs the spleen may become considerably enlarged and a state of cachexia develops. Where reinfection does not occur, for instance in an individual who has left the endemic area, after one or two relapses the patient's condition begins to improve and recurrences cease.

Relapses occur in untreated cases in which the malaria has eventually subsided spontaneously or in cases treated with schizonticides only (see page 32). The relapse usually begins with periodic fever and paroxysms, keeping the periodicity of the primary attack. It is usually milder and of shorter duration than the latter. The interval between the subsidence of one attack and the relapse is controlled to some extent by the strain of parasite involved (see page 35).

In individuals who have left an endemic area and are no longer exposed, relapses of *P. vivax* infection do not occur after 3 years.

Treatment. See page 57.

Ovale malaria (ovale tertian malaria; infection with *P. ovale*)

The pre-patent period is 9 days and prolonged latency is common, so that a primary attack may not develop until months or even years after infection.

In most respects the clinical course of this infection follows that of vivax malaria. The disease is relatively mild and no fatal case has been recorded. Febrile paroxysms are sometimes very severe, with high fever and considerable prostration. Since the parasites take about 50 hours to mature the periodicity is slightly longer than that of vivax malaria. The density of parasitaemia is low as reticulocytes are preferentially invaded. The spleen enlarges more slowly than in *P. vivax* infection and may not become palpable (i.e. about twice normal size) for several weeks in an overt attack. The liver may enlarge and become palpable. It is functionally involved, as in other malarias; jaundice has been reported.

The infection is easily suppressed by more dominant parasites, notably *P. falciparum*, and may appear in individuals with unsuspected mixed infections months after the latter have been treated successfully with schizonticides.

Quartan malaria (malariae malaria; infection with *P. malariae*)

The clinical picture is basically similar to that of vivax malaria, but there are differences.

The pre-patent period is longer than in other infections and is probably in the order of 13–16 days. The invasion of the erythrocytes builds up slowly, since the parasite differentially infects the older erythrocytes. Parasitaemias are consequently low.

The incubation period is very difficult to assess as it may be many weeks after infection before parasites can be found in the blood by ordinary diagnostic methods.

Febrile paroxysms may be already in existence before parasites can be found. The clinical onset is thus insidious.

The acute attack is often severe. There may be no initial period of intermittent or remittent fever so that the attack begins with a febrile paroxysm, and regular periodicity is immediately established. Quartan paroxysms are most commonly developed but there are some seven alternatives, including double quartan and quotidian periodicity. The periodicity tends to remain constant in a given attack, but variations may occur, for example, from quartan to double quartan and *vice versa*.

Febrile paroxysms occur during the day and usually in the afternoon. The paroxysms are similar to those of vivax malaria. The cold stage is sometimes severe and prolonged. True rigors are commoner in cases where there is quartan periodicity. The hot stage is also prolonged and may last for up to 6 hours. Cerebral symptoms, including delirium, are common. The sweating stage is similar to that in vivax malaria. The fall of temperature is rapid, and prolonged subnormal temperatures are common early in the interval, in which the patient may feel extremely prostrated.

Parasite numbers are low, seldom exceeding 20 000 per mm³. Over 70 000 per mm³ however, have been reported in a fatal case. All stages of parasites are seen in the peripheral blood, as in vivax infections.

Anaemia is mild and slow developing.

The *spleen* increases in size slowly and may not be palpable for several weeks. In long-continued infections the persistence of the parasites gradually leads to very considerable splenic hypertrophy. Functional liver disturbances can be demonstrated during the attack but there are no permanent effects and jaundice is rare.

In long-standing cases *oedema* of the ankles is

common and may be associated with depression of serum albumin.

Herpes labialis appears as in other infection.

In children a form of malarial nephrosis may develop as a complication, commonly called the nephrotic syndrome. This is the most serious complication of *P. malariae* infection (see page 55).

Quartan malaria is the most chronic and persistent of the human infections. Relapses have been reported many years after the primary attack. Parasites may remain for years in the blood without giving rise to clinical effects and without being detected by ordinary diagnostic procedures. The disease has been transferred by blood transfusion 20 years or more after the primary attack.

Falciparum malaria (malignant tertian malaria; subtertian malaria; infection with *P. falciparum*)

Falciparum malaria may be uncomplicated or complicated. These forms are discussed separately.

Uncomplicated falciparum malaria. The primary (and only) exoerythrocytic schizogony cycle takes about 6 days. Parasites are first detectable in the blood from about the tenth day, and the incubation period of the disease varies from 10 to 14 days.

Prodromal symptoms are common for the few days preceding onset. These include depression, severe headache, muscle pains, backache, especially in the lumbar and sacroiliac regions, gastrointestinal discomfort, nausea and irregular attacks of coldness and shivering.

The onset may be clearly defined or insidious. The first indication of trouble is usually fever. It may be accompanied by physical signs which are characteristic for the strains in certain geographical regions. Thus, diarrhoea is a common presenting sign in falciparum malaria in parts of West Africa.

The patient develops moderate fever with flushed or pale earthy skin, often damp with sweat. He may at this stage appear only moderately ill and the disease is at first easily mistaken for minor febrile conditions such as influenza. This appearance is deceptive, as at any time serious complications may appear. The patient is anxious and restless, and as the disease progresses becomes disorientated and confused. He is more prostrated than in vivax malaria and in cases where periodic fever has become established the feeling of refreshment and well-being which follows the sweating stage in the latter infection

is absent. At a late stage delirium is common and coma may develop. In light coma the patient can be roused and will drowsily answer questions. In deep coma he is unresponsive and usually incontinent (see *Complicated falciparum malaria*).

The fever is irregular at first, as in vivax malaria, without indications of periodicity. In many cases it remains irregularly remittent or intermittent and periodic febrile paroxysms do not develop. In others, tertian, subtertian or quotidian periodicity is established after a few days, with paroxysms resembling those of vivax malaria, but often of shorter duration. The cold stage tends to be short, with moderate rigors. The hot stage is often prolonged, so that what looked like becoming a paroxysm becomes a period of remittent fever. In cases where the paroxysm is well established, the peak of fever reached varies from episode to episode and may sometimes not be very high. The sweating is short and severe and may be aborted so that the skin remains moist throughout with periods of heavy sweating. In cases with high fever there may be no sweating. Sometimes double fever peaks resembling those seen in visceral leishmaniasis may occur. Even in severe attacks the fever reached may be only moderate. It tends to fall towards the end of the attack. In some cases, despite high parasitaemia, there may be little or no fever.

Parasites. In peripheral blood most of the parasites seen are early rings and young trophozoites, usually without pigment. The later stages of schizogony take place in the vessels of the deep tissues and schizonts are rarely seen except in very heavy infections and complicated cases. The number of parasites present varies considerably during the day, and the figure falls as the parasites retreat to the deep tissues for the late stages of schizogony. Nevertheless, as the infection progresses, the maximum numbers increase steadily until 15 to 20 per cent or more of the surviving erythrocytes may be infected. The characteristic crescentic gametocytes (which take no part in the pathogenesis of the disease) first appear about the tenth day and persist. The numbers rise for a fortnight or so, then subside.

Anaemia is severe. The parasites invade erythrocytes of all ages, leading to the destruction of large numbers of infected cells and haemolysis of uninfected erythrocytes. In cases of average severity the erythrocyte count falls in 10–14 days to 3.5 to 2.5 million cells per mm³. In the first few days there may be little obvious anaemia. The red cell count and the haemoglobin concentration at any stage may not give a faithful indication of the degree of anaemia, since they are often temporarily increased by haemoconcentration due to loss of circulating plasma volume. The anaemia is normocytic and the bone marrow response normoblastic and at first hyperplastic, later sometimes becoming hypoplastic.

In some cases catastrophic intravascular haemolysis occurs without warning and the haemoglobin liberated into the plasma is passed in the urine, giving rise to the syndrome of blackwater fever (see page 52).

There is usually a moderate leucopenia with a leucocyte count of 4000 to 6000 cells per mm³; granulocytes are reduced and there may be some increase in lymphocytes and lymphocytic macrophage cells.

In severe cases with high parasitaemia malaria pigment may be sometimes seen in the circulating macrophages and even in the polymorphonuclear leucocytes.

In many patients the *cardiovascular system* is disturbed from the outset, and the blood pressures fall to relatively low levels. Even in an uncomplicated case systolic pressures of 90 mmHg and diastolic of 40 or/50 mmHg are not uncommon. The pulse is full and usually fast to begin with, but after some days it may become slow in relation to the fever and in some cases persistent bradycardia may develop.

Abdominal signs and symptoms are common. Anorexia is the rule and nausea and vomiting common. There may be considerable epigastric discomfort or pain. Most patients have some degree of watery diarrhoea.

The *spleen* enlarges rapidly and is usually easily palpable by the tenth day. It continues to enlarge as the disease progresses. Where periodic fever is established it sometimes enlarges during the paroxysm and regresses in the interval. It is always tender and there is often tenderness in the splenic area before the organ can be felt. Pain over the splenic region and left lower rib cage is common and is usually worsened by respiration, giving the clinical impression of pleurisy or pneumonia. Sudden splenic infarction and localised perisplenitis may cause acute local pain, tenderness and muscular guarding in the left hypochondrium and referred pain in the left shoulder region. Surgical emergencies may occur as the organ may rupture, spontaneously or following a blow, or the pedicle may twist.

The *liver* is always affected in falciparum malaria. It becomes tender within a few days and is palpable by the end of the second week or earlier. Liver function is disturbed. 'Liver function' tests are deviated. Serum bilirubin is increased in most cases and there may be overt jaundice. Increased output of urobilinogen in the urine occurs, and in jaundiced cases bilirubin is excreted. Serum transaminase concentrations increase.

In the early stages there are few changes in serum protein concentrations, but as the disease progresses the albumin falls as a result of liver dysfunction and later, as immunity develops, the gamma globulins rise, reversing the albumin/globulin ratio.

The *respiratory system* may be severely affected. The respiration rate is usually increased and signs and symptoms of lung involvement may develop, including unproductive cough and scattered moist sounds and crepitations indicating some bronchopneumonia or pulmonary oedema. Pulmonary changes are more common in infections with some strains, such as those in eastern Europe and West Africa, than with others.

Renal function is seriously disturbed in some cases. Albumin and a few granular casts are usually present in the urine. The volume of urine discharged is low and the concentration of chloride diminished in patients who are sweating heavily and becoming dehydrated from diarrhoea and/or vomiting.

Severe renal involvement may develop, with marked oliguria, going on to anuria and acute uraemia (see pages 42, 43 and 64). In such cases the blood urea concentration rises rapidly. Even in apparently lightly involved cases, it may be above normal.

Occasionally a syndrome resembling acute nephritis may develop, with oliguria, frank haematuria and rising blood urea.

Herpes labialis occurs, as in other malarias, in about a third of cases.

Course and prognosis. The uncomplicated attack in the non-immune, if caught in time, responds very well to chemotherapy and proper management.

The untreated acute attack is of much shorter duration than that of vivax malaria. A fatal issue is common in 2 to 3 weeks. In some cases the infection is gradually subdued, presumably by the development of immunity, and the patient slowly recovers. Recrudescences due to the persistence and resurgence of the asexual E parasites are likely in such cases over the subsequent months, but they seldom develop after 12 months or 2 years at the most.

The treated case and the spontaneous survivor are usually severely anaemic on recovery. Restoration of the blood to normal is often slow and may require further treatment (see page 64).

Treatment is discussed on page 57 et seq.

Complicated falciparum malaria (pernicious malaria). Complications may appear at any stage in a primary attack or in a recrudescence in a non-immune individual. They usually appear in the late stages of an attack which has been untreated or after repeated and inadequately treated attacks. They occur in children indigenous of endemic areas but are rare in semi-immunes.

Pernicious signs are usually associated with high degrees of parasitaemia, but they may appear in light infections. They are common in persons with more than 5 per cent of the erythrocytes in the peripheral blood infected and in those who have been ill for some time and are already anaemic. In an untreated primary attack complications generally develop in the second or third week, but they may appear earlier and may even be the presenting signs.

Complications arise from the progress of the pathological processes initiated by the infection, which may involve certain tissues or organs in particular. The clinical classification is thus commonly arranged in terms of the organs involved. The commonest forms are cerebral malaria, hyperpyrexia, gastrointestinal complications and algid malaria. Blackwater fever is now regarded as a complication of falciparum malaria.

Clinical signs and symptoms related to the central nervous system are collectively grouped as *cerebral malaria*. The syndrome usually evolves over some days during the course of an attack in a non-immune, but it may come on rapidly and early in an attack or even be the first indication of the disease. The patient complains of severe headache, grows increasingly drowsy and confused and passes into light coma which soon becomes deep, with stertorous breathing, pupils contracted, often unequally, and deep reflexes abolished or exaggerated. In the late stages it may not be possible to rouse him from coma, but earlier he can be persuaded to talk and even answer questions. The developments may resemble those of the muttering delirium of typhoid and may be misdiagnosed as such in the febrile prostrated patient with diarrhoea.

In some cases there may be severe mental disturbances with disorientation and hallucination, sometimes maniacal violence. These signs appear some hours or even days before coma develops and may be difficult to assess, as the patient at this stage may not appear otherwise very ill. He may even be ambulant, and the picture may be mistaken for drunkenness, especially where alcohol has been consumed and the breath smells.

The neurological picture depends on the area of the brain functionally most affected. Localised signs may be present. Muscular twitchings, jerky or rhythmic movements of the head, neck and limbs and convulsions occur. Episodes closely resembling epilepsy are not uncommon. The clinical pictures are mixed and legion. Attempts have been made to classify cerebral malaria as epileptiform, meningeal, paretic and so forth depending on prevailing signs, but this is mere rhetoric. Multiple and disconcerted signs are to be expected in an infection which involves the whole central nervous system in general circulatory and functional disorder. The physician must learn to anticipate any or all kinds of mental or neurological disturbance in acute falciparum malaria.

In the vast majority of cases there is high parasitaemia with already pronounced anaemia. Ten per cent or more of the surviving erythrocytes may be infected, many of them with more than one parasite. Late pigmented trophozoites and schizonts are often present in the peripheral blood.

There is usually high remittent or intermittent fever, but complications may develop in a periodic attack. As they appear the fever becomes less pronounced in some, as a general toxic picture develops; in others it may rise to levels of hyperpyrexia.

Other features of a malarial attack including anaemia, splenic and hepatic enlargement, are, of course, present and progressive. Diarrhoea is common and the comatose patient is usually incontinent. General forms of complication may coexist.

The patient's life depends on rapid diagnosis and specific management and chemotherapy (see pages 56, 57 et seq.).

Hyperpyrexia occurs especially in individuals exposed to high ambient temperatures or who already display some evidence of cerebral involvement. The body temperature rises rapidly above 41°C and may reach 43°C or even higher. The clinical picture closely resembles that of heat hyperpyrexia. The most earthy skin becomes flushed and dry. Usually the whole body may be dry but there may be some sweating on the face, in the axillae and groins and the soles and palms. If signs of central nervous system disturbance are not present at the onset of the high fever, they rapidly become prominent; coma develops, usually with incontinence. The patient will die if the fever is not immediately dealt with by methods similar to those used in heat stroke. The blood contains many parasites and trophozoites and schizonts are commonly present.

Gastrointestinal syndromes. Abdominal pain and distension may occur, often with the frequent

passage of voluminous watery stools and sometimes with frequent uncontrolled watery vomit.
The picture resembles cholera or acute food
poisoning and very severe dehydration quickly
develops. Some patients present a syndrome
clinically undistinguishable from acute bacillary
dysentery with abdominal pain, tenesmus and the
passage of many small stools consisting largely of
blood and mucus or watery stools containing
blood and mucus. Dehydration is again rapid and
severe.

In some cases fulminating liver failure develops.
The liver enlarges in a few days until the very
tender edge may reach several fingers' breadth
below the costal margin. There is pain and tenderness over the liver. Jaundice appears within 36
hours and deepens rapidly. Bilirubin appears in
the urine. The patient passes into a low delirium
or light coma, which deepens; incontinence
develops and the patient dies in acute hepatic
failure. This complication is not now seen very
frequently, but it was once common in certain
holoendemic areas, particularly in West Africa,
where it was known as *bilious remittent fever*,
and was often mistaken for yellow fever.

In all of these complications parasitaemia is
high, multiple infection of erythrocytes is common
and late trophozoites and schizonts appear in
small numbers in the peripheral blood. The
patients are usually severely anaemic but this
may be masked by considerable haemoconcentration, particularly in the presence of pronounced
dehydration or shock.

Fever is remittent or irregularly intermittent,
occasionally periodic. In the late stages shock is
common and, with its onset, the temperature falls
rapidly below normal and the pulse rate rises
fast. This situation has a very serious prognosis.

Renal failure may develop in severe falciparum
malaria whether the disease appears complicated
or not. The pattern is basically that of renal
anoxia and results from overall reduction in the
renal blood flow. The syndrome may be present
in all stages. It begins with oliguria and some
increase in plasma urea concentration. It may
not go beyond this stage, but in some patients the
oliguria may worsen and relative anuria develops,
with high and rising plasma urea concentration.
The flow of urine may cease altogether, signs of
cerebral oedema develop, the patient passes into
coma and may die in acute uraemia. The picture
is essentially the same as that of the acute renal
failure so common in blackwater fever.

Medical shock may develop at any time in
falciparum malaria and is a common terminal
incident. The individual suddenly collapses and

rapidly passes into coma. The facies are drawn,
the eyes sunken, the skin cold, pale and clammy.
This condition is commonly called algid malaria
since the oral temperature may be normal or
below although the rectal temperature may be
slightly elevated. Breathing is fast and shallow.
Both systolic and diastolic blood pressures are
depressed; the latter is sometimes too low to
measure. The acute reduction in blood volume
and the commonly prevailing dehydration cause
haemoconcentration so that the erythrocyte
count and haemoglobin concentration are abnormally high, disguising the anaemia.

Parasitaemia is usually high, with schizonts
present in the peripheral blood.

Death follows if the patient is not immediately
treated both for the infection and the shock
(see page 61).

Blackwater fever. Acute intravascular haemolysis may occur in falciparum malaria under
certain conditions, causing haemoglobinaemia
and associated haemoglobinuria.

This complication is known as *blackwater
fever*.

It occurs most frequently in individuals who
have been exposed in endemic areas for at least
some months, often for years. Most patients have
a history of intermittent and inadequate treatment for attacks or recrudescences of falciparum
malaria and irregular chemosuppression, especially by quinine. They may also have been living
in areas where there is incomplete entomological
control.

The mechanism by which the intravascular
haemolysis is precipitated is not yet fully understood, but it is believed that irregular exposure to
the asexual parasites over some time creates in
the infected person some autogenous sensitivity
which causes a violent reaction to further overt
infection with the same parasite, particularly
when a period of quiescence or loss of parasitaemia occurs before the stimulating reinfection.
The haemolysis results from this antibody-
antigen reaction. It may develop without warning
or during an attack of falciparum malaria, whether
under treatment or not. Blackwater fever was
common in Caucasian troops exposed to *P.
falciparum* infection in West Africa in the early
days of World War II, occurring in the first days
of quinine therapy for an overt attack or in
individuals on irregular quinine chemosuppression or living in areas where entomological control
was intermittent. Later in the war, when West
African Negro troops returned home after long
periods in Burma where they were exposed to
strains of parasites not their own, blackwater

fever became common in them when they were infected with the local strains. It was shown in volunteers that such an infection could precipitate haemolysis. Recently, blackwater fever has followed recrudescence of chloroquine resistant infection after suppression for some time by only partly effective therapy.

There is some evidence that irregular suppression of parasites by quinine may predispose to the appearance of haemolysis, but it may occur after the use of any chemosuppressive agent which has been irregularly administered in inadequate dosage. The issue here is clouded by the fact that in rare individuals quinine may have some measurable direct haemolytic effect. What appears to be needed to precipitate the haemolysis is exposure to the antigen (the parasite) after a period of sensitisation by the same strain.

Haemolysis is rapid and severe, leading to gross anaemia. An erythrocyte count may drop from 4.0 million to fewer than 1.0 million cells per mm^3 overnight.

There may be only one haemolytic episode, which continues for several days, or there may be several waves of lysis. Haemolysis may be intractable from the start, and the patient may die from uncontrolled anaemia.

Haemoglobinuria rapidly follows the haemolysis. The urine is dark brown (methaemoglobin) if acid, red (oxyhaemoglobin) if alkaline or neutral. The first specimen after haemolysis may show little coloration, but the urine rapidly darkens, to lighten again and finally clear of pigment in a few hours. During the passage of the haemoglobin large amounts of fluffy sediment containing epithelial cells, casts and amorphous debris are passed in the urine and there is a heavy excretion of protein. In the non-haemolytic intervals the urine is clear, sediment is minimal and the content of protein falls notably. The urine is dilute, indicating functional damage to the renal tubules. The volume passed is low. Oliguria is common and signs of serious renal dysfunction frequently develop. The patient may become anuric with high and rising plasma urea concentrations. Acute uraemia occurs in about a third of fatal cases. This syndrome of acute uraemic renal failure is common to many acute conditions. It was first described in blackwater fever.

In contrast with other complications of *P. falciparum* infection, parasites are present but scanty in about half the cases examined during the early stages of the first lysis. They are usually absent thereafter but will return on recovery unless specific chemotherapy is given.

The diagnosis of blackwater fever is made on

the history of the patient, which must include exposure to falciparum malaria, and on the clinical evidence of acute intravascular haemolysis with haemoglobinuria. The syndrome must be distinguished from other causes of haemolysis and haemoglobinuria, particularly that caused by the use of 8-amino-quinolines in male hemizygotes with the erythrocyte glucose-6-phosphate dehydrogenase deficiency trait. A vicious form of haemolysis called *favism* due to sensitivity to the Fava bean is also linked with this enzyme deficiency.

Treatment. See page 64.

MALARIA IN SEMI-IMMUNE ADULTS

The vast majority of malaria attacks are seen in the indigenous populations of endemic areas, most of whom may be regarded as semi-immunes, who have acquired some immunity and resistance to superinfection as a result of repeated infection.

In general, the acquisition of immunity leads to considerable modification of the attack in infections with all species of parasite. The acute attack is of short duration and the symptoms are not severe. In the individual, overt malaria takes the form of mild febrile episodes, with some malaise, headache, backache, anorexia and sweating. The patient feels unwell and his working efficiency suffers.

The attacks become more severe if immunity is weakened by incomplete suppression with drugs or by the partial reduction of frequency of reinfection by incomplete entomological control measures. As pointed out above, in hyperendemic *P. falciparum* areas, such circumstances may lead to the appearance of blackwater fever. When immunity is completely lost as a result of treatment or after a long period outside the endemic area, new infection with the homologous strain will lead to acute attacks similar to those evoked in the non-immune. Infection with strains of the same species of parasite other than that to which immunity has been acquired may also lead to severe attacks.

Acquired immunity to a predominant strain in an endemic area is clearly a valuable and hard-won possession. It must not be lightly lost so long as the possibility of reinfection is sustained. Antimalarial control or eradication measures in an endemic area must therefore be assured and permanent. So far as the individual is concerned, since immunity is largely dependent on the continued, or at least frequent, presence of the parasites in the blood, treatment must be aimed not at the eradication of the E parasites, but at their control to subclinical levels.

The acute attack in the semi-immune is often only an episode in a long history of chronic ill health, brought about by almost continuous infection, with relatively high levels of parasitaemia in children and young adults, falling in older adults to the point where parasites are difficult to detect. In *P. falciparum* endemic areas in particular the individual sufferer is moderately or even severely anaemic, asthenic and often mentally dull. In holoendemic areas in which high degrees of immunity develop in the survivors from childhood, the picture may be relatively mild and the spleen is usually small and not palpable. In areas of lower endemicity the spleen is often considerably enlarged in the adults as well as in the children and anaemia may be pronounced and contain an element of hypersplenism. The liver is sometimes palpable and function tests may be deviated from normal. Similar pictures may develop in *P. vivax* and *P. malariae* infections. In the latter the spleen may become very large and hard.

This burden of chronic illness with occasional bursts of fever and mild attacks of malaria may be carried through life by the indigene of an endemic area and is one of the main physical causes of the social and economic backwardness which characterises so much of the world in which the disease is endemic.

MALARIA IN CHILDREN

It has been estimated that 5 to 15 per cent of deaths of children in malaria endemic areas result from the disease.

As pointed out elsewhere, malaria is rare before the fourth month of life in the breast-fed indigenous child, and the first overt attacks are often mild with low grade parasitaemia. Thereafter, in highly malarious regions attacks may become more frequent and more severe until the fourth or fifth year when immunity is well developed. This is most obvious where the infecting parasite is *P. falciparum*.

P. falciparum infections

Between the ages of 6
child in a holo- or hy
larly susceptible
which may en
generally
clinical
ren

resistance to reinfection with the homologous strain of parasite and the attacks of malaria caused by it become modified and mild. The child comes to terms with the infection and leads a moderately normal playful life, despite persistent and relatively heavy parasitaemia and considerably enlarged liver and spleen.

Children who are protected by chemosuppression during this period are liable to severe attacks if the treatment is discontinued or neglected.

The clinical picture of malaria in the indigenous child depends on whether it is suffering from an acute recent infection or from long-continued infection, or both. The severity of a given attack is determined by the degree of immunity already developed.

The acute attack of malaria is seen in the second 6 months of life and in the next few years while immunity is being built up. It is also seen in children who have been only partly protected by chemosuppression or by entomological control of transmission, who live in areas where malaria is seasonal or who are visitors to the endemic area.

The child is dull, listless and drowsy or irritable. It has no appetite and resents feeding; vomiting is common, especially after food. Fever is usual but not invariably present in the early stages. It may never be pronounced. It is usually irregularly remittent or intermittent and periodicity is uncommon. There is frequently abdominal pain and diarrhoea. The abdomen is distended and there is tenderness in the hepatic and splenic areas. The spleen is tender, enlarged and easily palpable; in children who have suffered numerous infections it may be very large and fill most of the abdomen. Infarction and perisplenitis may cause local exacerbation of tenderness and pain. Occasionally the organ may rupture or twist on its pedicle. The liver is moderately enlarged and tender along its edge.

Anaemia is often severe, especially after repeated untreated attacks. Haemoglobin concentrations of 5 g per cent or less are not uncommon. By the time this point has been reached parasitaemia may be light but in acute fresh infections 15 to 25 per cent of the erythrocytes in the peripheral blood may be infected. Usually only ring forms of parasites are seen but in severe cases schizonts may appear. Gametocytes are present about a week after the onset and persist.

If the malaria is not treated the condition becomes rapidly worse, complications may develop and the child may die. Sometimes it may temporarily recover with abatement of signs and symptoms until the next attack. After repeated attacks loss of weight becomes rapid, the limbs waste, the abdomen becomes more distended, the spleen and often the liver larger, and a state of progressive ill health with recurrent mild fever evolves which may end fatally or gradually regress as immunity develops. The listless, wasted child with skinny limbs and a huge protuberant abdomen is a common sight in highly endemic areas. The spleen is grossly enlarged and may present in the pelvis; rupture may follow external violence. If untreated, such children may become progressively worse and pass into a fatal cachexic state.

Complications are usually associated with high degrees of parasitaemia. As in adults, cerebral signs are common. In most severe attacks convulsions occur and the child may become comatose and occasionally hyperpyrexic. Gastrointestinal syndromes are common. The child may present with severe dehydration and diarrhoea with blood and mucus in the stools, a syndrome indistinguishable from bacillary dysentery. There may be persistent watery diarrhoea and vomiting resembling the picture of food poisoning. Sometimes fever and an enlarged tender liver are associated with progressing jaundice and the condition may be mistaken for infectious hepatitis.

In very severe attacks the child may become shocked and comatose. The picture then resembles algid malaria in the adult (see page 52) or that of acute adrenal insufficiency.

P. vivax and *P. ovale* infections

Ovale malaria is milder than vivax, otherwise similar.

Periodic fever (quotidian or tertian) is established within a week of onset, following a few days of irregularly remittent fever, but the characteristic febrile paroxysms seen in the adult are unusual. In general, the clinical picture resembles that of uncomplicated falciparum malaria but is milder. The spleen enlarges early in the disease and may eventually become grossly enlarged after repeated attacks. Anaemia is less pronounced than in falciparum malaria. Complications are rare, except for convulsions which are common when the fever is high. A fatal issue is rare, but has been reported in cases in which anaemia has become severe.

Parasitaemia seldom exceeds 2 per cent of erythrocytes. All stages of the schizogony cycle are present at some time between one febrile episode and the next.

Relapses occur as in the adult if the child is removed from the endemic area. In the endemic area it is not possible to distinguish relapses from reinfections.

P. malariae infections

In children quartan malaria may follow the same pattern as vivax malaria, except for the establishment of quartan periodicity.

This infection is associated with the appearance of a nephrotic syndrome in young children in endemic areas. The child presents with gross generalised oedema, massive proteinuria and severe hypoproteinaemia. The peak incidence is round about 5 years of age in both sexes. Renal biopsy shows tubular degenerative changes and glomerular lesions ranging from thickening of the basement membrane to fibrosis. Prognosis is poor.

MALARIA IN PREGNANCY

Malaria, especially *P. falciparum* infection, may cause abortion at any stage and premature labour in the last trimester.

In the late stages of pregnancy and following childbirth, mothers in holoendemic or hyperendemic areas of falciparum malaria lose some of their acquired immunity and may suffer from severe attacks, which are sometimes fatal if untreated.

In highly endemic areas *P. falciparum*-infected women often come to term with severe anaemia, which may be derived from mixed iron deficiency and folic acid deficiency. Loss of blood at delivery may exacerbate the condition and death may result. The pathogenesis of the anaemia is uncertain, but it is haemolytic in type and the haemolysis which occurs is greater than would be expected from the parasitaemia. In some cases an enlarged spleen or liver may obstruct the expansion of the uterus as the fetus develops and lead to abortion or difficult delivery. The chance of stillbirth is increased by *P. falciparum* infection in the mother.

Malaria in the pregnant woman must therefore be regarded seriously as a potential cause of abortion or complicated labour and puerperium. A postpuerperal fever in an indigenous mother should be considered as malaria unless proved otherwise. Antimalarial drugs should be given during pregnancy. In the doses recommended they do not affect the uterus. The severe anaemia can often be prevented by chemosuppression during pregnancy.

Congenital malaria. Malaria may be occasionally transmitted from the mother to the child across the placenta. This occurs more frequently when the mother is a non-immune, although massive parasitic infections of the placenta are common in semi-immunes.

DIAGNOSIS OF MALARIA

Parasitological diagnosis

Certain diagnosis can be made only by the identification of the asexual E parasites in the peripheral blood or elsewhere, as in the bone marrow. The presence of gametocytes only is not sufficient evidence of current active infection, since these forms of parasites remain in the infected erythrocytes for periods as long as 3 months, and may thus be present after cure and removal of the asexual parasites which are responsible for the clinical disease.

Blood films

The examination of stained thick blood films is sufficient for the diagnosis of the presence of asexual parasites. In many instances distinction can be made by this technique between infection with *P. falciparum* and with the other parasites. Differentiation of the latter usually needs examination of stained thin blood films.

If parasites are not easily found in blood films, examination of smears from bone marrow or other tissues is unlikely to help.

Thick films are prepared by placing a drop of blood from a needle prick in a finger or ear lobe on to a clean glass microscope slide and spreading it evenly over a circular area about 2 cm across. The film is dried quickly but thoroughly before staining (about half an hour in the tropics). Films should kept away from the ravages of ants or flies. For storage, films are best stained immediately or wrapped in plastic and kept in the refrigerator. The films are stained by immersion for 20 minutes face downwards in Giemsa's stain diluted 1 : 20 with distilled water buffered to pH 7.2. Alternatively, Field's stain may be used. The stained film is examined under oil with a 2 mm objective. The cytoplasm of the parasites stains blue and the nuclear chromatin red or reddish purple. The dehaemoglobinised erythrocytes are not stained, but the nuclei of leucocytes take up the blue and platelets stain a delicate pink.

Thin films are prepared and stained as for haematological examinations, except that the stain is buffered at pH 7.2. In these preparations the erythrocytes remain intact with the parasites stained (as above) within them. Differentiation of the infecting species depends on the appearance of the parasites. The finer distinctions, for instance separating *P. ovale* from *P. vivax* need expert knowledge. From the clinical point of view, however, the differentiation of *P. falciparum* parasites from the others is the most important diagnostic objective, and *P. vivax* and *P. malariae* are usually sufficiently characteristic to be separated.

Details of the morphology of the parasite species are given elsewhere (pages 33–37).

Usually only ring forms of the parasites are present in the blood in *P. falciparum* infections; occasional schizonts or late trophozoites may appear in cases which are complicated or in which a high proportion of erythrocytes are parasitised. In the other infections, all stages of the asexual phase will appear, the ring forms predominating in the immediate post-paroxysmal period and schizonts late in the cycle, at the beginning of the subsequent paroxysm.

A summary of parasite morphology is given in Table 1.

Failure to find parasites on a single examination or in a single film, thick or thin, is not significant. Repeated examinations, preferably morning and evening, should be made in a suspected case. This is particularly important in *P. falciparum* infections in which the numbers of parasites seen in the blood vary considerably over the day. If the patient is taking suppressive drugs these should be stopped if the clinical condition permits; it may be 24 hours or more before parasites can be easily found.

Clinical diagnosis

Malaria in an endemic area. In an endemic area malaria should be suspected in all febrile illnesses, until proved otherwise. Once periodicity has been established the succession of paroxysms and fever-free intervals is suggestive. The combination of anaemia and splenic enlargement is equally suggestive in indigenes of an endemic area. However, the clinical aspects of malaria are often very similar to those of other conditions and *examination of the blood for parasites is the only way of making the definitive diagnosis*. Where it is not immediately possible to examine blood slides, and particularly where falciparum malaria is suspected, antimalarial drugs should be given immediately and may be of some diagnostic value. In such circumstances films should be prepared before therapy is begun. The use of therapy as a diagnostic device is a thoroughly unwise procedure and no real faith can be put in it, since many fevers in the areas in which malaria is found are caused by other agents, especially arboviruses which are in any case self-limited and last only a few days.

Imported malaria. Malaria may appear outside endemic areas in travellers and immigrants. Importation of the disease is occurring all over the sophisticated world. It is very important to appreciate this as diagnostic errors are easily committed unless the disease is suspected. The patient's geographical history must be checked in order to identify endemic areas he may have visited or come from. Blood films should be made and examined as in a malarious region. In serious cases where falciparum malaria is suspected, treatment should be started immediately after the first films have been taken. It is important also to determine whether the patient has been taking suppressive drugs and when.

TREATMENT OF MALARIA

Treatment of malaria consists in the administration of specific drugs and in dealing with clinical problems which may arise, including anaemia, high fever, shock or dehydration.

Chemotherapy

Successful chemotherapy depends on using the right drug at the right time and in the right way. Few advances have been made in the last two decades in the provision of new drugs, but the appearance of parasite resistance to the major synthetic drugs has necessitated changes in usage and the administration of combinations of standard and new drugs.

Species of parasite. The rational application of chemotherapy in a given case depends on the species of parasite and on the status of the patient in regard to immunity and resistance to infection.

It is essential to determine the species of parasite because *P. falciparum* infection is dangerous and often fatal if unchecked, whereas the others are not and because the objectives of treatment and the chemotherapeutic regime adopted depend on the life cycle.

In *P. falciparum* infections only E forms of the parasite and inert gametocytes are present; there is no persistent infection in the liver. Hence the basic objective of chemotherapy is eradication (or control) of the asexual E parasites which are responsible for the clinical state of the patient. (In this context gametocytes are irrelevant.)

In *P. vivax*, *P. malariae* and *P. ovale* infections, asexual E parasites are present. In addition, there are persistent EE parasites in the liver cells. Hence, the ultimate aim of chemotherapy is eradication of both the E and EE forms.

Immune status of patient. Patients may be divided into:

1. *Non-immunes*, who have not been previously exposed to infection, were exposed a long time previously or were radically cured of infection sufficiently long ago to have lost any acquired immunity. Non-immunes are thus usually visitors to an endemic area from a non-endemic region or, sometimes, from a distant endemic area.

2. *Semi-immunes* (or immunes) in whom there is a history of long regular or intermittent exposure to the relevant parasite. Semi-immunes are usually indigenes of an endemic area or other persons (for example expatriate workers) in whom there is a history of frequent or continued exposure.

The objectives of chemotherapy are often different in the two groups. In non-immunes the aim is eradication of *all* phases of parasite in the host (excluding gametocytes), i.e. the E forms in *P. falciparum* infections and the E and EE forms in the other parasites. In immunes, eradication may not be desirable, since it is upon the presence of the E phase of the parasite that the integrity of the hard-won immunity depends, and chemotherapy is thus aimed at controlling rather than eradicating the parasites. These points will be discussed where relevant.

The following text concerns the chemotherapy and management of human malaria. The treatment of non-immunes and of semi-immunes is considered separately. Adult dosages of drugs are given on the basis of the dose required for a man of 60 kg body weight. Children in general readily tolerate antimalarial drugs in doses equivalent to the adult dose reduced in proportion to their body weight. Where relevant, tables of children's doses are given.

Drugs acting on asexual (E) parasites

Drugs which act on the E phase of the parasites (i.e. on the schizogony cycle in the blood) are called *schizonticides*. These are the compounds used in the clearance of parasites from the blood in all forms of malaria.

SCHIZONTICIDES. There are five main schizonticides: Quinine, the 4-aminoquinolines, mepacrine, proguanil and pyrimethamine. These compounds are discussed in detail below.

In the treatment of infection with a known species of parasite in an individual case or in members of a community exposed to infection, the choice of drug or drugs depends on many factors. The most important of these are: the immune status, the speed and reliability of action of the drug, its toxic effects, the method of administration required and the possibility of parasite resistance.

Quinine. A bitter colourless crystalline alkaloid prepared as bihydrochloride, hydrochloride and sulphate.

Preparations

Tablets contain 260 or 320 mg of the alkaloid as one or other of the salts. The hydrochlorides are readily soluble. The sulphate is much less soluble, especially when compressed as tablets and should therefore be avoided if possible, unless given in acid solution.

Ampoules, usually containing one of the hydrochlorides in powder form, in doses of 500 to 650 mg.

Ampoules, containing solutions of one of the hydrochlorides in doses of 500 to 650 mg.

Tablets for children, containing quinine ethylcarbonate (euquinine) or other less bitter salts.

Action on parasites. A powerful and rapid schizonticide, acting on the E phases of all parasites. Active as a gametocytocide in *P. vivax*, *P. malariae* and *P. ovale*, but not in *P. falciparum* infections.

Parasite resistance at a significant level has seldom been reported (see later).

Side effects and toxicity. In therapeutic dosage there may be tinnitus, some deafness and dizziness, sometimes nausea, occasionally vomiting. Rarely, sensitivity rashes may develop. Haemolysis and haemoglobinuria may be precipitated occasionally during the treatment of *P. falciparum* infection. Excessive dosage (well above that recommended) may cause abortion and sometimes blindness. In suppressive dosage some tinnitus and dizziness may develop.

4-Aminoquinolines. Bitter colourless crystalline compounds with a common 4-aminoquinoline base. The most widely used schizonticides. The diphosphate is called CHLOROQUINE (synonyms include Aralen, Resochin, Resoquine and Avlochlor). The sulphate is called NIVAQUINE. Other 4-aminoquinolines (with different side chains) include AMODIAQUINE (Camoquine), which is a dihydrochloride and certain experimental compounds with a piperazine group in the side chain, said to have greater and longer lasting tissue localization and persistence.

Preparations

Tablets containing 150 mg base chloroquine and nivaquine) or 200 mg base (amodiaquine).

Ampoules containing 200–300 mg base as powder or in solution for parenteral use. An example is Nivaquine Soluble which contains 200 mg base in 5 ml solution.

Action on parasites. Very active and rapid schizonticides. Gametocytocidal in *P. vivax*, *P. malariae* and *P. ovale* infections but not in *P. falciparum*.

Parasite resistance at highly significant levels occurs in some areas in falciparum infections (see below).

Side effects and toxicity. In therapeutic dosage there may be occasional gastrointestinal discomfort or pain, nausea and even vomiting immediately after taking the drug. These side effects are minimised by giving the drugs after food. Transient pruritus of palms and soles may also occur. Rarely, there may be some blurring of vision and even floating scotomata. Retinopathies have been reported, but only on doses much greater than those recommended for therapy of malaria and continued for much longer periods, or after administration of small doses (100 mg base) daily for several years. There is no evidence of retinopathy on the standard regimen for suppression (300 mg once weekly).

Mepacrine (synonyms include Atabrin, Atebrin, Chinacrin, Quinacrine). A bitter yellow acridine compound usually prepared as the hydrochloride or methane sulphonate.

Preparations

Tablets containing 100 mg base as the hydrochloride.

Ampoules containing the methane sulphonate equivalent to 300 mg of the hydrochloride ('musonate') as powder, for parenteral usage.

Action on parasites. An active and rapid schizonticide. Action on gametocytes is similar to that of 4-aminoquinolines. Still widely used, but replaced in many areas by 4-aminoquinolines.

Parasite resistance. Primary resistance has been reported. However, many parasites resistant to 4-aminoquinolines show cross-resistance to mepacrine.

Side effects and toxicity. In therapeutic dosage there are usually few side effects, other than mild gastrointestinal disturbances. In some individuals severe psychotic signs may develop, usually after the first 2–3 days of treatment. These are reversible on withdrawal of the drug. Very high doses (accidental or suicidal) may cause death. On suppressive dosage side effects are rare. Continued usage stains the skin yellow, especially pigmented areas, such as freckles; the hair may take up the pigment. Staining is prominent in skin areas exposed to light. Some brownish discoloration of the nails and irregular areas of the mucosa of the mouth and lips has also been reported after long usage at suppressive dosages. Bluish lesions similar to *lichen planus* have also been noted on the limbs. These effects are rarely significant.

Proguanil (synonyms: Paludrine, Chlorquanide, Chloroguanil, Proguanide). A colourless bitter biguanide, prepared as the hydrochloride. Seldom used for therapy but widely in use as a suppressive for *P. vivax*, *P. malariae*, *P. ovale* and as a suppressive and radical cure of *P. falciparum*.

Preparations

Tablets containing 100 mg hydrochloride.

Action on parasite. A schizonticide acting more slowly than quinine or mepacrine. It acts on the primary exoerythrocytic phase of some *P. falciparum* parasites (causal prophylaxis). It has no action on gametocytes but is sporontocidal, i.e. it inhibits the sexual cycle of *P. falciparum* in the mosquito.

Parasite resistance is widespread. Cross-resistance to pyrimethamine occurs.

Side effects and toxicity. In normal therapeutic dosage side effects are few and mild; there may be some gastrointestinal discomfort especially if the tablets are taken without water. Occasionally there is temporary nausea and vomiting; some episodes of haematuria have been recorded, especially in children.

Pyrimethamine (synonyms: Daraprim, Darapram). A colourless relatively tasteless crystalline compound closely related to the metabolite of proguanil.

Preparations

Tablets containing 25 mg base.

Action on parasite. Same as proguanil.

Parasite resistance is widespread. Cross-resistance to proguanil occurs.

Side effects and toxicity. Very slight in therapeutic or suppressive doses.

Two other groups of compounds are of special importance:

Cycloguanil embonate (Cl-501; Camolar; cycloguanil pamoate). A long-acting antimalarial compound composed of the embonate of the dihydrotriazine metabolite of proguanil. Action on parasites, as for pyrimethamine. Not used therapeutically. On trial as a suppressive.

Parasite resistance. Cross-resistance occurs with proguanil and sometimes with pyrimethamine.

Sulphonamides and sulphones. Sulphadiazine and the long-acting sulphonamides (sulphadimethoxine, sulphamethoxypyridazine and sulphormetoxine) and the sulphone, diaminodiphenylsulphone (Diaphenylsulphone, DDS), commonly used in the treatment of leprosy, all have moderate but often incomplete schizonticidal activity. They are not commonly used alone for therapy but have some value in special circumstances, as in chloroquine-resistant *P. falciparum* in combination with other drugs, notably pyrimethamine, which appear to potentiate them (see later). In glucose-6-phosphate dehydrogenase deficient individuals haemolysis may occur with larger doses than are recommended for treatment of malaria.

Drugs acting on tissue forms of parasites

Proguanil and **pyrimethamine** act on the primary exoerythrocytic cycle of *P. falciparum* and may be used for causal prophylaxis (see below). Proguanil has a much less pronounced inhibitory effect on the same cycle of *P. vivax*.

8-Aminoquinolines. Bitter colourless methoxyaminoquinolines. Three are in use: primaquine, pamaquine and quinocide. They are made up as follows:

PRIMAQUINE: *Tablets*, containing 7.5 mg or 15 mg of the active base.

PAMAQUINE: *Tablets*, containing 8 mg or 10 mg of the base.

QUINOCIDE: *Tablets*, containing 7.8 mg of the base.

Action on parasites. These drugs are poor and slow-acting schizonticides. They are highly active against the gametocytes of all species of parasites and are thus important in reducing transmission.

Their major importance in therapy is their activity against the primary exoerythrocytic phases of all parasites and against the secondary exoerythrocytic phases of *P. vivax*, *P. malariae* and *P. ovale*. In the latter infections, in combination with a schizonticide, they are used in obtaining radical cure.

Side effects and toxicity. Gastrointestinal disturbances, including colicky abdominal pain and the passage of frequent loose stools, are common in therapeutic doses. Mild cyanosis or blueness may appear, easily seen in the fingernail beds, due to development of methaemoglobin. In individuals, especially Negroes, with erythrocytes deficient in glucose-6-phosphate dehydrogenase, acute haemolysis accompanied by haemoglobinuria may occur; this is usually self-limited. Except when haemolysis appears, it is rarely necessary to withdraw the drug during treatment. There is little difference between the toxicity of primaquine and pamaquine. Properly used and with due regard to erythrocytic enzyme deficiency they are safe drugs if given under careful supervision. Where possible the patient should be at rest or, better, treated in bed.

Drugs acting on sexual forms of parasites

1. GAMETOCYTOCIDAL ACTIVITY. Gametocytes of *P. vivax*, *P. ovale* and *P. malariae*, but *not* those of *P. falciparum* are eradicated by therapeutic doses of quinine, 4-aminoquinolines and mepacrine. Proguanil and pyrimethamine are much less effective and also have no action on gametocytes of *P. falciparum*.

Gametocytes of *P. falciparum* and of all the other parasites are quickly eradicated by the 8-aminoquinolines.

2. SPORONTOCIDAL ACTIVITY. The development of the sexual cycle in the mosquito is inhibited by proguanil and by pyrimethamine but not by the other classical schizonticides.

The effect is observed in insects which have taken up blood containing gametocytes from patients taking therapeutic or suppressive dosage regimens. Sexual development is inhibited also when gametocytes and the drugs are taken up in separate blood meals. This serendipity has been used successfully in controlling transmission even in areas where the parasites are resistant to the drugs.

TREATMENT OF FALCIPARUM MALARIA
IN NON-IMMUNES

The chemotherapy and management of malaria caused by strains of *P. falciparum* which are not drug-resistant is described below.

The chemotherapy of drug-resistant strains is discussed on page 70 et seq.

CHEMOTHERAPY. The objective of chemotherapy is to eradicate the asexual erythrocytic (E) parasites as soon as possible.

The treatment of a primary attack and a recrudescence is the same.

For this purpose an active schizonticide is required. The drugs recommended are the 4-aminoquinolines (including chloroquine), quinine and mepacrine. Chloroquine is regarded as the most efficient. Proguanil and pyrimethamine are now seldom used.

In uncomplicated falciparum malaria the compound chosen is given orally. In complicated falciparum malaria it is given parenterally.

Uncomplicated falciparum malaria

4-Aminoquinolines. CHLOROQUINE (diphosphate), NIVAQUINE (sulphate).

Day 1: on admission 600 mg base (4 tablets)
       6 hours later 300 mg base (2 tablets)
Day 2: morning 300 mg base (2 tablets)
Day 3: morning 300 mg base (2 tablets)

In most cases treatment can now be stopped. The total dose is 1500 mg base. It may be continued for a further day (1800 mg base) or 2 days (2100 mg base).

Equivalent doses of amodiaquine (each tablet contains 200 mg base) may be used.

The patient must be treated in bed.

Apart from mild gastrointestinal discomfort and occasional nausea, side effects are few. If a good draft of water is not given after each tablet there may be some pain or soreness over the lower sternum as the tablets pass through the oesophagus into the stomach. Blurring of vision with scotomata occurs rarely on this dosage.

The patient must be watched for several hours after each dosage and all vomit examined, in case the drug is rejected. If it is, dosage should be repeated.

DOSAGE IN CHILDREN (in terms of chloroquine base)
Up to 1 year of age

Day 1	75 mg ($\frac{1}{2}$ tablet) repeated in 6–8 hours
Days 2–5	75 mg ($\frac{1}{2}$ tablet) once daily

1–3 years

Day 1	150 mg (1 tablet) followed by 112.5 mg ($\frac{3}{4}$ tablet) in 6–8 hours
Days 2–5	75 mg ($\frac{1}{2}$ tablet) once daily

3–6 years

Day 1	300 mg (2 tablets) followed by 150 mg (1 tablet) in 6–8 hours
Days 2–5	75 mg ($\frac{1}{2}$ tablet) once daily

6-12 years

Day 1	300 mg (2 tablets) followed by 150 mg (1 tablet) in 6–8 hours
Days 2–5	150 mg (1 tablet) once daily

12–15 years

Day 1	450–600 mg (3–4 tablets) followed by 150–300 mg in 6–8 hours (dose depends on weight of child)
Days 2 and 3	150–300 mg (1–2 tablets) once daily

Above 15 years Adult dose

Quinine (quinine hydrochloride, dihydrochloride, or sulphate) 650 mg (2 tablets) twice daily for 7–10 days. 650 mg may be given thrice daily for the first two days in heavy patients, then twice daily for 5–8 days.

Total dosage. 7 days: 9.10 g or 10.40 g
10 days: 13.00 g or 14.30 g

Note: In the treatment of chloroquine-resistant cases, the dosage is 650 mg *thrice* daily for 10 days.

Quinine can be given as the hydrochloride or bihydrochloride. The sulphate should not be used except in solution, since in tablet form it is often not dissolved in the intestine and tablets may be passed without absorption. Where there is doubt regarding absorption, the urinary content of the drug may be measured by the Tanret test.

Most patients will suffer from some tinnitus and deafness over the course of treatment. They often feel nauseated and may vomit.

It is better to avoid quinine as a routine for uncomplicated falciparum malaria. In patients with high parasitaemia and a history of repeated and inadequately treated attacks blackwater fever may be precipitated.

DOSAGE IN CHILDREN. Children tolerate the drug but find it very bitter. Quinine ethylcarbonate (Euquinine) which is much less bitter, may be substituted in equivalent dosage.

Up to 1 year of age: one tenth adult dose

More than 1 year old up to 15 years of age—

Dose is calculated as: $\frac{\text{age}}{20} \times$ adult dose, e.g.

5 years = $\frac{1}{4}$ adult dose, 10 years $\frac{1}{2}$ adult dose.

Note: In practice in rural areas it may be very difficult to be sure the child receives the drug. Under such circumstances it may be administered intramuscularly.

Mepacrine (mepacrine hydrochloride; Atabrin, Atebrine)

This drug is now seldom used, since it has been largely replaced by chloroquine which has less notable side effects. It is nevertheless very efficient and is useful if chloroquine is unavailable.

Day 1	300 mg (3 tablets) every 8 hours
Day 2	200 mg (2 tablets) every 8 hours
Days 3–7	100 mg (1 tablet) every 8 hours

Each dose should be given with a draft of water and is preferably taken with meals. By the second day the skin will become stained yellow, particularly noticeable in freckles and other pigmented areas. This coloration has nothing to do with liver dysfunction and can be distinguished from jaundice by the relative absence of staining of the conjunctiva. Some cases may be jaundiced; this should be ascertained by clinical study before therapy and by estimation of pre-treatment and subsequent serum bilirubin concentrations.

In highly strung individuals and in certain races, especially Singhalese and Malays, there is some risk of acute psychosis, which may occasionally lead to violence. This usually appears between the second and fourth day of treatment. It calls for immediate withdrawal of the drug. Recovery usually takes only a few days; permanent psychosis is rare.

By the time this serious toxic effect has developed the parasites have usually disappeared from the peripheral blood; further treatment, using chloroquine, should be given if they reappear.

DOSAGE IN CHILDREN. Experience has shown that it is better to avoid giving mepacrine to children. Where circumstances make this necessary it may be given as follows:

1–3 years	Day 1	3×50 mg
	Day 2	2×50 mg
	Days 3–7	50 mg
4–6 years	Day 1	3×75 mg
	Day 2	2×75 mg
	Days 3–7	75 mg
7–11 years	Day 1	3×100 mg
	Day 2	2×100 mg
	Days 3–7	100 mg

Adult dose may be given to children over 15 years of age.

Complicated falciparum malaria

Immediate specific chemotherapy is essential in complicated falciparum malaria. *The complications must be treated concurrently with the infection.* (See separate section, page 51.)

The chemotherapeutic objective, as in uncomplicated infections, is to eradicate the asexual E parasites as quickly as possible by using an efficient schizonticide. The drugs are given parenterally, either intravenously or intramuscularly. The compounds most commonly used are quinine and the 4-aminoquinolines. Mepacrine is used less frequently.

Choice of drug. Chloroquine may be used in infections caused by parasites which are not 4-aminoquinoline-resistant. Infections acquired in areas in which the parasites are known to be resistant or are possibly resistant should be treated with quinine. Where there is any doubt, use quinine. (Some authors advise quinine as a routine, since there is little time to spare in a complicated falciparum case, and chloroquine would not only be ineffective against a resistant strain but its administration would be wasting what time there was if, for example, the case in hand turned out to be the first resistant infection from an area, such as Africa, where chloroquine resistance has not yet been confirmed.)

The intravenous route is probably of slightly more immediate use, but effective continuous plasma concentrations of drugs are reached almost as quickly by intramuscular injection.

Intravenous administration may be performed either by syringe or via an intravenous saline drip or blood transfusion.

If given by syringe, the drug must be well diluted and given slowly. The usual method is to make up the dose provided in the chosen ampoules in 15–20 ml pyrogen free sterile physiological saline or water, and inject using a 20 ml syringe and small-bore needle. The injection should take about 10 minutes. In shocked patients the superficial veins may be collapsed and make the intravenous route difficult. In such circumstances the vein should be exposed and a saline perfusion set up. The needle of the syringe is then inserted into the tube near the cannula and the dose injected. This method is commonly used when a drip has been set up before chemotherapy is given.

It is usually advisable to give the first dose of an antimalarial intravenously by syringe. If the patient shows no sign of improvement after 6 or 8 hours, this process can be repeated. Subsequently, the dose of the drug can be added to the contents of a saline drip, provided the rate of flow at the time is not less than 500 ml in 2–4 hours.

Intramuscular injection is the alternative. Where the parasitaemia is moderate and the patient is not deeply comatosed or shocked, this method is usually successful. The drug is diluted under sterile conditions in 9 ml of sterile pyrogen-free saline or water and injected aseptically into the gluteal muscles.

Complications may result from parenteral drug therapy. Both chloroquine and quinine are hypotensive compounds and too rapid administration or excessive dosage may precipitate serious fall of blood pressures and lead to vascular collapse and shock. When shock is already present, the potential toxic levels of these drugs are considerably lower than in the normal individual and administration should be slowed by adding the drug to a saline drip.

Oral therapy should be substituted for parenteral as soon as possible on the basis of attaining the total dosage which would be given orally in an uncomplicated case, i.e. 1.50 g chloroquine in 3 days or 1.80 g in 4 days and 9.10 g quinine in 7 days or 13.00 g in 10 days.

Quinine. *Intravenously.* Quinine dihydrochloride 500–650 mg is made up in 15–20 ml sterile physiological pyrogen-free saline or water and injected or added to a saline drip as described above. The dose can be repeated if necessary—for instance if the patient is still comatose—in 6–8 hours and again 8 hours later. The total dose in 24 hours should not exceed 1950 mg of the salt.

Intramuscularly. The dose of 500–650 mg (usually the hydrochloride) is made up in 9–10 ml sterile pyrogen-free physiological saline or water and is injected into the gluteal muscles. Dosage as above. The injection is painful and may occasionally lead to abscess formation, which is commoner when the dihydrochloride is used, since this produces a much more acid solution than the hydrochloride.

DOSAGE IN CHILDREN. See formula on page 61. The drug is best given intramuscularly.

Chloroquine and nivaquine. *Intravenously.* 200 mg (base) made up in 15–20 ml saline or water and injected as described above. (A useful preparation is Nivaquine Soluble, prepared in ampoules as 200 mg base in 5.0 ml.)

Some authors recommend an initial dose of 300 mg (base), repeated after 12 hours if necessary or followed by 200 mg (base) 8-hourly to a maximum of 3 doses in 24 hours.

The second dose of 200 mg (base) may be given after 12 hours or, in very severe cases, after 6–8 hours, and the dose repeated in a further 8 hours. Not more than three doses should be given in the first 24 hours and it is seldom necessary to continue parenteral therapy beyond this.

Some authors advise up to 300 mg per dose, totalling not more than 900 mg in 24 hours. This higher dosage offers more risk of precipitating shock, and does not seem to offer better results.

Intramuscularly. 200 mg (base) are made up in 9 ml sterile pyrogen-free physiological saline or water and injected aseptically into the gluteal muscles. The dose may be repeated at 8-hourly intervals for the first 24 hours. It is seldom necessary to continue parenteral therapy beyond this period.

DOSAGE IN CHILDREN. Chloroquine should not be given parenterally to infants and young children. If circumstances demand it (for instance, if no other drug is available) the drug should be given intramuscularly and a single dose should not exceed 5 mg per kg body weight. Timing is as above.

Chloroquine has been given successfully to infants by the rectal route.

Mepacrine. This should be used only when other drugs are not available. It is given *intramuscularly only*.

Mepacrine should not be used in children.

In an adult, the dose is 375 mg mepacrine musonate (methane sulphonate) made up in the usual way in 9 ml sterile pyrogen-free physiological saline or water and injected aseptically into the gluteal muscles. A maximum of 3 doses 8 hours apart may be given in the first 24 hours.

MANAGEMENT OF UNCOMPLICATED FALCIPARUM MALARIA

The patient should be treated in bed, under close supervision. Blood films should be taken as quickly as possible after the patient is seen and morning and night thereafter until clinical cure has been established. Chemotherapy should begin as soon as the diagnosis is confirmed or immediately in a serious case when parasitological diagnosis is delayed, without waiting for confirmation. In the latter case blood films for subsequent examination should be taken before therapy is started.

In hospital the temperature should be recorded 4-hourly and the blood pressures should be checked periodically. The patient is encouraged to drink sweet fluids, soup, etc., freely and an input : output fluid account should be kept. The volume of each specimen of urine passed must be recorded and the urine examined for protein, bilirubin and renal casts. An account of the number and nature of stools passed should be kept. The haemoglobin concentration should be recorded on admission and daily thereafter during the acute attack. The blood should be grouped and the erythrocyte G-6-PD level estimated. Where possible, a check should be kept on serum concentration of bilirubin and plasma urea. Both are usually raised. In the early stages of renal dysfunction the blood urea concentration rises steadily and in renal failure may measure 300 mg or more per 100 ml.

However apparently mild the presenting signs are in a given case, it must be realised that serious complications may develop at any moment and the disease is thus potentially extremely dangerous to the infected individual. In the ordinary course of events it has little public health significance outside endemic areas. In some European countries it is a notifiable disease.

In many moderately severe and uncomplicated cases fluid loss by sweating and diarrhoea or vomiting is considerable and parenteral rehydration is necessary. Replacement of fluid and salt is carried out by intravenous drip. In uncomplicated cases this should proceed at about 500 ml in 4 hours and more than 1 to 1.5 litres is seldom necessary. Whatever fluid is given in this way must be included in the input : output fluid account.

MANAGEMENT OF COMPLICATIONS

When complications develop they must be treated concurrently with the infection. Treatment of hyperpyrexia, for instance, without treatment of the malaria is clearly useless, and *vice versa*.

Shock. This phenomenon is basically non-specific. It requires immediate infusion of fluid to restore the circulating blood volume. Physiological saline solution is commonly used by the intravenous route. Five hundred millilitres saline containing dextran or, alternatively, 500 ml plasma, is given rapidly in the first hour. This is followed by the slower administration of saline or a mixture of saline and isotonic glucose at the rate of about 500 ml every 4 hours. The blood pressures are recorded hourly. The volume of fluid needed is decided clinically.

Corticosteroids are sometimes given in the acute stage of vascular collapse with good effect. A common regime is hydrocortisone sodium succinate in an initial dose of 100 mg intramuscularly, followed by a similar dose in 8 hours. Up to three doses at 8-hourly intervals may be given during the crisis. Thereafter the dose is rapidly reduced.

Acute dehydration. Many patients with complicated falciparum malaria quickly develop severe loss of water and salt and replacement is essential. Parenteral replacement of water and salt is needed in cases which have developed choleraic diarrhoea (see above) and may be necessary in those with dysenteric syndromes. The fluid given in this way is included in the daily input : output account. The amount of intravenous infusion necessary in a given case is determined by clinical observation of the patient. If dehydration is severe a volume of 500 ml physiological saline is given in half an hour to an hour, as in shock; thereafter the same volume of saline or a 1 : 1 mixture of saline and isotonic glucose is given in the course of 4 hours and repeated until 3 to 5 litres have been infused. More than this is seldom needed. In severe dehydration there may be considerable loss of potassium. This is best replaced orally as potassium chloride; or 15 mEq potassium may be added to a litre of the infusion. Acidosis is rare in malaria complicated by dehydration, but it may develop in cases with intractable vomiting or during renal failure; in these circumstances a solution of physiological saline plus sodium lactate (50 mEq per litre) may be infused until the signs of acidosis cease.

Severe anaemia. Transfusion of cross-matched blood is necessary when the erythrocyte count falls below 2.0 million cells per mm³ (about 6 g haemoglobin per cent). Citrated blood is normally given at the rate of 500 ml in 4 hours. When there are signs of cardiovascular embarrassment the total volume of blood should not exceed 1 to 1.5 litres and the transfusion may be given slowly as packed cells. The amount of blood given must be included in the daily fluid input account.

In the treatment of severe anaemia in chronic or repeated infections, transfusion is seldom needed. Recovery usually follows treatment of the infection and the administration of ferrous iron (1 g per day in 3 divided doses) and restoration of the diet.

Blackwater fever. In the acute haemolysis of blackwater fever transfusion is required immediately. Some haemolysis of the infected cells occurs but this is unavoidable. Replacement of circulating erythrocytes is essential, and urgent. Great care is needed in cross matching donor and recipient bloods. Prednisolone phosphate may help contain the haemolysis in doses of 40–60 mg intramuscularly daily during lysis.

Where haemolysis is intense or repetitive the amount of blood needed may be considerable. Note must be kept of the volume used and the input should be graded accordingly.

The agglutinin patterns are disturbed in malaria and blackwater fever and the greatest care is necessary in choosing the donor's blood. Both cells and plasma must be cross-matched for each specimen of blood transfused. Blood must not be used on the basis of grouping alone, since cells of apparently the right group may in practice be incompatible.

Renal failure, hepatic failure, dehydration and shock are treated by standard methods.

Antimalarial chemotherapy is required only exceptionally in blackwater fever, since parasites are invariably few after haemolysis has started. Chemosuppression should be continued during and after the attack using proguanil, thus avoiding the hazards of quinine and of parasite chloroquine resistance; where proguanil-resistance is present, chloroquine should be given.

Renal failure. In practice the patient may be considered to be in acute renal failure when the volume of urine passed during the day is less than 400 ml and the plasma urea concentration exceeds 100 mg per cent. This arbitrary figure for output does not apply in a very hot ambient temperature in which urinary daily volumes of this order are common in normal people who are in a state of negative water balance; in these circumstances, however, the high blood urea is not present.

In order to determine the onset of the renal dysfunction it is essential to record from the beginning not only the 24-hour output of urine but the volume of each specimen. A strict record of input and output of fluid (including the volumes of saline infusions or blood transfusions) must be kept. The urinary specific gravity should also be measured, since in the oliguria of renal failure, unlike physiological oliguria, the urine is unconcentrated and the gravity low. The plasma urea concentration should be estimated at regular intervals.

The intake of fluid, electrolytes and protein is restricted. Once renal failure has developed the patient may be treated by standard methods.

If oliguria increases to the point of virtual anuria, with the passage of very small volumes of urine, and the plasma urea concentration is of the order of 200 mg per 100 ml per day and rising, dialysis should be considered. The need is urgent if there is hyperkalaemia, or if the patient has been overhydrated by excessive intraveous fluid administration. Where dialysis of the blood is not possible, peritoneal dialysis should be adopted, using a hypertonic solution of 6.3 per cent dextrose, containing 0.56 per cent sodium chloride; 3 mEq potassium per litre is added if hyperkalaemia is present.

Treatment of other complications

Cerebral malaria. There is no specific treatment for the cerebral syndromes. Prompt treatment of the malaria usually brings rapid relief. Corticosteroids are useful in comatose patients, for example 200–300 mg hydrocortisone intramuscularly on the first 24 hours or the equivalent doses of prednisolone, followed by half the dose the following day and subsequently descending doses.

Hyperpyrexia. This is treated in the same way as heat stroke. Treatment aims at lowering the body temperature and restoring sweating. This is done by bathing or spraying the body surface with cold water and aiding evaporation by fanning. Chlorpromazine (25–50 mg intravenously at the onset of treatment) is sometimes given to promote peripheral vasodilation and control restlessness and convulsions. The oral temperature is recorded every few minutes during cooling. When it reaches 38.8°C active treatment is stopped, otherwise the patient may pass into shock.

The temperature may now continue to fall to

normal or below. Fever may be re-established at subhyperpyrexial levels. This should be treated by sponging, and will subside with the treatment of the infection.

TREATMENT OF VIVAX, OVALE AND QUARTAN MALARIA

The following text deals with treatment of strains of parasites which are not drug-resistant. Treatment of drug-resistant strains is discussed on page 70 et seq.

The technique of administration is the same in all cases, since acute complications, as seen in falciparum malaria, do not normally occur.

The objective is to eradicate with a schizonticide the asexual E parasites in order to obtain a regression of the clinical malaria. In addition, radical cure aims at eradication of the persistent (EE) parasites in the liver parenchymal cells. An 8-aminoquinoline is needed for this.

The schizonticides commonly used in radical cure are 4-aminoquinolines (usually chloroquine or nivaquine) and quinine. Mepacrine is not used, since in combination with an 8-aminoquinoline the toxic properties of both drugs are potentiated. The 8-aminoquinoline most widely given is primaquine; pamaquine or quinocide are alternatives.

The treatment for a primary attack and for a relapse is the same.

Combined therapy is needed for radical cure. It offers about a 95 per cent chance of success. If it fails (i.e. if a relapse occurs subsequently), the treatment must be repeated.

There is some evidence that the schizonticide may potentiate the action of the 8-aminoquinoline. It is therefore customary to give the drugs simultaneously. As an alternative when chloroquine is used, the schizont may be administered first and then followed by the 8-aminoquinoline.

Suggested courses of treatment

A *Day 1*   Chloroquine 600 mg immediately, 300 mg after 6–8 hours
Primaquine 7.5 mg twice daily, morning and evening (a single dose of 15 mg may be substituted)
Day 2   Chloroquine 300 mg in the morning
Primaquine 7.5 mg twice daily
Day 3   As for Day 2

Day 4   As for Day 2 (optional so far as chloroquine is concerned but primaquine must be given)
Days 5–10 or 14   Primaquine 7.5 mg twice daily
B *Days 1–10*   Quinine 650 mg twice daily
Days 1–10 or 14   Primaquine 7.5 mg twice daily or in a single dose of 15 mg

Note: In the above regimes, pamaquine 8–10 mg base, thrice daily for 10 days may be substituted for primaquine. An alternative is quinocide, in doses of 7.8 mg of base thrice daily for 10 days.

The 8-aminoquinolines are unpleasant drugs to take and may be toxic. They usually produce some gastrointestinal discomfort, sometimes colicky abdominal pain and several loose motions in the day. Mild degrees of methaemoglobinaemia may develop, indicated by cyanotic blue discoloration of the blood visible in the fingernail beds.

It is preferable to treat the patient in bed or at any rate at rest while being given 8-aminoquinolines. He should be given plenty of fluids and a record kept of input and output of fluids. Each specimen of urine should be examined for haemoglobin.

In individuals with erythrocyte deficiency of glucose-6-phosphate dehydrogenase (G-6-PD) haemolysis followed by haemoglobinuria may develop after the first few doses. This phenomenon is commonly seen in Negroes. It tends to be self-limited but is usually regarded as an indication for stopping the administration of the drug.

Before starting combined therapy for radical cure in patients of Negro descent or in others in whom the enzyme deficiency is known to be common, it is advisable to test the enzyme level. If there is marked deficiency, the use of 8-aminoquinolines should be avoided. As an alternative, regular suppressive doses of chloroquine may be given after a full course of the schizonticide, but this assigns the individual to continued dosage for a period of 2–3 years.

Individuals with moderate G-6-PD deficiency will often take an 8-aminoquinoline without the development of overt haemolysis.

Treatment of children

Dosages of schizonticides may be given as for treatment of uncomplicated falciparum malaria. This will ensure clinical cure of all three infections. Children over the age of 4 may be given an 8-aminoquinoline for up to 10 consecutive days in the following doses (primaquine): *4–8 years old,* a total of 5.0 mg to 7.5 mg once daily or in two divided doses; *8–15 years*, 10 rising to 15 mg given as above; *over 15*, adult dose, given as 7.5 mg twice daily. Children in India have been successfully treated, with a moderate rate of radical cure, on dosages of 2.5 mg daily for 5 days.

If it is decided not to give an 8-aminoquinoline, an alternative is to place the child on a suppressive regimen for up to 3 years.

MANAGEMENT OF VIVAX, OVALE AND QUARTAN MALARIA

The patient should be treated in bed, preferably in hospital.

Blood films should be taken before chemotherapy is started and thereafter night and morning until cure.

Chemotherapy should begin as soon as diagnosis is established parasitologically.

Oral temperature should be taken 4-hourly. Fluids should be given freely and the volume of urine output recorded.

The haemoglobin concentration should be measured on admission and at intervals thereafter and the blood G-6-PD level ascertained. If there is pronounced enzyme deficiency the 8-aminoquinolines should be withheld.

Many individuals are already dehydrated by sweating and diarrhoea to some degree when first seen and intravenous replacement of fluid may be necessary.

During a paroxysm careful and patient nursing is essential.

MANAGEMENT IN SEMI-IMMUNES

In individuals repeatedly infected with any of the parasites the immunity developed to the infecting strain causes considerable modification of the clinical attack. The immunity will regress some months after successful treatment or if the individual has been for long enough outside the endemic area. It is often ineffective against strains of the same species of parasite in endemic areas other than that in which resistance was acquired. In such circumstances, attacks will be severe and the patient should be considered as a 'non-immune' and treated accordingly (see page 57 et seq.).

The modified attack in the semi-immune is treated in the same manner irrespective of the infecting species.

The objective of chemotherapy is to deal with the asexual E parasites and to contain them at non-clinical levels. In individuals still exposed in an endemic area this will allow the survival of the E parasite and so the hard-won resistance to the infection.

The aim is achieved by giving single large doses of an effective schizonticide, or occasionally, large doses on two consecutive days.

Where possible, a 4-aminoquinoline should be used. The recommended treatment for adults is chloroquine 600 mg base (4 tablets) given once only. Alternatives are (in single doses): amodiaquine 600–800 mg base (3 to 4 tablets); quinine 1.30 g or 1.95 g (2 to 3 tablets); mepacrine 300–500 mg (3 to 5 tablets); proguanil 300–500 mg (3 to 5 tablets) or pyrimethamine 500 mg (2 tablets).

Such dosage will usually provide rapid clinical cure. Occasionally it may need repeating on the following day.

Dosages for children are in proportion to their body weight (see above).

PROPHYLAXIS

Prophylaxis of malaria means complete protection against all stages of the life cycle of the parasite in man, including the sporozoite.

At present there is no compound capable of killing the sporozoites, so that true prophylaxis against malaria is not possible.

In *P. falciparum* infections the primary exoerythrocytic (PE) phase, initiated when the sporozoite penetrates the liver parenchyma cell, can be eradicated by proguanil and pyrimethamine, so that the asexual E phase of the parasite does not develop. In a sense this is a form of prophylaxis, and has been described as 'causal prophylaxis'. The drugs are said to produce the same effect in certain strains of *P. vivax*, but the evidence for this is not very convincing.

The 8-aminoquinolines eradicate the secondary exoerythrocytic liver phases of *P. vivax*, *P. malariae* and *P. ovale* and the primary exoerythrocytic parasites of all species.

SUPPRESSION

This means the control of the parasites after they have gained access to the human host. The word is usually regarded as referring to the suppression of the asexual E phase of the parasites to subclinical levels, or its complete eradication.

In most forms of chemotherapeutic control of malaria in practice the present aim is suppression. In *P. falciparum* infections, in which the asexual E phase of the parasite is the only form existing in the body of the host by the time clinical signs develop, successful suppression means, in effect, eradication, and the end result of suppression is therefore radical cure (apart from the inert gametocytes). In *P. vivax*, *P. malariae* and *P. ovale* infections, control of the E phase can be achieved easily by this means but radical cure is not obtained because of the persistent secondary exoerythrocytic parasites in the liver cells.

Non-immunes

The drugs available for suppression are the schizonticides, which deal with the asexual E parasites. All the standard drugs have been used successfully for this purpose. A major factor which has now to be considered is the development of parasite resistance to drugs (see page 68). Where this has appeared, the relevant compound is of no value and some other drug must be substituted.

In the absence of resistance, the schizonticides which are most successful are chloroquine, mepacrine, proguanil and pyrimethamine. All are extensively used.

For suppression of drug-resistant parasites see page 71.

In view of the superior action of chloroquine as a therapeutic agent and because of the possibility that wide and inefficient use of the drug may be one of the causal factors in the production of parasite resistance to it, under ordinary circumstances it may be better to use the other drugs for suppression and reserve this compound for chemotherapy.

There are inherent advantages in using proguanil or pyrimethamine for suppression of *P. falciparum* infections in that these drugs, in addition to suppressing the asexual cycle, inhibit the primary exoerythrocytic phase of the parasite, thus acting as causal prophylactics; they also inhibit the development of gametocytes in the mosquito, thus reducing the transmission. Unfortunately, the 8-aminoquinolines, which are highly successful in dealing with the tissue forms of all parasites, are weak schizonticides, and are too toxic for general use.

In the chemosuppression of malaria there are certain practical procedures which must be followed to ensure satisfactory results.

Suppressive therapy may be started immediately before or after entrance into the endemic area, except where mepacrine is concerned, the dosage of which must begin a fortnight before exposure in order to obtain a blood concentration adequate to suppress the parasites.

Whatever the regimen decided, it must be regularly and rigorously followed during exposure.

All drug dosages should be continued for at least a month after the individual has left the last endemic area before returning to a non-endemic region.

In the doses recommended the drugs are practically non-toxic. They cause no damage to the taker; they do not affect sexual potency; they have no effect on pregnancy and are not teratogenic. Their absorption is not hindered by reasonable intake of alcohol.

The most widely used compounds for suppression in non-immunes are chloroquine and other 4-aminoquinolines, proguanil and pyrimethamine. Quinine is also used but to a more limited extent. In areas where the parasites are not resistant these drugs are active against all species of parasite.

For dealing with drug resistance, see page 70.

Chloroquine or **nivaquine**: 300 mg base (2 tablets) once weekly or 150 mg base (1 tablet) twice weekly. Amodiaquine 400 mg base (2 tablets) as above.

The drug is taken first just before or on arrival in the endemic area and regularly thereafter and for a month after leaving the endemic area to return to a non-endemic area. Side effects are few (see page 58).

As pointed out above, in view of increasing parasite resistance, the drug is commonly restricted to chemotherapeutic usage.

DOSAGES IN CHILDREN (weekly dosage of chloroquine or nivaquine)

Birth–2 years	37.5 mg base ($\frac{1}{4}$ tablet)
3–5 years	75 mg base ($\frac{1}{2}$ tablet)
6–10 years	150 mg base (1 tablet)
Over 10 years	225–300 mg base ($1\frac{1}{2}$ to 2 tablets)

Proguanil: 100 mg (1 tablet) daily. The dosage is begun on arrival in the endemic area, continued regularly during exposure and for a month after leaving the last endemic area. Side effects are few (see page 59).

DOSAGE IN CHILDREN

Birth to 1 year	25–50 mg ($\frac{1}{4}$–$\frac{1}{2}$ tablet) daily
1-3 years	50–100 mg ($\frac{1}{2}$–1 tablet) daily

This drug or pyrimethamine is recommended for general usage and should be tried first in areas where parasites are resistant to chloroquine.

Pyrimethamine: 50 mg (2 tablets) once weekly. Dosage starts on entering the endemic area, continues throughout exposure and for 1 month after leaving the last endemic area. There are practically no side effects.

DOSAGE IN CHILDREN (once weekly)
Under 1 year   6 mg ($\frac{1}{4}$ tablet)
1–3 years   12 mg ($\frac{1}{2}$ tablet)
4–6 years   12-25 mg ($\frac{1}{2}$–1 tablet)
7–11 years   25 mg (1 tablet)
Thereafter rising to adult dosage

Quinine: 260–325 mg daily, as hydrochloride or dihydrochloride. Dosage starts on exposure, continues through exposure and for 1 month thereafter.

Quinine is regarded as less efficient as a suppressant than chloroquine, proguanil or pyrimethamine. It is used largely when other drugs are not available or in areas of parasite chloroquine resistance or for financial reasons, as it is cheaper in areas in which it is produced. Irregular usage may be a predisposing factor in blackwater fever.

Side effects are noticeable on this regimen. They vary in severity from person to person on the same dosage, and commonly include tinnitus, some dizziness and deafness; there may be occasional nausea and vomiting and, rarely, a skin sensitivity rash. Most people learn to live with quinine if they must.

DOSAGE IN CHILDREN
Up to 1 year   65 mg
1–3 years   130 mg
4–6 years   195 mg
7–11 years   260 mg
Thereafter   325 mg

Mepacrine: 100 mg hydrochloride daily. The dosage is started *14 days before exposure* in order to build up an active serum level of the drug. It is continued during exposure and for a month thereafter.

Side effects are slight. The skin is stained deep yellow and the drug is excreted in the hair. Women often object to the cosmetic effects. Late effects are rare. They include brown pigmentation of the nails, thickening and bluish coloration of exposed skin and eruptions, usually on the legs, resembling those of *lichen planus* (see page 58).

DOSAGE IN CHILDREN. Mepacrine is not given to infants and rarely to children. Where other drugs are not available, the recommended doses are:
1–3 years   25 mg ($\frac{1}{4}$ tablet) twice weekly
4–6 years   25 mg ($\frac{1}{4}$ tablet) daily
7–11 years   50 mg ($\frac{1}{2}$ tablet) daily
Thereafter   75 mg–100 mg (1 tablet) daily depending on body weight

Semi-immunes

Malaria in individuals exposed to repeated infection (usually the members of communities in endemic areas) who have acquired immunity to particular strains of parasite is relatively easy to suppress, provided there is no drug resistance.

Because of the risk of development of drug resistance and in view of their value as a therapeutic agent the use of the 4-aminoquinolines should be restricted where possible. When given, they are prescribed as in non-immunes: chloroquine 300 mg base (2 tablets) weekly; amodiaquine 400 mg base (2 tablets) or 200 mg (1 tablet) once weekly is a widely used alternative. These dosages provide a high degree of suppression, for example in labour populations, without unduly disturbing the level of immunity.

Other drugs are effective: proguanil 300 mg once weekly, pyrimethamine 50 mg weekly and quinine 650 mg once weekly.

PARASITE DRUG RESISTANCE

Resistance to antimalarial drugs has been established in parasites infecting man, monkeys and rodents. It has been defined as the 'ability of a parasite strain to survive and/or multiply despite the administration and absorption of a drug given in doses equal to or higher than those usually recommended, but within the limits of tolerance of the subject'. Resistance develops more easily against schizonticides acting by competitive enzyme inhibition on the folic acid–folinic acid cycle in the parasite (proguanil and pyrimethamine) than against compounds acting on the glycolytic cycle of the growing parasite before division (quinine, mepacrine and the 4-aminoquinolines). It is believed that resistance represents the usage or development of a metabolic bypass of the pathway blocked by the relevant drug.

Resistance is not absolute, but it may exist to the point where the relevant drug is ineffective up to the limits of the subject's tolerance to it. When resistance is strong, it can usually be demonstrated at all stages of the parasite life cycle and is transmitted cyclically from mammalian host to host via the mosquito.

In human malaria the degree of resistance often varies according to the strain of parasite as well as the species. For instance, resistance to proguanil may be evident when the drug is given in suppressive dosage but not at the more concentrated therapeutic dosage. On the other hand, a parasite may be clearly resistant to both therapeutic and suppressive dosage.

The factors involved in the development of resistance in man in endemic areas are not yet established. Resistance is most commonly found in regions of unstable endemicity and where the relevant drug is or has recently been readily available to the exposed community and not infrequently misused. This latter might well be an important factor, in view of the ease of experimental production of resistance to certain antimalarials in *P. berghei* infections in mice in the presence of repeated drug challenge. Mass migrations or immigrations of populations have also occurred in many of the affected areas.

Drug resistance has set some difficult chemotherapeutic problems since the relevant strains cause malaria indistinguishable from the disease resulting from normal strains.

At the moment resistance does not seem to have created serious difficulties in malaria eradication or control programmes, but its extension may do so in proportion to the dependence of such campaigns on the use of antimalarial drugs.

Resistance to proguanil and pyrimethamine

Resistance was first detected against proguanil and pyrimethamine in both *P. falciparum* and *P. vivax* infections. This is now widespread in Malaysia, Indonesia, East and West Africa and South America. Parasites resistant to one of these compounds are resistant to the other. There is no cross-resistance to the 4-aminoquinolines mepacrine or quinine, but cross-resistance to cycloguanil embonate exists.

Resistance of P. falciparum to 4-aminoquinolines

Resistance of *P. falciparum* to the schizontocidal action of the 4-aminoquinolines is now present in many parts of South-east Asia and South America. Other species of parasites are not so far involved.

In South-east Asia resistance to chloroquine and the other 4-aminoquinolines is widespread and mostly of grades I and II. Resistance at the grade III level is very uncommon.

Resistance was first noted by Tranakchit Harinasuta in Thailand, where it is now recognised as very common. It is also found in West Malaysia, in Cambodia and in South Vietnam, where, according to the district, a high percentage of non-immune military personnel infected with *P. falciparum* has been found to be infected with resistant strains.

F

Resistance to chloroquine, usually at the R I or R II levels, is present in South America, in Venezuela, Colombia and many areas in Brazil.

Although suspected in various parts of Africa, including Upper Volta, Liberia, Ghana, Malawi and Tanzania, there has so far been no case of insensitivity to chloroquine confirmed. It is thus generally agreed that falciparum infections are still sensitive to the drug in Africa.

The commonest evidence of resistance is recrudescence of the parasitaemia after a normal initial response to a full therapeutic course of chloroquine or other 4-aminoquinoline (grade I resistance). It is not known whether this response results from recent acquisition of resistance, since recrudescence rates have been seldom recorded in the past.

The reaction to chloroquine of the non-immune subject infected with a resistant strain differs in some respects from that of the semi-immune, in that he usually shows a less complete and slower parasite and fever response than the latter, who may quickly become symptom-free without much change in parasitaemia.

Cross-resistance. Strains of *P. falciparum* resistant to chloroquine are also resistant to other 4-aminoquinolines and usually to mepacrine. Some of them are resistant to proguanil and pyrimethamine, but others are not; it is probable that this resistance may have developed independently.

Some indication of R I resistance to quinine has been noted in a few chloroquine resistant strains from South-east Asia.

Determination of resistance. A gradient of response to a drug usually exists in the infected community in which drug-resistant parasites occur, ranging from full sensitivity to complete insensitivity. The search for further evidence of resistance, especially to chloroquine, in endemic areas is clearly important.

In order to classify the degree of resistance exhibited by a parasite, an arbitrary system of grading has been established, based on the resistance of the asexual (E phase) parasites of *P. falciparum* to the 4-aminoquinolines, but in general applicable to the grading of resistance to any schizonticide in any human malaria parasite.

Grading of resistance to therapeutic doses of antimalarial drugs is expressed as follows:

Sensitivity (S): Clearance of asexual parasitaemia within 7 days of the first day of treatment, without recrudescence.

Resistance: R I. Clearance of asexual parasitaemia as in sensitivity, followed by recrudescence.

R II. Marked reduction of asexual parasitaemia, but no clearance.

R III. No reduction of asexual parasitaemia.

It should be noted that measurement of resistance is made in terms of control or otherwise of parasitaemia and not of clinical effects. Parasitaemia and clinical signs of malaria, fever, for example, run parallel in non-immunes but may be increasingly divergent as immunity develops so that the appearance of the modified clinical response in the patient is related to higher levels of parasitaemia than in the non-immune individual. Thus, it often happens that in the continually exposed immune individual, clinical relief may be effected by a drug to which the parasites exhibit R I or R II resistance in terms of parasitological criteria.

The determination of the response of a malaria parasite to a drug must be carried out by standard procedures laid down by the World Health Organization and designed to cover certain variables and sources of error in the drug and its administration and in the response of the host.

In assessing the response of a *P. falciparum* infection to 4-aminoquinolines, a dose of chloroquine is given as follows:

Day 1 10 mg (base)/kg, e.g. 600 mg (base) for 60 kg adult

Day 2 10 mg (base)/kg, e.g. 600 mg (base) for 60 kg adult

Day 3 5 mg (base)/kg, e.g. 300 mg (base) for 60 kg adult

Total: 1500 mg (base)

The subject is kept under observation to make sure the drug is ingested and retained. The effect of the treatment on the parasitaemia (and clinical state) should be studied when possible over a period of 28 days. In an endemic area, the subject should preferably be placed in a hospital where reinfection can be excluded. Otherwise, he should be studied for at least 7 days. If resistance is suspected, the parasite should be examined further under experimental conditions, or the patient should be watched in a non-infective region. The activity of the drug on the parasite is finally determined in a non-endemic area in specialised reference centres by infection of volunteers. Resistance is classified as above.

Resistance to other drugs, including quinine, is studied in a similar fashion, using standard dosage regimens and following the effects for a period of 28 days.

During such experiments, drugs other than the antimalarial under observation should not be given to the subject.

Treatment of chloroquine-resistant *P. falciparum* infections

Quinine. The chloroquine-resistant parasites so far studied have all been found susceptible to large dosages of quinine. Some degree of 'resistance' to quinine has however been noted in certain strains from Vietnam. This has usually been grade I resistance, appearing in individuals given only small doses of the drug, for instance 6.4 g in 4 days or 9.45 g in 7 days (compared with the recommended dosage of 13.0 g in 10 days). Recrudescences have, however, been recorded in one strain after as much as 16.20 g in 10 days, though this infection was eradicated by a subsequent dosage of 22.68 g in 14 days.

For practical purposes, therefore, it seems legitimate to try quinine in doses of at least 1.3 g daily for 10 days in infections which have failed to respond to standard chloroquine therapy.

Combinations of sulphones or sulphonamides with pyrimethamine may eventually prove successful in chloroquine-resistant infections and perhaps in those infections which appear refractory to quinine.

The sulpha drugs are seldom used alone in chemotherapy because of their relatively limited and slow antiparasitic activity and the risk of evoking parasite resistance. They are, however, used to potentiate the action of other drugs, particularly pyrimethamine.

Combinations of pyrimethamine with sulphadiazine or long-acting sulphonamides such as sulphormetoxine or with diaminodiphenylsulphone (DDS) have been used with variable success in the treatment and suppression of both chloroquine- and pyrimethamine-resistant *P. falciparum* infections. They have also been used against normal strains of parasites since the development of resistance to either of the drugs in a given combination is likely to be slower and less intense than when the compounds are used separately.

For treatment of chloroquine resistant *P. falciparum* infections, Sulphormetoxine has been most often used, in a dose of 1.0 g with 50 mg pyrimethamine, and has proved highly successful in semi-immunes in Thailand. The same combination with a further dose of 50 mg pyrimethamine on the following day has also been successful in Brazil.

In Brazil, *P. falciparum* infections which did not respond to a total of 2.4 g chloroquine, were eradicated by a total dose of 1.5 g sulphormetoxine in 2 days, with 50 mg pyrimethamine on the first day.

In non-immunes with acute non-resistant *P. falciparum* infections combination of a single dose of 1.0 g sulphormetoxine and 50 mg pyrimethamine base in adults and 0.5 g sulphormetoxine plus 12.5 g pyrimethamine base in children have proved effective in clearing parasitaemia and relieving the clinical malaria.

No parasite resistance to the sulphonamide or to pyrimethamine has so far been reported from areas in which the combination has been used either for treatment or suppression.

Suppression of chloroquine-resistant *P. falciparum* infections

Proguanil and pyrimethamine in the usual doses will actively suppress chloroquine-resistant *P. falciparum* as long as the parasite is sensitive to them. Most are insensitive to mepacrine.

When, as in some South-east Asian strains, the parasite is insensitive to all four synthetic drugs, it may or may not respond readily to quinine. For example, quinine, in doses of 400 mg base daily from the time of the bites of infective mosquitoes did not prevent patency of an experimental infection with Vietnamese chloroquine-resistant strain of *P. falciparum* at the expected time.

Diaphenylsulphone (DDS) has shown some activity experimentally in preventing patent infection with two strains of chloroquine/pyrimethamine-resistant *P. falciparum* but was only partly successful in controlling chloroquine-resistant strains in Thai semi-immune patients.

Various combinations of drugs are being tested for suppressive activity against chloroquine-resistant *P. falciparum*. The most promising is the administration of sulphormetoxine and pyrimethamine in the doses quoted above. A combination of some potential is that of cycloguanil embonate and sulphadiamine (DADDS), which has shown some activity against chloroquine-resistant strains.

Treatment and suppression of other drug-resistant infections

Proguanil- and pyrimethamine-resistant *P. falciparum* and *P. vivax* infections respond to chloroquine or mepacrine (unless the former are also insensitive to the 4-aminoquinolines). They also respond readily to quinine.

Pyrimethamine-resistant strains of *P. falciparum* in some areas are sensitive to the combination of sulphormetoxine and pyrimethamine.

Proguanil-resistant strains of *P. falciparum* may respond to Cl 564 (cycloguanil embonate and DADDS) but resistant strains of *P. vivax* do not.

RECENT DEVELOPMENTS IN CHEMOTHERAPY

The appearance of parasite resistance to synthetic drugs has stimulated the search for other drugs with antimalarial activity.

New drugs and compounds under trial for various other purposes have been used for chemotherapy and suppression. These include the following.

Sulphones and sulphonamides

It has been known for many years that certain sulphonamides act as schizonticides when given alone. Sulphones share this activity. Both show some activity against strains of chloroquine resistant to *P. falciparum*, particularly in the semi-immune host.

Sulphormetoxine

Recently studies have been made on long-acting sulphonamides, particularly sulphormetoxine (Fanasil, sulformethoxine) a compound with a half-life of between 100 and 200 hours. Given alone in semi-immunes, this drug has a schizonticidal activity against some strains of *P. falciparum* equivalent to that of chloroquine. It has some action against *P. vivax* but no effect on tissue forms of parasites or on sporogony.

Its main potential as an antimalarial is its activity against the schizonts of chloroquine-resistant *P. falciparum*.

Toxic reactions to the long-acting sulphonamides may be precipitated by too frequent administration, as was recently demonstrated in Morocco, where this compound was used for the control of meningococcal meningitis. In the dosages recommended for control of malaria the risk is minimal.

Diaphenylsulphone (diaminodiphenyl sulphone: DDS)

This drug, which is widely used for the treatment of leprosy, has schizonticidal activity on

P. falciparum in single oral doses of 200 mg in semi-immune subjects. It is less effective against *P. vivax* infections.

In patients with erythrocytic deficiency of G-6-PD, DDS may induce haemolysis. This effect is undisturbed on addition of para-amino benzoic acid (PABA) which nevertheless inhibits the schizonticidal activity which is apparently due to interference with the incorporation of PABA in the formation of folic acid.

The schizonticidal activity of both sulphonamides and sulphones is slow, and there is danger that widespread injudicious use of the drug may lead to parasite resistance.

It has been shown, however, that the rate at which *P. berghei* acquires resistance to antimalarials as a result of combined treatment with two drugs (pyrimethamine and diaphenylsulphone) is slower than when either drug is used alone. This could indicate a means of delaying the appearance of resistance or of prolonging the period of effective use of drugs before resistance to them developed. Furthermore, in the above experiments the resistance to pyrimethamine acquired by administration of the drug alone was found to be substantially greater than that which developed when a 4-aminoquinoline was given simultaneously.

Moreover, it has been shown that sulphonamides and sulphones have a potentiating effect on the action of the biguanides and pyrimethamine.

It is the usual practice, therefore, to give the former in combination with more active schizonticides such as pyrimethamine. This combination is particularly useful in the treatment of some chloroquine-resistant strains of *P. falciparum* (see above).

It has also been used in combination with pyrimethamine (25 mg) in doses of 0.5 to 1.0 g weekly against pyrimethamine-resistant strains of *P. falciparum*.

Repository compounds

Depot substances capable of providing antiparasitic activity for long periods after a single administration are being studied, largely for use in eradication programmes.

The most widely used so far is *cycloguanil embonate*, the embonate of the dehydrotriazine metabolite of proguanil. This gives long-term protection against mosquito-borne infections. The dosage is 6 mg/kg body weight for adults and 5–15 mg/kg body weight for children, given intramuscularly as a suspension in oil. Protection

against *P. falciparum*, *P. vivax* and *P. malariae* infections continues for 3–4 months after a single dose. Its usefulness is limited in some endemic areas by its inactivity against proguanil- and pyrimethamine-resistant parasites.

Diacetyl diaminodiphenylsulphone (DADDS; sulphadiamine) is also successful in suppression of *P. falciparum* malaria in doses of 4–9 mg/kg body weight. It has been found active in *P. berghei* infections against strains of parasite resistant to cycloguanil, proguanil and pyrimethamine.

A combination of the two drugs (called at the moment Cl 564) given for therapy or for suppression and prophylaxis has been found active against some chloroquine- and proguanil-resistant *P. falciparum* strains, and inactive in proguanil-resistant *P. vivax* infections. Further studies are in progress.

Other drugs under consideration do not at the moment look very promising. They include: *4-aminoquinolines* with piperazine rings in the side-chain, said to be more tissue persistent than chloroquine, but without effect on chloroquine-resistant *P. falciparum*; *WIN 5037*, an 8-aminoquinoline with greater schizonticidal powers than primaquine but ineffective against chloroquine-resistant *P. falciparum*; *acridine dyes* similar to mepacrine but less effective; an *amidineurea* (nitroguanil), which is active but shows no advantages over proguanil; *naphthalene derivatives* inactive against chloroquine-resistant parasites and quinoline-methanols, which render the subject photosensitive.

Combinations of drugs

In attempts to obtain potentiation of schizonticidal activity or to provide an attack on more than one phase of the parasite, the following combinations of drugs have been used (World Health Organization, 1967).

Chloroquine and primaquine. In non-immune military personnel in Vietnam, as a prophylactic against *P. vivax* malaria: chloroquine 300 mg base, with primaquine (45 mg base) once weekly. In Central America a dose of chloroquine 450 mg base (or amodiaquine 450 mg base) has been used with the above dose of primaquine.

These regimes are unsuccessful against chloroquine-resistant *P. falciparum*.

Chloroquine and pyrimethamine. Chloroquine, 600 mg base together with pyrimethamine 500 mg base, has been used for presumptive treatment in malaria eradication campaigns (see later). It has also been given prophylactically at 3-weekly intervals. The efficacy of this mixture in mass chemoprophylaxis has not been confirmed.

Pyrimethamine and primaquine. Pyrimethamine 50 mg base and primaquine 40 mg base given together at intervals of 1 or 2 weeks has been tried in some areas because of the combination of the sporontocidal, gametocytocidal and schizonticidal properties of the drugs.

Pyrimethamine and quinine. Quinine 650 mg (2 tablets) thrice daily for 14 days; pyrimethamine 50 mg (2 tablet) for the first 3 days.

This regime is said to have reduced the number of recrudescences of *P. falciparum* reported in non-immunes in South-east Asia (DDS, 25 mg daily, has been added to this course of treatment).

Cycloguanil embonate plus DADDS. See above.

Chloroquine in table salt. The addition of 0.4 to 0.33 per cent chloroquine to salt has been widely used, concurrently with entomological control by residual insecticide spraying in Brazil, Guyana, Iran, Uganda and Tanzania. In spite of inherent disadvantages, including leaching out of the drug in stored salt, and the inadequate dosage of infants and young children, this method of parasite control has been reasonably effective. There is, however, a possibility of initiating drug resistance, which has already happened in similar trials with salt containing pyrimethamine. Pyrimethamine is now no longer used for this purpose.

FURTHER READING

ADAMS, A. R. D. and MAEGRAITH, B. G. (1971) *Clinical Tropical Diseases*, 5th edn. Oxford: Blackwell.

GARNHAM, P. C. C. (1966) *Malaria Parasites and other Haemosporidia*. Oxford: Blackwell.

MAEGRAITH, B. G. (1948) *Pathological Processes in Malaria and Blackwater Fever*. Oxford: Blackwell.

—— (1971) Medical progress 1970–71—Malaria. In *British Encyclopaedia of Medical Practice*, ed. Richardson, J. London: Butterworth.

PETERS, W. (1971) *Chemotherapy and Drug Resistance in Malaria*. New York: Academic Press.

WORLD HEALTH ORGANIZATION. *Technical Report Series on Malaria*.

3
African Human Trypanosomiasis

SYNONYMS. Sleeping sickness; Gambian sleeping sickness; Rhodesian sleeping sickness; *Trypanosoma gambiense* (or *T. rhodesiense*) sleeping sickness (or trypanosomiasis).

DEFINITION

African human trypanosomiasis is a disease resulting from infection by one or other of the trypanosome species known as *Trypanosoma gambiense* or *T. rhodesiense*. Both forms of the disease characteristically cause irregular fever, sometimes skin eruptions, progressive and finally severe damage to the central nervous system in the later stages, and, if untreated, death in all but extremely rare cases. The course of *T. gambiense* infections is more chronic and the period from infection to death in untreated cases may vary from about one to several years; in the later stages the chronic affection of the central nervous system leads typically to marked lethargy and 'sleeping'. The course of *T. rhodesiense* infections is more acute, death in untreated cases usually occurring within a period of from 3 months to 1 year and commonly within 5 to 9 months; the later stages are characterised more by symptoms of toxic effects on the central nervous system than by those of chronic destructive processes.

AETIOLOGY

Transmission

By far the commonest method of transmission of African human trypanosomiasis is by the bite of an infected tsetse.

The fly probes through the skin and, by the cutting action of the tip of its proboscis, usually ruptures small blood vessels, forming a pool of blood from which it feeds, intermittently ejecting into the area 'puffs' of saliva which, from an infected fly, contain metacyclic trypanosomes. Thus, these fully developed infective forms from the fly are deposited in the tissues and some, in all probability, escape directly into the circulation.

Relatively rarely the fly may probe directly into a blood vessel large enough to enable it to feed without forming a pool of blood and, should this happen, all the trypanosomes will be injected into the circulation and none be deposited in the tissues. It seems highly probable that this is the circumstance which determines whether or not a primary reaction develops at the site of the infective bite.

Although cyclical transmission is the cause of the vast majority of cases, direct or 'mechanical transmission by a tsetse or other biting fly disturbed while feeding on an infected person may occur but most experimental and field evidence suggests that its importance is negligible.

Congenital or transplacental infection of newborn infants has been shown to occur in both *T. gambiense* and *T. rhodesiense* trypanosomiasis but this is a relatively rare occurrence, probably because one of the early effects of the disease is to cause infertility or abortion in women of child-bearing age.

Infecting organisms

The two 'species' infective to humans are commonly spoken of as if they were quite distinct but, in fact, there is no clear-cut separation between them. However, because of epidemiological, clinical and chemotherapeutic differences, it still remains convenient to distinguish between them.

The features characteristic of typical *T. gambiense* are: relative lack of virulence—causing chronic infection in man and, in laboratory animals, either causing chronic infection or failing to infect; relative or great rarity of the occurrence of posteronuclear forms in infected laboratory animals; susceptibility to arsenicals, notably tryparsamide, and that the infection in man is typically associated with the *Glossina palpalis* group of tsetse.

Those of typical *T. rhodesiense* are: much greater virulence—causing much more acute infections in man and in laboratory animals, of which it consistently infects a wide range; the frequency with which posteronuclear forms are seen in certain phases of infections in laboratory animals, the maximum proportions of which may range from a few per cent to 30 or even over 50 per cent; resistance to arsenicals, particularly tryparsamide, and that human infections are typically associated with tsetse of the *G. morsitans* group.

However, strains intermediate in character can be found and there is both laboratory and field evidence that either type of trypanosome may be transmitted by either group of tsetse.

T. brucei is, by definition, a trypanosome which is not infective to man, and until the recent development by Rickman and Robson (1970a and b) of the blood incubation infectivity test (BIIT) could be distinguished from *T. rhodesiense* only by failure to infect in a direct test on a human volunteer. The fact that infectivity to humans alone separates *T. rhodesiense* from *T. brucei* has led to much debate on the relationships of these two species to each other and to *T. gambiense*. These relationships are likely to remain unsettled until it is known exactly what causes a trypanosome strain to be infective to man and whether this is a biologically stable property or not.

In passing, it may be noted that *T. brucei*-like organisms isolated from fly or an animal in a sleeping sickness area cannot be labelled *T. brucei* unless they have been tested on man or been clearly negative—and preferably repeatedly so— by BIIT. In specifying such strains the basis for identification as *T. brucei* should be given. Strains from non-human sources which are known, from tests on volunteers, to be non-infective to humans are sometimes identified as *T. brucei* (*sensu stricto*).

Space does not permit any discussion of the complexities of the systematics of the mammalian trypanosomes of Africa. Suffice it to say that those already mentioned may be classified as species of a subgenus, *Trypanosoma* (*Trypanzoon*) *brucei*, *T. (T.) gambiense* and *T. (T.) rhodesiense* (Hoare, in Mulligan, 1970), or as subspecies of a species, *T. brucei brucei*, *T. b. gambiense* and *T. b. rhodesiense*. For medical purposes, if the simplest nomenclature is considered inadequate, the former classification is to be preferred as avoiding any confusion between *T. brucei*, non-infective to man, and the other two.

Infections in laboratory animals

T. rhodesiense will readily infect all the ordinary small laboratory animals, mice, rats guinea pigs, rabbits and hamsters. The result of infection with a recently isolated strain is normally a relapsing parasitaemia, later changing to an irregular but steadily rising parasitaemia in the final stages before death. Albino rats normally die of such an infection in about 20 to 50 days though the period may be shorter or substantially longer. The length of life of mice tends to be shorter and that of guinea pigs and rabbits longer.

Less virulent strains cause an intermittent rather than relapsing parasitaemia, and as the characteristics of the strain tend more to those of typical *T. gambiense* the length of life and aparasitaemic periods become longer and the maxima of parasitaemia less intense. Typical *T. gambiense* strains either produce chronic infection in mice and rats which may last hundreds of days before death or, as is a common finding, they may fail to infect these animals at all.

Monkeys (*Cercopithecus* and *Erythrocebus* spp.) are much more susceptible to infection with *T. gambiense* and from them a strain can often be established in small laboratory animals. Another animal which is highly susceptible to infection with *T. gambiense* is the Gambian pouched rat (*Cricetomys gambianus*) but, though easily caught, this large rodent is difficult to manage unless bred in captivity and accustomed to being handled.

From the previous section, it will be clear that *T. brucei* infections of laboratory animals are exactly like those of *T. rhodesiense*.

Life cycle and morphology

The development of *T. brucei* group trypanosomes in tsetse may be summarised as occurring in four stages: if they succeed in becoming established in the fly at all, the first stage is of multiplication in the midgut within the peritrophic membrane; the second is invasion of the ectoperitrophic space, multiplication and conversion into the long, filamentous 'proventricular' forms; in the third these forms re-penetrate the peritrophic membrane at its anterior soft end and migrate via the oesophagus, hypopharynx and salivary gland ducts to the salivary glands, where they become crithidia; in the final stage there is further multiplication and transformation to the metacyclic forms capable of reinfecting mammalian hosts.

Failure of development may occur between any of the consecutive stages, and the chances of such failures combined with the chance of failure even to become established at first are such that, even in the best experimental conditions that are known at present, it is difficult to infect more than a very few per cent of flies.

When the metacyclic forms are inoculated by the biting fly into a mammalian host, they soon change into long slender blood forms and during the pre-patent period and the early stages of the first wave of parasitaemia, all the trypanosomes present are of the long slender type. As the parasitaemia approaches its peak, first forms intermediate between the long slender and short stumpy forms appear and then short stumpy forms in increasing proportion. During decrease of parasitaemia after the peak of the first wave, short stumpy trypanosomes predominate and their proportion may exceed 90 per cent. When these forms are present in large numbers, posteronuclear forms may be found, and their proportion may be high. The cycle of parasitaemia and morphological changes then repeats itself until separate waves can no longer be distinguished and the heavy parasitaemia contains a mixture of all forms.

Tsetse vectors

The genus *Glossina* comprises three groups of species. Of these, the *G. fusca* group, or forest tsetse, appear to be of no significance in the transmission of human trypanosomiasis since they very rarely, if ever, attack man.

The *G. palpalis* group, or riverine tsetse, are responsible for the transmission of *T. gambiense* throughout West and western Central Africa, and were in East Africa until eradicated by insecticides from some areas in recent years. The most important species are: in West Africa *G. palpalis* and *G. tachinoides*, and in western Central and East Africa *G. fuscipes* (previously often called *G. palpalis* or *G. palpalis fuscipes*).

The *G. morsitans* group, or savannah tsetse, are predominantly the vectors of *T. rhodesiense* wherever it occurs from Uganda to Botswana. The species responsible for far more transmission than any other is *G. morsitans* itself within its extensive distribution from North-western Tanzania, Rwanda and Burundi to Botswana. *G. pallidipes* is the main vector in South-east Uganda and a small part of western Kenya, and *G. swynnertoni* in some parts of Tanzania east and south-east of Lake Victoria.

As was mentioned above, it is very difficult to infect more than a few per cent of tsetse with the *T. brucei* subgroup trypanosomes, even under the best known laboratory conditions. In nature the proportion of flies infected with human-infective trypanosomes in areas of endemic sleeping sickness is likely to be of the order of 1 in 2000 to 1 in 10 000 and even in epidemic conditions is unlikely to rise above 1 in 500. It is still true that relatively little is known of the factors which determine whether or not a tsetse will become infected with trypanosomes after taking an infected blood meal.

EPIDEMIOLOGY

General features

There are two features of the epidemiology (and distribution) of African human trypanosomiasis that are well recognised and important. The first is that its incidence tends to be markedly focal and often localised to very small areas. Because of this fact, data giving the average incidence over a whole population are of very little value in assessing the risk of a greater outbreak; what is much more important is the highest single incidence in any one group of people, perhaps a single village, for it is this figure which gives some measure of the greatest rate of transmission and hence the chance of epidemic spread. Detailed knowledge such as this may allow epidemiologists responsible for the control of the disease to keep a close watch on small areas which will act as sensitive indicators of any tendency towards epidemic increase.

The second feature appears anomalous at first sight but has been explained in recent years. It is that although the disease is transmitted by tsetse its incidence is apparently unrelated to the abundance of the vector. For example, tsetse of the *G. palpalis* group are ubiquitous throughout the extensive forest areas of West and western Central Africa yet over very much of these areas the incidence of sleeping sickness is much lower than at the northern and southern fringes of the fly distribution where numbers are much lower.

The factors which limit the northern distribution of species like *G. palpalis* and *G. tachinoides* are heat and desiccation. At the height of the dry season the flies can only survive around isolated water holes in otherwise dry river beds. The flies are thus strictly limited in their distribution. Since the local human population are entirely dependent on the same water holes, isolated fly populations must feed again and again on the same restricted human populations. This extremely close man-fly contact has been variously described as 'recidivistic', 'personal' or 'intimate' and provides ideal conditions for the transmission of trypanosomiasis.

In the condition described above, man-fly contact arises from the unavoidable human activity of water collecting. Other activities of a more voluntary type may also be responsible. For example, in Sierra Leone (Hutchinson, 1954) it was found that people opening up new farms in the transitional zone between forest and savannah were exposing themselves to intimate and sustained contact with the fly. Johnstone, M. R. L. (personal communication) found the incidence of trypanosomiasis in some pagan tribes, who were developing new farms on one side of a river close to the Jos Plateau in Northern Nigeria and were dependent on the river for their water supply, was about ten times that in the established population on the other side of the same river where the villages had wells. The author has himself seen many newly developed farms in South-east Uganda and in part of South Nyanza, Kenya, which have been cut out of thicket infested with *G. pallidipes*, thus creating conditions of exposure to that fly and risk of *T. rhodesiense* infection.

There can be little doubt that in areas where *T. rhodesiense* is endemic, the main reservoir of infection is game animals and that man is infected only incidentally when he comes, or brings himself, into contact with fly infected from game. Hence, Apted *et al* (1963) suggested that an important factor determining the incidence and distribution of the disease might be 'sustained triple contact' between man, fly and reservoir animal.

An excellent example of factors operating to produce an explosive epidemic of *T. rhodesiense* infection was seen in Alego and surrounding locations in Central Nyanza, Kenya, during 1964. The epidemic was unique in being the only instance in which widespread transmission of *T. rhodensiense* was due to a fly of the *G. palpalis* group—*G. fuscipes*. This fly, whose normal habitat is riverine, had spread from the rivers and colonised the thick hedges of vegetation which are grown round small groups of huts in that area. Thus typical conditions of 'intimate' man-fly contact were produced and, in addition, as Onyango *et al* have since shown, cattle in the area were acting as a reservoir of infection so setting 'sustained triple contact' as well.

Other important general features of the epidemiology of African human trypanosomiasis are the relation of occupation to the incidence of the disease and the bearing that this has on its sex and age distribution. The disease is essentially one of underdeveloped rural areas since full agricultural development destroys all tsetse habitat and eradicates the disease. In underdeveloped or undeveloped areas, those whose occupations bring them most in contact with tsetse are at the greatest risk. In endemic areas of both *T. gambiense* and *T. rhodesiense*, travelling, hunting and fishing are occupations commonly associated with the disease. In addition to these, tin miners (in Nigeria), rail and road workers, and cocoa farmers may be at particular risk in West Africa, and honey and salt collectors in East Africa.

All these are occupations of adult males normally carried out at some distance from their homes. When it is seen that the incidence is predominantly in adult males, the inference may be drawn that the source of infection is at a distance from the homesteads or villages. If, however, a rising incidence is noticed in females and children, and particularly if they approach 50 per cent of the cases, it may be inferred that the source of infection is close to their homes, perhaps at water holes or at their area of cultivation. However, for such inferences to be valid, accurate knowledge of the habits of the local population is necessary.

Reservoir hosts

That animals may, and do, act as a reservoir of *T. rhodesiense* is established though quantitative data are lacking. There is only scanty evidence so far of any animal reservoir of *T. gambiense*, including some indications that the domestic pig may fulfil this role.

Comparative virulence

It is an established fact that human infective strains of trypanosomes may exist with all degrees of virulence from those causing chronic infections typical of classical *T. gambiense* to those causing acute infections typical of *T. rhodesiense*. Further, they may exist together in the same area.

On the basis of much laboratory experience, it may also be stated that, in general, the virulence of strains of *T. brucei* subgroup organisms in any one species of animal will be paralleled in most other species, infection (or not) and its course being governed by the natural resistance of the species. Thus to susceptible species typical *T. gambiense* will be infective and typical *T. rhodesiense* will be rapidly fatal, whereas less susceptible in species such as game animals normally contact with tsetse (Ashcroft, Burtt and Fairbairn, 1959) will not be infected by the mild *T. gambiense*-like strains but may be infected by a *T. rhodesiense*-like strain, perhaps for many months, before finally overcoming it.

The combination of these facts with the laboratory and field evidence that either type of trypanosome may be transmitted by either group of tsetse poses the problem of why the long-recognised associations of *T. gambiense* with the riverine, *G. palpalis* group tsetse, and of *T.*

rhodesiense with the savannah, *G. morsitans* group should have been so consistent. The present author (Willett, 1965) offered the following possible explanation. In areas infested with *G. palpalis* group tsetse, where man-fly contact is close and man is the main source of fly infection, the less virulent strains will persist longer in the human reservoir and, thus having a better chance of being re-transmitted, tend to become predominant, so producing the classical association of *G. palpalis* group tsetse with *T. gambiense*. On the other hand, in areas infested by *G. morsitans* group tsetse whose main source of food is animals, the less virulent *T. gambiense*-like strains, which, in general, will not infect animals with a high natural resistance, will be suppressed, leaving only the more virulent *T. rhodesiense*-like strains, and so producing the other association of *G. morsitans* group tsetse with *T. rhodesiense*.

DISTRIBUTION

African human trypanosomiasis is limited to the tsetse infested areas of the continent reaching as far as latitude 14°N in West Africa and as far south as the north-east corner of Botswana, in the Okavango delta.

Typical *T. gambiense* is not found outside the distribution of the *G. palpalis* group of tsetse and therefore has never occurred east of the eastern divide of the Great Rift Valley. Its furthest eastern occurrence was in Central and South Nyanza, Kenya, but with the eradication of *G. fuscipes* from those areas by insecticides, this form of trypanosomiasis has also been eradicated. Variable numbers of cases per year have occurred in Uganda, particularly in the central parts and West Nile Province, but the number of cases of *T. gambiense* sleeping sickness has declined sharply to almost none in the last few years. The one small focus in Tanzania, on Lake Tanganyika just north of Kigoma, was eradicated by insecticidal attack some years ago. Cases continue to occur in the Sudan, particularly near the border of the Congo and Central African Republic where tsetse belts extend into the southern Sudan, and along the Nile.

Otherwise, *T. gambiense* may be said to be almost ubiquitous in West and west Central Africa from Angola in the south through Zaire northwards to Caméroun and the extreme south-east of Chad, and thence westwards through Nigeria (except the north-east corner), Dahomey, Togo, southern Upper Volta and Mali, Ghana, Ivory Coast, Liberia, Sierra Leone and Guinea and Portuguese Guinea to southern Senegal and Gambia. Although the disease may be said to be ubiquitous there is a marked tendency, as has been mentioned already, for the incidence to be higher towards the fringe of the tsetse distribution.

In the period 1915–1940, an epidemic wave of *T. gambiense* trypanosomiasis spread from the Congo northwards and then westwards to Senegal. At present, owing to the complete breakdown of control which has followed the disturbed conditions in Zaire during recent years, there has been a great recrudescence of sleeping sickness and there would appear to be a risk of a repetition of the previous wave. However, in many countries there are still efficient control organisations—almost all of them stimulated by the 1915-1940 wave—and as long as these remain, the risk is accordingly lessened.

To the east of the Great Rift Valley human trypanosomiasis of the *T. rhodesiense* type is transmitted, in the main, by *G. morsitans*, but in South-east Uganda and Nyanza province, Kenya, by *G. pallidipes*, and in relatively small areas of North-west Tanzania, to the east and south-east of Lake Victoria, by *G. swynnertoni*. The main endemic area is the great belt of *G. morsitans* infestation which stretches from the Uganda-Tanzania border in the north (with an extension up the Kagera river into the lowlying area on the Rwanda-Burundi border) as far south as the Zambesi Valley in Rhodesia and the Okavango delta in Botswana. At the other end of its distribution, *T. rhodesiense* has recently been reported in a localised epidemic in South-west Ethiopia.

PATHOLOGY

Primary reaction

Relatively little work has been done on the primary reaction, or 'trypanosome chancre', at the site of the original infective tsetse bite, and there is a lack of detailed histological study of the reaction site. Gallais *et al* (1953) studied the reaction caused by inoculation of *T. gambiense* and found that only intradermal (and not snbcutaneous) inoculation resulted in the production of chancre. The paper includes photographs of the chancre at various stages.

With *T. rhodesiense* a chancre is normally produced either by fly-bite or inoculation of blood forms from a laboratory animal either intradermally or subcutaneously. The size of the chancre can be very variable, perhaps related to the degree of multiplication of trypanosomes in the tissues and the resulting tissue reaction. As much as is known at present indicates that there is lymphocytic infiltration, very large numbers of large mononuclear cells of histiocyte type with fewer eosinophils and macrophages and that trypanosomes may be limited to oedema fluid between tissue layers or occur throughout the chancre area.

Organs other than central nervous system

The lymph glands are involved very early in the course of the infection, particularly those in the lymph drainage of the area of the infected tsetse bite and chancre if one occurs. After this stage, involvement of lymph glands may be widespread or confined to localised groups. In *T. gambiense* infections, glands in the neck region are very commonly affected, particularly those in the posterior triangle, the swelling of which gives rise to the famous Winterbottom's sign. In *T. rhodesiense* infections, the glands most commonly affected are the epitrochlear, axillary and femoral, perhaps in relation to the site of the infective bite. Histologically there is hyperplasia with proliferation of lymphocytes, plasma cells and macrophages which pack the sinuses in large numbers. There may be small haemorrhages and trypanosomes are usually common so that they can be squeezed out in gland juice in a gland puncture. Much later in the infection the glands tend to become fibrous.

The spleen is commonly enlarged, though not usually more than moderately, and is congested. Lymphoid and reticuloendothelial hyperplasia are the main features. The Malpighian corpuscles are usually reduced in number and localised areas of necrosis may occur.

Anaemia of moderate degree is normal. In long-standing *T. gambiense* disease, it is often related to malnutrition and consequent iron deficiency. In more acute cases and *T. rhodesiense* infections, it is more toxic in origin. In the serum proteins there is an early fall in albumin—especially in *T. rhodesiense* infections—and later a marked rise in gamma globulins, particularly the IgM fraction. The bone marrow may show either gelatinous degeneration or areas of hyperplasia may be seen.

In the liver, particularly in *T. rhodesiense* infections, there are parenchymatous changes or degeneration which appears to be associated with abnormalities of hepatic function and the early serum changes (Robertson and Jenkins, 1959; Jenkins and Robertson, 1959). There is also infiltration of the portal tracts with mononuclear cells.

The main effect on the heart is to cause myocarditis, which may be mild and only detectable by careful examination in *T. gambiense* infections, or severe and dangerous in *T. rhodesiense* infections. In the latter, epicarditis may also be marked and pericardial effusions are common; these sometimes contain trypanosomes. The cardiac valves are not involved.

Effects on the reproductive system are often early and marked, causing amenorrhoea or abortion in women and impotence in men, but the mechanism of action is not known.

Central nervous system

After a variable length of time from first infection, the invasion of the central nervous system by trypanosomes begins and continues in the form of a progressive leptomeningitis until in the later stages irreversible damage is done to the brain tissue.

The progress of this pathological process is reflected in abnormal findings in the cerebrospinal fluid and examination of this fluid is essential to determine how far the disease has progressed.

Two stages of the disease are recognised by all authorities: the early or blood-lymphatic stage —before involvement of the central nervous system has begun—and the late or meningoencephalitic stage. Some people recognise a third intermediate stage which may be roughly described as that of early CNS involvement before the onset of irreparable damage.

Although the cell count in the cerebrospinal fluid increases steadily throughout the infection it is nothing like as reliable an indicator, quantitatively, of the degree of CNS involvement as the protein content of the fluid. By far the most commonly used method for CSF protein determination in the field of trypanosomiasis has been that of Sicard and Cantaloube, sometimes with slight modifications. Because it is so widely used, diagnosis of the stage of the disease will be discussed here in terms of protein determinations by this method.

The generally recognised normal maxima for cell counts and CSF proteins indicating no involvement of the CNS, are 5 cells per mm^3 and 25 mg per 100 ml protein. Some workers prefer 3 and 22 as safer criteria. Despite the fact that the normal maximum of protein in the CSF is usually given as 40 mg/100 ml, numerous authorities in many parts of Africa have quite independently found that in trypanosomiasis, no more than 25 mg/100 ml can be accepted as normal. This discrepancy may be due in part to the widespread use of the Sicard-Cantaloube technique since Gall, Hutchinson and Yates (1955), comparing this technique with determinations of protein by a sulpho-salicylic acid turbidimetric method, using the M.R.C. Grey-Wedge Photometer, found that true readings were obtained at about 20 mg/100 ml but that above this figure the readings were low, the Sicard-Cantaloube having a sensitivity of only about half a milligram per true milligram of protein. Nevertheless, most workers experienced in trypanosomiasis prefer not to accept CSF protein findings by any method as normal if above 25 mg/100 ml.

Recently Mattern (1964) has shown that in the CSF protein, there is an excess of the IgM fraction of gamma globulins (β_2-macroglobulin) the level, in relation to total amounts of protein present, being at least as high as that in the serum. This large proportion of IgM fraction in the CSF he regards as virtually pathognomonic of trypanosomiasis.

In the brain itself, the ventricles are distended with CSF and, as the disease progresses, the cortex becomes more congested and oedematous. The gyri become flattened and the dura mater may be thickened and adherent to both the scalp and arachnoid. Localised lesions, which resemble granulomata and are known as Dürck's nodes, may occur on the vertex or in the cortex.

With the generalised leptomeningitis there is widespread cellular infiltration with mononuclear cells. This is most pronounced under the pia mater and extends with it into the Virchow-Robin spaces along blood vessels and so gives rise to the perivascular cuffing which is so typical in the histology of cerebral trypanosomiasis. The infiltrating cells are lymphocytes, plasma cells and macrophages, and Mott's morula cells may be seen. These cells may be degenerate plasma cells and have a blue-staining eccentric nucleus with pink-staining vacuoles in the cytoplasm which give them their characteristic appearance.

The infiltration progresses until it is general throughout the white matter and focal areas of permanent and irreversible neuronal degeneration may occur with proliferation of glia cells and, sometimes, pinpoint areas of haemorrhage. The areas of the brain most affected are usually the frontal lobes, though cellular infiltration may be less than elsewhere, and the hypothalamus and basal ganglia.

SYMPTOMATOLOGY

Primary reaction

The primary reaction to infection with trypanosomes, at the site of the infected tsetse bite, must be clearly distinguished from any sensitivity reaction to the tsetse bite itself since the latter is common and of no importance whereas recognition of the former may permit positive diagnosis before patent parasitaemia. Sensitivity reactions to tsetse bites normally develop within minutes or hours and regress rapidly, at most in a very few days. Trypanosome chancres, on the other hand, rarely begin to develop before 5 days after the bite and then increase steadily in size. Therefore, only a progressively increasing swelling starting 5 or more days after exposure to tsetse can be the trypanosome chancre indicative of the earliest stage of infection.

Whether or not a chancre develops is most probably related to the method of feeding of the tsetse. The primary reaction is rarely seen in *T. gambiense* infections. It may be less common than with *T. rhodesiense* or it may be less conspicuous; again, it may be that, with the relatively mild onset, it is not identified as the earliest feature of an illness which itself is frequently not recognised as such until months or years later with the onset of nervous symptoms. It is much more frequently seen in *T. rhodesiense* infection. For example, Robertson (1958), treating sleeping sickness in South-east Uganda, saw no less than forty in 15 months; there it was recognised by fishermen as being the first symptom of sleeping sickness. There are also experimental data on its relative frequency of occurrence for Fairbairn and Burtt (1946) reported that 92 per cent of 206 volunteers infected with *T. rhodesiense* by the bites of *G. morsitans* developed trypanosome chancres.

If the exact site of the infective bite is known, the first sign of the chancre may be palpable as a small subcutaneous nodule not producing any visible swelling. This beginning is likely to occur at 5 to 10 days after the infective bite though the period may be less or substantially more. The subsequent rate of development is generally related to this 'incubation period' in that the shorter it has been, the more rapidly will the chancre develop. During the next 2 to 4 days or so, the chancre increases in size and produces visible swelling. On a pale skin it is pink at first and later deepens to purple in the centre. It may reach anything from about 1 inch to over 4 inches in diameter, and if large and on a limb is usually oval with the long axis along the length of the limb. It has a firm, rubbery consistency and a definite edge until it is nearly at its maximum stage. The edge then becomes indefinite and the impression is given that the swelling is diffusing into the surrounding tissues. It is usually at about this stage that pyrexia first begins and that parasitaemia becomes microscopically detectable. The region of the reaction is hotter than the surrounding skin and is also tender; it resembles an early subcutaneous cellulitis but is not usually as tender and never suppurates unless secondarily infected. As the chancre reaches full development, a central crop of small blisters may form which soon dry up and are succeeded by superficial desquamation which extends peripherally and may be repeated two or three times.

The primary reaction may resolve in about 3 weeks from its maximum stage or it may leave a hyperpigmented area for weeks or even months. The whole development of the chancre and its relation to the onset of pyrexia and patent parasitaemia give the impression that it is a violent local reaction to multiplication of trypanosomes which then escape to produce a rapid rise in the numbers in the general circulation. It may be possible to make a definite diagnosis from the chancre even 2 or 3 days before patent parasitaemia by puncturing it with a needle about halfway from centre to edge, stopping the bleeding from the puncture and then squeezing out some serous fluid in which trypanosomes may be found.

Early stage: blood-lymphatic

In the symptomatology of African human trypanosomiasis, no clear line can be drawn between *T. gambiense* and *T. rhodesiense* infections. In typical *T. gambiense* areas occasional very acute cases occur, resembling *T. rhodesiense* in every respect, and in *T. rhodesiense* areas occasional more chronic *T. gambiense*-like infections are seen. Therefore, in the following description it may be taken that the milder, more chronic manifestations will predominate in *T. gambiense* areas and the more severe and acute ones in *T. rhodesiense* areas.

The first symptom, other than the trypanosome chancre, is pyrexia which may vary from slight to hyperpyrexia and is usually accompanied by headache; the onset may be gradual or sudden. Shivering and sweating are common, particularly with a more severe onset. After a few days, the fever may abate to be followed by an apyrexial period of days or even weeks. Recurrent bouts of pyrexia are normal, being higher and with shorter apyrexial intervals the more severe the infection. As the disease progresses, pyrexia tends to decrease until in the stage of CNS involvement it is either low or absent.

Enlargement of lymph glands is also an early manifestation, the earliest being in the lymphatic drainage from the site of the infective bite. Later, generalised enlargement of lymph glands may occur, particularly in the more chronic cases. Typical *T. gambiense* seems most commonly to affect the glands in the neck—those in the posterior triangle (giving rise to Winterbottom's sign) and the superclavicular glands—whereas in *T. rhodesiense* infections the glands most affected are the epitrochlear, axillary and femoral. These differences may be related to the biting habits of the common vector species of tsetse. The swollen glands are firm and rubbery and freely mobile. Suppuration never occurs from trypanosome infection alone.

Another inconsistent, but sometimes valuable, finding is delayed hypersensitivity to deep muscular pressure, or Kerandel's sign. If the calf or other muscles are squeezed between the thumb and fingers, the patient may, after a brief delay, exhibit signs of pain quite out of proportion to the force used.

Tachycardia, of a degree inconsistent with the pyrexia, is a common finding, with ECG tracings indicative of myocardial involvement, though there may be a relative bradycardia without ECG abnormalities.

The typical rash of trypanosomiasis, if seen at all, usually appears a few weeks after infection. It consists of crops of macular erythematous patches often circinate or with the circles incomplete, commonly 3 to 4 inches in diameter but sometimes much larger. These usually last for a few days and then fade, to be replaced by another crop. They are readily seen on a white skin but extremely difficult to detect on a deeply pigmented skin.

Another marked and very common symptom of established trypanosomiasis is impotence in the male or amenorrhoea or abortion in the female of child-bearing age.

The spleen is usually found to be enlarged, though not more than moderately, and soft on palpation.

Late stage: involvement of central nervous system

The onset of this stage is gradual, the more so in the more chronic *T. gambiense*-type infections; it may begin within 2 to 4 weeks of first infection in the most severe *T. rhodesiense* cases but not until after several months or even 2 or more years with *T. gambiense*. The initial symptoms are unpredictable but headache is persistent and almost universal.

In *T. gambiense* infections in particular, the first signs of onset of the late stage may present as a psychological disturbance, often first noticed by relatives or close friends. Personality changes, variations of behaviour (sometimes sudden) or schizoid behaviour may be seen, and sometimes mania or convulsions though these are usually later manifestations.

Characteristic of the mental dullness that trypanosomiasis causes is the facial expression, so much so that the experienced worker can frequently pick out cases at a single glance. The main impression is of apathy; the patient appears to have no interest whatever either in himself or in his surroundings. As seen in mature women it has been described as 'silent grief', vividly summarising the impression of grief so profound as to shut out all feeling.

Another very characteristic sign, usually seen only in advanced cases, is pruritus which causes frequent and apparently aimless scratching, or leaves the marks of scratching; either of these should arouse suspicion of trypanosomiasis.

Tremor is common, especially of the hands or tongue, and choreiform movements, the last more especially in children. As involvement of the CNS progresses, rigidity often develops, and also the classical sleeping in the daytime. A far-advanced case may fall asleep in the middle of any activity, such as eating, and perhaps roll on his side with his limbs remaining in exactly the same relative position as when upright. Voracious appetite is common until the patient reaches the stage of being unable to feed himself sufficiently and the wasting, which is frequently seen despite the appetite, then rapidly increases. At this stage, death frequently occurs from intercurrent infections, of which pneumonia and dysentery are commonest.

In chronic *T. gambiense*-type infection, in which many months or even years may elapse before this stage is reached, it is not unusual for a patient to go downhill very rapidly and die within a relatively short time of the onset of the symptoms of central nervous involvement.

Some advanced sleeping sickness cases may present with a puffy, myxodematous appearance looking, at first sight, deceptively well nourished in contrast to the usual wasted appearance. In males, such cases may show some degree of gynaecomastia or other signs of endocrine imbalance. Despite their superficial appearance, these cases are often found to have reached an advanced stage of CNS involvement.

Many of the above symptoms or signs of chronic, progressive damage to the CNS are much more typical of *T. gambiense* than of *T. rhodesiense* which tends much more to cause acute toxic conditions. In the latter form there is obvious impair-

ment of the CNS and the dull, apathetic stage is common; the onset of lethargy is rapid but usually without the classical daytime sleeping. Convulsions and mania are more common. Wasting or the false well-nourished appearance may develop rapidly or the patient may die from toxaemia or as a result of severe myocarditis before advanced CNS involvement has been reached.

Symptomless cases or 'healthy carriers'

In foci of *T. gambiense* extremely chronic symptomless cases, apparently 'healthy carriers', may occur and they tend to be associated with old, long-established endemic foci.

Similar cases have been recorded from time to time in *T. rhodesiense* areas, for example by Ross and Blair (1956) despite the fact that the organism, when subinoculated into laboratory animals, behaved like *T. rhodesiense* rather than *T. gambiense*. Though some of these cases have been known to have been infected without apparent symptoms for many months, it is always open to question whether they can truly be called 'healthy carriers' since the final outcome of the infection is unknown. As occurs in *T. gambiense* infections, once the stage of CNS involvement was well established, their condition might deteriorate rapidly.

DIAGNOSIS

Parasitological

Demonstration of the infecting trypanosomes by one method or another remains the only positive proof of the diagnosis of trypanosomiasis.

The earliest stage at which trypanosomes can be found is in the primary reaction, or trypanosome chancre, or by puncture of a swollen gland in the lymph drainage from the area.

Once the infection has become general, other lymph glands become swollen and gland puncture is the most common means of diagnosing *T. gambiense* infections. Swollen glands in the posterior triangle of the neck or in the supraclavicular group are usually chosen. One is gripped firmly by the fingers and thumb of one hand, and after cleaning the skin over the gland, the point of a medium-sized hypodermic needle—without a syringe attached—is pushed into the substance of the gland. While it remains there the gland is 'massaged' between the gripping fingers and thumb, forcing gland juice into the lumen of the needle. The needle is then withdrawn; its contents are expelled with a syringe on to a clean microscope slide, covered with a coverslip and examined at once in the fresh condition.

T. rhodesiense infections are usually much easier to diagnose by finding the trypanosomes in the blood, in stained thick films. In a doubtful case these should be repeated daily for a week, particularly if there is a peak of pyrexia since these usually indicate peaks of parasitaemia which themselves tend to recur at about 7-day intervals. After centrifugation of blood, trypanosomes tend to be concentrated in the sub-buffy layer. Bone marrow smears may be positive when parasitaemia is subpatent.

Subinoculation to rats or mice will commonly reveal low parasitaemia with *T. rhodesiense* but often fail with the less virulent *T. gambiense*. Animals particularly susceptible to the latter are monkeys (*Cercopithicus* spp. and *Erythrocebus* spp.) and the Gambian pouched rat (*Cricetomys gambianus*).

The recent development of DEAE cellulose column separation of trypanosomes from blood (Lanham and Godfrey, 1970; Godfrey and Lanham, 1971) with concentration by centrifugation or millipore filtration is certainly far more sensitive than routine microscopy for detecting low parasitaemia, probably by a factor of 100 to 1000 times. Under laboratory conditions the technique is extremely efficient but certain practical difficulties in its application in the field have still to be finally eliminated (Lanham and Godfrey, 1972).

Once the central nervous system has been invaded, the organisms may be found in the CSF, either on direct examination, or after single, or sometimes triple, centrifugation. Air replacement during lumbar puncture has sometimes been used to obtain a larger volume of CSF and increase the chance of demonstrating trypanosomes, either in the centrifuged deposit or by subinoculation into a susceptible animal.

It is not uncommon, in mass surveys in the field where lengthy examinations cannot be conveniently carried out, to make presumptive diagnosis of 'clinical cases' on typical symptoms and to institute treatment, especially in remote areas which cannot be re-visited at short intervals. Improvement after specific treatment greatly strengthens the presumptive diagnosis and is frequently seen after such diagnosis by experienced field workers.

Serological

A complement fixation test has been developed using antigen prepared from the horse trypanosome *T. equiperdum*, and is claimed to give 95 per cent positive results in early cases though overall results are likely to be substantially less since the reaction decreases as the disease progresses.

There is a strong tendency in trypanosomiasis for the red cells to form long rouleaux and hence the erythrocyte sedimentation rate is usually greatly increased, but again this phenomenon is more marked in early cases and decreases later.

In the last few years, all older tests depending on changes in the serum proteins have been superseded by the demonstration, particularly by Mattern (1962, 1964) of the great increases in the IgM fraction of immunoglobulins, formerly known as β_2 macroglobulin. The level of IgM in the serum in trypanosomiasis is usually 8 to 16 times the normal and the rise to this level occurs very early in the disease, usually within 15 days. Similar serum IgM concentrations may be found in Waldenström's disease and in conditions of unknown origin vaguely known as 'hepatosplenomegaly'; therefore such exceptionally high levels of serum IgM cannot be taken as pathognomonic of trypanosomiasis but, in view of the earliness and consistency of the increase of IgM, low or normal levels virtually exclude the diagnosis.

There are several methods by which the serum IgM content can be estimated quantitatively by single or double diffusion techniques in agar gel, or by immunoelectrophoresis.

Recently, Cunningham, Bailey and Kimber (1967) have developed an extremely convenient modification of the single diffusion technique for the estimation of IgM in dried blood samples on filter paper, thus eliminating the need for separation or storage of serum.

A drop of blood, sufficient to make a 'blot' of about half an inch (12 mm) in diameter, is allowed to dry on Whatman No. 4 filter paper, the name or code number written beside it, and then stored between clean papers. Several specimens can be taken on one circular filter paper or a large sheet cut into small pieces for single samples and stapled together to form a book. The samples will retain their full activity for at least a week even if exposed to the full daily variations of temperature and humidity and for longer if preserved dry at room temperature. In the laboratory, a disc 3 mm in diameter is cut from the 'blood blot' with a standard leather punch and placed on the surface of agar incorporating 1 per cent anti-IgM. The whole is then incubated at room temperature in a saturated atmosphere for 48 hours and the diameter of the zone of precipitation read, preferably after staining with amido-black and drying. This technique has some outstanding advantages: it makes possible a postal screening service for trypanosomiasis mass surveys; it requires no difficult operations or bulky apparatus in the field, and it is extremely economical in the use of mono-specific anti-IgM serum; 1600 tests can be carried out using only 1 ml of the antiserum.

Zones of precipitation by this method of over 5 mm in diameter are regarded as 'positive' and indicating that the patient should be carefully examined for trypanosomiasis. Zones of 4–5 mm diameter are regarded as suspicious and a further sample from the 'blood blot' subjected to the following test.

Bailey, Cunningham and Kimber (1967) have described a method of applying an indirect fluorescent antibody test to the same dried blood samples. Trypanosomes from rats heavily infected with a strain of *T. rhodesiense* are used as antigen on to which blood from the dried blood discs is eluted allowing any trypanosomal antibodies to react with the organisms. The discs are then washed off and fluorescein-conjugated antihuman-IgM is added which will react with any antigen-antibody conjugate and show fluorescence under ultra-violet light. Resulting strong fluorescence enables suspicious results from the IgM test to be further screened. For full details of both techniques, readers should refer to the papers quoted.

Finally, Mattern (1962, 1964) has shown that appreciable increase of IgM in the CSF not only occurs early in the disease, even before increase of CSF cells and total protein, but also is virtually pathognomonic of trypanosomiasis. In his experience, levels of 100 μg per ml are always reached in meningoencephalitic trypanosomiasis and in no other disease.

DIFFERENTIAL DIAGNOSIS

Trypanosome chancre

The features which distinguish the developing trypanosome chancre from a reaction to a tsetse bite have already been mentioned in the preceding section. The only other condition for which it may be mistaken is an early subcutaneous cellulitis which it closely resembles. Even if demonstration of the presence of trypanosomes in serous fluid from the chancre fails, the fact that centre of a chancre never becomes fluctuant and never suppurates (in the absence of secondary infection) makes it readily distinguishable.

G

Early stage

Almost any condition which may cause a similar pyrexia, often with headache, needs to be distinguished from trypanosomiasis, particularly malaria, relapsing fever, visceral leishmaniasis, typhus or typhoid. Fever with glandular enlargement may also lead to confusion with tuberculosis or glandular fever. If demonstration of the parasites proves difficult, as it may often do in chronic cases of *T. gambiense* infection, the combination of high ESR with high IgM serum titres or raised IgM in the CSF may eliminate many of the alternative possibilities.

Late stage

At this stage other causes of chronic meningitis need to be distinguished, particularly tuberculosis, syphilis or cerebral tremor. Trypanosomes may be extremely difficult to demonstrate in blood or lymph glands but they may be found in the CSF by direct examination, perhaps after centrifugation or by subinoculation to susceptible animals. Again the high IgM levels in serum and CSF should provide a valuable distinguishing criterion.

TREATMENT

Curative

There are several drugs which are of value in the treatment of trypanosomiasis and some indication of their chemical and other properties needs to be given in addition to describing their use in the various stages or types of African human trypanosomiasis. All are organic compounds and they may be divided into two main categories, non-metallic and metallic (arsenical) compounds.

Non-metallic compounds. SURAMIN (Bayer 205, Antrypol, Moranyl, Germanin, or Naphuride) is a complex symmetrical derivative of urea with side chains ending in a naphthalene ring with three substituted sodium sulphonate groups. It is stable in the solid form and very soluble in water but it is unstable in solution and *must be injected immediately after the solution has been made up*. It is firmly attached to proteins in the body and very slowly excreted. Because of this fact, it may have a prolonged prophylactic effect but also, if injected too frequently, cumulative toxic effects may be produced.

The normal full single dose of suramin is 1.0 g intravenously in 10 per cent solution in distilled water or 20 mg/kg for patients under 50 kg in weight. Occasional severe reactions may follow the injection of a full dose, and may even result in death; the incidence of such reactions is variously estimated at 1 in 2000 to 1 in 5000 or even less. Such reactions are much more frequent in areas where onchocerciasis is present with trypanosomiasis and are very rare in areas without onchocerciasis. Because of these occasional reactions, it is normal to give a test dose of 0.2 or 0.25 g in 10 per cent solution on the day before starting full treatment. The full course of treatment for trypanosomiasis is five injections of 1 g, given on days 0 (start of full treatment), 2, 7, 14 and 21.

The commonest toxic effect of suramin is on the kidney tubules causing albuminuria and urine tests must always accompany treatment with this drug. So long as albuminuria remains mild, the treatment need not be interrupted, but if it becomes severe, or casts or red cells are seen in the urine, treatment should be interrupted for a time and then re-started with more frequent smaller doses. Because of the cumulative effect of the drug, the same therapeutic result can be obtained with doses of 0.5 g twice weekly, or 0.25 g on alternate days, instead of the full 1.0 g weekly.

It is very common, particularly in the treatment of *T. rhodesiense* sleeping sickness, for the first full dose of suramin to be followed by a pyrexial, Herxheimer-type reaction with the temperature often rising to 105°F (40.5°C) or sometimes higher. Apart from this reaction, which is probably the result of the rapid destruction of many trypanosomes and which does not justify suspension of treatment provided hyperpyrexia is controlled, a pyrexial reaction to the drug itself may occur, usually after later injections. An irritable, papular rash is sometimes seen, or desquamation, most commonly on the palms of the hands or soles of the feet. Joint pains, or tenderness of the soles, sometimes occurs. Exfoliative dermatitis is a possible serious complication, but is very rare if no more than five full doses are given at adequate intervals.

Suramin does not penetrate into the central nervous system and is therefore incapable of curing once CNS involvement is established. It is the drug of choice in early Rhodesian sleeping sickness, in which it is virtually 100 per cent effective; in the Gambian form it is a little less certain to cure the early stage of the disease. Although it will not cure late stage *T. rhodesiense* infections, it has a valuable place in the therapy of these cases. They are often in such poor condition that effective doses of melarsoprol would be extremely dangerous; suramin may often be used in separated doses of 1 g to produce a remarkable improvement in the patient's condition in 1 or 2 weeks, permitting the use of larger initial doses of melarsoprol.

PENTAMIDINE (Lomidine) is a symmetrical diamidine with the formula

$NH_2NH.C_6H_4O.(CH_2)_5.O.C_6N_4.CNH.NH_2(X)_2$

where X in the di-isethionate, or pentamidine, is $-CH_2OH.CH_2.SO_3H$ and in the dimethane sulphonate, or Lomidine, is $-CH_3.SO_3H$. For the purpose of calculating dosage, 1 g of active base is contained in 1.74 g pentamidine and in 1.56 g Lomidine.

The normal single full dose is 3 to 4 mg/kg of the active base in 10 per cent solution in distilled water; it is important to ensure complete solution before injection to avoid local reactions. The drug is given intramuscularly since its powerful hypotensive action makes intravenous injection dangerous. The full course of treatment consists of 7 to 10 injections given daily or every other day.

Patients should be kept at rest for an hour or more after each injection as the drug's hypotensive action may cause dizziness or fainting. Occasionally abdominal pain or even vomiting may occur soon after the injection, but after these transient effects have passed, long term toxic effects with pentamidine are very rare.

The drug is effective in the early stages of *T. gambiense* sleeping sickness but, like suramin, does not pass the blood-brain barrier and is therefore ineffective once there is established involvement of the central nervous system. Its use as a curative for *T. rhodesiense* sleeping sickness is not recommended; it has no advantages over suramin and there is some evidence that it may fail to cure even earlier in the course of the infection than suramin.

DIMINAZENE B. VET. C (Berenil) is a diamidine in which the active constituent differs from pentamidine only in the replacement of the central dioxypentane chain ($-O.(CH_2)_5.O-$) with a diazo-amino group ($-NH.N : N-$). Although primarily for veterinary use, since it is effective against *T. vivax* and *T. congolense* as well as the *T. brucei* subgroup, it has been shown to be effective in the treatment of human trypanosomiasis of either type.

Hutchinson and Watson (1962), using seven daily injections of 2 mg/kg active base in 2 per cent solution in sterile glucose (5 per cent), found the drug to be very effective against early *T. gambiense* infection. Recent work at the East African Trypanosomiasis Research Organization (de Raadt *et al*, 1966; Bailey, 1967) has also demonstrated its effectiveness against *T. rhodesiense*, both by intramuscular injection and by oral administration. Injections were of 5 mg/kg intramuscularly of a 5 per cent solution in saline. Since the drug, like the other diamidines, does not pass the blood-brain barrier, it is curative only in the early stage of the disease.

NITROFURANS. Nitrofurazone (Furacin) and furaltadone (Altafur) are both effective against both *T. gambiense* and *T. rhodesiense*, even after invasion of the central nervous system, but their action is unpredictable and toxic effects are frequent and may be very severe. Their use should therefore be limited to cases in which all other drugs have failed and they should, even then, be used only with appropriate precautions.

The dosage of nitrofurazone is 30 to 40 mg/kg daily, by mouth, divided into three or four doses, the maximum daily dose and course of treatment being 500 mg four times daily for a week. Up to three such courses can be given with a week's rest in between each. Furaltadone is given in a dosage of 30 to 60 mg/kg daily, divided into three or four doses. It is usually given by mouth, but may be given intravenously in 3.5 per cent solution in 5 per cent glucose.

Toxic effects of both drugs are common, the milder ones being headache, nausea, vomiting or pains in the joints. In patients with congenital glucose-6-phosphate-dehydrogenase deficiency (the incidence of which may be as high as 20 per cent in some African tribes) these drugs cause acute haemolytic anaemia. Therefore treatment with these drugs should invariably be preceded by a test for this deficiency. Disturbance of pyruvate metabolism may result in severe polyneuropathy which resembles beri-beri, and the 'burning feet' syndrome is not uncommon.

Metallic compounds. TRYPARSAMIDE, a sodium phenylarsonate derivative having the formula $NH_2 . CO . CH_2 . NH . C_6H_4 . AsO(OH)(ONa)$ or the very similar Orsanine,

$CH_3 . CO . NH . C_6H_3(OH) . AsO(OH)(ONa)$, have been for over 40 years the commonest drugs used in the treatment of *T. gambiense* infections, but have now been virtually superseded by the more active melamine compounds. Descriptions of their use and toxic effects are to be found in many text books and need not be repeated here.

MELARSEN was the first of the melamine group of drugs developed by Friedheim, and has the formula $(NH2)_2 . C_3N_3 . NH . C_6H_4 . AsO(ONa)_2$. It has been widely used in Nigeria for many years where it has been found not only to give a very high cure rate (over 90 per cent) in early cases of Gambian sleeping sickness, but also to be capable of curing infections resistant to tryparsamide. It is little or no more toxic than tryparsamide and optic complications are less frequent. However,

despite these advantages, it has been little used outside Nigeria.

Melarsen is given intravenously in 10 per cent solution in distilled water, which must be fresh, at a dosage of 15–20 mg/kg. The full course consists of eight to twelve injections at 5–7 day intervals and may be repeated after one month's rest.

Its toxic effects are very similar to those of tryparsamide, but have been found in Nigeria to have an incidence of less than 5 per cent. It has no place in the treatment of *T. rhodesiense* infections.

MELARSEN OXIDE, a trivalent compound closely related to melarsen and having the formula $(NH_2)_2 . C_3N_3 . NH . C_6H_4 . AsO$, was developed soon after melarsen and is highly active. However, it is so toxic that it has never found general use and has been completely superseded by its condensation product with dimercaprol, developed by Friedheim in 1949 in a particularly successful effort to release the therapeutic activity of the trivalent compound while reducing its toxicity.

MELARSOPROL (Mel B., Melarsen Oxice/B.A.L., Arsobal) is a trivalent arsenical, a melamine derivative of phenyl-arsenoxide condensed with dimercaprol and has the formula $(NH_2)_2 . C_3N_3NH . C_6H_4 . As :$

$$(SCH_2 . SCH)CH_2OH,$$

the arsenic being linked to both the sulphur atoms in the dimercaprol chain. Not only is it effective against all stages of *T. gambiense* infections and early *T. rhodesiense*, but its advent has also revolutionised the outlook for late cases of *T. rhodesiense* infection. Previously, once involvement of the central nervous system with *T. rhodesiense* was well established, there was no treatment which could hold out any hope of cure. Since the appearance of melarsoprol, even well advanced *T. rhodesiense* cases may be cured; in less advanced cases, but still after invasion of the central nervous system, cure rates as high as 90 per cent may be achieved. With this drug, there is only a narrow margin of safety when given at the required dosage, and serious toxic effects may occur; it should therefore be given only under strict medical supervision. However, since it offers the only hope for cure of late *T. rhodesiense* infections, it must be used in such cases despite the risk.

Melarsoprol is dispensed in 5 ml ampoules of 3.6 per cent solution in propylene-glycol and the full single dose is 3.6 mg/kg with a maximum of 5 ml, equivalent to this dose rate for a 50 kg man. The solution is unstable in contact with water and therefore dry sterilised syringes and needles must be used. Further, it is exceedingly irritant and must be injected with the greatest care, very slowly and *strictly* intravenously. The smallest leakage outside the vein will inevitably cause severe, painful, local inflammation with extensive, brawny swelling which resolves only very slowly.

Usual courses of melarsoprol consist of three or four daily injections with a rest period of at least 7 days between courses. Early cases of *T. gambiense* infection may be cured with a single course of three or four injections, but suramin is to be preferred for early *T. rhodesiense*. Late cases of either *T. gambiense* or *T. rhodesiense* may be treated with nine injections in three groups of three daily or eight in two groups of four with 7 day rests in between.

Because of the drug's value in late cases, particularly of *T. rhodesiense* infection, it may often be necessary to use it on patients in very poor condition and if treatment is started with full doses the risks of serious complications are very high. As a result, there has been a tendency to start with very small doses and work up gradually to a full dose, but, in the opinion of the author, such a regime entails serious risks of inducing drug resistance in *T. rhodesiense*, leading to relapse which will be extremely difficult to treat. Often the patient's condition may be strikingly improved by the preliminary use of suramin. Although this drug cannot cure a late infection, the elimination of the blood infection may produce a marked improvement in the patient's general condition in a period of a week or two and so permit the use of adequate starting doses of melarsoprol. The aim should be never to give less than half the full dose at the start.

Typical full treatments of late cases with melarsoprol are therefore: 2.5, 3, 4 and 5 ml on days 1, 2, 3 and 4; seven days rest and then 5 ml on each of days 12 to 15 inclusive; or three 3-day courses of, first, 2.5, 3 and 4 on days 1, 2 and 3, and 5 ml on each of days 11, 12 and 13, and 21, 22 and 23.

The risks from even slight leakage of melarsoprol injections have already been mentioned, but another aspect of the irritant properties propylene glycol solution is that it may cause burning pain up the arm or retrosternal pain, especially if injected too rapidly. Over-rapid injection is also liable to cause vomiting or abdominal pain.

Encephalopathy, which appears to be reactive in type, between the drug, the trypanosomes and the diseased brain, is not uncommon, its incidence sometimes exceeding 10 per cent. Its onset may be slow or sudden and its severity may vary from very slight to intense and fatal. Mental signs, varying from mild confusion to intense excitement or even mania, predominate, but other early signs are tremor, athetoid movements or aphasia. In more serious cases, convulsions or coma may result.

This reactive encephalopathy is most commonly seen during, or just after, the first course of treatment; it usually settles down gradually and is not repeated after further doses of the drug. Less frequently a hypersensitivity reaction to the drug is seen with nitritoid crisis, angioneurotic oedema or skin rashes, and this can only be overcome by reducing the dosage and gradually increasing it as the patient becomes desensitised. Dimecaprol may be of some help in the treatment of toxic effects.

In general, toxic effects of treatment with melarsoprol are more likely to be encountered the more severe the degree of involvement of the central nervous system.

TRIMELARSAN (Mel W., 9955 R.P) is a water soluble trivalent arsenical in which the mercaprol chain of Mel B. has been replaced by a dipotassium dithio-succinate group. Its only advantage over Mel B. is that it is much less irritant and can be given intramuscularly.

It is dispensed as a powder, in 200 mg ampoules, and is dissolved in 5 per cent solution in distilled water, saline or 5 per cent glucose. The full single dose is 4 mg/kg with a maximum of 200 mg, and the full course of treatment usually consists of two series of four daily injections separated by 7–10 days. In the first series, the starting dose should be half the maximum, increasing to the full dose at the end. The second series should consist of four full doses.

Toxic effects are similar to those seen with melarsoprol and reports of their incidence vary. Some workers have found it less toxic and very effective against *T. gambiense*, whereas others have reported more frequent toxicity and lower effectiveness. In the experience of Robertson (1963), using the drug against *T. rhodesiense* infections, toxic reactions were more frequent than with melarsoprol, and the cure rate definitely inferior. Relapses from treatment with trimelarsan can be expected to be resistant to melarsoprol and all other arsenical drugs.

Prophylactic

Only one drug, pentamidine, is of value in the prophylaxis of sleeping sickness and is effective, with any certainty, only against the Gambian type.

If given in doses of 4 mg/kg pentamidine will

protect against chronic *T. gambiense*-type infection for at least 6 months and has been used extensively for this purpose in many countries, drastically reducing the incidence of the disease. Its period of effectiveness for complete prophylaxis against *T. rhodesiense* infection is much shorter and is also more uncertain. It has been used, with good results, to cut short localised epidemics, but its use on a wide scale is liable to lead to suppression of the early symptoms of infection without affecting the time which the infection takes to become established in the central nervous system, so that the great majority of such cases as do occur are likely to present in the later stage.

For pentamidine prophylaxis to be fully effective, the whole population must be under sufficient control to ensure that adequate doses are given at regular intervals. These conditions can be met in, for example, a recruited labour force whose work exposes them to contact with tsetse in a sleeping sickness area, such as tin miners or railway workers in northern Nigeria. It is much more difficult, though, to ensure sufficient control of the whole population of a country or part of a country, particularly in the relatively sparsely populated conditions of much of the African continent and in the present political atmosphere of many of the newly independent countries.

Theoretically, if complete prophylactic coverage of a whole population is achieved and man is the only reservoir host of the disease, eradication should be achieved within a short time. The most thorough prophylactic campaigns have been carried out in French-speaking countries in Africa and eradication does appear to have been achieved in some areas. In the majority though, despite very remarkable reductions of sleeping sickness incidences, the disease has persisted at a very low endemic level. This persistence may be attributable to any of several possibilities, or a combination of them. One is that prophylactic coverage, despite the most careful organisation, may have fallen short of 100 per cent, allowing a few cases to escape. Again, some persons already infected may not have been diagnosed before the single prophylactic dose was given, and a single dose would be inadequate to achieve cure. Another possibility is the existence of a reservoir host other than man. Finally strains of trypanosomes might be present in an area against which pentamidine could not protect for the full 6 months between inoculations. It is possible that this last factor may have played a part in the recrudescence of human trypanosomiasis in Zaire since the breakdown of all organised prophylaxis against sleeping sickness. Not only has the recrudescence been much more rapid than was anticipated, but also it appears (Dr J. Burke, personal communication) that the disease pursues a more acute course than in the past, perhaps because the very thorough campaigns of prophylaxis previously organised by the Belgian authorities served only to eradicate the most chronic, typically *gambiense*-like strains.

PROGNOSIS

African trypanosomiasis is one of the few parasitic diseases that are almost inevitably fatal if untreated. Although instances have been recorded of apparent recovery without treatment, or of long-lasting infection without apparent ill effect ('healthy carriers') they are so few and far between that, in the normal course of events, the disease may be said to be invariably fatal.

If the disease is diagnosed and treated, the prognosis depends entirely on the type of the disease, whether of the chronic Gambian type or the acute Rhodesian type, and how far it has progressed. Whereas early Rhodesian sleeping sickness is virtually 100 per cent curable with suramin, the best cure rates of the early Gambian form are usually upwards of 95 per cent. After the onset of central nervous system involvement, the chances of cure remain high, of the order of 90 per cent at first, but steadily decrease as the condition of the patient deteriorates with increased damage to the brain.

The degree of brain damage also determines the final outcome even if cure is achieved. The onset of damage and degeneration is relatively late in the pathological processes, but once such degeneration has occurred, it is irreversible and even if completely cured, the patient will be left with permanent mental defect which may vary from very slight to severe.

REFERENCES

APTED, F. I. C., ORMEROD, W. E., SMYLY, D. P., STRONACH, B. W. and SZLAMP, E. L. (1963) *J. trop. Med. Hyg.*, **66**, 1.

ASHCROFT, M. T., BURTT, E. and FAIRBAIRN, H. (1959) *Ann. trop. Med. Parasit.*, **53**, 147.

BAILEY, N. M. (1967) East African Trypanosomiasis Research Organization Annual Report for 1966, p. 83. Entebbe: Government Printer.

BAILEY, N. M., CUNNINGHAM, M. P. and KIMBER, C. D. (1967) *Trans. roy. Soc. trop. Med. Hyg.*, **61**, 696.

CUNNINGHAM, M. P., BAILEY, N. M. and KIMBER, C. D. (1967) *Trans. roy. Soc. trop. Med. Hyg.*, **61**, 688.

FAIRBAIRN, H. and BURTT, E. (1946) *Ann. trop. Med. Parasit.*, **40**, 270.

GALL, D., HUTCHINSON, M. P. and YATES, W. (1955) *Ann. trop. Med. Parasit.*, **49**, 419.

GALLAIS, P. (1953) *Méd. trop.*, Numéro spécial, Dec. 1953, p. 799.

GODFREY, D. G. and LANHAM, S. M. (1971) *Bull. Wld. Hlth. Org.*, **45**, 13.

HOARE, C. A. (1970) In *The African Trypanosomiases*, ed. Mulligan, H. W., p. 950. London: George Allen and Unwin.

HUTCHINSON, M. P. (1954) *Ann. trop. Med. Parasit.*, **48**, 75.

HUTCHINSON, M. P. and WATSON, H. J. C. (1962) *Trans. roy. Soc. trop. Med. Hyg.*, **56**, 227.

JENKINS, A. R. and ROBERTSON, D. H. H. (1959) *Trans. roy. Soc. trop. Med. Hyg.*, **53**, 524.

LANHAM, S. M. and GODFREY, D. G. (1970) *Exp. Parasitol.*, **28**, 521.

—— (1972) *Trans. roy. Soc. trop. Med. Hyg.* (in press).

MATTERN, P. (1962) International Scientific Committee for Trypanosomiasis Research. Report of the 9th Meeting, Conakry, 1962. C.C.T.A. Publication No. 88, p. 377.

—— (1964) *Ann. Inst. Pasteur*, **107**, 415.

ONYANGO, R. J., VAN HOEVE, K. and DE RAADT, P. (1966) *Trans. roy. Soc. trop. Med. Hyg.*, **60**, 175.

DE RAADT, P., VAN HOEVE, K., BAILEY, N. M. and KENYANJUI, E. N. (1966) East African Trypanosomiasis Research Organization Annual Report for 1965, p. 60. Entebbe: Government Printer.

RICKMAN, L. R. and ROBSON, J. (1970a) *Bull. Wld. Hlth. Org.*, **42**, 650.

—— (1970b) *Bull. Wld. Hlth. Org.*, **42**, 911.

ROBERTSON, D. H. H. (1958) East African Trypanosomiasis Research Organization Annual Report for July 1956—December 1957, p. 3. Nairobi: Government Printer.

—— (1963). *Trans. roy. Soc. trop. Med. Hyg.*, **57**, 274.

ROBERTSON, D. H. H. and JENKINS, A. R. (1959) *Trans. roy. Soc. trop. Med. Hyg.*, **53**, 511.

ROSS, G. R. and BLAIR, D. M. (1956) International Scientific Committee for Trypanosomiasis Research, Report of the 6th Meeting, Salisbury, Southern Rhodesia, p. 9. C.C.T.A. Publication (unnumbered).

WILLETT, K. C. (1965) *Trans. roy. Soc. trop. Med. Hyg.*, **59**, 374.

FURTHER READING

MULLIGAN, H. W. ed. (1970) *The African Trypanosomiases*. London: George Allen and Unwin.

4
South American Trypanosomiasis

Chagas' disease is one of the few examples of an infectious disease of importance in man where the causative organism (*Trypanosoma cruzi*) was first observed in its arthropod vector. In 1907 Carlos Chagas found numerous flagellates in the hindgut of *Panstrongylus megistus* caught in the north of Minas State in Brazil. These flagellates readily infected a marmoset producing trypanosomes of a new species in the blood stream of this animal. Following up this lead, Chagas found similar trypanosomes in the blood of several sick children in the area (Chagas, 1909). It is of interest that one of these original patients, now a 60–70 year old woman, has been reinvestigated (Salgado *et al*, 1962) and the trypanosome recovered from her blood by xenodiagnosis. She is well and exhibits none of the complications of the chronic stage of this infection, but many infected people develop serious heart disease and die suddenly. This discrepancy as regards the affect of the parasite in man is not clearly understood.

Chagas believed that infection was acquired by the bug biting its mammalian host and introducing trypanosomes (anterior station transmission). He described flagellates in the body cavity and salivary glands of infected insects. Brumpt (1912) challenged these findings and showed that transmission was effected by the contamination of the hosts skin by bug faeces. Diaz (1934) confirmed Brumpt's experimental evidence and we now regard this infection as being an example of so-called posterior station transmission (Hoare, 1934).

Following these pioneer workers there was a period, as Van der Kuip (1966) points out, when interest in the infection waned. Chagas in his original reports noted that the infection had an acute and chronic phase and he described heart disease and dilatation of the gut as late complications of the infection. In the late thirties Mazza (1939) drew attention to the prevalence of this infection in Argentina and since then considerable evidence has accumulated to support many of Chagas' views as to the nature of this infection.

GEOGRAPHICAL DISTRIBUTION

From being a rather obscure infection Chagas' disease has recently risen to the standing of a serious public health problem. The World Health Organization estimates that 7 million people are infected and 30 million exposed to the risk of infection (W.H.O., 1960). The infection has been described as the most important cause of myocarditis in the world (*Lancet*, 1965).

T. cruzi infections occur in every country in South America (Romana, 1961) Human infections have been recorded in Central America and two such patients have been found who have never left Texas (Kagan *et al*, 1966). Nor is the Caribbean necessarily exempt for infected bugs have been found in Trinidad (Downs, 1963), Curaçao (Van der Sar and Vincke, 1965) and Aruba (Van der Kuip, 1966).

No authenticated instances of this infection occurring outside the western hemisphere are known to the author. Seventy-four of the 79 species of the subfamily Triatominae are found in the new world where they have developed an unusual avidity for mammalian blood. However, one species known to be capable of transmitting the infection, namely *Triatoma rubrofasciata*, is tropicopolitan. Other blood-sucking arthropods (Ornithodorus Cimex, Culex), can be infected in the laboratory, but it is doubtful whether they could transmit the infection in nature unless crushed into the skin or eaten.

In these days of rapid travel it is important to realise that theoretically *T. cruzi* could reach any country in the world in the form of an asymptomatic individual who nevertheless has a blood stream infection. Several batches of asian monkeys have been reported to harbour *T. cruzi* but in each instance it is likely that transmission occurred in the laboratory probably via bed bugs (Hoare, 1963).

Among the countries of South America, in Brazil, Argentina, Chile and Venezuela particularly, this infection poses a public health problem of the first magnitude. It has been estimated that there are 2.8 million individuals with this infection in Venezuela alone (Gomez Nunez *et al*, 1963). It should be noted, however, that such estimates are based on serological evidence of infection rather than actual disease (the important vectors vary according to the area). In Venezuela

Rhodnius prolixus is the main vector bug, in Brazil *Triatoma braziliensis* and *Panstrongylus megistus* are important in this regard, while *Triatoma infestans* is a scourge of the Argentine and Chile. In poor housing bugs breed easily in the cracks in the mud walls and the thatch. As much as a bushel of bugs have been taken from one dwelling. The species mentioned are readily domesticated and this accounts for their importance. Quite apart from the high standards of housing and the low virulence of North American strains the sylvatic habits of the vector bugs in North America (many of which are infected) may account for the rarity of human infections in the United States (Kagan *et al*, 1966).

ORGANISM

T. cruzi is a polymorphic trypanosome (15–20 μm long) and both slender and broad stumpy forms can be seen in peripheral blood films. The relative proportions of these forms varies in different strains (Brener, 1965). A very characteristic feature is the large oval posterior kinetoplast of such a size as to distort the cell. Electron microscopy reveals an investing double membrane, the inner layer of which is composed of spirally striated contractile protein fibrils. The blood stream trypanosome has never been observed to divide. Division by binary fission takes place intracellularly in the leishmanial phase in the vertebrate host. In the gut of the invertebrate host and in culture crithidial forms also divide by binary fission to give rise to other crithidia and a small proportion of metacyclic trypanosomes. The metacyclic trypanosome (formed between cycles) (Brumpt, 1913) in the faeces of the bug is the most infectious form of the organism.

T. cruzi can be cultured easily in a variety of media many of which consist of a blood agar mixture. Serum and haematin are usually necessary for growth (Bishop, 1967). The cultural forms appear to need purines and pyrimidines to make nucleic acid. Enzymes of the Krebs, Embden-Meyerhof and pentose pathways are present and dividing cultural forms consume much glucose (Warren, 1958). In contrast the blood stream trypanosome appears to utilise little glucose (Von Brand, 1966).

Temperature appears to exert a profound effect on morphology in tissue culture preparations. At 37°C leishmanial forms are common, but at 26°C both leishmania and stout trypanosomes are rare and replaced by slender trypanosomes.

It seems likely that a trypanosome population may be composed of several antigenic and biological variants (Lambrecht, 1965). Work on African trypanosomes has shown that antigenic variation occurs at frequent intervals even when an infection is induced by one organism (Gray, 1965). Differences in metabolism and ultrastructure have been noted in a population of African trypanosomes (Vickerman, 1965). Similar work has not yet been done in relation to *T. cruzi*.

Many strains of *T. cruzi* have been isolated and maintained in laboratory animals. They exhibit a wide range of pathogenicity as well as tissue trophism. Although cardiac muscle is invariably affected some strains show a greater tendency to involve the reticuloendothelial system or central nervous system of rodents (Von Brand *et al*, 1949). Antigenic differences have been noted between various strains of *T. cruzi* and man and bat seem to share similar strains (Nussenweig *et al*, 1963; Nussenweig and Goble, 1966).

A large number of mammals can be infected with *T. cruzi* and constitute important reservoirs of the infection. Apart from primates, marsupials, armadillos, bats and a wide variety of rodents domestic animals such as cats and dogs may carry the infection (Barretto, 1964). Farm animals may also harbour the organism (Diamond and Rubin, 1958) and in Bolivia a susceptible animal, the guinea pig, is an important reservoir since it is reared for food (Squires, 1968). In North America opossums and racoons are important reservoirs as well as 14 species of rodents and the infection is widely distributed as a zoonosis (Kagan *et al*, 1966). Many of these animals appear to harbour chronic benign infections but are nevertheless capable of infecting bugs. Moreover, the behaviour of a strain of *T. cruzi* varies in different animal hosts. An organism tolerated by an armadillo could be fatal to man. *T. cruzi* infections do not occur in birds and cold blooded animals have only rarely been infected (Ryckman, 1965).

The question arises as to whether the cruzi-like trypanosomes reported from so many mammals do in fact represent a single species. Barretto (1965) suggests that the following criteria be taken into consideration before identifying a newly isolated trypanosome as *T. cruzi*:

Morphological similarity.

Coincidence of biometric data particularly total length and mean nuclear index.

Infectivity to laboratory animals particularly young rats and mice.

Presence of leishmanial forms in the tissues of the vertebrate host.

Evolution in the digestive tract of triatomines with development of metacyclic trypanosomes in the hindgut.

Cultivability in blood agar media.

Presence of cross immunity.

The same criteria should be applied to flagellates in the faeces of wild caught bugs. Other members of the family Trypanosomidae can live in the gut of reduviids including *Trypanosoma rangeli* (D'Allessandro Bacigalupo, 1961) and *Trypanosoma conorhini* (Morishita, 1935) which also parasitise mammals.

In addition to these, Wallace (1966) lists 25 known isolations of insect trypanosomatid parasites from reduviidae.

VECTOR

The family Reduviidae contains the subfamily Triatominae of haemophagus insects which carry the disease. Several species populations have been shown to consist of a complex of subspecies which can be interbred to produce progeny of various degrees of fertility. A summary of the known chromosome complements in Triatominae is available (Usinger *et al*, 1966). Usinger (1944) lists over 40 species which have been demonstrated to incubate *T. cruzi* either naturally or under experimental conditions. In some areas of South America up to 75 per cent of bugs have been found infected.

These hemiptera have five instars, the larvae and nymphs resembling the adult insect but they are wingless. Even the youngest larval stage can feed through animal fur and in the laboratory immature forms feed more readily than adults. The apparent predilection for the face relates to the fact that this is the most frequently exposed area in sleeping man (Pick, 1959). As capillary feeders, they directly tap a suitable vessel and engorge rapidly (Lavoirpierre *et al*, 1959). A large insect may take up to 0.35 ml, of blood labelled with radioactive iron (De Frietas and Das Geudes, 1961). Bugs vary as to how soon they defaecate after commencing to feed and those bugs which defaecate late (e.g. *Triatoma protracta*) may be less important vectors in consequence (Wood, 1942). After defaecation the liquid bulk of the blood is reduced by the frequent passage of clear 'urine' (Wigglesworth, 1931).

After ingestion the trypanosomes form leishmania and crithidia which actively divide in the midgut of the bug. Flagellates are usually present in the faeces after 15-20 days but faeces may be infective as early as 7 days. (Phillips, 1958). The rate of development is influenced by environmental temperature. In contrast with *T. rangeli*, *T. cruzi* infection does not appear to shorten the life of the bug which may live for a year or more and remain infected. The flagellates only escape from the gut on the death of the bug in which event they can survive for many days in the haemocoele (Wood, 1951). There is no transovarial transmission of *T. cruzi*.

Clean bugs can become infected by feeding on the faeces of infected bugs (coprophagy) (Marinkelle, 1965) or by sucking blood from an engorged infected insect (Ryckman, 1951). It has been possible to identify some of the recent blood meals of wild bugs by precipitin tests on the stomach contents (De Frietas *et al*, 1960; Barretto, *et al*, 1964). In domestic bugs simultaneous presence of human and opossum blood has been noted.

There is no reason why any clinical unit concerned with the diagnosis of Chagas' disease should not maintain their own bugs. They are best kept at a temperature of 30°C, and a relative humidity of 50–60 per cent (Ryckman and Ryckman, 1966). They can be fed weekly on trypanosome-free mammals or birds and some will survive for many months without feeding. There is a little evidence that it may matter which species and strain of bug is used for xenodiagnosis and (Ryckman, 1965) if possible it is best to use clean bugs which are known vectors in the area concerned. It is a mistake to keep these bugs under too clean conditions in the laboratory since they may maintain their bacterial flora by coprophagy. There is some evidence that bacterial symbionts provide thiamine and folic acid for the host bug (Baines, 1956; Harington, 1960). A fungus *Nocardia rhodnii* is said to be essential for normal development of *R. prolixus* (Muhlpfordt, 1959).

PATHOGENESIS

Man is usually infected by the metacyclic trypanosome in the bug's faeces penetrating minute skin abrasions, mucous membranes, or the conjunctiva. However, human infection may arise from syringes contaminated with infected blood, or from infected blood used for transfusion. Gentian violet 1 : 4000 is added to blood 24 hours before transfusion in many blood banks in South America to kill the trypanosomes (De Rezende *et al*, 1965). Congenital infections have occurred in man (Rubio and Howard, 1963). Carnivorous animals can be infected by eating infected meat. In some of the many accidental laboratory infections of man the mode of transmission is not clear (Pizzi *et al*, 1963).

The incubation period before the onset of symptoms is about 10 days and trypanosomes can be detected in the peripheral blood from 14 to 28 days. Factors such as the route of infection and the number of organisms gaining access to the host will affect this period. Infections by blood transfusion are said to be particularly acute. There are probably many factors that influence the course of the infection, host factors such as the state of nutrition and the wide variations in virulence of the trypanosome itself. This is reflected in the pattern of the disease in man. Many individuals have positive serological evidence of *T. cruzi* infection suggesting they have encountered its antigens but exhibit no signs or symptoms of the disease. Others have all the signs of an acute infection on first encountering the organism. We are largely ignorant of the factors which determine which individual will go on to develop the late complications of Chagas' disease. The amount of visceral and autonomic nerve damage that occurs in the acute phase may pre-determine the changes that follow in later life (Koberle, 1963).

On entering the host cell the trypanosome assumes a leishmanial form and multiplies by binary fission until the cell is full of parasites (a so-called pseudocyst). Many leishmania assume a trypanosomal form before the cyst bursts. The released organisms circulate in the blood stream and invade further cells. The process of development of pseudocysts has been observed in tissue culture and takes 5 days. In man as well as laboratory animals this organism has an unexplained predilection for cardiac, smooth and striated muscle. Foci of leishmania have been detected in many other human tissues including brain, adrenals, testis, spleen and lymph nodes, and in experimental animals have been described from virtually every organ of the body.

If the course of the acute infection is studied in host tissues, it is found that after the first few generations of pseudocysts the hosts defensive cells make their appearance in the form of inflammatory cells, such as lymphocytes, histiocytes and plasma cells, which surround every focus of parasite multiplication. Granulomas which may even contain giant cells often form eventually with or without subsequent fibrosis. After a few weeks the cellular and humoral immune response of the host are such that parasitic multiplication is suppressed and trypanosomes become scanty in the peripheral blood. With time leishmania become difficult to find even in the heart, where all that remains is

chronic inflammation sometimes associated with acute focal necrosis. There may be haemorrhage, and hyalinisation and fragmentation of muscle fibres.

In the phase of parasitic multiplication and active inflammation in the heart and smooth muscle of the digestive tract, not only are the muscle fibres damaged but the important peripheral ganglia of the autonomic nervous system are also affected. The work of Koberle (1961) and his colleagues has drawn attention to the profound diminution of ganglion cells both in the wall of the right auricle in infected patients with cardiac disease and in the enteric plexuses of patients with chronic dilatation of the gut. Often in such patients parasites cannot be demonstrated in the vicinity of the degenerated ganglia (Mott and Hagstrom, 1965). In rats with acute infections a diminution in heart ganglion cells (Alcantcara, 1959) and anterior horn cell populations (Schwartzburd and Koberle, 1959) has been noted. This has led Koberle (1957) to postulate that a neurotoxin liberated at the time of pseudocyst rupture damages nerve cells remote from the site of parasitic multiplication. No such toxin has yet been identified. It is possible that by the time organ denervation is manifest, inflammatory lesions which may have been present near ganglion cells have disappeared. In laboratory animals a correlation between degenerative changes in ganglion cells and the local degree of inflammatory reaction has been noted (Andrade and Andrade, 1966). The extent to which dysfunction of the various muscular organs which are affected occurs may depend on the neuronal reserve of their autonomic ganglia.

Damage to the parasympathetic ganglia in the right atrium results in impaired sympathetic control with an increase in cardiac work followed by dilatation and hypertrophy. Thus it is possible that the high frequency of cardiac dilatation seen in this form of myocarditis is similar in mechanism to the chronic gut dilatations which occur following defective innervation due to ganglion cell destruction. Apart from the inflammatory effects the high frequency of conduction defects in the heart may be the result of defective oxygenation of the conducting system as well as the diffuse inflammatory myocarditis.

Apart from the myositis and destruction of autonomic ganglia, other factors may play a part in producing this cardiomyopathy. Okumura has noted arteritis in infected animals (Okumura *et al*, 1960) and similar arterial lesions have been seen post mortem in the hearts of patients with chronic chagasic myocarditis (Laranja *et al*, 1956).

Microscopic infarcts, the result of ischaemic lesions, have been reported in such hearts (Andrade and Andrade, 1955). Rosenbaum (1964) describes an acute pan-myocarditis in a fatal infection acquired by a research worker handling *T. cruzi*. He points out that for each fibre which contained parasites, there were many others that were damaged and had no parasites. He therefore postulates that the parasite must have had an indirect effect on such fibres and favours an immuno-allergic reaction suggesting that it may be possible to demonstrate heart autoantibodies in Chagas' myocarditis. Other workers have also suggested that cellular substances released by disintegrating infected cells produces an auto-immune type phenomenon (Jaffe *et al*, 1961). Okumura *et al* (1963) have reviewed the evidence for and against a toxic or allergic factor playing a part in the pathogenesis of this disease. Seneca and Peer (1966) have produced toxic effects and tissue lesions in mice with an extract of *T. cruzi*.

The hearts of patients dying from heart failure with the disease are larger and heavier than normal (Menezes and Koberle, 1965), but in places the myocardium may be very attentuated. Small apical ventricular aneurysms may appear due to slackening of the sinuospiral and bulbo-spiral ventricular muscle bundles of the heart (Migone, 1958; Raso, 1964). The pulmonary conus may be dilated for the same reason. Yet rupture of the heart is almost unknown probably because the myocardial contractility is so deficient. Thrombosis in the right auricle is common and there may be evidence of a pericarditis with the development of curious pericardial nodules along the lines of the coronary vessels. There may be circumscribed areas of endocardial fibrosis (Report, 1965).

Chronic inflammatory changes may also be found in the smooth muscle layer of the gut wall associated with damage to Auerbach's plexus. This plexus co-ordinates the activity of the smooth muscle of the digestive tract producing peristaltic waves. Interruption of normal peristalsis leads to incoordination or the wave-like motion with stagnation and retraction of solid residues and consequent dilatation. Aperistalsis is basically the malady resulting in enteromegaly. Megaoeso-phagus and megacolon may be more frequent because these parts of the gut contain large solid residues (Koberle, 1963). Megastomach, mega-gallbladder, megaduodenum, megajejunum, mega-appendix, megaureter and mega-bladder are also known. Bronchiectasis may follow dilatations of the bronchi in this disease (Koberle, 1959). The smooth muscle tissue of the walls of these muscu-

lar tubes regulates lumen size under normal conditions. There is a close correlation between serological evidence of infection, the existence of Chagas' myocarditis and the presence of mega-oesophagus (Report, 1965). 'Megas' have been shown to develop after long-standing infections in laboratory animals (Okumura and Correa Neto, 1961, 1963).

The frequency of chronic central nervous system involvement is not known. Meningo-encephalitis occurs sometimes in the acute invasive phase and small inflammatory foci may be seen throughout the brain associated with nests of leishmania. There may be perivascular cuffing. Chronic neurological syndromes could be a sequel to such damage and spastic paralysis mental deficiency, cord and cerebellar lesions have been attributed to chronic *T. cruzi* infections (Vieira, 1966). There have been few post-mortems, however (Jorg and Orlando, 1967), and the evidence for Chagas' infection in these chronic neurological cases often rests solely on the serological findings plus evidence of associated cardiomyopathy or megas. Atrophy of the cerebral cortex in long-standing infections has been attributed to hypoxia associated with chronic heart failure (Alencar, 1966). A reduction in the number of neurones in the cerebellum has been reported in chronically infected patients (Braudao and Zulian, 1966).

Further observations in man and laboratory animals confirm Chagas' view that there is an acute phase of this infection which is followed by a long latent period before the development of the chronic phase with cardiac damage and/or mega syndromes. Patients with chronic syndromes often give no history of the acute phase which may have been relatively asymptomatic or have occurred in childhood and been forgotten. Older children and adults may only have a mild febrile disturbance in the acute phase. In human experimental infection symptoms may be mild and the parasites never found (Yorke, 1937).

CLINICAL FEATURES

Acute phase (Canal Feijo, 1964; Lugones, 1964)

Patients identified at this phase of the disease are relatively rare even in endemic areas and are usually children. Initial local multiplication of the parasite may result in local inflammation with heat, redness and swelling. Such inflammation in the region of the eye is known as Romana's sign (Pick, 1954). Often local lymph nodes enlarge at the site of the portal of entry in *T. cruzi* infections. For instance periconjunctival infections are associated with pre-auricular node enlargement and even swelling of the lacrimal gland. Inflammation of the buccal fat pad occurs in young children (Jorg and Freire, 1961). There is some evidence that local oedema is produced by un-infected bug faeces alone in sensitised individuals (Lumbretas *et al*, 1959). There may be no visible lesion at the portal of entry.

General dissemination via the blood stream results in malaise, fever, sweating and muscular pains. Localised areas of inflammation and fat necrosis may give rise to multiple chagomas. Cutaneous eruptions of a morbilliform type also occur. Hepatosplenomegaly and lymphadenopathy heralds reticuloendothelial activation. Generalised oedema may be inflammatory in nature or associated with heart failure. Some degree of cardiac involvement occurs in every acute case. Although cardiac enlargement and a triple rhythm may occur a persistently raised pulse rate may be the only sign. Electrocardiographic abnormalities have been noted in 43.3 per cent of a large series of such patients (Laranja *et al*, 1956). Acute meningoencephalitis is a rare serious complication. Trypanosomes are rarely recovered from the cerebrospinal fluid.

In the early stages of the infection motile parasites are frequently seen in fresh blood films. After 6–10 weeks these become more scanty and xenodiagnosis, subinoculation of mice and culture may be necessary to find the organism. The complement fixation test becomes positive on about the thirtieth day; non-specific findings are a leucocytosis with a marked lymphocytosis, a raised erythrocytic sedimentation rate and a raised serum gamma globulin. There may be transient disturbances of liver function associated with fatty infiltration of that organ.

Ninety per cent of patients survive the acute phase but it is doubtful whether they ever eradicate their infection. What role re-infections have in the subsequent course of the infection is not known. Patients who have resided briefly in endemic areas may develop chronic Chagas' heart disease many years later. Usually after the acute phase, an asymptomatic period of 10–20 years ensues. During this time there may be transient swelling of lymph nodes, fever, and lymphocytosis. A subacute form of cardiac damage has been described where death from heart failure follows within a few years of initial infection (Andrade and Andrade, 1963).

Chronic phase

Chronic Chagasic cardiomyopathy. Eighty-two per cent of patients in a large series were between the ages of 11 and 50 years (Report, 1965), an important age group in society. Males are more frequently affected; this could be because their more strenuous cardiac work damages an already weakened heart.

The common presentation is with the signs of congestive cardiac failure. Since both ventricles are often involved there may be little pulmonary congestion. The heart may be grossly enlarged with the apex of the heart displaced to the left. Cardiac contractions are sluggish and an impalpable apical impulse and distant heart sounds may suggest a pericardial effusion. A third sound may be present. The inflammatory process does not affect the valves so that the only valvular lesions encountered are functional ones, the result of dilatation of the cardiac chambers. The murmur of functional mitral incompetence may be present. Signs of tricuspid incompetence, namely a pan-systolic murmur accentuated by inspiration, engorged neck veins transmitting a V wave and a pulsatile liver are sometimes seen. The pulse pressure tends to be low and the radial pulse small. It is often irregular.

The chest X-ray shows bilateral cardiac enlargement often with little evidence of pulmonary congestion. Screening may reveal diminished pulsation of the heart and abnormal contractions may be seen. The electrocardiogram is helpful since two thirds of such patients have some disturbance of cardiac rhythm (Rosenbaum and Alvarez, 1955; Pierretti, 1961) or conduction. Premature ventricular contractions and right bundle branch block are the commonest abnormalities. Some degree of atrioventricular block occurs in one third of cases with arrhythmia. Auricular flutter and fibrillation carries a poor prognosis and patients may die with ventricular fibrillation. Complete heart block occurs in 4–8 per cent of patients and may be associated with Stokes-Adams attacks.

Intractable heart failure and sudden deaths associated with acute cardiac arrest or ventricular fibrillation are common. Sudden death may be precipitated by undue exertion, infection, pregnancy or surgery. Mural thrombosis may be responsible for death associated with peripheral embolus, either into the lungs or systemic circulation. In one study of 503 Brazilian patients with chronic Chagas' disease of the heart, followed over a 6-year period, 96 died. There were 36 sudden deaths and 53 from chronic heart failure (Porto, 1962). The combination of an arrhythmia with a positive complement fixation test but without failure is often seen as an initial presentation.

Even in areas where *T. cruzi* infections are common, other forms of cardiovascular disease are more frequently responsible for failure. These include hypertensive, arteriosclerotic and rheumatic heart disease. These may of course coexist with *T. cruzi* infections and make diagnosis very difficult. The incidence of other forms of cardiomyopathy in endemic areas is beyond the scope of this chapter, but it may be noted that endomyocardial fibrosis has been reported from South America (Fagundes, 1963; Andrade and Guimares, 1964).

Mega syndromes. Although not commonly a cause of death, the dilatations of the gut or megas are a source of serious discomfort to the patient. Theoretically any hollow muscular viscus can be involved but megaoesophagus (Koberle, 1958) and megacolon (Koberle, 1958; Ferreira Santos, 1961) are by far the most common. Dysphagia is the symptom associated with megaoesophagus. Barium studies reveal a much enlarged oesophagus with poor peristaltic waves (Pessoa and Mesquitas, 1963). Megacolon presents as chronic constipation and manual evacuation may be necessary. Acute volvulus may be a complication if there is a mobile sigmoid loop.

Motility studies show abnormal weak intestinal contraction in such patients (Goma, 1967). Abnormal kymograph readings have been obtained in infected patients without megas (De Godoy and Vieira, 1963).

Endocrine and exocrine gland involvement. Although this occurs in experimental animal infections (Pizzi, 1945; Watkins, 1966), there is very little evidence to suggest that dysfunction of these glands ever poses a clinical problem. Abnormal glucose tolerance tests have been noted in infected patients Chagas described a parasitic thyroiditis (which has been noted in experimental animals (Goble, 1954) and believed it was responsible for the high incidence of goitre in some areas. Yorke (1937) reviewed the epidemiological evidence and came to the conclusion that endemic goitre due to iodine deficiency was present in many of the areas studied.

DIAGNOSIS

Isolation of the organism

As mentioned earlier, circulating parasites are found in the acute phase but after a few weeks become difficult to find. A drop of blood pressed to a monolayer film of cells under a coverslip and examined under the high power of a microscope will reveal motile trypanosomes. Giemsa-stained thick and thin films should also be examined. Various methods of concentrating small numbers of trypanosomes in the blood have been tried. Strout's method involves centrifugation of the supernatant from clotted blood (Flores, *et al*, 1966). Deane and Kirchner (1962) exploit the differential fragility of red cells and trypanosomes prior to centrifugation.

Xenodiagnosis first introduced by Brumpt (Brumpt, 1914) relies on the efficiency of reduviid bugs as the vector of this disease. At least 5 clean immature hungry bugs are fed on the patient and their rectal contents examined 30–60 days later for flagellates. At the site of bug feeding some patients exhibit a transient erythematous rash. Artificial feeding of bugs on the patient's blood through a suitable membrane can be used as an alternative (Harington, 1960). A recent modification of xenodiagnosis (Maekelt, 1962) involves homogenising the bugs. This homogenate is then filtered, the filtrate centrifuged and the deposit examined. Such a deposit can also be inoculated into mice. In the laboratory it can be demonstrated that apparently clean bug faeces from a bug exposed to infection will produce a patent infection in a mouse. Up to 20 per cent of patients with a positive complement fixation test have flagellates isolated by xenodiagnosis (Maekelt, 1964).

Subinoculation of susceptible strains of albino mice is yet another way of demonstrating the parasite. One millilitre of the patient's blood should be injected intraperitoneally into each of two mice and the tail blood examined at 7, 14, 21 and 28 days after inoculation. A higher proportion of isolations may be achieved by using cortisonised mice (Woody and Woody, 1961). Culture of the patient's blood on the type of media already referred to may be especially successful (Packchanian, 1943; Chiari and Brener, 1966). Horen (1960) has described a simple medium for use in field work and antibiotics may be added to reduce bacterial contamination. In the present state of our knowledge ideally all these methods should be employed to try and isolate the trypanosome, but in practice xenodiagnosis is the one most frequently used.

Leishmania may be demonstrated in lymph node biopsy material, splenic aspirate, or even in skin biopsies in the acute stage (Rodriquez, 1961). Skeletal muscle biopsy in the chronic stage of the disease is sometimes helpful. Even if no leishmania are seen granulomas of chronic inflammatory cells are suggestive of *T. cruzi* infection (Prata and Porto, 1966)

Serology

A precipitin test has been developed which is useful in the diagnosis of the acute stage (Muniz, 1947). In many patients who are regarded as having chronic Chagas' disease, the diagnosis has been arrived at on the basis of a suggestive clinical picture plus a positive complement fixation test (Chaffee *et al*, 1956; De Frietas, 1961). This test, often called the Machado Guerreiro reaction, was first introduced in 1913 (Guerreiro and Machado, 1913) but there are still difficulties in its interpretation and the antigen is not standardised. The antigen is best prepared from a freeze-dried extract of cultural flagellates. Positive titres of over 1 : 2 dilution have been regarded as significant and it is said that a positive test indicates live parasites (Report, 1965) but it is difficult to prove this statement. Apparently a positive C.F.T. seldom reverts to negative. *Leishmania donovani* infections can produce a positive reaction. About 80 per cent of patients with chronic heart disease due to T. *cruzi* have a positive C.F.T. while 90 per cent of patients with megaoesophagus have a positive reaction. In some areas of Brazil 10–23 per cent of people have a positive C.F.T. and 20–30 per cent of these may have cardiac signs (Report, 1965).

Recently alternative serological tests have been developed. An indirect fluorescent antibody test (Fife and Muschel, 1959) is more sensitive and correlated well with the C.F.T. (Camargo, 1966). Reliable results can be obtained using filter paper blood smears (Souza and Camargo, 1966). Haemagglutination tests are also more sensitive (Montano and Acros, 1965) and currently being investigated.

TREATMENT

This is most unsatisfactory at the present time. A number of drugs have been shown to be active against the blood forms but none is known which can attack the intracellular forms in the tissues (Goble, 1961). Clinical trials have been conducted with six groups of compounds, the bisquinaldines, trivalent arsenicals, phenanthridinums, 6-methoxy-8-aminoquinolines, nitrofurans and ribofuranocypurines. The bisquinaldines, 8-aminoquinolines and nitrofurans all have their advocates. Bisquinaldines are difficult to obtain.

Primaquin, a well known antimalarial, is the 8-aminoquinoline employed in an adult dose of 15 mg/day by mouth to a total of 500 mg. Of the nitrofurans, levofuraltadone has been shown to be effective in mice (Seneca *et al*, 1964). 30 mg/ kg/day for 15 days followed by 10 mg/kg/day for 3 months is one recommended dosage schedule (Hawking, 1964). Polyneuritis, a serious side effect of nitrofurazone therapy (Cancado *et al*, 1964), is less frequent with levofuraltadone. With both these groups of drugs it is important to exclude glucose-6-phosphate-dehydrogenase deficiency before therapy, otherwise a haemolytic anaemia may ensue. Both drugs are known bone marrow depressants. Even after combined therapy with primaquin and nitrofurazones, circulating trypanosomes have still been detected (Aronson, 1962). Some experienced physicians advise no treatment even in acute cases. As Goble (1961) suggests it is possible that treatment of acute cases with drugs which reduce parasitaemia may lower the subsequent foci of intracellular parasites. Tetracyclines are inactive and steroids are contraindicated. Several new drugs are under trial at the time of writing and of these Lampit (Bayer 2502) a new nitrofurazone compound is the most promising.

Symptomatic treatment must not be forgotten in patients with chronic complications. Heart failure may require digitalis, diuretics, salt restriction and rest. Patients with chronic Chagasic myocarditis may not respond as well as anticipated to such therapy. The sudden onset of cardiac arrthymias may require urgent therapy (Smith, 1960). Propranolol may be useful in controlling some paroxysmal arrhythmias (Sloman and Stannard, 1967). Intracardiac pacemakers may be of use in repetitive Stokes-Adams attacks (Bay and Sivertssen, 1967). Implantation of artificial pacemakers has been tried but is not always a success because of fibrosis and damage to the myocardium (Perretti *et al*, 1965). Mural thrombosis with peripheral embolisation may be an indication for anticoagulant therapy.

Mega conditions of the gut are difficult to manage. There is no curative treatment for aperistalsis since the destruction of the ganglion cells is permanent. Treatment is palliative and surgical (Ferreira Santos, 1961). Rectosigmoidectomy may be helpful, removing the dilated rectum and sigmoid but sparing the last 4-5 cm of rectum for the anastomosis. The Heller procedure may relieve obstruction at the gastro-oesophageal junction (Hawkins, 1967).

PREVENTION

Common sense and a knowledge of the dangers of acquiring the infection will help the individual and poster campaigns have made the inhabitants of endemic areas aware of the problem. Mosquito nets and night lights may prevent the bugs gaining access to man. In heavily infested dwellings faeces raining down from the ceiling may be a source of infection and such mosquito nets should have a cloth roof. Good housing and cleanliness will reduce the opportunities for bugs to become domesticated but bugs can enter the most modern dwellings via drainpipes and in clothes and food. It may not be possible to eradicate this infection from endemic areas in view of the host of animal reservoirs. Populations of domestic animals such as cats and dogs should be strictly controlled.

In general, prevention and control is equated with destruction of the vector bugs but this is not easy. Although DDT has been reported effective in some field trials (Pessoa, 1963), on laboratory testing it is disappointing (Rox *et al*, 1966). Some bugs have been shown to possess a DDT dehydrogenase (Fine *et al*, 1966). In one field study DDT may have actually increased the incidence of *R. prolixus* by killing off egg predators (Berti *et al*, 1960). Susceptibility of BHC (benzene hexachloride) has been demonstrated in the laboratory (Dias, 1965; Hack, 1966) and domestic bugs have been controlled with this insecticide (Gamboa and Perez Rois, 1966). Three applications a year of a house spray containing a 10 per cent solution of gammexane (1500 mg/m^2) is recommended. Dieldrin 1 g/m^3/year has been highly successful in some situations (Symes *et al*, 1962). Different instars have different susceptibilities to insecticides. Pifano *et al*. (1961) claim that control and even eradication of *R. prolixus* in Venezuela is possible using BHC, HCH and Dieldrin.

Gomez Nunez and co-workers (Gomez Nunez *et al*, 1963, 1964; Gomez Nunez, 1965) have investigated the susceptibility of *R. prolixus* to irradiation but sterilising doses inhibit mating. In consequence it does not appear that control by sterile male techniques using irradiated insects will work for *Rhodnius*. Valuable epidemiological data has been obtained by tagging *Rhodnius* with cobalt 60 and following subsequent intra- and extra-domestic distribution of bugs in the fabric of houses with the aid of a geiger counter. Unfortunately it appears that *Rhodnius* tends to concentrate in bedrooms and is present in high density near beds and hammocks. It is suggested that the emission of CO_2 and heat from the human body act as an attractant. Another useful sampling technique is to attach cardboard boxes to the walls as catching and breeding sites for the bugs. The degree of house infestation can be assessed by the number of bugs and eggs found in these boxes.

The potential of so-called third generation insecticides (Williams, 1967) in relation to the control of reduviidae remains to be seen but the concept of preventing maturation by exposure to analogues of the insect's growth hormone is an important advance. Initial experiments with *Rhodnius* have not been successful (Saxena and Williams, 1966). Certain insects readily parasitise reduviid eggs in the laboratory. There are several groups of predaceous bugs in the family reduviidae, e.g. reduvius species which will attack and kill the vectors of Chagas' disease (Wood, 1954; Ryckman and Ryckman, 1967). Although they do this readily in the laboratory no attempt has been made as yet to use them as a form of biological control.

Another possible approach to the prevention of human infection is the production of vaccine. It is possible to protect mice against a known fatal challenge with a virulent strain of *T. cruzi* by prior inoculation with a strain of mild pathogenicity (Kagan and Norman, 1961). The addition of actinomycin D to cultural flagellates inhibits multiplication but preserves motility and such a preparation can also immunise mice (Fernandes *et al*, 1965). In one situation rats surviving an infection produced serum antibodies which protected other rats, and there was some evidence of passive transfer of antibodies through the milk and placenta (Ryckman, 1965).

However in view of the impossibility of predicting the potential virulence to man of a *T. cruzi* strain avirulent to animals, only vaccines of killed organisms can be used at the present time. Formalin killed organisms have failed to produce antibodies but sonication or rapid freeze thawing of cultural forms has produced antigens capable of introducing protective effects when used with adjuvants (Johnson *et al*, 1963; Goble, 1964; Seneca and Peer, 1966).

Chagas disease has been further reviewed by Marsden (1971).

REFERENCES

ALCANTCARA, F. G. (1959) *Z. Tropenmed. Parasit.*, **10**, 296.
ALENCAR, A. (1966) *Anais Acad. bras. cient.*, **38**, 89.
ANDRADE, S. G. and ANDRADE, Z. A. (1966) *Rev. Inst. Med. trop. S. Paulo*, **8**, 219.
ANDRADE, Z. A. and ANDRADE, S. G. (1955) *Arch. bras. Med.*, **45**, 279.
—— (1963) *Rev. Inst. Med. trop. S. Paulo*, **5**, 273.
ANDRADE, Z. A. and GUIMARES, A. C. (1964) *Brit. Heart J.*, **26**, 813.
ARONSON, P. R. (1962) *Annals int. Med.*, **57**, 994.
BAINES, S. (1956) *J. exp. Biol.*, **33**, 533.
BARRETTO, M. P. (1964) *Rev. bras. Malar.*, **16**, 527.
—— (1965) *Rev. Inst. Med. trop. S. Paulo*, **7**, 305.
BARRETTO, M. P., SIQUEIRA, A. F. and DE FRIETAS, J. L. P. (1964) *Rev. Inst. Med. trop. S. Paulo*, **6**, 56.
BAY, G. and SIVERTSSEN, E. (1967) *Brit. med. J.*, **4**, 199.
BISHOP, A. (1967) *Advances in Parasitology* 5, p. 111. London: Academic Press.
BRAUDAO, H. J. S. and ZULIAN, R. (1966) *Rev. Inst. Med. trop. S. Paulo*, **8**, 281.
BRENER, Z. (1965) *Ann. trop. Med. Parasit.*, **59**, 19.
BRUMPT, E. (1912) *Bull. Soc. Path. exot.*, **5**, 360.
—— (1913) *Bull. Soc. Path. exot.*, **6**, 167.
—— (1914) *Bull. Soc. Path. exot.*, **7**, 706.
CAMARGO, M. E. (1966) *Rev. Inst. Med. trop. S. Paulo*, **8**, 227.
CANAL, FEIJO, E. J. (1964) *Rev. Fac. Med. Tucumán*, **3**, 227.
CANCADO, J. R., MARRA, U. D. and BRENER, Z. (1964) *Rev. Inst. Med. trop. S. Paulo*, **6**, 12.
CHAFFEE, E. F., FIFE, E. H. and KENT, J. F. (1956) *Amer. J. trop. Med. and Hyg.*, **5**, 763.
CHAGAS, C. (1909) *Mem. Inst. Osw. Cruz*, **1**, 159.
CHIARI, E. and BRENER, Z. (1966) *Rev. Inst. Med. trop. S. Paulo*, **8**, 134.
D'ALLESSANDRO BACIGALUPO, A. (1961) *Studies on Trypanosoma rangeli.* Ph.D. Thesis, Tulane.
DEANE, L. M. and KIRCHNER, E. (1962) *Rev. Inst. Med. trop. S. Paulo*, **4**, 407.
DE FRIETAS, J. R. and DAS GEUDES, A. (1961) *Bull. Wld. Hlth. Org.*, **25**, 271.
DE FRIETAS, J. L. P., SIQUEIRA, A. F. and FERREIRA, O. A. (1960) *Rev. Inst. Med. trop. S. Paulo*, **2**, 90.
DE GODOY, R. A. and VIERRA, C. B. (1963) *Rev. Goiana Med.*, **9**, 117.
DE REZENDE, J. M., ZUPELLI, W. and BAFUTTO, M. G. (1965) *Rev. Goiana Med.*, **11**, 35.
DIAMOND, L. S. and RUBIN, R. (1958) *Exp. Parasit.*, **7**, 383.
DIAS, J. C. P. (1965) *Rev. bras. Malar.*, **17**, 37.
DIAZ, E. (1934) *Mem. Inst. Osw. Cruz*, **28**, 1.
DOWNS, W. G. (1963) *J. Parasit.*, **49**, 50.
FAGUNDES, L. A. (1963) *Rev. Inst. Med. trop. S. Paulo*, **5**, 198.
FERNANDES, J. F., HALSMAN, M. and CASTELLANI, O. (1965) *Nature*, **207**, 1004.
FERREIRA SANTOS, R. (1961) *Proc. roy. Soc. Med.*, **54**, 1047.
FIFE, E. H. and MUSCHEL, L. H. (1959) *Proc. Soc. exp. Biol.*, **101**, 540.
FINE, B. C., LETELIER, M. E. and AGOSIN, M. (1966) *Exp. Parasit.*, **19**, 304.
FLORES, M. A., TREJOS, A., PAREDES, A. R. and RAMOS, A. Y. (1966) *Bol. chil. Parasit.*, **21**, 38.
GAMBOA, C. J. and PEREZ ROIS, L. (1966) *Bol. Inf. Dis. Malar. Sanaem Ambient*, **6**, 63.
GOBLE, F. C. (1954) *Amer. J. Path.* **30**, 599.
—— (1961) *Bol. Sanit. Panam.*, **51**, 439.
—— (1964) *J. Parasit.*, **50**, Supplement 19.
GOMA, A. H. (1967) *Rev. Hosp. Clin. Fac. Med. S. Paulo*, **22**, 137.
GOMEZ NUNEZ, J. C. (1965) *Acta cient. venez.*, **16**, 26.
GOMEZ NUNEZ, J. C., GALLIMORE, J. C., FERNANDEZ, J. M. and GROSS, A. (1963) *Acta cient. venez.*, **13**, 46.
GOMEZ NUNEZ, J. C., GROSS, A. and MACHADO, C. (1964) *Acta cient. venez.*, **15**, 97.
GRAY, A. R. (1965) *Ann. trop. Med. Parasit.*, **59**, 27.
GUERREIRO, C. and MACHADO, A. (1913) *Brasil-méd.*, **23**, 225.
HACK, W. H. (1966) *Z. Tropenmed. Parasit.*, **17**, 467.
HARINGTON, J. S. (1960) *Nature*, **188**, 1027.
—— (1960) *J. Parasit.*, **50**, 273.
HAWKING, F. (1964) *J. trop. Med. Hyg.*, **67**, 211.
HAWKINS, C. F. (1967) *Brit. med. J.*, **4**, 663.
HOARE, C. A. (1934) *Trop. Dis. Bull.*, **31**, 757.
—— (1963) *J. trop. Med. Hyg.*, **66**, 297.
HOREN, W. P. (1960) *J. Parasit.*, **46**, 456.

JAFFE, R., DOMINGUEZ, A., KOZMA, C. and GAVALLER, B. (1961) *Z. Tropenmed. Parasit.*, **12**, 137.
JOHNSON, P., NEAL, R. A. and GALL, D. (1963) *Nature*, **200**, 83.
JORG, M. E. and FREIRE, R. S. (1961) *Acta trop. (Basel)*, **18**, 318.
JORG, M. E. and ORLANDO, A. S. (1967) *Mem. inst. Osw. Cruz*, **65**, 63.
KAGAN, I. G. and NORMAN, L. (1961) *J. infect. Dis.*, **108**, 213.
KAGAN, I. G., NORMAN, L. and ALLAIN, D. (1966) *Rev. Biol. trop. (S. José)*, **14**, 55.
KOBERLE, F. (1957) *Rev. Goiana Med.*, **3**, 155.
—— (1958) *Gastroenterology*, **34**, 460.
—— (1958) *J. trop. Med. Hyg.*, **61**, 21.
—— (1959) *Z. Tropenmed. Parasit.*, **10**, 304.
—— (1961) *Bol. Sanit. Panam.*, **51**, 404.
—— (1963) *Gut*, **4**, 399.
LAMBRECHT, F. L. (1965) *Rev. Inst. Med. trop. S. Paulo*, **7**, 346.
LARANJA, F. S., DIAZ, E., NOBREGO, G. and MIRANDA, A. (1956) *Circulation*, **15**, 1035.
Lancet (1965) **1**, 1150.
LAVOIRPIERRE, M. M. J., DICKERSON, G. and GORDON, R. M. (1959) *Ann trop. Med. Parasit.*, **53**, 235.
LUGONES, H. S. (1964) *Rev. Fac. Med. Tucumán*, **3**, 239.
LUMBRETAS, H., FLORES, W. and ESCALLON, A. (1959) *Z. Tropenmed. Parasit.*, **10**, 6.
MAEKELT, G. A. (1962) *Arch. venez. Med. trop.*, **4**, 277.
—— (1964) *Rev. venez. Sanid.*, **29**, 1.
MARINKELLE, C. J. (1965) *Rev. Biol. trop. (S. José)*, **13**, 55.
MARSDEN, P. D. (1971) In *International Review of Tropical Medicine*, vol. 4, ed. Woodruff, A. W. and Lincicome, D. R. London and New York: Academic Press.
MAZZA, S. (1939) *Mission et Estudio de Pathologica Regional Argentina*, No. 40, Buenos Aires.
MENEZES, H. and KOBERLE, F. (1965) *O Hospital*, **68**, 139.
MIGONE, C. (1958) *Alguns Aspectos da Anatomia Pathologia da Cardite Chagasica Cronica*. Thesis, São Paulo.
MONTANO, G. and ACROS, H. (1965) *Bol. chil. Parasit.*, **20**, 439.
MORISHITA, K. (1935) *Jap. J. Zool.*, **6**, 3.
MOTT, K. E. and HAGSTROM, J. W. C. (1965) *Circulation*, **31**, 273.
MUHLPFORDT, H. (1959) *Z. Tropenmed. Parasit.*, **10**, 314.
MUNIZ, J. (1947) *Brasil-méd.*, **6**, 261.
NUSSENWEIG, V., DEANE, L. M. and KLOETZEL, J. K. (1963) *Exp. Parasit.*, **14**, 221.
NUSSENWEIG, V. and GOBLE, F. C. (1966) *Exp. Parasit.*, **18**, 224.
OKUMURA, M., BRITO, T., PEREIRA DA SILVA, L. H., CARVALHO DA SILVA, A. and CORREA NETO, A. (1960) *Rev. Inst. Med. trop. S. Paulo*, **2**, 17.
OKUMURA, M. and CORREA NETO, A. (1961) *Rev. Hosp. Clin. Fac. Med. S. Paulo*, **16**, 338.
—— (1963) *Rev. Hosp. Clin. Fac. Med. S. Paulo*, **18**, 351.
OKUMURA, M., FRANCA, L. C. M. and CORREA NETO, A. (1963) *Rev. Hosp. Clin. Fac. Med. S. Paulo*, **18**, 151.
PACKCHANIAN, A. (1943) *Amer. J. trop. Med.*, **23**, 309.
PIERRETTI, O. H., ROCHA, J. M., ACQUANTELLA, H., ANDERSON, R. and PIMENTEL, R. (1965) *Amer. J. Cardiol.*, **16**, 114.
PESSOA, J. and MESQUITAS, C. (1963) *Rev. Goiana Med.*, **9**, 29.
PESSOA, S. B. (1963) *Edemias Parasitorias da Zonas Rural Brasileira*, p. 568. São Paulo.
PHILLIPS, N. R. (1958) *Experimental Studies in Epidemiological Factors in the Transmission of American Human Trypanosomiasis*. Ph.D. Thesis, London.
PICK, F. (1954) *Acta trop. (Basel)*, **11**, 105.
—— (1959) *Bull. Soc. Path. exot.*, **50**, 234.
PIERRETTI, O. H. (1961) *El Electrocardiogram en la Cardiopatia Chagasica*. Thesis Caracas.
PIFANO, C. F., VAZQUEZ, A. D., MAEKELT, A., GUERRERO, L. MARTIN, G. G. and TINELLI, G. L. (1961) *Rev. venez. Sanid.*, **26**, 7.
PIZZI, R. (1945) *Biologia (Bratislava)*, **3**, 53.
PIZZI, T., NIEDMANN, G. and JARPA, A. (1963) *Bol. chil. Parasit.*, **18**, 32.
PORTO, C. C. (1962) *Arch. bras. Cardiol.*, **15**, 59.
PRATA, A. and PORTO, G. (1966) *Rev Inst. Med. trop. S. Paulo*, **8**, 193.
RASO, P. (1964) *Contrabuicao Ao Estudo da Lesso Vorticilar na Cardite Chagasica Cronica*. Thesis, Belo Horizonte.
REIS, L. C. F., DE OLIVEIRA, H. L. and VIEIRA, C. (1960) *Rev. Goiana Med.*, **6**, 155.
Report (1965) *Chagas Disease in Brazil* Pan Amer. Hlth. Org. Rep. 4/10, Washington D.C.
RODRIQUEZ, M. J. D. (1961) *Rev. ecuat. Hig.*, **18**, 49.
ROMANA, C. (1961) *Bol. Sanit. Panam.*, **51**, 390.
ROSENBAUM, M. B. (1964) *Prog. cardiovasc. Dis.*, **7**, 199.
ROSENBAUM, M. B. and ALVAREZ, A. J. (1955) *Amer. Heart J.*, **50**, 492.

H

Rox, I., Bayora, I. G. and Orozio, H. E. (1966) *Bull. Wld. Hlth. Org.*, **35**, 974.
Rubio, D. M. and Howard, B. J. (1963) *Biologica (Bratislava)*, **34**, 50.
Ryckman, R. E. (1951) *J. Parasit.*, **37**, 433.
—— (1965) *J. med. Ent.*, **2**, 93.
—— (1965) *J. med. Ent.*, **2**, 96.
—— (1965) *J. med. Ent.*, **2**, 105.
—— (1967) *J. med. Ent.*, **4**, 326.
Ryckman, R. E. and Ryckman, A. E. (1966) *Reduviid Bugs in Insect Colonisation and Mass Production*, p. 183.
     New York: Academic Press.
Salgado, J. A., Garcez, P. N., De Olivera, C. A. and Galizzi, J. (1962) *Rev. Inst. Med. trop. S. Paulo*, **4**, 330.
Saxena, K. N. and Williams, C. M. (1966) *Nature*, **210**, 441.
Seneca, H. and Peer, P. (1966) *Trans. roy. Soc. trop. Med. Hyg.*, **60**, 610
Seneca, H., Rees, P. M. and Reagan, J. W. (1964) *Exp. Parasit.*, **15**, 479.
Schwartzburd, V. H. and Koberle, F. (1959) *Z. Tropenmed. Parasit.*, **10**, 309.
Sloman, G. and Stannard, M. (1967) *Brit. med. J.*, **4**, 508.
Smith, S. (1960) *Brit. med. J.*, **1**, 638.
Souza, S. L. and Camargo, M. E. (1966) *Rev. Inst. Med. trop. S. Paulo*, **8**, 255.
Squires, F. A. (1968) *Pest articles News summaries, Sect. A*, **14**, 189.
Symes, C. B. Muirhead, Thompson, R. C. and Busvine, J. R. (1962) *Insect Control in Public Health*, p. 121.
     Amsterdam: Elsevier.
Trejos, A., Goday, C. A., Greenblatt, C. and Cedillos, R. (1963) *Exp. Parasit.*, **13**, 211.
Usinger, R. L. (1944) *U.S. Pub. Hlth Bull.*, **288**, 1.
Usinger, R. L., Wygodzinsky, P. and Ryckman, R. E. (1966) *Ann. Rev. Ent.*, **11**, 309.
Van der Kuip, E. J. (1966) *An Investigation into the Occurrence of T. cruzi in Aruba*. PhD. Thesis, Utrecht,
     Holland.
Van der Sar, A. and Vincke, B. (1965) *Trop. geogr. Med.*, **17**, 225.
Vieira, C. B. (1966) *Rev. Goiana Med.*, **12**, 31.
Vickerman, K. (1965) *Nature*, **208**, 762.
Von Brand, T. (1966) *Biochemistry of Parasites*, p. 88. New York: Academic Press.
Von Brand, T., Tobie, E. J., Kissling, R. E. and Adams, G. (1949) *J. infect. Dis.*, **85**, 5.
Wallace, F. G. (1966) *Exp. Parasit.*, **18**, 124.
Warren, L. G. (1958) *Exp. Parasit.*, **7**, 82.
Watkins, R. (1966) *J. Parasit.*, **52**, 958.
Wigglesworth, V. B. (1931) *J. exp. Biol.*, **8**, 411.
Williams, C. M. (1967) *Sci. Amer.*, **217**, 13.
Wood, S. F. (1942) *Amer. J. trop. Med.*, **22**, 613.
—— (1951) *J. Econ. Ent.*, **44**, 52.
—— (1954) *Bull. So. Calif. Acad. Sci.*, **53**, 174.
Woody, N. C. and Woody, H. G. (1961) *J. Pediat.*, **58**, 568.
World Health Organization (1960) *Tech. Rep. Ser.*, **202**.
Yorke, W. (1937) *Trop. Dis. Bull.*, **34**, 275.

5
Leishmaniases

This group of clinically differing diseases is due to infection with protozoa of the genus Leishmania and may be conveniently classified:

Visceral leishmaniasis (Kala-azar)
Cutaneous leishmaniasis (Oriental sore)
South American leishmaniasis
   Cutaneous (Bay sore, Chiclero's ulcer)
   Muco-cutaneous (Espundia)
Diffuse cutaneous leishmaniasis
Post kala-azar dermal leishmaniasis

AETIOLOGY

Leishmania occurring in the tissue cells of vertebrates is a small ovoid organism 2–4 μm in diameter, amastigote form or Leishman-Donovan (L.D.) body. It contains a trophonucleus, a rhizoplast and a vacuole, the various types being identical morphologically but differentiated antigenically. In culture or in invertebrates the promastigote forms appear. The reservoir of infection is commonly the domestic dog, but in some areas cats, jackals, monkeys, gerbils, ground squirrels, rodents and lizards are infected. In some parts of the world dogs are frequently infected but human disease is rare, in other parts canine infection cannot be demonstrated although the disease is endemic in man.

Leishmania donovani with reservoir in dog or man causes visceral disease. *Leishmania infantum* producing visceral disease in children, especially in the Mediterranean area, is considered by many authorities to be an identical organism to *L. donovani*.

Leishmania tropica causing cutaneous leishmaniasis is almost certainly always transmitted from animals.

Leishmania braziliensis causing South American leishmaniasis appears to have several subspecies: *L. mexicana* in cutaneous disease ('bay sore' type); *L. peruviana* causing 'uta'; and *L. braziliensis* var *americana* (or *L. pifanoi*) causing diffuse cutaneous leishmaniasis in Venezuela while the parasite in Ethiopia is believed to be *L. tropica*.

L. donovani, *L. tropica* and *L. braziliensis* have different antigenic structures but *L. donovani* and *L. infantum* are antigenically identical. Some strains of *L. infantum* are closely related antigenically to leishmaniae of canine origin. In man there is no cross-immunity between human and canine *L. donovani*. When live rodent strains from ground squirrels were injected intradermally into humans, kala-azar did not result but the leishmanin skin test became positive after 6 to 8 weeks. These people were thereafter immune to challenge with human strains. This was still so 3 years later. A positive leishmanin skin test means skin immunity. Adler and Gunders (1964) showed that patients recovered from oriental sore of the Middle East, were resistant to attempted experimental infection with *L. mexicana*—the parasite of 'bay sore' from the new world.

VECTORS

The vectors are female sandflies of the genera *Phlebotomus* and *Lutzomyia*, the males living on fruit juices only. The female after sucking leishmaniae requires a fruit juice feed before it becomes infective. *Phlebotomus* is a minute hairy fly (1.5–3.5 mm in size) whose usual biting time is about dusk or at night. The flying range is at most 50 yards (46 metres) in length and 70 feet (21 metres) in height. Sandflies are so tiny and light as to be very wind sensitive and may be carried up to 400 yards (366 metres). They usually exist at an altitude below 2000 feet (610 metres) except in certain mountain valleys; they require a mean temperature of above 45°F (7.2°C) and a mean diurnal range of less than 20°F (11°C) for at least 3 months of the year. A relative humidity of not less than 70 per cent is most favourable. In many parts of the world such conditions only occur during certain months of the year and then only in protected sites such as caves, cracks and crevices of ruins or of walls of buildings or in clefts in the ground. In such sites a favourable 'micro' climate exists. During the unfavourable season of the year larval forms remain in 'diapause' and adults cannot be found. The disease may therefore have a seasonal incidence of infection and may occur in small localised pockets as in South Arabia or East Africa, whereas in the Indian subcontinent infection may occur throughout the year and may be wider in distribution.

Although 'natural' transmission of leishmaniasis is by the sandfly, other modes of transmission have been reported; kala-azar by congenital infection of the child *in utero* from maternal kala-azar and by blood transfusion (Chung, Chow and Lu, 1948). Cutaneous lesions have been contracted from the bites of infected laboratory animals and by a laboratory assistant dropping an infected needle which punctured the foot (Martens, de Alencar and Magalhães, 1965). The strangest of all was the case reported by Symmers (1960) when a wife who had never left England developed on the vulva a leishmanial sore which was only diagnosed after much delay and difficulty. It was then found that the husband had had inadequately treated kala-azar some years before. Transmission during coitus was postulated.

Deliberate inoculation of material from a sore to normal skin of small children, on a site where disfigurement would be inapparent, is a form of protective vaccination used by 'wise women' in the Middle East, particularly Baghdad, for many centuries. This method, using promastigotes from culture, is also practised medically (see under *Prophylaxis*).

PATHOLOGY

Progmastigote forms of leishmania are injected into the skin by the biting sandfly and as amastigotes multiply by simple fission in the reticuloendothelial cells until the host cells are ruptured.

Visceral leishmaniasis. Rarely a primary skin papule may be noted (Central Asia, North Kenya and East Africa, but not in the Indian race) but more usually the leishmaniae spread throughout the reticuloendothelial system especially in the spleen, liver, lymph glands and bone marrow. The histological appearances in the human liver, as seen under electron microscopy, have been described by Miwa and Tanikawa (1965). Considerable enlargement of spleen and liver is invariable and in some varieties the lymph glands become enlarged. Parasites are found on rare occasions in the stool, in urine, in nasal secretions and in lymph glands. In acute kala-azar appearing in new areas or in non-immunes, e.g. North Kenya, parasites are found widespread in normally appearing skin. At autopsy, in skin sections from fatal cases, cells packed with leishmania are found below the dermis, in masses around sweat glands and arterioles and diffusely through the corium. This type of parasitic invasion has also been found experimentally in hamsters.

There is a marked pancytopenia, the white cells falling to about 2000 per mm³, but counts of 1200–2000 are found and not infrequently the total may be less than 1000. Platelets are markedly diminished. There is a profound anaemia with haemoglobin levels of 5–9 g/100 ml in 84 per cent of patients, and less than 5 g/100 ml in 1.5 per cent (Cachia and Fenech, 1964) and a frequently occurring reticulocytosis. Such haematological findings have in the past tended to be dismissed as 'marrow depression' or as a 'crowding out' particularly of the red cells series by proliferation of infected reticuloendothelial cells. More careful studies of the bone marrow however revealed that the erythropoiesis was hyperplastic with occasional megaloblastic reaction and that haemolysis was increased (Chatterjee, 1946; Rachmilewitz, Braun and de Vries, 1947; Cartwright, Chung and Chang, 1948). The mechanisms producing the anaemia have been studied by radioactive isotopic techniques (Knight, Woodruff and Pettit, 1967). The absence of gross abnormality in the ferrokinetic studies refuted the hypothesis that marrow hypoplasia is the main cause of the anaemia although the authors conceded that some degree of ineffective erythropoiesis could occur. It was further shown clearly that the red cell life span was greatly reduced—a mean red cell life of 21 days indicating that the red cells were being destroyed at 5.5 times the normal rate—with sequestration and probable haemolysis occurring in the spleen. A partly or wholly immunological basis for the mechanism of the haemolysis appears to exist.

A marked derangement of the plasma proteins, previously the basis of the classical serological tests (of Napier, Sia, Chopra), is now demonstrated very simply by paper electrophoresis when the gamma globulins may constitute 60–70 per cent of the plasma proteins. As the result of treatment the globulins return towards normal levels. Specific circulating antibody in the serum can be detected and measured by immunofluorescent techniques and microfluorometric measurements (Shaw and Voller, 1964; Duxbury and Sadun, 1964; Bray and Lainson, 1965). In positive tests the specific fluorescence can be seen on the test amastigote in the kinetoplast and also on the cell wall. Complement fixation tests either 'nonspecific' using an acid fast bacillus, or 'specific' using promastigotes from a culture or amastigotes from the spleen of an infected hamster as the antigen are also available. Fluorescent antibody and complement fixation tests may be positive in trypanosomal infections and therefore have limitations in areas where both diseases exist.

Cutaneous leishmaniasis. The initial lesion is a small papule slowly increasing in size, consisting of lymphocytes, plasma cells, and many enlarged reticuloendothelial cells engorged with leishmaniae. But a flat squamous lesion may also appear with scaling of the epidermis. The papule enlarges with thinning of the epithelium, central ulceration and secondary infection destroying the full thickness of the skin so that the base consists of granulomatous cells. The edge of the ulcer is a thickened mass of epithelial cell proliferation, the sulcus and base of the edge containing many reticuloendothelial cells full of parasites. Central healing seldom occurs with epithelial covering, therefore the neglected ulcer heals with considerable scar tissue formation and contraction deformity of the part.

South American cutaneous leishmaniasis results in more erosive and destructive skin lesions with less granulation tissue formation. The lesions are often papillomatous. Parasites are scanty and difficult to find.

South American muco-cutaneous lesions begin as papules or pustules. They show a marked perivascular infiltration leading to endarteritis and marked ulceration extending beyond the skin to mucous surfaces and eroding underlying tissues. Secondary infection is the rule. The leishmaniae are found in the advancing edge of the ulceration and in the perivascular infiltration.

Diffuse cutaneous leishmaniasis first described in Bolivia and Venezuela was later recognised widely throughout the Americas and in Africa (Convit and Kerdel-Vegas, 1965; Bryceson, 1969, 1970). Lesions are nodular and infiltrative but not destructive nor erosive and are most disfiguring. Amastigotes occur profusely and mainly in the macrophages which are numerically increased, but lymphocytes and epithelioid cells are scarce.

Post kala-azar dermal leishmaniasis produces multiple nodular infiltrations of the skin usually without ulceration. Leishmaniae are profuse in the nodules.

CLINICAL FEATURES

Visceral leishmaniasis. The onset of the illness, although generally insidious, may sometimes be surprisingly acute and the patient can present with a history of only a day or so and already show a high fever. The incubation period of kala-azar is usually 3 to 6 months, but it may be as short as 10 days and may often be much longer. Cases have been reported with extremely long latent periods; $2\frac{1}{2}$ years in one instance (Jopling, 1955) and even 10 years (Wright, 1959) in another.

Early in the illness symptoms may be minimal and fever the sole physical sign. In the fully developed illness the main symptoms are fever, sometimes with rigors, malaise and sweating, often more profuse at night. Loss of weight is a marked and constant feature. Less common and misleading symptoms are mild headache, cough and watery diarrhoea. On examination the most striking physical signs are fever, anaemia, wasting, splenomegaly of marked degree and hepatomegaly. In the early stages the liver and spleen may enlarge in equal degree but later the liver enlargement does not keep pace with that of the spleen, so gross splenomegaly without similar hepatomegaly is suggestive of the diagnosis. Fever is high up to 105°F, (40.6°C) intermittently swinging and frequently showing a double rise in 24 hours. Curiously the patient may remain ambulant and retains a clean moist tongue and good appetite even with a high fever. The patient is mentally clear and alert. Increased pigmentation (hence the name kala-azar or black fever) is noted earlier in fair-skinned races or in the lighter-hued Asians. The abnormal pigmentation is often first noticed on the dorsal surfaces of the hands and fingers and of the feet and toes particularly in Europeans. The face is also involved. In the dark-skinned races depigmentation occasionally is a feature and is strikingly manifested in post kala-azar dermal leishmaniasis. Enlargement of the lymph glands may be noted and certain types of the disease show only an afebrile lymphadenopathy. In the advanced stage of untreated illness, wasting, oedema, ascites, jaundice with multiple skin and mucosal haemorrhages, constitute the terminal clinical picture.

The combination of findings will vary with the stage of the disease, its acuteness or chronicity and indeed with the geographical variant of kala-azar encountered—Mediterranean, Transcaucasian, Sudanese, Indian, Chinese or South American. 'Infantile' kala-azar in children is the commonest form of the Mediterranean shores and islands and lymphadenopathy without evident visceral involvement has been recorded in young non-immune adults from the same area. Acute fulminating syndromes are common in the Sudan and adjacent parts of East Africa. Lymph node involvement is frequently seen in the Chinese variety.

Cutaneous leishmaniasis. The clinical presentation of this type is insidious, the incubation period usually being 2 to 3 months but varying from 2 weeks to 5 or more years. A painless reddish itchy papule appears on an exposed cutaneous site accessible to sandflies. On occasion the lesions are multiple. Most lesions are on the face or forearms and have been present for some time, often many weeks, before the patient reports to a doctor. Recognition is aided by a simple classification which also gives the stages of development —papular, papulo-necrotic, papulo-squamous, squamous, squamo-ulcerative and ulcerative. More than one lesion at different stages may be seen in the same patient.

Papular lesions become papulo-necrotic; multiple papular lesions may be difficult to recognise as leishmaniasis. The papulo-squamous lesions are flatter with heaped-up silvery scales easily detached, with a little central papule like a nipple. Solitary squamous lesions may be quite large and become squamo-ulcerative.

The fully developed ulcers, up to 10 cm or more in diameter should be recognised easily from their appearance, site and indolence. Attention should be paid to the shape—circular or oval—and to the rolled undermined scolloped edge of the ulcer. The violet-purplish hue of the narrow zone of indurated unhealthy skin surrounding the edge is distinctive and the demarcation from the surrounding healthy skin should be noted. Secondary infection produces a dirty slough on the base which on removal reveals a rough, red, granular appearance. The ulcers never heal centrally but after a year or more tend to heal with granular contraction, scarring and deformity, leaving a thin depressed pigmented unsightly scar. Infection may spread from the sore to related lymphatic vessels and glands producing secondary nodules while lupus-like lesions near old healed sores may persist (Leishmaniasis recidivans).

South American leishmaniasis. BAY SORE (Chiclero's ulcer) type usually affects the ear and lasts for many years. The lesion starts as a small papule enlarging to become ulcerative and erosive, finally destroying part or whole of the pinna. Cervical glands may be enlarged. The 'uta' type lesions are multiple, papillomatous and moist but do not ulcerate nor involve tissues other than skin.

MUCO-CUTANEOUS lesions of espundia commence as papulopustular swellings on the skin localised to the margins of the nostrils, mouth or eye, or widespread on the face, ears, elbows and knees. Local infiltration and swelling of the nose causes 'tapir nose'. Mucosal lesions may follow rapidly or many years later. Ulceration and erosion destroy the lips, soft palate and fauces, and the tissues of the nose. All soft tissue down to bone is eaten away, secondary infection is invariable, pain, suffering and mutilation being severe.

Diffuse cutaneous leishmaniasis produces widely disseminated thickening of the skin in plaques, macules or multiple nodules usually without ulceration. Lymphoedema and lymphadenopathy may appear and depigmentation may result in some patients.

Post kala-azar dermal leishmaniasis, seen most commonly in India and the Sudan, commences one to two years after apparent cure of visceral disease. Hypopigmented erythematous macules appear on any part of the body, later becoming nodular, especially on the face. The whole surface of face and body may be covered with exuberant lesions each of large size.

DIFFERENTIAL DIAGNOSIS

Leishmaniasis is often overlooked when it appears in non-epidemic areas, and this is particularly so after a long incubation period.

Visceral leishmaniasis. Malaria or pneumonia is usually first suspected and later typhoid fever or brucellosis. Reticulosis, tuberculosis or leukaemia may be suspected clinically. In the early stage with fever of recent onset the diagnosis can be elusive for a prolonged period, mainly because the disease is not suspected and is not considered until the patient has been ill for some time. The length of the incubation period adds to the difficulty. The condition must be considered when a patient presents with fever, splenomegaly, anaemia and wasting.

The first clue to the diagnosis may be the low total white cell count coupled with anaemia and paucity of platelets (see under *Pathology*). Increase in gamma globulin is demonstrated by paper electrophoresis. In the absence of a laboratory the formol-gel test may still have a place: 1 drop of commercial formaldehyde added to 1 ml of patient's serum produces solid opaque coagulation in about 20 minutes. If available, the 'specific' complement fixation test and fluorescent antibody test (page 104) are most useful, but in the former a parallel control test is required to exclude confusion with syphilis.

The demonstration of the parasite in suitably stained tissue material or in culture gives a definitive diagnosis. Sometimes L.D. bodies may be recognised in the mononuclear cells of the blood when appropriately stained or a positive blood culture may be found. But more usually they must be obtained by tissue puncture and aspiration. It is important when performing aspiration to use a perfectly dry needle and syringe since any trace of moisture will cause disintegration of the parasites. If lymph glands are enlarged aspiration of gland juice may provide material for smears and for cultures in special media (of Nicolle, Novy and MacNeal; of Adler; or of Lourie). An accessible lymph node may be removed for histological examination.

Aspiration of marrow bone from the sternum or iliac crest is the safest procedure but with careful microscopic and cultural techniques only 92 per cent of marrow specimens will be found positive. If splenic puncture is done on the failures the success rate in finding the parasite should be 100 per cent. Marrow aspiration is usually safe but fatalities have been reported from splenic puncture which should therefore be reserved for patients in whom the bone marrow has proved to be negative. Percutaneous splenic biopsy with the Menghini needle of 1 mm diameter yields a core of splenic tissue; a portion should be smeared and stained, the other portion being submitted to culture. Similarly by liver biopsy, material of positive histological or cultural properties may be obtained, but this procedure should seldom be necessary. In addition to smear and culture any material aspirated or obtained by biopsy should be injected into a hamster, this animal being very susceptible to leishmaniasis and developing the systemic disease quite rapidly.

Cutaneous leishmaniasis. Localised skin lesions such as staphylococcal furunculosis, rodent ulcer, yaws, leprosy and primary syphilis must be distinguished. The lesions should be recognised easily from the site, appearance and history of residence in an endemic area. The diagnosis is confirmed by finding the amastigotes of *L. tropica*. The organisms are very scanty in the papular and squamous types and must be sought by scraping the lesions in all parts after removal of scabs or scales and submitting material to microscopy and culture. When an ulcer is examined, leishmaniae are never found in the base but only in the edge or in the sulcus between the overhanging edge and base. From this site material is best aspirated by the insertion of a dry needle, with syringe attached, through healthy skin lateral to the rolled edge, the point of the needle slanting inwards towards the sulcus. Biopsy of the ulcer margin should not be performed but if undertaken in error, as has happened in the past, histological sections reveal scanty intracellular amastigotes.

The Montenegro skin test may be used but is only required if parasites are not found. Intradermal injection of 0.1 ml of antigen prepared from a culture of leishmaniae producing erythema and induration at the site after 48 hours is a positive reaction.

South American leishmaniasis. BAY SORE. Lesions of this type should be differentiated from rodent ulcer by the occupation of the patient, site of lesion, its chronicity and by the characteristic erosion of the pinna. 'Uta' resembles yaws, leprosy or fungal infection. Leishmaniae are very scanty in both forms therefore biopsy is usually required and the Montenegro test is useful.

ESPUNDIA. Early lesions may be difficult to differentiate from furunculosis, rodent ulcer, yaws, leprosy or fungal infection and the disfiguring advanced disease in the endemic area could be confused with leprosy, lupus vulgaris or gangosa. The diagnosis is confirmed as for bay sore.

Diffuse cutaneous leishmaniasis. Because of its close similarity to leprosy or generalised fungal infection of the skin this variety of the disease may not be considered. The possibility should be borne in mind in patients seen in or from South America or East Africa. In most cases the skin smear or biopsy teems with amastigotes.

Post kala-azar dermal leishmaniasis, described in India and Sudan, may well be diagnosed as leprosy but yaws, syphilis, lupus vulgaris, drug reaction or fungal infection may also cause confusion unless a previous history of treated visceral disease is obtained and the possibility borne in mind. Skin biopsy is essential.

TREATMENT

Visceral leishmaniasis. A variable response is noted according to the geographical type of disease, the Sudanese, East African and South American forms being less susceptible to the drugs available. In childhood, kala-azar is occasionally completely resistant to treatment with a rapidly fatal outcome. Sodium stibogluconate (Pentostam) is the drug of choice effective in most cases, and its dosage may be calculated as: initial dose 5 mg/kg body weight; subsequent daily doses 10–15 mg/kg body weight. A daily intravenous injection of 0.6 g for 10 days is a suitable course for an adult. (Commercially prepared ampoules of a solution containing 0.1 g/ml are recommended.) Then after a rest period of 2 to 4 weeks the course is repeated once or twice. In the more resistant forms three courses each of 10 days with rest periods of only 7 to 10 days are usually required. Children tolerate antimony well and therefore should be given a relatively larger dose than that used for adults.

If sodium stibogluconate fails, pentamidine isethionate (see page 108) or 2-hydroxystilbamidine isethionate should be used; seven daily intravenous injections of 5 mg/kg body weight in

10 ml sterile water may be repeated after an interval of 2 weeks. In persistently resistant cases such as are found in South America the fungicidal drug amphotericin B has been used. This drug being toxic and dangerous should not be the first choice and requires great care in administration. The intravenous infusion of a solution of nystatin has been used on rare occasions.

The severe anaemia requires specific consideration since it may worsen rapidly after treatment with antimony or may fail to improve. If, however, blood transfusion is given before antimony, the haemopoietic response is nil or only minimal. In anaemic patients the best results are obtained by leaving blood transfusion until at least the sixth day of antimony treatment or until the end of the first course if possible. The effect of treatment is assessed by reduction of the temperature to a normal level, increase in weight, diminution in the size of the spleen and liver, normal haemoglobin, red cell and platelet levels, and return toward normal levels of the plasma globulins. When the disease appears completely resistant to treatment (South American and childhood forms) with persistent splenomegaly and irremediable pancytopenia, splenectomy may be undertaken.

Cutaneous leishmaniasis. Since sores on the face may heal with considerable scarring and disfigurement it follows that such lesions must be treated early and carefully, especially in females and young people. The first step is to clean the ulcer to free it from pyogenic infection or to remove the scales from squamous sores. Electrothermal coagulation may be applied to certain lesions but should be used with care on the face and ideally only by an expert (Henderson, 1966). Such procedures require a general anaesthetic. The area is then covered with an occlusive dressing for a week or more. Other methods of local treatment used are application of a stick of carbon dioxide snow and superficial radiotherapy. Local injections are not now recommended. For all large, advanced or multiple sores and for those of the face, a course of sodium stibogluconate intravenously (see above) should be given. Dehydroemetine 100 mg orally daily for 10–21 days has recently been shown to cause rapid healing, but only a few cases have been treated by this drug. With these methods rapid complete healing with minimal scarring should occur.

South American leishmaniasis. BAY SORES and UTA should both be treated with parenteral sodium stibogluconate as detailed for visceral leishmaniasis above.

ESPUNDIA in its early stages may respond to sodium stibogluconate which is the drug of first choice. More advanced cases will require pentamidine isethionate or 2-hydroxystilbamidine, but amphotericin B by intravenous infusion may have to be given. Pyrimethamine is an alternative which has been used with success. Three courses each of 10 days are given, the daily dose in the first two courses being 50 mg, but in the third course only 25 mg, a rest period of 8 days being given between courses. Subsequent to drug therapy, plastic surgery with skin grafting will be required for destructive erosive lesions.

Diffuse cutaneous leishmaniasis is resistant to treatment and constantly relapses. Pentamidine isethionate and amphotericin B are the drugs of choice in Ethiopia but both have serious toxic effects (Bryceson, 1970). In Venezuela response to antimonials is better than to diamidines.

Post kala-azar dermal leishmaniasis should be treated as for visceral disease.

PROPHYLAXIS

Measures to be taken against the sandflies include destruction of breeding places by repair of cracks in buildings, especially of sandstone construction, and filling of crevices and fissures in the ground near inhabited areas, levelling of refuse and rubbish dumps and old buildings, and spraying of breeding places with insecticide. Personal protection can be achieved by the use of repellents, avoidance of sitting outside at dusk, use of a sandfly net at night or a mosquito net impregnated with insecticide. The air currents from an electric fan discourage sandflies.

In the endemic areas, known animal reservoirs should be destroyed, particularly dogs if emaciated, ill or with sores.

Treatment of all patients renders them non-infective to sandflies. Sufferers from post kala-azar dermal leishmaniasis and diffuse cutaneous leishmaniasis are particularly infectious to sandflies. Such individuals should be sought out, given energetic treatment and be kept under surveillance until cured.

No vaccine has so far been found effective against visceral disease but inoculation of promastigotes from a culture of *L. tropica* will produce a small ulcer and lasting immunity to oriental sore. Individuals so protected have also been found immune to attempted experimental infection with *L. mexicana*. If inoculation is performed on an inconspicuous site, ugly deformity can be averted. Inoculation with *L. mexicana* from culture prevents bay sore. Vaccination campaigns have been undertaken to protect non-immunes entering highly infected areas.

REFERENCES

ADLER, S. and GUNDERS, A. F. (1964) *Trans. roy. Soc. trop. Med. Hyg.*, **58**, 349.
BRAY, R. S. and LAINSON, R. (1965) *Trans. roy. Soc. trop. Med. Hyg.*, **59**, 535.
BRYCESON, A. D. M. (1969) *Trans. roy. Soc. trop. Med. Hyg.*, **63**, 708.
BRYCESON, A. D. M. (1970) *Trans. roy. Soc. trop, Med. Hyg.*, **64**, 369 and 380.
CACHIA, E. A. and FENECH, F. F. (1964) *Trans. roy. Soc. trop. Med. Hyg.*, **58**, 234.
CARTWRIGHT, G. E., CHUNG, HUI-LAN and CHANG, A. (1948) *Blood*, 3, 249.
CHATTERJEE, H. N. (1946) *Trans. roy. Soc. trop. Med. Hyg.*, **39**, 315.
CHUNG, H. L., CHOW, H. K. and LU, J. P. (1948) *Chin. med. J.*, **66**, 325.
CONVIT, J. and KERDEL-VEGAS, F. (1965) *Arch. Dermat.*, **91**, 439.
DUXBURY, R. E. and SADUN, E. H. (1964) *Amer. J. trop. Med. Hyg.*, **13**, 525.
HENDERSON, R. M. (1966). *J. roy. Army med. Cps.*, **112**, 36.
JOPLING, W. H. (1955) *Brit. med J.*, **2**, 1013.
KNIGHT, R., WOODRUFF, A. W. and PETTIT, L. E. (1967) *Trans. roy. Soc. trop. Med. Hyg.*, **61**, 701.
MARTENS, J. M., DE ALENCAR, J. E. and MAGALHÃES, V. B. (1965) *Rev. Inst. Med trop. S. Paulo*, **7**, 47.
MIWA, S. and TANIKAWA, K. (1965) *Rev int. Hépat.*, **15**, 489.
RACHMILEWITZ, M., BRAUN, K. and DE VRIES, A. (1947) *Blood*, **2**, 381.
SHAW, J. J. and VOLLER, A. (1964) *Trans. roy. Soc. trop. Med. Hyg.*, **58**, 349.
SYMMERS, W. ST C (1960) *Lancet*, **1**, 127.
WRIGHT, M. I. (1959) *Brit. med J.*, **1**, 1218.

FURTHER READING

BRAY, R. S. and BRYCESON, A. D. M. (1969) *Trans. roy. Soc. trop. Med. Hyg.*, **63**, 524.
GUNDERS, A. E., NAGGAN, L. and MICHAELI, D. (1972) *Trans. roy. Soc. trop. Med. Hyg.*, **66**, 235.
LAINSON, R. and SHAW, J. J. (1970) *Trans. roy. Soc. trop. Med. Hyg.*, **64**, 645.
WILLIAMS, P. (1970) *Trans. roy. Soc. trop. Med. Hyg.*, **64**, 317.
WORLD HEALTH ORGANIZATION (1969) *Wld. Hlth. Org. Tech. Rep. Ser.*, No. 423.

6
Amoebiasis

Amoebiasis describes the state of an individual who harbours *Entamoeba histolytica* irrespective of the presence or absence of symptoms.

AETIOLOGY

In 1875 Lösch, working in St Petersburg, observed amoebae in the stools of a patient suffering from a dysenteric illness. Succeeding years furnished further evidence of a causal relationship between amoebae and both dysentery and liver abscess culminating in the classical clinical and pathological study of Councilman and Lafleur (1891) in Baltimore which established the relationship beyond reasonable doubt.

A number of species of amoebae inhabit the human bowel, but only *E. histolytica* has been definitely shown to cause disease. Infection by this parasite, however, does not necessarily result in tissue invasion and it may live commensally in the lumen of the colon for long periods without giving rise to symptoms. The factors which cause it to enter the mucosa and destroy tissue are not definitely known but the disease occurs principally among the underprivileged where hygiene is poor and standards of nutrition low.

Infection takes place by swallowing cysts of *E. histolytica* which are circular, measure about 10–20 μm and contain up to four nuclei. In the gut excystation occurs and trophozoites establish themselves in the large bowel. These are actively motile amoebae which reproduce by binary fission. In symptomless infections they measure about 14–25 μm, while larger parasites 30–80 μm in diameter are usually seen in invasive amoebiasis. Under certain conditions trophozoites encyst and these cysts are passed in the faeces. In moist conditions they may survive for long periods to contaminate food or water and thus spread the infection. Patients with active intestinal disease pass trophozoites which only survive for short periods, but those whose infection is chronic and often symptomless pass cysts and are mainly responsible for the dissemination of amoebiasis.

EPIDEMIOLOGY AND DISTRIBUTION

E. histolytica has a world-wide distribution, but clinical manifestations are frequent only in areas where sanitation is poor and the standard of living low. Endemic areas of disease are for the most part in tropical or subtropical regions in Africa, Asia and South America. In communities in which symptomatic amoebiasis is common it is those living unhygienically and on poor diets who suffer most, while those who enjoy a high standard of living are, by comparison, seldom affected. Although it has been estimated that the parasite is present in as many as 5 per cent of the population of countries where the climate is temperate and public health highly developed, manifestations of disease due to the parasite are very rare. Epidemics, however, have been reported from such areas where it was shown that the water supply of those affected had been contaminated by sewage. It seems, then, that the weight of infection or repeated exposure may be important in determining whether tissue invasion will occur, but nutrition and the type of diet have been suggested as factors. As these possible causes usually coexist it is difficult to assess their relative importance.

Since infection with *E. histolytica* can present indefinitely without giving rise to symptoms there is no precise incubation period, but it is known that dysentery may follow infection by as little as 8 days. The interval is usually much longer; probably a month or more.

Symptomatic amoebiasis is commoner in males than in females, in the case of dysentery in the proportion of about 2 : 1 and in hepatic amoebiasis about 7 : 1. Most patients are in the third, fourth and fifth decades. The disease is much less frequent in childhood and then most patients are under the age of 5 years.

PATHOLOGY

When amoebae penetrate the mucosa of the colon a shallow ulcer is produced. If the lesion progresses the muscularis mucosae is penetrated and extension is then in a lateral direction forming the so-called flask-shaped ulcer with a relatively narrow mouth and neck in the mucosa and a much larger cavity undermining the mucosa. In severe cases shaggy sloughs are seen and occasionally tubular mucosal casts several inches long may be passed. Necropsy shows that the caecum is maximally involved and that lesions are nearly always present in the rectum. Occasionally the entire colonic mucosa is affected and rarely the terminal few inches of the ileum. In these extensive and severe cases the wall of the colon may be extremely friable and generalised peritonitis may supervene by seepage of infected material through the bowel wall or, more commonly, from perforation of an ulcer. When adhesions have formed, localised peritonitis may occur and sometimes walled-off abscesses are seen. Blood vessels of sufficient size to cause massive intracolonic haemorrhage may be eroded.

In most cases treatment is followed by healing without scarring, but severe colonic ulceration may give rise to strictures and sometimes a granulomatous reaction with the production of masses projecting into the lumen of the bowel, the so-called amoeboma. Sometimes ulcers fail to heal, leading to ulcerative post-dysenteric colitis.

Parasites which have penetrated the colonic mucosa may gain entrance to blood vessels, when they will be carried to the liver in the portal vein. It seems likely that this is a common occurrence, but the relative infrequency of hepatic amoebiasis compared with colonic infection suggests that they are often unable to survive. However, in the event of their survival and multiplication in liver tissue, cellular necrosis occurs with the formation of an abscess which is an expanding lesion with amoebae at its periphery destroying liver cells and necrotic debris with some exudate in the centre. Necropsy usually shows the abscess contents to be yellowish in colour. When pus is aspirated, however, there is frequently an admixture of blood which gives rise to the classical description of 'anchovy sauce' or 'chocolate' pus. Abscesses are mostly single, occasionally double and rarely multiple. About 90 per cent are in the right lobe of the liver. If untreated they may attain a considerable size: five or more pints of pus have been removed at a single aspiration. They do not provoke fibrous tissue formation and healing leaves little or no scarring.

An amoebic liver abscess may extend beyond the confines of the liver capsule, most commonly forming a right-sided subphrenic abscess. The diaphragm may be penetrated, usually with rupture of the abscess into the lung; sometimes the pleural cavity is involved, producing an amoebic empyema. Rupture into the lung is followed by drainage through the bronchi but pulmonary tissue may be destroyed with the formation of an amoebic lung abscess. Abscesses in the left lobe sometimes extend to the left lung or pleural cavity but may also rupture into the pericardium. After the lung and pleura the next commonest site of rupture is into the peritoneum causing generalised peritonitis, or less frequently a localised abscess. Liver abscesses may, in fact, involve any adjacent organ such as stomach, spleen, kidney and inferior vena cava.

Ulceration of the skin may occur, mostly in the perineal area, but fistulae, liver abscesses rupturing externally or infection of open wounds may rarely initiate the process. Blood-borne infection can reach the brain with abscess formation, or the lung may be involved in areas remote from a sub-diaphragmatic abscess. Ulceration of both male and female genitalia have been reported.

Lesions in tissues are due to trophozoites of *E. histolytica* and cysts are never seen in them.

INTESTINAL AMOEBIASIS

Symptomatology

It must constantly be borne in mind that most infections with *E. histolytica* are symptomless and that when symptoms do occur they are most often those of dysentery. Patients complain of diarrhoea with blood and mucus which is usually of moderate severity. Abdominal discomfort rather than pain is typical and this discomfort may also be felt in the lumbosacral area. Physical examination shows little beyond tenderness, often in both iliac fossae and there may be a low-grade fever. The toxicity and prostration associated with bacillary dysentery are conspicuously absent. This is the characteristic pattern of the disease but occasionally it is much more severe. Diarrhoea is almost continuous, faecal matter soon disappears from the motions, only exudate from the grossly diseased bowel being passed. Abdominal pain is more severe and tenesmus marked. The temperature may be high and dehydration and electrolyte loss are soon prominent features of the illness.

Although dysentery is the usual clinical manifestation of intestinal amoebiasis, patients harbouring the parasite are seen who complain of less well defined symptoms. Vague abdominal discomfort, intermittent diarrhoea, malaise, flatulence and many more are among the complaints listed under the term chronic amoebiasis. It is reasonable to suppose that an infection with *E. histolytica* may produce abdominal symptoms short of dysentery and that they will respond to specific treatment, and this is in accord with clinical experience, but it is not reasonable to attribute a wide range of symptoms remote from the bowel to a colonic infection with *E. histolytica*. Regrettably, this is sometimes done and when the patient fails to improve after specific therapy the conclusion is drawn that the parasites are resistant. Intestinal amoebiasis responds well to appropriate treatment and failure to relieve symptoms should prompt the physician to reconsider his diagnosis as infection with *E. histolytica* may coexist with any other disease, organic or psychogenic. A failure to bear this in mind may result in serious conditions such as carcinoma of the colon being missed.

Complications

Severe dysentery may cause generalised peritonitis either through seepage of infected material through a grossly diseased gut wall or by perforation of an ulcer. The onset is insidious. In an already gravely ill patient pain increases, abdominal distension supervenes and the belly becomes silent. Hiccough may be distressing and is a bad prognostic sign. Diarrhoea in the form of frequent passage of blood-stained exudate continues. Dehydration and electrolyte loss is severe. This type of disease runs a fulminating course with a high mortality. Occasionally peritonitis is localised, usually in the caecal or sigmoid region. There is tenderness and guarding in the affected area and an elongated mass representing thickened colon and adhesions may be felt. An abscess can result.

Following an attack of amoebic dysentery patients may complain of residual abdominal discomfort and intermittent diarrhoea although parasites are no longer present. This has been termed post-dysenteric colitis and is part of the irritable colon syndrome. There is no ulceration of the bowel and the condition is usually temporary. It should be distinguished from the more severe ulcerative post-dysenteric colitis in which although the preceding severe amoebic infection has been controlled, profuse diarrhoea, often with exudate, continues and may last for weeks or even months. The condition of the bowel resembles that seen in non-specific ulcerative colitis but differs in that recovery without relapse is the rule if the patient can be maintained, but there is a tendency to fibrous stricture formation.

The term amoeboma has been used to describe localised masses palpable in the course of the colon and associated with an infection by *E. histolytica*. These are granulomas and may project into the bowel lumen or form at its peritoneal surface in association with a deeply penetrating ulcer. Amoebomas are uncommon; when they occur they are usually a complication of severe dysentery, but may form after mild or even subclinical infections. They give rise to pain and tenderness, can easily be confused with another abdominal mass and their nature is established by evidence of amoebic infection, their rapid disappearance with specific treatment and biopsy when in range of a sigmoidoscope. Laparotomy is sometimes necessary to exclude the possibility of malignancy. Of similar pathogenesis to amoeboma are strictures which may occur anywhere in the course of the colon and cause considerable narrowing of the bowel lumen. In the rectum they can be felt and seen through the sigmoidoscope; in other areas they are demonstrable by barium enema. It is very unusual for these to cause obstruction and they respond to specific treatment although this may be a very slow process.

Intussusception, usually caeco-colic may complicate intestinal amoebiasis. An amoeboma may constitute the apex of the intussusception, but often it seems that thickening of the colonic wall is sufficient to cause this rather rare event. Its presence is suggested by a complaint of abdominal colic and examination shows an 'empty' left iliac fossa and a sausage-shaped mass in the course of the ascending or transverse colon. Periodic examination shows this to be moving and its nature is confirmed by radiological examination after a barium enema. These intussusceptions may reduce spontaneously or, indeed, appear and disappear alternately, but laparotomy is frequently necessary.

Erosion of a blood vessel by an amoebic ulcer may cause profuse haemorrhage into the colon requiring blood transfusion repeated until the bleeding stops.

A rare complication is the formation of fistulae, usually between colon and small bowel, by extension of an ulcer. Continued diarrhoea following treatment may arouse suspicion and suggest barium studies.

Rectal prolapse may occur in the course of severe dysentery and require repeated replacement. Ischio-rectal abscess perhaps occurs with undue frequency in patients with intestinal amoebiasis.

Diagnosis

Identification of the parasite is the cornerstone of diagnosis. In asymptomatic amoebiasis it will be found, usually in the form of cysts, in stools. If there is coincident diarrhoea trophozoites may be seen and these will not contain red blood corpuscles. Material should be examined directly in a drop of saline on a slide under a coverslip. Gram's iodine should be added to facilitate the finding of cysts and the search should always include a flotation method such as that with zinc sulphate. When difficulty in identification of amoebae occurs, stained preparations must be examined. In invasive amoebiasis examination of exudate on a slide in saline will usually reveal haematophagous trophozoites of *E. histolytica*. The presence of red blood corpuscles in the cytoplasm of the parasite is good evidence that the mucosa has been invaded.

Sigmoidoscopy is of value in identifying ulcers, granulomas or strictures and for obtaining exudate from ulcers for microscopy or biopsy material for histology. Beyond defaecation immediately prior to examination no preparation is required if the knee-elbow position is used. After the anal sphincter is passed the obturator is removed and the instrument passed under direct vision. In severe cases great care must be exercised as the wall of the colon may be very friable. In amoebic dysentery of average severity the mucosa appears red and oedematous and ulcers with irregular edges are seen which may be covered by yellowish exudate or have red granular bases. When exudate is present some should be removed with biopsy forceps for examination in saline; in its absence the base of the ulcer should be gently scraped to obtain material for microscopy. In typical cases one may say with some confidence that the abnormalities of the mucosa are due to amoebiasis, but there is a wide range and it may not be possible to differentiate from other dysenteric diseases on appearance alone. The great importance of the examination is that it provides an opportunity for obtaining material for microscopic examination in which, in the presence of ulceration, parasites can nearly always be demonstrated if untreated amoebiasis is the cause. The presence of very small mucosal pits and craters should be interpreted with reserve as it seems unlikely that they are strong diagnostic evidence of amoebiasis.

Anaemia is not a usual feature of invasive intestinal amoebiasis but about three quarters have a moderate leucocytosis. Of the serological tests available the gel diffusion precipitin method has given reliable results. It has been found to be positive in up to 40 per cent of cases of asymptomatic amoebiasis and in about 90 per cent of patients with amoebic dysentery. It is well to remember that such a test is evidence of past or present infection with *E. histolytica*, but not proof that present symptoms are necessarily due to this parasite.

Radiology plays no part in the diagnosis of the usual case of invasive intestinal amoebiasis but examination after a barium enema is necessary for the demonstration of strictures and amoebomas when these are beyond the reach of the sigmoidoscope. It will also confirm the presence of an intussusception and may demonstrate fistulae between large and small bowel as may a barium meal and 'follow-through' examination.

Differential diagnosis

When amoebiasis presents as dysentery it must be distinguished from other causes of this symptom and this can usually be done by the demonstration of actively motile haematophagous trophozoites of *E. histolytica* in stools or material obtained at sigmoidoscopy. Invasive intestinal amoebiasis can coexist with other dysenteric colonic disease, and failure of symptoms to respond to treatment when amoebae have disappeared from the stools should arouse the strongest suspicion of the presence of other disease.

The onset of bacillary dysentery tends to be more acute than amoebiasis, there is usually more systemic upset, stools contain more pus, there is no leucocytosis and shigellae can be grown on culture. In some reported series of amoebic dysentery a shigella has been isolated in about 5 per cent of cases and treatment for both conditions has been necessary. It is perhaps fortunate that tetracycline controls both diseases.

Infection with *Schistosoma mansoni* may cause diarrhoea with blood and mucus. This is usually a rather chronic condition, the appearance of the rectum is more granular than in amoebiasis and ova of *S. mansoni* can be found in rectal snips if not in the stools. In areas where schistosomiasis is endemic it is common to find ova in cases with colonic ulceration and demonstrable haematophagous trophozoites of *E. histolytica* in stools or scrapings from ulcers. In such patients it is almost invariably the amoebiasis which is causing the symptoms and specific anti-amoebic treatment will relieve them, the schistosomiasis being an asymptomatic infection.

Uncommon causes of dysentery such as infection with *Balantidium coli* or *Trichuris trichiura* in children and the mentally retarded can easily be distinguished by the presence of the causative organism and the absence of amoebae.

Non-specific ulcerative colitis can be confused with amoebic dysentery when the patient happens to have a coincident infection with *E. histolytica*. Under these circumstances the amoebiasis should be treated and lack of response should be one of the factors pointing to the correct diagnosis. Others are the appearance of the mucosa at sigmoidoscopy (amoebiasis seldom produces the velvety red mucosa of ulcerative colitis) and the characteristic radiological signs of the latter disease. It is perhaps more difficult to separate non-specific ulcerative colitis from ulcerative post-dysenteric colitis, but, in the latter, there will be the history of an attack of amoebic dysentery, the gel diffusion precipitin test will be positive and there will not be the same tendency to recurrence.

When intestinal amoebiasis causes rather non-specific abdominal symptoms without dysentery there is a very wide differential diagnosis which includes psychosomatic conditions. The main point of differentiation is that appropriate treatment will cure invasive amoebiasis. Its failure, when amoebae have been eradicated as they almost always can be, points to the presence of another malady.

The important condition to distinguish from amoeboma and colonic stricture is carcinoma. When the lesion lies in the lower sigmoid colon or rectum, histological examination of biopsy material will establish the diagnosis. When these narrowings or masses are more proximal, the radiological appearance of the barium-filled bowel are not diagnostic and laparatomy may be necessary. Where there is good evidence of invasive intestinal amoebiasis a trial of specific treatment is justified as an amoeboma may disappear with surprising rapidity, but in endemic areas it is not rare for patients with a carcinoma to have an infection with *E. histolytica* and failure of treatment completely to relieve symptoms and to restore the bowel to clinical and radiological normality should lead to laparotomy lest a carcinoma, amenable to surgical cure, be missed.

After the establishment of the amoebic aetiology of so-called tropical abscess of the liver at the end of the last century our knowledge of its clinical manifestations and treatment grew rapidly, largely due to the work of Sir Leonard Rogers which he summarised in his Lettsomian Lectures for 1922. Today liver abscess caused by *E. histolytica* is accepted by all, but there is still some controversy over other possible hepatic lesions due to this parasite.

HEPATIC AMOEBIASIS

Symptomatology

During an attack of amoebic dysentery the liver may be palpable and a little tender although a liver abscess is not present. If the intestinal amoebiasis is controlled by a drug, such as tetracycline, which has no action on amoebae in the liver, the hepatomegaly will regress and the tenderness disappear. The cause of this phenomenon is not known, but it has been suggested that it is a non-specific reaction due to substances or bacteria carried to the liver by the blood stream from an ulcerated gut. It is not amoebic hepatitis in the sense in which this term has been used.

The term amoebic hepatitis was introduced to describe a presuppurative phase in the formation of a liver abscess. This was a postulate, not based on a description of observed histological changes, and it came to mean a diffuse inflammatory reaction to amoebae scattered through hepatic tissue. The existence of such a condition was postulated to explain the clinical phenomenon of an acutely enlarged tender liver in which pus was not demonstrated, and probably represents early abscess formation. Unfortunately this concept has been extended to include patients who complain of chronic discomfort in the right hypochrondrium and who may have a slightly enlarged and tender liver. There is no convincing pathological proof that such an entity is due to invasion of the liver by *E. histolytica*; in fact, neither the study of the liver from patients dying of amoebic dysentery nor examination of material obtained by liver biopsy from patients who clinically appeared to have this condition showed any evidence of diffuse amoebic hepatitis. Either the liver was normal or an abscess was found. It is known that amoebic liver abscesses may resolve on specific treatment without drainage or rupture. The only lesion due to the presence of amoebae for which there is sound clinical and pathological evidence is an abscess. For these reasons the existence of diffuse amoebic hepatitis should be doubted and the following account of hepatic amoebiasis refers to amoebic liver abscess.

About half the patients suffering from an amoebic abscess of the liver give a previous history of dysentery. A small number develop abscesses during an attack of clinically overt invasive intestinal amoebiasis, but a substantial proportion have no history of infection so that amoebae may reach the liver during subclinical bowel infections.

The cardinal symptom of hepatic amoebiasis is pain, which is present in about 99 per cent of cases. It is usually felt in the right hypochondrium and right lower chest, but may be epigastric or even left-sided when the abscess is in the left lobe of the liver. The pain is continuous, may be severe and is made worse by jarring and sometimes by breathing or coughing. Quite frequently it is referred to the right shoulder or neck; rarely it is felt in the left shoulder. The patient may notice a mass in the right hypochondrium or epigastrium. Cough and non-specific diarrhoea are fairly common symptoms. In long-standing infections anorexia and weight loss may be prominent. Most patients seek medical attention within 2 weeks of the onset of their symptoms, but occasionally these are of several months' duration.

Eighty per cent of patients are febrile, the temperature usually ranging between 100° and 102°F (38° and 39°C). High fever is not particularly common. Except in long-standing or neglected cases when there may be emaciation, severe anaemia and swelling of the legs, the general condition of the patient is good. Jaundice occurs in less than 2 per cent of patients. A mass is sometimes seen in the right hypochondrium or epigastrium and the right lower chest is occasionally bulging. Such masses can be felt as smooth exquisitely tender swellings on the surface of or continuous with an enlarged tender liver. Irrespective of the occasional presence of such localised swelling the liver is enlarged, smooth, firm and tender in three-quarters of all cases and an area of localised extreme tenderness frequently overlies the abscess. Gentle pressure with the fingertips between the right lower ribs causes pain in over 90 per cent of patients and this intercostal tenderness is a very useful sign. Its location is valuable evidence of the site of the abscess. An amoebic liver abscess causes elevation of the right dome of the diaphragm in 60 per cent of cases and clinically this is reflected by diminished vocal fremitus, an impaired percussion note and diminished air-entry at the right lung base. Crepitations may be heard and occasionally a pleural rub. Rarely such signs are found on the left. Except for the occasional atypical case these symptoms and signs constitute a very characteristic clinical picture, and if the condition is kept in mind diagnostic errors should be few.

Complications

Most of these arise from extension to other organs and the commonest is rupture into the lung with the formation of a hepato-bronchial fistula and the expectoration of the abscess contents. There are usually, but not always, symptoms and signs due to the presence of the liver abscess itself followed often by a small haemoptysis and then the production of sputum which may be copious. This sputum has a characteristic appearance being reddish brown in colour and resembling the 'anchovy sauce' pus so frequently aspirated from liver abscesses. The signs of an elevated right hemidiaphragm are usually present and crepitations may be prominent, but occasionally these are surprisingly inconspicuous. Rarely these events occur on the left side. More uncommonly still bile-stained sputum may be expectorated. Sometimes the lung parenchyma is more extensively involved and the presentation is that of a rather chronic right basal pneumonia. Breakdown of tissue may occur with the formation of a lung abscess.

If the pleural surfaces have not become adherent a subdiaphragmatic liver abscess may rupture directly into the pleural cavity with the formation of an amoebic empyema. Very rarely there is sudden flooding of the pleura with a large quantity of pus causing profound shock and even sudden death; usually, however, such patients present with the signs of a pleural effusion and a history of insidious onset. There may be a history or signs suggestive of the underlying liver abscess, but the diagnosis is made by the aspiration of characteristic pus. A subphrenic amoebic liver abscess may cause a pleural reaction without frank rupture which leads to accumulation of straw-coloured fluid with a high protein content in the pleural cavity. This can be a prelude to empyema.

Generalised peritonitis results from the rupture of a liver abscess into the peritoneal cavity. In most cases this is an acute episode and the patient gives a history of sudden very severe pain, possibly preceded by symptoms suggestive of hepatic abscess. The signs are those of an 'acute abdomen' and laparotomy is necessary for both therapeutic and diagnostic reasons. Much less commonly liver abscesses leak into the peritoneum to produce walled-off abscesses. Rarely a chronic generalised peritonitis with adhesions and many loculated collections of pus occurs. The abdomen has the 'doughy' feel characteristic of tuberculous peritonitis but signs referable to the liver may point to the diagnosis.

Abscesses in the left lobe of the liver can involve the pericardium. A pericardial rub may be the only sign, or a straw-coloured pericardial effusion with or without signs of tamponade may occur, or the abscess may rupture into the pericardium producing purulent amoebic pericarditis. These events can succeed one another, the first two sometimes giving a timely warning of an impending and most serious complication. Rupture of an abscess into the pericardium causes central chest pain and there may be grave shock and even sudden death, but more often the onset is insidious and the patient presents with symptoms and signs of cardiac tamponade. The jugular venous pressure is raised, there is pulsus paradoxus, the blood pressure is low with a small pulse pressure, cardiac dullness is increased and the heart sounds are faint. Signs of a liver abscess may or may not be present and, moreover, eliciting them is difficult because the liver is frequently enlarged and tender due to increased venous pressure. Oedema of the legs and sacrum may develop and there may be ascites and pleural effusions.

The foregoing complications occur with some frequency but there are records in the literature of amoebic liver abscesses extending to involve gut, stomach, renal pelvis, spleen and inferior vena cava. A diagnosis is only made if symptoms and signs draw attention to the liver abscess, at laparotomy or at post-mortem. A liver abscess may precipitate thrombosis of the portal vein. External rupture can be the cause of cutaneous amoebiasis.

The great majority of amoebic liver abscesses are bacteriologically sterile, but bacteria may be introduced at aspiration, from the blood stream, through external rupture or from extension into the gut. When this occurs the temperature persists despite adequate treatment for the hepatic amoebiasis and the character of the pus removed by aspiration changes to a yellow or greenish colour and is frequently foul-smelling.

Diagnosis

Anaemia is common, particularly in long-standing cases. It is normocytic normochromic or normocytic and hypothromic. As in anaemia found with other infections the hypochromia does not indicate iron deficiency. It is usually of moderate degree but occasionally the haemoglobin may be as low as 3 or 4 g/100 ml. In 75 per cent of cases there is a leucocytosis and the erythrocyte sedimentation rate is almost invariably raised.

The amoebic gel diffusion precipitin test is positive in about 98 per cent of patients so that a negative result casts very serious doubt on a clinical diagnosis of liver abscess.

Postero-anterior and right lateral radiographs often give considerable diagnostic help. The right dome of the diaphragm is raised in more than 50 per cent of patients and there are often areas of discoid atelectasis in the lower lobe of the lung. The lateral film is helpful in localising the abscess. Rarely the changes are seen on the left side. When a hepatobronchial fistula is present there are usually changes in the right lower lung field but sometimes these are surprisingly slight. In endemic areas shadowing at the right base with or without elevation of the diaphragm should always arouse the suspicion of amoebiasis. Radiographs of the chest confirm the presence of pleural effusions, show lung abscesses and demonstrate enlargement of the heart shadow in pericardial effusions. Screening of the chest in liver abscess may show absent or diminished movement of the diaphragm and is of value in confirming that an enlarged cardiac outline is due to pericardial effusion as pulsation is commonly absent.

Electrocardiography provides evidence of pericarditis but has no features characteristic of amoebiasis.

It is sometimes very difficult to distinguish between primary lung disease and pulmonary changes secondary to an amoebic liver abscess. Help can be obtained by radiography after the introduction of carbon dioxide into the peritoneal cavity which outlines the upper surface of the liver and demonstrates the extension of an hepatic lesion to involve the diaphragm. Radiographs of the barium-filled stomach may show an indentation of its outline due to an adjacent liver abscess and is thus of value in localising the lesion.

Scintillation scanning of the liver following the administration of an isotope such as radioactive rose Bengal which is taken up by liver cells will demonstrate the site of liver abscesses, if of sufficient size, as these lesions do not take up the dye. In practice this examination only occasionally gives information which cannot be obtained by clinical means.

Aspiration of liver abscesses is a therapeutic procedure and should not be done unless the indications detailed in the section on treatment are present, but when a clinical diagnosis of hepatic amoebiasis has been made and aspiration of its contents is appropriate therapeutically, it will provide proof of the diagnosis. The pus withdrawn is very often characteristic. It is a rather glutinous brownish-red fluid with a slight musty but not unpleasant odour. Occasionally it is

I

yellow or green in colour and sometimes there is considerable admixture of blood. If pus is withdrawn before beginning specific drug therapy, which should be done, since there is no added risk in the procedure, *E. histolytica* can be identified in over 80 per cent of cases. In addition to direct examination, pus should also be cultured to exclude the presence of bacterial infection. Similar characteristic pus is obtained in amoebic empyema and suppurative pericarditis. When spread to the lungs is suspected, fresh specimens of sputum should be examined for the presence of *E. histolytica* before initiating treatment. It must be borne in mind that the common buccal commensal, *E. gingivalis*, may be seen in sputum but it can readily be distinguished from *E. histolytica* by an experienced observer.

Differential diagnosis

Conditions which cause enlargement and tenderness of the liver may simulate amoebic liver abscess and here serology, when it is available, can be of considerable help. A negative gel diffusion precipitin test goes far towards excluding hepatic amoebiasis as it is positive in so high a proportion of cases. Positive reactions may, however, be found in other diseases when there is, or has recently been a coincidental infection with *E. histolytica*.

Cirrhosis of the liver seldom causes as much tenderness as liver abscess, there is usually less fever, signs of increased portal pressure may be present, the spleen is often felt and there is seldom elevation of the right dome of the diaphragm. Liver function tests tend to be deranged in cirrhosis while they remain relatively normal in abscess. It may be very difficult to distinguish between a hepatoma and liver abscess. A localised very tender hepatic mass may be present in both, as may elevation of the right dome of the diaphragm. Masses tend to feel harder in new growth and jaundice is much commoner. Doubt can sometimes only be resolved by liver biopsy, which is safer than attempted aspiration as the latter procedure can lead to serious haemorrhage if the lesion proves to be a carcinoma. Infectious hepatitis seldom causes confusion as the onset with dyspeptic symptoms, the presence of jaundice, absence of leucocytosis and changes in liver function tests are all unlike liver abscess. Hydatid cysts are less tender, a thrill may be present, eosinophilia is frequent and immunological tests may be positive—if there is serious doubt it is safer to establish the diagnosis by laparotomy than to attempt aspiration. Pyogenic abscesses

may closely resemble the amoebic variety and can sometimes only be distinguished by the character of the aspirated pus. *Ascaris lumbricoides* may enter the liver along the bile ducts and lead to the formation of abscesses; jaundice is common and the abscess contents are not like those of an amoebic lesion.

Provided that the possibility of underlying liver abscess is kept in mind as a cause of pulmonary disease, the correct diagnosis will usually be made. Occasionally, however, only a trial of specific treatment demonstrates the probable aetiology by causing the resolution of a lesion which has been refractory to antibiotics. The character of the pus withdrawn from the pleura suggests the diagnosis, but it can sometimes be confirmed by the demonstration of amoebae. The amoebic aetiology of a serous pericardial effusion which occasionally is bloodstained can only be suspected if the history and physical signs indicate a liver abscess, but failure to make the diagnosis and give specific treatment will often lead to frank rupture of the abscess into the pericardium and characteristic pus will be withdrawn in which amoebae may be found.

Rarely amoebic liver abscesses cause neither pain nor hepatic tenderness and thus fall into the differential diagnosis of pyrexia of unknown origin. Sometimes anaemia is the only sign. A past history of dysentery, leucocytosis and positive serology may point to their presence and specific therapy may produce cure, but laparotomy should not be too long delayed as these abscesses can declare themselves by rupture, possibly with serious results.

AMOEBIASIS OF OTHER ORGANS

Cutaneous amoebiasis, while uncommon, usually extends from the anus to the perineum in patients with a bowel infection, but may result from a liver abscess rupturing externally or extending subcutaneously, from faecal fistulae and surgical wounds when specific therapy has not been given. It has been recorded following a burn. The lesion is an ulcer with undulating slightly undermined edges and a granulomatous base thinly covered with a grey-green exudate. Much sero-sanguineous fluid may exude from these ulcers and without treatment they can spread very widely. *E. histolytica* may be found in the exudate and histological examination of a biopsy specimen shows amoebae in the tissues.

Amoebae may be carried in the blood stream to the brain, where an abscess forms containing pinkish necrotic material. In most instances a liver abscess has been present but this can be a complication of intestinal amoebiasis. The condition may be suspected when a patient known to be suffering from invasive amoebiasis develops cerebral symptoms. The cerebrospinal fluid shows a rise in protein and a pleocytosis. Hitherto, amoebic brain abscesses have invariably proved fatal and their confirmation has been at necropsy.

Ulceration of both male and female genitalia due to infection with *E. histolytica* has been recorded by a number of observers. These ulcers have been seen on the glans penis, vulva, vagina and cervix uteri and their nature established by examination of biopsy material.

E. histolytica has been found in the urine and its presence there is due either to fistulae between bladder and infected bowel or rupture of a liver abscess into the renal pelvis. Infection of the urinary tract does not persist unless an intestinal or hepatic source is maintained.

The term primary pulmonary amoebiasis has been used to describe lung lesions in the absence of direct spread from a liver abscess. They are not in fact primary as an intestinal infection still precedes them. Lung lesions without evidence of the presence of a liver abscess are very rare, but there have been some well-documented examples.

A large number of conditions including arthritis, bronchitis, nephritis, dermatitis and urticaria have been attributed to infection with *E. histolytica*, but the evidence is unconvincing and they should not be included in the symptomatology of amoebiasis.

AMOEBIASIS IN CHILDHOOD

Although similar, there are some differences between the manifestations of amoebiasis in the young and in adults. In children it is a more acute disease; the rather vague symptoms associated with the term chronic amoebiasis have very seldom been reported. The sex incidence of both intestinal and hepatic disease is equal. Amoebic liver abscess has a more fulminant course and the prognosis is much more serious.

The same drugs may be used for treatment with suitable reduction in dosage.

TREATMENT

A great many drugs are available for the treatment of amoebiasis, and particularly among those acting in the bowel lumen there is considerable room for personal preference. In the following account a relatively small number has been selected on the basis of efficacy, safety and tolerance, in an attempt to present a simple and effective scheme of management. Omission does not necessarily imply lack of therapeutic effect.

Emetine. Ipecacuanha was used during the nineteenth century to treat dysentery and tropical abscess, but its value in amoebiasis was not at once fully appreciated because of failure to distinguish this condition from bacillary dysentery. In 1912 Vedder showed that its derivative emetine was amoebicidal and, in India in the same year, Rogers successfully treated both hepatic and intestinal amoebiasis with emetine hydrochloride. Emetine hydrochloride is given by intramuscular or subcutaneous injection in a dose of 1 mg per kg body weight per day for 10 days. The daily dose should not exceed 60 mg. It is rapidly absorbed from the site of administration and concentrated in the tissues, particularly the lungs and liver where it is actively amoebicidal. It is slowly excreted and thus cumulative.

Emetine is a striated muscle poison and reaches a sufficient concentration in the myocardium to produce electrocardiographic changes in a substantial proportion of patients. These are mainly flattening or inversion of T waves, but widening of the QRS complex and a variety of arrhythmias may be produced in susceptible individuals. Sinus tachycardia is the earliest sign of toxicity and hypotension is quite frequent. Weakness of skeletal muscle sometimes occurs (usually with overdosage) and nausea and vomiting may be caused by a central mechanism. Emetine is an irritant and can cause pain and even necrosis with the formation of sterile abscesses at the site of injection.

Despite the foregoing rather formidable catalogue of toxic actions emetine is, in practice, a safe and reliable drug provided appropriate care is taken during its administration. It remains the most effective tissue amoebicide which can be given parenterally. Suitable reduction in dosage must be made for the young, the elderly and the underweight. When possible, it should be avoided during pregnancy. Patients receiving emetine should be kept in bed but allowed toilet privileges and the pulse rate must be watched because a progressive rise which cannot be accounted for by the disease is an indication for stopping the drug. The presence of heart disease is a relative contraindication to its use. Strenuous exertion should be forbidden for a month after a course.

Emetine finds its greatest use for the treatment of liver disease and other tissue lesions. Alone it is inadequate for dysentery because it will destroy amoebae in the bowel lumen in only about 50 per cent of cases.

Recently dehydroemetine has been introduced. It is a synthetic preparation which is more rapidly excreted than emetine hydrochloride, and although its pharmacological properties are similar it is probably less toxic. The dose is 1.5 mg per kg body weight per day by intramuscular injection for 10 days. It is unnecessary to exceed a daily dose of 80 mg. Dehydroemetine has been shown to be, therapeutically, as effective as emetine hydrochloride and is now to be preferred. The same precautions should be observed during its administration and it has the same therapeutic indications.

Chloroquine (Aralen, Nivaquine, Resochin), an antimalarial, is also of value in the treatment of hepatic amoebiasis. It is given by mouth in the form of the sulphate or phosphate in a dose of 600 mg of the base *statim*, followed by 300 mg 6 hours later and then 150 mg twice daily for 28 days. Serious toxicity like ocular damage should not occur with such short courses, but nausea and vomiting can be troublesome. They are, however, usually temporary and can be controlled by anti-emetics when the drug may be continued without further gastric intolerance. This drug is of no value in the treatment of intestinal amoebiasis as it is rapidly absorbed and concentrated in the liver. Used alone it is inferior to emetine, but the two drugs used together are very effective and this regimen obviated the necessity for a second course of emetine which would otherwise be necessary.

Metronidazole (Flagyl) is a very recent addition to the drugs used for amoebiasis. It is unique in that it is effective in both hepatic and intestinal forms, appears to be devoid of serious toxicity and is well tolerated. Its main disadvantage seems to be that it cannot be given parenterally. Evidence for its efficacy in the treatment of all the complications of intestinal and hepatic amoebiasis is not yet available, but it seems likely that it will become the drug of choice whenever oral medication can be used in the treatment of all forms of amoebiasis.

Metronidazole is well absorbed and reaches the liver and other tissues. Probably because the quantity in the lumen of the gut is small it must be given in high doses for intestinal amoebiasis. In amoebic dysentery 800 mg thrice daily for 5 days is effective. For hepatic disease a single dose of 2.4 g or 400 mg thrice daily for 5 days is adequate. Clearly, if invasive intestinal amoebiasis and liver abscess are to be treated in the same patient the higher dose must be used. There is occasionally some gastrointestinal intolerance.

Tetracycline. A large number of antibiotics have some therapeutic effect in amoebic dysentery but tetracycline, chlortetracycline and oxytetracycline are much the most effective. It is worth noting that dimethylchlortetracycline is relatively inactive, and that antibiotics are of no value whatever in amoebic liver abscess.

Tetracycline is not directly amoebicidal and is thought to work in amoebic dysentery by modifying the bowel flora which are necessary for the growth and multiplication of *E. histolytica*. In a dose of 250 mg 6 hourly for 10 days it is a very effective remedy for amoebic dysentery but a tissue amoebicide should be given as well to prevent hepatic disease.

Diiodohydroxyquinoline (Diodoquin, Embequin, Savorquin, Yadoxin) is given by mouth in a dose of 600 mg thrice daily for 20 days. It is not absorbed and is practically devoid of side actions. Used alone it may suffice for the treatment of asymptomatic amoebiasis, is inadequate for amoebic dysentery but is useful in combination with other remedies because of its activity in the lumen of the gut.

Diloxanide furoate (Furamide), although absorbed, seems to be most useful in the treatment of asymptomatic and chronic intestinal disease. It is inadequate, alone, for acute amoebic dysentery and has no value in hepatic amoebiasis. The dose is 0.5 g thrice daily for 10 days. It is non-toxic but mild gastrointestinal intolerance has been reported.

MANAGEMENT OF INTESTINAL AMOEBIASIS

Particularly in endemic areas, asymptomatic bowel infections should be treated. A non-toxic preparation such as diiodohydroxyquinoline or diloxanide furoate should be used and the stools examined after treatment and then at monthly intervals for 2 months to ensure that cure has been achieved. In the event of failure the preparation not used in the first instance should be tried.

For the efficient treatment of invasive intestinal amoebiasis, amoebae must be killed both in the wall and in the lumen of the bowel; in addition, liver involvement must be prevented or controlled. These ends may be achieved in several different ways and the following drug regimens will be found adequate for the management of the great majority of patients:

A. *Metronidazole* 800 mg thrice daily for 5–10 days.

B. *Tetracycline* 250 mg 6 hourly for 10 days. *Diiodohydroxyquinoline* or *diloxanide furoate* in the doses recommended above.

Chloroquine 150 mg of base twice daily for 15 days.

The three drugs are started concurrently.

C. *Dehydroemetine* for 10 days.
Tetracycline for 10 days.
Diiodohydroxyquinoline or *diloxanide*.
The drugs are given together.

An attack of amoebic dysentery of average severity will respond to any of the above schedules, the cure rate being over 95 per cent. Regimens A and B have the advantage of avoiding injections and can be given to ambulant patients. In the unusual event of parasitic cure not being achieved with one schedule, an amoebicide, not already given, should be tried. The symptoms will determine whether hospitalisation or domiciliary care is appropriate. Diet does not seem important and, if need be, a drug such as codeine phosphate can be given to control diarrhoea in the early stages.

When amoebic dysentery is very severe and there is distension of the abdomen, oral remedies are not practicable since it is necessary to use a nasogastric tube and suction for decompression. Dehydroemetine and parenteral tetracycline are given under these circumstances. Dehydration and electrolyte loss must be corrected by intravenous fluids and these must be continued while gastric suction is necessary and copious diarrhoea persists. If peritonitis supervenes, nothing is gained by surgery as the colon is too friable to repair and a drain confers no benefit. The treatment for such patients is the same as for severe dysentery. Hiccough usually responds well to chlorpromazine.

It is these seriously ill patients that tend to suffer from ulcerative post-dysenteric colitis. Here, although dysentery or diarrhoea persist, parasitic clearance has been achieved and repeated courses of amoebicides are useless unless stool examination, which should be done at weekly intervals, shows the presence of *E. histolytica*. Patients suffering from ulcerative post-dysenteric colitis should receive as high a calorie diet as possible, parenteral fluids may be necessary and drugs such as codeine phosphate sometimes control the diarrhoea to some extent. A course of an insoluble sulphonamide may help. Both local and systemic steroids have been tried but are often disappointingly ineffective. The condition is a temporary one and, if the patient can be maintained on conservative treatment, recovery without relapse is the rule. For this reason radical surgery such as colectomy is almost invariably contraindicated.

Amoebomas and strictures should be treated with dehydroemetine, tetracycline and diiodohydroxyquinoline or diloxanide furoate. Amoebomas may regress and disappear with surprising speed, but strictures can sometimes persist for long periods. When *E. histolytica* can no longer be demonstrated, repeated courses of amoebicides do not accelerate regression. Obstruction by strictures is very rare and surgery seldom necessary.

Massive haemorrhage into the colon is treated by blood transfusion and the appropriate amoebicides. Very large quantities of blood are sometimes required. Surgical treatment is not indicated.

It has been pointed out that an intussusception may reduce spontaneously, but waiting for this event must not be prolonged as the blood supply of the bowel is threatened and surgical reduction often necessary.

All patients who have suffered an attack of invasive intestinal amoebiasis should be kept under out-patient surveillance for a period of 2 months after apparent cure as 'parasitic relapse' may occur. Stools should be examined after treatment and at monthly intervals as the reappearance of parasites often heralds symptomatic relapse and treatment must be given to eradicate *E. histolytica*.

Despite apparently successful treatment it sometimes happens that patients suffer a number of recrudescences of their intestinal amoebiasis. It should not be assumed that these are necessarily relapses as repeated reinfection may be the cause. A contaminated food or water supply may be the reason and if these seem blameless, stools from the other members of the household should be examined lest one or more of them have asymptomatic amoebiasis.

MANAGEMENT OF HEPATIC AMOEBIASIS AND ITS COMPLICATIONS

Emetine, metronidazole and chloroquine are effective in the liver; the other drugs previously listed are not. Metronidazole can be used alone and if given in a dose of 800 mg thrice daily for 5 days it will also control coincident intestinal amoebiasis. When given in one of the recommended lower dosages it should be combined with diiodohydroxyquinoline or diloxanide furoate, and if dysentery is present tetracycline should be given as well. A course of dehydroemetine 80 mg daily for 10 days combined with chloroquine, 600 mg of the base *statim* then 300 mg 6 hours later followed by 150 mg twice daily for 28 days is curative for hepatic disease, but diiodohydroxyquinoline or diloxanide furoate should be added to control intestinal infection, and tetracycline is also required if the patient suffers from dysentery.

Some patients with an amoebic liver abscess will respond to drug therapy alone, but the majority require drainage of the pus by aspiration, the indications for which are as follows: the presence of a visible or palpable, tender mass; an enlarged liver over the surface of which there is a localised area of exquisite tenderness; localised severe intercostal tenderness; signs of a markedly raised diaphragm. Under these circumstances aspiration can be done immediately before starting specific therapy as *E. histolytica* can then frequently be found in the pus, but it sometimes happens that indications for aspiration only appear some days after initiating drug therapy. Less commonly still, although there is no localised tenderness, patients fail to respond fully to drug treatment. A search for pus can then be made with the aspirating needle which is best introduced through the ninth intercostal space in the mid or anterior axillary line. Experience has shown that this closed drainage by means of aspiration is preferable to open surgical drainage as the mortality is lower and there is less chance of introducing bacterial infection. Surgical intervention in amoebic liver abscess is seldom necessary, the main indications being inability to find pus or failure of response despite repeated (about five) aspirations.

Aspiration is done with a syringe through a wide-bore needle after the injection of local anaesthetic. A two-way tap facilitates the procedure. As much pus as possible should be withdrawn. It usually leads to considerable lessening of pain and tenderness and should be repeated if local tenderness or swelling recurs and in any case if more than 250 ml of pus have been withdrawn. Failure to obtain pus should not lead to frequently repeated attempts at many different sites, the needle being introduced in various directions; it is better to resort to laparotomy if there are clinical indications that pus is present which cannot readily be withdrawn by aspiration.

Specific drug treatment and aspiration are the most important factors in treatment, but severe anaemia must be corrected by the transfusion of packed cells and in the first few days many patients will require analgesics. When assessing cure it must be remembered that the diaphragm may remain elevated for months and that this does not necessarily indicate persistence of an active abscess. Following aspiration of subcostal abscesses an area of induration may persist for weeks. With the above methods of treatment,

failure in uncomplicated cases is very rare. If relapse occurs it is nearly always within 2 months and is usually due to inadequate drainage. For this reason patients should be seen twice at monthly intervals following their discharge from hospital.

When amoebic liver abscesses rupture into the lung, drainage through the bronchi is usually adequate and should be assisted by posture and physiotherapy. Specific drug treatment should, of course, be given. This also produces resolution of lung abscess.

Amoebic empyema requires treatment with emetine and chloroquine (the place of metronidazole has not yet been established) and repeated aspiration of as much pus as possible at intervals if not more than 48 hours. If large quantities of pus are still being withdrawn after about a week or there are still radiological signs of a considerable effusion, drainage through an in-dwelling tube introduced intercostally must be considered. There may be considerable residual pleural thickening, but serial radiology over a period of months shows that this will eventually resolve.

When a liver abscess ruptures into the peritoneum and presents the clinical picture of an 'acute abdomen', laparotomy should be undertaken without delay after resuscitation if this is indicated. Laparotomy is necessary because it is very difficult to make a confident clinical diagnosis and it enables pus to be removed from the peritoneal cavity. As soon as the diagnosis is known, dehydroemetine must be given and chloroquine added when the patient can take oral medication. Chronic peritonitis is treated conservatively although sometimes laparotomy is necessary to establish the diagnosis. Localised intraperitoneal abscesses should be drained.

When amoebic pericarditis presents with a rub or a serous effusion treatment is by drainage of the liver abscess (by aspiration if possible, by surgery if not) and the administration of dehydroemetine and chloroquine. Purulent pericarditis requires, in addition to these drugs, relief of cardiac tamponade by frequent pericardial aspiration. It is customary to give digitalis, and diuretics are useful to control oedema. Surgical drainage is contraindicated and conservative measures must be persevered with as the natural history of this condition is for complete resolution to occur even after signs of constriction have been present for many weeks. Pericardectomy should only be undertaken when it seems that the patient's life is threatened by progressive cardiac embarrassment.

Secondary infection of liver abscesses by bacteria will usually respond to an appropriate antibiotic given systemically and, when possible, locally too. Occasional cases require surgical drainage.

Cutaneous and genital lesions respond well to emetine and chloroquine. Large ulcers may require skin grafts.

PROPHYLAXIS AND PREVENTION

Although *E. histolytica* has been able to survive in all parts of the world, invasive disease is rare except where living standards are low. Hence, the most effective means of prevention is sound hygiene.

There is some evidence that the regular ingestion of a non-absorbable drug such as diiodo-hydroxyquinoline has some prophylactic value against infection. Such a measure might be justified under exceptional conditions such as war or civil disturbance when it is known that drinking of faecally contaminated water is probable. Under normal conditions, however, drug prophylaxis seems neither desirable nor necessary since those who are likely to take the drug are also those who live under sanitary conditions which make invasive amoebiasis very improbable.

PROGNOSIS

The outlook for lasting cure in cases of invasive intestinal amoebiasis of average severity is excellent. There is no sound evidence for strains of *E. histolytica* becoming resistant to treatment and with the drugs now available patients can be cleared of their infection. It is only in those infrequent cases where the disease is very severe, particularly when peritonitis occurs, that the mortality rate is high.

Amoebic liver abscess can be a fatal disease, the mortality rate in adults being between 3 per cent and 5 per cent. In uncomplicated cases recovery can be confidently expected but rupture into the pericardium or peritoneum are dangerous events. In the former, with conservative treatment, the majority should recover and in the latter, provided that diagnosis is timely, deaths should be infrequent. Rupture into the lung carries a very good prognosis but empyema is more serious particularly when diagnosis and treatment have been delayed. Very large abscesses or multiple lesions worsen the outlook. Rarely, patients present with severe dysentery, multiple liver abscesses and often jaundice. Such cases have a poor prognosis.

Despite the fact that an amoebic liver abscess may attain a very large size with destruction of much liver tissue, successful treatment is not followed by any impairment of liver function and scarring is minimal.

In summary, it may be said that almost all forms of invasive amoebiasis are amenable to treatment, that subsequent impairment of function is rare and that complete cure is the rule.

REFERENCES

COUNCILMAN, W. T. and LAFLEUR, H. A. (1891) *Johns Hopk. Hosp. Rep.*, **2**, 395.
LÖSCH, F. (1875) *Virchows Arch. path. Anat.*, **65**, 196.
ROGERS, L. (1912) *Brit. med. J.*, **1**, 1424.
—— (1922) *Lancet*, **1**, 463, 569, 677.
VEDDER, E. B. (1914) *J. Amer. med. Ass.*, **62**, 501.

FURTHER READING

CRAIG, C. F. (1944) *The Etiology, Diagnosis and Treatment of Amebiasis*. Baltimore: Williams and Wilkins.
MANSON-BAHR, P. (1944) *The Dysenteric Disorders*. London: Cassell.
OCHSNER, A. and DE BAKEY, M. (1943) Amebic hepatitis and hepatic abscess; analysis of 181 cases and review of the literature. *Surgery*, **13**, 460, 612.
WILMOT, A. J. (1962) *Clinical Amoebiasis*. Oxford: Blackwell.
WOODRUFF, A. W. ed. (1970) *Alimentary and Haematological Aspects of Tropical Disease*. London: Edward Arnold Ltd.

7

Toxoplasmosis

When Nicolle and Manceaux (1908) in Tunis and Splendore (1908) in Brazil simultaneously and independently found *Toxoplasma* in wild and domestic rodents respectively, neither investigator realised the human importance of the organism, and *Toxoplasma gondii* remained a zoological curiosity for the next 30 years. However, during this interval, two cases of suspected toxoplasmosis in man were reported. Castellani, in 1914, identified the organism in a boy in Ceylon who died of an obscure fever associated with splenomegaly, and in 1923, Janku found 'pseudocysts' of *Toxoplasma* in the retina of a hydrocephalic child in Prague.

In 1939, cases of congenital toxoplasmosis were described in the United States, and soon afterwards, the Sabin-Feldman dye test was discovered and was eventually shown to be highly specific for the detection of antibodies against the organism. In the next few decades, the clinical features of the disease in man became recognised, and the wide distribution of the infection in the animal kingdom, including man, was revealed. Many studies have been made about the epidemiology of toxoplasmosis, but the complete life cycle of the parasite and its coccidial nature have only been revealed in the last few years.

THE ORGANISM

Toxoplasma gondii is a protozoan of warm-blooded vertebrates, and belongs to the class Sporozoa. It is small (about 5–7 μm in length), curved like a bow but rather stumpy and possessing a single nucleus; under the electron microscope, a wealth of ultrastructure is revealed, the nature of which is strikingly similar to that of malaria parasites and coccidians. The terminology of the different stages is in a confused state, each investigator employing new terms. Hoare (1972) has suggested the use of simple, logical names and these are given here.

As seen in man, the parasite is found in two forms—the proliferative stage (or pseudocyst) and the cyst. On entry into the body, the organism, in the aberrant or exoenteric cycle, invades lymphoid-macrophage cells, where multiplication by a peculiar form of binary or multiple fission (endogeny) takes place, with the production of a *pseudocyst* containing about twenty or more endozoites. The pseudocyst bursts and neighbouring cells become infected, or the parasites are carried by the blood or lymph to distant organs, including the lungs, tonsils, lymph nodes and placenta, to develop as *proliferative* forms of the parasite or as *cysts*, the latter lasting in the brain and muscle for months or years. The cysts grow to a size of up to 100 μm and contain hundreds of cystozoites packed within the thin but resistant cyst wall: no reaction is provoked in the surrounding tissue and the cysts apparently cause no signs or symptoms. On the other hand, the acute proliferative disease is accompanied by extensive damage to the brain, terminating, in congenital toxoplasmosis, in calcifications which are clearly visible in skiagrams of the head.

The cycle in the cat (the definitive host) is briefly described under *Transmission*.

DISTRIBUTION

The incidence of the infection on human populations has been determined by serological surveys or, less accurately, by means of skin tests with toxoplasmin. The surveys reveal the great frequency of infection in many countries. In certain tropical islands, such as Tahiti, Trinidad and Tristan da Cunha, the rate may be as high as 90 per cent in people over 20 years of age. On the other hand, in some isolated groups, such as the inhabitants of the oases in the 'New Valley' of Egypt, amongst the Navajo Indians of the U.S.A. and in Iceland, the incidence of infection is very low. But in many places, e.g. Great Britain (Beattie, 1964) and other countries of Europe, and the United States of America, the rate in adults is up to 30 per cent. as shown by a positive Sabin-Feldman reaction.

The infection is commonest in people with special habits. It is frequent in meat handlers of any sort, such as butchers, slaughterhouse workers, skinners or laboratory workers using experi-

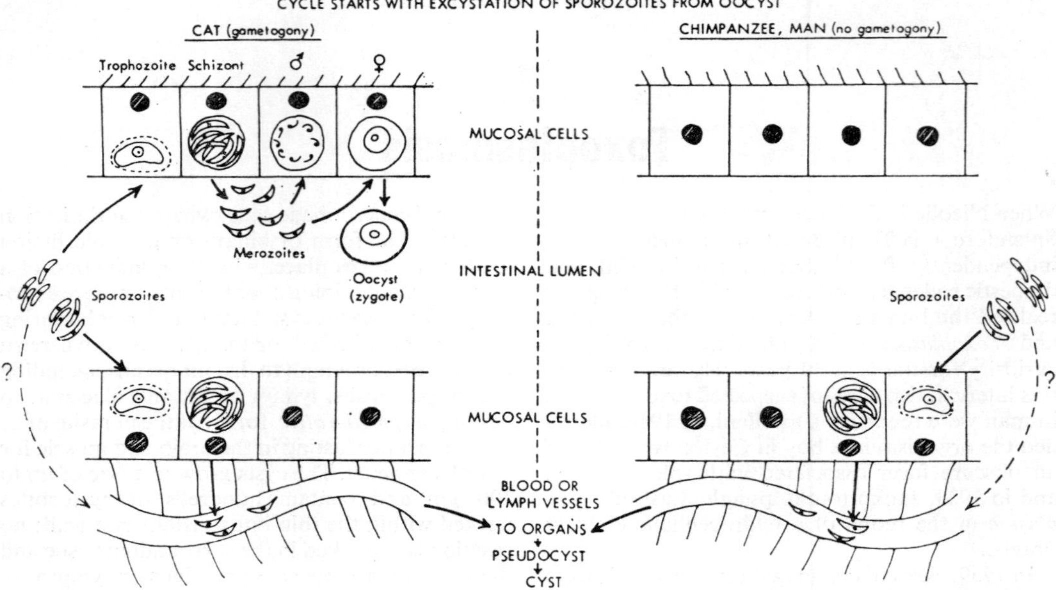

FIG. 7.1.   Possible developmental cycles of toxoplasma in different hosts. (*From* Draper *et al*, 1971.)

mental animals; wounds on their hands become infected with the organism present in the meat. Oral transmission is common in places like Paris where infants and young children are fed on raw meat juice, and the incidence of the infection then rapidly mounts to nearly 100 per cent (Desmonts *et al.*, 1965). On the other hand the rate in vegetarians is about the same as in meat-eaters in many parts of the world.

Toxoplasmosis occurs in almost all domestic animals and is responsible for epizootics in sheep and chickens, while it may practically exterminate colonies of animals such as rabbits, mink, etc. kept in overcrowded conditions. The organism has been found in the greatest variety of wild animals, and although strains vary in virulence, there is only one species, *Toxoplasma gondii*, as described originally from the gondi, a small rodent living in semi-desert conditions in Tunisia.

TRANSMISSION

A variety of methods exists for the transference of *Toxoplasma gondii* from one animal to another. Congenital transmission via the placenta is a well-established route. Contamination of a wound is another method, and the consumption of uncooked mutton commonly leads to infection in certain circumstances, though the lightest cooking is enough to destroy the organism (Garnham and Lainson, 1960). Aerial transmission of pseudocysts or cysts is a possibility, as these stages of the parasite exist in the lungs and coughing will result in their dissemination, either from person to person or from an infected cat to a child, though infection is unlikely to follow. (Fig. 7.1 and Plate 1.)

Cats. The natural or biological method of transmission was only elucidated in recent years, after the fundamental discovery by Hutchison in 1965 that cats pass infective faeces after being fed on mice suffering from chronic toxoplasmosis. *Toxocara cati* was at first thought to be the agent which carried the infective form, but both Jacobs (1967) and Hutchison *et al* (1968) soon discovered that *T. gondii* could be transmitted by the faecal route in the absence of nematodes. It was not until 1969 that Hutchison and his Danish colleagues demonstrated the enteric cycle of the parasite. They showed first that it took the form of typical coccidian oocysts (of an *Isospora* type) and then (1970, 1971) they discovered the complete asexual and gametogonic cycles in the intestinal mucosa. This work was quickly confirmed by North American investigators (Frenkel *et al*, 1970; Sheffield and Melton, 1970) and by others in Germany, Holland, U.S.S.R. and elswhere. The parasite was shown to develop in the tips of the villi of the ileum in cats fed on *T. gondii*-infected material. The oocysts themselves are both extraordinarily resistant and long-lived; they are highly infective and several laboratory infections are known to have occurred.

Chimpanzee. So far only cats and other felines (Frenkel, 1972) have been shown capable of producing oocysts. In all other animals, including probably man, the infection is limited to asexual multiplication in the enteric phase, even though flagrant exoenteric development may take place. Failing the use of human volunteers, Draper *et al* (1971) administered heavily infected brains of mice to a chimpanzee. Its faeces were carefully watched for over a month for the appearance of oocysts, but none appeared; however, its serum showed a progressive rise in titre of the dye test from nil to a high level in the following weeks while the blood was shown to contain parasites on the seventh day as was also an enlarged lymph node a few days later. The animal however never became ill.

Man. Such probably is the usual course of the natural infection in man. Probably he ingests the oocyst from cats' faeces, brought into the house on its paws or fur and easily passed to the child or adult in various ways. Ruiz and Frenkel (1972) have actually shown that peridomestic earth and sweepings from plantations contain viable oocysts of *T. gondii*.

DISEASE IN MAN

Toxoplasmosis may occur in the acquired or congenital form.

Acquired infection is usually latent and no symptoms are recognised though possibly a transient fever or a condition of being slightly 'off-colour' is the body's reaction to infection. This is the prelude to the acquisition of immunity as shown by the various serological reactions.

The next most common form (*Siim's disease*) is lymphadenopathy usually accompanied by pyrexia and sometimes by a sore throat or a rash. All groups of lymph nodes may become moderately enlarged; the nodes are soft and usually painless. This condition is relatively mild, though it may persist for weeks. The disease is often confused with infectious mononucleosis, but the latter is easily recognised by the presence of a positive Paul-Bunnell reaction; probably about 10 per cent of patients suspected of having 'glandular fever' but with a negative reaction are suffering instead from toxoplasmosis.

A more malignant type of the disease is *meningoencephalitis*, and this is sometimes the terminal event in Hodgkin's disease, leukaemia or cancer, where the patient's resistance to an accompanying but latent infection with *Toxoplasma gondii* has been lowered by irradiation or immunosuppressant drugs. The organism then undergoes the proliferative stage and multiples, as in a tissue culture, in the brain and meninges; there is extensive necrosis and the patient dies rapidly in coma. A typhus-like syndrome has been described and also bronchopneumonia, polymyositis, and heart failure, but these varieties of toxoplasmosis are rare. Beverley (1971) emphasises the effect of stress on *T. gondii* infections, and refers particularly to measles and vaccination with its virus in children, and to distemper and vaccination in dogs. Toxoplasmosis may then flare up with hepatosplenomegaly and focal hepatitis.

Ocular toxoplasmosis may be either congenital or acquired, and sometimes it is difficult to be sure of the origin of the condition. The typical lesion is a focal chorioretinitis and necrosis which usually extends to the macula; much scarring follows and pigment-ringed scars, often peripheral in distribution, present a characteristic picture. It seems likely that the organisms persist in the eye for prolonged periods. Thus Hogan *et al* (1958) recovered them from the eye of a man of 20 years of age who had almost certainly been congenitally infected. It seems probable that recurrent attacks of retinitis which occur in some affected patients result from survival of organisms in the retina in this way.

Congenital toxoplasmosis is the result of the mother acquiring the infection in the first trimester of pregnancy. The fetus then becomes infected; it may die and an abortion take place, or the baby may be born at term, dead, severely damaged or with the latent disease. Fortunately, the mother is only infective to the fetus on this single occasion and she can be assured that the infection will be absent in subsequent children. There is, however, an unconfirmed impression that habitual abortion may be due to toxoplasmosis, and it has been shown in mice that the infection may pass through eight or more generations (Beverley, 1959).

The congenital disease is manifested by a tetrad of signs; hydro- or microcephalus, chorioretinitis, cerebral calcifications, and mental deficiency. These conditions vary in severity, but are usually so pronounced that the child dies within a short time after birth. Microcephaly is caused by gross necrosis of cerebral tissue, and hydrocephaly is the result of blockage to the flow of cerebrospinal fluid from the ventricles. Paraplegia and cranial nerve palsies, generalised convulsions, twitching of individual muscles, tremor of groups of muscles and nystagmus may all result from damage to parts of the motor cortex or cerebellum.

TREATMENT

No specific drug exists for the certain cure of toxoplasmosis, but the synergistic effect of pyrimethamine (Daraprim) and sulphadiazine is well known in experimental animals and is the standard therapy in man. Unfortunately, these substances must be given in high dosages for a prolonged period; pyrimethamine should be pushed up to 50 mg a day and sulphadiazine to 1–2 g. The treatment should be continued for up to 6 months in severe forms of the disease, or in otherwise intractable cases of uveitis (for which prednisone is also recommended). With this dosage of pyrimethamine, the white blood count should be estimated at frequent intervals in order to watch for signs of damage to the bone marrow; if they appear, the drugs should be stopped immediately. It is advisable in cases where prolonged treatment is necessary to interrupt chemotherapy for a week at a time. Throughout treatment, folinic acid should be given regularly (5 mg tds). Antibiotics have been shown to have an antitoxoplasmic effect *in vitro*, e.g. Spiromycin (in doses of 4–5 g daily in 4 divided doses for 10–14 days), and various tetracyclines. If treatment is stopped prematurely, a severe relapse may occur months later.

None of these drugs produces a certain cure, and several infections of laboratory origin which have received immediate treatment have proved fatal.

Pregnancy. A difficult problem is to decide upon the correct procedure to adopt in pregnancy accompanied by toxoplasmosis. If the active disease is diagnosed in the mother during the first 5 months, a full course of treatment should be given or, in certain circumstances, therapeutic abortion might be considered justifiable.

If the disease occurs later, treatment again should be administered for the sake of the mother. The significance of the presence of a positive serological reaction in the mother has to be carefully assessed. If by chance a sample of serum taken before or very early in pregnancy is available and this gives a negative dye test, to be followed by a positive reaction during pregnancy, it may be assumed that active infection has taken place at the critical time when transmission to the fetus is occurring; in these circumstances, the mother should be treated. If, on the other hand, the dye test was positive before pregnancy or if no such sample were available, and the sera in pregnancy showed *no rise in titre* of a positive reaction, treatment of the mother would be unnecessary. It should be remembered that probably 30 per cent of all women will have a positive serological reaction and its significance must be weighed according to the factors mentioned above, and others.

An important consideration in the prevention of congenital cases of toxoplasmosis is to ensure that no female workers of child-bearing age are employed in laboratories on work involving the live organism, unless they already have a positive Sabin-Feldman reaction.

DIAGNOSIS

The disease is best diagnosed by isolating the organism, but this may prove to be impossible in non-fatal human cases. At autopsy, *T. gondii* may be recovered from the brain or other organs, or it may be recognised in the cystic or proliferative stage in sections or suspensions of suitable material. In man, the organism has to be distinguished from pseudocysts of *Trypanosoma cruzi*, *Histoplasma capsulatum*, *Leishmania donovani*, *Sarcocystis lindemanni* and *Pneumocystis carinii*.

In life, the organism may be recovered from enlarged lymph nodes by inoculation of suspensions into mice, from cerebrospinal fluid, from diseased organs (e.g. the eye) or even from the saliva (Cathie, 1954). Several 'blind passages' in mice may be required before the organism becomes easily apparent.

Sabin-Feldman dye test. This remains the most widely used diagnostic test and results from it are very reliable. The test depends upon the fact that endozoites exposed to *Toxoplasma* antibodies do not stain with methylene blue whereas those not so exposed will do so. A dye test, positive in serum diluted 1/16, is often taken to be indicative of active infection although a positive test at any titre indicates infection at some stage or other in the patient's life. In those with overt disease, titres of one in several thousand are commonly encountered. The dye test becomes positive early in the course of infection, probably after 2 or 3 weeks and remains positive for many years though at a diminishing titre. For certain diagnosis it is highly desirable to take at least two samples of blood at 3–4 week intervals in order to observe the rising titre of the reaction in active cases of the disease.

Serology. Complement fixing antibodies develop later in the course of the illness and disappear sooner than do those responsible for the dye test. A positive complement fixation test is therefore a valuable indication of active disease.

Fulton's agglutination test is sensitive and accurate, and does not require the use of live organisms; the same applies to the indirect haemagglutination test. The indirect fluorescent antibody test is becoming increasingly popular; it is easy to perform and can be used either on the immune serum or for confirmation of the nature of a cyst in the tissues.

The delayed hypersensitivity reaction following the intradermal injection of toxoplasmin has been widely employed in surveys, and is easy to carry out, but it is not as reliable as the serological reactions.

REFERENCES

BEATTIE, C. P. (1964) *Roy. Coll. Phys. Edinb.* Pub. No. 28.

BEVERLEY, J. K. A. (1959) *Nature*, **183**, 1348.

—— (1971) *J. med. Wom. Fed.*, **53**, 73.

CATHIE, J. A. (1954) *Lancet*, **ii**, 115.

DESMONTS, G., COUVREUR, J., ALISON, F., BAUDELOT, J., GERBEAUX, J. and LELONG, M. (1965) *Ref. fr. Etud. clin. biol.*, **10**, 952.

DRAPER, C., KILLICK-KENDRICK, R., HUTCHINSON, W. M., SIIM, J. C. and GARNHAM, P. C. C. (1971) *Brit. med. J.*, **2**, 375.

FRENKEL, J. K. (1972) *Amer. J. trop. Med. Hyg.* (in press).

FRENKEL, J. K., DUBEY, J. P. and MILLER, N. L. (1970) *Science*, **167**, 893.

GARNHAM, P. C. C. and LAINSON, R. (1960) *Lancet*, **ii**, 71.

HOARE, C. A. (1972) *J. trop. Med. Hyg.*, **75**, 56

HOGAN, N. J., ZWEIGART, P. and LEWIS, A. (1958) *Arch. Ophthal.*, **60**, 548.

HUTCHISON, W. M. (1965) *Nature*, **206**, 961.

HUTCHISON, W. M. DUNACHIF, J. F. and WORK, K. (1968) *Acta. path. microbiol. Scandinav.* **74**, 462.

HUTCHISON, W. M., DUNACHIE, J. F., SIIM, J. C. and WORK, K. (1969) *Brit. med. J.*, **4**, 806.

—— (1970) *Brit. med. J.*, **1**, 144.

HUTCHISON, W. M., DUNACHIE, J. F., WORK, K. and SIIM, J. C. (1971) *Trans. roy. Soc. trop. Med. Hyg.*, **65**, 380.

JACOBS, L. (1967) In *Advances in Parasitology* 5, p. 1, London: Academic Press.

NICOLLE, C. and MANCEAUX, L. (1908) *C. R. Acad. Sci.*, **147**, 763.

RUIZ, A. and FRENKEL, J. K. (1972) *Amer. J. trop. Med. Hyg.*, **21**, 513.

SHEFFIELD, H. G. and MELTON, M. L. (1970) *Science*, **167**, 892.

SPLENDORE, A. (1908) *Rev. Soc. Sci. (S. Paulo)*, **3**, 109.

FURTHER READING

The bibliography of toxoplasmosis is enormous (see *A bibliography of toxoplasmosis and Toxoplasma gondii*, Federal Security Agency, N.I.H. Washington, 1952 and 1st Supplement, 1954), but a detailed account of the subject is given by C. Beattie in *Recent Advances in Medical Microbiology*, 1967, edited by A. P. Waterson. London: Churchill, and by L. Jacobs in *Recent Advances in Parasitology*, 1967, New York: Academic Press.

8
Intestinal Protozoa Other Than
Entamoeba histolytica

In addition to *Entamoeba histolytica*, fifteen species of parasitic protozoa may live in the alimentary tract of man. They form a rather heterogeneous group and comprise seven species of amoebae (*Entamoeba coli, E. hartmanni, E. polecki, E. gingivalis, Endolimax nana, Iodamoeba bütschlii* and *Dientamoeba fragilis*); six flagellates (*Trichomonas homonis, T. tenax, Giardia intestinalis, Chilomastix mesnili, Retortomonas intestinalis* and *Enteromonas hominis*); one ciliate (*Balantidium coli*) and one coccidian (*Isospora belli*). Two of these species, *E. gingivalis* and *T. tenax*, inhabit the oral cavity; they are especially prevalent in persons with poor dental hygiene; neither species form cysts and transmission is usually by direct oral contact. Their role in the causation of periodontal disease is doubtful, but they probably live in a symbiotic relationship with the rich bacterial flora found in infected periodontal tissues. *E. gingivalis* very closely resembles *E. histolytica* and as the former is often found in sputum specimens it may cause confusion in patients with suspected pulmonary amoebiasis.

Of the remaining species, *G. intestinalis* and *I. belli* inhabit the small intestine while all the others live in the large bowel. They are all transmitted by the faeco-oral route, usually by the ingestion of viable cysts except in the case of *D. fragilis* and *T. hominis* in which no cystic stage is known and infection is by the ingestion of trophozoites. In population surveys the latter two species are likely to be overlooked unless fresh wet preparations of formed as well as unformed stools are examined; even if this is done the examination of a permanently stained preparation will be necessary to differentiate *D. fragilis* from other small amoebae such as *E. hartmanni*. Since the epidemiology of all these intestinal protozoa is similar, the finding of any one of them in a patient's stool should arouse the suspicions of the clinician that the patient may also be infected with *E. histolytica* and further stool specimens should be examined. High prevalence rates for many of these protozoa are often found in situations in which faecal con-tamination of the environment is particularly great, as occurs in orphanages and homes for the mentally backward.

Except for *B. coli* and *Entamoeba polecki*, both of which are probably normally pig parasites, these protozoal infections are believed to be derived from human sources. However, parasites morphologically identical to several of the other parasites have been reported from primates, domestic animals and livestock; the extent to which cross-transmission occurs with these parasites is not known.

E. polecki is the most recently recognised addition to the list of human intestinal protozoa; its exact taxonomic status is still under debate. It is probably identical with the species referred to as *E. suis* in pigs. Surveys suggest that up to 70 per cent of pigs may be infected and human infection may not be uncommon, especially in pig-handlers. It is important to differentiate it from *E. histolytica* as no treatment is necessary. In size the cysts and trophozoites are similar to those of *E. histolytica*. However the mature cyst is uninucleate with a moderately large, somewhat eccentric karyosome and rather coarse and irregular peripheral chromatin; the chromatoid bodies are angular with pointed ends and often a large rounded or oval inclusion mass of unknown composition is present in the cytoplasm. The trophozoites of this species cannot be differentiated from *E. coli*.

B. coli, G. intestinalis and *I. belli* are probably the only species pathogenic to man; however some consider *D. fragilis* to be occasionally pathogenic. Although in most respects it behaves like an amoeba, recent electron microscopic work suggests that *D. fragilis* may be a flagellate. It is believed to inhabit the large bowel in man and as there is no cystic stage, transmission is by ingestion of the trophozoite. In a wet stool preparation the trophozoites may show several lobose pseudopodia. The protozoon measures 7–16 μm in diameter and a permanently stained preparation will usually show two nuclei each with a large fragmented but clumped karyosome but no peripheral chromatin. Culture is the most sensitive method of diagnosis and prevalence rates of 5 per cent are not unusual. Evidence for the pathogenicity of this parasite is largely based on self-infection experiments by several research workers who have developed recurrent bouts of loose stools sometimes containing mucus and associated with flatulence, abdominal distension and intestinal colic; infection can persist for at least 2 years. Kean (1966) reported a series of 100 patients whose symptoms improved following the successful treatment of this parasite. There are several reports of the finding of this parasite in surgically removed fibrotic appendices but a causal relationship is very doubtful. More studies are needed before this parasite can be definitely regarded as a human pathogen but in view of our present inability to find a cause in many cases of short diarrhoeal illnesses, it would be foolish to dismiss the possibility that it may be responsible for some of them. In the past patients have been treated with tetracycline or carbasone but metronidazole may become the drug of choice.

BALANTIDIASIS

In many parts of the world including Britain, 50–80 per cent of all pigs are infected with a species of *Balantidium* morphologically identical with the human parasite. Human strains have been successfully transmitted to the pig but so far porcine strains have not been successfully transmitted to man; however, epidemiological evidence very strongly suggests that man is normally infected from the pig. In New Guinea where pig/man contact may be fairly intimate, high prevalence rates have been reported. In most parts of the world the prevalence is less than 1 per cent but in several countries in South and Central America the figure may exceed 5 per cent. High figures have been reported from mental institutions.

Cultural methods usually give higher prevalence rates; in asymptomatic patients parasites are often scanty and despite their large size are probably often missed, as both cysts and trophozoites are present in the stool and the latter will not be detected by concentration techniques. *In vitro* culture is relatively easy and horse serum diluted in physiological saline together with some added rice starch will usually be successful.

In both the pig and man the infection is usually asymptomatic. However, in both a severe and sometimes fatal disease may develop. Cysts remain viable in the soil for many months, encyst-

ment may take place outside the body. The use of pig excrement as a fertiliser for vegetables may be an important source of human infection.

Pathology

In symptomatic cases severe ulcerative lesions of the large bowel may occur, especially in the rectosigmoid. Macroscopically the ulcers rather resemble those of amoebiasis, but they may penetrate more deeply, causing intestinal perforation, or they may coalesce within the bowel wall, causing extensive sloughing of the mucosa. Microscopically the lesions are seen to be necrotic in the centre and the trophozoites are seen at the periphery of the lesion; most of the lesion shows an extensive infiltration of lymphocytes and neutrophils but the parasites themselves may be surrounded by a narrow clear zone. At autopsy parasites have been found in the mesenteric lymph nodes. Recently a convincing case of balantidial liver abscess has been described from Venezuela and in an autopsy in Costa Rica there was pulmonary involvement.

Clinical features, diagnosis and treatment

Balantidial dysentery is clinically indistinguishable from amoebic dysentery and the sigmoidoscopic appearances are similar. Milder forms of the disease with recurrent bouts of bloodstained loose stools also occur. In symptomatic cases trophozoites are usually easy to demonstrate in sigmoidoscopic scrapings or stool specimens. The trophozoites are unmistakable oval bodies, 50–150 μm in length, which swim with corkscrew movement due to the somewhat spirally arranged longitudinal rows of cilia. In asymptomatic carriers, either the trophozoites or cysts may be passed; the cysts are 50 μm in diameter, nearly spherical and have a thick wall. The parasite may retain its cilia within the cyst wall for some time; usually the kidney-shaped macronucleus is visible.

Antibodies have been demonstrated in the serum of symptomatic patients using either an indirect fluorescent antibody or trophozoite immobilisation test. Serology at present is not used in diagnosis but it may be that in the past liver involvement has been mistaken for an amoebic liver abscess; if this is the case, then perhaps serological techniques will become important.

Both tetracycline and ampicillin have been successfully used to treat balantidiasis; but it is very likely that in future metronidazole will become the drug of choice. There would seem to be no justification now for using arsenicals such as carbasone.

ISOSPORIASIS

Several coccidian parasites have been found in human faeces. In many cases these are spurious infections resulting from the ingestion of food containing the oocysts of non-human parasites: thus *Eimeria sardinae*, *E. steidae* and *E. dublieki* may be present in sardines, herrings, rabbit liver and pig sausage-skins respectively. True human infection occurs with *I. belli* which is similar morphologically and may be identical with the dog parasite *I. bigemina*. The pathological changes and complete life cycle in man have recently been described from small bowel biopsy specimens (Brandborg *et al*, 1970). Following oocyst rupture the organism undergoes a limited number of schizogonic cycles within the epithelial cells of the small bowel. This is followed by gamete formation and eventually the liberation into the bowel lumen of oocysts which are then passed into the external environment. The oocysts are very resistant indeed and remain viable in the soil for many months; they may be immature when passed in the stool and sporogony is perhaps only completed in the presence of oxygen. The mature *Isospora* oocyst contains 4 sporozoites and a residual body within each of the two sporocysts. The oocysts of the human species are oval in shape and measure about 29 by 13 μm.

Isospora hominis has in the past been regarded as a separate species but it is likely that the oocysts attributed to this species are merely more mature oocysts of *I. belli* (Zaman, 1968). Sometimes free sporocysts may be found in the stool if the oocyst wall has ruptured. Infections are best diagnosed by flotation techniques either using a saturated salt solution or zinc sulphate; this is because of their very low specific gravity which makes sedimentation difficult. Besides being found in the stool, oocysts have been found in duodenal aspirates. For accurate identification the cysts must be mature and it may be necessary to incubate them in 2 per cent potassium dichromate solution in a shallow dish for 4–5 days in order to allow this to occur. *Eimeria* oocysts can be differentiated by the fact that they contain four sporocytes each with two sporozoites; in addition, being spurious infections, they will be passed in the stool over a much shorter period. To see the internal structure of an oocyst, iodine staining must be used. Another difficulty is that being very light, they float up under the coverslip and may be missed.

Because of the difficulties in diagnosis most recorded prevalence rates of *I. belli* are probably underestimates. The parasite has a cosmopolitan distribution and figures of 3 per cent have been reported from Chile and Colombia, in mental institutions in the latter country prevalence rates of 18 per cent have been recorded. Recently, using special techniques, a figure of 7 per cent has been recorded in Holland (Smitzkamp *et al*, 1966).

Human infection is definitely associated with a short diarrhoeal illness but this is self-limiting and no specific treatment is required. In experimental infections the incubation period is about 7 days and the main clinical features are low fever, malaise, colicky abdominal pain and a moderately severe diarrhoea. The stools may be pale and often contain mucus and undigested food. The symptoms may last for 2 or 3 weeks but excretion of oocysts may continue for up to 80 days.

GIARDIASIS

Giardia intestinalis is a common and cosmopolitan parasite; prevalance rates of up to 25 per cent are by no means uncommon in the tropics. Its epidemiology is very similar to that of *E. histolytica*. The cysts, which are the infective stage, can survive for up to 3 months in water, but they are very susceptible to desiccation. Infected food handlers are probably important and quite extensive outbreaks have been described in which piped drinking-water supplies have been contaminated with sewage (Moore *et al*, 1969).

While many, perhaps the majority of infections are asymptomatic, there is now no doubt that it can cause a disabling illness in adults as well as children; the infection may persist for several years and during this period recurrent bouts of illness may be interspersed with long periods of apparently normal health. An association with kwashiorkor has been noted by several workers, especially in Africa. It is postulated that the deleterious effects of this parasite on intestinal mucosa may be sufficient to tip the patient over into overt malnutrition.

Only recently has this parasite been successfully cultivated *in vitro* (Karapetyan, 1961); culture is difficult and at present it can only be done in the presence of a yeast organism. Many domestic and laboratory mammals harbour *Giardia* parasites but until more cross-infection studies have been done the relationship of these to the human parasite remains unknown.

K

Pathology

Excystment and trophozoite multiplication takes place within the lumen of the duodenum, jejenum and upper ileum; it is believed that the parasites normally attach themselves to the intestinal mucosa by means of their ventral sucker and obtain nutriment directly from the epithelial cells. Some histological studies however suggest that trophozoites may actually enter epithelial cells (Morechi and Parker, 1967).

Duodenal and jejunal biopsies show a variable picture. Asymptomatic patients usually show no mucosal changes, but in other patients partial villous atrophy and a quite extensive cellular infiltrate of lymphocytes, plasma cells and polymorphs occurs within the lamina propria. The parasites are seen especially in the intervillous spaces. The epithelial cells may show an increased number of mitotic figures suggesting an increased cell turnover; the number of goblet cells may be increased.

The mechanism by which functional changes are produced is not clear; the simplest hypothesis is that when the trophozoites are very numerous, they may reduce the absorptive area of the mucosa. However it is likely that the mucosal cells are in fact damaged since it has been shown that the amounts of lactase and other disaccharidases within the epithelial cells is reduced in some patients, suggesting that microvillar function is affected. Moreover, an increase in protein loss into the gut has recently been demonstrated.

The functional effects of these small bowel changes are a malabsorption of fat, vitamin A, xylose and probably folic acid. Absorption of iron and vitamin B_{12} is usually normal and in any case the functional changes do not persist long enough for a deficiency of these substances to develop. The parasite has been found in the gallbladders of a few patients undergoing cholecystectomy for gallstones but a causal relationship is very unlikely.

Clinical features and diagnosis

The most common symptoms are poorly localised upper abdominal discomfort, sometimes with colicky pain, borborygmi, flatulence and frequent loose and rather pale stools which may contain mucus. These symptoms may be related to meals, and a diarrhoeal stool immediately after breakfast is rather characteristic. In more severe cases the stools may be manifestly steatorrhoeic and contain up to 15 g of fat daily; such patients may lose weight, become anorexic and suffer considerable malaise and lethargy. Symptoms are more common in children but adults, especially those visiting the tropics from temperate regions, may also develop a quite disabling and prolonged illness. The factors which determine whether an infection will be symptomatic are not very clear but at least in European adults visiting the tropics it appears that a poor diet, poor living conditions and perhaps even the taking of cannabis may upset the host-parasite equilibrium.

Diagnosis is usually relatively easy, cysts being found in formed stools and trophozoites in unformed stools or duodenal aspirates. The cysts when mature have four nuclei and measure 9–13 μm in length. They are elliptical in shape and usually two longitudinal fibrils can be seen. The trophozoites are unmistakable flattened pear-shaped bodies, 12–18 μm in length, with eight flagellae, two nuclei and a large anteriorly situated ventral sucker. The number of parasites found in a stool specimen probably does not give a reliable indication of the number of trophozoites living in the small bowel. The finding of only a few cysts in a stool does not necessarily mean that the parasite is not the cause of the patient's symptoms; in fact, even in some patients with malabsorption, the parasites may only be demonstrable by duodenal intubation. If jejunal biopsy is carried out on a patient with malabsorption, the trophozoites if present can easily be found in material taken from the luminal aspect of the specimen.

In children giardiasis may simulate coeliac disease and in adults confusion with tropical sprue and even idiopathic steatorrhoea may arise. However although serum folate levels may be somewhat reduced, anaemia does not occur and the absence of glossitis, stomatitis, tetany and bone changes help in the clinical differentiation. In those cases without steatorrhoea, giardiasis may give symptoms similar to cholecystitis with intolerance to fatty foods and post-prandial-dyspepsia. But perhaps the irritable bowel syndrome is the most important differential diagnosis in these cases; here the response to therapy will be the best guide as to whether the parasite is causally related to the patient's symptoms.

Treatment

A single 8-day course of either mepacrine or metronidazole will cure about 80–90 per cent of infections: suitable dosages for an adult are mepacrine 100 mg three times daily and metronidazole 200 mg three times daily. If treatment with one of these drugs fails, the other should be tried.

The decision whether or not to treat asymptomatic patients will depend on the circumstances; in highly endemic areas food handlers at least should be treated. In areas of low endemicity, perhaps all infections should be treated in order to prevent transmission to other persons particularly children.

REFERENCES

BRANDBORG, L. L., GOLDBERG, S. B. and BREIDENBACH, W. C. (1970) *New. Engl. J. Med.*, **283**, 1306.

KARAPETYAN, A. E. (1961) *Med. Parasit. (Moskra)*, **30**, 691.

KEAN, B. H. (1966) *Amer. J. digest. Dis.*, **11**, 735.

MOORE, G. T., CROSS, W. M., McGUIRE, D., MULLOHAN, C. S., GLEASON, N. H., HEALY, G. R. and NEWTON, C. H. (1969) *New Eng. J. Med.*, **281**, 402.

MORECHI, R. and PARKER, J. G. (1967) *Gastroenterology*, **52**, 151.

SMITZKAMP, H. and OEY MULLER, E. (1966) *Trop. geogr. Med.*, **18**, 133.

ZAMAN, A. (1968) *Trans. roy. Soc. trop. Med. Hyg.*, **62**, 556.

9
Primary Amoebic Meningoencephalitis

Recently it has been recognised that certain free-living soil amoebae, in particular of the genus *Naegleria*, can cause a rapidly fatal infection of the central nervous system in man. This condition is now usually designated as primary amoebic meningoencephalitis. It must of course be distinguished from the rare cases of invasion of the brain by *Entamoeba histolytica* in which brain involvement results from haematogenous spread usually from a liver or lung amoebic abscess.

It has been known for some time that free-living amoebae can contaminate bacterial or tissue cultures; paradoxically one of these contaminates was thought initially to be a virus and was named the Ryan virus, only later did microscopy reveal that the organism infecting these particular monkey kidney tissue cultures was in fact an amoeba. Similar amoebae have on occasion been isolated from the nose and throat swabs of persons both with and without upper respiratory symptoms; the significance of these isolations is not clear but it is not impossible that relatively asymptomatic human infection may be quite common.

Culbertson *et al* (1961) showed that several species of soil amoebae produced a fatal infection of the brain and spinal cord when injected intranasally into mice and monkeys. In 1965 Fowler and Carter described the first definite case of fatal human disease from Australia. There are now 57 proved cases in the literature together with 12 possible cases (Carter, 1972); the latter include the two cases of unusual cerebral amoebiasis which had originally been attributed to *Iodamoeba butchlii*. Other possible cases are those described by Symmers (1969) who re-examined the brain specimens of two patients who died in Britain in 1909 and 1937 respectively and found amoebae resembling *Naegleria* in sections of brain tissue.

AETIOLOGY

While many species of free-living amoebae belonging to several genera have been shown to invade the brain of experimental animals following intranasal inoculation, it is not yet clear how many of them can cause disease in man. In stained histological sections or stained preparations of cerebrospinal fluid, the trophozoites of the several genera and species look very similar. They are nearly spherical and measure 10 to 25 μm in diameter. The nucleus is characteristic and rather resembles *Iodamoeba*, having a large discrete central karyosome surrounded by a clear zone which separates it from a very thin ring of peripheral nuclear chromatin. The species can only be differentiated in culture; the structure of the mitotic spindle and the nuclear membrane during cell division are important taxonomic characters. Encystment can be induced in various ways, perhaps the easiest being to grow the amoeba on a colony of the bacterium *Escherichia coli*. Cyst structure is also very helpful in taxonomy.

So far, with one doubtful exception, all the pathogens cultured from man have been identified as *Naegleria*, in particular *N. gruberi*. The other genus which has been incriminated is *Hartmanella* (syn. *Acanthamoeba*). *Naegleria* trophozoites are usually smaller than *Hartmanella* and under unfavourable conditions, e.g. when placed in distilled water, they assume a flagellate form with two or four flagellae. There is a recent report from New Zealand (Mandal *et al*, 1970) in which the amoebae cultured from the cerebrospinal fluid of one patient developed hyphal-like structures and spores under certain conditions; this organism has been provisionally identified as a *Myxomycetale* or slime mould.

EPIDEMIOLOGY AND DISTRIBUTION

So far the clinical reports of this condition have come from scattered parts of the world, including Czechoslovakia, Britain, southern United States of America, Australia and New Zealand. However, the species of *Naegleria* and other soil amoebae probably have a world-wide distribution. Their normal habitat is in the film of water surrounding soil particles, but they may also be found in fresh and brackish water especially if it is muddy. Growth occurs rapidly between 25 and 30°C. Encystment occur at lower temperatures and when their environment dries up. Dispersal may occur by wind-borne cysts.

Most of the human patients give a history of diving, swimming or bathing in water; children and young adults have usually been affected and it appears that children playing even in rain puddles may become infected. Some reports have described small outbreaks in which several persons have been infected simultaneously in the same water. Evidence from animal work and also the severe pathology seen in the region of the olfactory bulb of the brain in human cases suggests that the infection crosses from the mucosa of the roof of the nose, through the cribriform plate, into the skull and subarachnoid space.

PATHOLOGY

At autopsy the brain is oedematous with flattening of the cerebral gyri, the meninges are opaque and there is usually a bloodstained purulent exudate in the subarachnoid space, especially in the basal cisterns. Vascular dilatation and congestion is present on the brain surface and within the brain substance there are areas of cerebral softening which may be haemorrhagic; these areas are located especially in the midbrain, pons, medulla and the olfactory bulbs.

Microscopy shows vascular congestion, petechial haemorrhages, neuronal degeneration and demyelinisation; a neutrophilic inflammatory exudate extends into the grey matter from the subarachnoid space. Significant involvement of the spinal cord has not been reported in man. Amoebae are most numerous in the grey matter and are usually found somewhat ahead of the advancing edge of a necrotic lesion. They are situated perivascularly and are not associated with much local inflammatory reaction.

Outside the nervous system little specific pathology has been found although pulmonary oedema and an acute diffuse myocarditis with scattered areas of haemorrhage and focal necrosis have been reported. In one patient amoebae were cultured from the spleen, liver and lungs and were seen microscopically in blood from the heart; such dissemination is presumably terminal.

SYMPTOMATOLOGY

The incubation period is uncertain but symptoms probably begin 2–14 days after exposure. Mild upper respiratory symptoms and headache occur initially but within a few days the patient becomes severely ill with an acute meningitic syndrome with fever, neck rigidity, coma and later convulsions; localising neurological signs are usually absent. Death occurs within 2 to 5 days although some patients have been kept alive for longer periods on a respirator. In several reports the nasal and faucial mucosae have been congested and inflamed. It is not impossible that mild self-limiting infections occur; in one of the recent British cases—a child whose brother developed the typical fatal illness—the only clinical findings were mild neck stiffness and upper respiratory symptoms, yet amoebae were found in the cerebrospinal fluid which was otherwise normal.

DIAGNOSIS

At present this rests entirely on the cerebrospinal fluid findings; no serological methods have so far been developed. At lumbar puncture or ventricular tap the cerebrospinal fluid is usually turbid, bloodstained and under considerably raised pressure. Microscopy reveals considerable amounts of amorphous debris, numerous red cells and often several thousand white cells per cubic millimetre; the white cells are predominantly neutrophils. The protein level is high and in some reports the glucose level has been reduced. Amoebae may number up to several hundred per cubic millimetre of fluid, but unless they are specifically looked for they may easily be missed or mistaken for macrophages.

In fixed preparations stained with conventional stains, the amoebae appear as ill-defined smudges. However, with an iron haematoxylin stain the details of nuclear structure can be seen. Examination of a fresh wet unstained preparation kept at 25–37°C is essential; ideally phase contrast microscopy should be used. Many of the amoebae contain ingested red blood cells. Culture is relatively easy using media suitable for *E. histolytica* or plain agar seeded with live *Escherichia coli* but as a diagnostic measure this is too slow if there is to be any hope of successful therapy. For accurate generic and specific identification, however, culture is essential.

Unless amoebae are seen, the clinical and cerebrospinal fluid findings may closely resemble an acute pyogenic bacterial meningitis. However, the absence of bacteria revealed by Gram's stain should arouse suspicion. Cryptococcal and other mycotic meningitides should also be considered in the differential diagnosis. Moreover, the initial cellular reaction in both tuberculous and viral meningitis may sometimes be predominantly polymorphonuclear.

TREATMENT AND PROGNOSIS

Conventional amoebicidal drugs such as emetine, chloroquine and metronidazole have no definite effect on these organisms. In laboratory animals sulphonamides have some effect on *Hartmanella* but not *Naegleria* infections. At present the only drug known to be effective against *Naegleria* is amphotericin B; there is as yet no information as to whether this drug is also effective against *Hartmanella*. At the time of writing only two patients with primary amoebic meningoencephalitis are known to have survived and one of these cases is of doubtful validity as the patient had a relatively mild aseptic meningitis syndrome and recovered without treatment although *Hartmanella* had been cultured from the cerebrospinal fluid. The other patient, a child with proved *Naegleria* infection whose brother had died of the disease, was treated with amphotericin B, 0.25 mg/kg intravenously for 8 days; this success may well have been related to early diagnosis since the patient was fully conscious when treatment was started (Apley *et al*, 1970). In several other patients who have been given this drug, amoebae have been shown to disappear from the cerebrospinal fluid although the patients have died.

In the present state of our knowledge and bearing in mind that *Hartmanella* could be pathogenic, it would appear justifiable to start treatment with both sulphonamides and amphotericin B as soon as the diagnosis is made. Intrathecal amphotericin B should certainly be considered and a dosage similar to that used in cryptococcal meningitis would seem appropriate: 0.5 mg of the drug is diluted in 5 ml of cerebrospinal fluid which has already been mixed with 20 mg of hydrocortisone succinate and this fluid is then injected into the spinal theca. This procedure can be repeated two or three times weekly.

As clinical awareness of this condition increases it is likely that more cases will be diagnosed at a less advanced stage, and with earlier treatment one hopes that the present gloomy prognosis will be improved.

REFERENCES

APLEY, J., CLARKE, S. K. R., ROOME, A. P. C. H., SANDRY, S. A., SAYGI, G., SILK, B. and WARHURST, D. C. (1970) *Brit. med. J.*, **1**, 596.

CARTER, R. F. (1972) *Trans. roy. Soc. trop. Med. Hyg.*, **66**, 193.

CULBERTSON, C. G., OVERTON, W. M. and REVEAL, M. A. (1961) *Amer. J. clin. Path.*, **35**, 195.

DERRICK, E. H. and WENGON, C. M. (1948) *Trans. roy. Soc. trop. Med. Hyg.*, **42**, 191.

FOWLER, M. and CARTER, R. F. (1965) *Brit. med. J.*, **2**, 740.

KERNOHAN, J. W., MOGATH, T. B. and SCHLOSS, G. T. (1960) *Arch. Path.*, **70**, 576.

MANDAL, B. N., GUDEX, D. J., FITCHETT, M. R., PULLON, D. H. H., MALLOCH, J. A., DAVID, C. M. and APTHORP, J. (1970) *N.Z. med. J.*, **71**, 1.

SYMMERS, W. St C. (1969) *Brit. med. J.*, **4**, 449.

Helminthic Diseases

Cestodes

Hydatid Disease

Intestinal Nematode Infections

Schistosomiasis and Other Trematode Infections

Filariasis

10
Cestodes

Cestodes or tapeworms are ribbon-shaped segmented worms which are found exclusively in the intestine. A tapeworm consists of a head or scolex and a body or strobila. The head is equipped with suckers and also sometimes with hooks by means of which the worm is attached to the intestinal wall. The posterior part of the head is a proliferating area which continually supplies young segments which grow to form the body. There is no alimentary canal; food is absorbed through the surface of the worm. Each mature segment or proglottis has testes, which are usually numerous, an ovary, a uterus which contains ova, glands, ducts and excretory vessels. The eggs are passed in the stools or extruded from ripe segments which may appear either singly or in chains. Segments of large tapeworms may wriggle out through the anus. From the egg, *only a larva* can develop, the host of the larva being infected by swallowing the egg.

Larval forms. The egg hatches in the small intestine, the intermediate host releasing an embryo, which has six hooks (hexacanth embryo) with which it bores its way into the intestinal mucosa. In most cases the larva is then carried in the blood stream to the tissues where it develops, and the main or adult host becomes infected by swallowing mature larvae in the tissues of the intermediate host. Larvae of a few species (e.g. *Hymenolepis nana*) mature in the intestinal villi.

There are many thousands of species of tapeworm but the life cycle has been worked out accurately in only about one hundred. Of those affecting man, *Diphyllobothrium latum* requires three hosts, *H. nana* and other dwarf tapeworms require only one, and the rest require two hosts.

There are various types of cestode larvae. They are mainly in two forms; bladder larvae and solid larvae. Of the bladder larvae, the cysticercus is simple with one head which is readily evaginated by pressure, the cysticercoid has a poorly developed bladder, the coenurus has a single bladder and many heads, and the hydatid produces thousands of heads in brood capsules and daughter cysts. In the case of the solid larvae, there is no central liquefaction and the embryo develops into a form known as a plerocercoid or sparganum.

Adult cestodes

Man is the only main or definitive host of two tapeworms, *Taenia saginata* and *T. solium*. *H. nana* and other dwarf tapeworms which infect man are normally found in rats and mice. *Dipylidium caninum* is a common parasite of dogs and cats which sometimes infects man. *D. latum* is found in the small intestine of many other vertebrates besides man.

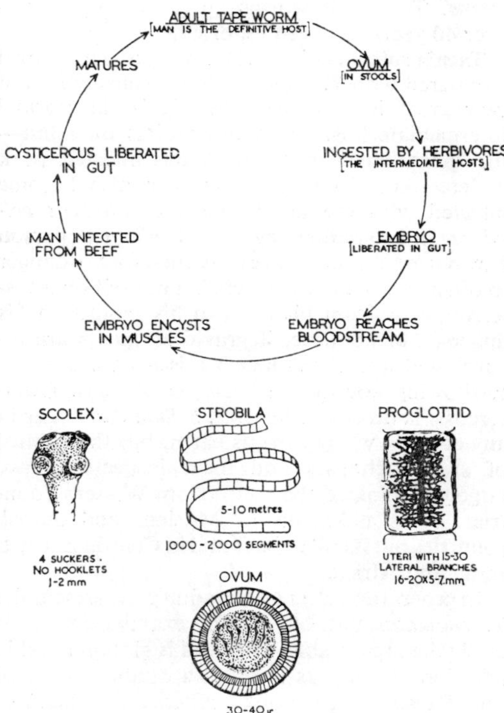

FIG. 10.1. *Life cycle of* Taenia saginata.

Taenia saginata. (Fig. 10.1): the commonest tapeworm infecting man. It is known as the 'beef tapeworm', since man becomes infected through eating under-cooked beef containing the larval form (*Cysticercus bovis*). Its distribution is world-wide and it is particularly common in parts of the

Middle East and in Ethiopia, where multiple infections are very common.

The worm usually measures several metres in length, sometimes attaining 10 m with thousands of segments. The head is pear-shaped, about 1–2 mm in diameter, with four suckers but no hooks. Gravid segments measure some 2 × 1.4 cm. The uterus has twenty to thirty-five compound lateral branches in each side. The egg measures about 36 μm in diameter and has a thick brown radially striated shell which is often ruptured and lost. It contains a hexacanth embryo. Cattle become infected with cysticerci through swallowing eggs or segments passed in the faeces of man on their pasture land. The cysts measure about 9 × 5 mm. When they are swallowed by man the bladder is digested and the head attaches itself to the wall of the small intestine and gives rise to segments, developing into an adult in some 6 weeks. The adult worms are very long-lived— over 40 years has been reported.

Taenia solium. (Fig. 10.2): an uncommon worm compared with *T. saginata*, but medically it is of very great importance. The pig is the normal intermediate host and man acquires the adult— the 'pork tapeworm'—by eating infected pork undercooked. Man, however, can also become infected with the larval stage, *Cysticercus cellulosae*, if he swallows eggs of *T. solium*. A person harbouring an adult worm is therefore a danger to others and can also autoinfect himself by transferring eggs from his anus to his mouth on his fingers. Furthermore, if gravid segments are regurgitated into the stomach this is equivalent to swallowing countless thousands of eggs. Cysticercosis is described later. *T. solium* can occur in any country where pork is eaten, but the control of slaughterhouses and meat inspection have largely eliminated the worm from Western countries. It is unknown in Moslem and Jewish countries but is still to be found in Central Europe, India and Africa.

In general appearance, the adult worm resembles *T. saginata*, but on careful examination it is easily distinguishable. The head is globular and in addition to suckers it bears a double crown of about twenty-eight hooks, whereas the head of *T. saginata* is bare. The worm can also be distinguished if a gravid segment is examined with a hand lens, for in *T. solium* the uterus has only eight to ten coarse lateral branches whilst in the case of *T. saginata* there are about three times as many fine branches. The eggs of *T. solium* and *T. saginata* are identical in appearance. The pig becomes infected with cysticerci by swallowing eggs or mature segments passed in human faeces.

'Measly pork' is honeycombed with cysts which are about the size of a pea. They can usually be seen under the tongue of an infected animal; 'langueyage' was first used by meat inspectors in France.

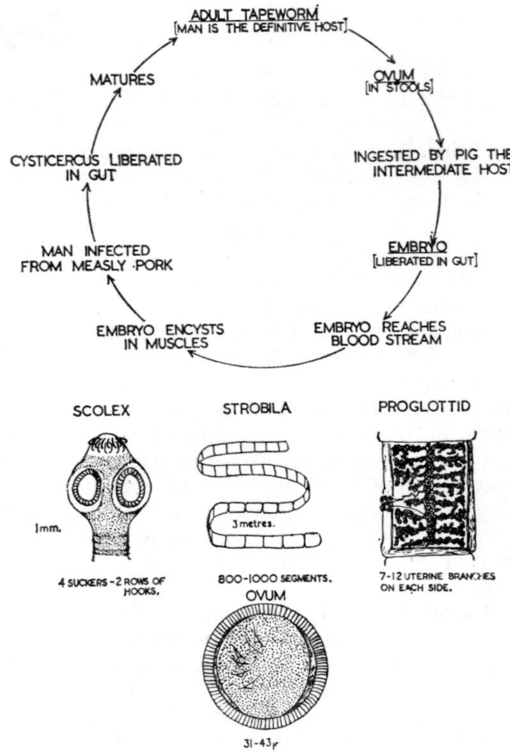

Fig. 10.2. *Life cycle of* Taenia solium.

Hymenolepis nana. This is one of a large group of dwarf tapeworms which are common parasites of rats and mice. Three of these—*H. nana*, *H. diminuta* and *Drepanidotaenia lanceolata*—may be found in large numbers in man in the tropics and subtropics. *H. nana* infection is common in parts of the U.S.A.

The worm lives in the small intestine. It is small and thread-like, about 1–3 cm long with over a hundred proglottides which are short and broad. The head is globular with four suckers and a single crown of hooklets. The egg measures about 50 μm and has an outer and an inner vitelline membrane. When it is swallowed, the hexacanth embryo escapes and penetrates a villus where it develops into a cysticercoid larva. This matures and ruptures the villus, returning to the lumen of the intestine. The head becomes attached to the intestinal wall and gives rise to segments. There is no intermediate host and man becomes infected by swallowing the eggs in food or water polluted by rats or by infected persons.

Dipylidium caninum. This is a common parasite of dogs, cats, foxes and jackals. It occurs all over the world and sometimes is found in man. The worm measures about 30 cm in length. The head has four elliptical suckers and three to four rows of hooklets. There are several hundred narrow segments. It has a round egg measuring about 40 μm. The eggs are eaten by larval fleas and lice in which minute cysticerci develop. Man is infected by accidentally swallowing infected fleas.

Diphyllobothrium latum. This large worm, known as the 'broad tapeworm' or 'fish tapeworm', is discussed on page 147.

Symptoms

The average patient with tapeworm infection is symptomless. The first indication of the presence of one of the larger worms is usually the passage of segments in the stools. Mature segments often wriggle out through the anus and are discovered in the bed or on the underclothes. There may be vague abdominal discomfort and loss of weight. The appetite may be voracious, but anorexia, vomiting, diarrhoea and anaemia sometimes develop in debilitated patients and in children. In rare instances *T. saginata* has caused severe enteritis and malabsorption which has proved fatal. Massive infections with dwarf tapeworms, at times numbering thousands, can cause abdominal pain, diarrhoea with mucus and convulsions in children. *Diphyllobothrium* produces severe anaemia if it is attached high up in the small intestine in the duodenum or jejunum where it can absorb vitamin B_{12} from the intestinal contents before the host is able to do so. Eosinophilia is variable in tapeworm infection, but it is rarely pronounced.

Treatment

Many different drugs and native remedies have been used in the treatment of tapeworm. The object is to expel the whole of the worm. In the case of *T. saginata*, *T. solium* and *D. latum* infections, if the head is not recovered from the stools following treatment the patient should be followed up for 3 months. If no eggs or segments are passed again during this time, cure has been achieved; if they do appear, treatment must be repeated. It should be remembered that multiple infections with these large tapeworms are not unusual. The following are the principal drugs in use. They are effective against all tapeworms.

Male fern. This time-honoured remedy gives good results provided attention is paid to the preparation of the patient, who should be well purged and fed on fluids only for 48 hours before treatment. Filix mas is the rhizome of the male fern and contains filicic acid and aspidin, which are both anthelmintics. The liquid extract can be given as a draught, which is nauseating, through a duodenal tube or in capsules by mouth. Provided the capsules are fresh and dissolve readily, they are very satisfactory. Starting first thing in the morning two capsules, each containing 1 ml of liquid extract of filix mas, are given at intervals of 15 minutes for six doses. Two hours later the worm and the drug are removed with a saline purge such as 15–30 g of magnesium sulphate. Castor oil should not be used because fats aid the absorption of the drug, which may cause toxic effects such as peripheral neuritis. All stools are saved for the next 24 hours, strained through muslin, and searched against a dark background for the minute head of the worm.

Mepacrine. This is equally effective after the same preparation as for treatment with filix mas. One gram (ten tablets) is administered first thing in the morning, followed 2 hours later by a purge. When the worm is evacuated it is stained bright yellow. Mepacrine is an extremely bitter substance and is liable to cause vomiting, especially, if it is given in a draught. It is better avoided for patients infected with *T. solium*, since vomiting may cause ripe segments of the worm to be regurgitated into the stomach: liberation of the many thousands of ova which they contain might lead to a massive infection with cysticerci.

Dichlorophen (Anthiphen) has been widely used since its introduction in 1955. The great advantage of this drug lies in the fact that no special preparation is necessary. It kills the worm in the intestine and the parasite may disintegrate in the bowel before it is passed, so that the head may not be recognised in the stools. Cures, therefore, cannot be claimed until the patient has been followed up for 3 months. The drug is given in a single dose of twelve tablets (0.5 g each) for adults and four to eight tablets for children, taken with a drink before breakfast. The drug has a laxative effect, so that no purge is necessary.

Niclosamide (Yomesan) is a very effective new anthelmintic. No preparation is necessary. Two tablets (0.5 g each) are chewed first thing in the morning on an empty stomach, washed down with water, and two more tablets are taken after an hour. There are no side effects. After 2 hours a saline purge is given or alternatively, an intramuscular injection of pituitrin, 5 units. The worm is then passed, usually complete with its head and stained faintly yellow.

CYSTICERCOSIS

The larval forms of a number of tapeworms can invade the tissues of man, often with serious consequences. Hydatid disease (page 153) and cysticercosis are common forms of somatic taeniasis. Other rarer examples are sparganosis (page 150) and infection with *Coenurus cerebralis*, the larva of *Multiceps multiceps*, a canine tapeworm. This larva occurs commonly in the brains of sheep and other herbivorous animals and is a rare cause of cerebral symptoms in man. The coenurus cyst is a vesicle, usually the size of a walnut, which contains clusters of scolices. Larvae of other species of *Multiceps* are at times found in human muscles.

Cysticercosis is the name given to the accidental somatic infection of man by the larval or bladder-worm stage of *T. solium*. As already stated, the adult *T. solium* is a parasite of man alone and normally the larval stage is passed in the pig, the parasitised flesh being known as 'measly pork'. The disease has been reported from most parts of the world. It was once common in Germany, where the popularity of uncooked ham favoured the survival of *T. solium*. It now occurs mainly in Central Europe, Central and South America, Africa, the Far East and India, where most of the patients diagnosed in Britain became infected during military service.

Aetiology

An individual harbouring the adult worm passes hundreds of thousands of eggs in the stools, for a gravid proglottis *T. solium* contains some 40 000 eggs. Man can become infected with cysticerci by swallowing eggs in water, uncooked vegetables, salads and other articles of food which have been contaminated directly or through the agency of flies. In addition, autoinfection is common in hosts of the adult worm, either by transferring eggs from the anus to the mouth on the fingers or by the regurgitation of gravid segments from the small intestine into the stomach. In most heavily infected patients, in which there may be countless thousands of cysticerci, there is usually a history of tapeworm.

Hexacanth embryos liberated from the eggs penetrate the intestinal mucosa and are carried in the blood stream to their final habitat, usually the voluntary muscles and the brain, where they prefer the grey matter. Any tissue or organ may, however, be affected; cysts have been found in the eye, heart, liver, lungs, pancreas and peritoneum. The full development of the cysticercus takes about 3–4 months. Except in the brain the cysticercus becomes enveloped in a fibrous capsule. In the brain there is a proliferation of surrounding neurological tissue together with cellular reaction. As a rule, as long as the cysticercus is alive no ill-effects are produced, although massive infection of the brain may prove fatal at any early stage.

When it dies, it acts as an irritant foreign body and a cellular reaction is set up, and in addition the cyst wall becomes distended with fluid and pressure may occur. The life span of the cysticercus varies greatly. Many parasites die off between the third and sixth years but they may continue to live for much longer periods. Dead cysts become calcified and eventually, after some years, can be seen on X-ray examination. Cysts in the brain show less tendency to calcify than those in the muscles; intracranial calcification can be demonstrated in about 30 per cent of patients with cerebral symptoms (Plate 2a).

Symptoms

The most characteristic clinical features of cysticercosis are palpable subcutaneous cysts and epileptiform attacks. However, these are by no means invariable. Fulminating cases may occur in which massive infection of the brain proves rapidly fatal in the early stages, the clinical picture being one of acute encephalitis. In other cases there may be symptoms of a rapidly expanding intracranial lesion leading to coma and death.

Premonitory symptoms. At the time of invasion of the tissues there may be fever, generalised muscular pains, headache and urticaria accompanied by eosinophilia. Such premonitory symptoms are not constant, but they have been noted in patients harbouring adult *T. solium* who have later developed cysticercosis.

Incubation period. This is often impossible to assess. The majority of patients develop symptoms of cysticercosis within 7 years of the probable time of infection. Recorded incubation periods vary from a few months to as long as 30 years. The disease may remain symptomless in some cases.

Established disease. The first indication is usually an epileptiform attack. Fits are present in over 80 per cent of patients and are the sole symptom in some 30 per cent. These attacks are extremely variable. They may resemble major epilepsy so closely that patients have been kept under treatment for grand mal for many years before the true aetiology has been recognised. Other attacks may simulate petit mal, or there may be series of

Jacksonian attacks starting from different foci in the same patient.

Epilepsy is not the only disease simulated. Symptoms and signs may suggest disseminated sclerosis or cerebral tumour. A cysticercus arising from the leptomeninges in the basal cisterns may develop in a racemose form and may cause intermittent or permanent hydrocephalus with symptoms of meningoencephalitis and cerebellar dysfunction. There may be alterations in the psyche and in the behaviour pattern, and some patients are diagnosed as hysterics. A cysticercus in the pituitary fossa can produce the syndrome of panhypopituitarism.

Nodules. Palpable or visible subcutaneous cysts occur in about 50 per cent of cases. These may appear and disappear so that the patient may form the impression that they can migrate from place to place. They may be as small as a grain of rice or as large as a pigeon's egg. They are not tender and they may be difficult to find. Careful palpation of the whole body is an essential part of the examination of a patient suspected of cysticercosis. They are more frequently felt in the pectoral and abdominal muscles than in the limb muscles. They may antedate or follow the onset of fits. Multiple cysts in the muscles may cause pseudohypertrophy.

Some infected individuals may remain free from symptoms and calcified cysts may be revealed in healthy individuals at routine X-ray examinations. The mortality from cysticercosis is low; about 8 per cent of cases are fatal. Individual prognosis is very difficult, but in the average case the fits tend to lessen after about 10 years (Dixon and Hargreaves, 1944).

Diagnosis

Cysticercosis should be considered in all cases of epilepsy in which the patient has lived in an endemic area, especially India. A careful search for nodules should be made and if one is found it should be excised. It is then freed from its fibrous capsule, when gentle pressure will cause the head to evaginate. Radiological examination is the only other certain means of diagnosis. It is only positive when the cysts have become calcified. The films should include all the muscles of the body and the skull. The small opaque nodules are characteristic and may be present in small numbers or in thousands (Plate 2b).

Treatment

This is very unsatisfactory and consists of palliative measures. Anticonvulsant drugs are given as for epilepsy. Surgery is useful in only a very small number of selected cases. Excision of cerebral cysticerci for focal epilepsy rarely affects the course of the disease. Decompression for intracranial hypertension has proved worthwhile in some instances.

DIPHYLLOBOTHRIUM LATUM

Aetiology

Parasite. The adult worm *Diphyllobothrium latum* is a ribbon-like segmented tapeworm 3–10 m long and 1 cm broad. It is greyish white in colour. The head (1–5 mm) is shaped like a spatula with two lips in the form of elongated suckers. These are the bothria, one ventral and the other dorsal. Behind the neck begin a series of segments or proglottides which number 3–4000 in all. Each is hermaphrodite and, when mature, greatly swollen at the centre which bulges from the accumulation of eggs within the uterus which shows as a black spot. Male and female genital orifices occupy a common papilla near the anterior border of the proglottis. Behind this lies the uterine pore or tocostome. Egg-laying begins in the middle segments; those at each end do not separate off forming fragments, but break up individually.

Definitive host. The tapeworm lodges itself in the duodeno-jejunal portion of the small intestine. Like other tapeworms, it absorbs food by osmosis and possesses both an excretory apparatus and a rudimentary nervous system. Unlike *Taenia saginata* and *solium*, infection is not just a question of a single worm. Man can harbour more than ten worms, whose overall length might amount to 60 metres. This multiple parasitism argues against any form of immunity or premunity.

In a case reported by Riley (1914) the lifespan of diphyllobothrium was estimated at 13 years. Other mammals such as the dog, cat, fox, leopard, pig, bear, seal, etc., can act as the definitive host, but in practice they represent less favourable hosts than man. In cats, the worm only reaches a length of 60 cm, 1 per cent of its eggs are viable and its lifespan is a few months. In dogs, 50 per cent of the eggs are viable.

Development (Fig. 10.3). Eggs are deposited in the faecal matter of the human intestine and excreted at a rate of a million eggs per tapeworm per day. The eggs are similar to those of the fluke, operculated, measuring about 70 by 45 μm. They are not embryonal at the egg-laying stage but must develop in water. After 10–15 days at 15–25°C, a ciliated hexacanth embryo is formed—the oncosphere or miracidium. For its subsequent development, diphyllobothrium requires two intermediate hosts.

Primary intermediate host. The miracidium must adapt its underwater environment. Since it can only exist for 24 hours, it has to be ingested by a freshwater copepod crustacean—*Cyclops* or *Diaptomus*—whose species vary greatly from country to country. Once in the digestive tract of the crustacean, the miracidium loses its cilia and relies on its hooks, invading the intestinal wall and developing in the haemal cavity. After 2–3 weeks it becomes a procercoid of 500 μm, with hooks at its caudal end.

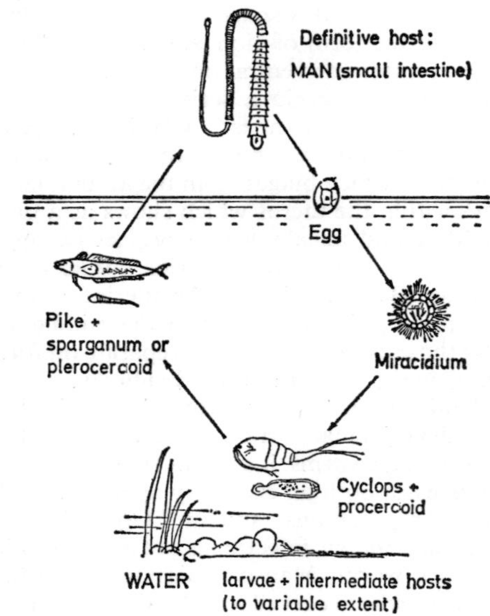

FIG. 10.3. *Life cycle of* Diphyllobothrium latum.

Secondary intermediate host. Cyclops is then ingested by a fish. The procercoid penetrates the intestinal wall and settles in various organs, especially muscle. Here it becomes a plerocercoid or sparganum, 1–2 cm long, 2–3 mm broad, worm-like but non-segmented and milky white in colour. The extreme anterior end is invaginated but has no scolex. It often happens that a small fish already infected is swallowed by a larger fish. The plerocercoids then become encapsulated within the muscles of their new host (burbot) or within the abdominal viscera (pike). The fish which are most commonly infected, at least in Europe, are pike, burbot, perch, salmon, trout, lavaret, char, pope, and in southern Africa, barbel.

Mode of entry. Man becomes infected by eating uncooked or inadequately cooked fish which con-tains plerocercoids. Once in the small intestine, these develop into adult diphyllobothria 5 weeks later.

Distribution

Diphyllobothrium or fish tapeworm is a wide-spread parasite whose distribution is continually extending. It is encountered mostly in cold or temperate lake regions, though it also exists at certain altitudes in the tropics, for instance in southern Africa around Lake N'gami. It is found in Central Africa too, in Uganda, Madagascar and the Congo. The most important European foci are the Scandinavian countries, the rivers of the Baltic, and Rumania at the delta of the Danube. Switzerland offers an example of its uneven distribution between lakes; while the pike, perch and burbot of Geneva, Bienne and Neu-châtel (occasionally Maggiore and Como) are carriers of sparganum, those of Lugano, Lucerne and Constance are free of infection.

In Asia, *D. latum* occurs in Palestine, Turkestan, Siberia and Japan. In the United States the para-site has been introduced by immigrant carriers crossing from Canada, particularly to Minnesota. Cases from South America have only been des-cribed during the last 12 years, in Chile, apparently the result of importing live trout for breeding. Normally trout do not exist in the southern hemisphere.

Cases of infection may be encountered outside the country of origin from consumption of im-ported fish, caviare for example from pike. There seems to be no significant variation in suscepti-bility nor any form of immunity or premunity. Infection depends on individual eating habits, occasionally on inadequate preparation of fish. Females have a higher incidence of worm infec-tion because the housewife often tastes her dish before it is fully cooked.

In countries like Finland, where infection is endemic, the definitive host is usually man, but the comparative rarity of human cases in Switzer-land and Italy makes it more likely that the role is here taken by other fish-eating animals such as the dog or cat.

Clinical features

1. In the great majority of cases, diphyl-lobothriasis remains latent and is discovered by chance during faecal examination.

2. In a few rare cases, the parasite causes vague *digestive, nervous,* or more *generalised* symptoms. Their variable nature causes them to be attri-buted more often to the temperament of the

patient than the pathological effect of the cestode. Sometimes these upsets are digestive in type—nausea, vomiting, meteorism, anorexia, boulimia; alternatively diarrhoea and constipation, or pain mimicking ulcer, appendicitis, biliary colic, etc.

It occasionally gives rise to nervous disorders—choreiform convulsions, meningitic symptoms, sensory disorders, e.g. vertigo. Allergy may manifest itself in itching, urticaria or asthmatic crises. General emaciation is rare.

3. A very characteristic sign of diphyllobothriasis is *anaemia*, usually of moderate severity, but occasionally progressing to simulate severe pernicious (Addisonian) anaemia. It presents as pallor of the skin and mucous membranes without jaundice, together with dyspnoea of effort, palpitations and tachycardia. Glossitis is rare, the nails are normal. There is no fever or oedema, nor any neurological or psychiatric signs.

It is hyperchromic and macrocytic in type, sometimes megaloblastic. It responds favourably to liver extract, vitamin B_{12} and folic acid. An essential feature is that in recovery the blood picture is maintained once the worm has been expelled.

The existence of parasitic anaemia is often challenged by assertion of certain paradoxical facts: compared with the widespread geographic distribution of diphyllobothrium, that of the anaemia is limited to the Scandinavian countries; even in these countries the proportion of anaemic patients is small when compared with the total number infested; finally, the severity of anaemia does not parallel the severity of infestation.

On the other hand, defenders of parasitic anaemia, notably Von Bonsdorff, put forward the following points:

(*a*) Diphyllobothrium takes up large amounts of vitamin B_{12}. Von Bonsdorff and Nyberg find the B_{12} content of diphyllobothrium to be fifty times (2–3 μg) that of *T. saginata*. Nyberg, making use of labelled Vitamin B_{12}, finds that in infected subjects 44 per cent of the vitamin is absorbed by the worm as against 0 per cent in *T. saginata*. In 1962, the same author showed that *D. latum* is able to denature, break down and utilise combined extrinsic and intrinsic factors. The serum level of cyancobalamin in a patient with diphyllobothriasis is diminished (100 mg/ml instead of 275 mg/ml in a healthy subject).

(*b*) This parasitic affinity for vitamin B_{12} is favoured by a site high in the intestine, e.g. jejunum, and antagonised by positions lower down, e.g. ileum.

(*c*) The number of worms harboured by an individual seems to be less important than the pathogenicity of certain species of diphyllobothria.

(*d*) Yet even in Scandinavia, the only area where this complication is seen, anaemia does not occur in all infected subjects. Only those whose worms are situated high in the intestine are susceptible, and are particularly so if undernourished before they become infected. Perhaps this has a similar basis to the anaemia described by Immerslund (1962).

Diagnosis

The diagnosis of diphyllobothriasis is easily established by faecal examination since the eggs of *D. latum* deposited in the intestine will be mixed with faecal matter. They are often confused with eggs of the liver fluke *Fasciota hepatica*, but may be distinguished by their size and profusion. In North America it is difficult to differentiate the eggs from those of *D. cordatum* (70 × 50 μm), and in Japan from those of *Diplogonoporus grandis*. It is essential for diagnosis to examine for worms after administration of a purgative.

Treatment

Tapeworm infection is treated with the classical purgatives such as male fern extract, or with niclosamide used in a single dose of 2 g. Such treatment may be employed both in the individual case and for large numbers of patients.

Mass prophylaxis must be directed towards the principal definitive host, man. Latrines and sewers must avoid contaminating lakes, pools and other fresh water.

Individual prophylaxis lies in protecting the healthy subject from consuming raw or poorly cooked fish.

OTHER DIPHYLLOBOTHRIA

Compared with the frequency of infections with *D. latum*, other species play a minor role, limited both by their low incidence and their non-tropical distribution. We may mention:

D. cordatum is a small tapeworm (1 m) which exists in North America and Japan. The definitive hosts are dogs, bears and pinnipeds; very rarely man. The secondary host is a saltwater fish.

Diplogonoporus grandis can attain a length of 10 m. The definitive hosts are cestaceans, and in Japan occasionally man. The plerocercoids are found in teleostean marine life.

Diphyllobothrium pacificum is a tapeworm of seals and man. Specimens found in man are bigger (10–196 cm) than those found in the seal. Human cases have been encountered along the north

L

coast of Peru in subjects who have never left the shores of the Pacific or ingested freshwater fish. Infection arises from the consumption of a Peruvian delicacy called 'lebice' made of raw seafish minced and soaked in lemon. The eggs of *D. pacificum* are found about once in every thousand faecal specimens examined.

PLEROCERCOIDOSIS OR SPARGANOSIS

Cestodes most commonly responsible for cases of plerocercoidosis in man belong to the genus *Spirometra*, in particular the two species *S. erinacei europaei*, which occurs throughout the world, and *S. erinacei mansoni* which is confined to Asia, especially tropical areas.

The definitive hosts are cats and dogs, either domestic or wild. Man does not seem to be susceptible.

The primary host is a small copepoda of the genus *Cyclops*.

The secondary hosts are batrachia (adult or larval), reptiles and even small mammals. The mode of transmission to man is considered below.

Sparganosis induced by penetration of body surface

These cases are seen especially in Indochina and Hong-Kong, less commonly in Africa. They present as subcutaneous sparganosis involving the eye and eyelids.

The traditional medicine of the Far East includes a special form of anti-inflammatory treatment—a freshly skinned frog is applied to the inflamed surface, say the conjunctiva of the eye, and this produces a cool soothing sensation.

Unfortunately the frog is often a carrier of sparganum, the secondary larval stage of *S. erinacei mansoni*, a parasite of dogs and members of the cat family. By true biotropism, the parasite abandons the dead frog and enters the eye, a migration accomplished without any painful reaction; it ends by encapsulation of sparganum. After a latent period of 6–12 days, an oedematous swelling, inflamed and irritant, appears in the orbital region. The face is disfigured and super-infection often occurs leading to loss of the eye.

Ocular sparganosis, well known to ophthalmologists in the Far East, is amenable to surgical treatment, that is, incision of the pseudocyst and removal of the larva which measures 3–5 cm by 5 mm.

Sparganosis involving other organs has been observed occasionally after the application of skinned frogs to the male or female genitals. The parasite responsible always seems to be *S. erinacei*

mansoni. The mechanism of encapsulation in induced sparganosis has been fully worked out and confirmed by experimental studies.

Spontaneous sparganosis

Apart from a few cases in Africans and Australians, 41 cases of spontaneous human sparganosis have been reported during the last 10 years in the United States, 14 in Louisiana and 5 in Florida. Swartzwelder (1964) has published some 23 cases (16 female, 7 male) aged about 35 years from both rural and urban areas. The swellings were subcutaneous or muscular, occasionally involving mucous membranes, peritoneum or epididymis. They contained sparganum, some of which had remained alive for several years, some as many as 20 years.

Riwlin (1968) writes of an amateur fisherman of 37 in Florida. A painless mobile swelling in the region of the left zygoma reached the size of a walnut in 2 months resembling a sebaceous cyst or lipoma. After excision, histological examination revealed a worm in the dermal layer surrounded by a histiolymphocytic reaction. It proved to be a plerocercoid of *S. erinacei*.

The mode of infection in spontaneous sparganosis remains obscure as do the larval stages, procercoid and plerocercoid, presumably responsible for the infection. Several theories have been advanced.

1. Encapsulation of sparganum after penetration of the skin, for which there is no evidence.

2. Internal spread of sparganum followed by encapsulation after ingesting inadequately cooked fish, frog, reptile or game. This would be due to the parasite rejecting man as the definitive host. A more plausible explanation is that the man accidentally swallowed a tadpole. Questioning often uncovers the fact that the patient drank swamp water while out shooting. Bonne, and Galliard, have shown that the adult frog *Rana tigrina* is not susceptible to procercoids formed in *Cyclops*. But when the frog swallows an infected tadpole, the larvae encapsulate.

3. Another possibility is accidental ingestion of *Cyclops* in drinking water. H. Kokayashi has shown that the plerocercoids of *S. erinacei mansoni* will readily develop in some homothermal vertebrates, for instance rats, mice and even man who as incidental host then acts as substitute for the secondary intermediate host.

Also puzzling is the origin of *Sparganum proliferum* whose adult stage is unknown. A few cases have been observed in Japan and Florida. It presents as a giant larva, dividing and growing in the manner of a malignant tumour and capable of invading the subcutaneous tissues, intermuscular septa, intestinal wall, mesentery, kidney, lungs, heart and brain.

Is this the teratological behaviour of a larval form of *D. mansoni,* as J. E. Mueller thinks, or that of a different species altogether whose definitive host remains obscure?

Treatment and final diagnosis. Treatment consists of incising the tumour containing the parasite and removing it intact and living. By feeding it to a dog or cat, the development of the cestode to its adult stage allows an accurate diagnosis of the species to be made. This is the first essential if we are to elucidate the mode of infection in spontaneous plerocercoidosis of man.

REFERENCES

BONNE, C. (1942) *Amer. J. trop. Med.,* **22,** 643–645.
BRUMPT, E. (1950) *Précis de Parasitologie,* ed. Masson. Paris.
DIXON, H. B. F. and HARGREAVES, W. H. (1944) *Quart. J. Med.,* N.S. **13,** 107.
EUZEBY, J. (1964) *Les Zoonoses Helminthiques,* ed. Vigot Frères. Paris.
FAUST and RUSSELL (1964) *Clinical Parasitology,* ed. Lea and Fibiger. Philadelphia.
GALLIARD, H. and NGU, D. V. (1946) *Ann. Parasit.,* **21,** 246–253.
GRASBECK, R., NUBERG, W., SAARNI, M. and VON BONSDORFF, B. (1962) *J. Lab clin. Med.* **59** (3),419–429.
MUELLER, J. F., HART, E. P. and WALSH, W. P. (1963) *J. Parasit.,* **49,** 292–296.
RYWLIN, A. M., BECK, J. W. and SNYDER, G. B. (1968) *Arch. Derm.,* **97** (4), 425–427.
SWARTZWELDER, J. C., BEAVER, P. C. and HOOD, H. W. (1964) *Amer. J. trop. Med,* **64** (13), 43–47.

11
Hydatid Disease

Hydatid disease or echinococcosis is the clinical term given to the existence of a hydatid cyst, the larval stage of *Echinococcus granulosus*, in the tissues of man.

PARASITE

E. granulosus is a small tapeworm that varies in length between 2.5 and 9 mm. It is formed of a head with four suckers, a short slender neck, and three or four body segments. It lives in the small intestines of canine species such as dogs, wolves, foxes and jackals. Intermediate hosts include sheep, cattle, camels and dogs, but man may also be an intermediate host (Fig. 11.1.)

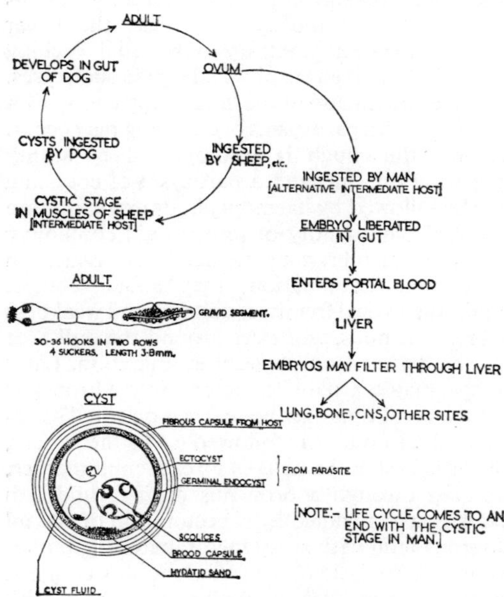

FIG. 11.1 *Life cycle of* Taenia echinococcus.

Transmission of infection to man is through the ingestion of eggs usually conveyed by uncooked vegetables or water contaminated with infected canine faeces. Contamination of the hands through playing with infected dogs is another important method of human infection.

PATHOLOGY AND PATHOGENESIS

Ova are swallowed by the intermediate host, the egg shell is digested in the duodenum and the six hooked oncosphere escapes into the lumen of the jejunum. The released oncospheres then penetrate the intestinal wall and invade the portal blood stream, being carried passively in the blood until they reach a capillary filter. The first such filter is the mass of small intrahepatic branches of the portal vein where the majority of oncospheres become implanted. This explains why the liver is the most common site of hydatid disease. The next filter is in the lungs, where further arrest occurs. A small proportion of oncospheres pass the lungs and these may lodge in any organ of the body. Such larval forms are attacked by the host's defence mechanisms and large numbers are destroyed. However, surviving embryos increase rapidly in size. Vacuoles develop in their cytoplasm and within 3 weeks they become vesicular and visible to the naked eye. After 3 months a hydatid cyst attains a diameter of 5 mm, and within 5 months it doubles this size.

Hydatid cysts are usually solitary but sometimes more than one may be detected. About the fifth month, when the cyst has reached 4 cm in diameter, its wall becomes differentiated into the classical internal granular layer or *endocyst*, and an outer cuticular laminated non-nuclear layer, the *ectocyst*. The tissues of the host react by forming an enveloping *fibrous capsule*. The cavity of the cyst contains hydatid fluid with daughter cysts, brood capsules and scolices.

From the germinal layer, brood capsules arise as small buds which grow and become vacuolated and later develop stalks. Brood capsules may become separated from the mother cyst wall and lie free in the cystic cavity. They may develop internal buds, which ultimately form scolices with suckers and hooks, or rupture and liberate scolices into the hydatid fluid. Both brood capsules and free scolices which lie in the fluid of the hydatid cyst are commonly referred to as *hydatid sand.* Herniation of part of the mother cyst wall may occur after trauma or pressure resulting in endogenous daughter cysts. Exogenous buddings also occur, especially in bones.

In some cases brood capsules and scolices fail to develop and a sterile *hydatid cyst* forms. This type of cyst is unilocular, but there are two other important varieties, the *osseous* and the *alveolar*. The osseous hydatid is a simple unilocular cyst which is prevented from assuming the usual spherical form by the dense surrounding tissues. It travels along the bony canals and erodes the osseous tissue, sometimes invading the medullary cavity.

The alveolar hydatid is a malignant metastasising form with an irregular reticulate outline and little fibrous adventitia. The cyst is formed of a spongy mass with multiple vesicles, which are frequently sterile or undergoing degeneration or calcification. They contain instead of cystic fluid a jelly-like matrix. This alveolar hydatid is now known to be the larval stage of another species, *E. multilocularis*.

The liver is the chief site of cyst formation but other organs such as the lungs, abdominal cavity, muscles, subcutaneous tissues, pleura, heart, brain or spinal cord may become involved. The following incidence of hydatid cysts in the different organs has been reported by various observers: liver, including secondary peritoneal involvement, 63.3 per cent; lungs, 24.5 per cent; muscle and fascia, 4.6 per cent; bones, 2.6 per cent; kidneys, 2.2 per cent; spleen, 1.3 per cent; brain, 0.9 per cent; heart, 0.3 per cent; breast, 0.1 per cent; parotid, prostate and pancreas, 0.1 per cent. In another series the incidence was reported as: liver, 57–76.6 per cent; lungs, 3.8–14 per cent; omentum and peritoneum, 1.37–18.2 per cent; pleura, 0.7–0.9 per cent; skin, subcutaneous tissue and muscles, 0.7–9.1 per cent; spleen, 1.2–9.1 per cent; brain, 0.9–2 per cent; spinal cord, 0.8–0.9 per cent; kidneys, 1.6–6.1 per cent; pelvis, 0.2 per cent; bones, 0.8–9.1 per cent; other organs, 2.8–4.2 per cent.

A hydatid cyst of the left ventricle has been known to lead to a fatal paroxysmal tachycardia. In a personal case of hydatid cyst of the lung, much was coughed out and led to a temporary spontaneous cure, but 2 years later the same patient came back with extensive hydatid disease of the right lobe of the liver. This terminated in rupture of the cyst and death of the patient from allergic shock. In another personal case where multiple cysts were present in the spleen, liver and lung, a large hydatid cyst occupying the upper half of the spleen was diagnosed only after pneumoperitoneography.

The symptoms of a hydatid cyst depend upon its type, size and location in the body. It may remain asymptomatic throughout the patient's life, to be discovered only at autopsy. On the other hand, symptoms may be absent until the cyst becomes large enough to cause irritation or pressure on neighbouring organs or until rupture or suppuration supervenes.

A history of recurrent attacks of urticaria has been noted by the author in several patients who later proved to be suffering from hydatid disease. The urticaria was relieved by antihistaminic drugs and an intradermal test would have directed attention to the exact aetiology of the disease in the early part of its course.

In hydatid disease of the liver, indefinite symptoms such as vague abdominal pain may continue for a long time until the nature of the disease is discovered. Nausea may occur soon after meals and may be followed occasionally by vomiting which gives transient relief. On examination, bulging of the right hypochondrium or epigastrium due to gross hepatic enlargement may be seen. The swelling moves on respiration and is more marked if the cyst lies near the lower border of the liver. Contrary to the usual teaching a hydatid thrill is a rare physical sign in such cases.

In hydatid disease of the lung, recurrent pyrexia associated with paroxysms of coughing may occur. At first, the cough is accompanied by scanty expectoration, but later a paroxysm of coughing may be followed by haemoptysis or expectoration of a variable quantity of serous fluid containing shreds of membranous tissue. This tissue, on microscopic examination, may show scolices. Diminished vocal fremitus, dullness and weakness of breath sounds, and rales around the dull area may be detected on physical examination. Later the cyst may evacuate its contents into a bronchus and the condition may be relieved or cured spontaneously. In one case followed up by the author, a hydatid cyst of the lung, in an expectant mother, ruptured through a bronchus during childbirth and was accompanied by expectoration of 500 ml of serous fluid with spontaneous cure. In another instance, a hydatid cyst of the lung was coughed up, but 2 years later the patient came back with a large hydatid cyst in the right lobe of the liver.

In hydatid disease of the spleen, the cyst not uncommonly occupies the upper pole of the organ, projects backwards and is masked by the apparently normal anterior margin of the spleen. This renders clinical diagnosis impossible. Such cases can be detected radiologically only after diagnostic pneumoperitoneography. This procedure may be valuable in revealing the nature of lesions responsible for vague abdominal symptoms.

Osseus cysts usually develop slowly and, because of their insidious nature, are difficult to diagnose early. The commonest sites are the upper end of the femur, tibia or humerus, the vertebrae and the ribs. They may present with long-standing bony pain or with spontaneous fracture of a long bone. They are usually diagnosed radiologically. Spinal involvement may present clinically as a vertebral infection.

COMPLICATIONS

Rupture of the cyst, either spontaneously or during surgical interference, is accompanied by anaphylactic shock with vasomotor collapse, oedema, urticaria and respiratory distress. If the cyst ruptures into a blood vessel, dissemination of hydatid disease into other organs will occur in addition to anaphylactic shock. A hydatid cyst of the lung may rupture into a bronchus, resulting in spontaneous cure. A cyst of the liver may rupture into the peritoneal cavity or, after the development of adhesions, it may rupture into a bronchus, stomach, colon or any other adjacent hollow organ.

Suppuration of a hydatid cyst leads to symptoms of a liver or lung abscess. The commonest sites of such an abscess are the inferior border of the right lobe of the liver and the base of the right lung respectively.

Calcification of a hydatid cyst may lead to spontaneous cure.

DIAGNOSIS

A *history* of contact with dogs, the occasional detection of a hydatid thrill, together with recurrent attacks of allergic manifestations may suggest the diagnosis of hydatid disease. *Blood examination* shows a moderate eosinophilia. This is also suggestive but not diagnostic of hydatid disease, since it is present in other helminthic infections. The diagnosis is confirmed by the following laboratory examinations.

Serological tests

Intradermal test (Casoni's reaction). The antigen needed for this test, as well as for other serological investigations for the diagnosis of hydatid disease in man, is prepared from hydatid fluid obtained aseptically from cysts of infected cattle, sheep, hogs or man. Fluid from cysts degenerating or contaminated with blood or serum is discarded. Several samples are pooled. The fluid is filtered through a Seitz filter, incubated to ensure sterility, sealed in ampoules and stored at 4°C. It may or may not be preserved with 0.5 per cent phenol. It retains its antigenic properties for several months. It should be tested for antigenicity against normal persons to exclude pseudo-positive reactions due to animal proteins, as well as against persons with known echinococcus infection.

The test is performed by injecting intradermally 0.2 ml of 1 : 1000 dilution of the antigen in one forearm, and at the same time 0.2 ml of physiological saline in the other forearm as a control. Two types of reaction may occur. An *immediate reaction* appears within 20 minutes in the form of a wheal surrounded by erythema and induration. The area of the wheal should not be less than double that of the wheal initially raised by the injection before the test is considered positive. A *delayed reaction* occurs after 6 to 12 hours. Reports of 14 investigators between 1920 and 1929 indicate that about 86 per cent (58 to 100 per cent) of infected persons give positive reactions. Uninfected persons, as a rule, do not give positive reactions although the test involves a group reaction for taenial worms. The immediate reaction is positive more commonly than the delayed reaction. Care should be taken to exclude pseudo-reactions due to sheep serum in the antigen and traumatic sensitivity of the skin.

Complement fixation test. This is positive in 60 per cent of cases of hydatid disease. Complete calcification or death of the cyst may result in a negative reaction.

Precipitin test. One millilitre of serum from a suspected case is mixed with 1 ml of hydatid fluid in a test tube. The mixture is incubated for 3 hours at 37°C. Thick, fine or microscopic flocculation may be shown in a positive case. This test is of value in less than 50 per cent of cases.

X-ray diagnosis

Roentgenological examination is particularly useful in diagnosis and in locating cysts. The cysts are identified by their fluid content, spherical shape, the dense outline of the adventitia and alteration of the normal contour of the invaded organ. Shadows due to calcification of the cyst wall may be seen. Stereometry is the best method for localisation. However, the appearance of pulmonary cysts may simulate other conditions.

Laboratory diagnosis

This includes the finding of scolices, brood capsules, or daughter cysts in the fluid from a ruptured hydatid cyst. Exploratory puncture for the purpose of obtaining hydatid fluid is contra-indicated, since leakage may cause an immediate anaphylactic shock and secondary echinococcosis.

TREATMENT

Ideally the treatment of a hydatid cyst is surgical. The location and nature of the cyst determine the mode of surgical interference. Unilocular cysts are usually inoperable. Whenever possible, the cyst should be enucleated. Preliminary marsupialisation of the cyst, because of its safety, is the operation of choice especially with infected cysts.

Most workers consider that the chances of spontaneous cure are unpredictable and that cysts in the lung should be removed as early as possible. Lobectomy is usually the treatment of choice, as simple enucleation will not eliminate pulmonary suppuration if the lung parenchyma is badly damaged. Cysts in the liver, when removed, leave a large raw area and postoperative complications and death are not uncommon. Most cysts of the liver are best left alone.

Allergic manifestations of hydatid disease can usually be controlled by antihistamines. For severe allergy, oedema of the glottis or collapse from rupture of a cyst, corticosteroids and particularly dexamethazone in intravenous dosage of 10–20 mg may be life-saving.

PREVENTION

Since the dog is the chief source of human infection, attention should be directed towards reducing canine infection and to limiting contact between man and dog. In endemic areas, dogs should be barred from slaughterhouses and should not be fed on uncooked offal; the refuse from slaughtered animals should be burned or sterilised. Stray dogs should be killed and all dogs should be given a taeniafuge once or twice per year. Arecoline hydrobromide 4 mg per 5 kg body weight eliminates 95 per cent of *Echinococcus* from dogs, and three doses usually eliminates all the worms as well as *Dipylidium caninum* if present.

Personal cleanliness, proper hygenic conditions, proper cooking of vegetables and boiling of drinking water or ensuring that the supply is safe are all important.

12
Intestinal Nematode Infections

Aetiology

Parasite. Ascariasis in man is caused by infection with *Ascaris lumbricoides*, a nematode of which the male measures 150–310 mm and the female 200–350 mm by 4–6 mm. The male is distinguished from the female not only by its smaller size but by the marked ventro curvature of its posterior extremity and by two spicules which are contained within the terminal part of the ejaculatory duct. The ova measure 35–70 by 35–50 microns and are covered by an irregular albuminous coat within which there is a relatively thick transparent chitinous layer and within this again there is a delicate vitelline membrane. Infertile ova are not uncommonly found in faeces of infected persons; they are longer and narrower than are those which are fertile measuring 88–94 microns by 39–44 microns. They occur not only in those infections in which only female worms are present but also in ordinary infections in which up to about a fifth of the ova passed may be infertile. Infections in which all the worms are of one sex are invariably light for if any considerable number are present it is virtually certain that both sexes will be represented.

Development and life cycle. Ova are relatively resistant to desiccation and to antiseptics; they withstand 8 months' exposure to 2.4 per cent formaldehyde but are killed by solutions of 7.4 per cent. They are very resistant to cold and survive for long periods in snow during winter. Dryness and excessive moisture inhibit development of ova in soil, the optimum temperature for development being approximately 25°C. The larva moults within the ovum, it becomes infective and on being swallowed is liberated in the small intestine. It then burrows into the intestinal wall, reaches a blood vessel or lymphatic and is carried to the lungs. In the lungs it burrows through tissue until it reaches a bronchiole up which it migrates until it reaches the epiglottis. It is then swallowed in food or saliva and on reaching the small intestine again, develops into an adult (Fig. 12.1).

Those larvae which enter lymphatics are carried through the mesenteric lymph nodes from which they may eventually drain into the thoracic duct and thence into the subclavian vein and blood passing to the right heart. Alternatively they may find their way to the liver or burrow through the lymph node and so reach the peritoneal cavity from which they may also pass to the liver. Most

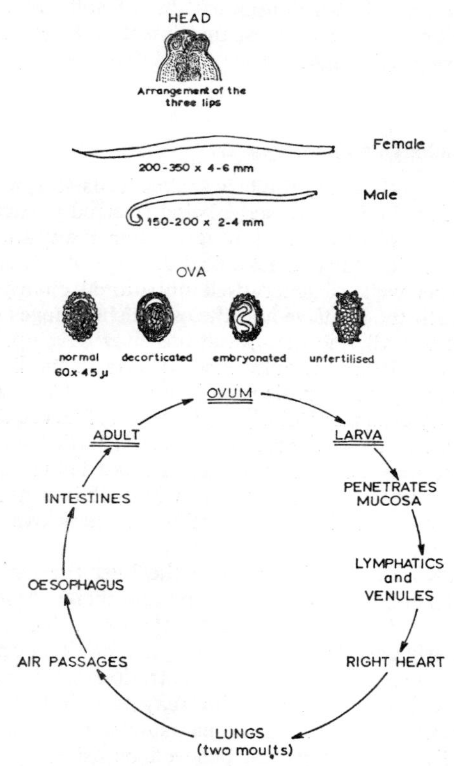

Fig. 12.1 *Life cycle of* Ascaris lumbricoides.

of those larvae reaching the liver will eventually be taken in blood to the lungs. The incubation period from the ingestion of the ova to maturation of the worm in the intestine is between 25 and 30 days.

Epidemiology

It follows from the life cycle of the parasite that consumption of food contaminated with soil containing ova of the worm is a common source of infection. Salad vegetables and others grown on contaminated soil and then eaten without being cooked are probably the commonest source of infection in adults. In children infection commonly occurs as a result of crawling or playing in earth and then putting the fingers to the mouth. Water-carried sanitation does much to reduce the incidence of the infection.

A. lumbricoides is encountered throughout the tropics and subtropics and in some temperate regions. Its prevalence varies widely from region to region and locality to locality; rates of 70 per cent or more may occur. In that part of some towns in the tropics inhabited by the poorer socio-economic classes contamination of soil around dwellings may be intense and infection rates correspondingly high.

Pathology and pathogenesis

The path which the larva takes leads to symptoms in the invasive stage being referred particularly to the liver and lungs. After maturation worms may cause mechanical damage to the viscera as well as generalised nutritional changes. In both the invasive and the established stages of infection allergic manifestations may develop.

LIVER. In and around larval tracks in the liver there may be necrosis with infiltration of inflammatory cells particularly eosinophils. If larvae die in the liver, a small granulomatous focus develops. There may be some enlargement and tenderness of the liver among those in whom it is heavily invaded following consumption of many ova at one time.

LUNGS. In the lungs as in the liver the larval tracks are haemorrhagic at first and then necrotic with much infiltration of inflammatory cells, particularly eosinophils. Areas of pneumonitis occur and there may be increased secretion within the bronchi; bronchial secretion may contain larvae.

BRAIN. In the brain, changes similar to those in the liver and lungs are believed occasionally to occur during the larval, invasive stage.

Histological reactions to Ascaris larvae. The changes in mesenteric lymph nodes invaded by *Ascaris* larvae were investigated by Tukumo (1956), and consisted of proliferation of reticulum and mononuclear cells, plasma cells and eosinophils; neutrophil leucocytes were scanty. The picture was that of a generalised mesenteric lymphadenitis. It was postulated that this resulted from four factors: (*a*) reaction to parasitic toxin, (*b*) the production by wandering larvae of physical and chemical destructive effects, (*c*) an allergic factor and (*d*) stimulation of the lymphatic nodes by unknown factors brought about by attachment of worms to the intestinal mucosa. Tukumo undertook this study because he had been confronted by many patients who complained of inconstant digestive symptoms and ill-defined abdominal pain and he concluded that the mesenteric lymphadenopathy demonstrated could well be the cause of such symptoms.

Pathology produced by adult *A. lumbricoides*. The main pathological changes produced by the adult worms are those resulting from mechanical obstruction to the intestinal tract or to ducts entering the tract. Others result from nutritional defects which may be precipitated by the infection. Obstruction to the small intestine may occur if the worms form into a bolus. This is most often encountered when young children are heavily infected and doubtless the relatively small size of the small intestine predisposes to this complication. Children who crawl on contaminated earth are also liable to develop particularly heavy infections.

NUTRITIONAL EFFECTS. Many clinical observations indicate that those infected with *Ascaris* or certain other helminths become stunted in growth provided the infection is heavy enough and persists for long enough. Laboratory confirmation of interference of *A. lumbricoides* with nutrients is, however, limited. There is good evidence from veterinary work that animals heavily infected with nematodes may use only as little as 40–60 per cent of the protein in their diet, and that as infections become lighter utilisation of the protein improves. In man Venktachalam and Patwardhan (1953) showed that *A. lumbricoides* interfere with the digestion and absorption of dietary protein. It is probable that in part this nutritional effect derives from the requirements for growth of the worms themselves and in part from production by the worms of enzymes which interfere with digestion of protein in the host's intestinal tract.

It has long been known that extract of *A. lumbricoides* inactivates trypsin and Collier (1941) isolated and purified an antienzyme factor from *Ascaris* and demonstrated in it both antitryptic and antipeptic properties, an observation suggesting that the antienzymes protect the worm from digestion by the host's intestinal ferments and at the same time are responsible in part for worms assisting in the production of malnutrition. Some of the enzymes produced by helminths are known to possess antigenic properties. Thus it has been shown that from an enzyme derived from

Ancylostoma caninum an antiserum may be produced which will inhibit and suppress the helminthic infection itself (Thorson, 1956). It was also shown by Koppisch and Oliver Gonzalez (1959) that extracts of cuticle, muscle, intestine and coelomic fluid of *A. lumbricoides* var *suum* are capable of producing autoagglutination of erythrocytes in experimental animals inoculated with the tissue extracts. This autoagglutination is mediated, it was suggested by alpha-2 isoglutinins, normally present in the animal's sera and which react with the injected antigen.

Competition between the helminth's and the host's supplies of vitamins may result in vitamin deficiencies and Scudmore *et al* (1961) using radioactive cobalt (^{60}Co) demonstrated a small uptake of vitamin B_{12} by *A. lumbricoides*.

Clinical features

Invasive stage. Although all *Ascaris* larvae pass through the lungs during their migration to the intestinal tract, not all of those who develop even heavy *Ascaris* infection give a history of having had symptoms referable to the lungs. This is explicable on the basis of a small number of larvae in the lungs at any one time being incapable of producing symptoms; however if small numbers of ova are swallowed at frequent intervals, a heavy infection would ultimately build up although not more than a few larvae would have passed through the lungs at any one time and such a small number would not give rise to symptoms.

The ability of the larvae, however, to produce severe clinical manifestations was demonstrated by Koino (1922) in what was a classical experiment on himself. He swallowed 2000 mature *A. lumbricoides* ova and 6 days later developed a fever of 104°F (40°C) which persisted for 7 days. He developed pneumonic symptoms and signs with dyspnoea and some cyanosis. There was profuse sputum and from the eleventh to sixteenth days after infection, this was saved and 202 *Ascaris* larvae were recovered from it; 50 days after swallowing the ova an anthelmintic was taken and 667 *A. lumbricoides* were passed in the faeces. Thus, of 2000 ova, 869 were accounted for either as larvae or as adult *A. lumbricoides*, leaving 1131, most of which had probably disintegrated in the tissues or failed to mature; some may have been discarded before the collection of sputum was commenced. The eosinophilia which so commonly follows the invasive stage of *Ascaris* infection doubtless results from disintegration of invading larvae in the tissues.

The invasive stage of *Ascaris* is thus known to be capable of producing pneumonitis or pneumonia with sputum, fever and eosinophilia. As is mentioned in the section on pathology, there is also a suggestion that ill-defined abdominal symptoms may result from larval invasion of mesenteric lymph nodes and the liver. Meningeal involvement as a result of invasion by *A. lumbricoides* larvae was suggested by Rodriguez and Zulian (1960).

Symptoms due to adult A. lumbricoides. In most light or moderately heavy infections there are few recognisable symptoms directly attributable to the parasites. There may be intestinal colic and occasionally worms are passed in the faeces. In such infections, and more particularly in heavy infections, they may migrate into orifices such as those of the appendix, Meckel's diverticulum or the common bile duct and be a cause of inflammatory disease. Occasionally they may migrate into the stomach and be vomited, and still less frequently they may reach the pharynx and nares. They have been known to enter and obstruct the Eustachian tubes. One of the most important complications of heavy infection is intestinal obstruction caused by a bolus of worms; this is most likely to develop in young children whose intestinal lumen is relatively small. It presents with signs and symptoms of intestinal obstruction often associated with fever caused by inflammation of the peritoneum covering the affected gut. Jaundice may be caused by the worms when they obstruct the common bile duct but this, although much described, is rare.

Expulsion of *A. lumbricoides* from children may speedily be followed by striking increase in weight, as was reported by Jelliffe (1953), and this is thought to be a manifestation of the benefits which follow removal of the adverse effects which *Ascaris* have on nutrition.

Treatment

The best treatment currently available for the infection is with piperazine. The drug paralyses the worms which are then passed in the faeces and their expulsion is aided by a small dose of purgative administered 1–2 hours after the anthelmintic. It has been claimed that a single dose is sufficient to expel the worms, but practice reveals that two or sometimes even three doses at intervals of 24 hours or more are necessary. Piperazine may be given as an elixir and this is particularly suitable for children. Of piperazine citrate elixir (Antepar, Burroughs Wellcome & Co.) 5 ml is equivalent to 750 mg of piperazine. For all persons weighing 20 kg or more, the recommended single dose is 30 ml and for those less than this weight 20 ml. A second dose after 24–48 hours is usually necessary to ensure a complete cure. Tablets of piperazine phosphate are also available each containing the equivalent of 500 mg piperazine; of these the adult dose is 4 g (8 tablets), and for those less than 20 kg in weight 3 g (6 tablets). Piperazine adipate (Entacyl B.D.H.) is produced in tablets containing 300 mg and 5 g of this salt are equivalent to 4 g piperazine. For adults and all over 6 years of age 4.8 g (16 tablets) are prescribed.

Toxic effects of piperazine include unsteadiness and vertigo of central nervous origin. Such symptoms are particularly liable to occur in persons

flavouring agent. It is very effective and has the advantage of cheapness, but stimulates the worms to considerable activity prior to killing them and fears have been expressed that this activity may cause damage to the bowel wall; as far as is known, however, there is no recorded incidence of this having happened.

Bephenium hydroxynaphthoate (Alcopar) is as effective against *Ascaris* as it is against hookworms and is given in doses of 5 g, washed down with a draught of water; no ensuing purgative is necessary.

Pyrantel pamoate (Combantrin) is effective in single doses of 10 mg per kg of the patient's body weight. Side effects are seldom encountered and it is also very effective against hookworms.

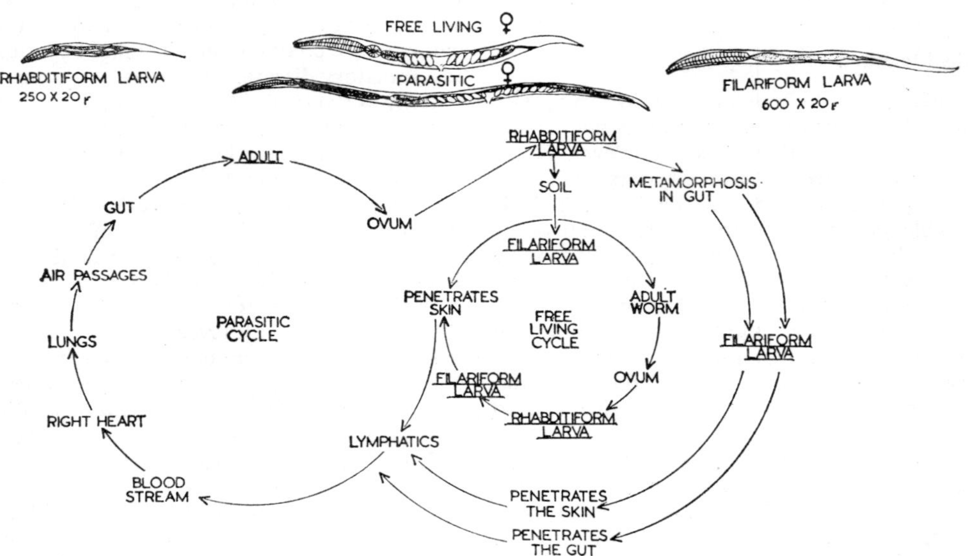

FIG. 12.2. *Life cycle of* Strongyloides stercoralis.

with impaired renal function and in others who are specially predisposed.

Tetramisole is given orally in a single dose of 2.5–5.0 mg per kg of the patient's body weight and is very effective and free from toxicity. The laevorotatory isomer of tetramisole (Levamisole) is also effective and is given in doses of 40 mg for those up to the age of 3 years; 60 mg between 3 and 9 years, and 80 mg for those of 9 years and over.

Tetrachlorethylene is much used for treatment of ascariasis, adults being given 3 to 4 ml, those of 8–14 years, 2 ml, and under this age 1 ml. It is best emulsified with mucilage and given as a draught flavoured with peppermint or other

Prognosis

The prognosis, both as regards termination of infection and recovery from complications, is excellent.

STRONGYLOIDIASIS

Definition

Strongyloidiasis is infection in man with the nematode *Strongyloides stercoralis*.

Aetiology

Life cycle of parasite. Acquisition of infection in man is by penetration of tissues with filariform larvae but the larvae which emerge from the ova produced by parasitic females are rhabditiform. These rhabditiform larvae must therefore develop into filariform larvae if they are to produce infection and they may do so either in a direct or indirect manner. If the direct pathway is followed, the rhabditiform larvae transform into the filariform after leaving the host and these will develop into adults if they succeed in penetrating the tissues of man. If the indirect pathway is followed, rhabditiform larvae in the faeces develop into free-living male and female adults. These produce ova from which rhabditiform larvae and some filariform larvae develop (Fig. 12.2).

The adult parasitic female measures 2.2 mm by 0.04 mm and has a slender tapering anterior extremity and a short conical pointed posterior. There are four indistinct lips to the buccal cavity and a long slender oesophageal pharynx which continues into the intestine. The free-living female measures only 1 mm by 0.06 mm and has a muscular oesophageal pharynx with two bulbs.

The parasitic and free-living adult males are similar to one another measuring 0.7 mm by 0.04 mm and having a ventrally curved tail. There are two copulatory spicules and a gubernaculum but no caudal alae.

The uterus of the parasitic female contains 8–12 thin-shelled ova measuring 50–58 microns by 30–34 microns.

Mode of infection. Filariform larvae which may have arisen from rhabditiform larvae either outside the body or within the intestinal tract, penetrate the intestinal mucosa or the perianal skin. They reach venules or lymphatic tracts which eventually empty their contents into the circulation and are carried to the right side of the heart whence they reach the lungs. In the lungs they pass through their third and fourth stages of development and usually pass up the bronchial tree to the pharynx. They are then swallowed in food and reaching the intestine mature into adults.

Autoinfection. Autoinfection plays an important part in the life cycle of the parasite and in its persistence as an infection in man. The rhabditiform larvae must change into filariform larvae before they can develop further and this may occur within the body as well as outside of it. The filariform larvae so produced may penetrate the perianal skin or the intestinal wall. It is also possible for the rhabditiform larvae that have invaded the tissues to develop into larvae of the filariform type. Each of these events may be followed by migration of the larvae to the lungs and ultimate development into adult form. Infection may persist for many years in man and autoinfection facilitates such prolonged persistence.

Epidemiology

The parasite is present in tropical and subtropical countries, more particularly among the warmer and more humid of them. *S. stercoralis* was first observed in Cochin-China, and the Far East remains one of the more highly endemic regions; it is also common in West Africa. Poor sanitation and contamination of soil by human faeces in areas of high rainfall are particularly liable to lead to transmission.

Pathology

Pathological changes may be produced at the site of penetration of the larvae in the skin, along their route of migration to the lungs and in the lungs themselves. Adult worms and larvae may give rise to pathology in the intestine.

Skin. The track of the penetrating filariform larvae may contain erythrocytes and inflammatory cells and be surrounded by acute inflammatory changes. Some persons who have been sensitised by previous infection may exhibit a considerable allergic response to invasion of the skin by larvae and oedema and erythematous wheals may then occur.

Lymph nodes. Tracks of parasites may be seen in invaded lymph nodes, and haemorrhage within and around the tracks may occur along with infiltration of inflammatory cells among which eosinophils are prominent. Areas of eosinophilic degeneration are not uncommon as a result of larval migration of this and other parasites.

Lungs. Migrating larvae produce areas of pneumonitis in which in addition to haemorrhage there is infiltration with leucocytes, particularly of the eosinophil variety. Local bronchi may become blocked with secretion and lobular areas of consolidation develop. Bronchial secretion may contain larvae which may either be following an invading migratory pathway or which may result from adults which have matured in the lungs. Tropical pulmonary eosinophilia constitutes a group of disorders in which radiological mottling of the lung is associated with eosinophilia and cough and it may be associated with a variety of helminthic infections of which *S. stercoralis* is one.

Intestine. In the mucosa and submucosa of the upper small intestine, adult females form cyst-like lesions and produce larvae which in heavy infections may lead to extensive honeycombing.

Larval tracks may be associated with haemorrhage and infiltration with inflammatory cells and catarrhal inflammation with sloughing may occur, the degree and extent of the changes depending upon the heaviness of the infection. In very heavily infected patients granulomatous masses may develop. From such regions of the intestine larvae may radiate widely to other parts of the intestine, the liver, gall-bladder, lymphatics, pancreas, mesentery and other organs and tissues. Heavy infections with honeycombing of the intestinal wall have been associated with malabsorption and a sprue-like syndrome (Alcron and Kotcher, 1961).

Blood. An instance in man in which *Escherichia coli* were disseminated by filariform *S. stercoralis* larvae was reported by Wilson and Thompson (1964). In this case *E. coli* and filariform larvae were removed at operation from a mesenteric lymph node. The patient later died from *E. coli* meningitis and the organism was found to be the same as that isolated from the lymphatic node. It appeared highly probable that the filariform larvae migrating from the intestinal tract to the lymphatic nodes had taken with them *E. coli* which by causing a septicaemia had resulted in the meningitis from which the patient died. This case underlines the importance of larvae, which migrate from the intestinal tract to other tissues, as sources from which intestinal organisms may reach the blood and produce septicaemia or viraemia. Woodruff (1968) drew attention to helminths as vehicles and synergists of microbial infections.

Clinical features

Symptoms arise from the presence of larvae in the skin and their migration through tissues to the lungs where both larvae and adults may give rise to clinical manifestations. Most symptoms however are related to the intestinal tract, where both larvae and adults may also be responsible for them.

Experiments with human volunteers have revealed (Desportes, 1944; Tanaka, 1958) that approximately 6 days after larvae have penetrated the skin, cough develops; it may be followed in 2 to 4 weeks by hunger pains, indigestion and more abdominal pain which may persist for several weeks. After approximately 4 weeks, diarrhoea may commence and be associated with blood and mucus in the stool. Mild fever and malaise are common during the invasive period.

Bronchitis and lobular areas of pneumonitis, caused, either by larval migration or by development of adults in the lungs, may be associated with cough, fever and sputum, either as an acute episode or as one persisting in a chronic form. The combination of cough, eosinophilia and radiological mottling of the lungs which may occur makes strongyloidiasis one of the causes of 'tropical pulmonary eosinophilia'. Asthma may occur in those who become sensitised to the larvae, the worms or their products and is usually associated with marked eosinophilia.

As has been mentioned in the section on pathology, there is evidence that the migration of larvae from the bowel to lymph nodes and other tissues may result in coliform and other intestinal organisms being taken from the bowel to the invaded tissues and blood with resultant septicaemia. This mechanism should be considered in those with unexplained pyrexia and of these there are always many in tropical practice. In such patients steps should be taken to confirm or exclude a diagnosis of strongyloidiasis.

Symptoms arising from invasion of the intestinal wall by the parasites are often absent even in heavy infections. Attacks of diarrhoea or intermittent looseness of the stools are however common and there may be intermittent colic or more diffuse abdominal pain. Epigastric discomfort and hunger pains simulating a duodenal ulcer are known to occur, as is pain and discomfort in the lower abdomen and right iliac fossa. Occasionally there may be nausea and vomiting and in heavy infections associated with malabsorption, abdominal distension and flatulence. Lymph node involvement may increase any tendency there is to malabsorption by obstructing lacteals and it may also be a contributory factor in the causation of abdominal pain. Cholecyctitis may result from invasion of the gallbladder and biliary tract by larvae.

Diagnosis

Rhabditiform larvae of *S. stercoralis* may be found by direct examination of the stools; more rarely filariform larvae or even adult female worms may be present. Concentration techniques such as that of Allen and Ridley (1970) greatly increase the probability of recovering larvae from faeces of those who are lightly infected.

Aspiration of juice from the duodenum provides a useful method of obtaining larvae, often when it is difficult to do so by other means. The predilection of the worms for the upper small intestine favours recovery of larvae from this situation. A variation on this technique is the use of string composed of brushed nylon. This is attached to a plastic capsule, and swallowed; the capsule takes it into the upper duodenum and small intestine where its presence may be detected radiologically and from which it is later withdrawn. Juice is squeezed from the string on to a slide and examined for larvae. This method appears to yield rather more positive results than does duodenal aspiration and is very often positive in light infections when stool examination is negative.

Complement fixation tests carried out for filariasis may give cross-positive reactions in patients with strongyloidiasis so that when such positive reactions are encountered, both diagnoses should be considered.

Treatment

The most effective and readily available remedy is thiabendazole which is given orally in a dosage of 25 mg/kg body weight twice daily for 3 days. Nausea, vomiting, diarrhoea and dizziness are side effects that may be encountered. Thiabendazole is 2-(4-thiazolyl-n(butizimidazine). Following treatment the usual prognosis is good, Symptoms in some cases may continue for months or years if treatment is not given.

TOXOCARIASIS

SYNONYM. *Visceral larva migrans*. This term, which embraces all conditions in which larvae migrate in the viscera, is one which it has been possible to replace with a more precise aetiological designation in most cases following the introduction of effective diagnostic methods for toxocariasis.

Definition

An infection in man with larvae of *Toxocara canis* or *T. cati*. The larvae migrate in the tissues in which they cause damage but do not, except with the greatest rarity, develop into adults.

Aetiology

The original identification of the parasite now known as *T. canis* is attributed to Werner in 1782, but until recently there has been great confusion between it and related species, particularly *Toxascaris leonina*, which was not clearly differentiated from *T. canis* until described by Lieper (1907). The full development of these worms was not studied until recently by Sprent (1958).

Adult *T. canis* measure 3 to 5 in (7.5 to 12.5 cm) and live in the intestine of dogs and cats. They produce eggs which after maturing are infective to other dogs and cats and to man. When dogs, cats or man swallow infective eggs, the larvae are liberated in the intestine and burrow into the intestinal wall. When this occurs in puppies under the age of 5 weeks the larvae can go on to mature into adult *T. canis*, probably pursuing a cycle of development similar to that of *A. lumbricoides* in man; that is, being taken to the liver or lung in the blood and there leaving the blood vessels to migrate up the bronchial tree and re-enter the intestine. The most usual method of infection of dogs, however, is prenatally; when older dogs swallow *T. canis* eggs, the larvae resulting migrate in the tissues and persist in the second stage for long periods. From these tissues, particularly the retroperitoneal tissues, larvae from the pregnant bitch probably enter the fetus by a route the details of which are not known. The result is that puppies are very commonly infected with *T. canis*, the older dogs less commonly so.

In cats prenatal infection does not often occur, and probably the commonest mode of infection in them is for older cats to swallow eggs or larvae contained in the tissues of mice which then pursue a full cycle of development leading to the presence of *T. cati* in the animals' intestinal tracts. Eggs of *T. canis* and *T. cati* are swallowed by mice, rats, monkeys and a wide variety of animals, and develop into second stage larvae just as they do in cats and dogs, but in these animals they do not go beyond the second stage. If, however, dogs or cats should eat meat of rats or mice containing second stage *T. canis* or *T. cati* larvae respectively, these larvae will then develop into adults. When ingested in this way larvae of *T. cati* develop into adults in cats more readily than do those of *T. canis* in dogs (Sprent, 1958).

The ova of *T. canis* measure 0.080 mm by 0.070 mm and have a pitted outer surface. There is a thin inner shell. The ovum of *T. cati* measures 0.070 mm–0.065 mm and it is not so deeply pitted as is the surface of *T. canis* ova.

When infective *T. canis* or *T. cati* eggs are swallowed by man, larvae emerge from the eggs in the human intestine, penetrate the bowel wall, and are taken in portal blood to the liver and lungs and usually beyond them to other tissues throughout the body. Sprent (1955a) deduced that it is the size and shape of the body of the larva which determines the kind of vessel it enters and hence how it proceeds along its migratory pathway. Once in a vessel the larva appears to leave it at a point at which its body approaches the diameter of the vessel. This is indicated by the occurrence of haemorrhages at specific sites, such as those on the surface of the brain in mice experimentally infected with *T. canis* (Sprent, 1955b). This is also likely to explain the somewhat uniform position of granulomata caused by larvae of *T. canis* emerging from retinal blood vessels (Duguid, 1961a and b). It explains, too, why ascaris larvae are filtered out of the circulation in man in the liver or lung and do not pass, in the blood, beyond these organs to other parts of the body. A week after infection, *A. lumbricoides* larvae reach a diameter of 0.038 mm, whereas at the same stage *T. canis* larvae are only 0.02 mm in diameter.

Epidemiology

Surveys of the prevalence of the infection in dogs have revealed that it is cosmopolitan, that in south-eastern Britain about 10–20 per cent are infected, and that in tropical Africa a peak incidence of 37.5 per cent is found in Nigeria (Wiseman and Woodruff, 1971). In Calcutta a prevalence rate of 82 per cent has been reported (Maplestone and Bhaduri, 1940). There is less information of the prevalence of *T. cati* infection in cats but in south-eastern England approximately 20 per cent have been found to be infected (Woodruff, 1970).

The high prevalence of infection with the adult worms in dogs and cats renders it probable that very considerable numbers of humans become infected, and although it is only since 1952 that it has been known to occur in man, evidence points to it being responsible for much morbidity and pathology hitherto regarded as being of idiopathic or of undetermined origin.

Pathology

Granulomatous lesions in which leucocytes, particularly eosinophils, are prominent occur around larvae which die in tissues. These tissues include the liver, lungs, heart, brain and eye. It seems probable that almost all tissues in the body may be invaded.

Eosinophilia is usual during the early phase of infection and probably represents a reaction to metabolic products from larvae and from their protein after their death and absorption. Humoral antibodies are produced early after infection and antibodies soon become fixed on skin cells (Woodruff, 1970). There is also evidence that the infection may predispose to poliomyelitis and epilepsy, the former either by conveying virus from the alimentary tract to the central nervous system or by damaging the central nervous system and thus facilitating growth within the damaged area of circulating virus. Epilepsy is likely to arise from scarring and granulomatous foci caused by the larvae in the brain (Woodruff, Bisseru and Bowe, 1966).

Larvae of *T. canis* have been recovered from the myocardium; it is therefore possible that the infection may give rise to myocarditis and that it may be a factor in the causation of endomyocardial fibrosis in Africa.

Clinical features

A history of close contact with a dog or cat is common but not invariable. There may be a history of soil eating or of eating sandwiches and similar articles of diet without washing the hands after gardening.

In most cases of proved toxocariasis, it is the eye which has been involved and often the sight in the affected eye becomes lost or markedly impaired, the deterioration in vision usually occurring during days or weeks. Very rarely is there more than one eye involved; the granuloma raises the retinal surface so that the clinical features are those of a unilateral raised lesion in the retina, very often in the macular vicinity but sometimes anteriorly just behind the ciliary body.

The liver is invaded and the granulomata within it may give rise to symptoms of hepatitis and mild hepatomegaly. Cough and asthmatic attacks may result from larval migration in the lungs and the sensitivity which they provoke. Epilepsy in those in whom there is evidence of toxocaral infection may be of any variety, either grand mal or petit mal—the type probably depending on the number and distribution of the larvae and resulting granulomata in the cerebral cortex.

During the first months or years of a toxocaral infection an eosinophilia is usual; as the infection becomes chronic however, the eosinophilia usually disappears.

Otherwise unexplained epilepsy should be investigated as possibly being of toxocaral aetiology.

Diagnosis

The definitive diagnosis depends on the identification of the larvae in the tissues. The probability of this being possible in any given instance is small for the granulomata produced measure only a millimetre or so in diameter and many sections may have to be cut in order to find the larva.

The fluorescent antibody test gives good results

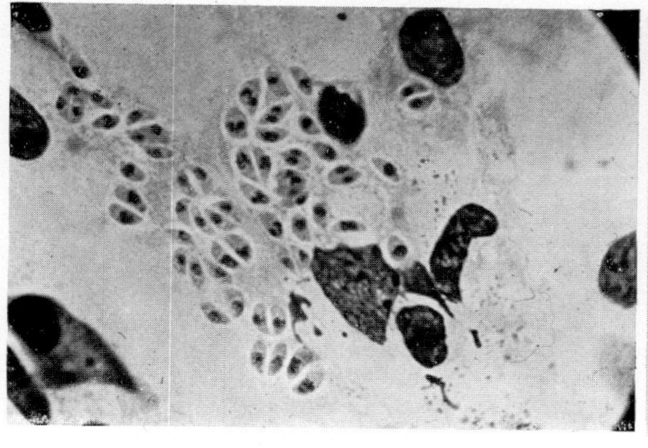

CHAPTER 7

A

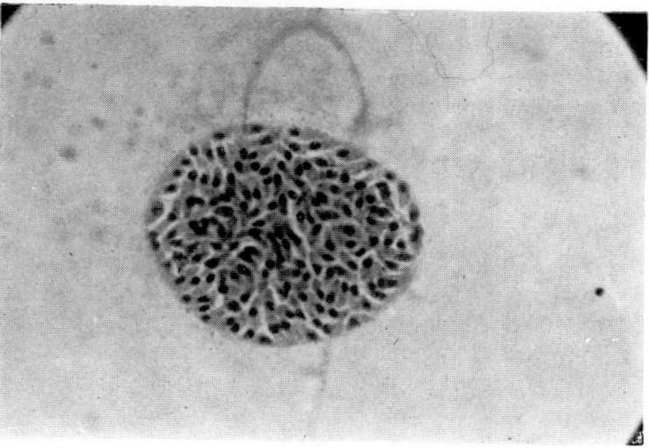

B

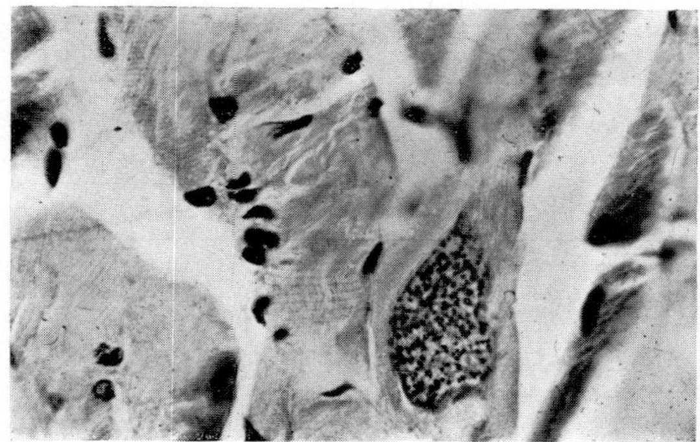

C

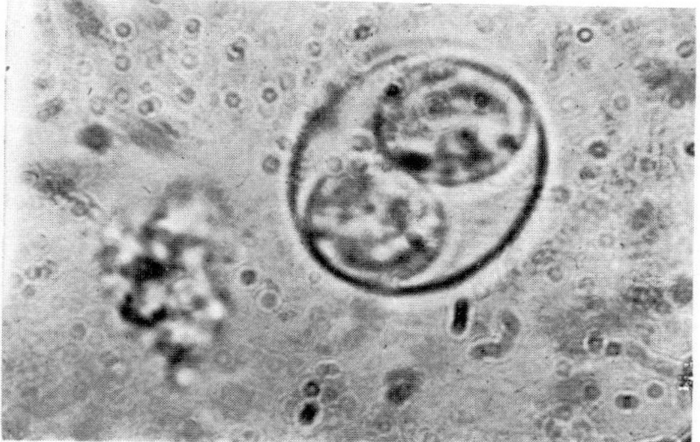

D

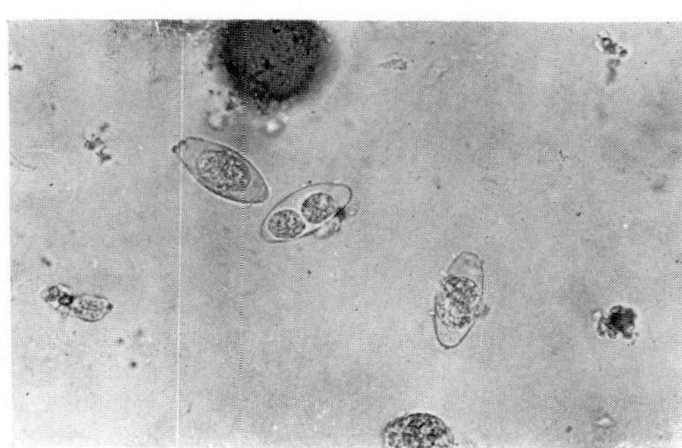

E

Plate 1

A Toxoplasma gondii. *Endozoites ruptured from pseudocyst (osmium fixed, Giemsa stained).* ×1000

B Toxoplasma gondii. *Cyst in mouse brain filled with cystozoites (osmium fixed, Giemsa stained).* ×750

C Toxoplasma gondii. *Cyst in muscle (section).* ×500

D Toxoplasma gondii. *Oocyst containing two sporocysts.* ×2500

E Isospora belli. *One sporulated oocyst between two unsporulated.*

(A & B: From material supplied by R. Lainson. C: From Garnham & Lainson, 1960. D: From cat material supplied by W. M. Hutchison. E: From human material supplied by W. P. Stamm.)

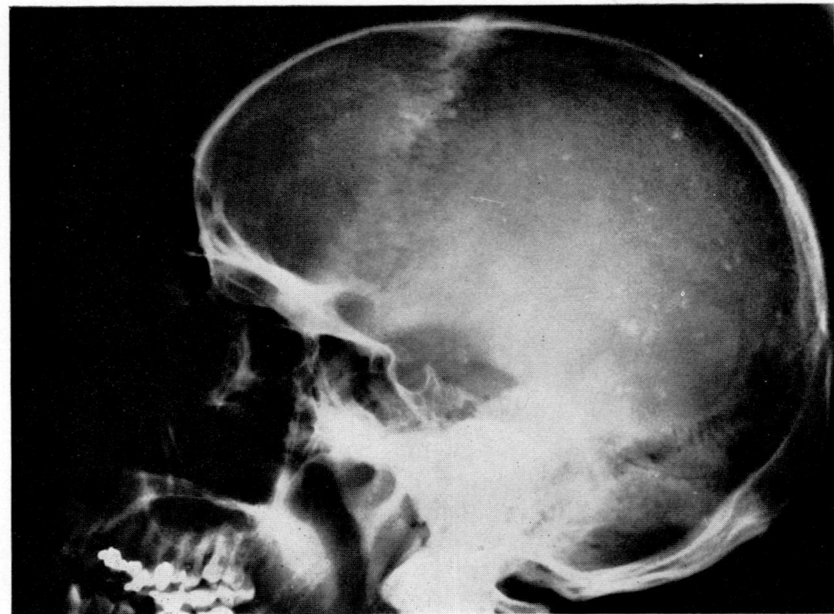

CHAPTER 10

PLATE 2 A *Calcified cerebral cysticerci in an African.* (Courtesy of Major-General W. H. Hargreaves.)

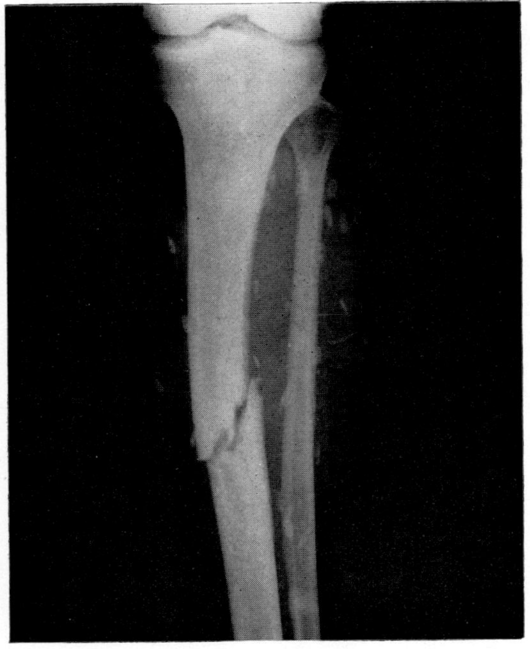

PLATE 2 B *Calcified cysticerci in the calf muscles of an ex-soldier who developed fits after serving in India. Cysticercosis was diagnosed accidentally when his leg was X-rayed after a fracture.* (Courtesy of Major-General W. H. Hargreaves.)

and although cross-reactions with serum of patients with *A. lumbricoides* may occur clear differentiation is possible if the serum is absorbed with *Ascaris* extract (Woodruff, 1970).

A skin test using a dilute extract of *T. canis* adult worms, the extract containing not more than 20 μg protein nitrogen/100 ml gives good results and few cross- or false-positive reactions (Woodruff, 1970).

Treatment

Diethylcarbamazine is probably the most satisfactory drug available and is given in doses of 3 mg/kg body weight thrice daily for 21 days. This maximal dosage level should be worked up to over 3–5 days. In heavy infections more than one course of treatment may be necessary. Thiabendazole in standard dosage of 25 mg/kg body weight twice daily for 3 days appears to be less satisfactory (Wiseman *et al*, 1971).

Prognosis

The prognosis appears to be good after treatment and new lesions or marked progression of existing lesions appears to be uncommon. Damage already done to the retina cannot, of course, be expected to heal without scarring.

OTHER ANIMAL NEMATODES
CAUSING VISCERAL LESIONS

The larva of *Gnathostoma spinigerum* a nematode which normally infects dogs, cats, tigers and other wild animals in the East, may affect man as the result of eating infected raw fish. The immature worm migrates to the subcutaneous tissues where it causes swelling and pruritus. During migration the worm may cause damage to the lungs, kidneys, eyes and other organs. Eosinophilia occurs. The adult worm, some 3 cm long, can sometimes be detected under the skin and removed surgically. Fatal cases of gnathostomiasis have been reported in Thailand where immature male worms have been identified in the brains of patients dying of eosinophilic myeloencephalitis.

Other animal nematodes are known to invade man. The larvae of *Anisakis marina*, the herring-worm, give rise to eosinophilic granulomas in the bowel, sometimes with obstruction and perforation. Anisakiasis was first reported from the Netherlands, where for centuries feasting on fresh herring in the spring has been traditional. The disease is now known to be common in Japan. *Angiostrongylus cantonensis*, a lung nematode of rodents, the larval stage of which develops in molluscs and freshwater shrimps, is an important cause of eosinophilic meningitis in the Far East, South-East Asia and the Pacific Islands. Angiostronglyiasis is acquired by eating infected shrimps, crabs and snails or by swallowing infected slugs on unwashed vegetables or fruit. Eosinophils, giant cells and sometimes young adult worms are found in the CSF which has a high protein and low sugar content.

ANCYLOSTOMIASIS

Ancylostomiasis or hookworm infection is rife in tropical countries where it is associated with poverty, insanitary habits and lack of education. Hookworm anaemia is a disease of major importance economically since it incapacitates people for work. Stoll estimated in 1947 that the world-wide incidence of infection was over 450 million. In temperate countries it can occur among workers in mines and tunnels where there is a suitable temperature and imperfect sanitation.

Aetiology

Human ancylostomiasis is caused mainly by two species of nematodes belonging to genera of the family *Ancylostomidae*. These are *Ancylostoma duodenale*, the so-called 'old world' hookworm, and *Necator americanus*. Their respective distribution is difficult to define as they have often been confused in the past. Both species occur in most affected countries and both are often present in the same patient. *A. braziliense* and *A. caninum*, which normally cause hookworm disease in cats and dogs, occasionally invade man. Their larvae produce 'creeping eruption' of the skin but do not attain the adult form in man. *A. malayanum*, another parasite of animals, has been found in rare instances to develop fully in man.

Life cycle. The life histories of *A. duodenale* and *N. americanus* are identical. The adults are small worms, about 8–10 mm long, *N. americanus* being the smaller of the two. The anterior end is hooked dorsally. The buccal cavity has ventral teeth (*Ancylostoma*) or chitinous cutting plates (*Necator*). The worms inhabit the small intestine, mainly the jejunum, and attach themselves to villi which are sucked into the buccal cavity. They feed on blood, secreting a toxic fluid which has an anticoagulant effect and when they migrate they leave bleeding points behind them. The eggs measure some 60×40 μm. They are oval and

M

contain, when freshly passed in the faeces, an ovum which has segmented into four cells. There is a clear space between the ovum and the egg shell (Fig. 12.3).

When ova are deposited on warm, moist soil or in water larvae hatch out in less than 24 hours. The newly hatched larva has a rhabditiform (short and bulbous) oesophagus. It lives on faecal matter and moults twice, the oesophagus becoming long and filariform. Filariform larvae may remain viable for 3–4 months in warm damp soil

worm load of about one hundred ancylostomes seldom produces anaemia. Recent investigations have shown that past assessments of the amount of blood loss caused by hookworms were grossly excessive; some estimates were as high as 1 ml per worm daily. Isotope studies with ^{51}Cr have demonstrated that the amount of blood lost in *N. americanus* infection is about 1 ml daily for twenty worms, or 0.05 ml daily per worm. In *A. duodenale* infection the blood loss is somewhat higher; it is a larger worm, armed with teeth, and it is more

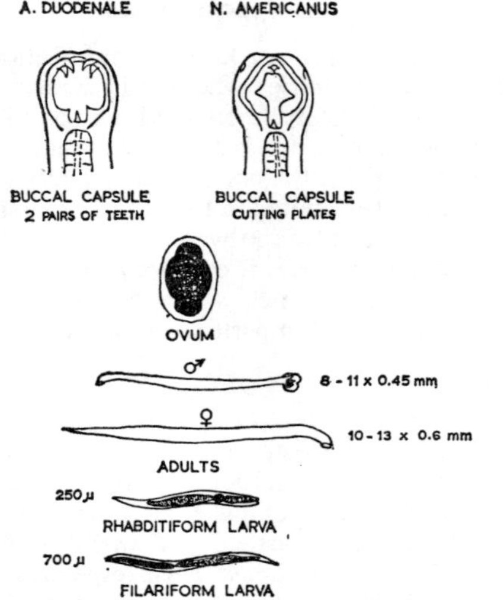

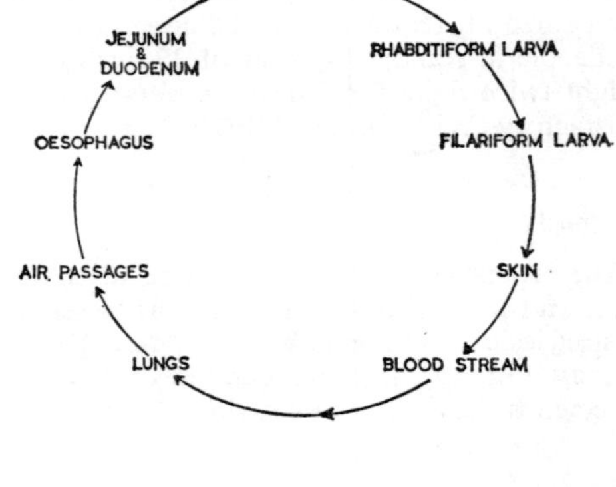

FIG. 12.3. *Life cycle of the common hookworms.*

or faecal matter. They are infective and penetrate the unbroken skin, usually of the feet. They bore their way to the blood stream in which they are carried to the heart and lungs. There they reach the alveoli and bronchi and make their way up the trachea and larynx into the oesophagus and thence to the stomach and small intestine, where they mature. After copulation the female produces eggs which appear in the faeces 7–10 weeks after infection. It is also possible for infection to take place when the larvae are swallowed, but by far the more common route is through the skin.

Hookworm anaemia

Whether or not hookworm infection produces anaemia depends mainly upon the intensity of the infection and the state of nutrition and iron storage of the infected individual. Another factor is the presence of associated disease. The average

migratory, leaving more bleeding points. Worm loads of two to three thousand may cause a daily blood loss of 250 ml. In addition to the loss of red cells, albumin is also lost into the gut; when anaemic patients are treated with iron alone the haemoglobin may return to normal but the serum albumin content does not become normal unless the patients are wormed.

Clinical features

The average infected individual is symptomless in spite of considerable numbers of ancylostomes in the small intestine, and in many tropical countries incidental ancylostome infection is present in the majority of hospital patients, whatever their complaints.

Ground itch often occurs initially after the penetration of the larvae. This is a dermatitis which usually affects the feet, particularly the interdigital clefts. There is intense itching and scratching causes secondary infection. Infected vesicles break down to form an impetigenous infection. In extreme cases dermatitis has covered the whole of the back after sunbathing on the bank of a river, following after some weeks by acute hookworm anaemia of severe degree.

This initial dermatitis may be followed shortly afterwards by *bronchitic* symptoms caused by the passage of larvae through the lungs to the bronchi. This was known as 'miner's bronchitis' among the workers in the tin mines of Cornwall. Also at this early stage the patient begins to suffer from *gastrointestinal* symptoms, varying from vague digestive disturbances to burning epigastric pain which is intermittent or constant. There may be anorexia or the appetite may be ravenous and depraved with dirt-eating or 'pica'. The stools sometimes contain flakes of blood-tinged mucus, but melaena and frank blood in the stools are rare.

Anaemia. This usually develops insidiously, although massive infections may at times cause sudden symptoms of blood loss. The commonest complaints are lassitude, pallor, dyspnoea, syncope and swelling of the legs. Some patients have anginal symptoms and pain in the calves and thighs on walking. Impotence is common.

The physical findings are variable, depending upon the degree and chronicity of the infection. Severe chronic cases have a characteristic appearance. There is no obvious wasting. The face is usually pale and puffy, the skin being smooth, silky and sparsely haired. Fair-skinned patients develop extreme pallor with dusky pigmentation over the face in a butterfly distribution. Darker patients tend to show depigmentation. The mucous membranes and tongue become almost white. Koilonychia is a common finding, and there is often general oedema and pot-belly. There are changes in the colour and texture of the hair which becomes fine and sparse. This is particularly evident in children, who often show retarded mental and physical development, which may be followed by infantilism. Signs of anaemic heart disease are usually found; high pulse pressure, capillary pulsation and raised venous pressure. There may be gross cardiac dilatation with loud haemic murmurs which, together with the low-grade fever and retinal haemorrhages which are sometimes present, may suggest the diagnosis of infective endocarditis.

Diagnosis

It is wise to remember in tropical practice that the discovery of hookworm ova in the stools does not necessarily indicate that the patient's symptoms are due to ancylostomiasis, and before this diagnosis is made other causes of iron deficiency anaemia should be excluded. Oedematous cases may closely simulate such conditions as nephrotic syndrome and beri beri. There is usually eosinophilia which may be profound in acute cases, but it may be absent when ancylostomiasis is complicated by malaria or kala azar. The degree of infection can be assessed by counting the number of ancylostome ova in the faeces. In a survey in western Nigeria by Gilles *et al* in 1963 patients were presumed to have hookworm anaemia if they had a haemoglobin level of 6 g or less per 100 ml and if the faeces contained more than 20 000 ova per g. Heavy infections of long standing may cause intestinal malabsorption.

Treatment

This consists essentially of the correction of the iron deficiency and the administration of anthelmintics. An easily assimilable high protein diet is advisable. Severe hookworm anaemia will benefit greatly from an initial blood transfusion, but this is not practical when dealing with large numbers and the response to iron therapy is usually rapid. Ferrous sulphate, 400 mg t.d.s. should be given by mouth and continued for 3 months after the haemoglobin concentration has risen to 12 g per 100 ml. On this treatment alone patients may become relatively free from symptoms but when it is stopped they will quickly relapse if they have not been wormed, and in addition it has been found that if the worms remain the serum albumen concentration remains low. Modern anthelmintic drugs are comparatively non-toxic and can be given at the start to debilitated patients.

Tetrachloroethylene is the most widely used drug. It is given in a single dose of 0.1 ml/kg body weight emulsified with mucilage and flavoured with peppermint. Capsules may not disseminate their contents until they have passed the duodenum and upper jejunum where most of the worms are situated. The drug is given in the morning on an empty stomach. Purgation is not necessary.

Bephenium hydroxynaphthoate (Alcopar) has been found to be highly effective against hookworms and free from side effects. It is given on an empty stomach, 5 g daily on 3 consecutive days, without purgation. For children weighing less than 10 kg half this dose is given. It is more effective for *A. duodenale* than for *N. americanus.*

Thiabendazole, 25 mg/kg daily for 3 days, has

given high clearance rates in *A. duodenale* and *N. Americanus* infections.

Dichlorvos, an organophosphorus compound, given in a resin formulation in a single dose of 12 mg/kg, has proved very effective against *N. americanus* in preliminary trials.

The worm load can be recovered by washing and sieving the stools. Clearance tests are carried out 1 week after treatment, which can be repeated if necessary.

Control

Health propaganda and education are all-important, together with the use of footwear and sanitary measures. Wide-scale vermifuge campaigns and fortification of the diet with iron should be adopted in endemic areas.

TRICHOSTRONGYLIASIS

Several species of *Trichostrongylus*, a nematode which is normally a parasite of the small intestine of sheep, goats and camels, not uncommonly infect man in agricultural districts of tropical countries, especially in Iran. Semi-filariform larvae enter the body through the skin or the mouth. The ova are easily mistaken for those of ancylostomes but they are somewhat smaller. Both ova are often found in the same specimen of stool. Trichostrongyliasis, which responds to treatment as for ancylostomiasis, is usually symptomless but there may be secondary anaemia in heavy infections.

CUTANEOUS LARVA MIGRANS
(CREEPING ERUPTION) *included here for convenience*

This is caused by the invasion of the skin by larvae of various animal hookworms, most often *A. caninum* and *A. braziliense* which are parasitic in dogs and cats. These larvae tunnel in the skin but do not develop any further in man. The infection is acquired by contact with infected ground, particularly bathing beaches which have been fouled by dogs or children's sandpits in which cats or dogs have defaecated. Whole families have been infected during a day's outing on a beach. Another source of infection is clothing which has been spread out on the ground after laundering, a common practice in the Far East. The condition is encountered in most countries with warm climates, particularly in Africa, the Americas and the East.

The larva moves through the skin, progressing at a rate of 2–3 cm daily, causing a linear erythe-

matous reaction along its track, which is often serpiginous (Plate 3). At the head of the track there is a bleb or nodule indicating the situation of the larva. There may be multiple lesions and extreme pruritus which may cause insomnia.

The treatment consists of freezing the active end of the tunnel with ethyl chloride or CO_2 snow. Thiabendazole (Mintezol), 50 mg/kg twice daily by mouth for 2 days, relieves the symptoms and halts the tracks. Mintezol is available as chewable tablets (0.5 g) and as an oral suspension (1 g per 5 ml). Topical use of the latter has proved successful. If untreated, the infection dies out in a matter of months. Preventive measures consist of excluding dogs from bathing beaches and covering children's sandpits when they are not in use.

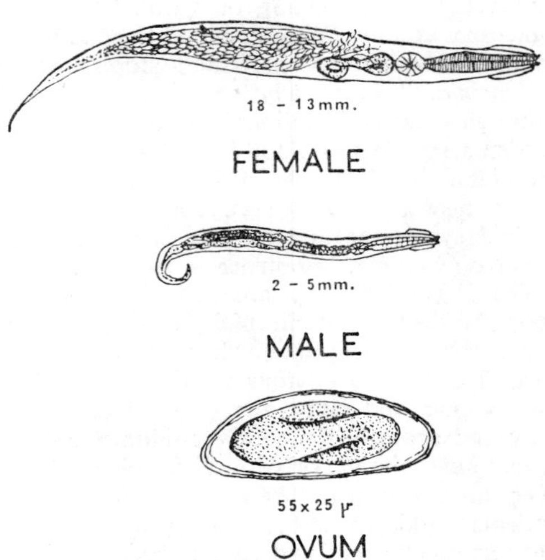

FIG. 12.4. *Adult* Enterobius vermicularis *and ovum.*

ENTEROBIASIS

Enterobius vermicularis (*Oxyuris vermicularis*), the threadworm or pinworm, has a wide distribution throughout the world. It is a common parasite of man, especially of children. It is a small white worm easily visible to the naked eye, the female being about 1 cm and the male about 4 mm in length (Fig. 12.4). The ova are colourless and asymmetrical, one side being flattened, and measure about 55×25 μm. They are deposited outside the body on the perianal skin and contain tadpole-like larvae. When eggs are swallowed by man the larvae escape and after moulting become adult in the small intestine, where the female is fertilised by the male which then dies. The male worm is rarely seen in the stools. The fertilised female migrates to the rectum and, during the night, passes out of the anus and deposits her eggs on the perineum, usually giving rise to intense itching so that the patient scratches the anal region and eggs are carried on the fingers to the mouth, causing reinfection. Retroinfection can also occur; larvae sometimes hatch in the perianal region and crawl back through the anus to mature in the bowel. If untreated, the infection becomes cumulative in one person and is readily transmitted to others. Children with threadworms tend to be irritable. Insomnia is a common symptom in adults.

Diagnosis

Ova are not often found in the stools but are most easily detected by taking perianal swabs using transparent adhesive tape which is placed on a microscope slide. If children are examined at night when asleep, worms may be seen by torch-light around the anus.

Treatment

Careful hygiene alone will break the cycle of reinfection and cure the condition since the worms only live for 3–6 weeks. Nails should be cut short and hands washed carefully after stool and before eating. Antiseptic ointment applied locally at night will prevent retroinfection.

Piperazine compounds are specific against threadworms. The citrate, phosphate and adipate are given in the form of syrup or tablets (Antepar, Entacyl) in a dosage of 75 mg/kg daily for a week, repeated after 1 week's interval. A single dose treatment with Pripsen, a granulated preparation containing piperazine phosphate and senna, has proved effective. Children aged 2–5 years receive three teaspoonfuls and those of 6–12 years four teaspoonfuls. Vyprynium embonate (Vanquin), 5 mg/kg, is an alternative single-dose treatment.

TRICHINOSIS

This infection is caused by *Trichinella spiralis*, which is essentially a parasite of rats. Pigs become infected by eating diseased rats and man acquires trichinosis by eating undercooked pork.

The adult worms live in the small intestine. The male measures 1.5 mm and the female, which is viviparous, about 3 mm (Fig. 12.5). The male dies after fertilising the female, which burrows into the intestinal mucosa where several hundred larvae are liberated into the blood stream over the course of a few weeks. The larvae are carried in the circulation to striated muscles all over the body, where they curl up and become encysted, surrounded by a fibrous capsule derived from the host. The cysts measure about 800×300 μm, and are particularly numerous in the muscles of the diaphragm, chest wall, neck, limbs, larynx, tongue and eye. The encysted larvae remain alive for some years and eventually die and become calcified. Man becomes infected by eating the larvae

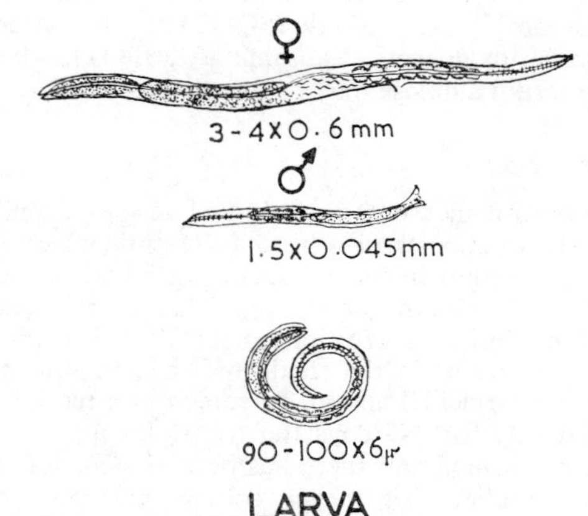

FIG. 12.5. *Adult* Trichinella spiralis *and larva.*

in infected pork, uncooked sausage meat being an important source of infection.

Symptoms

These are very variable, depending upon the intensity of the infection and the situation of the larvae. Light infections are symptomless. A day or two after eating infected meat there may be abdominal pain, vomiting and diarrhoea, which may be severe. The stools may contain blood. These symptoms are caused by the invasion of the bowel wall by female worms. Soon there are symptoms of larval invasion. Fever, tachycardia and oedema of the face, eyelids and conjunctivae are common. Muscular pains occur, especially in the chest wall. Involvement of the diaphragm causes pain, cough and dyspnoea. The limbs may be stiff and painful and the muscles of the mouth are often affected. A typhoid-like state may develop with mental changes and meningeal irritation. Splinter haemorrhages under the nails are common. Profound cachexia may ensue with oedema of the face and extremities. Death may occur from myocardial damage by migrating larvae.

Diagnosis

This is very difficult but it may be suspected from the symptoms. It is more obvious if the condition affects several people who have all eaten the same pork. There is usually leucocytosis with eosinophilia. Biopsy from the deltoid or gastrocnemius may show encysted larvae, and cysts may be demonstrable in the infected meat if it is still available. Precipitin and intradermal tests may prove helpful. Transaminase estimations may show a moderate rise of the serum glutamic oxaloacetic transaminase (SGOT) and the serum pyruvic oxaloacetic transaminase (SPOT), while the serum aldolase may be greatly increased.

Treatment

General measures include bed rest and analgecsis. Corticosteroids have a dramatic effect on the symptoms in severe cases. Clinical trials with *thiabendazole* are promising. This broad-range anthelmintic, in addition to its effect on adult female worms in the small intestine, appears to have a larvicidal action. In some cases receiving 25 mg/kg for 2–5 days the symptoms and fever have subsided and there has been a reduction of eosinophilia. The longer course may produce side effects: anorexia, nausea, vomiting, giddiness, headache and drowsiness. Some patients may excrete a metabolite in the urine which has a strong odour like that which occurs after eating asparagus.

TRICHURIASIS

This cosmopolitan infection is caused by *Trichuris trichiuria*, the whipworm, so called because of its shape (Fig. 12.6). The posterior end is stout, the anterior end hair-like, resembling the lash of a whip. The male measures some 4 cm and the female 5 cm in length. The adults inhabit the large bowel, particularly the caecum. The eggs are brown and barrel-shaped with a plug at each end. In water or damp soil an infective larva develops inside the egg. Infection of man usually takes place from the pollution of water or vegetables. When infective ova are swallowed they hatch in the intestine and the larvae mature into adults which fix themselves to the intestinal wall by means of the fine anterior end which is inserted into the mucosa.

Most infections are symptomless but there may be vague abdominal pain and diarrhoea. Worms can sometimes be seen on the wall of the bowel during sigmoidoscopy.

In undernourished children heavy infections

may cause bloody diarrhoea, anaemia, volvulus and prolapse of the rectum.

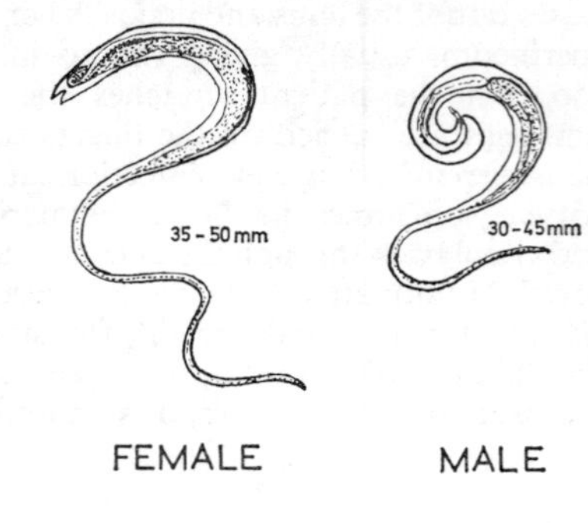

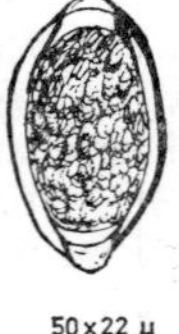

FIG. 12.6. *Adult* Trichuris trichiuria *and ovum.*

Treatment

Trichuris is a very difficult worm to eradicate. Dithiazanine and thiabendazole, given as for strongyloidiasis, have some effect, but the most promising results have been obtained with *dichlorvos*, given in a single dose of 12 mg/kg in a slow-release resin formulation: complete clearance has been reported in over 90 per cent of patients with heavy infections.

CAPILLARIASIS

In 1967, in northern Luzon in the Philippine Islands, there was an extensive outbreak of severe enteritis with a high mortality rate. This was found to be caused by *Capillaria phillipensis*, a minute whipworm of about the same size as *Strongyloides*, which invades the crypts of the jejunum and produces a protein-losing enteropathy with extreme malabsorption. It is acquired by eating infected fish and crustaceans; the latter are often eaten alive in 'jumping salads'! Eradication of the worm has proved very difficult but prolonged courses of thiabendazole have been used with success: as much as 25 mg/kg daily for 1 month, continued on alternate days up to 6 months.

REFERENCES

ALCRON, M. O. and KOTCHER, E. (1961) *Sth. med. J.*, **54**, 193.
ALLEN, A. V. H. and RIDLEY, D. S. (1970) *J. clin. Path.*, **23**, 545.
COLLIER, H. B. (1941) *Canad. J. Res.*, **19B**, 91.
DESPORTES, C. (1944) *Ann. Parasit. hum. comp.*, **20**, 160.
DUGUID, I. M. (1961a) *Brit. J. Ophth.*, **45**, 705.
—— (1961b) *Brit. J. Ophth.*, **45**, 789.
JELLIFFE, D. B. (1953) *Docum. Med. geogr. trop. (Amst.)*, **5**, 314.
KOINO, S. (1922) *Jap. Med. Wld.*, **2**, 317.
KOPPISCH, E. and OLIVER GONZALEZ, J. (1959) *Proc. Soc. exp. Biol. Med.*, **100**, 829.
LIEPER, R. T. (1907) *Brit. med. J.*, **1**, 1296.
MAPLESTONE, P. A. and BHADURI, N. V. (1940) *Indian J. med. Res.*, **28**, 595.
RODRIGUEZ, R. and ZULIAN, G. (1960) *Mal. Infett.*, **12**, 428.
SCUDMORE, H. H., THOMPSON, J. H. and OWEN, C. A. Jnr. (1961) *J. Lab. clin. Med.*, **57**, 240.
TANAKA, H. (1958) *Jap. J. exp. Med.*, **28**, 159.
THORSON, R. E. (1956) *J. Parasit.*, **42**, 21.
TUKUMO, A. (1956) *Hiroshima J. med. Sci.*, **5**, 21.
VENKTACHALAM, P. S. and PATWARDHAN, V. N. (1953) *Trans. roy. Soc. trop. Med. Hyg.*, **47**, 169.
WILSON, S. and THOMPSON, A. E. (1964) *J. Path. Bact.*, **87**, 169.
WISEMAN, R. A. (1971) *Trans. roy. Soc. trop. Med. Hyg.*, **65**, 591.
WISEMAN, R. A. and WOODRUFF, A. W. (1971) *Trans. roy. Soc. trop. Med. Hyg.*, **65**, 591.
WOODRUFF, A. W. (1968) *Trans. roy. Soc. trop. Med. Hyg.*, **62**, 446.
—— (1970) *Brit. med. J.*, **3**, 663.
WOODRUFF, A. W., BISSERU, B. and BOWE, J. C. (1966) *Brit. med. J.*, **1**, 1576.

FURTHER READING

Soil-transmitted Helminths. World Health Organization Technical Report Series No. 277, 1964.
Control of Ascariasis. World Health Organization Technical Report Series No. 379, 1967.

13
Schistosomiasis and Other Trematode Infections

The term 'schistosomiasis' or 'bilharziasis' covers a group of diseases caused by certain digenetic trematode worms of the family *Schistosomatidae* (Looss, 1899). The adult worms inhabit the veins of the portal system, the mesenteric and pelvic veins, the females passing eggs which escape from the human body in the urine or faeces. Oviposition leads to urinary or dysenteric symptoms, and serious complications with marked visceral manifestations may occur later as the disease passes into the chronic stage.

Haematuria is known to have existed in Egypt since ancient times. It is referred to as (â a â) disease, in Eber's papyrus written about 1500 B.C., as well as in other papyri written at later dates. Ruffer (1910) found calcified *Schistosoma haematobium* eggs in the kidneys of two Egyptian mummies of the XXth dynasty (1200–1190 B.C.). It seems that vesical bilharziasis also has an ancient history in Mesopotamia, its symptoms being described in Babylonian inscriptions and in mediaeval Arab literature.

Bilharz (1852) discovered the worm which he called *Distomum haematobium* and identified it as the cause of endemic haematuria in Egyptian patients. In 1856, the worm was named 'Bilharzia' by Meckel von Hemsbach, who recognised it as a separate genus, but the International Commission on Zoological Nomenclature decided in 1954 that the generic name of the group to which the human blood flukes belong is that of *Schistosoma* designated by Weinland in 1858, and the worm discovered by Bilharz is thus named *Schistosoma haematobium*. The same body recommended that the term 'bilharziasis' should continue to be used for the disease which the schistosomes cause in man.

Though Bilharz (1852) also noted lateral spined eggs, and Patrick Manson (1903) described them in the faeces and suggested that there might be two species of human schistosomes, it was Sambon (1907) who named the hypothetical species with lateral spined eggs *Schistosoma mansoni*. This matter was finally settled by Leiper (1918), who proved the morphological distinction between the two species. Katsurada (1904) described the ova of *Schistosoma japonicum*, and this he followed by the discovery of the adult worms in the portal system of some domestic animals.

Four species of schistosomes are normally parasitic in the circulatory system of man, namely:

1. *Schistosoma haematobium* (Bilharz, 1852; Weinland, 1858)
   SYNONYMS: *Distomum haematobium* (Bilharz, 1852)
   Bilharzia haematobia (Meckel von Hemsbach, 1856)
   Gynoecophorus haematobius (Diesing, 1858)
2. *Schistosoma mansoni* (Sambon, 1907)
   SYNONYM: *Schistosoma americanus* (Da-Silva, 1909)
3. *Schistosoma japonicum* (Katsurada, 1904)
   SYNONYM: *Schistosoma cattoi* (Blanchard, 1905)
4. *Schistosoma intercalatum* (Fisher, 1934)

S. haematobium is the causative agent of urinary bilharziasis, in which the adult worms live in the portal system, in the pelvic veins, particularly the vesical plexuses, and sometimes in the veins of the rectum. The eggs are excreted in the urine and occasionally in the faeces. The adult worms of the other three species, which are the causes of intestinal bilharziasis, inhabit the portal system, the mesenteric veins, especially the superior and inferior branches, and the haemorrhoidal plexus. The eggs are passed in the faeces and are rarely found in the urine.

Some species of schistosomes, normally parasitic in other mammalian hosts, have been reported from man. *S. mattheei* (Veglia and Le Roux, 1929), whose natural hosts include sheep.

cattle and horses as well as a wide range of antelopes, has been recorded from man in South Africa, where it causes serious epizootics in stock and where the extent of human infection is believed to be not insignificant. Ova of *S. bovis* (Sonsino, 1876) which naturally infects sheep and cattle, and is also reported from camels, horses and donkeys, have been occasionally described in the faeces and more rarely in the urine of humans in North, Central and South Africa. The recorded human infections with *S. bovis* were transitory and symptomless, being apparently incidental infections. Those with *S. mattheei* seem to have a mild pathogenicity. *S. rodhaini* (Brumpt, 1930), a species closely related to *S. mansoni* and believed to be a parasite of wild rodents has been once recorded from man in the Congo (Haenens and Santele, 1955).

S. faradjei (Walkiers, 1928), which Le Roux (1933) called *S. margebowiei*, is a common parasite of antelopes in Central Africa, where its japonicum-like eggs have been described in the faeces of some individuals; in all probability these represented spurious infections as a result of ingestion of infected animal tissues. The human cases of infection by *S. spindale* (Montgomery, 1906)—normally parasitic in cattle, sheep, goats, water buffaloes and antelopes in southern Asia—which were represented by Gawston (1925) and Porter (1926) in Africa, are believed to represent abnormal ova of *S. bovis* or *S. mattheei*, as *S. spindale* has not been recorded from animals in Africa. Ova of *S. incognitum* (Chandler, 1926) were discovered in supposedly human faeces in India; both eggs and parasites, however, were later found in Indian pigs (Saunders, 1934).

Some workers believe that *S. intercalatum* is nothing more than a hybrid of *S. haematobium* and some animal schistosome, while others claim that it is an adaptation to man of *S. mattheei*. These suggestions appear to be unlikely as relatively high infectivity rates with *S. intercalatum*, which always occurs as a pure infection, were found in man in areas where there was no *S. haematobium* infection. Moreover, *S. mattheei* infection in man has almost on all occasions been found in association with *S. haematobium* or *S. mansoni*.

Parasites

The adult worms have separate sexes. The female is slender and filiform, while the shorter male has a cylindrical anterior portion bearing the suckers, and a broader posterior portion, the sides of which are incurved ventrally to form the gynae-cophoric canal which holds the female. The outer surface of the integument of the male is provided with spines or tuberculations in *S. haematobium*, is grossly tuberculate in *S. mansoni* and non-tuberculate in *S. japonicum*, while the surface of the female is smooth in all species. The mouth opening is situated in the oral sucker, there is no pharynx, and the short oesophagus terminates posteriorly in a bifurcation which forms the intestinal branches. These again join to form a single slender tube terminating near the posterior end of the body.

The male reproductive organs consist of several testes, a number of vasa deferentia joining to form a vesicula seminalis, an ejaculatory duct and a genital pore situated posterior to the ventral sucker. The female reproductive system includes a single elongate ovary, an oviduct, vitelline glands, shell glands, and an ootype in the central canal which passes forwards to the uterus. The uterus, a straight or slightly sinuous tube, leads to the genital pore just behind the ventral sucker. The excretory system consists of a number of flame cells joined to a series of collecting tubes.

The male of *S. haematobium* measures 10–14 mm in length and 1 mm in width; there are three to five testes. The female is 16–20 mm in length and 0.25 mm in width and the ovary is situated in the posterior third of the body. The eggs, which pass in the urine, are elongated and oval in shape with a terminal spine, and measure 112–170 by 40–70 μm.

The male *S. mansoni* is 6–12 mm in length and 0.45–1.2 mm in width; there are six to nine testes. The female measures 7–17 mm in length and 0.25–0.3 mm in width and the ovary is situated in the anterior half of the body. The eggs, which pass in the faeces, are elongated and oval in shape with a prominent lateral spine and measure 114–175 by 45–68 μm.

In *S. japonicum* the male worm measures 10–20 mm in length and 0.5–0.6 mm in width, and there are six to eight testes. The female measures 14–28 mm in length and 0.3 mm in width and the ovary is located in the middle of the body. The eggs pass in the faeces, are oval to rounded in shape with a small lateral hook and measure 70–100 by 50–65 μm. The eggs of *S. haematobium* and *S. japonicum* are passed in groups, while those of *S. mansoni* are passed singly.

Schistosoma intercalatum is distinguished from *S. haematobium* only by the shape of the eggs which are larger and narrower with a longer and sharper spine and measure 140–240 by 50–85 μm.

The miracidium which hatches from the egg is an ovoid ciliated free-swimming organism. The anterior extremity is marked by cone-shaped papillae. A rudimentary intestine is found close to the anterior papilla and lateral to it lie two groups of penetration or salivary glands with ducts opening into the mouth. The nervous system is made up of a mass of cells situated posterior to the gut, with extending nerve filaments. The excretory system consists of flame cells provided with ducts which merge into a common collecting tube opening on the outside. A number of germ cells lie in the posterior body cavity.

The cercaria which emerges from the snail intermediate host consists of a body and a tail trunk branched at the posterior extremity so as to form two furci. The surface is covered with small spines. It has an anterior pyriform oral sucker containing the mouth opening and a smaller circular ventral sucker located in the posterior quarter of the body. There is a functionless digestive system consisting of a thin-walled canal extending posteriorly from the oral sucker and ending blindly. The penetration glands are relatively large bodies situated laterally to the ventral sucker and are provided with ducts which pass forwards to the oral sucker.

The excretory system in either *S. haematobium* or *S. mansoni* consists of four pairs of flame cells arranged along the margins of the body of the cercariae; only three pairs are found in *S. japonicum* cercariae. There is another pair in the tail stem in all species, and all these flame cells are connected to a common excretory duct. The length of the body and tail of the cercariae varies between 0.33 and 0.45 mm for *S. haematobium*, 0.36 and 0.53 mm for *S. mansoni* and 0.25 and 0.32 mm for *S. japonicum*.

Life cycle

In the egg-laying operation, the female worm, after leaving the male, proceeds down against the blood stream to the terminal venules and oviposits immediately adjacent to the walls of the urinary bladder in the case of *S. haematobium*, or the walls of the intestine in the case of *S. mansoni*, *S. japonicum* or *S. intercalatum*. Occasionally females of *S. haematobium* reach and deposit their eggs in the vessels of the intestinal walls, while more rarely females of the other three species reach the bladder wall where they oviposit. The eggs are not fully embryonated when they are laid, and a completely developed miracidium is formed after about 10 days. The escape of the eggs from the host body is accomplished through contractions of the muscular layers of the bladder or intestine and the excretion of cytolytic ferments

by the miracidium. By the time the eggs are finally passed in the urine or faeces the miracidium contained within the ovum has reached maturity and is ready to hatch if the egg reaches water. Some eggs may be unable to escape being held up in the tissues of the walls of the bladder or intestine by local inflammatory reactions.

The miracidium moves in water by means of its cilia. It seeks out and attacks the suitable intermediate host which is a freshwater snail. In the event of failure to contact this host, the miracidium dies usually in less than 24 hours. In penetrating the snail host, the miracidium finds its way to the head, foot, mantle, tentacles or other locations where it loses its cilia and transforms into a sacculate sporocyst. The sporocyst, in turn, produces within its cavity a second generation of sporocysts which migrate to the digestive gland of the snail where they develop into cercariae.

When mature, the cercariae emerge from the snail to attack the suitable mammalian host. The time which elapses between penetration of the snail by the miracidium and emergence of cercariae is usually about a month. Generally only one or two miracidia proceed with their development inside each snail, and many thousands of cercariae may be produced by a single miracidium.

Cercarial penetration of the skin of the definitive host is achieved through the combined action of the anterior spines and the action of lytic ferments, secreted by the cephalic glands, and believed to contain collagenase-like enzymes and hyaluronidase (Levine *et al*, 1948; Stirewalt and Evans, 1952). Penetration may also be assisted by evaporation of a surface film of water, especially after emergence of the host from infected water. The cercariae which fail to contact the mammalian host usually die within 48 hours.

The process of penetration, during which the cercaria loses its tail, is effected quite rapidly and may occur within 10 minutes. The cercariae finally reach a small lymph vessel or venule and are eventually carried by the venous circulation to the heart. Via the pulmonary artery they reach the lungs, and from there cross the capillary bed to reach the arterial circulation through which they are transported to various parts of the body. It is only those cercariae which are carried to the arteries of the abdominal viscera and are able to pass to the mesenteric veins that continue their development and reach maturity. Except in rare instances, those cercariae which reach other locations never develop further.

From the mesenteric veins, the schistosomulae, as they are termed, reach the intrahepatic vessels where they continue to develop until they become sexually mature. Depending on the species, the adult worms then migrate to the mesenteric veins (*S. mansoni*, *S. japonicum*, *S. intercalatum*) or to the veins of the pelvic plexuses (*S. haematobium*) where natural egg production begins. The period between infection, i.e. cercarial penetration of the skin, and recovery of eggs from the stools or urine of the definitive host is usually 30–40 days, but may be much longer.

Intermediate hosts (Plate 4)

The snail intermediate hosts of *S. japonicum* were the first to be discovered, by Miyairi and Suzuki in Japan in 1913. Those of *S. haematobium* and *S. mansoni* in Egypt were identified by Leiper in 1915 and 1916. This was followed by recognition of the intermediate hosts by many workers in other parts of the world where the disease was endemic.

The intermediate hosts of *S. haematobium*, *S. mansoni* and *S. intercalatum* belong to the molluscan family *Planorbidae* (superfamily, *Hygrophila*; order, *Basommatophora*; subclass, *Pulmonata*; class, *Gastropoda*). These are freshwater, non-operculate hermaphroditic snails whose gills have disappeared and have been replaced by lungs. The male and female genital organs are separate, and each snail has one pair of tentacles with the eyes placed at their bases. The snails belonging to this family are characterised by the presence of haemoglobin in their blood which renders it red or pink in colour.

The intermediate hosts of *S. haematobium* and *S. intercalatum* are members of the subfamily *Bulininae* being distinguished by their ovate shells. They are included in the genus *Bulinus* which is naturally divided into two subgenera, *Bulinus s.s.* (*sensu-stricto*) and *Physopsis*, each of which includes a number of the snail vectors.

All the known intermediate hosts of *S. mansoni* are of the genus *Biomphalaria* belonging to the subfamily *Planorbinae* whose members have characteristic disc or lens-shaped shells.

A species of the genus *Ferrisia*, belonging to the family *Ancylidae*, is suspected to act as an intermediate host for *S. haematobium* in India. These are relatively very small snails with low shield-shaped shells.

The snail intermediate hosts of *S. japonicum* belong to another subclass of gastropods, *Prosobranchia*, which includes unisexual snails which have gills instead of lungs. The genus *Oncomelania* (family, *Hydrobiidae*; order, *Mesogastropoda*) comprises various geographical species which are involved in the transmission of the

disease. These are operculate freshwater prosobranchs with conical or turriculate shells which are also adapted to live on land.

The different genera, subgenera and species of the snail intermediate hosts are differentiated from each other by the morphological characteristics of their shells and the differences in their soft anatomy (Mandahl-Barth, 1957).

GEOGRAPHICAL DISTRIBUTION

The available data on the geographical distribution of the human schistosomes and their snail intermediate hosts are still restricted and subject to many limitations. Undoubtedly there are endemic foci of bilharziasis which remain to be discovered, especially in isolated areas which still lack health facilities particularly in Africa, and much needs to be learned about the identification and distribution of the molluscan hosts. The species of snails to be mentioned include those involved in the transmission of the disease on the basis of natural or experimental infection, or epidemiological evidence.

Schistosoma haematobium

This species is widely distributed in Africa, as shown below. Foci with variable endemicities are found in every country in that continent, with the exception of Gabon where the disease has not been as yet recorded.

North Africa	United Arab Republic (Egypt), Libya, Tunisia, Algeria and Morocco.
West Africa	Mauritania, Senegal, Gambia, Mali, Portuguese Guinea, Guinea, Sierra Leone, Liberia, Ivory Coast, Upper Volta, Ghana, Togo, Dahomey, Niger, Nigeria, Caméroun, Gabon, Congo (Brazzaville), and Angola.
Central Africa	Chad, Sudan, Central African Republic, Congo (Kinshasa), Uganda, Zambia, Rwanda and Burundi.
East Africa	Ethiopia, Somalia Kenya, Tanzania, Malawi and Mozambique.
South Africa	Rhodesia, Republic of South Africa, Lesotho and South-west Africa.

In South-west Asia, *S. haematobium* is reported from Aden, Saudi Arabia, Yemen, Israel,

Lebanon, Syria, Turkey, Iran and Iraq. In the Indian ocean it occurs in the islands of Madagascar (Malagasy Republic) and Mauritius. Two small foci are present in southern Portugal and in Maharashta state, India respectively.

Bulinus (Bulinus) truncatus truncatus is the intermediate host of *S. haematobium* in North Africa. *Planorbarius metidjensis*, which serves the same role in Portugal, is also incriminated in the transmission of the disease in northern Morocco. With the exception of Aden, where *Bulinus (B.) reticulatus* and *Bulinus (B.) beccarii* are the vectors of *S. haematobium, Bulinus (B.) truncatus truncatus* is again the recognised intermediate host in the other countries of South-west Asia where the disease is endemic as well as in northern and central Sudan. Other *Bulinus (B.)* snails proved to play a part in the transmission of the disease include *Bulinus (B.) senegalensis* and *Bulinus (B.) geurnei* in Gambia and Senegal, *Bulinus (B.) cernicus* in the Mauritius, *Bulinus obtusispira* in Madagascar, *Bulinus (B.) sericinus* in Ethiopia, and *Bulinus (B.) truncatus rohlfsi* which is widely distributed in some countries in West Central Africa and transmits the disease in Ghana and Angola.

Bulinus (Physopsis) globosus is the principal intermediate host of *S. haematobium* in all African countries south of the Sahara with the exception of Ethiopia, Somalia, and most of the Sudan. Other *Bulinus* snails of the subgenus *Physopsis* which act as intermediate hosts include *Bulinus (Ph) nasutus* (Kenya, Tanzania, Uganda), *Bulinus (Ph) jousseaumei* (Gambia, Senegal, Portuguese Guinea) and *Bulinus (Ph) abissinicus* (Somalia). *Bulinus (Ph) africanus* is widely distributed in eastern Africa and westwards to the eastern Congo. It is a definite intermediate host in Kenya and Mozambique and is possibly involved in the transmission of the disease in Tanzania, Zambia and South Africa. *Ferrisia tenuis*, a small snail belonging to the family *Ancylidae*, is the alleged intermediate host of *S. haematobium* in the focus located in India.

Schistosoma mansoni

This species is distributed throughout Africa and is present in the island of Madagascar. Endemic foci occur in South-west Asia and in some countries in the western hemisphere.

In general, *S. mansoni* has a limited distribution in Africa, as compared to that of *S. haematobium*, the latter being the predominant species in North, West, East and South Africa. In Central Africa, however, *S. mansoni* seems to be more widely distributed, particularly in the Central African Republic, in the Congo (Kinshasa) and in Uganda. In North Africa the disease has a limited distribution, being present in Egypt, where it is endemic in the Nile Delta, and in Libya. *S. mansoni* has not been reported yet from Mauritania, Portuguese Guinea, Niger and Congo (Brazzaville) in West Africa, or from Somalia in East Africa, but is endemic in the other countries of those regions.

In South-west Asia, *S. mansoni* is found in Aden, Saudi Arabia and in Yemen, being again less widely distributed than *S. haematobium*. No autochthonous infection with *S. mansoni* has been reported from Iraq, Iran, Syria, Lebanon or Turkey.

In the western hemisphere, *S. mansoni* is endemic in Brazil, Surinam and Venezuela in South America. Foci are found in some islands along the northern and eastern boundaries of the Caribbean Sea, namely the Dominican Republic, Puerto Rico, Vieques, St Martin, Antigua, Guadeloupe, Martinique and St Lucia.

In Africa, four groups of *Biomphalaria*, each of which comprises several or few species, act as intermediate hosts of *S. mansoni*. Snails of *Biomphalaria pfeifferi* group are the most important intermediate hosts in East, West, Central and South Africa, and are solely responsible for the transmission of the disease in South-west Asia and in the island of Madagascar. The *Biomphalaria sudanica* group, acts as an intermediate host in Central Africa, and is suspected to be involved in transmission in Ghana, Tanzania and Ethiopia. Members of the *Biomphalaria alexandrina* group have a limited distribution acting as intermediate hosts in North America, while the fourth group, *Biomphalaria choanomphale*, comprises few forms which are restricted to the great lakes in Uganda and Tanzania where they are responsible for local transmission.

Biomphalaria glabrata is the most widely distributed intermediate host of *S. mansoni* in the western hemisphere, being responsible for transmission of the disease in all endemic foci in that region. *B. straminae*, found in north-eastern Brazil, is, however, a much more important vector in that area than *B. glabrata*. *B. tenagophila* is another intermediate host with a limited distribution in southern Brazil.

Schistosoma japonicum

This species occurs in some countries in the Far East. In China, it is found in the Yangtze valley to the north and south of the river, the southern limit of the endemic area being considerably extended by the presence of three large lakes, Tung-Ting, Poyang and Taihii, around which the disease is prevalent. Other foci of endemicity are found in several localities around the coast, particularly in coastal river basins. The endemic area covers one municipality (Shanghai), one autonomous region (Kwangsi) and ten provinces (Kiangsu, Chekiang, Hupeh, Hunan, Kiangse, Anhwei, Kwantung, Fukien, Szechwan and Yunan). In the Philippines, endemicity of *S. japonicum* is established in six of the main thirteen islands of the archipelago, namely, Luzon, Mindoro, Samar, Leyte, Mindanao and Bohol. In Japan, the endemic areas are well defined and are limited to either the main island of Honshu or the southern island of Kyushu. Other foci of *S. japonicum* have been located in the Central Celebes around the west shore of Lake Lindoe, in eastern and southern Thailand, and in southwestern Laos.

There are three geographical species responsible for transmission of *S. japonicum: Oncomelania hupensis* (China), *O. quadrasi* (Philippines), and *O. nosophora* (Japan). The molluscan intermediate hosts in the Celebes, Thailand, and Laos have not yet been discovered.

Schistosoma intercalatum

This species is the fourth in importance with regard to infectivity of schistosomes in man. It is endemic in certain areas of the Democratic Republic of the Congo (Kinshasa), where the intermediate host, verified by experimental infection is *Bulinus (Ph.) globosus. Schistosoma intercalatum* cases have also been reported from Gabon.

Schistosomes causing dermatitis

The cercariae of certain species of the family *Schistosomatidae*, normally parasitic in birds or mammals other than man, may penetrate the human skin and cause a form of sensitisation reaction resulting in an intense itch and pruritus which occurs within a few minutes of exposure. The cercariae themselves are locally destroyed in the skin, though the symptoms may continue for a few days being increased by scratching. This form of dermatitis, also known as swimmer's itch, occurs in lakes, swamps, irrigation channels and beaches with vegetation which provides protection and food for the snail intermediate hosts of the incriminated schistosomes (Olivier 1949).

Some of the important schistosome species known to be involved in the causation of this form of dermatitis are:

Trichobilharzia ocellata (Brumpt, 1931). This is a schistosome complex comprising certain species which are normally parasites of ducks in Europe and North America.

Trichobilharzia physellae (Talbot, 1936), another parasite of ducks in North America.

Schistosomatium douthitti (Cort, 1914), a parasite of rats and mice in North America.

Schistosoma spindale (Montgomery, 1906), a parasite of wild animals, sheep and goats in southern Asia.

Gigantobilharzia sturnioe (Tanabe, 1951), a parasite of various species of birds in Japan.

EPIDEMIOLOGY

The evolutionary origin of human schistosomes is a matter of speculation. Some authors claim that it seems reasonable to assume that vesical bilharziasis originated in the Tigris and Euphrates valleys, and that it has spread through the Middle East to Egypt and then southwards and westwards to other parts of Africa, its distribution being materially influenced by population movements, migrations, wars and similar factors. On the other hand, judging from the extent of animal infections with schistosomes in East, South and Central Africa, and the fact that the intermediate hosts of both *S. haematobium* and *S. mansoni* definitely belong to the Ethiopian malacological fauna which practically covers the whole of Africa, it seems likely that *S. mansoni* and probably *S. haematobium* evolved with man in Africa being originally parasitic in his anthropoid ancestors. In all probability *S. mansoni* was introduced into the western hemisphere through the slave trade. It should be said that the evolutionary origin of *S. japonicum* is still obscure.

The epidemiology of schistosomiasis represents an extremely complex series of phenomena. Some of the factors which play an important role in the transmission of the disease have not yet been completely elucidated, and much remains unknown about the bionomics and ecology of the snail intermediate hosts. In general, it could be said that schistosomes exist in a certain locality through the common presence of their intermediate and definitive hosts. The establishment of endemicity is governed by factors related to the definitive host, to the parasite itself, to the intermediate host, to reservoir hosts if present, and to climatic conditions.

Human factors influencing transmission and spread

Human infection is acquired through the skin in the vast majority of cases. Drinking water may be contaminated with cercariae and infection may occur through the mucous membranes, but bathing, swimming or working in infested water provide the most frequent opportunities for infection. Children frequently acquire the disease early as soon as they are able to play in water. Agricultural practices contribute to a great extent to the spread of infection; rice farming is particularly important in this respect as it requires frequent contact with water. The practice of irrigation by farmers exposes them to infection as the snails find optimum ecological conditions in irrigation channels, especially secondary and tertiary canals, and in drains. Other occupational exposures include fishermen and boatmen in inland waters, and the washing of clothes and utensils, mainly female activities, in streams, pond and lakes. Human habits such as passing excreta near water, particularly that used for ablution, or the practice of using night soil as fertiliser in parts of the Far East, contribute materially to the cycle of transmission.

The density of the population and the nature of water supply within a locality are closely correlated with the prevalence of infection. There is evidence to show that where safe waters are supplied for washing and drinking the incidence of *S. mansoni* tends to drop; but unless safe bathing is also provided *S. haematobium* incidence is not much affected. Where safe drinking and washing water are available and infested canals are located at a respectable distance away, the incidence, in general, greatly drops. If infested bathing waters are available to children the incidence of *S. haematobium* is equal in scattered populations and densely congregated farms. Heavy congregation of people without proper sanitary arrangements leads to a very high incidence of *S. mansoni*.

The introduction of new irrigation schemes in the form of canals, drains, storage dams and reservoirs is an important aspect of economic development. Unfortunately, every species of the intermediate hosts of human schistosomes has been found to be able to take advantage of the extra water introduced into such areas. This increase in the snail population leads to the establishment of endemicity or even hyperendemicity of the disease. An outstanding example is recorded in certain localities in Upper Egypt where the incidence of *S. haematobium* among the population increased from 3–7 per cent to 70–80 per cent within 3 years after the change from 'basin' to 'perennial' irrigation in these areas (Khalil, 1938).

The highest prevalence rates of infection are usually found in children and adolescents. These younger persons may be more susceptible to infection, or suffer more intense and more frequent exposure, or are more susceptible because they had no opportunity to build up resistance against infection. Undoubtedly, there are some individuals who may have some natural resistance against bilharzial infection although there is no sound evidence for racial or regional immunity. There is also circumstancial evidence that as a result of infection with schistosomes, man may develop acquired immunity to subsequent exposures, though this immunity may not be absolute and appears to take a long time to develop. In experimental animals partial or complete resistance to reinfection can be achieved. There is little evidence relating to the mechanism of this resistance, it is suggested that it is produced by an antigen which is secreted or excreted by the worms, or alternatively, an unstable antigen which is present only in living schistosome cells (Vogel, 1958; Smithers, 1962).

Though much has yet to be learned concerning the role of nutritional factors in determining the relations between schistosomes and their host, experimental studies thus far indicate that with diets deficient in certain amino acids and vitamins the worms do not undergo normal development and the sexually immature worms do not produce eggs. Since eggs are the major cause of tissue damage, the pathological consequences of infection are greatly reduced. It might appear that protein-deficient diets might explain, in part, some of the differences in pathological manifestations of the disease in various parts of the world (De Witt, 1962).

Parasitic factors influencing transmission and spread

The hazards involved in completing that part of the life cycle between the miracidia and the vector snails are enormous, a risk which is compensated by the great number of eggs produced by the worm. Eggs may be held up in the tissues of the definitive host and never reach the outside; in some cases eggs are not viable and will never hatch. There is evidence to show that there are significant differences in hatchability of eggs from patients of different ages; in general, the percentage of the number of hatchable eggs decreases in older age groups, a phenomenon probably related to immunity.

Mortality among miracidia increases with

miracidial age, reaching 100 per cent after about 9 hours. The ability of miracidia to penetrate the snails decreases also with age, and the greatest penetration occurs within the first 2-hour period, after which it rapidly declines. Some loss of larval stages occurs during the period when the infection in the snail is still immature, and schistosome infections are known to cause increased death rates in the snails as compared with uninfected controls.

The number of cercariae produced increases proportionately to the size of the respective snail intermediate host. Thus *Biomphalaria glabrata*, the largest host of any human schistosome, yields an average of 2000 cercariae per day, while the relatively smaller African species of *Biomphalaria* yields an average of 250–600 per day. The respective average numbers recorded for some species of *Bulinus* and *Oncomelania* are 200 and 15, the latter snails being much smaller than most of the other intermediate hosts. The ability of the cercariae to penetrate the skin of the definitive host is considerably lessened with increasing age, this decrease in penetration being reported to start after only 8 hours.

The rate of egg laying by female schistosomes is an important factor influencing epidemiology. Experimentally, the daily egg production for *S. mansoni* and *S. japonicum* has been estimated to range from 250 to 350 eggs for the former species and from 1400 to 3500 eggs for the latter. *S. haematobium* seems to have an egg-laying rate intermediate between those of the other two species. The life span of adult schistosome worms has been estimated by different workers to vary between 2 and 18 years or even more.

Certain biological differences between the three main species of human schistosomes seem to have their bearing upon the epidemiology of the disease. There is hardly any experimental evidence to indicate that infectivity varies in the different species, though there is a strong suspicion that the infectivity of certain strains of the parasite is at a lower rate than other strains.

There are distinguishing differences in the pathogenicity of the three species; these being mainly ascribed to differences in egg production, since it is known that deposition of eggs in the tissues is the major cause of the pathology. It is claimed that *S. mansoni* eggs always produce more sclerosing granular tissue with marked fibroplasia than *S. haematobium*. Moreover, within the species itself, there is evidence of variation in ability to produce disease; with *S. japonicum*, it was shown that the Japanese strain is more virulent than the Chinese. The relative response to chemotherapy with certain drugs is another biological difference; it is well known that with both antimonials and lucanthone, *S. haematobium* responds more satisfactorily than *S. mansoni*, and the latter more so than *S. japonicum*.

Factors related to intermediate hosts

Snail habitats may be and often are extremely varied, there being differences between snail species in their habitat requirements. Nevertheless, the ranges of tolerance greatly overlap, the optimum conditions being similar for all species but extremes are tolerated better by some species than by others (Abdel Malek, 1958). In general, vector snails show considerable adaptability to changing light conditions; they, however, seem to prefer lightly shaded areas. Similarly, all species favour stagnant or slow-flowing water; *B. truncatus* is not established where the flow rate is more than 15 metres per minute, and the same is true for the other aquatic species within moderate variations.

Floods wash the snails downstream and alter the whole ecological situation. None of the vector snails favours deep water; they prefer shallow waters near the shore, rarely exceeding 2 metres in depth. With regard to salinity, there is a wide range of tolerance; *Biomphalaria glabrata* is not inhibited by sodium chloride content until it reaches 6000 parts per million whereas the maximum limit for *Bulinus truncatus* is 4000 ppm. A certain amount of calcium is needed for shell formation. The snail vectors are tolerant to a wide pH range (4.8–9.8). A certain amount of organic pollution is favourable for snails, but gross pollution is detrimental, as are densely turbid or muddy waters. Water plants form a desirable, but not an entirely essential factor in the ecology of the snail intermediate hosts.

The intermediate hosts of *S. japonicum* are amphibious and spend a major portion of their time out of the water. They favour the moist soil at the margins of slow-moving streams, at ditches, irrigation canals and overflow areas richly supplied with vegetation.

Climatic factors

Bilharziasis is confined to an area between 36°N and 34°S latitude as the snail vectors are found only within tropical or semi-tropical countries where the water temperature will average 25–30°C. The general breeding threshold for the various snail hosts is in the range of 18–22°C. In nature, where the vegetation is dense and water

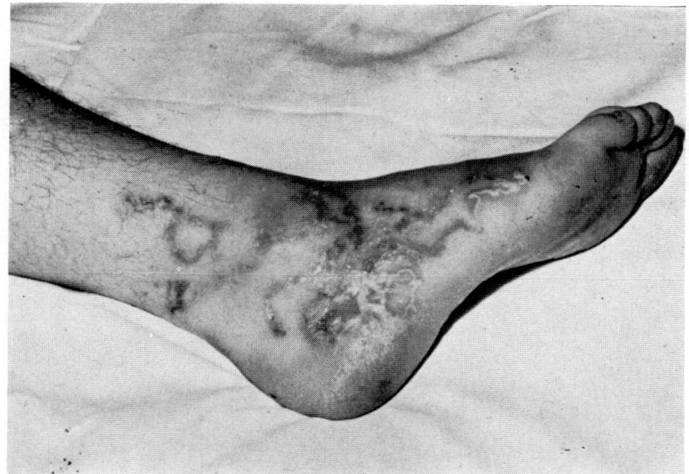

PLATE 3 *Cutaneous larva migrans, showing the typical circinate erythema.*

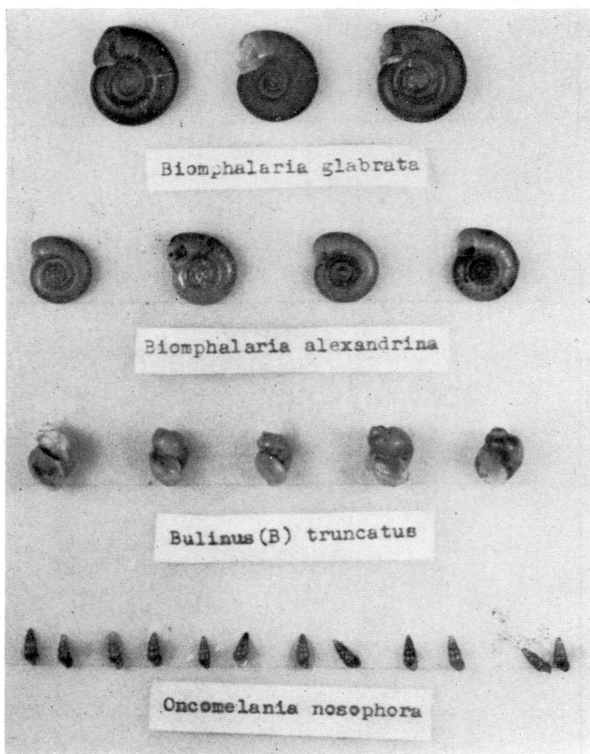

PLATE 4   Intermediate hosts.

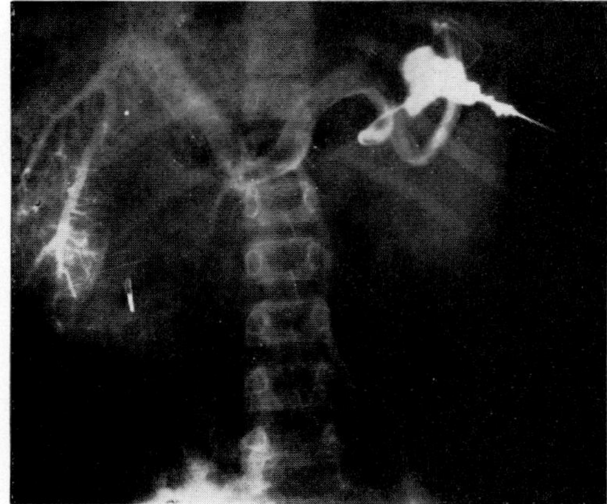

PLATE 5   *Lienoportography in a moderately hypertensive hepatosplenic bilharziasis.*

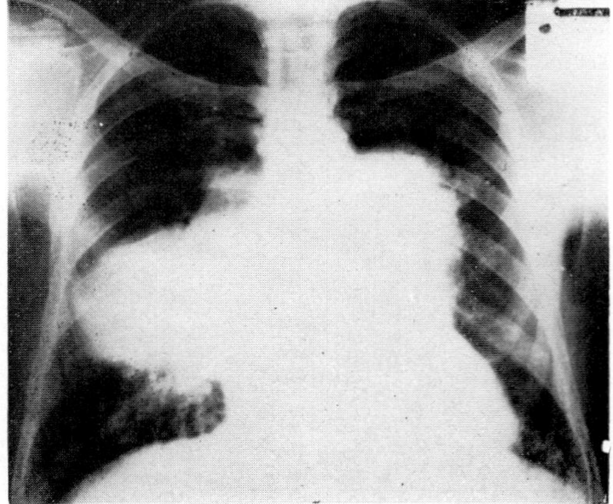

PLATE 6   *X-ray of cor pulmonale grade 3 in cardiopulmonary schistosomiasis.*

current minimal, surface temperature may reach 35°C for several hours in the afternoon in some situations, and it may reach 40°C in paddy fields in the Far East. The vector snails show considerable resistance to cold, particularly those belonging to the genus *Oncomelania*, which survive refrigerator temperature for about 30 days. Possibly this tolerance is related to the long term survival of *Oncomelania* in cracks and crevices where it is more protected. Variations in temperature, particularly when they abruptly occur, affect the incubation of snail eggs, the development of young snails, and the life span of the species.

Mature ova survive in the faeces or urine for less than 24 hours at 22°C. At lower temperatures they survive longer, i.e. 7–10 days at 7–10°C, and they succumb in 1–2 days at the usual warm tropical temperature, a maximum viability of 8 days being recorded under the most favourable tropical conditions. The miracidia are most active between 28°C and 33°C, and the cercariae are rapidly killed by temperatures above 50°C. Both miracidia and cercariae are rapidly inactivated or killed by freezing.

In endemic areas where the seasonal changes in rainfall are minor, or where the habitats consist of large bodies of water that are relatively unaffected by such changes, snail population may be remarkably stable. In other areas, however, with heavy rainfall, snail population decreases as snails are flushed out of their habitats. Where there is marked seasonal rainfall followed by a dry season, the desiccation results in heavy mortality of the snail population, though some of them manage to survive in temporary habitats passing the dry season out of water in the protection of debris and vegetations, and rapidly producing new generations with the return of the rains.

Animal reservoir hosts

There are very few records of natural infections with *S. haematobium* in mammals besides man, these included a mangabey (Cobbold, 1859), sea lions (Ezzat *et al*, 1958), baboons and monkeys (Nelson, 1962) and domestic pigs (Hill and Onabamiro, 1960). The present evidence suggests that *S. haematobium* is maintained in nature by man and that animal infections are incidental and are of no significance as far as the epidemiology of the human disease is concerned.

In the Congo, Kenya, South Africa and South America, an imposing number of species of rodents, a few insectivora (shrews) and some mammals were found naturally infected with *S.*

mansoni (Stijns, 1952; Martins *et al*, 1955; Kuntz, 1958; Pitchford, 1959). A high rate of natural infection with *S. mansoni*, was reported from baboons (papio doguera) in Kenya (Nelson, 1962). The real significance of these animals as reservoir hosts of *S. mansoni* has not yet been assessed; it should be proved that a certain strain infects humans and animals, and that animal infections increase transmission to man.

With *S. japonicum*, the situation is quite different and true reservoir hosts are known. This species of schistosomes occurs naturally in a wide variety of lower animals, dogs, cats, pigs, horses, cattle, water buffaloes, deers and various rodents. It has been estimated that in some areas of the Philippines 75 per cent of bilharzial infections come from human sources and 25 per cent from animal hosts. In Formosa (Taiwan), only zoophilic strains of *S. japonicum* exist which are not infective to man.

Morbidity and mortality

At present, the available data on the incidence and prevalence of bilharziasis tend to show that the disease is spreading and increasing in prevalence in most countries where it is known to exist, or is more prevalent than previously thought. It appears reasonable to place the present estimate of the population infected at 150–180 million.

The severity of the disease caused by *S. haematobium* is well recognised in some countries; in the U.A.R. (Egypt) for instance, it is regarded as one of the major health problems (Khalil, 1941; Makar, 1955). This infection, however, was not considered to be a cause of significant morbidity and was denied particularly any role in the mortality recorded in other countries of Africa and the eastern Mediterranean. Recent studies, however, carried out in some areas of East and West Africa have shown the high incidence of severe lesions revealed by intravenous urography (calcified bladder, ureteric deformities, hydronephrosis) in the youngest age groups; as high as 45 per cent of school children infected with *S. haematobium* in some localities (Forsyth and MacDonald, 1965). By comparing figures obtained from areas of different levels of endemicity, it was clearly established that these lesions are due to bilharziasis and that their prevalence was related to the weight of infection as measured by egg output in the urine.

The occurrence of such serious lesions in children and adolescents suggests that urinary bilharziasis might be the cause of considerable mortality in economically vital groups of the population. *S. haematobium* can cause pulmonary

N

arteritis progressing to cor pulmonale, which is an irreversible and fatal condition; in Egypt 58 per cent of total pulmonary bilharzial involvement was considered to be due to *S. haematobium* infection alone (Shaw and Ghareeb, 1938). In Egypt, Nigeria and other parts of Africa there is evidence to show some relation between the occurrence of cancer of the bladder and urinary bilharziasis. This type of bladder cancer is usually met with at a relatively younger age and various mechanisms have been postulated to explain its relationship with bilharziasis (Hashem, 1961; Abul-Fadl and Khalafallah, 1961).

The severity of the disease due to infection with *S. mansoni* or *S. japonicum* is now generally recognised in all endemic areas. Both species are responsible for obstruction to portal blood flow and the relation of these infections to Symmer's pipe-stem fibrosis is well established. Schistosomal obstruction of the pulmonary arteries and arterioles, ending eventually in heart failure, can result from these infections, usually in patients with portal hypertension and portasystemic collateral circulation. Such severe and often fatal disease of the liver and lungs is common in some localities.

In an endemic area in Brazil where the overall death rate of the population over 10 years was found to be 13.7 per thousand, 11.3 per cent among them presented enlarged bilharzial spleens (Kloetzel, 1962). When patients with chronic bilharzial splenomegaly were followed up for a total of 678 man-years, 58 per cent of the deaths occurring during the study were attributed to *S. mansoni* infection (Kloetzel, 1967). In an endemic area in the Philippines (Farooq, 1963) 62 per cent of the infected population were classified as asymptomatic carriers and 38 per cent with mild, moderate or serious manifestations. In Japan, the disease has no doubt clearly declined in recent years as a result of control measures adopted, with considerable decrease in morbidity and mortality, the majority of the infected cases being described as asymptomatic.

It appears that the disease caused by *S. intercalatum* is usually mild; hepatic and hepatosplenic involvement may occur, but pulmonary manifestations are not met with.

Despite the many detailed descriptions of the various morbid manifestation of bilharziasis, its sequelae and related pathological conditions, the proper assessment of ill health and mortality in this disease is still an open issue. The foundations for such an accurate assessment have recently been laid (W.H.O., 1967) and cross-sectional studies have already started in some endemic areas to estimate the prevalence and intensity of infection and the nature and prevalence of the lesions present. These lesions have to be followed up in longitudinal studies together with the complications and related pathological conditions that may develop, and the magnitude of the resulting disease is expressed in clinical and pathological terms. The data could thus be properly expressed in terms of sickness disability or death.

GENERAL PATHOLOGY

The fundamental pathological lesions of human schistosomiasis are similar in the three species and are produced either by cercariae, schistosomulae, adult schistosomes, ova or their circulating metabolites. Man suffers according to the number of cercariae which can successfully penetrate his skin and survive to maturity in the pelvic veins. Although the main pathological lesions of this disease are found in the urogenital and digestive organs, any system or organ in the body including the cardiopulmonary, nervous, ocular, endocrinal, tegumentary and reticuloendothelial systems may be involved.

It is a common observation that the richer the part in venules, the more likely is it to be affected with schistosomal lesions, for it then affords a greater opportunity to the female worms to reach the part and deposit ova.

The pathological lesions produced by schistosomes vary according to the stage of infection, the tissue response and the number of invading cercariae. They may be classified as follows:

Stage of invasion and maturation
Stage of localisation and oviposition
Stage of ulceration and repair
Pathological lesions related to allergy or immunity
Relation to malignancy

Stage of invasion and maturation

After penetration of the skin by cercariae, erythematous, petechial or papular rashes may occur due to vasodilatation of the dermal capillaries associated with cellular infiltration by eosinophils and neutrophils. After an incubation period of 2–4 weeks, transient congestion of lung capillaries with focal oedema or haemorrhages usually occurs around circulating schistosomulae associated with bronchiolitis, interstitial pneumonitis and rarely thrombosis of pulmonary vessels. Other viscera may be similarly affected, especially liver, spleen and intestines, causing slight enlargement of these organs during the maturation stage of the surviving schistosomes.

Stage of localisation, oviposition and elimination of ova

Live adult schistosomes do not produce lesions in the veins they inhabit, but dead worms produce severe allergic reactions which are manifested by necrosis of the vascular walls and surrounding tissues and dense infiltration of eosinophils, neutrophils and large mononuclear cells. A schistosomal pigment is excreted into the blood and is deposited in the reticuloendothelial cells of the liver, spleen, bone marrow, intestines and mesenteric lymph nodes. Although the ova are delivered fully embryonated they take at least 10 days to become fully mature and remain alive for a further few weeks before being eliminated, otherwise they die *in situ*. The extent of damage to the tissues is proportional to the number of ova trapped within them and this in turn depends on their number and species. For every ovum of the *S. mansoni* female, 20 to 30 are laid by the *S. haematobium* and more than 50 by *S. japonicum*.

Ova deposited by female worms are eliminated through vesical or intestinal mucosa partly by the action of lytic enzymes from miracidia, and partly by the action of the spines which engage on the capillary wall and cause contraction and rupture of vessels. The resulting trauma from rupture of vessels and penetration of ova through the mucous epithelium, causes hyperaemia of the mucosa, submucosal haemorrhages and minute epithelial erosions.

An undetermined number of ova extruded into the tissues fail to escape into the lumen of the intestinal or urinary tracts and are trapped *in situ*. Such ova bring about the development of local granulomatous lesions as well as some general reactions.

Around the ova, large mononuclear cells and a small number of lymphocytes and plasma cells collect in the form of schistosomal tubercles. Tissue eosinophilia is associated with blood eosinophilia, though this may not develop if there is a severe septic process in the body producing neutrophilic leucocytosis. The miracidia of the ova degenerate and become amorphous and gradually undergo calcification, while the chitinous shells remain unchanged. Commonly some of the foreign body giant cells are found engulfing the collapsed ova or their remains.

Later a fibroblastic reaction follows leading to a process of lamellar fibrous whorls beginning at the periphery of these follicular lesions. Necrosis of the cellular infiltrate or the parenchymatous cells may appear in the vicinity of the ovum. In solid organs such as the liver or pancreas diffuse infiltration produces thickening of the portal tracts. Polypoid formations occur in hollow organs when the delicate unstable connective tissue internal to the muscularis mucosa is infiltrated with vascular granulation tissue which raises the mucosa above the surface. The epithelial covering also shows evidence of hyperplasia, which help in producing polypi.

Ova of *S. mansoni* or *S. japonicum* produce lesions mainly in the intestines, gall-bladder and pancreas, but those which fail to engage in the vascular walls are carried by the portal blood as emboli to the liver where they produce different lesions according to their number and severity.

Ova of *S. haematobium* produce lesions in the bladder, ureter, kidneys, urethra, seminal vesicles, spermatic cords, epididymis, vulva, vagina, uterus, uterine tubes and ovaries. Vesical, prostatic and uterine plexuses drain into the inferior vena cava; thus emboli of ova may reach the lungs.

S. mansoni ova and adults easily reach the lungs through the portasystemic collaterals which result from portal hypertension in the late stages of hepatic involvement. Some of the embolised ova may bypass the lungs and reach different parts of the body. The conjunctiva, skin, spinal cord, brain, heart, thyroid and adrenals are among the ectopic sites in which ova and the lesions they produce have occasionally been found. Worms may have reached some of these ectopic sites via the vertebral system of veins.

Stage of ulceration and tissue repair

Most granulation tissue is transformed in time to scar tissue, and this continues to contract, causing narrowing of the lumen of hollow organs. As a result vessels become constricted and most papillomata slough off, giving rise to multiple ulcers. The ulcers heal by scarring unless secondary infection supervenes when healing may be protracted and sinus formation results. The nearer an organ is to the exterior, the earlier will secondary infection be likely to occur and to initiate the formation of papillomata. Stasis of tissue fluid due to fibrosis leads to chronic infection and further spread may be in an ascending or disseminated form.

Some of the severe lesions of the disease, especially those in the liver and lungs, are believed to be caused or modified by treatment which brings about a shift of worms or ova. The nutritional state of the individual also modifies visceral symptoms which are less obvious in malnourished subjects.

Pathological lesions related to allergy and immunity

It has long been noted that infection is usually mild among patients in middle or old age, while in children it is commonly severe. In hyperinfected hosts, immunity may be readily demonstrable simulating that of bacterial or viral infections, but milder or infrequent infection confers little or no resistance.

The main antigens responsible for immunity are connected with the production of eggs in host tissues. Experimentally, it is found that in the late stages of the disease, the lesions of repeated re-infection are frequently few in number and extent. Severe exudative reactions observed around disintegrated ova or worms are most probably allergic in nature. Fluorescent antibody techniques and certain serological tests demonstrated such reactions clearly. The possibility of an autoimmune response was also shown in some organs.

Relation to malignancy

There is much evidence to indicate an aetiological relationship between cancer of the bladder and bilharziasis of this organ. No such relation has been found with cancers of colon, liver, lungs, pancreas or other organs. It is believed that cancer of the bladder is dependent for its initiation on specific humoral carcinogenetic factors related to the infection or to altered metabolites in the urine. In addition, there is no regenerative hyperplasia in solid organs affected by the disease as the lesions are essentially interstitial and ischaemic and thus do not predispose to neoplastic formation.

GENITOURINARY SCHISTOSOMIASIS

On the basis of anatomical and experimental evidence, *S. haematobium* worms are believed to proceed along the mesenteric veins to reach the genitourinary system, and thence along anastomotic channels to reach either the superior or inferior mesenteric veins. As this type of infection is very prevalent in the Nile Valley, genitourinary bilharziasis plays an important role in the life of the Egyptian peasants. The infection is primarily urinary and the genitalia are usually infected secondarily.

The site and degree of infiltration in any organ of the genitourinary system determine the pathological lesions and their complications. The ova are usually deposited either submucously or deep in the tissues. Submucously they stimulate epithelial and mesodermal changes; in deeper tissues mesodermal changes only ensue. The pathological processes involved are either proliferative (hyperplastic), degenerative (hypoplastic) or atrophic; sometimes metaplasia occurs, especially in the epithelial lining. The presence of secondary pyogenic infection causes more severe reactions than that in closed lesions which are not open to infection.

Kidney

Primary affection of the kidney is rare. However, this organ suffers considerable damage secondary to ureteric and vesical involvement.

Pathology. Ova may be deposited in the renal parenchyma or in the submucous tissue of the renal pelvis and calyces. The former lesions are usually detected accidentally in routine pathological examination of the kidneys as they present no gross pathological characteristics. In the submucous lesion of the renal pelvis, greyish-white bilharziomata, patches of hyperaemia which show dark fresh haemorrhages, sandy greyish-yellow patches, different forms of papilloma, small cysts or ulcers may be encountered. Phosphate concretions, renal calculi, or pyelonephritis may complicate the picture. The kidneys may also suffer secondarily to affection of the ureters or bladder, leading to hydro- or pyonephrosis resulting from strictures and calculi in the urinary outflow. Malignant transformation may be encountered.

Clinical features. The intrarenal lesions produce little or no obstructive symptoms, but their presence predisposes to septic infection and the formation of stones, mostly of calcium phosphate. Hydronephrosis, usually bilateral, is a very common complication of bilharzial ureteritis and among rural inhabitants in the Nile Valley causes many deaths by renal failure. Management of such cases is usually medical. The urologist is confronted with them when a fixed pathological state develops; examples include stenotic lesions, epithelial changes, fistulae and infection following back pressure. Indications for surgical intervention are discussed below.

Diagnosis. Scanning renography using isotopes is helpful in cases with renal failure and may show filling defects due to renal bilharziomata or suspected malignancy. Angiography whether aortic or femoral is helpful in demonstrating the distribution of the renal blood supply in cases complicated by hydronephrosis.

Ureter

Schistosomiasis of the ureters is common and in most cases disease occurs concomitantly with active infection of the bladder. It is usually bilateral with preponderance of infection on one side more than the other. It may be unilateral with predilection for the left side since anastomosis between mesenteric and ureteric veins is more extensive on the left side.

Pathology. The transitional epithelium undergoes hyperplasia or even metaplasia into squamous type. Downward prolongation of the epithelium with formation of glandular ureteritis may occur, as well as cystic ureteritis due to mucoid degeneration of the nests of Von Brunn. Malignant transformation of the epithelium leading to carcinoma of the ureter is liable to follow, especially when there is obstruction of the urinary outflow.

Proliferation of the connective tissue of the submucosa leads to formation of polypi which increase in size, partly due to retardation of fluid drainage as a result of narrowing of the venous lumen by cellular infiltration. Hypertrophy of the muscle coats occurs hand in hand with the sclerosing stenotic lesions, usually seen in the distal parts of the ureter, where degeneration of muscle and fibrosis ensue. Secondary infection and encrustations may occur leading to calcification, hydronephrosis and pyonephrosis. Primary and secondary ulceration or sandy patches may result from diminished blood supply, escape of ova due to desquamation, or atrophy of the epithelium overlying larger numbers of calcified ova.

Chronic periureteritis leading to fibrosis and thickening of the periureteral tissues occurs to a marked degree in the pelvic segments and to a lesser extent proximally. These changes may be so marked as to cause the ureter to resemble an intestinal tube with calcification involving part of its length.

Clinical features. In cases in which the vesical symptoms are so mild that the ureteral manifestations predominate, the main symptoms are haematuria, ureteric colic and tenderness along the course of the ureter.

Haematuria tends to diminish as the lesions responsible become chronic and less vascular. When the source of bleeding is situated high up in the ureter, the blood passed is mostly coagulated in worm-like filaments, producing clot colic. In lower ureteric lesions, the blood is mostly liquid and the pain less severe. By turning the recumbent patient towards one side in order to displace the intestine, the affected ureter can be compressed directly against the brim of the pelvis. Pressure by the examining hand elicits pain along its course and a desire for micturition. Palpation of the last ureteric segment by a finger in the rectum or vagina may be followed by a similar sensation.

The patient then suffers from dull aching pain in the loins, and every now and then some exacerbation of renal colic occurs. In some cases, symptoms of hydronephrosis or pyonephrosis develop due to supervention of fibrosis and secondary infection. This is especially so in adult males and may be detected by urography.

The attacks of renal colic, though simulating those of stones and non-schistosomal lesions, are not so painful, so frequent or so lasting as the latter. Later, unless the condition becomes complicated, the attack becomes less frequent and less severe.

Primary renal calculi are essentially non-bilharzial and are mostly related to intestino-hepatic, metabolic or constitutional derangements favouring crystallisation.

Diagnosis. As in the case of the schistosomal bladder, cystoscopy and radiography are the most important diagnostic methods. Chromocystoscopy and ureteric catheterisation give further information.

Prognosis. Despite an apparently benign outlook as regards fistulae and malignant transformation, ureteric cases are examples of latent uraemia, and many pass into a state of severe uraemia after an accidental or minor surgical intervention, e.g. ureteric catheterisation or cystoscopy.

Specific therapy with antibiotics and intermittent diuresis, supplemented sometimes by physiotherapy, are helpful in non-complicated or late cases.

Management. Specific medical treatment is indicated for active infection before resorting to the following surgical procedures.

Stricture of the upper third is treated by ureterolysis in most cases; occasionally a longitudinal incision with transverse suture is performed or the stenosed area may be excised with subsequent spatulation of the cut ends or end-to-end anastomosis.

Stricture of the lower third may be treated by closed or open dilatation, ureterovesical meatoplasty, pull-through nipple ureteroneocystotomy, partial nippling, sleeve resection or ureterocystotomy according to the site, length and tightness of the stricture, with proper and adequate control of secondary infection before and after surgery. No force is used to dilate a stricture, otherwise surgery is adopted and nephrostomy is recommended in some cases.

In cases of epithelial enclosures, especially diagnosed radiologically as calcified ureteritis calcenosa, repeated catheterisation or ureterolithotomy with scraping of the interior of the ureter with a blunt curette is indicated.

Nephrectomy may have to be performed as a last resort when the surgeon cannot employ any of the previous surgical procedures. When either kidneys are hydronephrotic, nephrostomy may be done on one side, on the better kidney, or on both kidneys, depending on the condition of the patient and the state of his kidney.

Bladder

The trigone is the commonest part affected; in heavy infections the fundus is also affected.

Pathology. Lesions in the bladder wall mainly result from ova. Living worms inhabit the veins and do not provoke specific reaction unless they die when they induce a severe allergic reaction with necrosis and heavy eosinophilic reaction. Ova are deposited either in the submucosa or in the muscle coats in few or excessive numbers. The tissues react to their presence either by nodular or diffuse reaction with a hyperplastic or a proliferative effect.

The epithelium becomes heaped up in several layers and may undergo metaplasia into stratified squamous cells with downward prolongation into the submucosa in the form of pseudo-epitheliomatous masses. Leukoplakia with hyperkeratinisation is sometimes met with. Glandular cystitis is a common finding and opinions differ as regards its pathogenesis or formation and whether there is central degeneration of the epithelial cell nests, secretory activity of these cells or invagination of the hyperplastic mucosa with inflammatory closure of their necks. It is considered to be precancerous. The connective tissue also undergoes proliferation, pushes the epithelium in front of it, leading to formation of polypi which may be sessile or pedunculated, single, multiple or branching (villous).

It is probable that the presence of worms in the polyp itself or its pedicle may be related to the characteristic formation of these polyps, especially if the worms are arrested in the main vessels of the pedicle and continuously feeding it with ova.

The muscles undergo mechanical adaptive hypertrophy, especially when there is obstruction at the neck of the bladder. Ulceration and sandy patches develop in different sizes and shapes, and secondary pyogenic infection may set in leading to cystitis and aggravation of damage to the tissues.

Cystitis cystica which is considered to be a degenerative change in the mucosa may also be seen. Haemorrhage, and schistosomal pigments are sometimes seen in the cyst which may occasionally rupture. Encrustations with phosphates oxalates and urates are a common finding pre-disposing to calculus formation. Finally dense collagenous tissue is seen in the various layers of the bladder, including muscle, leading to contraction and calcification of the bladder wall.

Clinical features. The clinical manifestations may present in an acute or chronic form.

ACUTE VESICAL SCHISTOSOMIASIS. The main complaints are haematuria, dysuria and frequency of micturition which may be vague or lacking in mild infection. Haematuria is terminal and is due to the passage of schistosome ova through the congested vesical mucosa, exacerbated by contraction of the bladder musculature hyperaemia and oedema of the mucous membrane, and the presence of vascular papillomata or ulcers. Bleeding is usually so slight that it does not worry the patient. Strenuous body exercise, riding or motoring on rough ground, trauma to the hypogastrium and excessive heat or cold aggravate it. The patient experiences little difficulty in passing urine but has a feeling of discomfort and perineal heaviness at the termination of micturition.

CHRONIC VESICAL SCHISTOSOMIASIS. Supervention of secondary infection leads to persistence and extension of the ulcerative process which is helped by diminished vascularity of the bladder wall. In the presence of this and other complications, e.g. stone formation, dysuria is considerably enhanced. Pain is usually referred to the glans penis. Pain or tenderness may also be felt suprapubically or perineally over the region of the bladder and of the prostatic urethra respectively.

Because of the increase in excitability of the mucous membrane, the patient passes his urine more frequently, especially at night; later due to contraction of the bladder wall and secondary infection, strangury persists. Rarely a state of schistosomal muscular atony leads to urinary retention.

In advanced cases, the sphincters become involved and incontinence follows with dribbling of foul-smelling purulent urine. Stone formation, fistulae, uraemia and malignancy may supervene adding to the patient's misery.

Complications. PRIMARY SUBPERITONEAL VESICAL INFILTRATION. This is rare, but occurs not uncommonly as an extension of schistosomiasis of the ureters, prostate and seminal vesicle. Areas of infiltration are hard and may be detected suprapubically and *per rectum*. They persist unless sepsis or malignant disease reaches them from the bladder, when they undergo softening or suppuration.

FISTULAE. Fistulae between the bladder and the skin or bowel may result. Trauma may act as a causative factor. Rarely the fistulous tracks reach the ischiorectal fossa giving rise to an abscess and later to urinary fistulae.

Fibrosis occurring near the internal meatus, helped by the presence of papillomata, or by prostate or seminal vesicle involvement, leads to bladder neck obstruction.

Diagnosis. Examination usually reveals manifestations of the disease elsewhere than in the bladder. Examination of the urine and serological tests for schistosomiasis are important. Cystoscopy and biopsy remain the key to the diagnosis unless the lesion is wholly muscular.

Bladder neck obstruction exhibits shortening and sacculation of the superior part of the posterior urethra, approximation of the orifices of the trigone and altered mobility of the bladder neck.

Only when large numbers of ova calcify do they show on the plain X-ray as white shadows. These are at first patchy but later the patches coalesce to form a line which will demonstrate the shape and size of the bladder which is usually contracted at this stage of the disease. Later this calcification may become so extensive that the whole bladder appears as a dense calcified bag; associated or complicating stones are usually clearly seen.

Radiological changes of bladder neck obstruction demonstrable by urography are increasing elevation of the base of the bladder so that it becomes globular and balloon-like in shape, and dilatation of the bladder, ureters and finally the pelvis of the kidney. Cysts and papillomata show as filling defects which need further investigation to exclude malignancy. A micturating cystogram will demonstrate the presence of any ureteric reflux resulting from obstruction to the urinary outflow or pathological changes of vesicoureteric function.

In doubtful or complicated cases radiological examination by urography whether ascending or descending is of great help and kidney function tests also reveal the degree of obstructive uropathy present.

Management. In addition to specific antischistosomal and antimicrobial therapy, surgical interference differs according to the prevailing pathology and whether the surgery is for epithelial change or fibrosis.

ULCERATION. When acute and multiple, ulcers respond to electric cauterisation but surgical excision usually proves more successful. Chronic deep ulcers need partial cystectomy.

EPITHELIAL CHANGES. Metaplasia in the form of leukoplakia is better removed as it may pave the way to malignancy. Polyposis resists antischistosomal therapy; perurethral resection is possible if the polyps are localised and limited to the bladder,

otherwise removal by open surgical excision is required.

BLADDER NECK OBSTRUCTION (due to dense fibrosis of the subtrigonal plate). Dilatation with ironing of the posterior lip or its excision with or without lateral sphincterectomy is needed. In advanced cases trigonectomy with total excision of the trigonal plate is required. The hazards of excisional treatment are internal insemination and temporary sterility, and occasionally temporary incontinence. Attempts to modify such complications, especially the former, include subtrigonal plate excision.

CONTRACTED BLADDER. *Vesical denervation* (presacral or pudendal) whether by injection or by neurectomy is indicated.

Supravesical urinary shunt either by bilateral nephrostomy, bilateral ureterocutaneous implication, ureterocolic or ureteroiliac transplantation may be resorted to.

Mechanical extension of bladder capacity using an ileal loop whether closed or open, a pedicled skin graft, or both followed by cystoplasty, are lines of management.

Overdistension under anaesthesia with perivesical injection of a fibrolytic agent combined with short wave therapy may be tried.

Urethra

The route of infection is through the arborisation which links the vesicoprostatic plexus with the pudendal plexus, the latter receiving venous blood from the urethra and penis through the deep dorsal vein. The intensity of infection varies according to the richness of the local venous supply. In the bulbous urethra, infection occurs near the roof, whereas in the penile urethra infiltration is denser in the floor.

In females, the shortness of the urethra, its wide calibre and greater distensibility, make such complications as urinary obstruction, periurethral abscesses and fistulae rare.

Pathology. Lesions occur in the usual three stages: infiltration, ulceration and cicatrisation. During the infiltrative stage, polypi may form in the navicular fossa of the penile urethra. Again the verumontanum in the prostatic urethra may be hypertrophic and exhibit thick oedematous lips. In the ulcerative stages, superficial ulcers are formed which may heal by scarring of the penile urethra, except in the bulbous part.

Secondary infected ulcers lead to formation of periurethral abscesses. The pus tracks along the lines of least resistance and may ultimately point in the perineum, scrotum and penis forming fistulous tracks which may be branching and associated with pseudo-elephantiasis of the penis, although this is nowadays becoming rare.

Clinical features. Bilharziasis of the penis or prostatic urethra may be noticed in adult patients who have a severe degree of infection. A sensation of urethral discomfort or even retention and impotence may occur when associated with perineal or scrotal fistulae, in addition to sequelae of urethral obstruction including pseudo-elephantiasis.

Diagnosis. Urethroscopy is helpful. A micturating cystogram carried out under fluoroscopy or urethrography to determine the site of a urethral obstruction or fistulous track or any suspected urethral calcification is needed.

Management. In addition to antischistosomal, antibiotic and chemotherapeutic drugs, suprafistulous urinary shunts may be needed in case of gross pyuria with resistant organisms. The shunt is advised, or suprapubic cystectomy, in cases of a fistulising mass and perineal cystectomy in cases of fistulising tracks. Any persistent fibromatous mass should be excised, followed by a course of repeated dilatation to obviate post-urethritis strictures which are prone to occur after the operation.

Prostate and seminal vesicles

Adults are the most commonly affected and the main manifestations in the early stages are partly urinary and partly sexual. The route of infection is particularly through the anastomosis of the rectal veins and those of the vesicoprostatic plexus. It is not unlikely that worms invade the prostate and seminal vesicles while the venous pathways to the bladder are obstructed by the disease.

Pathology. Ulcerative and cicatrising lesions predominate. In the infiltrative stages ova are deposited in the interstitial tissue, submucous and muscular coats leading to enlargement of the organs affected. Their vascularity is increased and there is hyperplasia of the endothelial lining of the vesicles. Escape of ova in the secretions of the prostate and seminal vesicles leads to alteration of the glandular mucosa, haemospermia associated with priapism, and later impotence.

In the fibrotic stage, localised or diffuse narrowing or actual obliteration of the lumina may be associated with diminution in size and increased firmness of the organs and adherence to the base of the bladder.

Calcification is frequently coincident with fibrosis. Muscular hypertrophy due to incomplete or intermittent obstruction frequently occurs and ends in fibrosis.

Clinical features. Frequency of micturition due to associated cystitis may occur but is not necessarily nocturnal. The stream of urine is apt to be thin, interrupted or weakened and there may be terminal dribbling. A sensation of discomfort, heaviness or even pain related to micturition, coitus or constipation may be felt in the perineum or suprapubically and may be referred to the rectum or sacrum. Haemospermia. is mostly related to affection of the seminal vesicles and there may be sexual hyperexcitability, night dreams, sterility or impotence.

On rectal examination the findings vary with the stage of the disease. In the congestive stage the vesicles and prostate are palpable, nodular and tender. It is not always possible to feel the median prostatic sulcus, and the prostatic margins may be overlapped by the enlarged seminal vesicles. In the fibrotic stages 'boggy' or fluctuating cysts can be felt with no marked tenderness unless secondarily infected or complicated, as they may rarely be, by malignancy.

Diagnosis. Schistosomal ova in spermatic fluid may be found, especially in cases with haemospermia. The endoscopic appearance of the prostatic urethra will elucidate the source of sanguinous semen.

In late involvement of the seminal vesicles they appear radiologically oval in outline with a comb-like pattern. They are situated on either side of the midline in a position higher than that of the trigone and internal to the position of the shadows usually produced by calcified schistosomal ureters.

Management. Massage and diathermy after specific therapy may diminish the congestion in early cases. Surgery may occasionally be called upon to drain pus when the approach is through the perineum as in the case of ordinary periprostatic abscesses. Excision of the vesicles or prostate is rarely resorted to except in cases associated with bladder neck obstruction.

Spermatic cord, epididymis and testis

The schistosomal worms progress from the abdomen and pelvis to the intrascrotal structures along venous channels, probably the internal spermatic and deferential veins respectively.

Pathology. The testicle and tunica vaginalis seem to possess a remarkable immunity against schistosomal infection; very rarely they are involved in an extension of severe epididymal infection. In the epididymis, miliary, solitary or massive nodular lesions may occur. Although the vas deferens is adherent to surrounding tissues, its lumen is patent unless involved in inflammation of the seminal vesicles.

Schistosomal funiculoepididymitis may be accompanied by a small hydrocoele as a result of fibrosis affecting the lymphatics. The scrotum is not affected unless involved by nearby sepsis.

Clinical features. The chief complaint is swelling in the scrotum with some discomfort locally or referred to the testes. Patients are often worried lest a venereal or malignant condition is present and their sexual ability may be affected.

Diagnosis. Biopsy is very helpful in diagnosis and vesiculography may be needed to exclude any luminal obstruction of the vas deferens or to choose the line of treatment.

Management. If the patient is worried and also in late cases not responding to specific therapy, surgical removal, avoiding injury to the testicle and vas deferens, may be needed.

Female genital organs

This is comparatively rare in endemic areas for the route of infection is through the pelvic veins anastomosing with the mesenteric veins. The body of the uterus is rarely involved, for shedding of the endometrium monthly with menstruation does not allow the ova to remain *in situ*, though a few cases have been known to be accompanied by bleeding or even with pregnancy or malignancy. The cervix uteri, when affected, exhibits friable polypoid mass giving rise to bleeding and simulating carcinoma. Ovarian involvement is mainly at the hylum and luteinisation occurs normally. Fibrosis leading to amenorrhoea and sterility is described in certain localities but is not common. In the vagina polypoid masses and diffuse sclerosis may occur and malignant change may become superimposed.

Vesicovaginal fistulae may occur. The vulva shows marked epithelial hyperplasia histologically, with pseudo-epithelial appearances and rarely ulcers. Ova may be recovered in vaginal scrapings, endometrial biopsy or rarely in menstrual fluid. Colposcopy may reveal lesions in the form of sandy patches on vaginal mucosa, ulcers, nodules or leukoplakia which may be verified as schistosomal by biopsy or by taking scrapings. Calcification of the female genital organs has not been recognised radiologically to be of any diagnostic importance, though it should be suspected in female patients with abnormal pelvic shadows.

Cancer of bladder in relation to schistosomiasis

Schistosomiasis is associated with cancer of the bladder to a statistically significant degree and it has a potentiating effect on the pathogenesis of cancer of that organ. The geographic distribution of cancer of the bladder in Egypt and other places runs parallel with that of schistosomiasis. A significant reduction in its incidence in Egypt was seen in autopsies carried out between 1934 and 1950 compared with that seen during a similar period from 1909 to 1930 in the same areas. This decline is in all probability related to the reported decrease in the incidence and intensity of the disease.

Cancer of the bladder in Egypt accounts for 0.65 per cent of total malignancy and 7.9 per cent of all carcinomata. It also arises at an earlier mean age than that of other organs in the same patients. In such cases the age incidence follows by about a decade the age distribution of schistosomal infection, and the incidence of both decreases gradually after the fourth decade.

In the case of non-schistosomal bladder cancer, the incidence increases steadily as age advances. The sex ratio is about nine males to one female, possibly as the latter are less exposed to infection during adolescence.

Pathology. Histologically three types are recognised; squamous carcinoma accounts for 60 per cent, transitional cell carcinoma for 35 per cent and adenocarcinoma for 5 per cent. It has been clearly demonstrated that systemic haematobiasis can produce hyperplastic and metaplastic changes in mouse bladder epithelium in the absence of local deposition of schistosomal ova. Such changes with the addition of a small dose of a bladder carcinogen led to the induction of numerous benign and malignant neoplasms. These findings suggest that some toxic factors influence the bladder epithelium either via the blood stream or because they are concentrated in urine.

Alternative theories put forward to explain the relationship between bladder cancer and schistosomiasis are as follows:

1. Cancer results from prolonged irritation of bladder epithelium by the presence of schistosomal ova beneath it, during their passage through it, or as a result of a reparative process which progresses beyond normal limits and proceeds to hyperplasia and then to malignancy.

2. Cancer results from sepsis and consequent alkalinity of an inflamed schistosomal bladder. The marked destruction of the muscle coat in schistosomal cystitis, and later fibrosis with bladder neck obstruction,

would certainly interfere with evacuation and result in urinary stasis. In almost all autopsied cases, cancer of the ureter or renal pelvis is associated with schistosomal fibrotic stenosis below the site of the neoplasm.

3. Cancer results from the presence of carcinogens in the urine. It has been found that urine in schistosomal cases contains large amounts of the enzyme glucuronidase which in the presence of stasis, secondary infection and alkaline urine may release carcinogenetic substances from harmless conjugated forms. Furthermore, the level of the enzyme is highest in cases of schistosomiasis complicated by bladder cancer or suffering from nutritional deficiencies, especially vitamin B_6 deficiency. The carcinogenetic metabolites of tryptophan in urine are reduced by administration of vitamin B_6 which is needed for the growth, maturation and oviposition of the schistosomes in the portal system. This effect is possibly related to a change in liver activity.

Clinical features. The onset usually develops insidiously over 10 or more years in schistosomal cases. In some the first warning may be an attack of severe haematuria without important previous symptoms of bladder irritation or increased frequency. Dysuria is aggravated by ulceration of the growth, and later by sepsis, and leads to insomnia, anxiety, toxicity and cachexia. Symptoms of renal insufficiency may supervene and cause rapid deterioration. The pain is felt at first in the glans penis, later it may be felt in the hypogastrium or be referred to the perineum, rectum, or along the thigh where it simulates sciatica.

On examination, the kidneys may be palpable and an indefinite or a hard mass may occupy the hypogastrium. Anal examination will show the extent of the growth and its fixation to neighbouring structures. Secondary deposits may appear locally in liver, lung, or elsewhere. Acute perforation rarely occurs.

Diagnosis. Cystoscopy will reveal the growth and enable a biopsy to be taken. Examination of the urinary sediment for exfoliative cytological changes also helps as a screening test.

In cases in which there is calcification of the bladder, inequalities of the calcified outline should arouse suspicion of malignancy. Intravenous pyelography or ascending cystography will show an irregular filling defect at the site of the lesion.

Prognosis. This is usually bad as the general condition and kidney function deteriorate rapidly.

Treatment. PROPHYLACTIC. Prophylactic treatment is the most important and consists of early specific therapy, treatment of secondary infection and early removal of papillomata, glandular cystitis, leukoplakia and ulceration.

RADICAL. Radical anterior pelvic exenteration is indicated in operable cases. The bladder, prostate, seminal vesicles, vas deferens, pelvic vesical fascia and pelvic lymph nodes are removed *en bloc*. In the female, the bladder, uterus, vagina, adnexa, pelvic vesical fascia and pelvic lymph nodes are dissected out. Invasion of the rectum is a contra-indication to operation, as is old age, poor kidney function or poor general condition of the patient. Such operative measures are associated or preceded by ureterocolic diversion.

Partial cystectomy. This is done only in precancerous and early cases. It is usually associated with diversion of the ureters into the sigmoid colon.

PALLIATIVE. In cases in which there are contra-indications to surgery, presacral neurotomy, electrocoagulation of the growth, or implantation of radium or radioactive isotopes may be helpful. Therapy with deep X-rays or cobalt beam may give better results.

ALIMENTARY SCHISTOSOMIASIS

Schistosomal lesions are more common in the distal than in the proximal alimentary tract but may occur at any point, including the stomach, small intestine, appendix, colon or rectum. Lesions have also been encountered in the gall-bladder and pancreas.

Stomach and small intestine

The stomach and small intestine are rarely the sites of schistosomal involvement in *S. mansoni* and *S. japonicum* infections, but may form submucous or subserous nodules which are difficult to diagnose preoperatively. Peptic-like ulcerations with haematemesis have been recorded. Papillomata have been reported in the ileum, and schistosomal ulcerations which perforate through adhesions between loops of small intestine forming palpable tumours have also been reported. Examination soon after death is necessary in order to avoid post-mortem autodigestion and disappearance of lesions. Serial autopsies on stomach and small intestine of cases of *S. mansoni* infection reveal a higher incidence of such lesions. Gastric and jejunal biopsy with a Crosby capsule is now utilised for that purpose and reveals a high incidence of lesions with minimal reaction around deposited ova.

Appendix

This is a common post-mortem and postoperative finding; however, the infrequency of acute appendicitis in such cases needs explanation. The following pathological lesions have been described in the three types of schistosomiasis:

1. Schistosomal non-obliterative appendicitis.
2. Schistosomal obliterative appendicitis.
3. Schistosomal stenotic appendicitis which may lead to suppurative appendicitis.

Hard plastic subperitoneal nodules may be encountered in the region of the appendix with heavy deposition of ova which produce fibrosis of the submucosa extending to adjoining lymph glands. Such changes are mostly found in areas in which *S. haematobium* is the predominant endemic infection.

Colon

The changes in the colon are mainly present in the descending part, sigmoid and rectum; however, in severe infections higher levels are involved even in *S. haematobium* infection.

Pathology. The colon may show any stage of schistosomal lesion, whether localised or diffuse. If diffuse, the lesions may be so extensive as to lead to marked infiltration of all coats and filling of the lumen with papillomata, thickening of the mucosa and hypertrophy of the muscular layers. The subserosa, appendices epiploica and layers of mesocolon are densely infiltrated with specific granulation tissue having a remarkably abrupt edge. Papillomata occur in 5–20 per cent of cases. They are due to deposition of ova in the superficial layers of the submucosa where the connective tissue is loose and allows larger accumulations of granulation tissue. Later the muscularis mucosa becomes involved and the overlaying mucosa undergoes adenoid hyperplasia.

Rectal and anal polyposis with primary or secondary ulcers may be complicated by anal fissures, fistulae or pseudo-elephantiasis of perianal region. Some cases may be associated with pericolonic masses, but this is rare, and may lead to perforation or intestinal obstruction. Carcinoma of colon has been variously reported to be associated with the presence of schistosomal lesions, suggesting a causal relationship but may well be coincidental.

Clinical features. Four clinical types exist:

1. LATENT. Although there is no subjective evidence of colonic involvement, there is thickening of the colon, diffuse or patchy hyperaemia of the rectosigmoid region and this on healing may leave patches of submucous fibrosis and small sessile papillomata. Living ova are detected in stools, in rectal swabs or in biopsies.

2. RECURRENT DYSENTERIC. This type manifests itself as bouts of diarrhoea or dysentery alternating with bouts of constipation. Bleeding per rectum is a common feature and prolapse of anal mucosa may occur. Anaemia may be moderate or severe in long-standing cases and clubbing of the fingers or osteoarthropathy may be noticed in chronic cases with secondary bacterial ulcerations of the colon. Melaena, flatulence and tenesmus are not common. The spleen and liver are not markedly affected in such cases.

3. COLONIC PAPILLOMATOUS. As the disease progresses, polypoid formation predominates and the polyps vary in size from tiny outgrowths to large masses almost blocking the lumen of the bowel. Such papillomata may be sessile or pedunculated and vary in number from one or two to very many involving the whole lower gut. They may occur in clusters with healthy intervening mucosa, or may affect only a narrow collar of gut. This may be dependent on the arrangement of the veins in the area. The polyps bleed easily on touch, and often have greyish necrotic tips. Rectal polyps may sometimes prolapse through the anus as cauliflower masses.

4. CHRONIC ULCERATIVE. Schistosomal ulcers have been described as resulting from fibrosis of old flat submucous lesions strangulating the blood vessels.

Complications

1. Prolapse of rectum may occur from persistent straining.
2. Fistulae may track from the wall of the rectum to perianal tissue.
3. Intussusception of gut may occur in right-sided lesions with papillomata.
4. Subacute intestinal obstruction may be caused by a larger group of polyps.
5. Perforation into peritoneum is a rare complication possibly resulting from excessive fibrosis.
6. Malignancy is rare in comparison with its occurrence in urogenital lesions. It is usually of the adenocarcinomatous type and mostly in the rectum.

Diagnosis of schistosomiasis of the colon depends on demonstration of ova either in stools or mucosa obtained by examining snip mucosal biopsy taken at proctoscopy. At least three specimens of stools are examined as the output of ova may be intermittent or irregularly mixed with stools and, since such examination is more difficult and less reliable than that of urine, the specimens are preferably taken from the surface of the faecal mass, especially if it contains blood and mucus. This improves the chance of finding ova, especially if larger quantities are examined. The method employed should be quantitative, standardised, dependable and consistent. In order to detect small numbers of eggs, it is necessary to concentrate them from faecal material, produced by sedimentation or by filtration or both. In judging the viability of the ova sound methods should be adopted, either screening the moving miracidia or resorting to hatching techniques.

Proctosigmoidoscopy is not only used for diagnosis but also for detecting any associated or complicating conditions. The mucosa is inspected for congestion, ulcers or papillomata. A swab or biopsy is taken and examined directly under the microscope for ova and other parasites; and if a biopsy specimen is taken a portion should be sent for histopathology.

RADIOLOGY. A barium enema helps to demonstrate lesions, if present, especially in the form of filling defects.

Management of intestinal schistosomiasis

Specific antischistosomal therapies differ in the response they induce in intestinal lesions which are mostly due to *S. mansoni* and *S. japonicum* infection. Oral drugs and certain antimonial preparations such as mercaptosuccinate which produce only a small worm shift to the liver, give better results than other standard antimonial preparations.

Symptomatic treatment for control of rectal bleeding and associated malnutrition are essential and should precede specific therapy in some cases. Antibiotics and intestinal antiseptics play only a minor role in the management of these cases. In view of the importance of removing most of the polypi from the lower gut to prevent symptoms such as bleeding and prolapse, and to avoid the possibility of malignant degeneration, it is essential to apply simple measures for the purpose. These include snaring and applying the diathermy or galvanocautery through the sigmoidoscope. If these measures fail, resort to further surgical measures must be had.

The first attempt at cure of schistosomal lesions of the large intestine by surgery were those of Richards (1910) before the discovery of medical treatment of the parasite by antimony compounds. Fahmy and Dolby (1924) were the first to emphasise that schistosomal polyps do not respond to specific medical treatment. They recommended and practised excision of a tube of the entire rectal sigmoid mucosa with the contained polyps followed by suture of the normal mucosa above to the skin of the anal canal. Later authors did not recommend this operation as it causes severe haemorrhage and there is a possibility of intractable stricture of the rectum or anal incontinence developing. El-Afifi (1961) found that a temporary defunctioning type of transverse colostomy will lead to resolution of the mass in 3–6 months, thus making subsequent resection of the pelvic colon easier.

As schistosomal strictures are very rare and are impossible to differentiate at laparotomy from constricting carcinomata, they should be considered malignant and treated as such. Complete prolapse of rectum is a problem, and treatment by proctosigmoidectomy from below is a dangerous procedure except in the hands of certain surgeons because of its difficulty and the risk of the anastomosis breaking down.

Pancreas

It was not until 1916 that the first instance of pancreatic schistosomiasis was reported by Ultra and Silva. Day in 1924 mentioned a case of glycosuria with schistosomal ova in the urine which disappeared after a course of antimony. In 1928 Sorour stated that *S. mansoni* ova were often found deposited in the pancreas, producing significant fibrosis. Again Erfan (1933) described a case of diabetes mellitus with *S. mansoni* infection, cured by specific therapy. Carcinoma of the pancreas with schistosomal pancreatic infection was reported by Abu-Ghareeb (1941) and later by others. Arafa and Hasham (1962) described the histopathological findings of schistosomiasis of the pancreas. They found the organ to be the seat of schistosomal lesions in 6 per cent of their autopsies on infected patients and that 42 per cent of patients with intestinal schistosomiasis had pancreatic lesions. Most cases are associated with intestinal and hepatic involvement.

Pathology. The pancreas usually show no gross changes and is adherent to surrounding tissues. Its surface is nodular, the capsule thick and opaque, the enlargement diffuse or localised and any part of it may be affected and simulate a neoplasm. It is firm and sometimes cartilaginous and the cut surface simulates the fine and coarse schistosomal fibrosis of the liver. Interlacing bundles of diffuse reticulated scar tissue divide the gland into islands of pale pancreatic tissue. A scraping from the cut surface may show ova.

Microscopically ova may be seen in various stages of degeneration, mainly in the inter-lobular connective tissue but occasionally in the parenchyma where they excite the production of schistosomal granulation tissue. Either focal or diffuse fibrosis with atrophy of adjoining paren-chymal tissue may be present. There is correspond-ing atrophy of the nearby islets of Langerhans, while others hypertrophy. Ova may be found in the wall of the pancreatic duct causing marked thick-ening. The peripancreatic lymph glands are sometimes enlarged, very firm and adherent. Schistosomal worms may be found inside the venules of the pancreas and the peripancreatic tissue.

Clinical features. Usually schistosomal involve-ment of the pancreas remains symptomless and unsuspected until detected accidentally during operation or at autopsy. In severe cases, such symptoms as diarrhoea, flatulence and passage of bulky pale fatty stools associated with loss of weight are suggestive but not conclusive. Intestinal and hepatic symptomatology usually mask the pancreatic symptoms. Regarding the internal secretory function of the pancreas, the presence of glycosuria, although suggestive of involvement, may be an unrelated association. A favourable response to treatment raises the possibility but schistosomal diabetic patients may fail to respond if islets have been irreparably damaged. Only cases of advanced pancreatic involvement exhibit pancreatic enzymatic dysfunction.

Diagnosis. The following signs are suggestive of pancreatic invasion:

1. Loss of weight with no apparent cause.
2. Dyspepsia with left hypochondriac discom-fort.
3. Glycosuria which may decline after specific therapy.
4. Chronic hypoglycaemia with symptoms of hyperinsulinism.
5. Lowering of serum lipase with secondary steatorrhoea and disturbed amylase level.
6. Tumour in the region of the pancreas sub-siding on specific therapy.
7. Evidence of cancer of the pancreas in a highly endemic area—a very rare finding.
8. Lowered tryptic activity.

Management. This is wholly medical, both specifically and non specifically.

Gall-bladder

Cases of true schistosomal cholecystitis are rare and genuine cases diagnosed on purely clinical data have not been reported. Most cases are only suspected and proof is obtained by pathological examination after removal of the gall-bladder.

Pathology. Schistosomal ova have been found in all layers of the gall-bladder and have even penetrated to its lumen. The ova may induce marked thickening of the wall and may be asso-ciated with acute inflammatory reaction.

Clinical features. Schistosomal involvement of the gall-bladder usually gives rise to no specific symptoms and few cases are suspected. It paves the way for secondary bacterial infection and even gallstone formation. The physical signs do not differ from other cases of cholecystitis and may be masked by intestinal and hepatic involve-ment.

Management. Duodenal intubation may help in demonstrating schistosomal ova and evidence of gall-bladder involvement. Otherwise management is wholly medical, unless there is secondary infec-tion and gallstones in which case cholecystectomy is indicated.

Omentum and peritoneum

Terminal spined ova are those most prevalent in the omentum. Many cases of generalised peri-toneal schistosomiasis have been recorded in which the peritoneum has been studded all over with round nodules creamy-white in colour and varying in size from a pea to a small nut. Histo-logically these are schistosomal angiomatoid granulation tissue rich in endothelial cells. The deposition of ova may involve also the fatty tissue of the mesocolon.

Occasionally one or more large masses form along the side of the sigmoid and less often the descending or transverse colon, or caecum. A large mass may wrap itself round a large sector of the circumference of the gut. In the great majority of cases such masses are associated with other lesions such as polyps or ulcers; the presence of the mass handicaps surgical management.

Diagnosis is based on associated signs of vis-ceral schistosomiasis, their response to specific therapy if still in the fibrocellular stage and in some cases exploratory laparotomy.

Management. It has been found that these masses are cured in a few months by temporary defunctioning transverse colostomy; otherwise other surgical management is directed to asso-ciated papillomatosis or chronic ulceration if these resist medical treatment.

HEPATOSPLENIC SCHISTOSOMIASIS

This forms a distinct clinicopathologica pattern. It is caused by the presence of any of the schistosomes or their products in the liver, predominantly *S. mansoni* and *S. japonicum* and less frequently in *S. haematobium*. Liver involvement was first described in Egypt by Kartulis (1885), followed by Symmers (1904) and then by Day and Ferguson (1909), based mostly on clinical and autopsy material. Later Sorour (1928) studied the pathology of the disease in detail and found that the structure of hepatic lesions is different from other forms of cirrhosis, being an interstitial hepatic fibrosis, mainly concentrated around the smaller and larger tracts.

Pathology

The pathology of the disease is predominantly a periportal cellular infiltration followed by fibrosis and associated with vascular changes in the intrahepatic portal tributaries. In the early phases, ova are impacted in and around the fine, medium or main portal tracts exciting histocytic and eosinophilic cellular reactions which are gradually replaced by fibroblasts, tapering towards similar lesions in neighbouring portal tracts. There is also hypertrophy and hyperplasia of Kuppfer cells with dilatation of sinusoids which persist through the different stages of the disease. Schistosomal pigment is seen engulfed by the reticuloendothelial elements and differs slightly in its chemical characteristics from other blood pigments. The parenchymal liver cells show no signs of fatty infiltration, degeneration, necrosis or regeneration.

In the advanced stage of the disease there is thickening of the portal tracts, with mild cloudy swelling and wasting of liver cells at the periphery of lobules resulting from progressive portal ischaemia. The lobular pattern of the liver, though preserved, may show some distortion by fibrous tissue; whether fine (diffuse) or coarse (pipe-stem) fibrosis results, appears to depend on which of the smaller or larger portal tracts are mainly involved. This in turn may be related to the rate and number of ova or worms deposited. Very often they are combined and sometimes even one lobe shows periportal and the other diffuse fibrosis. Lack of excessive regeneration of the hepatic cells in this disease explains the rare incidence of primary hepatic cancer.

In the early stages of active hepatic schistosomiasis there is a progressive enlargement of the spleen due to hyperplasia of the splenic reticular tissue in response to schistosomal toxins associated with active congestion and cellular infiltration, while ova or worms are rarely found in the splenic pulp. Later, the hyperplastic reticulum gives way to diffuse fibrosis associated with marked destruction of musculoelastic tissue of the trabeculae and capsule, leading to a diminution of elasticity and excessive distensibility of the spleen induced by progressive portal hypertension. As a result of excessive congestion and occasionally of thrombosis of the smaller vessels, haemorrhage occurs which on healing results in fibrosiderotic nodules and pericapsular adhesions. Rarely prehepatic portal or splenic vein thrombosis occurs and aggravates the enlargement and splenic congestion.

Pathogenesis

As early as 1923 the relation between *S. mansoni* infection and this syndrome was suggested by El-Kadi and later by Day (1924, 1933), mainly on the parallel incidence of the two conditions based on epidemiological, clinical and therapeutic data. In areas heavily infested with *S. mansoni* in Egypt, 50 per cent of the rural population show hepatic affection, while this only occurs in about 15 per cent of the inhabitants in areas where *S. haematobium* predominates. The latter incidence was explained by supposing an occasional faulty habitat with *S. haematobium* delivering its ova in the portal tract, or may be as a late finding when collateral anastomosis occurs between caval and portal systems allowing free communication. Khalil (1928) was not in favour of the schistosomal origin of hepatic involvement and was inclined to regard intestinal schistosomiasis as a predisposing factor provoking the absorption of toxins from the intestinal canal. Girgis (1930) attributed the hepatic lesions to toxins released by male worms only.

Lea (1928) found that unisexually infected Chinese hamsters never developed cirrhosis of the liver after the schistosomal infection had lasted for 3 years. Hashem (1947) studied experimentally the effect of schistosomal worm extract injected intraperitoneally into rats and through the portal veins of rabbits as well as into the portal veins of dogs by *S. haematobium* ova suspensions. The worm extract produced no significant changes, while the eggs resulted in pathological lesions exactly similar to those seen in the evolution of the human disease. Dead ova were found to cause little or no reaction. Melleney *et al* (1953) described the histopathological lesions produced in bisexual infections with *S. mansoni* in experimentally infected mice, hamsters, rats, guinea pigs and rabbits and compared them with those produced by *S. japonicum* and *S. haematobium*. They concluded that most of the pathology was produced by fertilised eggs and dead worms forming localised lesions which, if numerous enough, lead to extensive scarring.

The early periportal cellular infiltration in the liver is interpreted as an allergic phenomenon resulting from the presence of worms in the portal mesenteric veins. It decreases as the infection continues and does not appear to contribute significantly to ultimate cirrhosis of the liver. Hamilton *et al* (1959) stated that antischistosomal therapy probably has an important influence on the production of liver fibrosis through dead adult worms inducing thrombophlebitis and causing associated embolism of living ova. However, Cameron and Ganguly (1964) found that as long as infection in mice continues with *S. mansoni*, fresh ova lodge in the liver inducing formation of granulomata which become confluent and give rise to broad irregular fibrocellular bands enclosing groups of liver lobules closely similar to the pipe-stem fibrosis of human schistosomiasis.

Humberto (1963) used dead adult schistosome worms as emboli in the portal system of mice and obtained lesions similar to those already described with the usual cercarial infection, thus providing evidence that dead worms can produce hepatic lesions. Menzes (1967) emphasised also that the worms not only obstruct the vascular lumen but cause destruction of the vessel walls, inducing an inflammatory reaction with proliferation of the subintimal connective tissue. Deposition of ova in newly opened capillaries only contributed, in his opinion, to increased fibrosis.

Filho (1959) found in albino mice experimentally infected with *S. mansoni* that in addition to focal intimal reaction in pulmonary vessels containing the necrotised worms, there is a diffuse intimal reaction in other vessels free from any ova or worms. This was more common during reinfection than in primary infections and thus suggested a toxic allergic reaction to circulating schistosomulae during the development of immunity. In this connection, Andrade *et al* (1961) were able by immunocytochemical methods to demonstrate antigen-antibody complexes in the liver of mice infected with *S. mansoni*, thus providing support for the immunological nature of the self-perpetuating hepatic involvement in schistosomiasis.

Raslavicus (1965), in his studies of parabiotic mice, only one of which was infected with *S. mansoni*, demonstrated that diffuse parenchymal changes do not occur in the livers of unexposed animals. Stenger *et al* (1967) studied the liver of mice infected with *S. mansoni* 8, 11, 33 and 12 weeks after infection with *S. mansoni cercaria* by electron microscopy. In the early phases of the disease, paragranulomata and hepatocytes displayed subcellular alterations indicative of hepatocellular injury, but at later intervals hepatic cells revealed no major ultrastructural abnormality. Such data corroborated the evidence that schistosomal ova are the primary factor in the pathogenesis of overt hepatosplenic *S. mansoni* infections. They also revealed that the schistosomal pigment is different from that of malaria in its distribution and ultrastructure.

Erfan *et al* (1957) concluded that the aetiology of hepatic disorders among rural inhabitants is schistosomal in 70 per cent of cases in Egypt; half of these are purely schistosomal, as shown by liver biopsy, and the other half are complicated mostly by nutritional defects or the sequelae of viral hepatitis—the latter is of common occurrence among patients having repeated antimonial therapy.

Dewitt (1958) showed in experimental animals that diets deficient in certain amino acids and vitamins have a profound effect on the course of *S. mansoni* infection. In some cases the worms did not undergo normal development and were sexually immature and unable to deposit eggs. Since eggs are the major cause of tissue damage, the pathological consequences of the infection were greatly reduced. Hashem *et al* (1961) were able experimentally to produce pure hepatic schistosomiasis in animals on a normal diet with an ample supply of protein and vitamins. They also studied the effects of various deficient diets on the evolution of the disease in animals and concluded that dietary deficiency may make the liver more vulnerable to schistosomal infection in its early stages, but in late stages deficiency of diet creates an unfavourable medium for the proper development and reproduction of worms during the infection. In the terminal stages, the fibrosis consequent on fatty metamorphosis due to protein deficiency appears to accentuate that resulting from healing of schistosomal granulomatous lesions.

Warren (1961), after studying the effects of both unisexual and bisexual schistosomal infections on both well-fed animals and animals kept on deficient diet, concluded that ova are the primary factor in the production of liver fibrosis in schistosomiasis.

Clinical features

The disease occurs at all ages between 10 and 70 years, but the incidence gradually rises after the age of 15 to reach a maximum in the fourth decade, after which its incidence gradually diminishes.

Among those affected, males predominate in the proportion of nine to one due to more frequent exposure to infection, reinfection and treatment.

The main presenting symptoms are weakness, gradual loss of weight, epigastric discomfort and abdominal distension after meals with a dull aching pain in the left hypochondrium. The liver is at first enlarged and not markedly tender with a smooth surface and a well-defined edge. The spleen is also enlarged, firm and not tender. Enlargement of these two organs, usually starting early in life and progressing over several years, leads to widening of the subcostal angle, separation of the recti and a barrel-shaped chest. Later the liver shrinks until it may become impalpable, becoming firm with a fine granular edge and surface.

Diarrhoea, swelling of the lower limbs and abdomen with occasional haematemesis or melaena supervene. The spleen may reach a huge size, but with the onset of ascites, usually diminishes. The relative size of the liver and spleen, though helpful in grading the disease clinically, cannot be relied upon when cases are complicated or associated with vascular, nutritional or parenchymal hepatic involvement. Ascites appears towards the end and may be very extensive; the fluid has the characteristic of a transudate with low specific gravity, moderate protein content and a higher cellular count than is usually met with in other transudates.

Clubbing of the fingers is occasionally observed, when associated with intestinal polyposis or chronic ulcers. Endocrine changes in the form of gynaecomastia, alopecia, palmar erythema, arteriolar spiders, etc., may be met with especially in malnourished patients late in the disease. Portosystemic encephalopathy may occur in patients with extensive collaterals or when there is associated parenchymal damage. Gastro-oesophageal varices are demonstrable by endoscopy in many cases and may lead to haematemesis and melaena.

The introduction of needle biopsy, haemodynamic studies of the liver, in addition to the battery of liver function tests, have thrown light on the aetiology, pathology and degree of dysfunction of such cases. The presence of schistosomal ova in the liver and intestine can be easily demonstrated by the transparency technique. Splenic puncture is only carried out when reticulosis or aleukaemic leukaemia is suspected.

Biochemistry

As would be suspected in a disease which affects mainly mesenchymal tissues of the liver and spares the parenchyma until very late, liver function tests usually reveal little impairment of hepatocellular function. The serum albumin is slightly lowered in non-ascitic cases and more so in those with ascites. Some globulins, on the other hand, are raised mainly in the gamma fraction reflecting reticuloendothelial activity so that the albumin/globulin ratio is markedly reduced or inverted.

The hippuric acid test, prothrombin synthesis and carbohydrate metabolism are usually normal. Occasionally hypoprothrombinaemia occurs and is easily corrected by vitamin K administration. The dysproteinaemia of schistosomal hepatic fibrosis is responsible for positive seroflocculation tests. Transaminases and other hepatic enzymes rise in parallel with the course and activity of the disease; antischistosomal therapy results in a further rise. Cholangiolar involvement is rare and occurs late, but the alkaline phosphatase is moderately raised in 30 per cent of non-ascitic cases. The bromsulphthalein test is normal in early, and moderately affected in advanced cases.

Finally liver function tests show further deterioration with the onset of ascites or after a bout of haematemesis. Serum sodium and potassium levels are within normal in non-ascitic cases, but the former tends to rise with the onset of ascites, unless this is controlled by diuretics or tapping when the serum sodium tends to fall and the blood ammonia to rise. 17-ketosteroids are reported to be low, while the FSH level is markedly diminished in cases with endocrine disturbances. They are related to either prolonged malnutrition or to insufficient inactivation of certain hormones, especially antidiuretic hormone, aldosterone and oestrogens, with secondary inhibition of pituitary function.

Haemodynamics

The nature of portal hypertension in hepatosplenic schistosomiasis has been worked out by Mousa *et al* (1959), who were able to demonstrate the discrepancy between the hepatosinusoidal pressure and the portal pressure. They concluded that the obstruction of the portal circulation in the schistosomal liver is at a presinusoidal rather than at a sinusoidal or postsinusoidal level, as is well known Laennec's portal cirrhosis. The intrasplenic pressure was also found to correspond roughly to the pressure in the portal vein as is seen in cases studied during surgical interference.

The more advanced the stage of the disease, the greater the hypertension tends to be, unless complicated by recent haematemesis. In some cases the portal pressure rises temporarily during an intensive course of specific therapy, while ascites is rapidly accumulating after excessive drinking of fluids or after strenuous exercise. The intrasplenic pressure can be modified by the action of vaso-active or diuretic drugs which are utilised for control of potential, impending or recurrent haematemesis.

Probably either functional or structural factors operate to produce portal hypertension, and vaso-active agents endogenous or otherwise may behave differently at different levels of the portal vasculature. Catecholamines, histamines and serotinin in excess are considered to play an important role in such mechanisms

Intravariceal pressure measurement during oesophagoscopy as reported by El-Rooby (1966) approximates to the intrasplenic pressure more closely than when measured through dilated abdominal vessels. Such an approach has been found useful in splenectomised patients for following the progress of the disease. The total plasma volume has been found to be higher than that of normal controls. This is attributed to dilated portal tributaries, enlargement of the spleen and a tendency to water retention.

The portal circulation time is initially prolonged but shortens later with the establishment of collateral circulation. The effective hepatic blood flow, estimated either by the bromsulphthalein clearance test or by isotopic methods, is found to be slightly reduced, the degree of reduction paralleling the size of the liver and its pathological changes as well as the extent of the portosystemic collaterals. In cases with portosystemic collaterals, it is recommended that one should depend upon the hepatic uptake of radiogold rather than blood clearance in estimating the effective hepatic blood flow.

A barium swallow is essential for visualising the gastro-oesophageal and sometimes duodenal varices if oesophagogastroscopy is not available. Portal venography using the percutaneous intrasplenic route shows the degree of portal hypertension, the intrahepatic portal vein pattern, portosystemic collaterals and any prehepatic portal or splenic vein thrombosis. Splenic and superior mesenteric artery angiography may be utilised before and after portal surgery, especially if associated with splenectomy (Plate 5).

Haematology

A mild normocytic hypochromic anaemia without macrocytosis is common. Malnutrition, bleeding from piles, oesophagogastric varices and associated intestinal or urinary bleeding or ancyl-

ostomiasis are usually the cause of any severe degree of anaemia present. Leucopenia and mild thrombocytopenia encountered in moderate and advanced stages of the disease are speculatively attributed to a humoral splenic factor either unchecked because of a failing liver or by passing through portosystemic shunts affecting the bone marrow directly.

Eosinophilia is common in the early stages of the disease or when associated with active pulmonary schistosomiasis. The bone marrow is mostly hyperplastic, and eosinophilia is a constant finding even in absence of eosinophilia in the blood. The blood coagulative mechanism is normal or only slightly affected in late cases. Splenectomy does not improve the anaemia in every case, although Woodruff et al (1963), by a study of the red cell half-life and organ uptake of the spleen by ^{51}Cr, in patients with anaemia and gross splenomegaly showed some shortening of the erythrocytic lifespan related to hypersplenism. Saoad (1965) noticed early hypoplasia of bone marrow in experimental *S. mansoni* infections with no relation to the size of the spleen.

Diagnosis

The demonstration of schistosomal ova or specific lesions in the liver is the only sure method of diagnosis. This may be facilitated by taking a needle biopsy or wedge biopsy during abdominal surgery. A specimen may be removed through a laparoscope. In addition to the histopathological transparency technique, histochemical fluorescent antibody methods and tissue digestion can be also utilised. By repeated biopsies, one can follow the evolution of the disease and correlate the clinical with the pathological progress, with special reference to different means of management. Electron microscopy may also be used.

According to haemodynamic and functional studies the following classification may be adopted:

A. *Compensated*
B. *Decompensated*
   1. Haematemesis (vascular)
   2. Hepatic failure (parenchymal)
   3. Ascites (parenchymo-vascular)
C. *Complicated or mixed*
   1. Vascular: portal or splenic vein thrombosis and cardiac cirrhosis
   2. Parenchymo-vascular:
     —portal and toxic cirrhosis
     —post-viral
     —nutritional

O

Prognosis

The course is slowly progressive unless the disease is arrested by early management. The prognosis is better in cases with mild infection or when the patient is transferred to a non-endemic area and is not further exposed to infection. If cases are neglected, exposed to repeated infection and therapy the prognosis is bad, and the disease will follow a progressive course with well-established hepatic failure and portal hypertension with its serious sequelae.

Management

This varies with the clinical picture and whether the disease is active or arrested. The slow method of antimonial therapy (Atta and Mousa, 1959) and the hypotensive effect of chlorothiazides and their analogues have helped modern surgical techniques in hypertensive cases.

At the early normotensive or mildly hypertensive stages, antischistosomal therapy is indicated with widely spaced administration of the antischistosomal drug—at most twice weekly in hospitalised cases and weekly for ambulant cases. Antiallergic measures or small doses of steroids are given to those patients showing toxic or allergic reactions.

In haematemesis, a high protein, low salt diet is indicated especially in malnourished cases. In the early stages prophylactic splenectomy with or without vasoligation or splenic artery ligature have been found useful in Egypt in patients liable to be repeatedly exposed to infection. The removal of the spleen or splenic artery ligature will obviate the excessive portal blood inflow reflected by the portal pressure through the dilated intrasplenic sinusoids. Vasoligation of the coronary veins will divert blood from the dangerous zone at the oesophagogastric junction to other portosystemic collaterals. Such operations at this stage have a minimal operative risk and requirement for technical skill and do not prevent further surgical operations when needed. Follow-up of such cases has demonstrated an improvement in hepatic and general condition with absence of haematemesis for longer periods than in control cases. Possibly surgery by itself is the best stimulus to the patient, and even to other members of the family, for proper education against the serious risks of exposure to polluted water.

In hypertensive cases with no or mild haematemesis, splenectomy with vasoligation and gastric transection is needed and specific therapy must be given cautiously in small doses, at widely spaced intervals and associated with deportalising measures such as use of oral diuretics. Dietetic measures with selected restriction must be advised.

In cases with repeated haematemesis or mild ascites, granted that there is no gross parenchymal involvement, shunt operations in the form of end-to-side anastomosis and lienorenal shunt may be employed. The moderate diminution of extrahepatic blood flow in those cases with marked collaterals present, indicates that the liver adapts to some deprivation of portal blood and no fatal deterioration will occur after shunt operations. Specific therapy is contraindicated in such advanced cases whether before or after operation, as it increases the risk of pulmonary and cardiac complications.

In decompensated or some complicated cases, conservative measures have to be adopted and specific therapy is avoided. Hepatic artery ligature has been tried in some cases with the object of inducing hepatic revascularisation from the diaphragmatic vessels, but the results are not always predictable. Peritoneosaphenal and peritoneopleural drainage were tried with temporary effect in some cases necessitating repeated paracenteses. Hepatic restorative measures, including administration of antibiotics in addition to widely spaced oral diuretics, are the main measures to be applied in such desperate cases.

CARDIOPULMONARY SCHISTOSOMIASIS

This results from involvement of the lungs by schistosomal ova and worms. These reach the lungs via the pulmonary arterioles and result in fibrosis and obstruction of the pulmonary circulation with eventual hypertrophy and strain of the right side of the heart. This may end in pure right ventricular failure and may or may not be associated with other pulmonary manifestations.

Pathology

Shaw and Ghareeb (1938) demonstrated in their study of pulmonary lesions due to schistosoma ova that 33 per cent were due to *S. haematobium*, 3.6 per cent to *S. mansoni* and 11.1 per cent were mixed. However, *S. mansoni* produced vascular lesions and hence usually more advanced stages of the disease than *S. haematobium*. Worms of both species were present in the lungs in 3.6 per cent of all cases and in 10.5 per cent of cases with pulmonary involvement, while schistosomal cor pulmonale was diagnosed in 2.1 per cent of all cases and in 6.3 per cent of cases with pulmonary involvement.

Schistosomal cor pulmonale has been reported

frequently from Egypt and Brazil, while broncho-pulmonary and early grades of cardiovascular schistosomiasis have been found predominantly in other endemic areas in Africa and the Far East. This may be related to the high incidence in Egypt and Brazil of both *S. haematobium* and *S. mansoni* infections as well as to the high incidence of advanced stages of hepatic schistosomiasis with opened portosystemic collaterals.

The lungs may be affected by cercariae in their migration during the invasive stage of the disease and this may cause patchy congestion associated with transient bronchitis—larval pneumonitis. This phase takes 4 to 6 weeks and is usually mild in indigenous inhabitants, possibly due to developed immunity, but it may be severe especially in expatriates. Embolised worms may be found in the lung vessels but produce no lesions unless they die. After specific therapy they may produce an acute focal necrotising verminous type of pneumonia. The foci of this so-called verminous pneumonia appear as small area of consolidation heavily infiltrated with eosinophils and macrophages. Foreign-body giant cells may attach dead worms; later, however, the exudate is absorbed and cicatrisation occurs while the dead worms become encircled by fibrous tissue and may undergo calcification.

Large granulomata in lungs simulating tumours supposed to be due to healed embolised worms and ova have been reported by Mallah and Hashem (1953). The more important pulmonary lesions are, however, caused by the ova which reach the lungs as emboli from the normal habitat of the worms and become impacted in the pulmonary arterioles causing necrotising arteriolitis which leads to destruction of the media. Hence the ova will be able to pass to the extravascular space forming the characteristic tubercles which are formed by ova surrounded by eosinophils, round cells and giant cells. When the ovum dies it calcifies and the tubercle becomes invaded by fibroblasts and new capillaries leading to a nodular scar. Healing of the arterioles will lead to thickening of the intima, narrowness of the lumen and destruction of the media. Later, in advanced cases, canalisation occurs, new vessels dilate producing angiomatoids in which the muscle coat is absent. Widespread pulmonary arteritis will lead to cor pulmonale and right ventricular hypertrophy.

Marchand (1957) stressed in his pathological studies three groups of pulmonary vascular changes. The first included the organic changes produced by schistosomal tubercles. The second was toxic-allergic in nature leading to arteritis with intimal fibrinoid degeneration similar to that of collagen diseases with destruction of the media and production of hyaline thrombi in the pulmonary vessels. The third change resulting from pulmonary hypertension included medial hypertrophy of the pulmonary vessels, diffuse intimal arteriolar proliferation and premature atheroma of the large pulmonary artery. Occasional schistosomal tubercles may be found inside the alveoli surrounded by areas of emphysema and may also be seen inside the bronchioles, causing partial or complete obstruction of their lumen. However, affection of the bronchioles is only occasional and can hardly produce bronchiectasis or generalised emphysema.

The myocardium is occasionally involved with schistosomal ova which become surrounded by miliary foci of fibrosis as reported by Clark and Graef (1935), but this is a very rare type of affection. Gazayerli (1969) demonstrated schistosomal worms in the coronary vessels at autopsy; however, advanced cases of cor pulmonale are characterised by right-sided heart failure with no left ventricular affection. Failure of the myocardium in these cases may be precipitated by sudden strenuous exercise, gross pulmonary embolism, bronchopneumonia or mal-administered specific therapy.

Pathogenesis

For many years the dying ova embolising from their original site of deposition were considered to be the main aetiological factor in producing the pulmonary arteriolar lesions. These were thought to be due specifically to liberated miracidial toxins since ova killed by heating are not able to produce such lesions. However, Caelho (1954) found in naturally infected rats endarteritis in the lungs directly related to dead worms present in the arterial branches. Filho (1959) in mice experimentally infected with *S. mansoni* found a different intimal reaction in the pulmonary arteries which seemed to be produced by toxic products. He concluded that pre-immunised mice were able to retain the schistosomulae in their pulmonary capillaries and arterioles. The death of many of these parasites induced a diffuse inflammatory reaction.

Abdin in 1962 concluded that the pathological process in the pulmonary arteries, instead of being due to impaction of ova, might be due to toxins produced by embolised worms which die in such arteries since the maximal lesion has been observed in those arteries with a wide lumen compared with the size of the ova ($60 \times 150 \ \mu$m). It was suggested that these worm toxins probably act on the walls of the pulmonary arteries, producing antigen which combines with specific antibodies to produce its maximal effect on such vessels. Menzes (1965) was able to produce pulmonary obliterative endarteritis by injecting dead worms in the pulmonary arteries of dogs.

Bronchopulmonary manifestations of schistosomal infection have been related pathogenically to the toxic effect of the dying parasites, to the development of allergic reactions to infection, to the effect of repeated specific therapy and possibly to the effect of secondary infection.

Clinical features

The syndrome of cardiopulmonary schistosomiasis is classified into three clinical types: cardiovascular, bronchopulmonary, and mixed.

Cardiovascular. Cases belonging to this group can be classified according to their progress into three grades, mostly based on radiological findings:

GRADE 1. In this grade there are segmental arterial lesions. These cases are usually met with accidentally during routine X-ray of the chest since they exhibit neither symptoms nor signs referrable to the heart or lungs. The vascular changes are limited to the peripheral pulmonary vessels. The resting pulmonary artery pressure remains normal but may rise on exercise. The ECG is also normal. The plain X-ray of the chest shows focal perivascular nodulation due to tubercles. Ova appear in the sputum in about 20 per cent of cases. Eosinophilia is usual and occasionally eosinophils may be found in the sputum.

GRADE 2. Here there are hilar pulmonary arterial lesions. These cases start to show evidence of mild pulmonary hypertension with signs of low fixed cardiac output. The patient may complain of moderate grades of giddiness, weakness and even syncope on slight exercise.

Clinical evidence of pulmonary hypertension and of pulmonary artery dilatation will be present. Plain X-ray of the chest will show dilatation and sclerosis of the hilar vessels with moderate dilatation and hypertrophy of the right ventricle limited to its overflow tract. Angiocardiography will show a pattern characteristic of schistosomal arterial change. The pulmonary artery is dilated and the segmental vessels are tortuous and irregular with abruptly commencing obliteration of the second and third grade arterioles. A diagnostic feature of this disease is the discrepancy between the angiocardiographic pattern done selectively for the pulmonary arterioles—especially of the right base —and their shadows in the plain film.

GRADE 3. *Cor pulmonale.* This condition is characterised by marked limitation of exercise tolerance, palpitation, fatigue and cardiac pain. Cough and occasionally haemoptyses may be met with while giddiness, transient dimness of vision and syncopal attacks on effort are late features. Fully developed cases present with right ventricular hypertrophy and dilatation of the pulmonary artery; hepatosplenomegaly is usually present.

The pulse is usually small and regular; arrhythmia, mainly auricular fibrillation, is occasionally seen. The venous pressure may show giant waves due to pulmonary hypertension or exaggerated y descent in cases complicated by tricuspid regurgitation. Precordial pulsations are noticed with left parasternal lift due to right ventricular hypertrophy, which may also cause epigastric pulsation. The apex may not be clearly defined, being pushed backwards by the hypertrophied right ventricle. Pulsations in the pulmonary area are usually seen and felt and a diastolic thrill may be present in advanced cases with pulmonary regurgitation.

On auscultation, an ejection systolic murmur is heard maximally in the pulmonary area. The second sound is split and behaves normally with respiration; its pulmonary element is markedly accentuated. In advanced cases, an early diastolic murmur will be detected in the left second and third spaces due to pulmonary regurgitation and shows a hilar dance on screening. A long pansystolic murmur maximally heard on inspiration at the tricuspid area may be present in cases complicated with tricuspid regurgitation. The latter may induce increased flow to the right ventricle and thus cause a mid-diastolic flow murmur similar to that produced by mitral stenosis. In advanced cases a gallop may be present; this may be presystolic due to a right atrial sound which indicates an increased resistance to right ventricular filling secondary to pulmonary hypertension. The sound may be protodiastolic and in reality be an audible third heart sound produced by the rapid ventricular filling phase which occurs especially in patients with tricuspid regurgitation.

Plain chest X-ray (Plate 6) will show the pulmonary conus and trunk to be markedly dilated; they may reach aneurysmal sizes, producing a picture simulating mitral stenosis. Perivascular nodulations are no longer present and both lungs look oligaemic. Tortuosity and a beaded appearance of the medium-sized arteries are usually seen in the middle and basal lung zones. In many cases aneurysal dilatation of the right hilar vessels may be seen in contrast to the markedly narrowed segmental vessels giving a radish root appearance. Angiographic study of such cases may show filling defects suggesting mural thrombosis. The right oblique view will show evidence of right ventricular hypertrophy.

ECG tracings will show evidence of right ventricular hypertrophy and cor pulmonale. Occasionally incomplete right bundle branch block may be encountered due to right ventricular hypertrophy. The pulmonary artery pressure will be raised and may reach systemic levels, particularly in cases with right ventricular failure. The pulmonary vascular resistance will be increased as well, while the wedge capillary pressure will remain normal. The cardiac output will be either normal or slightly diminished, indicating that it is an obstructing type of cor pulmonale. The circulation times may be prolonged, particularly in grades 2 and 3 and when complicated with right ventricular failure. Cyanosis is absent in most cases belonging to this group and arterial oxygen saturation is usually maintained within normal limits or very slightly diminished. In some cases, however, cyanosis may be manifest in the absence of heart failure with relative arterial hypoxia which does not improve on breathing 100 per cent oxygen, indicating the presence of bronchopulmonary shunts. Evidence of such shunts was obtained by Zaki *et al* (1962), who injected Evans blue into the aorta and were able to recover it by a catheter placed in the pulmonary artery, within 1.5 seconds.

Pulmonary function tests will show evidence of mild obstructive and/or restrictive ventilatory insufficiencies with hyperventilation.

Differential diagnosis of cardiovascular schistosomiasis

Schistosomal cor pulmonale has to be differentiated from other causes of pulmonary hypertension. Since the pulmonary artery pressure is the product of pulmonary blood flow multiplied by pulmonary resistance, cases of pulmonary hypertension will be related to (*a*) increased pulmonary blood flow or (*b*) increased pulmonary resistance.

Increased pulmonary blood flow. The normal pulmonary blood flow is 5 litres per minute but may be increased up to 20 litres in cases with left to right shunt. Such congenital heart conditions include:

Atrial septal defect. This can be differentiated by the wide fixed splitting of the second sound over the pulmonary area, by the pulmonary plethora and hilar dance, and by complete bundle branch block as shown in the ECG.

Ventricular septal defect may be differentiated by a pansystolic murmur, a systolic thrill over the third and fourth spaces, and by the biventricular hypertrophy.

Patent ductus arteriosus is distinguished by high pulse pressure and machinery murmur, hilar dance, and evidence of left ventricular hypertrophy in the ECG.

Eisenmenger's complex is associated with cyanosis.

Oxymetric determination of blood samples taken from the various chambers of the heart and great vessels will confirm the above cases.

Increased pulmonary resistance. The normal pulmonary resistance is 50 dynes/s/cm^2. An increase to 100 or more will result in pulmonary hypertension. According to the site of obstruction in the lung and its relationship to pulmonary capillaries, these cases may be divided into (*a*) post-capillary, (*b*) capillary and (*c*) pre-capillary pulmonary hypertension.

(a) *Post-capillary pulmonary hypertension* occurs in the following disorders:

Mitral stenosis
Mitral regurgitation
Double mitral disease
Left ventricular failure

The wedge capillary pressure in these cases will be increased (normal 5–8 mmHg), and the left auricle will be enlarged and shown to be compressing the filled oesophagus with barium in the right oblique position.

(b) *Capillary pulmonary hypertension.* This group is encountered in cases with lung disease, the most important of which are emphysema and pulmonary fibrosis. Besides the clinical picture, pulmonary function tests will show ventilatory or diffusion defects, both of which are not features of pure schistosomal cor pulmonale. Arterial saturation of oxygen will also be diminished in these but not in schistosomal cases.

(c) *Pre-capillary pulmonary hypertension.* Here the obstruction is before the pulmonary capillaries. It is seen in:

1. Recurrent pulmonary embolism.
2. Schistosomal endarteritis obliterans causing pulmonary hypertension.
3. Primary (essential) pulmonary hypertension. In this group the pulmonary artery pressure is raised but there is normal wedge capillary pressure and normal cardiac output. The differentiation of such cases in endemic areas may be helped by the associated gross bilharzial visceral manifestations.

Management of cardiovascular schistosomiasis

Specific antischistosomal therapy may be given cautiously in grade 1 but not in grades 2 and 3. Antimonials are known to produce more pulmonary hypertension and derange the already strained right ventricle, precipitating failure. Oral drugs like lucanthone may be tried in such cases. Associated anaemia should be corrected as well as other parasitic infections. In the case of right-sided heart failure digitalisation and diuretics should be used cautiously.

Bronchopulmonary schistosomiasis

Bronchopulmonary manifestations occurring in cases suffering from schistosomiasis may or may not be related to their schistosomal infection. In most cases the schistosomal nature of the lesion is very difficult to establish except after pathological examination of the affected lung.

We may classify the pulmonary manifestation of schistosomiasis into the following forms.

1. **Larval pneumonitis.** This condition was first described by Lawton (1918) and later by Fairley (1919–22). It is characterised by irregular low-grade fever of gradual onset, mild cough and minimal expectoration. The symptoms may persist for 2 to 4 weeks but the general condition is fair, especially in natives. Careful questioning will elicit a history of exposure to infection; cercarial dermatitis or urticarial rash may be reported.

A few crepitations, mostly basal, are present and scattered wheezes may be heard later. The liver is always enlarged, soft and tender; the spleen may be palpable and generalised adenopathy has sometimes been noted. The blood picture will show definite leucocytosis with marked eosinophilia. The cutaneous antigen test is strongly positive. Radiologically there is mottling, mostly at the bases. Specific treatment is not indicated in this condition since it subsides spontaneously. Specific treatment will be indicated when there is evidence of active infection.

2. **Verminous pneumonia.** This condition is mostly due to embolised worms dislodged into the lungs either accidentally or during administration of antischistosomal therapy. The condition is often complicated by secondary infection. The clinical picture is either that of acute broncho-pneumonia or pneumonitic affection of varying severity. It is characterised by the sudden onset of dyspnoea, cough and basal pleuritic pain or right hypochondrial ache. There is moderate remittent fever which lasts for about 2 to 3 weeks. On examination, patches of consolidation are easily detected. Radiologically there are areas of dense patchy infiltration in either or both basal lobes, sometimes associated with pleural effusion. The condition usually subsides slowly, except

in very severe fatal cases. However, some will be left with varying degrees of fibrosis in either the lung or the pleura, or both. Treatment is symptomatic; antischistosomal therapy should be stopped until all signs and symptoms abate.

3. **Reactionary pneumonitis** (Loeffler-like syndrome). This condition is due to flaring up of schistosomal lesions in the lungs or to further embolisation resulting from specific therapy. It was mostly seen when intensive courses were used. Clinically, the condition is characterised by the development of fever and cough with little expectoration during the course of antischistosomal therapy. If the reaction is severe, dyspnoea, mild cyanosis and rarely jaundice may develop.

On examination, a few patches of consolidation in both lungs will be demonstrated as patchy bronchovesicular breathing, crepitations and rales. Radiologically, the chest will show veiling of the lung fields with patchy infiltration and exaggerated bronchovesicular markings; mild pleural effusion may also be found. The high blood eosinophilia and the markedly positive cutaneous test may help in its differentiation from other pneumonitic affection. The condition usually subsides in a few days; however, it is preferable to stop specific therapy until all signs and symptoms subside.

4. **Miliary, nodular and granulomatous infiltrative lesions.** These lesions are usually silent and only detected accidentally by radiography or at autopsy. However, large granulomata may simulate bronchogenic carcinoma. Their parasitic nature will not be established except after microscopical examination of the removed lobe or mass.

5. **Asthmatic bronchitis.** Asthmatic conditions in schistosomal cases may or may not be causally related to the parasitic infection. However, sensitisation of the lung to schistosomal antigen does occur during the invasive stage of the disease, when larval stages of the parasite circulate in the lung before they reach the adult stage in the portal vascular bed. Later, allergic manifestations can be detected in some schistosomal subjects due to liberated toxins formed by the dying parasites whether this death occurs in the lung or in the normal habitat of the adult worms in other abdominal viscera.

The parasitic nature of the process can be deduced from various findings; amongst these are the presence of ova in sputum, the relationship to antischistosomal therapy and the focal nature of the condition. High degrees of eosinophilia and a strongly positive cutaneous response may also be helpful.

6. **Emphysema.** There is a high incidence of

emphysema occurring early in adolescent schistosomal cases in the absence of other organic lung disorders. It is usually mild as the disease is primarily vascular rather than parenchymal. The early enlargement of the liver and spleen in childhood in *S. mansoni* infection expands the subcostal and upper abdominal regions and aggravates the signs of the emphysematous chest already present. The condition is also aggravated in cases with bronchial asthma and bronchiolectasis. In some cases localised emphysema is noticed due to obliterative bronchiolitis or to pressure exerted by dilated hilar vessels compressing the adjoining bronchi.

Management of bronchopulmonary schistosomiasis

Besides symptomatic and general supportive measures, specific therapy if given in modified form, either widely spaced or in fractionated doses, usually ameliorates the symptomatology of these forms of schistosomal affection. Some advise steroid administration in association with specific therapy in order to suppress possible toxic-allergic reactions.

ECTOPIC SCHISTOSOMIASIS

Ectopic lesions in schistosomiasis were defined by Faust (1948) as those specific local reactions to the worms or their eggs occurring outside the portacaval venous circulations, including extension of the latter into the pulmonary arterioles.

Various theories have been put forward to explain how schistosomal ova or worms can reach these ectopic sites. Diamantis (1928) suggested that cercariae enter the skin and mucous membrane and develop directly into adults in nearby veins, but this was denied when intrahepatic portal vein development was found to be essential. Other workers postulated a patent foramen ovale to explain how eggs reach such ectopic sites. A third possibility is that eggs which are deposited by the parent worms in the usual sites filter through the capillary barrier in the liver and lungs or get into the general circulation to be filtered out in the terminal blood vessels.

One theory suggests that adult worms migrate from their habitat and travel against the venous blood stream. Another depends on the vertebral venous system and postulates that its connections with the veins of the body cavities at each intervertebral space and with the veins of the girdles, the azygos system of veins, the veins of the brain, skull and thoraco-abdominal wall and the rich anastomoses within the pelvic viscera are the

vehicles of the ova. Development of collaterals in hepatic fibrosis would assist distribution of ova by this complex.

Most ectopic lesions are due to affection of the brain and spinal cord, the eyes and the skin.

Brain and spinal cord

The lesions of the brain and spinal cord are caused by ova, not by worms. The ova are found either sporadically, being deposited as emboli, or in a circumscribed area causing relatively large granulomata. The specific pathological picture produced by such deposition is similar to that elsewhere in the body.

The clinical picture varies according to the type of lesion, whether it is cerebral or spinal and whether the granuloma is localised or diffuse. All three species can produce such lesions, but *S. japonicum* is responsible for about 60 per cent of the reported cases. This may be due to the fact that *S. japonicum* produce more and smaller eggs than other schistosomes.

Convulsions and epileptiform seizures form the commonest presenting symptoms in cerebral schistosomiasis. Next to these are headache, vomiting, optic field defects, difficulty of speech, mental changes and occasionally loss of consciousness. There may be also tremors, clumsiness of movements, muscle weakness and reflex changes. In some cases, however, no abnormality is detected. Occasionally the optic discs are injected and there may be papilloedema. X-ray of the skull is usually normal. Sometimes ventriculography helps in the diagnosis by showing a space-occupying lesion causing a shift of the ventricular system. Electroencephalography may show dysrythmia suggesting a focal abnormality. The cerebrospinal fluid is usually normal, the tension however may be slightly raised and its proteins and cells (mainly lymphocytes) may be increased. Alves (1958) is believed to be the only person to have recorded schistosomal ova in the cerebrospinal fluid.

The most common presenting picture of spinal schistosomiasis is that of transverse myelitis. Pain in the back, root pains, sphincteric disturbances and paraplegia with a level or a Brown-Sequard syndrome will be the end-result of such involvement. The cerebrospinal fluid may be under moderately increased pressure, its cells and proteins may be slightly increased while myelography may show evidence of obstruction of the spinal canal.

Clinical diagnosis of such cases can only be presumptive; definite diagnosis cannot be made except after histological examination of biopsy or autopsy material. The schistosomal nature of the lesion can be suggested from the history of exposure, eosinophilia of the blood, evidence of a space-occupying lesion and the therapeutic response to specific schistosomicidals.

In such cases, specific therapy should be tried. Patients with a localised granuloma in the brain or spinal cord should be treated surgically.

Eye

This is a rare site of ectopic schistosomiasis, only reported in Egypt and usually affecting male children. The actual lesion in the ocular tissues, which is usually unilateral, is a granuloma. It appears as a polypoid or diffuse swelling, or as multiple pinpoint or larger discrete nodules. *S. haematobium* ova only have so far been responsible for such lesions; in some cases the adult worms have been discovered in nearby veins. Lesions are found in the palpebral or bulbar conjunctiva or in the caruncle. No lesion has been reported on the globe, lacrimal passages, lacrimal gland or orbit. Other ocular manifestations such as retrobulbar haemorrhage (Noronha, 1947), urticaria and oedema of the lids during the systemic invasion of the parasite have not been recorded in Egypt.

Treatment of ocular schistosomiasis is surgical removal of the lesion followed by antischistosomal therapy to prevent recurrence. The nature of the tumour will be determined by the discovery of schistosomal ova amid the tissue reaction.

Skin

Schistosomal affection of the skin can be classified (after El Mofty and El Zawahry, 1962) into the following categories:

1. *Cercarial dermatitis* (swimmer's itch). These lesions are due to penetration of the cercariae into the skin. Any part of the body may be affected, but the legs and arms are the commonest sites. Different rashes in the form of erythemata, urticarial lesions and itchy papules occur and after a week papules, if present, disappear leaving pigmented spots. All human as well as non-human species of schistosomes can produce these lesions, however the human species will produce milder dermatitis especially in those who have developed some immunity.

2. *Late non-specific allergic* manifestations in the parasitaemic stage are caused by the products of schistosomes. The lesions are mainly anaphylactoid reactions with erythemata and pruritus accompanying a feverish state and occurring 2 to 6 weeks after the original infection. Joint pains, headache, enlargement of the liver and spleen and eosinophilia are common manifestations of this stage.

3. *Perigenital infiltrative granulomata* may appear late in the disease and are produced by schistosomal ova, provoking an inflammatory and fibrotic reaction.

4. *Extragenital infiltrative* lesions are very occasionally caused by the deposition of schistosomal ova in the dermis in foci on the trunk. They are of multiform appearance, fresh lesions exhibit groups of small firm rounded or oval papules with the same colour as the skin or little darker. Older lesions aggregate and form papules and nodules of rough granulomatous appearance. These masses are asymptomatic, neither itchy, tender nor painful.

The diagnosis of the last two infiltrative lesions can easily be made by scraping and spreading the material on a slide when schistosomal ova will often be revealed.

DIAGNOSIS OF SCHISTOSOMIASIS

The first step in investigating a patient with schistosomiasis is to diagnose the presence of active infection. In some cases the infection may have died out but have left residual pathological lesions which need retrograde diagnosis to prove their nature. Further investigations should be done to assess the degree of structural damage caused by the infection and its effect on function of the organ concerned. The investigations to be performed will vary with the presentation, the system affected and the clinical condition of each patient.

The diagnosis of the active schistosomal infection may be direct or indirect. By direct methods it is implied that the parasite or one of its stages is demonstrated in the excreta or in tissue obtained by biopsy. The search for ova is the most common method used for diagnosis. Adult worms can only occasionally be demonstrated by filtering the portal blood during surgery or by finding the adult worm in a rectal polyp.

The ova count in epidemiological work has become an essential for assessment of the morbidity of the disease and the response to control measures.

Indirect methods are serological techniques which may either involve recognition of antibody circulating in the serum or fixed on tissue cells. The latter methods are sensitive, easy to perform and rapid, so are therefore commonly used for epidemiological studies. However, some may be non-specific and some may remain positive long after parasitological cure. Attempts are being made to quantify these tests, which would then be of enhanced value for the follow up of patients after treatment.

The assessment of cure is sometimes difficult, as absence of ova does not necessarily indicate complete elimination of the adult worms. A relapse with the passage of ova may wrongly be considered a reinfection.

Urine examination

Sedimentation. The urine of the patient is put in a conical glass and left to sediment for at least 15 minutes. A drop of the sediment is taken in a pipette, spread on a glass slide and examined microscopically under low power. By this method most positive cases can be detected, but if ova are scanty, the examination of a 24-hour urine collection will increase the percentage found positive provided that the last drops of urine expressed during micturition have not been missed. Exercise or excessive diuresis are said also to increase the percentage found to be positive.

The viability of the ova should be confirmed as only living ova imply active infection. Living ova are clear and transparent. Under higher magnification the miracidium contained inside the shell can be seen with its flame cells moving. Ova that are surrounded by erythrocytes or leucocytes, so called beaded ova, are usually living. By contrast, dead ova are dark, do not exhibit clear structure and no moving flame cells can be demonstrated within them. In doubtful cases it is not easy to differentiate between the living and dead ova, and resort should be had to hatching techniques.

Sedimentation and hatching. A few drops of sediment obtained by the above technique are put on a watch glass, distilled water at room temperature is added and the sample left for 15–20 minutes. It is then examined by a hand lens for the presence of swimming miracidia.

Centrifugation. The urine is left to stand in a conical glass for 15 minutes. The supernatant fluid is decanted and the sediment transferred into a centrifuge tube with saline. After slow centrifugation for a few minutes, the supernatant fluid is decanted and the last drops left in the tube are put on a glass slide, to be examined microscopically. The addition of a few drops of ether or chloroform will clarify the sediment and make examination easier.

In cases in which the urine is very dilute as in diabetes insipidus, the ova may hatch in urine. The specimen should be cooled and centrifuged immediately after voiding.

The examination of urine is sometimes difficult due to associated pathology which masks the ova. In severe haematuria with blood clots, addition of cold distilled water to the sediment will lead to haemolysis of the erythrocytes. Saline should be added to the distilled water after 5 minutes so as to allow the ova to hatch; the specimen should then be recentrifuged. The urine may also be first passed through a sieve before sedimenting.

In research work, the urine after being passed through a wide-mesh sieve is passed through another of only 40 mesh and schistosomal ova all collect above the sieve, can be suspended in normal saline and the contents of 24-hour urine specimen can be counted. Repeated washing with normal saline and centrifuging will destroy pus cells and unmask ova in cases with severe pyuria. Acidifying the urine with acetic acid will clear the urine of phosphate crystals. Addition of fat solvents such as ether, chloroform or xylol to chylous urine will dissolve the fat and facilitate the demonstration of schistosomal ova.

If in spite of all these methods, urine examination reveals no ova and there is still a suspicion that the patient is infected, resort should be had to one of the following methods:

1. *Rectal massage of the base of the bladder.* This is especially valuable if done against a metal catheter in the bladder.
2. *Irritation of the bladder by dilatation.* A 40–50 Higgar dilator may be used and the urine examined afterwards.

Stool examination

Simple smear. A small quantity of faeces is emulsified in a drop of water or saline on a glass slide and examined under low power. The proper choice of the part to be examined, and examination of more than one smear increases the percentage of positives.

Emulsifying, straining and sedimentation. Faeces is emulsified with concentrated salt solution, usually 1–2 per cent. It is then strained through a sieve, left to sediment, and the sediment examined for ova. If the fluid is not clear the process is repeated. Addition of ether, formalin or dilute hydrochloric acid clears the ova.

Hatching. Sediment, obtained by the above technique, is diluted with distilled water, left in bright light and examined with a hand lens for swimming miracidia.

Formalin-ether technique. About 2 g stool is mixed with saline and strained through gauze into a centrifuge tube. A few millilitres of saline are added to make up to 10 ml. The tube is centrifuged at 2000 rpm for 1 minute. The supernatant fluid is then decanted and the precipitate washed; 9 ml of 10 per cent formalin are added and then 3 ml of ether. The tube is plugged and agitated for 1 minute. The plug is removed and the tube recentrifuged. The layer between the ether and formalin is rimmed off, the whole contents are decanted except the precipitate which is examined under the microscope.

Measurement of daily egg output (Bell's technique). A 24-hour stool collection is weighed, mixed with 10 per cent formalin solution and made up to a litre with tap water. It is then mixed for 15 minutes using an electric stirrer and 50 ml is decanted into a screw-capped container in which, if necessary, it may be stored until counted.

For counting the ova 1 ml is removed from the container, using for the purpose a wide-bore pipette and siliconed syringe. It is passed through a sieve to remove large particles and drawn through a filter paper by suction, usually from a water pump. Rinsing both sieve and filter ensures that all eggs reach the paper.

The eggs may be stained with ninhydrin (triketohydrindene hydrate) which forms Ruhemann's purple with certain amino acids contained in the miracidia, which thus take on a purple colour if the filter paper is incubated with an aqueous solution of ninhydrin at 37°C for 12 hours. The filter paper is dried and equal parts of it are mounted on a 3 × 2 inch glass slide moistened with saline, after which the eggs are counted using an eyepiece containing a rectangular graticule to ensure that the whole area of the paper is scanned. Three such papers are scanned and the mean number of eggs per paper approximates to the daily output of eggs in thousands. The papers may be preserved for future reference (Bell, 1963).

Rectal swab. The soap-lubricated gloved finger is introduced into the rectum. The rectum is massaged, the material obtained is spread on a glass slide, emulsified in saline and examined for ova.

Rectal biopsy

A proctoscope is introduced and with a Harrison's cutting curette 1–3 small snippets of mucose are removed and examined unstained microscopically under low power.

Serological methods

The diagnostic procedures based upon the detection of parasite in the excreta have many limitations. Immunological means have been adopted in recent years. Much diversity of opinion has developed regarding the relative value of demonstrating the ova and applying immunological tests with follow-up of schistosomal cases. The serological tests are rapid, easy and economical. Patients with constipation or who cannot submit stools for some other reason may be tested serologically. However, the high percentage of false positives and false negatives reported in some series limit the wide application of these tests at present. Advances in methods of preparation and purification of antigens will increase the value of these serological methods of diagnosis.

Intradermal test (I.D.T.). Patients with schistosomiasis become positive only 4–8 weeks after infection. The test is a sensitivity test of the immediate reaction type, being read 15–20 minutes after the injection. Many types of antigen are used by various workers, but the one most commonly used now is the whole adult worm antigen. Other antigens prepared from ova, miracidia, infected snails or even metabolic exogenous antigen are also used. Reactions in infected patients are obtained with all species of adult schistosomal worms. *Fasciola gigantica* antigen gives more or less similar results.

The antigen is injected intradermally into the forearm, usually in amounts of 0.05 ml. A similar dose of merthiolate solution is injected into the other forearm as a control. The test is read after 15–20 minutes and the size of the two wheals noted. The size of the wheal may be measured by a special stencil plate issued by the World Health Organization. Chinese and many other workers do not inject any control and are satisfied by comparing the size of the wheal immediately following the injection and again 15–20 minutes later.

A positive result means that the patient is or has been infected with schistosomiasis. The test usually remains positive for many years after successful treatment and this can be one of its disadvantages.

Circumoval precipitin test (C.O.P.). This test has the advantage of turning negative shortly after successful therapy and thus can be used for the follow-up of patients. It can, moreover, be used in a semi-quantitative manner. It depends on the presence of antibodies against ova. Viable bilharzia eggs from the patient's own urine or from any other patient are incubated at 37°C with the patient's serum for 24 hours and viewed under the low power of the microscope. If antibodies to the ova are present in the patient's serum, globules or digital projections are formed around the ova. The test is thought to be specific for the oviposition stage and for each species. The antibodies involved in this test are present in the α-globulins.

Complement fixation test (C.F.T.). Various antigens have been used, including aqueous and alcoholic extracts of cercarial and infected snail liver, adult worms or other trematoda.

An advantage of the test is that it is easy to read and it is more strongly positive in acute cases.

Cercaria-Hullen reaction. This test becomes positive early after infection, even if unisexual, and turns negative 4–21 days after successful therapy. The cercariae when incubated with a patient's serum become surrounded by a membrane. The antibodies responsible for the test are present in the γ globulin fraction of the serum.

Cercaria agglutination test. The test is positive 80 days after infection, then gradually fades.

Miracidia immobilisation test. This test is positive in the acute stage. The antibodies responsible for the immobilisation are different from that involved in the complement fixation test as it is inactivated by heating at 56°C for 30 minutes.

Precipitin test. Precipitation can be demonstrated both in the urine and serum of infected patients, especially in the acute stage. The test is considered positive if precipitation occurs after dilution up to 1 : 800. The titre may rise to 1 : 3200 in the serum.

Flocculation test. The antigen used in this test is an extract of adult *Schistosoma* adsorbed on cholesterol lecithin crystals. This antigen when added to sera of patients produces flocculation. The extent of flocculation can be divided into stages.

Haemagglutination test. In this test sheep erythrocytes are used as an indicator. Antigen is formed by adsorbing schistosomal extract on sheep's erythrocytes treated with tannic acid. If the serum is positive and incubated with these cells, agglutination occurs.

Fluorescent antibody test. Cercariae are most commonly used as antigen, are exposed to various dilutions of serum from patients and then to fluorescein-labelled anti-human globulin and viewed under ultra-violet light. Those cercariae that have been exposed to serum containing anti-cercarial antibodies are then seen to fluoresce brightly. Anticercarial antibodies are to be found in the serum of patients with schistosomiasis.

This technique is of great value in field surveys as most of the work can be performed in a central laboratory and enough serum for the test may be obtained by extraction of a drop of patient's blood adsorbed on filter paper.

Soluble antigen can be adsorbed on small filter papers and the amount of fluorescence read by a fluorimeter instead of using the microscope as when working with cercaria.

TREATMENT OF SCHISTOSOMIASIS

The first step towards finding a specific remedy for schistosomiasis was the use of emetine, which was first suggested by Tsamis (1913) and was later advocated by Mayer (1915) Diamantis (1916) and many others in Egypt and in the Far East. Emetine hydrochloride solution was widely used in Egypt during the next 15 years. Injections were administered intramuscularly or intravenously every other day thrice weekly for a period of 4 weeks, the total dose given for an adult patient varying from 1.09 to 1.12 g. Symptomatic relief was rapid and an apparent cure rate of 33 per cent was recorded among the patients treated (Khalil, 1931). The toxicity of the drug and its low therapeutic value in the treatment of schistosomiasis greatly limited its use particularly after the introduction of tartar emetic and other antimonial drugs.

The synthetic and less toxic 2-dehydroemetine has been used for the treatment of schistosomiasis (Gelfand, 1962). It appears that this drug has to be administered in a prolonged course and with maximally tolerated doses in order to be an active schistosomicide, though still much less effective in this respect than antimonial drugs.

In 1918 Christopherson published a series of articles on the value of tartar emetic treatment in schistosomiasis, and a copious flow of literature on the subject soon followed confirming the marked efficiency of the drug in all forms of the infection. Since that time, tartar emetic has been and still is the most widely used antischistosomal compound in endemic areas where mass treatment is carried out.

Difficulties encountered with the use of tartar emetic arise mainly from the prolonged course of treatment, the strictly intravenous route of administration, and the potential toxicity of the drug. These have long stimulated the desire to find a better method of using antimony for the treatment of schistosomiasis. Since 1928 other complex trivalent antimony compounds have been introduced and are considered less toxic than tartar emetic and can be administered intramuscularly. Courses of treatment with them are appreciably shorter than when tartar emetic is used. The compounds include sodium antimony–III-bispyrocatechinol disulphonate of sodium (Stibophen), lithium antimony thiomalate (Anthiomaline), sodium antimonyl gluconate (Triostam), and sodium antimony meso-dimercaptosuccinate (Astiban).

In 1938 an important advance was achieved in the chemotherapy of bilharziasis when Miracil D was found to be effective in eradication of the worms when administered orally to animals experimentally infected with *S. mansoni*. Chemically this new compound is the hydrochloride of I - methyl - 4 - B - diethylaminoethylaminothioxanthone, and it is of proved effectiveness when given by mouth to humans infected with *S. haematobium* (Blair *et al*, 1947; Halawani *et al*, 1948). In recent years many other oral antischistosomal compounds have been subjected to clinical evaluation, and two among them, namely Niridazole (1-(5-nitro-2-thiazolyl)-2-imidazolidinone), and Amphothalide (1-p-aminophenoxy-5-phthalamidopentane), are now used in some endemic areas.

Worm response

In experimental animals infected with *S. mansoni* receiving adequate doses of schistosomicides the worms leave their location in the mesenteric veins and migrate to the small branches of the portal vein in the liver. These damaged worms lose muscle tone under the effect of the drug, the couples separate, and are probably carried passively by the blood stream to the liver. The worms cease to feed and obvious degenerative changes begin to appear. The walls of the vessel in which the worm lies become thickened and fibrosed, the worm then dies and its tissues are invaded by leucocytes. Should the dose of the drug fall below the muscle-paralysing level or should drug elimination be accomplished before worm degeneration has proceeded to an appreciable extent, then a process of regeneration sets in. Such worms regain muscle tone, begin to feed, paired worms migrate again to the mesenteric veins and once they start egg-laying a 'relapse' is established (Standen, 1953).

Presumably a similar hepatic shift occurs in the human host with intestinal schistosomiasis. In *S. haematobium* infection, where the adult worms reside in the vesical plexus, it is speculated that, under the influence of treatment, worms that are not caught up in the venous network of this plexus traverse the internal iliac vein and the inferior vena cava and eventually are carried to the lungs.

Evaluation of therapy

Parasitological cure from bilharzial infection is considered to have occurred when there is complete disappearance of viable eggs from the excreta for at least 6 months after treatment in the absence of exposure to reinfection. Multiple examination of the excreta is necessary after treatment, preferably on three consecutive days. Eggs that appear black, discoloured and partially opaque are clearly dead and may be passed for several months or even years after successful therapy, especially in urinary schistosomiasis. Rectal biopsy is of considerable value for post-treatment assessment, particularly in *S. mansoni* and *S. japonicum* infections.

Antimonial drugs

TARTAR EMETIC. Potassium antimonyl tartarate contains 36 per cent of trivalent antimony, while the sodium salt, also used in some countries, contains 39.5 per cent. Tartar emetic solution in distilled water or in 5 per cent glucose, is prepared for intravenous injection in different concentrations varying from 1 to 6 per cent. A daily dose of 2 mg/kg body weight is administered on alternate days for a period of 3–4 weeks. The maximum individual dose should not exceed 130 mg (2 grains) and a total dose of 25–30 grains (1.5–1.95 g) is recommended. It is usual to begin with 30 mg (0.5 grain) and to increase gradually by 30 mg (0.5 grain) at a time until the maximum individual dose is reached. In Egypt, a 6 per cent solution is used for mass treatment and the injections are given on alternate days three times weekly for 4 weeks; with this concentration, a small amount of the solution is injected each time, and the individual dose is easily calculated as 1 ml of solution contains 1 grain (65 mg) of tartar emetic.

STIBOPHEN. (Synonyms: Fouadin, Repodral, Neoantimosan). This drug which contains 13.5 per cent of trivalent antimony is administered as a 6.3 per cent solution by intramuscular injection. Each ml contains 8.5 mg antimony. An individual dose of 5 mg/kg body weight on the average is recommended with a maximum of 315 mg (5 ml). It is usual to begin with one-third and two-thirds of the calculated dose on the first and second days of treatment respectively. The first three doses are administered on consecutive days, to be followed by injection on alternate days up to a total of 10–14 doses (45–60 ml).

ANTHIOMALINE. This compound contains 16 per cent of trivalent antimony. It is supplied in 2 ml ampoules of a 6 per cent solution (or 0.01 g of antimony) and is injected intramuscularly or intravenously, with an average individual dose of 4 mg/kg body weight (maximum dose 4 ml = 240 mg) on alternate days up to a total of 10–12 doses.

SODIUM ANTIMONYL GLUCONATE (Triostam). The formulation should only be administered intravenously. It contains 36 per cent of trivalent antimony and is supplied in ampoules containing 190 mg of the powder which has to be dissolved in 3.5 ml of distilled water before use. A total adult dose varying from 20 to 25 mg/kg body weight is administered in equally divided doses over 6–8 consecutive days.

ASTIBAN. This compound, which is preferably administered by the intramuscular route, contains 25 per cent of trivalent antimony. It is supplied in the form of a lyophilised powder which is dissolved in distilled water or in physiological saline before injection. A 10 per cent solution is usually prepared and a dose of 8 mg/kg body weight (maximum 500 mg) is injected daily or on alternate days up to a total of five doses.

Excretion and storage of antimony. Results of studies carried out on the behaviour of antimony in the body indicate that the principal organ of excretion is the kidney, and only very small amounts of the injected dose (1–4 per cent) are excreted in the stools. The urinary excretion of antimony is initially rapid after injection, but then becomes relatively slow and small amounts can be detected in the urine until 2 months after the end of treatment. It is also known that some organs of the body, the liver being first in this respect, have a great ability to retain considerable amounts of antimony for prolonged periods; the thyroid gland and the heart also retain appreciable quantities (Goodwin and Page, 1943; Bartter *et al*, 1947; Abdallah and Saif, 1962).

Side effects and toxic manifestations. Nausea, vomiting, paroxysmal cough, rheumatic muscular pains, a metallic taste in the mouth and momentary giddiness may occur during treatment with antimony compounds, being more frequent and more intense with the drugs injected intravenously, and particularly when short courses of treatment, as with Triostam or Astiban, are employed. Electrocardiographic changes, mainly flattening or inversion of the T wave, in one or more leads frequently occur during treatment; these are, however, reversible within 2–4 weeks after treatment (Mainzer and Krause, 1940). Signs of intolerance which necessitate withdrawal of the drug include persistent vomiting or tachycardia, diarrhoea and diminution in the amount of urine. Accidents or sudden death during treatment are occasionally reported. Two fatal syndromes have been recognised: one pattern involves primarily the heart with the development of fatal cardiac arrhythmias; the second pattern, which predominantly occurs when the intramuscular route of administration of antimony is used, involves a shock-like syndrome that has many of the characteristics of anaphylaxis (McKenzie, 1932; Halawani *et al*, 1956).

Contraindications. These include organic heart disease, renal insufficiency, parenchymatous liver damage, advanced pulmonary disease, pregnancy and febrile and anaemic conditions. Treatment with antimony compounds should not be repeated without a lapse of 6 months.

Results. In general, *S. haematobium* responds more satisfactorily to therapy with antimony than *S. mansoni*, and the latter more so than *S. japonicum*. Children are presumably rapid excreters of antimony and their tolerance to treatment is better than adults, though relapses among them are relatively more common. Their liver is also larger in comparison with their body weight and presumably absorbs a greater proportion of the infected dose. The tartar emetic course of treatment with a total dose of 20–21 grains usually results in very high cure rates (90–100 per cent) in cases of *S. haematobium* not exposed to reinfection. Less favourable results are obtained in infections with either *S. mansoni* or *S. japonicum* to whom the maximally tolerated doses should be administered. Similar results are reported with the use of Triostam or Astiban, but the prescribed courses of treatment with those two compounds are not tolerated by an appreciable percentage of the patients in endemic areas. Anthiomaline and Stibophen are generally less effective in curing schistosomiasis, especially *S. mansoni* and *S. japonicum* infections, than the other antimony compounds, and relapses are more common with their use.

Non-antimonial compounds

LUCANTHONE (Synonyms: Miracil D, Nilodin, Tixanthone). This drug is supplied in the form of sugar-coated tablets each containing 200–250 mg. A daily dose of 10–20 mg/kg body weight is prescribed, being divided into two or three equal fractions and taken after meals. The smaller daily dose is repeated for 10–20 days and the larger one is administered for 7–10 days. Though this compound is practically devoid of toxicity, yet it very frequently causes gastrointestinal disturbances, giddiness, headache and insomnia which are variably tolerated by individual patients. It also results in a yellow coloration of the skin which disappears within a few days of the end of treatment. With the different dosage schemes applied, the therapeutic value of this drug is inferior to that of antimony compounds particularly in *S.*

mansoni infection. It has hardly any effect in *S. japonicum* infection.

The addition of 5 mg Extractum belladonna siccum (B.P.) to each tablet helps to diminish the severity of the side effects, and cure rates of 75 per cent and 37 per cent of infections with *S. haematobium* and *S. mansoni* respectively are claimed after the administration of such tablets with a maximum total dose of 12 g over a period of 20 consecutive days. The use of lucanthone hydrochloride tablets coated with cellulose acetate phthalate is said to alleviate to a considerable degree the frequency of the gastrointestinal side effects of the drug (Halawani *et al*, 1957; Alves, 1958; Lees, 1967).

AMPHOTHALIDE (Schistomid). Many compounds of the para-aminophenoxyalkane series have been found to possess significant schistosomicidal activity in experimental animals, but at the same time to be responsible for ocular disturbances, particularly choroidoretinitis. Amphothalide, however, is one of those compounds which is devoid of such toxicity though it retains some antischistosomal effect. It is supplied in 500 mg tablets and administered in a total dose of 300–400 mg/kg body weight over a period of 5–10 days. Side effects are not infrequent, mainly nausea, anorexia and vomiting, and pain in the loins with strangury may occur during treatment. The therapeutic value of the drug is limited to *S. haematobium* infection in which cure rates of 40–50 per cent have been reported by different workers (Standen, 1953; Ashton, 1957).

NIRIDAZOLE (Ambilhar). This compound has been extensively tried in the past few years in different countries where the disease is endemic. Undoubtedly it exerts a remarkable schistosomicidal activity against the three main human species of the parasite. The drug is orally administered in 500 mg and 100 mg tablets, and various schemes of treatment have been applied in different groups of patients. The daily dose is usually divided into two fractions administered at 12-hourly intervals; there is evidence that when the drug is given in single daily doses it results in cure rates comparable with those obtained with the fractionated dose method. The available data indicate that an average daily dose of 25 mg/kg body weight given for 7 consecutive days is sufficient to cure 80–100 per cent of infections with *S. haematobium*. In *S. mansoni* and *S. japonicum* infections, similar or less favourable cure rates have been reported.

This drug, however, causes various side effects which have limited its use to individual therapy. Anorexia, vomiting and abdominal pains are frequent, sometimes necessitating a temporary withdrawal of the drug. Lassitude, muscle pains and skin eruptions are less frequent, and occasionally epistaxis may occur. Electrocardiographic changes, mainly diminished amplitude or inversion of the T wave, commonly occur during treatment; these are transient and disappear within an average of 3 weeks from the end of treatment. The most important side effects are those related to the central nervous system which include headache, insomnia and dizziness, all of which are common; muscular tremors and psychotic episodes develop less frequently and rarely there are epileptiform seizures. These neuropsychic manifestations predominantly occur in cases of hepatosplenic bilharziasis; and some recent studies have shown that 20–30 per cent of such patients may develop mental disorientation, hallucinations, muscular tremors or spasms, or epileptiform convulsions during treatment with niridazole.

The onset of these manifestations is usually on the third to the fifth day of treatment, being frequently preceded by severe headache, nausea and vomiting. It is suggested that the presence of collateral and vascular shunts in those patients may allow a certain amount of the unmetabolised drug to pass to the central nervous system and produce these effects. Potential liver dysfunction preventing complete metabolism of the drug in such cases is also postulated as a possible factor (Jordan, 1966; Wolfe, 1967).

At present, it seems that the use of niridazole with the recommended dosage schemes is contraindicated in the following conditions: decompensated disease, advanced schistosomal hepatosplenic involvement, decompensated organic heart disease, renal insufficiency, latent or manifest psychoses, neuroses or epilepsy, central nervous system disorders, clinical malnutrition and pregnancy.

ETRENOL (Hycanthone). A relatively new schistosomicide is administered intramuscularly, as a single dose of 3 mg/kg of body weight. A significant number of cures has been reported and the drug may find an established place for mass therapy but hepatotoxicity is a problem with it and the cure rate is too low for general use.

Other methods of treatment

Intensive therapy. In an attempt to shorten the course of treatment of schistosomiasis intensive therapy was introduced. In one course 360–480 mg (6–8 grains) of tartar emetic were divided into three equal doses administered in one day at 3–4 hourly intervals. The more usually employed intensive course was of 2 days and involved the injection of a total dose of 12 mg/kg body weight in equally divided doses thrice daily 3 hours apart on each of the 2 consecutive days. Another scheme was to administer 120 mg (2 grains) tartar emetic or 5 ml of Stibophen twice daily to adult patients for 5 consecutive days. The short courses prescribed for treatment with Triostam and Astiban could also be regarded as aiming towards the same goal (Alves and Blair, 1946; Halawani, 1946; Talaat and Shoaib, 1953). Though high parasitological cure rates were claimed serious toxic effects were frequent, particularly with the drugs injected intravenously. In endemic areas where other parasitic infections, malnutrition and anaemic states are prevalent, only a minority of the schistosomal patients could tolerate intensive antimony therapy and those only if they could be treated and followed up for a few days as in-patients (Halawani *et al*, 1957).

Spaced dosage therapy. In endemic areas where mass treatment of the infected population is carried out, the use of the 'classical' courses of treatment by antimony compounds is often hampered by the frequent occurrence of side reactions. Studies carried out on the behaviour of antimony in the human body have suggested that the timing of the individual doses could be so arranged that the drug exerts its therapeutic effect and, at the same time, the patient is saved from the side reactions which occur with frequent dosing at short intervals. Experience with the use of tartar emetic in doses of 2 mg/kg body weight repeated at weekly intervals for 12–16 weeks has shown that about 50–58 per cent respectively among the treated patients are apparently cured with negligible side reactions. When the same dose of the drug is administered twice weekly for a period of 6 weeks, the cure rates obtained are comparable with those reported when 'classical' tartar emetic courses are applied, and the side reactions were comparatively very few. Similar instances of good tolerability and satisfactory response to therapy are noted when 5 mg/kg body weight of Stibophen are administered twice weekly for 4–5 weeks, or when a dose of 8 mg/kg body weight of Astiban is injected once or twice weekly until a total of five doses has been reached. These spaced dosage schemes of treatment also called 'slow treatment methods' are in routine use for mass treatment in Egypt (Mousa and Ata, 1960; Abdallah and Saif, 1964).

Suppression. Fredheim and De Jongh (1959) reported that single doses of 0.3–0.5 g of TWSB, an earlier formulation of Astiban, could prevent excretion of viable ova for 1 month. Other workers confirmed this or found a reduction of egg output with different antimonial drugs; some have reported that the eggs shed after single injections contain 'pathological' miracidia which cannot infect the snail vectors. When such doses are repeated at monthly intervals, a percentage of the treated individuals will be parasitologically cured, the cure rate increasing parallel to the number of doses administered (Salem and Sherif, 1960). Lees (1967) found that a total dose of 60 mg/kg body weight of lucanthone hydrochloride coated with cellulose acetate phthalate administered in fractionated doses twice daily during 3 days to patients with *S. mansoni* results in a mean overall reduction of 80 per cent in egg output and a 16 per cent cure rate; the reduction in egg output was maintained for 4 months.

Suppression is defined as the ability of a drug to cause a temporary reduction or a complete inhibition of eggs for a time. This reduction in egg output apparently reduces the extent of the pathological changes in the individual or prevents their development. On the community level, suppressive management may prove its importance in control projects; it is speculated that suppressive therapy may lead to arrest of transmission by preventing infection of snails, or, at least to a reduction of the infection rate of snails.

CONTROL

Total eradication of schistosomal infection from a locality involves both the prevention of transmission and the cure of all infective patients. The tools and methods now at hand are not adequate to ensure the attainment of this objective in most endemic areas. On the other hand, control implies the reduction of schistosomiasis to a prevalence where it is no longer a major health problem, and the prevention of transmission with the greatest possible reduction of the load of infection in the affected people. The available methods of schistosomal control include the prevention of human contact with water, environmental sanitation, mass treatment of all infected humans, and snail control.

Prevention of human contact with water

It is true that schistosomiasis could be prevented if man did not come into contact with water; such contact involves both pollution of water by the excreta, and infection of man. So long as primitive irrigational and agricultural practices and lack of industrialisation remain in endemic areas, this contact with water is difficult to eliminate. Some human habits, particularly passing excreta near water and children swimming and playing in water, have to be altered, and this can only slowly be achieved. Avoidance or prevention of contact in older population groups has only little beneficial effect since initial contact almost invariably occurs in childhood, and children are the most important source of the infection.

Environmental sanitation

In most schistosomal areas, facilities for the disposal of human excreta are either inadequate or completely absent. The construction of sanitary privies and the provision of potable water and safe washing, bathing and recreation facilities, particularly to entice children away from snail habitats, will undoubtedly contribute materially to the control of the disease. Public health education is also more effective in localities with improved sanitation.

Sanitation has its limitations, however, especially in restricting the transmission of *S. japonicum* and *S. haematobium*. With *S. japonicum*, animal reservoir hosts tend to maintain the infection in the snails even in the absence of infection from human hosts. With *S. haematobium* the eggs are passed in the urine, and the provision of facilities for disposal of the excreta has less effect than with faecal-borne diseases.

Mass treatment of all infected patients.

Attempts to conduct mass treatment campaigns have limitations; a relatively large number of the patients discovered do not complete the courses of treatment, mostly because of the unpleasant side effects of the available drugs, and a number of those completing treatment suffer relapses. As multiple examinations are necessary if all infected cases are to be detected, and these are often impracticable, large numbers of patients are usually missed. The relapsed and missed patients will maintain transmission of the disease, and, in *S. japonicum* areas, the animal reservoir hosts will continue to supply eggs for the infection of snails.

In endemic areas where mass treatment is carried out, as in Egypt, it is difficult to assess the relative efficacy of chemotherapy in comparison with other control measures. There is reason to believe that drug treatment on the extensive scale employed has contributed to reduction in the severity of the disease and its complications. Until more effective and better tolerated drugs become available, mass therapy will have only a small part in any control programme.

Suppressive treatment, already referred to, is currently applied in some control projects to evaluate its effect on the transmission of the disease.

Snail control

The biggest concentration of effort in the field of prevention of schistosomiasis is now undoubtedly directed to snail control by the application of chemical molluscicides. Environmental control by engineering methods is also carried out; it involves modifications to the environment of both the human and the snail host. Biological control of snails is another approach to the problem which has not as yet had widespread practical application.

Before the start of any snail control programme, it is essential to delineate the exact distribution of the intermediate hosts and to identify the zone in which transmission of the disease can occur. The establishment of these geographical limits must be carried out at regular intervals for 1 year since there may be considerable variation in the snail population from season to season. The time and places of transmission should be identified through a systematic study of the bionomics of the intermediate hosts. Climatic factors, including seasonal variations in rainfall, its amount, daily and seasonal temperature variations and humidity should also be known. With such background knowledge at hand, the best method of snail control can be chosen. Quantitative data required for evaluation of the results must be collected; these include prevalence of the snail hosts and the prevalence of schistosome infection in the human population, particularly the younger age groups. It is by their effect on these two indices that the efficacy of the control measures must be judged.

Chemical control

Molluscicidal compounds are used to produce rapid reduction in snail populations. It is essential to ensure that the application of the chemical to bodies of water in the concentration used to kill snails and their eggs will not result in harm to the human or animal population. It should also be relatively stable, reasonably safe in the hands of trained workers, usable with simple durable equipment, and at a cost enabling it to be employed economically. The nature of any snail habitat dictates the selection of the molluscicide to be used and its method of application. In general, these habitats are either dry or moist soil areas, shallow inundated areas, static water of various extent or flowing water, and different techniques and specialised equipment have to be used for each habitat in order to obtain effective control (W.H.O., 1965). The number of molluscicide applications per year depends upon seasonal variations in snail populations, climatic factors, and the proper choice of the time of application and of the place to be treated. The following preparations are the commercially available molluscicides currently in use in control programmes.

5, 2 - DICHLORO - 4 - NITRO - SALICYLIC - ANILIDE (ethanolamine salt): *Bayluscide, Bayer 73*. The compound is supplied in the form of a wettable powder; it quickly acts in low concentrations with concentration-time products of 2–7 ppm/hour. Direct sunlight and high water hardness reduce its efficiency; it is also slightly adsorbed on mud and colloidal particles. It can be applied by water carriage to canals and streams and it is also effective in moist soil habitats. At present, it seems to be the molluscicide of choice to be used in most snail habitats.

SODIUM PENTACHLOROPHENATE (Na PCP). This compound is irritating to the skin and mucous membranes and suitable precautions should be exercised in this respect. It is applied at the rate of 10 ppm for 8 hours in flowing water, i.e. a concentration-time product of 80 ppm/hour. It is less effective as an ovicide in amphibious snail habitats (oncomelania), and its effectiveness is also generally reduced by high alkalinity and by adsorption on mud.

COPPER SULPHATE ($CuSO_4$). This is usually applied as a solution with a concentration of 30 ppm to aquatic habitats only. It is stable and easy to handle, but its effectiveness is reduced in the presence of organic matter, certain types of dissolved solids and a high pH. Reports of its ovicidal properties are variable.

2-CYCLOHEXYL-4, 6-DINITROPHENOL (DNCHP). It is supplied in the form of a wettable powder and gives the best results in moist soil habitats of amphibious snails when applied at the rate of 0.1–5.0 g/m^2. In aquatic habitats the concentrations used must be maintained for 24 hours to be effective.

AQUALIN (85 per cent acrolein). This compound was originally used as a herbicide to control aquatic vegetation with a concentration-time product of 30–75 ppm/hour, and it was found to be ovicidal and molluscicidal. It is volatile and irritating, and has to be handled with care. Application is made by water carriage, but the volatility of the compound, particularly when the temperature is high, may require a series of booster applications in long canal systems. The cost of this compound seems to restrict its use to areas where control of both snails and submerged aquatic vegetation are combined.

P

Environmental control

The object, in the case of human hosts, is to alter their habitats in such a way that they no longer come into contact with infested water, or to lessen the chances of such contact to a minimum. For intermediate hosts, the ecology of the waters in which they live has to be changed so that there are no suitable habitats.

New villages should be sited as far away as possible from infested streams; a minimum distance of 500 metres is recommended, otherwise it is necessary to flank the stream by high walls or fences, through the village and for a distance of 500 metres on either side, or to enclose the stream completely within the same limits in a long culvert or underground channel. Provision of latrines and of adequate waste disposal facilities are essential, as is the construction of bathing pools separate from any other bodies of water. The pools should be filled with clean chlorinated water.

Various methods have been devised for the elimination of the snail intermediate hosts. In some endemic localities, where marshes and low-lying areas contiguous to streams are important breeding places, land reclamation has been employed to great advantage. Changing the course of streams in order to increase the flow rate is a valuable tool where it can be done in keeping with agricultural conditions and practices. Straightening of banks, elimination of pockets, cementing of canals and clearance of aquatic vegetation have also been employed, among many other methods. In the planning of irrigation schemes in endemic areas, the possibility of creating snail habitats should be carefully considered and avoided.

Biological control

The use of disease agents to infect snails, certain insects or their larvae which prey upon or parasitise molluscs, or certain freshwater fish which utilise molluscs as a source of food, have all been tried as possible means of biological control of the snail intermediate hosts (Dias and Cruz, 1953; Dias and Dawood, 1955; La Grange and Fain, 1952; La Grange, 1953; Dechiens and Lamy, 1954; De Bondt, 1956). Promising results have been obtained with the introduction of other predator or competitor snails. An ampullarid snail, *Marisa cornuareitis*, was found to affect *Biomphalaria glabrata* in at least two ways: (*a*) as a competing voracious feeder, and (*b*) by devouring both the egg masses and the young of the intermediate hosts (Chernin *et al*, 1956; Oliver

Gonzales *et al*, 1956). *Marisa* is not known to serve as an intermediate host for any important parasites affecting man or domestic animals.

Another snail competitor is the planorbid *Heliosoma tenue*, which very rapidly multiplies and competes for survival with the intermediate hosts and finally replaces them in laboratory experiments (Mandahl Barth, 1965).

Any successful predator-prey relationship involves the introduction of a species previously foreign to a particular area, and harmful effects may result. The extension or practical application of biological control can thus only be carried out after prolonged and careful study.

Personal prophylaxis

Drinking water, if drawn from infested streams and if not chlorinated, has to be boiled or filtered through a Seitz filter before consumption. If bathing water is allowed to stand for 60 hours, or if it is heated at 50°C for 3 minutes it is safe for use. An ointment containing 20 per cent benzyl benzoate, or an ordinary insect repellent (e.g. dibutyl phthalate) incorporated into a suitable ointment base prevents skin penetration by the cercariae. Impregnation of uniforms with a 5 per cent emulsion of any of these chemicals will also provide protection, as will the employment of rubber footwear.

Artificial immunisation has been studied by many workers, but since it has been shown to depend on the attainment of full maturity by the invading worms, the use of viable material for human immunisation would be completely contraindicated (Hsu and Hsu, 1961; Hunter *et al*, 1962). Research on this subject is in progress.

OTHER TREMATODES

CLONORCHIASIS

Clonorchiasis or Chinese liver fluke disease is caused by infection of the biliary passages by *Clonorchis sinensis*. This worm belongs to the superfamily *Opisthorchoidea*, medium-sized transparent flukes which produce operculated ova containing miracidia. They have two intermediate hosts; an initial larval stage is passed in snails and a second in various fresh-water fishes.

Distribution

Clonorchiasis is a common disease of fish-eating mammals in the Far East, affecting in particular dogs, cats, pigs and man. Fish-raising

areas of Japan, Korea, China and Indo-China are highly endemic regions. The infection has been recorded in Chinese inhabitants of India, Mauritius and Cuba.

Aetiology (Fig. 13.1)

C. sinensis measures about 11–20×3–4 mm. The eggs, which resemble those of *Heterophyes* and *Opisthorchis*, measure some 30×16 μm. They are carried down the common bile duct to the duodenum and are passed in the stools. On reaching water they hatch after being ingested by a suitable snail, e.g. of the genus *Bythnia*. The miracidium then makes its way into the visceral mass of the snail and changes into a sporocyst which gives rise to numerous slender rediae. These multiply and produce cercariae which leave the snail,

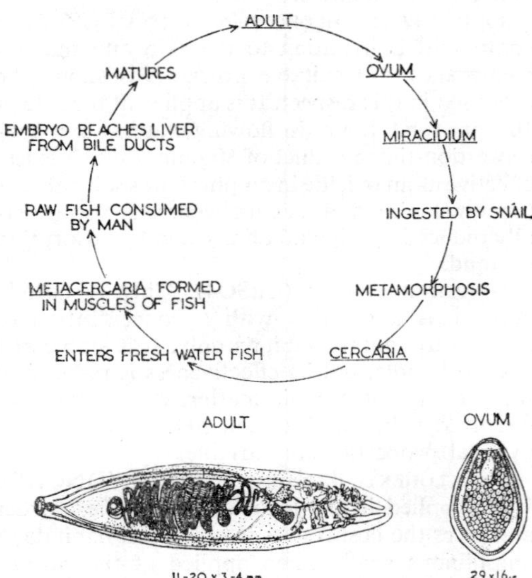

FIG. 13.1. *Life cycle of* Clonorchis sinensis.

swim in the water, and are swallowed by the second larval host, a freshwater fish, in which, after several weeks, they produce cysts which are infective for the definitive host. The infective or metacercarial stage can develop in the musculature of more than forty species of fish belonging to the families *Cyprinidae*, *Anabantidae*, *Salmonidae* and *Gobiidae*, and these may harbour hundreds of cysts per g body weight.

The fish ponds of China are the main source of the infection. Man and other mammals are infected by eating uncooked fish; the Chinese are particularly fond of dipping raw fish into Soya bean sauce and eating them. The cysts are digested and the parasites are set free in the duodenum from which they migrate through the ampulla of Vater into the common bile duct and then into the smaller biliary radicles.

Pathology

Adult *C. sinensis* inhabits the bile ducts and sometimes the pancreatic ducts. It tends to localise in the distant bile passages, especially those of the left lobe of the liver. The biliary epithelium proliferates and in the larger ducts there is gradual dilatation into large cyst-like cavities or diverticula. Biliary cirrhosis and suppurative cholangitis may develop. The liver becomes much enlarged and malignant changes may supervene.

Symptoms

These depend upon the degree of the infection; individuals harbouring a few worms may be symptomless. Chronic diarrhoea with intermittent attacks of jaundice, progressive hepatomegaly and oedema are common symptoms. There is leucocytosis with eosinophilia. Cachexia and extreme jaundice are found in advanced cases. The diagnosis depends upon finding the eggs in the faeces or in fluid obtained by duodenal intubation.

Treatment

Many drugs have been used in the past with little success. Sodium antimony tartrate given intravenously was found beneficial in early cases. Chloroquine is now the drug of choice in a dosage of 600 mg (base) daily by mouth for 6 weeks.

FASCIOLIASIS

This is caused by the presence of the sheep liver fluke, *Fasciola hepatica*, in the bile ducts or liver parenchyma. It is essentially a disease of sheep, goats and cattle, in which it produces 'liver rot'. The parasite is widely distributed throughout the world; British interest in the human disease was stimulated by an outbreak in Hampshire in 1960.

Aetiology (Fig. 13.2)

F. hepatica is a large fluke measuring about 3.5×1.2 cm. The eggs are operculated and measure about $140 \times 80 \mu$m. They are passed in the faeces of the infected person or herbivorous animal. In water, the miracidium hatches out in about a month and enters a freshwater snail.

Limnaea truncatula and many other molluscs are suitable intermediate hosts in which sporocysts, rediae and cercariae develop. The cercariae escape from the snail and encyst on aquatic vegetation. When ingested by the main host the parasites excyst in the intestine and migrate through the intestinal wall. Some reach the liver through the portal circulation and others pass into the peritoneal cavity and penetrate the liver capsule.

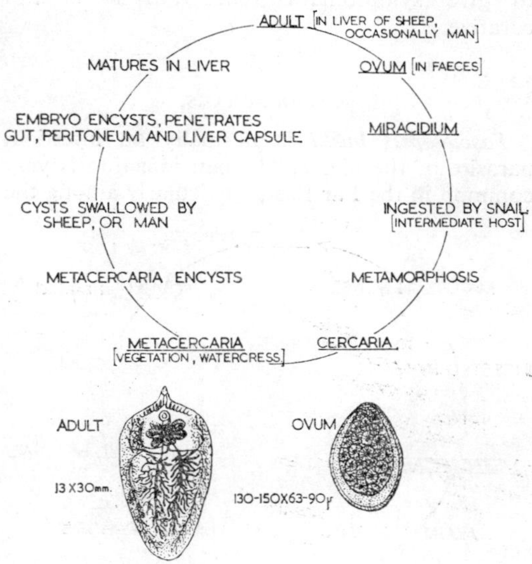

FIG. 13.2. *Life cycle of* Fasciola hepatica.

They mature on reaching the bile ducts. Man usually contracts the infection by eating watercress from meadows frequented by sheep.

Clinical features

There are usually three distinct phases; after the phase of invasion there is a latent period followed by an obstructive phase. The invasive phase produces serious symptoms. There is high fever lasting many weeks with general symptoms and wasting. Commonly there is pain over the liver which is enlarged and tender. Shoulder pain is frequent. There is usually urticaria and eosinophilia. Immature parasites may occasionally settle in sites other than the liver—'ectopic fascioliasis'. They may appear in the pharyngeal wall, spleen, abdominal muscles and lungs. The latent phase, which may last for months or even years, occurs after the larvae have reached the liver. The obstructive phase is due to adult flukes in the bile ducts which cause epithelial proliferation and lead to biliary cirrhosis. Ova are not found in the faeces for the first 3–4 months following infection, and this makes early diagnosis particularly difficult.

Treatment

As in the case of clonorchiasis, chloroquine is at present the drug of choice. It has been found to give symptomatic relief but it is not curative.

FASCIOLOPSIASIS

Fasciolopsis buski is normally an intestinal parasite of the pig, but human infection is very common in the Far East, particularly among the

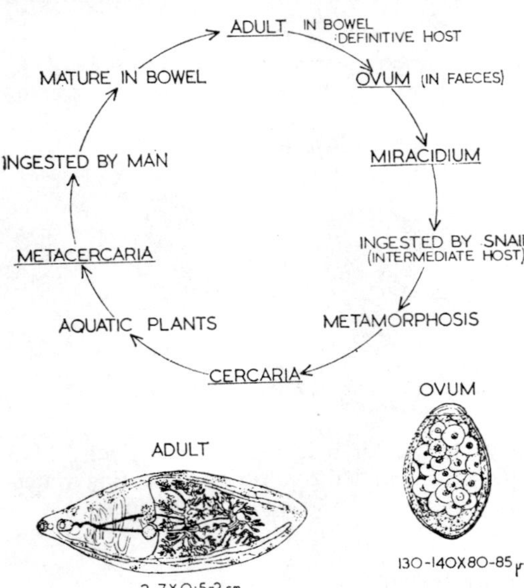

FIG. 13.3. *Life cycle of* Fasciolopsis buski.

Chinese. It is a large fluke, 2–7 × 0.5–1.4 cm, resembling *F. hepatica* in appearance (Fig. 13.3). It inhabits the small intestine and its eggs, measuring 140 × 80 µm or more, are passed in the faeces. They are usually very numerous, for each worm can lay 25 000 eggs per day. They hatch in water after 16 days and the miracidia enter snails of the genus *Planorbis*, forming sporocysts, rediae, daughter rediae and cercariae. The cercariae encyst on aquatic plants such as the water-caltrop or water chestnut which is cultivated in ponds and fertilised by human faeces. The tubers of this plant are eaten raw by the Chinese. As many as

1000 cysts have been found on the surface of one nut and infection occurs from peeling it with the teeth. The metacercariae excyst in the duodenum and attach themselves to the wall of the small intestine.

Clinical features

Light infections are symptomless but large numbers of flukes give rise to alternating diarrhoea and constipation, the stools being pale and offensive. Abscesses in the intestinal wall may give rise to haemorrhage. There may be nausea and vomiting and in advanced cases there is general toxaemia, oedema and ascites. Fatal cases have been reported.

Treatment

The drugs used in the treatment of ancylostomiasis are effective.

PARAGONIMIASIS

Human infection with the lung fluke is confined to the Far East. *Paragonimus westermani* and other allied species are found in the lungs, pleura, bronchi and occasionally the liver, spleen and other organs of man, dog, wolf, leopard, tiger, cat, pig, otter and mink.

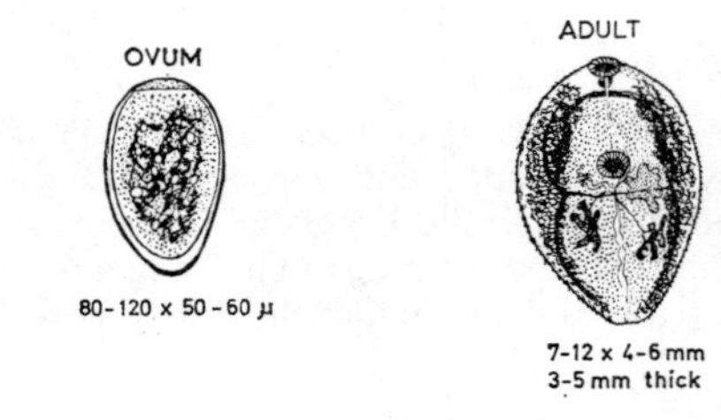

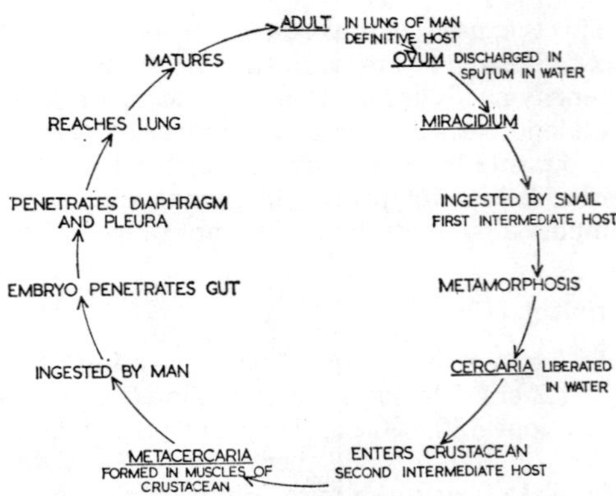

FIG. 13.4. *Life cycle of* Paragonimus westermani.

The adult *Paragonimus* is a fleshy worm, reddish-brown in colour and resembling a split pea in shape. It measures about 7–12 by 6 mm. The eggs, 70×45 μm, contain a fertilised unsegmented ovum when found in the sputum or faeces. They hatch in fresh water after a few weeks and the miracidium infects the snail *Melania* in which it forms sporocysts, rediae and young cercariae (Fig. 13.4).

Metacercariae develop in various fresh-water crabs and crayfish. Infection is acquired during their preparation for cooking or by eating raw crab. In China, raw crab meat cut into strips and soaked in alcohol is a popular delicacy known as 'drunken crab'. The larvae penetrate the wall of the intestine and migrate via the peritoneal cavity through the diaphragm into the pleural cavity, burrowing into the lungs. There they produce tunnels and cystic cavities containing flukes. Tunnelled tumours may also be found in the liver, intestine, skin, testes, muscles, spinal cord and brain. Hundreds of flukes have been found in abscesses.

Clinical features

The onset is gradual with chronic cough, discomfort in the chest and abundant sputum containing large numbers of eggs, which are also found in the faeces. The main symptom is haemoptysis; this may be frank or more often the sputum is rusty and pneumonic. Clubbing of the fingers is common but the signs in the chest are usually indefinite. Radiologically there may be opacities and infiltration, and the great difficulty lies in the exclusion of pulmonary tuberculosis which is very frequently associated with paragonimiasis; if ova are found in the sputum examinations must be made for *M. tuberculosis*. There may be abdominal symptoms; diarrhoea and pain with hepatomegaly. Adenitis, prostatitis and epididymitis are quite common. Parasites in the brain may cause Jacksonian attacks and other focal symptoms. Transverse myelitis and cutaneous ulceration have been recorded.

Treatment

Bithionol, 2,2'-thiobis (4,6-dichlorophenol), a tasteless white powder previously used in cosmetics and for the treatment of chicken tapeworm and liver fluke in cattle, has been found effective. Single daily doses of 30 mg/kg are given by mouth for 10–15 days. Chloroquine has been used with some success, as in clonorchiasis and fascioliasis. Previously, courses of parenteral emetine were given. Improvement has followed the injection of lipiodol into the bronchi. Localised lesions have been cured by lobectomy.

HETEROPHYIASIS

Heterophyes heterophyes is a very minute fluke, measuring less than 2 mm, which is commonly found in large numbers in the small intestine of man, dog, wolf and cat in Egypt and the Far East. The eggs, 30×16 μm, resemble those of *Clonorchis*. They are passed into the faeces and the miracidium enters the snail *Pironella conica*. Metacercariae develop in the mullet and other fish which produce the infection in man when not properly cooked.

Clinical features

Even when present in large numbers these worms may be harmless but very heavy infections may give rise to diarrhoea and deposits of ova have at times been found in the heart, brain and spinal cord.

Treatment

Tetrachloroethylene, as in the treatment of ancylostomiasis, is effective.

REFERENCES

ABDALLAH, A. and SAIF, M. (1962) *Ciba Foundation Symposium on Bilharziasis*, p. 287.
—— (1964) *J. Egypt. med. Ass.*, **47**, 427.
ABDEL MALEK, E. (1958) *Bull. Wld Hlth Org.*, **18**, 785.
ABDEL-SHAFI, M. (1940) *Roy. Egypt med. Ass.*, **23**, 1.
ABDIN, F., FATTAH, Y. and SHAFEIK, N. (1959) *Gaz. Egypt. Soc. Gynaec. Obstet.*, **11**, 1.
ABDIN, F. H. (1962) *Proc. 1st Int. Symp. Bilh. (Cairo)*, **2**, 429.
ABU EL-FADL, M. (1962) *Proc. 1st int. Cong. Bilh. (Cairo)*, **1**, 700.

ABU EL-NASR, A. L. (1962) *Proc. 1st int. Cong. Bilh. (Cairo)*, **1**, 68.
ABUL-FADL, M. and KHALAFALLAH, A. S. (1961) *Brit. J. Cancer*, **15**, 479.
AFIFI, S. (1962) *Proc. 1st int. Cong. Bilh. (Cairo)*, p. 61.
ALVES, W. (1949) *S. Afr. med. J.*, **23**, 428.
—— (1958) *Bull. Wld Hlth Org.*, **18**, 1109, 1092.
ALVES, W. and BLAIR, D. M. (1946) *Lancet*, **1**, 9.
ANDERSON, R. (1960) *J. trop. Med. Hyg.*, **9**, 299.
ANDERSON, R. and NAIMARK, D. (1960) *Amer. J. trop. Med. Hyg.*, **9**, 600.
ANDERSON, R., SADUN, E. and WILLIAMS, J. (1961) *Exp. Parasit.*, **11**, 111.
ANDRADE, Z. A. *et al* (1961) *Amer. J. trop. Med. Hyg.*, **14**, 100.
ARAFA, M. A. (1952) *Ann. Inst. Med. trop.*, **9**, 1177.
ASHTON, N. (1957) *J. Path. Bact.*, **74**, 103.
ATTA, A. A. and MOUSA, A. H. (1959) *J. Egypt. med. Ass.*, **42**, 285.
AZAVEDO (1954) *Ann. Soc. belge. Med. trop.*, **34**, 738.
BADR, M., ZAHER M. and FAWZY, R. (1958) *J. Egypt med. Ass.*, **41**, 624.
BARTTER, F. C., COWIE, D. B., MOST, H., NESS, A. T. and FORBUSH, S. (1947) *Amer. J. trop. Med.*, **27**. 403.
BAYOUMI, M. (1962) *Proc. 1st int. Cong. Bilh. (Cairo)*, **1**, 449.
BELL, D. R. (1963) *Bull. Wld Hlth Org.*, **29**, 525.
BIGGAM, A. G. and ARAFA, M. A. (1930) *Trans. roy. Soc. trop. Med. Hyg.*, **24**, 2, 187.
BILHARZ, T. (1852) *Z. Wissensch. Zool.*, **4**, 72.
—— (1856) *Wien. med. Eschr.*, **6**, 49, 65.
BLAIR, D. M., HAWKING, F. and ROSS, W. F. (1947) *Lancet*, **2**, 911.
CAMERON, I. and EL-TERAI (1950) *Brit. med. J.*, **1**, 1117.
CAWSTON, F. G. (1937) *J. trop. Med. Hyg.*, **40**, 15.
CHAFFEE, E. F., BAUMAN, P. M. and SHAPILO, J. (1954) *Amer. J. trop. Med. Hyg.*, **3**, 905.
CHANDLER, A. C. (1926) *Indian J. med. Res.*, **14**, 179.
CHERNIN, E., MICHELSON, E. G. and AUGUSTINE, D. L. (1956) *Amer. J. trop. Med. Hyg.*, **5**, 297.
CLARK, E. and GRAEF (1935) *Amer. J. Path.*, **11**, 693.
COBBOLD, T. (1859) *Trans. Linn. Soc. Lond. (Zool.)*, **22**, 364.
CORT, W. N. (1950) *Amer. J. Hyg.*, **52**, 251.
DAY, H. B. (1924) *Trans. roy. Soc. trop. Med. Hyg.*, **9**, 121.
—— (1933) *J. trop. Med. Hyg.*, **36**, 17.
DAY, H. B. and FERGUSON, A. R. (1909) *Amer. J. trop. Med. Parasit*, **3**, 379.
DE BONDT, A. F. (1956) *Ann. Soc. belge Med. trop.*, **36**, 667.
DECHIENS, R. and LAMY, L. (1954) *Bull. Soc. Path. exot.*, **47**, 809.
DE WITT, W. B. (1962) *Ciba Foundation Symposium on Bilharziasis*, p. 157.
DEWITT, W. E. (1958) *Amer. J. trop. Med. Hyg.*, **12**, 741.
DIAMANTIS, A. (1928) *J. Egypt. med. Ass.*, **11**, 212.
DIAS, E. and CRUZ, D. (1953) *Trans. roy. Soc. trop. Med. Hyg.*, **47**, 581.
DIAS, E. and DAWOOD, M. M. (1955) *Mem. Inst. Osw. Cruz.*, **53**, 13.
DOLBY and FAHMY, I. (1924) *Lancet*, **2**, 1, 87.
EL MOFTY, M. A. and EL ZAWAHRY, M. (1962) *Proc. 1st int. Symp. Bilh. (Cairo)*.
ELWI, A. M. (1955) *J. Egypt. med. Ass.*, **38**.
ELWI, A. P. (1959) *Textbook of Pathology*. Anglo-Egypt. Bookshop, Cairo.
ERFAN, M. (1940) *J. Egypt. med. Ass.*, **14**, 1, 61.
ERFAN, M., ERFAN, H., MOUSA, A. M. and DEEB, A. A. (1949) *Trans. roy. Soc. trop. Med. Hyg.*, **42**, 477.
—— (1957) *Gaz. Kasr El-Aini (Cairo)*, **23**, 1.
EZZAT, M. A. E., TADROS, G. and ABD EL HALIM, M. I. (1958) *Bull. Vet. Lab. Res. Admin. Agri. Egypt.*, No. **285**, 1–20.
FAIRLEY, N. H. (1919) *Proc. roy. Soc. Med.*, **13**, 1, 1.
—— (1919) *J. Path.*, **23**, 289.
—— (1927) *Trans. roy. Soc. trop. Med. Hyg.*, **20**, 236.
FAROOQ, M. (1963) *Ann. trop. Med. Parasit.*, **57**, 323.
FAUST, E. C. (1948) *Amer. J. trop. Med.*, **28**, 175.
FAUZI, R. M. (1962) *Proc. 1st int. Cong. Bilh. (Cairo)*, **1**, 607.
FERGUSON (1913) *Glasg. med. J.*, **79**, 14.
FILHO, A. M. (1959) *Amer. J. trop. Med. Hyg.*, **805**.
—— (1959) *Amer. J. trop. Med. Hyg.*, **32**, 18.
FORSYTH, D. M. and MACDONALD, G. (1965) *Trans. roy. Soc. trop. Med. Hyg.*, **59**, 171.
FREDHEIM, E. A. and DE JONGH, R. T. (1959) *Ann. trop. Med. Parasit.*, **53**, 316.
GAWSTON, F. G. (1925) *J. trop. Med. Hyg.*, **28**, 406.

GAZAYERLI, M. (1939) *J. Egypt. med. Ass.*, **22**, 34.
GAZAYERLI, M. and KHALIL, H. A. (1954) *J. Egypt. med. Ass.*, **37**, 1, 86.
GELFAND, M. (1949) *Afr. med. J.*, **33**, 255.
GELFAND, M., REID, E. T. and SIMPSON, B. E. (1962) *Trans. roy. Soc. trop. Med. Hyg.*, **56**, 77.
GELFAND, M. and ROSS, W. F. (1953) *Trans. roy. Soc. trop. Med. Hyg.*, **47**, 215.
GARHAB, M. H. (1957) *Alex. med. J.*, **3**, 13.
GIRGIS, R. (1930) *J. trop. Med. Hyg.*, **33**, 7.
—— (1931) *J. trop. Med. Hyg.*, **34**, 65.
GOODWIN, L. G. and PAGE, J. E. (1943) *Biochem. J.*, **37**, 482.
HABIB, M. A. (1966) MD Thesis, Ein Shams.
HAENENS, G. D. and SANTELE, A. (1955) *Ann. Soc. belge Med. trop.*, **35**, 497.
HALAWANI, A. (1946) *J. Egypt. publ. Hlth Ass.*, **21**, 219.
HALAWANI, A. and BADRAN, A. (1958) *J. Egypt. med. Ass.*, **41**, 439.
HALAWANI, A. E., WATSON, J. M., NOR-EL-DIN, G., HAFEZ, A. and DAWOOD, M. (1948) *J. Egypt med. Ass.*,
  31, 272.
HALAWANI, A. E. and ABDALLAH, A., SHAKER, M. W. and SAIF, M. (1956) *Lancet*, **1**, 190.
HALAWANI, A. E. and ABDALLAH, A. and SAIF, M. (1957) *Z. Tropenmed Parasit.*, **8**, 134.
HAMILTON, P. K., HUTCHISON, H. S., JAMISON, P. N. and JONES, J. R. (1959) *Amer. J. clin. Path.*, **32**, 18.
HASHEM, M. (1931) *J. Egypt. med. Ass.*, **14**, 461.
—— (1947) *J. roy. Egypt. med. Ass.*, **30**, 48.
—— (1947) *J. roy. Egypt. med. Ass.*, **40**, 1.
—— (1961) *J. Egypt. med. Ass.*, **44**, 857.
HASHEM, M. and ARAFA, M. (1951) *Pri. Int. Soc. Gastroentro.*, Bologna, Italy.
HASHEM, M., ZAKI, S. A. and HUSSEIN, M. (1961) *J. Egypt med. Ass.*, **44**, 579.
HASSEEB, N. M. (1964) MD Thesis, Ein Shams.
HILL, D. H. and ONABAMIRO, S. D. (1960) *Brit. vet. J.*, **116**, 145.
HSU, S. and HSU, H. (1961) *Science*, **133**, 176.
HUMBERTO, M. (1963) *Amer. J. trop. Med. Hyg.*, **12**, 741.
HUNTER, G. W., CRANDALL, R. B., ZICKAFOOSE, D. E. and PURVIS, Q. B. (1962) *Amer. J. trop. Med. Hyg.*,
  11, 17.
HUTCHINSON, H. S. (1928) *Amer. J. Path.*, **4**, 11.
ISHAK, K. (1957) *J. Egypt. med. Ass.*, **40**, 461.
JORDAN, P. (1966) *Brit. med. J.*, **5482**, 276.
KAGAN, I. (1958) Rice Institute Pamphlet, **45**, 151.
KARTULIS, S. (1885) *Lancet*, **2**, 346.
KHALIL, M. (1928) *Proc. roy. Soc. trop. Med. (Cairo)*, **3**, 270.
—— (1931) *Arch. Schiffs. trop. Hyg.*, **31**, 1.
—— (1938) *J. Egypt. med. Ass.*, **21**, 95.
—— (1941) *J. Egypt. med. Ass.*, **24**, 439.
KHATTAB, M. *et al* (1959) *J. Egypt. Soc. Endocr.*, **5**, 1.
KLOETZEL, K. (1962) *Amer. J. trop. Med. Hyg.*, **11**, 472.
—— (1967) *Trans. roy. Soc. trop. Med. Hyg.*, **61**, 803.
KUNTZ, R. E. (1958) *Proc. helm. Soc. Wash.*, **25**, 37.
LA GRANGE, E. (1953) *Ann. Soc. belge Med. trop.*, **33**, 227.
LA GRANGE, E. and FAIN, A. (1952) *Ann. Soc. belge Med. trop.*, **32**, 53.
LAMBERT, C. R. (1966) *Acta Tropica*, **32**, 137.
LAWTON, F. B. (1918) *J. roy. Army med. Cps.*, **31**, 6, 472-479.
LEA, C. V. (1928) *In* HASHEM, M., 1947, *J. roy. Soc. med. Ass.*, **30**, 48.
LEES, R. E. (1967) *Trans. roy. Soc. trop. Med. Hyg.*, **61**, 806.
LEIPER, R. T. (1918) *J. roy. Army med. Cps.*, **30**, 117.
LE ROUX, P. L. (1933) *J. Helminth.*, **11**, 57.
—— (1954) *J. Helminth.*, **48**, 3.
LEVINE, M. D., GAZOLI, R. F., KUNTZ, R. E. and KILLOUGH, J. H. (1948) *J. Parasit.*, **34**, 158.
MADDEN, F. C. (1969) *J. trop. Med. Hyg.*, **12**, 24, 370.
MADEN, F. C. (1918) *Urol. cutan. Rev.*, **22**, 677.
MAGDI, T. and HEFNAWY, F. (1950) *Bilharzia of Female Genital Organs*. Cairo: Sch. Press.
MAHFOUZ, M. M. and EL-DEEB, A. A. (1962) *Proc. 1st int. Cong. Bilh. (Cairo)*, **1**, 767.
MAHFOUZ, N. (1939) *Atlas of O.B.T. Gynaecology*. London: Sheral.
MAINZER, F. and KRAUSE, M. (1940) *Trans. roy. Soc. trop. Med. Hyg.*, **33**, 405.
MAKAR, N. (1955) *Urological Aspects of Bilharzia*. Cairo: Soc. Orientale de Pub.
—— (1955) *Urological Aspects of Bilharziasis in Egypt*.
MALLAH, S. and HASHAM, M. (1953) *Thorax*, **8**, 148.

MANDAHL-BARTH, G. (1957) *Bull. Wld Hlth Org.*, **16**, 1103.
—— (1957) *Bull. Wld Hlth Org.*, **17**, 1.
MARCHAND, J. E. *et al* (1957) *Arch. int. Med.*, **100**, 965.
MARTINS, A. V., MARTINS, G., BRITO, R. DE SIEBRA (1955) *Rev. Bras. Malar.*, **7**, 269.
MAZHAR, K. and SHAABAN, H. H. (1962) *Proc. 1st int. Cong. Bilh. (Cairo)*, **1**, 659.
McKENZIE, A. (1932) *Trans. roy. Soc. trop. Med. Hyg.*, **25**, 407.
MEHREZ, H. E. *et al* (1953) *Amer. J. trop. Med. Hyg.*, **2**, 883.
MEHREZ, I. (1958) *Gaz. Kasr El-Aini Fac. Med.*, **24**, 208.
MENZES, H. (1965) *Rev. Inst. Med. trop. (São Paulo)*, **70**, 2, 65.
—— (1967) *Bilharziasis*, p. 175. Basle: Springer verlag.
MORALES, F. H. (1942) *Bull. publ. Hlth trop. Med.*, **18**, 1113.
MOUSA, A. H. *et al* (1957) *Gaz. Kasr El-Aini (Cairo)*, **23**, 1.
MOUSA, A. H. and EL-GAREM, A. (1959) *J. Egypt med. Ass.*, **42**, 444.
MOUSA, A. H. and ATA, A. A. (1960) *J. Egypt. med. Ass.*, **43**, 846.
MOUSA, A. H. and GAREM, A. A. (1963) *Proc. 7th int. Cong. trop. Med. (Rio de Janeiro)*.
NELSON, G. S. (1960) *Trans. roy. Soc. trop. Med. Hyg.*, **54**, 301.
—— (1962) *Ciba Foundation Symposium on Bilharziasis*, p. 127.
NORONHA (1947) *Bull. Soc. Ophtal. Paris*, **3**, 409.
OLIVER-GONZALEZ, J., BAUMAN, P. M. and BENENSON, A. S. (1956) *Amer. J. trop. med. Hyg.*, **5**, 290.
OLIVIER, L. (1949) *Amer. J. Hyg.*, **49**, 290.
OZAWA (1928) *Jap. J. exp. Med.*, **95**.
PALMER, F. (1947) *Amer. J. trop. Med.*, **27**, 45.
PITCHFORD, R. J. (1959) *Trans. roy. Soc. trop. Med. Hyg.*, **52**, 213.
PORTER, A. (1926) *S. Afr. J. Sci.*, **23**, 661.
RASLAVICUS, F. A. (1965) *Amer. J. trop. Med. Hyg.*, **14**, 100.
RUAS, A. and FRANCO, A. L. T. (1966) *Acta trop. Suppl.*, **9**, 203.
RUFFER, A. (1910) *Brit. med. J.*, **1**, 16.
SADUN, E. WILLIAMS, J. and ANDERSON, R. (1960) *Proc. Soc. exp. Biol. Med.*, **105**, 289.
SAFWAT, M. (1961) *J. Egypt. med. Ass.*, **44**, 8.
SALEM, H. and SHERIF, A. (1960) *J. Egypt. publ. Hlth Ass.*, **35**, 95.
SAMBON, M. F. (1907) *J. trop. Med. Hyg.*, **11**, 3, 44.
SAMI, A. (1962) *Proc. 1st int. Cong. Bilh. (Cairo)*, **2**, 448.
SAOAD, M. (1965) Ph.D. Thesis, London.
SEBAEI, I. (1961) *Kasr El-Aini J. Surg.*, **2**, 183.
SHAMMA, A. H. (1965) *Bilharzial Hepatic Fibrosis*. Baghdad.
SHAW, A. F. B. and GHAREEB, A. A. (1928) *J. Path. Bact.*, **46**, 401.
—— (1938) *J. Path. Bact.*, **47**, 115.
SHOEB, S. and BASMY, K. (1967) *J. Egypt. med. Ass.*, **50**, 3.
SMITHERS, S. R. (1962) *Ciba Foundation Symposium on Bilharziasis*, p. 239.
SOROUR, M. F. (1928) *Proc. Cong. int. Med. trop. Hyg. (Cairo)*, **4**, 322, 367.
STANDEN, O. D. (1953) *Ann. trop. Med. Parasit.*, **47**, 26.
—— (1955) *Brit. J. Pharmacol.*, **10**, 191.
STEIN, H. B. (1938) *S. Afr. med. J.*, **12**, 297.
STIJNS, J. (1952) *Ann. Parasit. hum. comp.*, **27**, 385.
STIREWALT, M. A. and EVANS, A. S. (1952) *J. infect. Dis.*, **91**, 191.
SYMMERS, W. ST (1904) *J. Path. Bact.*, **4**, 237.
—— (1908) *C.R. 1st Egypt. med. Cong. (Cairo)*, **2**, 18.
TALAAT, S. M. and SHOAIB, S. (1953) *Trans. roy. Soc. trop. Med. Hyg.*, **47**, 425.
TOPOZADA, H. K. (1962) *Proc. 1st int. Cong. Bilh. (Cairo)*, **1**, 667.
TOUSSAINT, A. and ANDERSON, R. (1965) *Appl. Microbiol.*, **13**, 552.
ULTRA and SILVA (1916) *Trans. Confer. (Buenos Aires)*.
VOGEL, H. (1958) *Bull. Wld Hlth Org.*, **18**, 1097.
WARREN, K. S. (1961) *Amer. J. trop. Med. Hyg.*, **10**, 670.
WOLFE, H. L. (1967) *Lancet*, **18**, 350.
WOODRUFF, A. W. *et al* (1963) *7th int. trop. Med. Malar. (Rio de Janeiro)*.
WORLD HEALTH ORGANIZATION (1965) *Wld Hlth Org. Techn. Rep. Ser.*, No. 229.
—— (1965) *Wld Hlth Org. Monogr. Ser.*, No. 50.
—— (1967) *Tech. Rep. Ser.*, No. 349.
ZAHER, M. F. *et al* (1956) *J. Egypt. med. Ass.*, **39**, 48.
ZAKI, H. A., EL-HENEIDY, A. R. and FODA, M. T. (1962) *Brit. Med. J.*, **1**, 367.
ZAYAT, M. A. and GAAFER, A. (1959) *Alex. med. J.*, **2**, 61.

14
Filariasis

Definition

A disease caused by infection with the filarial worm *Loa loa* and characterised by repeatedly occurring swellings of the subcutaneous tissue and the occasional appearance of adult *L. loa* beneath the skin and less commonly the conjunctiva.

Aetiology

Causative organism. Adult male *L. loa* measure approximately 3 cm in length by 350 μm in breadth; the female measures 5–7 cm in length by approximately 500 μm in breadth. The worms are creamy-white in colour, and viewed microscopically, the cuticle is seen, except at the anterior and posterior extremities, to be covered with knob-like processes known as cuticular bosses.

Adults live and travel widely in subcutaneous tissues; the females produce microfilariae which are sheathed and measure approximately 250 by 8 μm. When stained, they have a curiously irregular outline as contrasted with microfilariae of *Wuchereria bancrofti*. The nuclei within the microfilariae extend to the tip of the organism, unlike those of *W. bancrofti* in which the nuclei stop some distance short of the tip.

Epidemiology

Distribution. The infection is, it seems, transmitted only in parts of tropical Africa, the most highly endemic area being that bordering on the Gulf of Guinea, particularly Cameroun. It occurs, however, over much of West Africa, in the Congo, south-western Sudan and parts of Uganda. Occasionally transmission has been suspected in non-African tropical regions, but enquiry has invariably shown that patients affected have resided at some time in tropical Africa.

Vectors. The infective larvae of *L. loa* are transmitted by flies of the genus *Chrysops*, which breed on the floors of streams covered by sand, fine mud and decaying leaves and in the mud around such streams which usually flow through dense forests. In West Africa the species most concerned with human transmission are *C. silaca* and *C. dimidiata*, although *C. zahria* has been found to be infected in southern Nigeria, and in the southern Sudan *C. distinctipnnis* and *C. longicornis* have also been found to be naturally infected. In Cameroun *C. longicornis*, *C. langi* and *C. griseicollis* may also at times be vectors, but it is believed that they usually transmit only the siminian form of the disease. All these *Chrysops* flies normally live in the canopy of high rain forest trees and usually obtain their blood meals from monkeys, but *C. silaca* and *C. dimidiata* will descend to ground level if in need of a blood meal and will then obtain it from man. In these flies the larvae develop more rapidly than in *C. longicornis*, *C. langi* and *C. griseicollis*, so that they form the most useful vectors of the human infection.

Transmission. The smoke from wood fires is attractive to the flies, and those who are frequently exposed to an atmosphere of this smoke are particularly liable to be bitten by them; this is of course of particular relevance to indigenous inhabitants of endemic areas who very often live in huts in which there is an open wood fire. *Chrysops* flies do not bite in darkness, semi-darkness and direct sunlight; the interiors of well-lit houses are therefore places in which the flies commonly seek a blood meal. Movement is attractive to them, particularly when it occurs in groups of persons, and the flies have been noted to congregate around such groups.

The distance between man and the edge of the forest in which flies are living markedly affects the probability of the flies having access to human blood meals. It has been found that a clear space of 1000 to 2000 yards may be sufficient to prevent flies penetrating from their breeding areas to those in which they can feed on man and that the further a village is away from the forest fringe, the lower is the incidence of loiasis among those living there. Only female *Chrysops* are blood feeders.

Pathology

The bites which the *Chrysops* inflict on man are almost invariably deeply situated in the subcutaneous tissues and cause a small area of local haemorrhage. It is in this situation that the infective larva is deposited and migrates along fascial planes. The great majority of evidence suggests that it is in these fascial planes that the worm, once mature, remains throughout its life, and extensive observations in wild monkeys infected with monkey loiasis did not reveal worms elsewhere than in subcutaneous tissue (Gordon *et al*, 1950). Other workers have, however, reported the finding of an occasional worm in the brains of dogs and monkeys, and Kivits (1942) reported four fatal cases of encephalitis in humans whose cerebrospinal fluid contained microfilariae of *L. loa*, although it was not contaminated with blood, thus suggesting that the microfilariae had not entered the cerebrospinal fluid in blood resulting from trauma caused by the aspirating needles. It seems possible, therefore, that in man the microfilariae are either able to pass through the choroidal plexus or that worms occasionally reach the subarachnoid space. Microfilariae appear to be unable to pass the placental barrier, for congenital filariasis is not known.

The reasons underlying the periodicity of microfilariae in the blood are imperfectly understood in spite of much work within recent years. Variations in the diurnal concentration of oxygen and carbon dioxide are generally considered to be insufficient to account for the periodicity of the microfilariae. It appears that they are thermosensitive and that small variations in body temperature probably act as a trigger mechanism precipitating movement of the microfilariae, but why this mechanism should be effective is unknown.

The pathological changes responsible for the typical Calabar swellings which occur in loiasis have not been worked out. It seems that they are a form of allergic response, but it is not known with certainty whether this response is occurring around a worm situated in or near the swelling or whether the tissues are sensitised generally by adsorption of antibodies to *L. loa* and the swelling in sensitised tissues then occurs as a result of an additional mechanism interfering with stability of the tissues; in this connection such a mechanism might involve muscular exercise and accumulation of products of metabolism. Certainly, Calabar swellings are well known to occur in the vicinity of joints following vigorous exercise; it is not uncommon for a swelling to commence in the hand, wrist or elbow following vigorous use of the arm in carpentry or sport and similar activities.

Immunological changes. In loiasis, as in other helminthic infections in which the worms or their larvae invade the tissues or blood, some increase in the gamma globulin faction of the serum is usually found. Antibodies resulting from infection circulate in the plasma for as long as parasitaemia is present and for a variable time, commonly up to 6 months, after successful treatment with eradication of the infection. During this period they may be detected by a complement fixation test in which the antigen has been prepared from various filarial worms. The test is not species-specific and this has resulted in a considerable variety of such worms being used as antigen. When infection is no longer active the complement fixation test reverts to negative, presumably as a result of cessation of antibody production and breakdown or elimination of that which had been present in the plasma. As is the case in many infections, antibodies may be present in higher concentration in the plasma shortly after a successful course of treatment, and this is thought to result from the death of the parasites, their absorption and the consequent response of the antibody producing tissues to the availability of such amounts of antigen.

Antibody is adsorbed on skin cells and its presence there is the basis of a skin test which may be performed by injecting intradermally a sterile solution in saline of antigen. The most usual solution is of one part dried worm antigen in 1000 parts sterile physiological saline. Following incubation the antigenic solution is sterilised by filtration through a Seitz filter or a Millipore filter. It is important to standardise the antigen and to adjust the nitrogen content, usually to between 10 and 15 μg/100 ml. 0.1 ml of such a solution is injected and the size of the wheal raised measured; a positive result is usually taken to be doubling in the area of the wheal within 20 minutes. Those who exhibit a positive skin test usually continue to do so for many years after the infection has ceased to be present, presumably because antibody adsorbed on the skin cells is eliminated only very slowly. The skin test, like the complement fixation test, is genus-specific but not species-specific.

The antibodies responsible for the complement fixation test and the skin test do not appear to possess any protective function.

Clinical features

The main clinical manifestations of the infection consist of the appearance of swellings, commonly known as Calabar swellings, and from time to time of the appearance of adult worms beneath the skin of various parts of the body or beneath the conjunctiva. In addition there may, in some cases, be occasional attacks of fever, particularly when a Calabar swelling is present, and, rarely neurological symptoms develop which have been attributed to the presence of the worm or microfilariae in nervous tissue. Toussaint (1965) produced evidence that microfilariae of *L. loa* may occasionally cause choroidoretinitis.

Calabar swellings. These are the commonest and most distinctive clinical feature of loiasis. They usually consist of distinctly puffy tissue affecting the face, particularly the region of the orbit, or the limbs where the hand, wrist and forearms are most affected. There is a tendency for the swellings to occur around the medium sized joints. They may be pink from injection; they are not well circumscribed but fade gently into their contiguous tissues. They may be uncomfortable but are not painful. Their frequency varies widely in different patients and at different times; thus for a period of months some patients may seldom be without one, others or the same patient at another time may have one at only intervals of a year or so. Each swelling usually persists for from a few hours to a day or two and disappears slowly. Those on the limbs are often preceded by vigorous use or movement of the affected part. At times mild fever accompanies the swellings.

Adult worms. Most patients see and feel adult worms beneath the skin at some time during the course of the infection. The worms not uncommonly remain in a locality for several days and appear from time to time during this period. They will be visible beneath the skin for some minutes or an hour or two and then work their way into deeper tissues. They appear to be positively thermotropic and it is not uncommon for those who have been sitting in front of a fire to encounter the worms beneath the skin of the warm shin. Peripheral neuritis, affecting respectively the median and ulnar nerves, has been attributed to migration of the worms in the region of the carpal tunnel and medial epicondyle at the elbow. More serious neurological damage has been reported by Kivits (1952) and by Bertrand-Fontaine (1948). The former described four fatal cases of encephalitis in which microfilariae of *L. loa* were found in the cerebrospinal fluid. The presumptive evidence that loiasis was the cause of the encephalitis was strong but the author admitted that a viral encephalitis could not be ruled out with certainty. Bertrand-Fontaine also reported presumptive evidence that *L. loa* adults or microfilariae had produced bilateral hemiplegia. The patient he described was only 31 years of age, free from hypertension and syphilis, and ventriculography had shown no sign of a cerebral tumour. The patient made a complete recovery following treatment of the loiasis. Migraine has also been attributed to loiasis.

When the adult loa appear beneath the conjunctiva, they usually take a minute or so to wriggle from one side of the eye to the other before disappearing into the orbital tissues. During their passage they cause considerable discomfort and the patient is not uncommonly aware of movement in the orbit and discomfort for some days.

Some degree of leucocytosis with eosinophilia is usual during the course of loiasis.

Diagnosis

Identification of the microfilariae or adult worms is the most satisfactory means of diagnosis. As the microfilariae have a diurnal periodicity, blood is best taken during the day for this purpose. When microfilariae are scanty 2–3 ml blood may be laked with water, centrifuged and the deposit examined. An estimation of the number of microfilariae present in the blood may be obtained by spreading a measured amount, commonly 20 mm^3 on one or more microscope slides, staining with Leishman's stain and examining the whole. Various filtration techniques are also utilised. Adult *L. loa* can occasionally be removed from under the skin, more particularly when they have died in that situation during diethylcarbamazine therapy. They are also occasionally removed from beneath the conjunctiva, but except in skilled hands this procedure is hardly justifiable.

Adult female *L. loa* range in size from 5 to 7 cm in length by 0.5 mm in breadth. Males vary from 3 to 3.4 cm by 0.35 to 0.45 mm. The microfilariae range from 250 to 300 μm.

A complement fixation test using for the purpose an alcoholic extract of *Dirofilaria immitis* or other filarial worm is used in a number of specialised laboratories. It gives valuable results, particularly when taken in association with the clinical features and the presence or otherwise of eosinophilia. Weak cross-reactions may occur with serum from patients with *Strongyloides stercoralis*, but a strongly positive filarial complement fixation test in association with clinical features suggestive of the disease is of great diagnostic significance.

Skin test. A sterile aqueous solution of filarial protein may be used for an intradermal diagnostic test. Such a solution usually contains between 10 and 20 μg of helminthic protein per ml. An intradermal injection of 0.1 ml of the solution is made and a positive test is usually taken as one in which the initial wheal doubles its area within 20–30 minutes.

Eosinophilia. Some degree of eosinophilia which is usually present during the active phases of the *L. loa* infection may provide a general guide to the presence of helminthiasis.

Treatment

The only really effective drug for the treatment of loiasis is diethylcarbamazine, but fortunately it is highly satisfactory in its action against this parasite so that other drugs are not required. It is administered orally as the citrate or hydrochloride salt, and proprietary preparations of it are known as Banocide, Hetrazan, Notezine and Carbilazine. An initial dose of 0.25–0.5 mg drug per kilogram of the patient's body weight is given and if this is well tolerated the dose is administered thrice on the following day; thereafter the dose is doubled each day until 3 mg per kg body weight is being administered thrice daily. At this level the dosage should continue for 21 days.

Immediate effects of treatment include the development of urticarial wheals, headache, nausea and in some cases fever. The latter may occasionally be severe enough to require interruption of treatment. These symptoms occur simultaneously with the disappearance of microfilariae from the blood; usually very few can be found 24 hours after the administration of a dose of 3 mg per kg body weight. The full course of treatment will however ensure complete eradication of the microfilariae and of adult worms. The headache and skin manifestations occur at the same time as microfilariae are disappearing from the blood or shortly after they have done so. They are results of the death and disintegration of the microfilariae; they are not toxic effects of the drug itself for if therapeutic amounts of the drug are given to non-infected persons such symptoms do not develop.

Within the first 2–3 weeks after commencing treatment the white cell count rises, sometimes to 20 or 30 000 per mm^3 and the proportion of eosinophils also greatly increases and may reach 60–70 per cent. In some patients adult *L. loa* may die beneath the skin, where they form linear protuberances. Antihistamines may be required for control of the allergic symptoms occurring during treatment. These symptoms are of course akin to a Herxheimer type of reaction; they settle down within days, but eosinophils if present may not disappear for 2–3 months.

Following treatment relapses are very rare, a complete cure being almost invariable. A weakly positive or negative complement fixation test may become positive during or shortly after treatment and may take some months to revert to negative. A filarial skin test however, once positive, usually remains so for many years.

In some areas and with some patients, reactions to treatment may be severe, but with a cautious approach and the use of antihistamines interruption of treatment is very seldom necessary. Steroid therapy may very occasionally be needed to diminish allergic responses during therapy.

Prognosis

The prognosis in treated patients is excellent. Reinfection may occur among those who continue to live in an endemic area but relapses are of the greatest rarity among those who following treatment reside in a non-endemic region.

Prevention

The best method of prevention is to avoid the bites of the vector *Chrysops*. Fly-proofing of houses and the wearing of clothing that covers the limbs as well as the body will do much towards this end.

Chemoprophylaxis has been carried out on an experimental scale using diethylcarbamazine in doses of 200 mg taken on three successive days at monthly intervals.

DIPETALONEMA PERSTANS INFECTIONS

Dipetalonema perstans also occurs only in Africa where it is frequent in those areas in which loa loa and bancroftian filariasis are common. The adult worm frequents the mesentery, the perirenal areas, the retroperitoneal tissues and the pericardium. The microfilariae do not inhabit the skin. Infection produces positive serological and skin tests for filariasis but does not cause symptoms.

Trichlorophone has been used with success in Mexico. It is given in fortnightly doses of 10 mg/kg a total of four doses is given. It is said to kill both adult worms and larvae. Toxic effects are slight but nausea, colicky abdominal pains and diarrhoea may occur.

WUCHERERIA BANCROFTI INFECTIONS

NOMENCLATURE. *Wuchereria bancrofti* (Cobbold, 1877) has in the past also been known as *Filaria sanguinis hominis* (Bush, 1872); *Filaria bancrofti*

(Cobbold, 1877); *Filaria nocturna* (Manson, 1891); *Filaria philippinensis* (Ashburn and Cray, 1906). The disease it causes is commonly referred to as bancroftian filariasis.

Epidemiology and distribution

W. bancrofti is the most widely distributed of the human filarial parasites and occurs in many regions throughout the tropics and subtropics; it is found between 30° north and 30° south in the western hemisphere and 41° north and 28° south in the eastern hemisphere. It is heavily endemic in many parts of India and the Far East, tropical Africa and the tropical Americas. Very high prevalence rates have been reported from many Pacific islands, and from these during World War II large numbers of troops were invalided because of filariasis.

In Africa, the East African High Commission Filariasis Research Unit during the years 1951–54 found high prevalence rates in the hot damp parts of Tanzania where microfilariae were encountered in the blood even in infants under the age of 1 year and in some localities up to 60 per cent of the adult population were shown to have microfilaraemia. Similarly Hammon *et al* (1967) report that 'the economic development of African states implies rural and environmental changes and large movements of population which, if no action is taken, will result in a wide spread of the vectors and permit the appearance of new foci of bancroftian filariasis'. They point out that though bancroftian filariasis is widespread in tropical Africa, especially in coastal areas and in lowland savannahs, its distribution in forested areas is very patchy and there the disease has perhaps recently been introduced.

W. bancrofti surveys in tropical Africa have never been carried out on a routine basis and discrepancies in its distribution and prevalence are probably linked to the lack of comprehensive investigations in many areas. Similarly, infection with *W. bancrofti* in man has, it is thought, increased as a result of urbanisation in parts of India (Joseph and Prasad, 1967). The parasite has been found to be important in Rangoon, where much work on it has been carried out under the aegis of the World Health Organization (*Bull. Wld. Hlth. Org.*, 1967). In particular the vector there, *Culex pipiens fatigans*, its bionomics and means of control have been studied in detail.

Vectors. The principal vector is *Culex fatigans*, which is well adapted to transmission in that many strains feed on human rather than animal blood and breed in close proximity to man. Thus its larvae thrive in contaminated water in receptacles such as cisterns, septic tanks, old tins and broken bottles, calabash shells and the like found around human dwellings. *C. fatigans* readily enters houses and control of it is possible by residual spraying, but this should include the upper as well as the lower surfaces of walls. *Anopheline* mosquitoes which have been found to be naturally infected include *A. funestus* in Congo and Tanzania, *A. gambiae* and *A. funestus* in parts of East Africa, *A. gambiae* and *A. maculipennis* in Rhodesia, and *A. gambiae* and *A. melas* in Ghana. Members of the genus *Aedes* have also been found naturally infected, as for example *A. scapullaris* in Brazil, *A. polypnesiensis* in the Central and South Pacific and *A. fijiensis* and *A. pseudoscutellaris* in Fiji. Experimentally infection with larvae of *W. bancrofti* has been induced in a wide variety of mosquitoes.

Aetiology

Causative organism. The adult male is approximately 4 cm long by 0.1 mm in diameter; the adult female is approximately twice this size, being 8–10 cm in length and 0.24–0.3 mm in diameter. The anterior extremity tapers bluntly so that the parasites have a rounded end. The vulva is situated close behind the anterior extremity of the female. The male is equipped with two spicules measuring 0.6 and 0.2 mm.

Habitat. The adult worms live in the lymph nodes and vessels and the females produce embryonated ova containing first-stage larvae, or microfilariae. The latter become active at or just before liberation from the worm and soon escape from the ovum to appear as sheathed microfilariae in the blood in which they have nocturnal periodicity. The microfilariae, on being taken up in the blood meals of vector mosquitoes, develop into larvae infective to man. These are not capable of penetrating the unbroken human skin but presumably enter the tissues via the puncture mark made by the mosquito in biting. The posterior extremity of the microfilariae tapers gradually and the tip is free from nuclei.

Pathology

The earliest pathological changes recognised in man occur it seems several months after the infective larvae have been introduced into the tissues. During this period the patient has usually been infected on a number of occasions and has had an opportunity therefore to become sensitive to the larvae and the developing worms and their products. The lymphatics are principally affected and the changes within them may be divided into acute, subacute and chronic stages. During the acute stages there is inflammation in the vicinity of the worm which may be found tightly coiled within a lymphatic. These acute inflammatory changes are marked by the presence of many polymorphonuclear cells among which eosinophils predominate; there is oedema and proliferation of reticuloendothelial cells. Similar changes have been produced experimentally by the injection of *D. immitis* antigen.

The acute changes merge in a period of a week or so into those of the subacute stage. There is granulomatous reaction and enlargement of the lymphatic nodes and sinuses in which numerous macrophages, reticuloendothelial cells, eosinophils and foreign body giant cells are to be found. Proliferation of the endothelium of the lymphatics occurs, the lymphatic wall becomes thickened and oedematous and its lumen narrowed. Around the worm a cellular exudate occurs and tissue necroses. Adult worms lie tightly coiled in dilatations of the lymphatics and lymph nodes, particularly in the cortical part of the nodes.

In the chronic stage, the inflammation is replaced by fibrosis and maybe cicatrisation. Later there is absorption of granulomatous tissues and possibly hyalinisation or calcification of scar tissue, particularly around dead or degenerating worms. Varicosity of lymphatics develops in some places and other lymphatics are replaced by fibrous strands. There is evidence that the affected lymphatic channels first become varicose, and later fibrose and atrophy, perhaps becoming totally obliterated.

In elephantiasis there is much extracellular fluid which is comparatively rich in protein which amounts to approximately 2 per cent instead of the normal 0.02 per cent found in extracellular fluid. There is much hypertrophy of hypodermal and dermal connective tissue and proliferation of collagen.

Pathogenesis of elephantiasis. The classical view is that obstruction of the lymphatics, particularly as they pass through lymphatic nodes, impedes the flow of lymph and causes it to be retained in the affected limb. It has however also been shown that fluid in elephantoid limbs contains more protein than does that in normal tissue. Lymphography in elephantoid limbs reveals that there is first dilatation and tortuosity of the lymph channels and stasis of the fluid within them; later the channels atrophy. Phlebographic studies have shown that in such limbs there is often some venous as well as lymphatic stasis.

The increased protein in the lymph in elephantoid limbs may result from disintegration of macrophages, microfilariae and erythrocytes. There is much fibrous tissue generally in these limbs and this by contracting and obstructing lymph channels which have not been already obstructed by fibrosis caused by lymphangitis all adds to the picture of lymphatic obstruction. Much work on this subject was done in the period shortly after World War II and this work is reviewed by Woodruff (1961). Valuable lymphographic studies of elephantoid limbs were done by Cohen *et al* (1961).

The site of the lymphatic involvement determines in large measure the part of the body to become elephantoid or oedematous. From comparative studies of elephantiasis and hydrocoele in patients infected with *W. bancrofti*, it has been concluded (Jordan, 1955) that in patients with hydrocoele, the obstruction is in the para-aortic nodes and in those with elephantiasis of the leg, it is in the inguinal or iliac group of nodes. The lymph from the leg drains into the superficial and deep inguinal nodes between which there is little communication, and all the lymph from them passes to the external iliac group situated at the bifurcation of the common iliac arteries. Obstruction to lymph passing through them causes elephantiasis of the legs. Lymphatics from the scrotal skin also pass through the superficial inguinal nodes, lesions of which give rise to elephantiasis of the scrotum.

Lymph from the tunica vaginalis, the epididymis and spermatic cord, however, drains into the para-aortic nodes though some from the tunica vaginalis and the tail of the epididymis reaches these nodes after first passing through the external iliac group. Lesions of the para-aortic nodes cause obstruction, therefore, to fluid passing through the tunica vaginalis, and thus cause hydrocoele but not oedema of the scrotal skin which drains into the superficial inguinal group. If both hydrocoele and elephantiasis of the scrotum are present, it is believed that both groups, i.e. the superficial inguinal and para-aortic, are involved.

Persons with elephantiasis seldom exhibit microfilariaemia, but microfilariae are more commonly found in association with filarial hydrocoele. Jordan (1955) found microfilariae in only 4.3 per cent of 259 persons with elephantiasis but found them in 25 per cent of 957 persons with filarial hydrocoeles. Among 59 who had elephantiasis of a leg and hydrocoele, microfilariae were found in the blood of only 2 (i.e. 3 per cent).

Immunology. Complement-fixing antibodies

develop in persons infected with *W. bancrofti* and these have been used as a basis for a diagnostic complement fixation test. This gives positive reactions, particularly during the first few years following infection, but as the duration of infection increases the proportion of positive reactors diminishes. The strength of the complement fixation test may be paralleled by the degree of eosinophilia present.

Since it became possible to identify and quantify immunoglobulins in serum and other tissues, it has been shown that in filarial infections generally serum IgM is significantly increased. This immunoglobulin is especially directed against and able to destroy many surfaces foreign to the individual.

Particulate antigens act as potent stimuli to the production of IgM, especially when these antigens are continuously presented to the blood stream (Hobbs, 1968). Molecules of appropriate IgM are capable of attaching themselves to the foreign surface, fix and activate complement and cause a hole to be made in the surface. This process plays an important part in the causation of lysis.

Periodicity of microfilariae. The periodicity of microfilariae of *W. bancrofti* continues to pose considerable problems. Many theories have been put forward, and among those current during recent years have been sensitivity to changes in oxygen and carbon dioxide tension occurring in peripheral as contrasted with central blood. McFadzean (1952) showed that in infected monkeys exposure to an atmosphere of 60 per cent oxygen resulted in migration of microfilariae from deeply placed lung vessels to the peripheral blood and that even during the microfilariaemia occurring at night, such exposure can augment the number of microfilariae in the peripheral blood. The changes in oxygen tension occurring in the blood of man during the night as contrasted with the day, however, are not sufficient to bring about the changes in the distribution of microfilariae which can be observed experimentally.

There appears to be no doubt the deep vessels, particularly those of the heart and lungs, are those in which the microfilariae of *W. bancrofti* congregate during the day and from which they migrate to the peripheral blood at night. This receives support from the findings of Rowlands (1956), who showed that the lungs and heart muscle of a man who died in Ghana during the day contained many more microfilariae per unit volume of blood than did that of peripheral organs. Hawking *et al* (1967) have published a series of detailed studies of microfilarial periodicity; no final answer to this periodicity can be given, but it appears that the microfilariae are sensitive to diurnal thermal changes.

Clinical features

W. bancrofti gives rise to widely differing clinical features among different persons infected in one endemic focus and the predominating clinical features may also differ between one focus and another. This variability has been explained by Beaver (1970) as resulting from disturbances in the host-parasite relationship. He states that most indigenous populations have evolved a relationship which is satisfactory to the parasite and tolerable to the host but that the introduction of infection into new geographic regions inhabited by different types of people, or the immigration of different peoples into those areas with established filarial endemicity, could introduce unsatisfactory and poorly tolerated combinations of host and parasite. He points out that areas of undisturbed endemic infection without evident disease are common.

An early symptom is the appearance of lymphangitis which very often affects the leg, sometimes the scrotum, less commonly the arm. Much study of these early symptoms was carried out among United States troops in endemic areas in the Pacific during World War II. Among these troops it was found that symptoms never occurred until at least 5 months after the first possible date of infection and the usual incubation period was between 5 and 18 months (Wartman, 1947). The lymphangitis causes swelling of the nodes draining the affected area, and these in order of frequency with which they may be detected by clinical examination are the inguinal, femoral, axillary and epitrochlear. A red streak appears on the affected part, usually in association with some malaise or fever which can be severe and disabling. Early attacks of the lymphangitis may be associated with puffiness of the scrotum or limb; in later attacks there usually is more definite oedema. The oedema disappears after the initial attack, but if attacks are repeated it becomes more permanent. In males the scrotum, testes and penis are commonly involved and become swollen and inflamed, the testis may become double its normal size and the vas stands out as a thick cord.

When attacks have been recurring for a year or two, oedema may become permanent, the legs, scrotum and penis being the organs most commonly affected, and less commonly the vulva, arms or breasts. The skin of the scrotum may become filled with vesicles distended with lymph. It then has a soft velvety feel when touched and the condition is known as lymph scrotum; it is a variant of the process leading to elephantiasis. Leakage from lymphatics into the genitourinary tract may result from lymphatic blockage, distension and later rupture of the lymphatics of the genitourinary tract which ramify with those conveying absorbed material, particularly fatty chyle, from the gastrointestinal tract. The urine then becomes milky or chylous in appearance. This chyluria may persist for weeks or months but more often lasts only for a few days at a time; it is, however, commonly recurrent over years. Sometimes the chyle is tinged with blood and presents a pinkish appearance. If the urine is allowed to settle in a conical urine glass, it is not uncommon to find a deposit of cellular material in the bottom of the glass. Chylous effusion into the peritoneal cavity, though rare, may result from similar lymphatic damage and, still rarer, chylous effusion into the pleural cavity has been reported.

Hydrocoele is a common complication of bancroftian filariasis when the para-aortic nodes are involved in the filarial process. As explained in the section on pathology, hydrocoele is not likely to be associated with oedema of the scrotal skin unless the superficial inguinal group of lymph nodes is also involved.

Elephantiasis may be steadily progressive and sometimes become enormous. There are usually recurrent attacks of inflammation affecting the elephantoid part. Some of these attacks may be of true filarial origin, others result from secondary bacterial infection. The latter is particularly likely to occur when sebaceous material and dirt accumulate in infolded skin of the affected part. The attachment of skin to the ligaments of the ankle in particular causes deep folds in this situation and these are common sites for the collection of such debris.

An important aspect of filarial infection is its psychological counterpart. The fear of progressive, chronic deformity, particularly that affecting the genitals, is a potent stimulus to the development of anxiety and other psychological states. Fortunately, in those with limited exposure and in those who have permanently left endemic areas, it is usually possible with justification to give an optimistic prognosis.

Blood. Particularly during the early phase of the infection leucocytosis with eosinophilia is usual; however, when the infection has been present for many months or years the white cell count is to be expected to return to normal.

In most patients the disease takes a prolonged and chronic course during much of which it may be asymptomatic but be punctuated by episodes of lymphangitis or local inflammation, some of which will be associated with fever.

Diagnosis

The pattern of clinical features and particularly recurrent attacks of lymphangitis associated with fever and lymphoedema, strongly suggest a diagnosis of *W. bancrofti* infection. Resort to the diagnostic procedures discussed below will usually greatly assist in confirming a suggestive diagnosis. Diagnostic investigations of particular value include (*a*) a search for eosinophilia which if present may give a general indication to the presence of an helminthic infection, (*b*) demonstration of microfilariae in the blood, (*c*) serological investigation and (*d*) intradermal tests.

Eosinophilia. Demonstration of eosinophilia gives no more than a general guide to the possible presence of an helminthic infection. It is a valuable and often overlooked investigation. It may be particularly helpful in pointing to an helminthic aetiology in patients with recurrent lymphangitis when not only this but also bacterial infection has to be considered.

Demonstration of microfilariae. These are not usually readily found in blood until the second or third year of infection; they are scanty or absent in the earlier stages and also in long-standing infections in which the adult worms have died but pathological changes persist. Examination of 20 mm³ of blood, measured in a simple haematological pipette and spread on one or more microscope slides, is a more convenient method and the measurement of the amount of blood being examined enabled comparisons to be made of the density of microfilariae at different times in one patient or between patients and groups of patients. After spreading on the slide the film is allowed to dry, is dehaemoglobinised and stained with Giemsa or Leishman's stain. Blood taken between 10 p.m. and 2 a.m. is most likely to exhibit microfilariae.

Various concentration techniques are employed to demonstrate microfilariae, and of these one of the most convenient is to lake 1–2 ml of blood with 10 ml water or dilute formalin solution. The resultant mixture is centrifuged and the deposit stained and examined. Larger quantities of blood may be dehaemoglobinised with nine times its volume of distilled water and passed through a filter such as one made from steel wire of 23 microns mesh or through filter paper. Microfilariae on the wire are rinsed into a watch glass or other suitable container in which they are searched for by a low-power microscope. Filter paper is dried and stained before being examined.

Serological investigations. The complement fixation test carried out with an alcoholic extract of *D. immitis* or *Setaria equina* is perhaps the most valuable of the immunological investigations. It may, however, become negative after the infection has been established for a year or two and there is evidence that cross-positive reactions at low but not at high dilution may be obtained with serum from patients with *Strongyloides stercoralis* infection. The test is of course a group one, but this does not impair its usefulness, for if a filarial infection is indicated by it, the species or type of infection could be indicated by clinical means or by isolation of the parasite. The test may be very valuable in lightly infected patients and in the prepatent period of the infection.

Intradermal test. Various filarial antigens are used intradermally for the diagnosis of filariasis and positive reactions tend to persist for long periods. Care must be taken to ensure that any particular antigen used does not give a significant proportion of cross-positive or false-positive reactions in patients with other helminthic infections.

Biopsy. Histological identification of adult worms in tissues gives, of course, a precise diagnosis, but biopsy for purely diagnostic purposes is not to be generally recommended. Worms can very seldom be located except in large lymphatic nodes and their excision will predispose to or aggravate lymphoedema. Thus biopsy of these lymphatic nodes as a diagnostic procedure can only be accomplished at the expense of making the patient's prognosis worse.

Radiology. Occasionally calcified worms will be found in X-ray films and have obvious diagnostic value.

Differential diagnosis

Hereditary lymphoedema or Milroy's disease. This is among the more difficult conditions to distinguish from filarial elephantiasis. In it, however, a history of involvement of other members of the family would be obtained and it is virtually always bilateral whereas bancroftian filariasis is more commonly unilateral. Although exceptions occur, Milroy's disease seldom gives rise to enormous elephantiasis.

Lymphangiography using the technique of Kinmonth (1954) may enable differentiation between Milroy's disease and filarial lymphoedema, for in Milroy's disease there is usually hypoplasia of the lymphatics which appear as straight atrophied lines on the lymphangiogram.

Such hypoplasia is present from a very early stage in the disease, but in filariasis at the stage of lymphoedema, lymphatic trunks are dilated, tortuous and more are apparent than in a normal lymphogram. As the disease becomes more long-standing, however, and elephantiasis develops, the lymphatics atrophy and fewer are apparent so that in both diseases the late picture may be similar (Cohen *et al*, 1961).

Lymphoedema from other causes. The associated history or presence of other diseases will usually provide evidence on which a satisfactory differential diagnosis can be made. Thus chronic lymphoedema may follow surgical removal of lymphatic nodes for cancer as for example in block dissection of the axilla for carcinoma of the breast. It may also occur in onchocerciasis when other features of onchocerciasis will provide a diagnostic clue. In Ethiopia and other parts of Africa a chronic lymphoedema of the legs has been described and attributed to prolonged exposure to soil and earth containing irritant minerals.

Venous thrombosis. This is usually easily distinguished from filarial lymphoedema by its more sudden onset, often during a period of illness and confinement to bed from some other cause. It causes the leg to be pale, white and to pit much more easily on pressure than with filarial lymphoedema—probably because in the latter chronic irritation and fibrous tissue render the limb resistant to pressure.

Lymphangitis. Lymphangitis caused by micro-organisms, fungal infections and other non-filarial agents is seldom recurrent as in filariasis. The clinical and laboratory features of filariasis are absent and the infection is not usually associated with eosinophilia.

Prognosis

Treatment during the early stages of bancroftian filariasis can be relied upon with a high degree of certainty to eradicate the infection, and if at the time elephantiasis has not developed, it is very unlikely to do so at a later date. In those who have elephantiasis at the time of treatment it is unusual for it to progress markedly, although some progression may have to be anticipated. In untreated patients with elephantiasis steady increase in size of the part may occur but in the majority of patients the downward progress is slow.

Treatment

Treatment with diethylcarbamazine will rapidly kill the microfilariae and will more slowly but

Q

nevertheless effectively kill adult *W. bancrofti*. Many studies have now shown that those so treated lose their microfilariae permanently unless re-infected; so that the adult worms must have been killed. The usual commencing dosage is 0.25 mg diethylcarbamazine per kilogram of the patient's body weight on the first day. The drug is administered orally and the dose increased according to tolerance up to 3 mg per kg body weight given thrice daily, at which level it is continued for 21 days. If no untoward reactions occur, the period between the initial small dosage and the maximal dosage may be reduced to 4–5 days.

Particularly during the early stages of treatment the patient may develop headache, fever, nausea, painful swellings of the lymph nodes and along lymphatics, and sometimes urticarial wheals. The generalised symptoms may be alleviated by the use of an antihistamine such as Phenergan in doses of 10 mg once or twice daily, but if the dosage of diethylcarbamazine is increased only gradually marked symptoms are unusual. Occasionally, however, high fever will develop and treatment should then be interrupted. Such interruption is preferable to coincident administration of corticosteroids which may interfere with the mechanism whereby the worms are killed and which can of course give rise to other sequelae. Following treatment of this kind with diethylcarbamazine, it is usual to find that microfilariae disappear from the blood within days or 2–3 weeks at most. Relapses occasionally occur after a few months.

The reactions which develop during treatment are a result of death, disintegration and absorption of microfilariae and/or adult worms and their products and these give rise to an allergic response on the part of the patient. Such reactions do not occur if a healthy person is given diethylcarbamazine in usually administered doses.

Elephantiasis. Treatment with diethylcarbamazine does not improve the patients with elephantiasis for this represents the end-result of a process initiated by the worms which however, in some instances, may be no longer living. The damage done unfortunately is all too often irreversible. If evidence of activity of infection is still present—such evidence being usually no more than eosinophilia for microfilariae are very seldom found in the blood of patients with elephantiasis—then a course of treatment with diethylcarbamazine is advisable. It is also advisable if the patient has not previously had a course of treatment because the worms may survive many years and continued production of microfilariae and other products by them might be expected to give rise to accumulating tissue damage.

Management of elephantiasis *per se* consists mainly of attempting to reduce the size of the affected part by supportive treatment. If the part is gross, however, plastic surgery may have to be considered.

In providing supportive treatment for elephantoid parts, the patient should remain in bed with the part elevated and if the leg or legs are affected the foot of the bed should be elevated as much as possible. Usually after a week or more the size of the part will have reduced considerably and if it is a leg that is being treated a closely fitting elastic stocking should then be used. It should be put on before the patient gets out of bed in the morning and not taken off until retirement at night. For scrotal elephantiasis a suspensory bandage will be used. These measures and selection of suitable employment where possible will do much towards increasing mobility of the patient and alleviating discomfort. Employment to be avoided for those with oedema of the dependent parts is that which involves prolonged standing such as working as a shop assistant or in a similar occupation.

Surgery in elephantiasis. Elephantiasis of the genitals can usually be treated very satisfactorily by surgery. Oedematous tissue is removed and flaps of relatively healthy skin are used to reform the scrotum or vulva. Surgery in elephantiasis of the limbs, however, is difficult and requires resources of a properly equipped department for plastic repair. Such repair is most often done for elephantiasis of the leg. Flaps of healthy skin are then prepared, beneath them lymphoedematous tissue is removed and the flaps then applied to the deep fascia. In successfully operated patients a functional limb results but a good cosmetic result can, of course, not be anticipated. Operations of this kind should only be recommended where the size of the limb is such that the patient's mobility is so restricted that the quality of their life or their ability to earn a living is severely reduced.

BRUGIA MALAYI INFECTIONS

These infections so closely resemble those caused by *W. bancrofti* that they do not merit a separate description. Only the important differences are recorded.

Distribution

The disease is common in Malaya, the East Indies, southern India and Ceylon. It exists as a zoonosis in cats, monkeys and other animals. Transmission to man from these animal sources, though suspected, has never been proved. There exists in Malaya a filarial worm, *B. pahangi*, which is closely similar to *B. malayi*. It has been found in many species of wild animal and is strongly suspected of infecting man in addition to its main role of maintaining a zoonosis.

Aetiology

Adult worm. Both sexes are slightly smaller than *W. bancrofti*.

Vector. The genera *Culex*, *Mansonioides* and *Anopheles* are the principal vectors. These mosquitoes breed in water which frequently contains the water lettuce, *Pistia*.

Clinical features

The onset of symptoms following exposure is more rapid than in *W. bancrofti* infections. Cases are on record in which symptoms developed within 3 months. The upper limbs are more frequently involved than in bancroftian infections. It is sometimes held that scrotal involvement is rare in the Malayan form. This is not so as recent survey work has shown.

ONCHOCERCIASIS

SYNONYMS. Onchocercosis, blinding filariasis, river blindness.

Definition

Onchocerciasis means a complex of dermal, nodular, ganglionic and ocular manifestations caused by the host reaction to the presence of *Onchocerca volvulus* introduced by black flies of the *Simulidae* family.

Aetiology

Morphology. *O. volvulus* (Leuckart, 1893; Raillet and Henry, 1910) is a white, transparent filarial worm parasitic in man, with a cuticle showing a distinct transversely striated appearance. Both extremities are rounded, but bearing anteriorly one pair of lateral and four pairs of minute submedian papillae on a single ring and posteriorly a number of perianal and caudal papillae.

Sexual dimorphism is very marked. The adult male ranges from 20 to 40 mm in length and 0.13 to 0.21 mm in diameter. It is provided with two copulatory spicules and 3–4 pairs of pedunculate perianal papillae and a few sessile caudal papillae. The adult female is much longer, ranging from 330 to 550 mm in length and 0.27 to 0.40 mm in diameter. The vulva opens posteriorly to the oesophagus. The existence of different strains, such as a forest and savannah type, has been postulated (De Leon and Duke, 1966).

Life cycle. ADULT STAGE IN MAN. The tissue-inhabiting adult worm lives free in subcutaneous tissues, or males and females may be interlaced within encapsulating nodules. Man is the only known reservoir.

REPRODUCTION IN MAN. After fertilisation the females produce embryos or first-stage larvae which will be found in the fluid of the nodules, in the tissues and lymph spaces of the skin, and the peripheral connective tissue in the neighbourhood of the worm localisation.

The microfilariae are unsheathed, gracefully curved, making non-progressive, twisting movements. Their size varies from 200 to 350 by 7–8 microns, distributed between a small (200–290, mean 254 microns) and a large form (295–358, mean 332 microns). The cephalic cone is thickened, the nuclei are coarse, the posterior part narrows abruptly and ends in a sharply pointed recurved tail of which the caudal nuclei do not reach the tip.

O. volvulus microfilariae show no periodicity, but their density varies with a maximum at 22–24 hours.

DEVELOPMENT IN THE VECTOR. The microfilariae are chemotactically attracted by the salivary secretions of the specific vectors, belonging to the *Simulidae* family. They are taken up from the infected host with the blood meal. The majority of the ingested larvae are imprisoned by the peritrophic membrane and digested with the blood. The few remaining outside the membrane pierce the digestive wall and proceed to the muscle of the thorax, where development will take place. After 6–10 days and two moults they become active, mobile, filiform, infective third-stage larvae. They migrate through the haemocoele to the insect head, enter the proboscis and await the opportunity of a meal to invade a new host. There is no multiplication of the parasite in the vector.

DEVELOPMENT IN THE HUMAN HOST. The infective larvae actively escape from the tip of the proboscis and, being unable to penetrate intact skin, enter the host through the puncture made by the vector. Not much is known about the further development of these minute larvae. They penetrate the subcutaneous lymphatics and proceed to their maturation sites. It is likely that they undergo two more moults before becoming sexually mature, which requires about 15 months, the duration of the prepatent period, for the forest strain, although one child under 1 year has been found positive in the savannah.

How far and for how long a period the infective larvae can migrate is still unknown. Facts about maturation and about the incentives to encapsulation at definite bodily sites are yet lacking.

The lifespan of the microfilariae, although not necessarily the same for all strains, may be estimated for the forest strain at about 2 years (6 months–3 years), being the time to reconstitute the pretreatment level. A microfilarial population deprived of regeneration declines to zero by natural mortality in the thirteenth month.

The length of life of the adult worm may be estimated at about 10–15 years. One female worm produces 1 million microfilariae per year.

Epidemiology

Geographical distribution. In tropical regions of both the old and the new world, human onchocerciasis reservoirs are known.

In the western hemisphere this filariasis has been identified, sometimes surprisingly late in several countries. In Mexico the disease is restricted to the states Oaxaca and Chiapas, and is believed to have been introduced by Sudanese soldiers of the Army Corps of Bazaine. In Guatemala two foci have been identified so far in eight regions. The northern one (Huehuetenango) is adjacent to the Chiapas focus; the other includes Guatemala, Suchitepequez, Sololà, Escuintla, Chimaltenango, Santa Rosa, Jutiapa. In Venezuela, onchocerciasis was first detected in 1948 and is known to be present in nine states: in the northeast, Sucre and Monagas; in the central-north, Anzoategui, Aragua, Carabobo, Cojedes, Guárico Mirandas and Yaracuy, all of them along the Cordillera de la Costa. In Colombia the disease was identified in 1965 in a narrow coastal zone between the Cordillera de los Andes and the Ocean. In Surinam aboriginal cases have been seen.

In Africa, onchocerciasis may be present from latitude 15°N to 13°S, or from Casamance (Senegal) to Ethiopia in the north and from Angola to Tanzania in the south.

The whole of West Africa is heavily infected, especially in the forest region and the Sudanese savannah, the Volta basin being one of the worst and most extensive foci. In Central Africa it occurs from Cameroun and the Congo to the Sudan and the Central Graben. In East Africa, foci have been found in Ethiopia, Sudan, Uganda, Kenya and Tanzania and in the south-east of the Arabian peninsula and Yemen. In the whole world 20 million people are estimated to harbour the parasite and as a result more than 250 000 parasitised individuals are blind.

Vectors. The vector distribution is related to the biology and ecology of the aquatic stages and the adults of the *Simulium* genus. A correct knowledge of *Simulium* biology is therefore the indispensable background for any control measures to be taken against the different biospecies of the vector.

BIOLOGY AND ECOLOGY OF AQUATIC STAGES. The African vectors are members of the *S. damnosum* (Theobald) and *S. neavei* (Roubaud) groups.

The eggs of *S. damnosum* are deposited by the gravid fly partly submerged in irregular clusters on rocks, stones, twigs, aquatic plants, whenever water breaks over an obstruction, in large as well as in small rivers, both in forest and savannah. They hatch shortly after deposition and the larva migrate to somewhat (± 15 cm) deeper water or, under unfavourable circumstances, to another more suitable base over limited distances. The length of the larval life varies from 8 to 14 days according to environmental conditions and the pupal life from 2 to 4 days. The larvae hang with their head downstream and have for growth several basic needs, such as well-aerated water with a definite oxygen content, running at a velocity of 60–250 cm/s at an altitude between 0 and 1500 m and an adequate food supply, although they are indiscriminating feeders.

The ovipositing of *S. neavei* occurs in batches of ± 100 on vegetation near rocky falls or cascades of perennial streams, in woodlands or forest in which freshwater crabs of the *Potamon* species, suitable for a phoretic association, live. The larvae migrate to the crabs and live on their carapace, bases of legs, mouth-parts and eye stalks. They spin their cocoon and pupate on the crab host.

The American vectors are *S. ochraceum* (Walker), *S. metallicum* (Bellardi), *S. callidum* (Dyar and Shannon) and *S. exiguum*. The breeding sites are, for *S. ochraceum*, very small streams not in completely open country and at altitudes between 500 and 1500 m; for *S. metallicum* and *S. callidum*, large rivers at altitudes between 250 and 3000 m. *S. exiguum* breeds both in large and small streams, but not in the major ones.

BIOLOGY OF ADULT STAGES. Adults of the black flies being more directly related to *O. volvulus* transmission, their habits and dynamics have been studied by way of control projects.

S. damnosum includes several biospecies (sibling species), some of which do not attack man. The haematophagy of females is the main epidemiological feature, but even the anthropophylic may feed on goats, dogs, donkeys, game, birds. The blood meal of the nulliparous takes place after about 24 hours, and there will be only one such meal per gonotrophic cycle. Ingestion of sweet plant juices or nectar occurs before the blood meal. Biting activity is diurnal with a peak in the morning and a second in the late afternoon, but the rhythm is conditioned by the outside temperature and the physiological state of the fly. They do not enter habitations to feed and prefer the lower extremities of man since only 2 per cent of the bites are above the waist.

The black-fly has a reduced longevity, varying from a few to 20 days, the lifespan being on the whole longer in savannah than in forest areas, so that paradoxically individuals living under the best ecological conditions have the shortest life, which may be simply related to a more sedentary life. One troublesome problem of great practical importance is the dry-seasonal survival under adverse conditions: at what stage or in what unusual breeding sites?

The flight range is from 10 to more than 80 km (maximum 150 km and effective 25 km) being either linear along the river or following paths and roads, or a radial dispersion at random. In any case the density decreases with the distance from the breeding sites and furthermore seasonal variations are marked in the savannah, such as upstream migration from permanent breeding places at the beginning of the rainy season. *O. volvulus* parasitism does not markedly impair the flight capacity.

The *S. neavei* complex is anthropophilic, but not strictly. Some, although a definite nuisance, are non-vectors. The adults bite in the open in bright sunlight the lower extremities, but also the upper parts. The adults, being more sensitive to climatic conditions, gather after hatching, mostly in dense forest galleries with high humidity or well-wooded banks of hills, sometimes at distance from breeding places.

Their lifespan is not well known, but must be of more than 10 days. The usual range of flight has been recorded as 50–650 m, with a maximum of 29 km. *S. neavei*, *S. woodi* (de Meillon) and *S. vorax* are the possible vectors of this complex.

S. ochraceum, the main American vector, is characterised by a short flight range (maximum 12 km) and its close association with coffee plantations on mountain slopes. The fly, the coffee and the villages are accommodated along small streams in hilly regions at altitudes from 500 to 1500 m. *S. ochraceum* is markedly anthropophilic (98 per cent), very aggressive (100–1000 bites/hour) and 60–80 per cent of its bites are above the waist. Although rather sedentary it is an efficient

vector capable of an intake of several hundred microfilariae without any appreciable reduction of the probability of survival.

S. metallicum lives in open valleys of mountainous regions (800–1500 m) along the river banks of small rapidly flowing rivers, at a main temperature of 22–24°C and 1200–1600 mm precipitation. Less specifically anthropophilic (23 per cent), it tends to bite low (about 30 per cent of its bites are above the waist) with an activity peak in the morning and a second in the afternoon. It is a poor vector with a low intake of microfilariae. Its lifespan approaches 85 days.

S. callidum is found alongside larger rivers at altitudes of 250–2000 m, anthropophily is reduced to 3 per cent with only 5–8 per cent of bites above the waist and a very low intake of microfilariae (10 per fly).

S. exiguum is ecologically bound to both large and small rivers, but never major streams.

Parasite-vector relationship. It is well known that the importance and the pattern of onchocerciasis is changing according to the bioclimatic conditions prevalent in the zone concerned. At least in Africa, two distinct prototypes exist, the forest and the savannah.

The *rain forest* type foci are widespread, and mostly continuous with adjacent foci. The vectors are a nuisance, being present throughout the year but in low density. They have a shorter life, a certain lack of contact and poor transmission potential. Repercussions are common but severe infestation of man rare.

The *savannah* type foci (Sudan type) are characterised by sparse distribution and concentration of vectors in the vicinity of their breeding places, separated by large non-infected areas. The vectors live longer, are in frequent contact with man, and their 'transmission potential' is up to 30 times higher. Their nuisance may lead to evacuation of villages in fertile valleys, a very high parasite load in man and important clinical manifestations. Foci in the Guinea-type savannah (Isoberlinia woodland savannah) and in the forest savannah mosaic represent transition gradients between these two distinct dividing lines. Differences in 'transmission ability' will vary with rainy and dry seasons.

The epidemiological consequences of differences in the ecology of the vector in the major African bioclimatic zones has been clearly demonstrated. Duke and his colleagues put forward the hypothesis of two distinct '*O. volvulus–S. damnosum*' complexes in forest and savannah areas, based on cross-development of forest *O. volvulus* in savannah *S. damnosum* and vice versa. But genetically

S. damnosum of forest and savannah zones are identical in West Africa, and the variations in size are insignificant in the forest and season-dependent in savannah foci.

Transmission depends on man-fly contact, and thus on the density of the vectors, their seasonal variations, anthropophily, longevity, feeding behaviour, and the size of the man-biting infective *Simulium* population and its transmission potential.

The 'infectivity' rates have been found to be, for *S. damnosum* in the Sudan savannah, 2–6 per cent, in the Guinea savannah 2.5 per cent, and 1.5 per cent in the rain forest: when the density of the flies decreases, the infection rate rises. A 'transmission index' or the number of infective stage larvae which may be transmitted in a given number of bites is a better index.

Human host factors. The human host also influences transmission. Several biological factors such as age, nutritional state (vitamin A deficiency) concurrent diseases and genetic factors may have an effect on the transmissibility. Seasonal migrations and changes of habits are not without consequences for transmission. The effects of clothing habits in determining the localisation of the *Simulium* bites is well known. Immunological status and intervals between exposure and re-exposure are possible limiting factors.

Man-made factors. The construction of dams for combating water shortage, for irrigation schemes, for hydroelectric plants, and traffic, creates artificial breeding sites in spillway and downstream sections, but reduces their number to some extent by flooding upstream breeding places. Engineering modifications to dam spillways are investigated in order to check the multiplication of *Simulium*.

Increased industrial and other water pollution factors reduce in part the breeding possibilities. Deforestation and bush-clearing may be useful against vector species bound to a thick bush cover or may harm by increasing the flight range possibilities of other vectors.

The distance of human dwellings from breeding places influences the seriousness of the onchocerciasis situation, more especially in the savannah foci. The first-line villages are those most affected.

Pathogenesis

The adult worm and, to a certain extent, its microfilariae, are well tolerated by the host. As Sharp in 1927 and Mohammed in 1931 pointed out, *O. volvulus* normally lives free in the connective tissue of the host without provoking tissue reaction, but giving rise to detectable humoral antibodies. After fertilisation, the female produces large numbers of microfilariae which move in the surrounding skin, and also penetrate the eye, the lymph nodes and all organs, though in smaller numbers. Heavy loads of microfilariae may be found in the absence of any cellular reaction.

A regular immunologic response will be provoked, which is both humoral antibody-mediated and cell-mediated in type. A dual balance existing at the host-parasite interface implies that *O. volvulus* may use certain immunologic defence mechanisms against the vertebrate host or its aggressors in order to assure its survival. Whether adaptation to the host implies the building of a defence barrier, lowering of the threshold level of available antigenic information and/or the degree of induced paralysis for self-recognition by the host, change in the immunobiological identity of the parasitic antigen, the production of anti-enzyme, or other systems is not known.

Allergic sensitisation is frequently associated with helminthic infections having a parenteral phase of development, and prolonged tissue infection will elicit an immediate type hypersensitivity. It is induced by some metabolic products or enzymes and is mediated by IgE related skin-sensitising 'reagins'. Reagin-like homocytotropic antibodies have indeed been demonstrated in rats infected with *Litomoscides carinii*.

The IgE has the property of adhering to mast cells or tissue basophils which are in ready supply in connective tissue. The mast cell loaded with IgE will combine with the corresponding antigen and will, due to some mechanism, degranulate and release heparin, histamine, serotonin and other vasoactive substances. The liberated basophil material is taken up amongst others by fibroblasts, inducing sensitisation of the connective tissue.

A variety of allergic as well as immunologic reactions may appear during the natural course of the infection. The early cutaneous symptoms which were attributed at first only to the bites of the *Simulidae*, may in fact be related to the interreaction of antigens and immunologic systems producing an allergic inflammatory reaction. The invasion of the human host by infective larvae will, after a short period of latency, unlatch at least in hyper-reactive individuals a hypersensitivity reaction. This cutaneous reaction is of the immediate local anaphylactic type. A similar wheal-and-flare response may be elicited in the infected by intradermal injection of an homologous antigen.

The presence of immature worms may be

accompanied by hypersensitivity of a cell-mediated type, characterised by local redness, oedema and pruritis.

Again when microfilariae appear, more reactions may be observed. Microfilariae have their own secretions and metabolism. They may temporarily remain a foreign hapten for the host's proteins or foreign proteins for the host's hapten, at any rate until certain metabolic processes trouble the equilibrium or as long as disintegrating whole microfilariae do not induce a dispersion of antigens. The presence of such antigens in the connective subcutaneous tissues will attract a certain cellular response, such as the antigen-sensitive scouting T-lymphocytes. These circulate incessantly, identify the antigens through their immunological memory and release soluble factors which activate macrophages. The macrophage ingests the antigen and breaks it down to immunogenic fragments which attach themselves to RNA. These will stimulate small lymphocytes to become effector cells in the perivascular infiltration and increased vascular permeability typical of the delayed, cell-mediated hypersensitivity reaction. The antigen-antibody complexes attract to the reaction site polymorphs and eosinophils, followed by the local liberation of more enzymes (cathepsin, beta-glucuronidase, nucleases, etc.) and the adherence of eosinophils to the microfilariae.

The best known reaction against the adult worm is the eventual inflammatory reaction leading to encapsulation. It has not yet been proved whether the walling off starts only around a worm segment or a degenerating helminth. *O. volvulus* is living in connective tissue, in which it stimulates mastocytosis, as many other helminths do. Lately more attention has been focused on the fluctuating numbers of mast cells in the loose connective tissue of all organs.

In the skin, the fibroblastic reactivity induced by the antigen-antibody complexes originated by the microfilariae and to a certain extent the macrofilariae produces a scleroderma-like infiltration with atrophy of glands and sclerosis. In the lymph nodes, especially rich in mastocytes ($8000/cm^2$), a fibroblastic sclerosing reaction is also met with. In the eye, inflammatory fibrinous reactions and vascular changes occur.

The worms become encapsulated in subcutaneous nodules by a coarse, low-grade fibroblastic reaction.

In the pathogenesis of onchocerciasis several mechanisms are certainly involved. Some are related to the reactivity proper to the host, amongst which the possible rôle of hetero-allergic sensitisation should never be neglected. Others are connected with the life cycle of the helminth including simultaneous humoral- and cell-mediated reactions of both of an immediate and a delayed type.

Many pathogenetic assumptions have had their vogue: direct mechanical effect, anatomical localisation, elaboration of toxins, vitamin A and/or B deficiencies, toxoplasma, rickettsiae, genetic factors. The present-day fashion calls on self-markers, cellular immunity, cell-membranes, connective tissue diseases, autoimmune reactions. None of these stop-gap surmises may be correct, but every one may initiate further progress towards more accurate knowledge.

Pathology

Skin lesions. The presence of numerous free-living microfilariae in the dermis does not induce by itself inflammatory reaction. Their number and more superficial localisation reflect to a certain degree the intensity and duration of the infection. Nevertheless, some fundamental histopathological changes are there from the earliest stage: slight hyperkeratosis, spotty parakeratosis, some hypogranulosis.

As the infection continues, the hyperkeratosis will increase, the epithelial layer atrophy, the elastic fibres degenerate, the dermal connective tissues hypertrophy, an eosino-lymphohistiocytic perivascular infiltration commence. Gradually, by a spontaneous or treatment-induced succession of quiescent and exacerbation periods, the subcutaneous tissues will increase two or three times in thickness and this hypertrophic stage will progress unavoidably to atrophic changes and presbydermia.

In long-standing onchocerciasis the pigmentation process, disturbed at first, around the hair follicles and in the vicinity of coiled microfilariae, will become completely disorganised due to the dysfunction and even the absence of melanoblasts. Repigmentation may occur just as hyperpigmentation may develop after treatment.

The Central American 'mal morado' and 'erisipela de la costa' are epidermal, oedematous, erysipeloid relapsing reactions against microfilariae.

Nodules. Live adult worms may become inextricably coiled up and surrounded by a thin fibrous envelope expanding into a labyrinth of cellular tunnel walls filled with a viscous greyish-yellow substance, which takes shape in about 8 months. Several nodules may coalesce into larger ones. The thickness of the capsule increases with age and in later stages the nodules become completely fibrosed and some even calcified.

Not enough information is available about reliable criteria for assessing the age of the nodules and the signs of ageing and viability of the worms. Up to 50 per cent of the nodules of untreated patients may contain only necrotic segments or worms, and it is also known that good preservation may be compatible with recent death. In evaluating macrofilaricidal drug activity the examination of nodules is the only available criterion, and successful activity has been claimed on the finding of 60 per cent non-viable nodules in treated patients.

On histological examination, the peripheral fibroblastic reaction consists of honeycombing at the centre, enclosing in the most capricious arrangements worm sections surrounded by countless live microfilariae. As degeneration sets in, the last identifiable remnant being the cuticle, microfilariae become rare, degenerate and disappear altogether. The vascular and cellular reaction will also gradually decrease and vanish. Complete fibrosis is the usual end-point.

Lymphadenopathy. Microfilariae present in the lymph spaces will gradually induce a plasma cell infiltration of the trabeculae, followed by proliferation of the connective tissue and some lymph stasis. This process is followed by diffuse fibrosis and sclerosis of the enlarged lymph nodes lying in loose connective tissue under inelastic atrophic skin. They may thus sag down and produce a so-called 'hanging groin' or 'pseudo-Hottentot apron'.

Genital elephantiasis. The skin of external genitalia is thick, tough and white and the sub-dermal tissues are hypertrophic, jelly-like and yellowish. The epidermal hyperkeratosis is often accompanied by loss of pigmentation. The dermal hypertrophic fibroplasia, in which microfilariae and scarce cellular elements are seen, is accompanied by a loss of elasticity. The subsequent lymphoedema will increase until balance is reached.

A close association of parasites and a given symptom does not in itself imply an aetiological relationship, but may indicate a 'cause favorisante'.

Onchophthalmia. Healthy microfilariae have been found in all eye tissues. As long as they do not disintegrate, the host-parasite balance will, up to a certain threshold, tend towards a mechanism of tolerance.

The histopathological manifestations around dead microfilariae consist of an inflammatory infiltration by round cells, plasma cells, lymphocytes and eosinophils accompanied by hyper-trophy, oedema and vascular changes in the tissues concerned. This may be found around those lying below the epithelium of the conjunctiva, in the limbus, the substantia propria of the cornea, the iris-ciliary body and in the anterior chamber.

The microfilariae are scanty or even absent in the lesions of the posterior segment. This is no more remarkable in chronic uveitis than in presby-dermic skin. The exudative and degenerative chorioretinitis is very typical, due to a curious irregular pigmentation, sclerosis of the choroid, vascular occlusion and optic atrophy.

Clinical features

Early symptoms. Some individuals are hyper-sensitised to *Simulium* bites and react immediately with a non-specific cutaneous reaction of short duration. Others react to the invasion and development of infective larvae, as can be demonstrated by experimental infections in volunteers. In the latter a pruriginous oedematous zone centred on the *Simulium* bite will appear and enlarge gradually to the zone concerned, e.g. from the ankle to the whole of the foot. After about 2 months an urticarial rash may extend over the whole of the affected limb and even to the entire body. This reaction is accompanied by fever (38°C) and eosinophilia, in the absence of as yet immature microfilariae.

Dermal onchocerciasis or onchodermatitis. The skin invasion by microfilariae may, in some trigger off an acute maculo-papular rash often localised to the lower back, the buttocks or upper arms with extension to more distal parts. The accompanying pruritis of varying intensity will be the dominant symptom and induce scratching. According to the degree of reactivity of the patient, this chronic condition, which is characterised by alternating periods of quiescence and exacerbations, will produce a scabies-like condition, including pustulation and crusting, often described as 'filarial craw-craw' or 'gale filarienne'.

By each exacerbation the skin becomes more thickened. The deepening of the folds and the dilated pilo-sebaceous pores give a shagreen skin, also known as 'pig-skin' appearance, covering large areas but most typical on the abdominal wall. Gradually the skin becomes more fibrous and, losing its lustre, develops a pachydermic appearance. Eventually scleroderma succeeds the pachyderma; the by-now dry, wrinkled skin has been compared with 'lizard or crocodile skin'.

The final loss of elasticity is such that the skin has an appearance like crumpled paper, the well-known presbydermia or scleroderma. Years ago

Ouzilleau described this as follows: 'Youths look like old people and the elderly like lizards'.

The Latin American 'erisipela de la Costa' (Robles) is a reaction, mostly in patients under twenty, made up by a painful, itchy, deep red swelling of the face, oedema of the eyelids, photophobia, conjunctival injection, iritis, periorbital pain and fever: this erysipeloid reaction inducing a 'blood-hound' facies relapses periodically.

The 'mal morado' is a purplish reaction occurring in plaques, not unlike lichen planus, or in papules. Its site includes head, neck, pectoral region and arms in those over twenty.

Browne has observed similar conditions in African adults. Non-immune adults suddenly exposed to *Simulium* may develop, outside the bitten areas, localised brawny, pricking, burning swelling of the lumbar region, buttocks or thighs resembling and reacting as neurodermatitis. Recurrences of this 'erisipela de la Costa' type of reaction are frequent. Their localisation is apparently related to the pelvic girdle and lower limb preponderance of nodules in Africa.

In the early stages of massive onchocercal infection in African adults a dark purplish-brown plaque-like skin reaction of the 'mal morado' type may also be seen. Plaques are localised typically on the anterior aspect of the middle third of the thighs and related to the proximity of coincident nodules in the paratrochanteric region. The 'sowda' of Yemen features an intensely itching hyperchromic dermatitis of the lower limbs with an accompanying inguinocrural lymphadenopathy.

In dark-skinned patients hyperpigmentation may occur in the first stages; however, the pretibial depigmentation of long-standing onchocerciasis is more typical. Disappearing papules leave achromic macular spots in their centre with sharply defined borders, which may coalesce to leucodermal plaques. Islets of normally pigmented skin remain scattered throughout the achromic areas giving a mottled 'leopard skin' appearance. The groin, the fossae iliacae and the chest are other depigmentation sites.

Nodules or onchocercomata. One of the main features of onchocerciasis is the presence of palpable nodules. For a long time it was considered almost the only one. Nowadays, however, it is acknowledged that 10–40 per cent of parasitised persons remain nodule-free. The nodules may appear in less than 1 year and take 3–4 years to attain their full size—a grain of wheat to a walnut, most often a hazelnut—although larger dimensions can be attained by the clustering of several nodules. They are usually localised at pressure points where bony prominences lie under the skin; they are firm and mobile, unless fixed by fascia or periosteum or erode into the skull bones. The onchocercomata are painless, except transiently when swelling, redness and itching occur and are ascribed to transient escape of microfilariae or to a needle aspiration. Eventually they become fibrous, calcify and even disappear, and only very occasionally will they turn to an abscess.

The topographical distribution differs somewhat in Africa and in America. In central and tropical America the head, suboccipital region, shoulders, upper limb and trunk are the most common sites, although the pelvic girdle may be the first choice in certain foci, as it is in tropical Africa. The iliac crest, trochanter and sacrum are there the favourite sites, followed by the trunk (ribs, acromion, scapula), but the knee, the elbow and also the skull may be involved.

The number of nodules increases with exposure to infection and well over one hundred have been recorded. Nodules have been known in an infant only 8 months old. Their prevalence is usually greater in males than females.

Ocular symptoms or oncophthalmia. Ocular onchocerciasis is a serious condition since it may result in loss of vision and blindness. Its prevalence depends on the site of dwellings in relation to *Simulium* breeding places.

The ocular manifestations may start acutely with a sensation as of the presence of a foreign body or with pain, photophobia, lacrimation, oedema of the eyelids and tonic blepharospasm. It fades gradually into a chronic conjunctivitis. A chronic limbitis with brownish pigmentation is frequently present.

Microfilariae may be present in the cornea, where they are easily detected with a slit lamp and corneal microscope. Alive they cause little harm but when they disintegrate they give rise to punctate, fluffy opacities, always beginning close to the limbus in a temporal and/or nasal equatorial situation. This punctate keratitis may become nummular, even vascular, and become confluent towards the lower half of the cornea.

Microfilariae may be seen, with a slit lamp, swimming around in the anterior chamber. They invade the iris and ciliary body and induce a chronic fibrous iridocyclitis, characterised by the loss of the lower part of the pupillary pigmented ruff and by sluggishness of the pupil. Eventually the latter becomes pin-point, fixed, ectopic and pyriformly distorted. The occluded pupil interrupts the passage between anterior and posterior chambers and results in glaucoma.

The lesions of the posterior segment are not so

regularly associated with the presence of micro-filariae. Their onchocercal aetiology is neverthe-less unquestionable even if the pathological mechanism may be obscure. The first danger signals are an early bilateral loss of peripheral vision and night blindness. The fundal appearance of a 'mottled tigroid' or 'dapple' choroidoretinitis results from pigment migration exposing the choroid. This state evolves towards sclerosis and the 'dried-mud' picture of Ridley. There follows narrowing and sometimes sheathing of the retinal arteries as they leave the disc, and finally there may be optic atrophy.

Although it may be difficult to assess the causes of blindness, it is obvious that 'an increas-ing incidence and intensity of onchocercal infec-tion in a community is associated with a dramatic rise in incidence of blindness . . .' (Budden). According to the British Empire Society for the Blind, the prevalence is 0.25 per cent in Europe, 0.5 per cent in trachomatous regions and from 1.5 to 30 per cent in onchocercal foci.

Lymphadenopathy or onchoadenitis. A non-painful enlargement of lymphatic glands may be observed in the infected zone. Localisation of the worms in the upper part of the body results in lymphadenopathy in the cervical and occipital groups; worms on the thoracic wall in axillary adenitis, and in the legs, lymphadenopathy mainly in the crural and inguinal regions. Chronic slight inguinocrural adenopathy is common and related to several causes including recurrent pyogenic conditions of the legs. On puncture of lymph nodes which are not too sclerosed, microfilariae may be aspirated and their numbers are in accord-ance with the intensity of the infection. Micro-filaricidal treatment induces an 'allergic' reaction.

The usually bilateral fibrosis of the inguino-crural glands is accompanied by minimal lymph stasis and periadenitis, but the lymph nodes may agglomerate to masses which sag down by their own weight in the surrounding inelastic, gelatin-ous connective tissue and atrophic skin. Such pendulous skin may reach an enormous size, occasionally even reaching knee-level and weigh-ing up to 2–3 kg. This is the 'pseudoadenolympho-cele' (Rodhain) or 'hanging groin' (Nelson) associated with long-standing infection.

Tropical elephantiasis. The significant incidence of genital elephantiasis in certain hyperendemic areas (Uele, Central African Republic, southern Sudan) and its obvious absence in others (Kasaï, Sankuru, West Africa, East Africa, Latin America) has resulted in some supporting and some oppos-ing the views that a causal relationship exists between onchocerciasis and elephantiasis.

Where elephantiasis is present, the scrotal skin becomes thickened, rugous and deeply furrowed, and a jelly-like condition of the underlying con-nective tissue develops. The lesion is sharply confined to the scrotal skin and neither invades the contents nor extends to the abdomen. Similar changes may also occur on the corona of the penis or the labia. The evolution of these lesions is characterised by recurrent attacks of inflammatory reaction followed by an increase of the swelling which may attain a large or even enormous size.

Elephantiasis of the legs is comparatively rare in onchocercal regions, as is localisation to arms, breasts or face.

Miscellaneous manifestations. Hydrocoele, funi-culitis and orchitis are not aetiologically asso-ciated with onchocerciasis, although microfilariae may be found in hydrocoele fluid.

Synovitis, especially of the knee, is common in onchocerciasis, as well as in other filarial infections and is characterised by recurrent attacks (Wanson). Nodules are frequently attached to the joint capsule and microfilariae migrate into the synovial fluid, which may contain specific antibodies. Administration of microfilarial drugs may cause an allergic type of reaction in the joint.

Cerebral manifestations, including giddiness and epileptiform convulsions, have been attributed to the pressure of onchocercal nodules, which have been demonstrated on the meninges and optic nerve (Rodger). Microfilariae of *O. volvulus* have commonly been found in the cerebrospinal fluid but have been attributed to accidental introduc-tion by the aspirating needle.

On the evidence available it seems unlikely that onchocerciasis is causally related to endemic dwarfism (Nakalanga syndrome) of Uganda, or to repeated abortion.

A curious calcinosis of the scrotal wall, charac-terised by small, rounded, hard, movable masses mainly near the raphé and containing *O. volvulus* has been described by Browne who also focused attention on the appearance of papillomata in onchodermatitic skin.

Diagnosis

Clinical. The most common *dermal lesions* are pruritis, craw-craw or 'gale filarienne', skin atrophy leading to scleroderma or presbydermia, mottled depigmentation or 'leopard skin'. In Central America one may add 'erisipela de la costa' and 'mal morado'.

The subcutaneous nodules or *onchocercomata* in typical localisations have to be differentiated from fibromata, lipomata, dermoid cysts, juxta-articular nodules of yaws, and other cysts.

The *lymphatic lesions* include lymphoedema, lymphadenopathy and pseudo-adenolympho-coele or 'hanging groin'.

The *eye lesions* include keratitis punctata, sclerosing keratitis, chronic iridocyclitis, pyriform deformation of the pupil, choroidoretinitis with migration of pigment and sclerosis, and optic atrophy.

Parasitological. The demonstration of the *adult worms*, free in tissues or enclosed in nodules is definitive proof of the diagnosis.

The detection of specific microfilariae in tissues or fluids is also definitive proof of the aetiology: microfilariae can be sought in the skin and, using a slit lamp, in the eye.

Examinations should be repeated if necessary after an interval of some days.

Skin biopsies yield the highest return of positive results. The correct identification of microfilariae is imperative; microfilariae of *D. streptocerca* should be carefully distinguished from those of *O. volvulus* and confusion with blood-borne microfilariae, especially *A. perstans*, should be avoided.

SKIN. *Skin-snips* may be taken either by cutting off with a razor-blade a cone of skin elevated on the sharp end of a needle or by use of a punch biopsy drill with a 2 mm bite; the clear-cut or torn-out snips are mounted in saline under a coverslip, allowed to stand for 15–30 minutes and examined under a microscope using a magnification of ×100. Alternatively the snips may be teased in 5 ml saline and centrifuged (Browne). Snips may be weighed on a torsion balance and the microfilariae in them expressed on a quantitative basis. In this way evidence of the distribution of the microfilariae in the body can be found. In order to avoid possible errors resulting from diurnal fluctuations in the position of the microfilariae, serial observations should be taken at the same time each day.

The sites containing the highest numbers of microfilariae are the shoulder (deltoid-scapular) in the Americas and the pelvic girdle, buttocks and external aspect of the thigh in Africa. However in early infections and in localised light infections the site of election will be that in which the dermatitis is most marked. At least two snips should be taken and in chronic cases five or six if possible. In dry atmospheric conditions care must be taken to avoid desiccation.

Scarification (d'Hooghe, 1934). The skin is scratched with a needle and blood-tinged fluid is squeezed out between thumb and finger, dried and stained. Alternatively smears can be made of the cut surface after taking skin shavings. The method is easy to apply but cannot be used for quantitative comparison and because microfilariae from the blood will, if present, contaminate the preparation, cannot be used for critical work.

The site with the greatest number of microfilariae and the highest recovery rate is the periumbilical, but the best sites are the same as for the snips.

EYES. *Conjunctival biopsy* is not routinely advisable. It should be performed only by those with ophthalmological training. It has been noted that possibly due to some kind of chemotaxy the microfilarial count in the conjunctiva rises after instillation of cocaine.

Direct examination of the anterior chamber, either with a slit lamp or ophthalmoscope after fully dilating the pupil, may visualise the microfilariae. Eye massage may ease the detection of the microfilariae.

Immunobiological tests. INTRACUTANEOUS OR SKIN SENSITIVITY TESTS. These are performed with lipid-free antigens, prepared from different filariae (mostly *Dicrofilariae immitis*).

The cutaneous reaction on the volar surface of the arm is tested. The response is mainly of the immediate type and usually read within 15 to 30 minutes. In positive tests the wheal raised by the injection at least doubles its original size. Variations in results are disturbing and can only be overcome by adequate standardisation of the criteria for reading the test and by developing a standardised antigen.

SEROLOGICAL TECHNIQUES. The *complement fixation test* is a very valuable diagnostic tool. Lack of agreement on its usefulness and reliability results from variability in the nature and specificity of the antigens used and a lack of standardisation of the procedure. In competent hands it is superior to the skin test and is especially useful in the detection of the lightly infected. Cross-reactions exist with several helminths, more especially for strongyloidea.

Precipitation test. This test to date has been unreliable in onchocerciasis and cannot be recommended.

Indirect fluorescent antibody test. Results of this test are too controversial and inconclusive, mostly due to autofluorescence, to be of any value at this stage.

Soluble antigen fluorescent antibody test. With the use of a lipid-free somatic adult worm antigen (*D. immitis*), a satisfactory degree of sensitivity and specificity may be obtained. The test, using only minute amounts of dried blood, is useful for the study of large numbers of individuals. As with the other serological tests, false negatives occur in the recently infected and cross-reactions may be observed with sera from patients with other parasitic infections.

PRAUSNITZ-KUSTNER TEST. Reagin-like antibodies have been found in a proportion of parasitised persons.

MAZZOTI TEST. The administration of a dose of diethylcarbamazine produces in the microfilarial carrier an allergic response 1–2 hours after administration due to liberated foreign protein from the destroyed microfilariae. The positive reaction is characterised by pruritis, papular rash and oedema of the skin, headache, fever, swelling of the lymph nodes and arthralgia. This test can be misleading as positive reactions occur in streptocerciasis and other filarial infections and cannot therefore be used for critical work. Its use by destroying some microfilariae hinders accurate diagnosis.

Treatment

Chemotherapy. This aims both at treatment of the individual and, in endemic areas, interruption of transmission by elimination of the microfilarial reservoir. All the antihelminthic and many other antiparasitic drugs have been tried on onchocerciasis with no or very transitory results: only very few drugs are effective.

MACROFILARICIDAL PREPARATIONS. *Suramin* (Bayer 205, Antrypol, Germanine, Moranyl), a complex urea derivative, is consistently active against the adult worm when used in schedules at an optimum dosage. It also clears the microfilariae from the skin in a proportion increasing with dosage. Unfortunately even standard dosage results in prolonged albuminuria and renal damage in some cases.

Administration is intravenous and the dosage is 1 g a week (after a test dose of 0.1 g or 0.2 g) to a total of 6 g. Higher dosages might be slightly more parasiticidal but become *pro rata* alarmingly toxic.

An Herxheimer-type immediate reaction occurs rarely, but temporary albuminuria is a common toxic manifestation. Other side effects include febrile reactions, exacerbation of skin symptoms, muscle pain, arthralgia and chronic degeneration of the adrenal cortex.

Melarsonyl (Mel W, Trimelarsan). Pentylthiarsophenyl melamine, a trivalent arsenical preparation, did not fulfil the expectations originally held of it neither for individual, nor for mass use. A single intramuscular dose of 7.5 to 10 mg/kg body weight, with a ceiling of 500 mg, is not uniformly active but may be toxic. In a significant number of persons, not less than 1 in 1500, an

absolutely unpredictable fatal encephalopathy may develop. Spreading the administration over two to four doses of 200 mg does not eliminate the risk of encephalopathy (Duke).

Microfilariae persisting after the injection are normally transmissible. Decrease in toxicity resulting from combining treatment with promethazine (phenergan) is being assessed.

Melarsonyl, although a valuable macrofilaricide, is too dangerous for use. In a non-fatal disease the use of a potentially deadly drug is never justifiable.

MICROFILARICIDAL PREPARATIONS. *Diethylcarbamazine* (DEC, Hetrazan, Banocide, Notezine, Carbilazine), a piperazine derivative, is a highly effective microfilaricide and has a less marked effect on adult worms. The therapeutic dosage is 2 mg/kg body weight three times a day for 21 consecutive days or three to four 10-day courses with an interval of 2–3 weeks. Unpleasant reactions, allergic in character (cf. Mazzoti test), are so common that it is advisable to commence with a third of the daily dose under cover of antihistaminics. The increase in dosage should be carefully and individually adjusted according to the reaction. A proportion of those so treated have no further symptoms so that some adult onchocercal worms must be killed by the drug. The proportion increases with repeated courses of treatment.

If the eye is involved, particular caution must be exercised and the use of corticosteroid cover may be advisable. It is worthwhile mentioning that diethylcarbamazine inhibits the antigen-induced release of slow-reacting substance and that Latin American authors claim that antiserotonin drugs (Deseril) are effective.

Several *antimonial preparations*, both tri- and penta-valent—tartar emetic, stibogluconate (Pentostam), ethylstilbamine (Neostibosan), Astiban, stibocaptate (TWSb), MSbE—are microfilaricidal, blocking embryogenesis in adult female *O. volvulus*, and this eventually kills the adults. The parasiticidal activity too varies considerably from one patient to another. Antimonials are often ill tolerated; untoward reactions attributable to the toxicity of antimony and microfilaricidal activity contraindicate their use.

COMBINED MACRO- AND MICRO-FILARIAL TREATMENT. Suramin is active on macrofilariae and at the recommended dosage may produce severe allergic reactions, including fever, headache, pruriginous rash, involving eventually the eye. It is advisable therefore to start with a microfilaricidal drug at a low dosage and under cover of antihistaminics or corticosteroids, at least for the first few days.

Preliminary elimination of the microfilariae

may be achieved by starting with a dose of 1 mg/kg body weight of diethylcarbamazine on the first day, gradually increasing each day, according to the reactivity of the patient, by 0.5–1 mg/kg until the active daily dose of 6 mg/kg is reached, this dosage being divided over three doses. Full dosage will be continued for 1 week. After an interval of 2–3 weeks this procedure may be repeated or one may proceed immediately to the 100–200 mg test dose of suramin, followed by weekly doses of 1 g to a total of 6 g to kill the adult worms. Careful observation for nephrotoxicity and other toxic effects is absolutely essential.

In untreated patients spontaneous disappearance of microfilariae may take up to 15 years.

Nodulectomy. Surgical removal of nodules has long been practised in Central America where mass campaigns have been effective in controlling 'erisipela de la Costa' and the incidence of blindness.

Nodulectomy is also popular and asked for in parts of Africa. It is however not a reliable control measure since by its means small and deep-seated nodules are missed as are the free-living adult worms. As an individual therapeutic measure it should be limited to nodules on the head which lead to invasion of the eye. Intranodular injection of substances such as thymol and gentian violet, and even mechanical disruption have been tried without success. It is painful and ineffective if the nodule is composite.

Chemoprophylaxis. While 200 mg diethylcarbamazine taken once a month on 3 consecutive days has been used as a prophylactic measure against *Loa loa*, this schedule is not effective against *O. volvulus*. Considering that microfilariae may reinvade the skin within a month after diethylcarbamazine treatment, only regular treatment would be efficacious, but this is impracticable. Furthermore, as diethylcarbamazine is inactive against the infective larvae, casual prophylaxis would have limited value.

Mass treatment. To date mass therapeutic campaigns have not been feasible. As an alternative, selective use of diethylcarbamazine has been recommended in order to reduce the onchocercal reservoir and impair transmission. A weekly dose of 50 mg diethylcarbamazine on 6 successive weeks has been recommended and does not produce untoward side reactions. This administration has to be repeated twice or thrice a year, according to the prevailing endemicity.

Assessment of therapy. The assessment of a drug's action on *O. volvulus* is difficult, because the parasitological criteria are uncertain. To date the only reliable criterion is the continued absence of microfilariae from the skin over a period of years.

DIPETALONEMA STREPTOCERCA INFECTIONS

The filarial worm exists only in Africa, its distribution corresponding to that of onchocerciasis. It is generally conceded that the worm does not produce symptoms in human beings. Its presence gives rise to positive complement fixation and intradermal skin tests and this may lead to confusion in diagnosis. The microfilariae inhabit the skin but can be distinguished from those of *O. volvulus* by the presence of a 'walking stick handle' curve of the tail.

MANSONELLA OZZARDI INFECTIONS

This parasite occurs only in the New World, in Northern Argentina, the Amazon Valley, the Northern Coast of South America, in Central America and some West Indian Islands. The microfilariae are non-periodic unsheathed and resemble those of *A. perstans* but the nuclei do not quite reach the tip of the posterior extremity as they do in the case of those of *A. perstans*. Various species of Culicoides appear to be the main vectors but *Simulium* and *Tabanus* flies have been found naturally infected. Pathogenicity in man has not been clearly proved but hydrocoeles and lymphadenopathy have been reported in infected persons. Diethylcarbamazine appears to be without therapeutic effect in this infection.

DRACUNCULUS MEDINENSIS
(GUINEA-WORM)

Distribution

The guinea-worm is the oldest known human parasite. It appears to be referred to by Moses (*Numbers*, Chap. XXI) as the fiery serpents that molested the Israelites on the shores of the Red Sea. The disease is common in Africa, especially along the west coast. It also is encountered in the Sudan, in India, Arabia and in the Caribbean islands and in South America. The disease may be cleared from an area in times of drought.

Adult worm

Dracunculus medinensis is the largest filarial worm. The female attains a length of 3 feet or more whilst the male seldom measures more than 4 cm. The uterus occupies most of the body of the female worm and may contain up to 3 million embryos. There is a pronounced hook towards the tail and it is sometimes asserted that this is used by the organism to obtain attachment to the tissues and to resist removal. The vulva is situated towards the cephalic end. After copulation the male worm is thought to die. It is seldom encountered in human tissues. The female does not inhabit the lymphatics but lives in the subcutaneous tissues.

When the pregnant female is ready to discharge embryos it comes to lie close under the skin. A

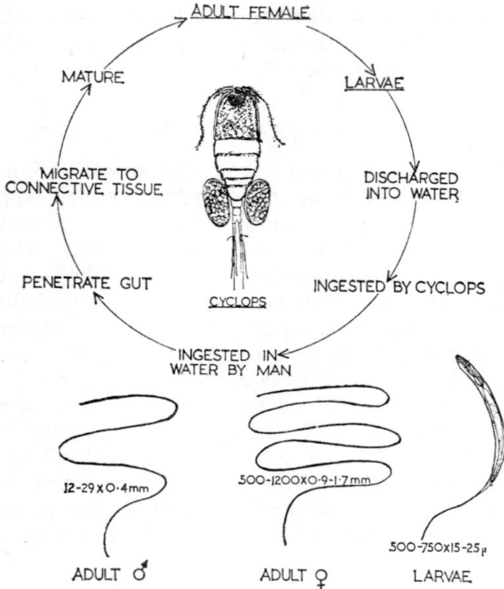

FIG. 14.1. *Life cycle of the guinea-worm.*

secretion from the head glands in the worm contains a toxin which causes a blister to form. This produces an irritation and the patient frequently scratches open the vesicle. The next stage requires the presence of water for further development. This is not infrequently provided by the patient as he bathes the blister to alleviate irritation. In the presence of water the uterus of the worm expels the embryos. The embryos are often discharged into wells or muddy puddles where they may be available to the intermediary host, *Cyclops*, a minute crustacean which is just visible to the naked eye. *Cyclops* is attracted by the jerky movements of the embryos and proceeds to engulf them.

Man becomes infected with guinea-worm by swallowing water which is contaminated with infected *Cyclops*. The cyclops is digested by the

gastric juice and the freed larva then pierces the mucosa and eventually works its way to the subcutaneous tissue. It takes about 1 year to develop sexual maturity.

Clinical features

Symptoms only occur when the female worm is ready to discharge embryos. General symptoms of allergy may appear at this stage. They consist of local erythema, extensive itching, fever, urticaria and occasionally asthma or collapse. They can be produced experimentally by the injection of an extract of the worm. In many patients the history of allergic manifestation is absent.

A minute vesicle appears in the skin. This is usually situated on areas that come into frequent contact with water. The leg or foot are the most frequent sites. The hand is not uncommonly selected. In Indian water-carriers the back is often affected. The breast or scrotum are occasionally attacked. The vesicle ruptures disclosing a small opening into which a probe can be inserted. If the lesion is douched repeatedly with water the uterus will be extruded. A thin milky fluid will then be discharged from the wound and if it is examined under the microscope myriads of larvae will be seen.

Occasionally cellulitis is caused by a secondary infection spreading around the worm. The neighbouring joints may show swelling and increase of synovial fluid. Sometimes a guinea-worm may be palpated as a fine cord as it lies superficially under the skin. It can be demonstrated radiologically after the injection of opaque material. Calcified worms are not infrequently disclosed in a limb in an X-ray taken for some other purpose. Guinea-worms have been described within a hernial sac.

Treatment

The worm may be extracted by means of a matchstick or a piece of split bamboo. This manoeuvre is a knack often acquired by medical orderlies in preference to medical officers. It is a tedious business and requires patience and practice before one becomes adept. The presenting portion of the worm is threaded through a slit in the matchstick which is rotated several times without causing undue tension. Frequent douches of cold water or the application of a cold compress is necessary before the next attempt. Day by day more and more of the worm is uncoiled until it is finally removed. If too much

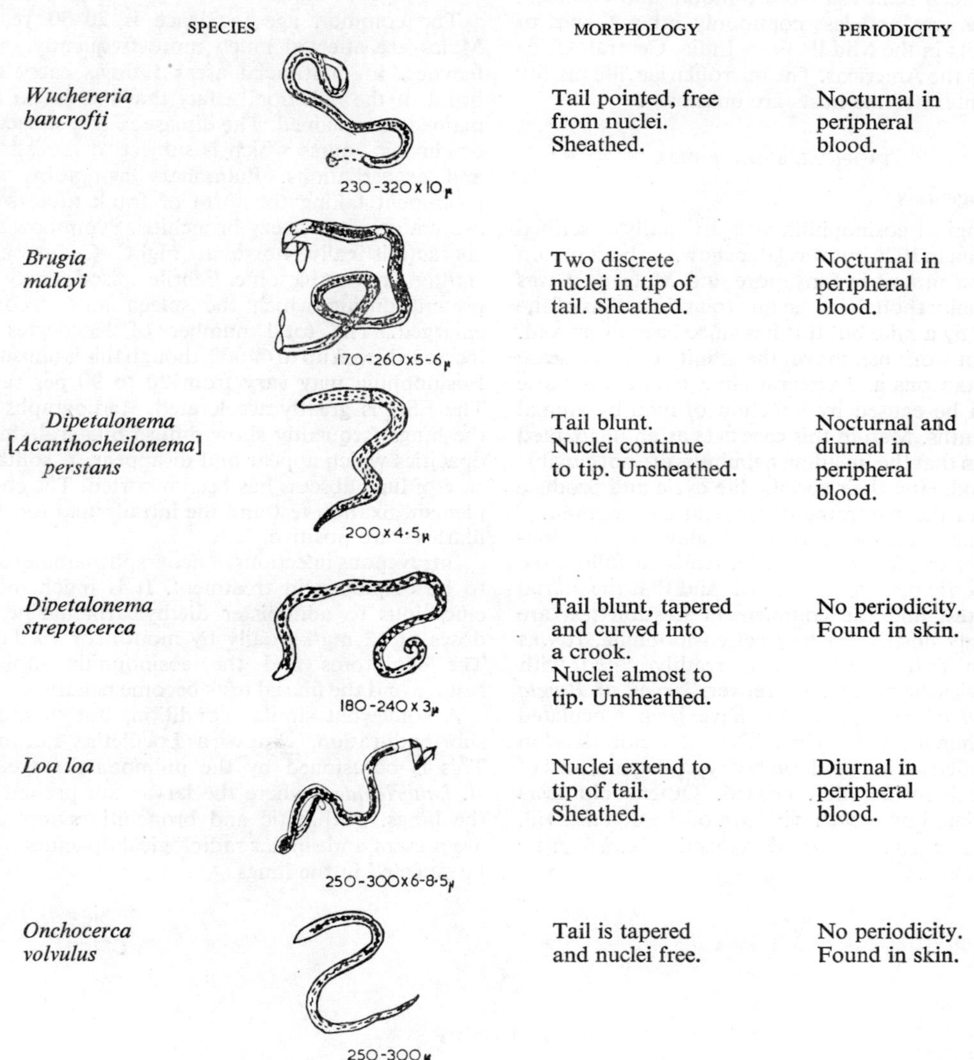

FIG. 14.2. *Summary of the main differences between the microfilariae of the filarial diseases.*

tension is applied the worm will break and acute allergic symptoms are likely to ensue or sepsis occurs and results in cellulitis.

The alternative is to remove the worm by open operation in which case several incisions may be required. Diethyl carbamazine is not effective in curing adult worms but is said to prevent infection in those who have ingested infected *Cyclops.*

OTHER FILARIAL INFECTIONS

Occasional infections in man have been reported with *Dirofilaria immitis* and cough and chest pain have been ascribed to it. *Dirofilaria conjunctivae* have been removed from tumours and abscesses of the eyes and less commonly other tissues of patients in the Middle East, India, Central Africa and in the Americas. The microfilariae, life history and intermediate hosts are unknown.

TROPICAL EOSINOPHILIA

Pathogenesis

Tropical eosinophilia was originally described in India in 1940 but was later shown to be common in Ceylon and in Singapore and Malaya. It was originally thought to be due to an infection of the lungs by a mite but this has since been disproved. Recent work has shown the affinity of this disease to cutaneous and visceral larva migrans because it can be caused by infection of man by animal helminths. Man in this case acts as an unadapted host in that the invading helminths are not capable of producing their specific life cycle and produce instead the syndrome of tropical eosinophilia.

It has been shown that in Malaya the distribution of tropical eosinophilia tends to follow the geometric pattern of filariasis and that the filarial skin test and the complement fixation test are strongly positive in tropical eosinophilia. It was shown that the disease is readily cured with diethylcarbamazine. Moreover, larvae of *Brugia malayi* of monkey origin have been inoculated into human volunteers. They did not develop microfilariae in the blood but typical symptoms of tropical eosinophilia ensued. Other volunteers inoculated by mouth with ova of the dog ascarid, *Toxocara canis*, also developed characteristic symptoms.

Clinical features

The common age incidence is 20–30 years. Males are affected much more frequently than females. In multiracial areas Indians carry the brunt of the infection, a fact that has so far remained unexplained. The disease runs a subacute or chronic course which is subject to remissions and exacerbations. Pulmonary symptoms are prominent taking the form of frank attacks of asthma or of a wheezy bronchitis. Symptoms are characteristically worse at night. Cough and sputum are troublesome. Febrile episodes may be present during which the spleen may become enlarged. The total number of leucocytes is increased, even up to 60 000, though this is unusual. Eosinophilia may vary from 20 to 90 per cent. The ESR is greatly accelerated. Radiographs of the lungs frequently show diffuse bilateral small opacities which appear and disappear. A solitary case of lung abscess has been reported. The complement fixation test and the intradermal test for filariasis are positive.

Intravenous injections of neoarsphenamine used to be employed in treatment. It is much more efficacious to administer diethylcarbamazine in doses of 12 mg/kg daily by mouth for 10 days. The symptoms and the eosinophilia rapidly resolve and the filarial tests become negative.

A somewhat similar condition, but of much shorter duration, is known as Loeffler's syndrome. This is occasioned by the pulmonary stage of *A. lumbricoides*, where the larvae are present in the lungs. Asthmatic and bronchitic symptoms are present and similar radiological opacities may be detected in the lungs.

REFERENCES

BEAVER, P. C. (1970) *Amer. J. trop. Med. Hyg.*, **19**, 181.

COHEN, L. B., NELSON, G., WOOD, A. M., MANSON-BAHR, P. E. C. and BOWEN, R. (1961) *Amer. J. Trop. Med. Hyg.*, **10**, 843.

DE LEON R. J. and DUKE, B. O. L. (1966) *Trans. Roy. Soc. trop. Med. Hys.*, **60**, 735.

HAMMON, J., BURNETT, G. F., ADAM, J. P., RICKENBACH, A. and GERJEBINIE, A. (1967) *Bull. Wld Hlth Org.*, **37**, 217.

HAWKING, F. and CLARK, J. B. (1967) *Trans. roy. Soc. trop. Med. Hyg.*, **61**, 817.

HAWKING, F., MOORE, P. GAMMAGE, K. and WORMS, M. J. (1967) *Trans. roy. Soc. trop. Med. Hyg.*, **61**, 674.

HOBBS, J. R. (1968) *Brit. med. J.*, **4**, 42.

JORDAN, R. (1955) *J. trop. Med. Hyg.*, **58**, 113.

JOSEPH, G. and PRASAD, B. G. (1967) *Ind. J. med. Res.*, **55**, 1259.

KINMONTH, J. B. (1954) *Ann. roy. Coll. Surg. Eng.*, **15**, 300.

MCFADZEAN, J. A. (1952) *Brit. med. J.*, **1**, 1106.

ROWLANDS, A. (1956) *Trans. roy. Soc. trop. Med. Hyg.*, **50**, 563.

Toussaint, D. P. (1965) *Arch Ophth.*, **74**, 470.
Wartman, W. B. (1947) *Medicine*, **26**, 333.
Woodruff, A. W. (1961) *Recent Advances in Tropical Medicine*, 3rd edn., ed. Fairley, N. H., Woodruff, A. W. and Walters, J. H. London: J. & A. Churchill Ltd.
World Health Organization (1967) *Tech. Rep. Ser.*, No. 359.

FURTHER READING

Nelson, G. S. (1970) In *Advances in Parasitology*, Vol. 8. Academic Press, London and New York.
World Health Organization. *Tech. Rep. Ser.*, No. 335.

Bacterial Diseases

Bacillary Dysentery

Diarrhoea of Travellers

Cholera

Typhoid Fever and Other Salmonella Infections

Plague

Brucellosis

Leprosy

15
Bacillary Dysentery

Bacillary dysentery is an acute infectious enteritis caused by members of the genus *Shigella*. It is usually characterised by the sudden onset of frequent mucosanguineous stools accompanied by colicky abdominal pain, tenesmus and fever. The large bowel and frequently the terminal ileum show extensive inflammation, superficial necrosis and hyperplasia of lymphatic nodules. Gradual improvement with early and complete recovery is the usual course, but the disease may terminate abruptly in death or pass into a subacute or chronic phase. Man is the principal host, and his intestine is the natural habitat of *Shigella*; the primary route of transmission is faecal-oral. Distribution is world-wide but prevalence is greatest under conditions of crowding and poor hygiene.

AETIOLOGY

Epidemics of dysentery have been recorded throughout history and descriptions have been attributed to both Hippocrates and Herodotus. The amoebic and bacillary forms were not differentiated, however, until the last quarter of the nineteenth century. Lösch in Russia isolated trophozoites of *Entamoeba histolytica* from dysenteric stools in 1875, and by 1890 amoebae were established as the cause of a particular form of dysentery characterised by chronicity, undermining ulcerations of the colon and occasional concomitant hepatic abscess formation. It was not until 1896, however, that Shiga, in Japan, isolated a causative bacillus (later designated *Shigella dysenteriae*) and demonstrated that these organisms agglutinated with sera of 34 of the 36 dysenteric patients of his study. This work was later confirmed in the Philippine Islands by Strong and Musgrave (1900) and by Flexner (1901). Flexner isolated an organism differing from Shiga's bacillus in its ability to produce acid in mannite media (*Sh. flexneri*). Other strains were later described by Sonne in Denmark (*Sh. sonnei*) and by Boyd in India (*Sh. boydii*).

The classification of the *Shigella* has been a matter of extreme complexity. In general it can be said that the genus *Shigella* consists of Gram-negative, non-motile, non-sporulating rods, corresponding to *Sh. dysenteriae* in staining properties and morphology. All members ferment glucose, some ferment mannitol, and with few exceptions none produce gas from fermentable substances. They are aerobes and facultative anaerobes and grow well on relatively simple media at 37°C. They can be distinguished from most coliform bacilli by their selective growth on media containing bile salts (SS and desoxycholate).

It is practical to divide the members of the genus *Shigella* into four subgroups: A (*Sh. dysenteriae*), B (*Sh. flexneri*), C (*Sh. boydii*) and D (*Sh. sonnei*). Within these subgroups there are individual serotypes, those belonging to subgroups B and D most commonly causing disease in the United States and Great Britain. Unfortunately the more virulent organisms of subgroup A (*Sh. dysenteriae*) still account for a significant proportion of bacillary dysentery in many tropical and subtropical areas of the world.

EPIDEMIOLOGY AND DISTRIBUTION

Man is the primary host and only significant reservoir of *Shigella*, and direct and indirect faecal-oral transmission is responsible for spread. While food and water-borne transmission occasionally occur, the resulting epidemics are generally slowly evolving rather than explosive. Simian primates and, rarely, dogs may be infected but have not been shown to play a role in transmission to man. The disease is not limited to any particular region of the world. Its distribution is determined more by conditions of personal hygiene and environmental sanitation than by geographical considerations, and its prevalence in a community depends primarily on the opportunity for infected faeces to be transferred from one individual to another.

Outbreaks of dysentery have been the scourge of troops at war and of displaced persons in war zones. During World War I it was a major problem in all the armies, and the defeat of the British at Gallipoli has been attributed to shigellosis. As

Zinsser (1935) has expressed it, 'Typhus with its brothers and sisters—plague, cholera, typhoid, dysentery—has decided more campaigns than Caesar, Hannibal, Napoleon and all the inspector generals of history'. It was only with the advent of improved sanitation and the use of sulphonamides during World War II that bacillary dysentery ceased to be a bane of military campaigns. Nevertheless, outbreaks of dysentery responsible for almost 2000 deaths occurred at American prisoner-of-war camps in South Korea during a 14-month period in 1950–51. Of almost 1000 United States Marines hospitalised recently for diarrhoea in Vietnam, infection with *Shigella* spp. was the cause in at least one-third (Forman *et al*, 1971).

The mild nature of most infections makes it difficult to arrive at a true estimation of frequency, but there is no question that bacillary dysentery is a significant cause of morbidity and mortality throughout the world. In the United States there were 12 180 reported cases in 1968, and in England and Wales there was notification of more than 23 000 cases in 1969. It has been noted that for each case of acute bacillary dysentery there are 8–10 convalescent or passive carriers, and on the basis of a study in the southern United States it has been calculated that perhaps less than 1.0 per cent of infections are detected and reported to public authorities. That there is a striking variation in detectable infection among the general population is shown by positive cultural isolations of less than 1 per cent of asymptomatic persons in a survey in New York City and of greater than 10 per cent in areas in the south-western United States. As would be expected, the incidence of bacillary dysentery is greatest in the lesser developed areas of the world, but meaningful data are unavailable.

Prevalence is low in infants younger than 6 months of age but rises rapidly at about 1 year of age with a peak at about the fifth year of life. Asymptomatic infection is much less common in children than in adults and partially accounts for the preponderance of infection recorded under the age of 10 years. Crowding and poor personal hygiene account for the inordinate frequency of infection in institutionalised children.

In the United States, *Sh. sonnei* and *Sh. flexneri* 2 account for more than 60 per cent of isolates, while in England and Wales *Sh. sonnei* alone accounts for 98 per cent. Infection with the more virulent *Sh. dysenteriae* is at present unusual in temperate areas, and although not uncommon in the tropics there has been an indication that its incidence is declining throughout the world.

Shigella organisms are extremely sensitive to sunlight and drying and do not persist in water as well as the hardier *Salmonella*. During the acute phase of the illness the nature and frequency of the stools subject attendants to contamination, but the convalescent and asymptomatic carrier states are probably responsible for most instances of spread (Mata *et al*, 1966). The factors of mild, asymptomatic, and relatively prolonged infection are important epidemiologic considerations. Mechanical transmission of *Shigella* organisms by flies is an important determinant of prevalence of infection in some areas, and may account for wide seasonal variations.

PATHOLOGY

Bacillary dysentery is characterised by inflammation of the large bowel and not uncommonly the terminal portion of the ileum; if examination is made at the proper stage, *Shigella* organisms are demonstrable both in the bowel mucosa and among the contents of the lumen. Electron microscope studies have shown that following penetration of epithelial cells the shigellae enter the lamina propria and incite inflammation at that site (Dammin, 1968).

In the early stages there is a diffuse hyperaemia of the mucosa with moderate oedema and diffuse hyperplasia of lymphatic nodules and Peyer's patches. As the disease progresses the mucosa becomes progressively inflamed, with superficial coagulation necrosis, erosion and haemorrhage. The lymphatic nodules may undergo central necrosis. The submucosa is infiltrated with large numbers of inflammatory cells, is haemorrhagic, and the bowel wall becomes thickened and indurated. The mucosa may be covered by a 'diphtheritic' membrane composed of mucus and necrotic debris. At this point the disease may subside or proceed to further necrosis and ulceration.

The ulcers are characteristically superficial but may extend to the muscularis; they are non-undermined, are surrounded by inflamed, congested mucosa and tend to involve free folds of the intestine in a longitudinal pattern. The most severe lesions are frequently seen in the distal colon, the ileum being rarely involved to an equal degree. Perforation and peritonitis are rare sequelae, and probably in most instances result from superimposed pyogenic infection. Chronic dysentery produces further induration, thickening and occasional strictures. Epithelial cyst-like structures containing mucus and viable *Shigella* organisms have been found in the intestinal wall of persons with long antecedent dysentery.

SYMPTOMATOLOGY AND CLINICAL CHARACTERISTICS

Clinical expression of infection varies tremendously, ranging from the asymptomatic carrier state to that of an abrupt, fulminant and fatal course. The incubation period is usually 24 hours to 7 days and the consequent clinical states may be generally divided into the following:

1. Mild or subacute dysentery
2. Acute dysentery
3. Fulminating dysentery
4. Relapsing dysentery
5. Chronic dysentery.

As noted earlier, undetected *Shigella* infection frequently occurs, and the diagnosis should be entertained in nearly every acute diarrhoeal disease. The majority of *Shigella* infections probably present as mild diarrhoea and go undetected. The mild attack may be characterised by the onset during the first day of illness of several loose stools which become less copious and more frequent during subsequent days. There may be no fever, mild tenesmus, only small amounts of blood or mucus in the faeces, and the symptoms may subside in a few days.

The acute form starts more abruptly with rapid development of a diarrhoea progressing to frequent small movements of mucosanguineous stool accompanied by colicky pains, marked tenesmus, fever as high as 40°C and abdominal tenderness. Nausea and vomiting are not unusual and anorexia is the rule. The patient may appear toxic and dehydrated. Untreated, the dysenteric symptoms may persist for a week or more, may end abruptly, subside slowly, or pass into a subacute or chronic phase.

Fulminating dysentery likewise presents with an onset of cramping abdominal pains, urgency and diarrhoea, but the symptoms may progress to an awesome state which includes extreme toxicity with fever and chills, delirium, dehydration and prostration. The number of stools may exceed forty in a 24-hour period, the patient suffering from a continuing agonising urge to defaecate even though passage of faeces through the inflamed rectum may produce severe burning pain and provide only transient relief of the abdominal colic. The stools rapidly lose their faecal character, becoming mucosanguineous in type, of small volume, and containing the characteristic inflammatory cell exudate. Alarming bloody discharges may occur but are unusual. General abdominal tenderness with mild guarding may be present. The course may terminate in hypothermia, hypovolaemic circulatory collapse and death. In those who recover, less severe diarrhoea may persist for several weeks before remission. Fulminant dysentery is rarely produced by subgroups other than *Sh. dysenteriae* but does occur in infants, the elderly and the malnourished.

Chronic bacillary dysentery characterised by persistence of a mild diarrhoea with recurrent moderate exacerbations of original symptoms over a period of months or years has become uncommon since the introduction of antibiotic treatment. The chronic state may be confused with idiopathic ulcerative colitis or regional enteritis. Felsen (1945) described the development of chronic non-bacterial ulcerative colitis in persons previously involved in a clearly established epidemic of dysentery caused by *Sh. flexneri*. Symptoms of an irritable colon may persist for many months following an initial episode of shigella dysentery.

We have avoided the use of terms such as 'relapse' and 'recrudescence' inasmuch as these are as often bacterial as clinical. Occasionally, patients, following the initial episode, will have a return of symptoms with or without the presence of stools positive for *Shigella*. On other occasions, stools may become positive again without any clinical manifestations. The reasons for these phenomena are unclear. Fortunately, these episodes are uncommon; each must be handled on an individual basis, for generalisations are not productive.

Shigella infections are distinguished by intestinal localisation of disease even though occasional septicaemic states have been documented. All shigellae produce an endotoxin, similar to that of salmonellae and coliforms, which if injected into rabbits or guinea pigs produces diarrhoea, inflammation and necrosis of the bowel. That a similar process operates in man is, however, a matter of conjecture. *Sh. dysenteriae* type 1 alone produces in laboratory animals a potent exotoxin with neuropathic properties which has been postulated to be partially responsible for meningismus and convulsions in infants and for rare instances of peripheral neuritis. Other extraintestinal lesions include occasional acute pyelonephritis. conjunctivitis and an acute arthritis usually involving elbows, knees or ankles. The arthritis occurs in the active or convalescent phase of the dysentery, is self-limited, and the joint fluid rarely contains *Shigella* organisms.

DIAGNOSIS

The diagnosis of bacillary dysentery is firmly established when there is laboratory isolation and identification of *Shigella* organisms cultured from the stool or from a swab sample of rectal or colonic mucosa.

During the acute phase of the disease the stools contain large numbers of organisms, and if cultured promptly will yield positive results in a majority of patients; rectal swab techniques have, however, been clearly shown to be superior, and are strongly advocated. Material must be promptly transferred to culture media and this is best done at the bedside. Selective media which allow prompt differentiation from coliform organisms are of great advantage; however, some combinations of selective media inhibit the shigellae themselves and should be avoided (Taylor and Harris, 1965).

Agglutination, haemagglutination and immunofluorescent techniques have been described but their usefulness is limited. Cultural isolation of organisms from the blood stream is unusual. Microscopic examination of the stool may be extremely helpful in making a tentative diagnosis, especially when amoebiasis is a possibility. Many microscopists have been impressed by the large number of polymorphonuclear leucocytes present in the stools of patients suffering from bacillary dysentery, and have used the presence of faecal leucocytes as a clue to rapid diagnosis while awaiting the results of bacterial cultures (Harris *et al*, 1972). Proctoscopy provides direct definition of ulcer type, allows swabbing of areas of high bacteriologic yield, and is useful in evaluating therapeutic response.

DIFFERENTIAL DIAGNOSIS

The differential diagnostic possibilities include amoebic and balantidial dysentery, salmonellosis, enteropathic coliform disease in children, salmonellosis, the 'diarrhoea of travellers', staphylococcal enterocolitis, schistosomal dysentery and idiopathic ulcerative colitis. Amoebic and balantidial colitis are usually less abrupt in onset and produce fewer signs of systemic toxicity; they may be distinguished by proctoscopy, stool examination and culture. The delayed incubation period, prominence of headache, fever and gastric complaints, and the presence of splenomegaly and rose spots may help to differentiate salmonellosis; occasionally bacteriologic confirmation is required.

Other causes of bacterial colitis are distinguished by stool culture. Blood and mucus are not characteristics of the 'diarrhoea of travellers' and the stools are free from usually recognised pathogens. Schistosomal dysentery in the acute phase of established infection is frequently accompanied by a high eosinophilia, allergic manifestations and ova in the stools or rectal mucosa. An acute toxic megacolon may be indistinguishable from fulminating bacillary dysentery in its presentation and require stool cultivation for differentiation.

TREATMENT

The principal aim in therapy is the establishment and maintenance of normal physiological homeostasis—attempts to eradicate the offending agent with antibiotics are of much less importance. The patient and his bowel should be put to rest. Small and frequent feedings of bland soft foods and liquids (rice, apple sauce, tea, fruit juices) are given until diarrhoea is checked. Fluid and electrolyte replacement and maintenance are of utmost importance in the prevention of dehydration, hypovolaemia and circulatory collapse in the severely ill patient. Transfusion of blood may be necessary in the unusual instance of frank haemorrhage. Paregoric and morphine should be used with caution. Fortunately *Shigella* infections are generally self-limited and mortality is low without specific antimicrobial therapy.

The sulphonamides were the first agents found to be specifically effective and were widely used with success during World War II. They were replaced by broad-spectrum antibiotics following extremely successful trials with tetracycline and chloramphenicol in outbreaks of dysentery in prisoner-of-war camps in South Korea (Hardy *et al*, 1952).

Ampicillin then became the drug of choice because of its efficacy and relative safety. Favourable results were also described with other drugs including aureomycin, oral polymyxin, naladixic acid, carbenicillin, the cephalosporins and aminoglycosides such as streptomycin, kanamycin, gentamicin, and neomycin.

The extensive battery of useful drugs is now blockaded in good part by the development of drug resistance which is often multiple in character. This resistance has been found to be mediated by a cytoplasmic DNA particle (R factor) that replicates independently of the host chromosome and is capable of transfer from cell to cell among various species of Gram-negative bacilli (Watanabe, 1966). The incidence of antibiotic-resistant *Shigella* is therefore a reflection of the presence of antibiotic-resistant intestinal bacteria in the community (Barrett-Connor, 1966).

Since 1955, when drug resistant *Shigella* were described in Japan, more and more reports of a similar nature have appeared in various parts of the world including England (Datta, 1965) and the United States. Almost every drug used in the treatment of shigellosis has been incriminated including the important 'stand-bys' tetracycline, chloramphenicol, and ampicillin. Resistance to these preparations and others appears to have been influenced by the frequency with which they had been used in a particular area. For example, chloramphenicol widely used in Japan is no longer effective there (Watanabe, 1963, 1966). The resistance to ampicillin increased from 6 to 95 per cent in Washington, DC in a 4-year period (Ross, Controni and Khan, 1972), but remained at a low level in Atlanta (Farrar and Eidson, 1971). In London, ampicillin resistance approximated 90 per cent during the period 1967–69 (Davies *et al*, 1970). The result has been that it is no longer possible to make a general recommendation on which drugs should be used in the treatment of shigellosis but every case must be considered separately with evaluation of the following factors: the age, state, and medical status of the patient; the severity of the infection; the strain of the organisms and their response to or resistance to various antibiotics *in vitro*; and the local information available in regard to resistance.

Many patients require no treatment at all, but from a public health standpoint, the rapid elimination of the organism from the stool is desirable. It is our own policy to treat all patients with tetracycline, 2 g daily in divided doses for 3–5 days. If further therapy is necessary, ampicillin, 2–3 g daily, or chloramphenicol in the same dosage may be substituted for 3–5 days.

Both serum antibodies and coproantibodies are easily demonstrable in patients with shigellosis, and some persons in endemic areas apparently are partially immune. The true role of immune mechanisms in *Shigella* infection is not yet defined, and serotherapy has generally been disappointing. Negative results have been more impressive than positive ones (Higgins *et al*, 1955; Mel *et al*, 1965). Dubos (1946) described the preparation and experimental use of a toxoid derived from the exotoxin of *Sh. dysenteriae*, but its efficacy in man is unproved. Treatment with bacteriophage has likewise been disappointing. Prophylactic antimicrobial therapy has been generally unsatisfactory. Prevention is a matter of carrier reduction, contact control, improved environmental sanitation and personal hygiene.

An accurate statement regarding prognosis is not possible, since there is such great variability of clinical severity among outbreaks, among individuals within the same outbreak and in disease produced by the different subgroups. In general, morbidity and mortality are greatest at the extremes of age and are increased by malnutrition and concomitant illness. The most severe disease is usually produced by *Sh. dysenteriae*. Death is rare in a patient receiving close supportive care.

REFERENCES

BARRETT-CONNOR, E. (1966) *J. Amer. med. Ass.*, **198**, 717.
DAMMIN, G. J. (1968) *Resident Physician*, **14**, 57.
DATTA, N. (1965) *Brit. med. Bull.*, **21**, 254.
DAVIES, J. R., FARRANT, W. N. and OTTLEY, A. H. C. (1970) *Lancet*, **2**, 1159.
DUBOS, R. J. and GEIGER, J. W. (1946) *J. exp. Med.*, **84**, 143.
FARRAR, W. E. and EIDSON, M. (1971) *J. infect. Dis.*, **123**, 477.
FELSEN, J. (1945) *Bacillary Dysentery, Colitis and Enteritis*. Philadelphia: W. B. Saunders Co.
FLEXNER, S. (1901) *J. Amer. med. Ass.*, **36**, 6.
FORMAN, D. W., TONG, M. J., MURRELL, K. D. and CROSS, J. H. (1971) *Amer. J. trop. Med. Hyg.*, **20**, 598.
HARDY, A. V., MASON, R. P. and MARTIN, G. A. (1952) *Ann. N.Y. Acad. Sci.*, **55**, 1070.
HARRIS, J. C., DUPONT, H. L. and HORNICK, R. B. (1972) *Ann. intern. Med.*, **76**, 697.
HIGGINS, A. R., FLOYD, T. M. and KADER, M. A. (1955) *Amer. J. trop. Med. Hyg.*, **4**, 281.
MATA, L. J., CATALAN, M. A. and GORDON, J. E. (1966) *Amer. J. trop. Med. Hyg.*, **15**, 632.
MEL, D. M., TERZIN, A. L. and VUKSIC, L. (1965) *Bull. Wld. Hlth. Org.*, **32**, 647.
ROSS, S., CONTRONI, G. and KHAN, W. (1972) *J. Amer. med. Ass.*, **221**, 45.
STRONG, R. P. and MUSGRAVE, W. E. (1900) *J. Amer. med. Ass.*, **35**, 498.
TAYLOR, W. I. and HARRIS, B. (1965) *Amer. J. clin. Path.*, **44**, 476.
WATANABE, T. (1963) *J. Bact. Rev.*, **27**, 87.
——(1966) *New Engl. J. Med.*, **275**, 888.
ZINSSER, H. (1935) *Rats, Lice, and History*. Boston: Little, Brown and Co.

16

Diarrhoea of Travellers

The diarrhoea of travellers is an acute, self-limited disease of unknown aetiology, most commonly affecting travellers who have recently arrived in tropical or semi-tropical countries.

The following synonyms give some idea of the geographic distribution of the disease, and the wry respect in which it is held in various parts of the world:

Acclimatisation diarrhoea, apricot sickness, Aztec two-step, Basra belly, Casablanca crud, Delhi belly, GI's, 'Gyppy' tummy, Egyptian tummy, hill diarrhoea, Hong Kong dog, turkey trot, Lower Burmas, Montezuma's revenge, Poona poohs, Simla trots, San Franciscitis, squitters, travellers' diarrhoea, tourist diarrhoea, tourist trots, turista.

Readers will undoubtedly be able to add others.

AETIOLOGY

Although various aetiologies have been ascribed to the diarrhoea of travellers, its cause remains obscure. Changes in water, alcoholic indulgence, tension of travel, altitude, climate, highly seasoned food, cooking oils are a few of the non-infective factors which have been cited as possible causes. There is no scientific evidence for incriminating any of these.

The syndromes caused by viruses, *Salmonella* spp., *Shigella* spp., enteropathogenic *Escherichia coli*, and the protozoa (especially *Entamoeba histolytica* and *Giardia lamblia*) frequently have been confused with the diarrhoea of travellers. Attempts to incriminate viruses as the cause of the diarrhoea of travellers have been uniformly unsuccessful. In parts of the world where the diarrhoea of travellers is common, *Salmonella* spp., and *Shigella* spp. are not uncommonly isolated from local inhabitants but are rarely found in visitors with diarrhoea.

Evidence that varieties of enteropathogenic *Escherichia coli* are responsible for attacks of the diarrhoea of travellers is accumulating and is in harmony with early clinical and epidemiological observations in Mexico.

At first the evidence was solely statistical but there have been several isolations of 'new' strains of enteropathogenic *E. coli*, some with toxogenic qualities from patients with a syndrome resembling tourist's diarrhoea. It is likely that there will be intensive work on this aspect of the problem within the next few years. A factor favouring such an association is the efficiency of antibiotics such as the sulphonamides in preventing the disease (Rowe *et al*, 1970; Editorial, *J. Amer. med. Ass.*, 1971).

Amoebiasis and giardiasis are easily distinguished from the diarrhoea of travellers by stool examination. Several convincing studies have indicated that the parasites causing these diseases are not present during the acute attack.

More recently the possibility has been considered that alterations in bacterial populations of the small and large bowel may be responsible for the diarrhoea of travellers. The delay in development of symptoms would tend to support this theory. However, since studies on quantitative gastroenterologic bacteriology are complicated, tedious and difficult, it may be some years before current studies in this field are completed.

EPIDEMIOLOGY

Although the attack rate of the diarrhoea of travellers is evidently great in many parts of the world, e.g. Cairo, Delhi, Madrid, Brazzaville etc., there are no accurate studies of the incidence of the disease. It is difficult to collect the data from individual travellers or even from groups visiting these cities. The most extensive work has been done in Mexico City, where the attack rate among visiting students from the United States was evaluated. Over a 5-year period, in a series of studies that eventually included approximately 4000 individuals, the attack rate varied from 25 to 35 per cent. In Hawaii, which was used as a control, only 7 per cent of visitors developed diarrhoea.

Turner reported that the incidence of diarrhoea of travellers in BOAC personnel and their families (1100 out of 1883) travelling abroad was as follows: Africa 25.9 per cent, Middle East 23.5 per cent, South Europe 16.9 per cent, North and Central Europe 15.6 per cent, Asia (including

India and Pakistan) 15.4 per cent, South America and the Caribbean 12.6 per cent, Australasia 11.3 per cent, North America 7.7 per cent.

Another study indicated that almost half of the young, healthy United States students who went to Europe for a 2 month summer vacation had attacks of diarrhoea. The prevalence of diarrhoea was twice as high in those who visited the Mediterranean areas as in those who visited Northern Europe. According to Dandoy, 'To ascertain whether foreign visitors to the United States experience the diarrhea of travelers, 215 foreign students matriculating at the University of California, Los Angeles, were interviewed. The attack rate of diarrhea was 14.0 per cent during the first month after arrival in the United States. In a comparison group of 238 U.S. students, the attack rate of diarrhea in one month was 8.4 per cent. The difference in attack rate was not statistically significant.'

Time of onset

The diarrhoea of travellers does not usually occur within the first 2–3 days after arrival. One study in Mexico showed that 90 per cent of those who developed turista became ill within a fortnight of their arrival; the peak was reached on the eighth day. In another investigation in Mexico, the key day was the fourteenth. In other parts of the world, peak times vary from the seventh to the tenth days.

Age

The incidence of turista in Mexico is higher in adolescents and young adults than in older individuals. It is possible that this represents a development of immunity with age. The variation, however, is probably due to the fact that the young are less likely to take sanitary precautions and to get sufficient rest, and are more likely to live in poorer circumstances. In Mexico, the diarrhoea of travellers occurred more frequently among students who could only afford the boarding houses and private homes, rather than in those who resided in the larger luxury hotels.

Sex

Turista occurs more frequently in men, simply because they travel more. In groups of travellers there is no difference between the sexes in the incidence of diarrhoea.

Season

The data are confused, inasmuch as summer diarrhoea and other entities which have specific causes (e.g. viral diarrhoea in children and salmonellosis) are often confused with the diarrhoea of travellers. No good evidence has established a seasonal difference for this entity.

Immunity

The incidence of diarrhoea is considerably less among individuals who have travelled extensively and who have had one or two previous attacks. Whether this represents the development of an immunity or is due to the greater precautions of the experienced traveller is not known. Approximately two thirds of those who develop diarrhoea while visiting Mexico have one attack but one third has two or more attacks. The question of whether permanent residents of a country develop the same disease as afflicts recently-arrived visitors has been studied in Mexico, without definite conclusions. However, the evidence suggests that they do acquire the same syndrome but at a lesser rate. In a recent survey of participants in an international congress of tropical medicine held in Iran, it was found that diarrhoea developed in a significantly greater number of those travelling from temperate areas than in those from countries in tropical areas (where infectious causes of diarrhoea are considered to be more common). If immunity is responsible for this difference, this would support the infectious hypothesis for the origin of travellers' diarrhoea. The fact that diarrhoea does not usually recur as an individual continues in the new environment may not be due to immunity but to a wisdom gleaned from prior experience.

PATHOLOGY

Proctoscopic examination during the acute phase discloses a surprisingly normal mucosa, free from ulceration. It is usually pale, but on occasion somewhat hyperaemic, and there is no excess mucus.

Rectal biopsy discloses a slightly flattened mucosa, slight oedema of the submucosa, and a barely recognisable cellular infiltrate of neutrophils. Clinico-pathologic studies of the blood are negative except for changes expected with varying degrees of dehydration.

Almost nothing is known about the pathologic changes high in the bowel, for the illness is brief and the rare death is due only to complications.

Stool examinations invariably are negative; the watery specimens contain few cells and are without diagnostic pattern.

SYMPTOMATOLOGY

Whether the attack occurs in Mexico City, Madrid or Madras, the clinical pattern is essentially the same and may be illustrated by the following case history:

The patient was awakened with a start, desperately aware of the need to move his bowels. He traversed the bed-to-bathroom distance in record time and relieved himself of a totally watery bowel movement which was accompanied by slight 'transverse colon' cramps. The patient returned to bed stunned, only to discover that he was immediately constrained to leave again. These spasms were repeated at 15 minute intervals, with the patient exhibiting progressive weakness, profound malaise, increasingly severe cramps, almost constant nausea, and several episodes of vomiting.

He remained afebrile and had no chills, but had 10 bowel movements in 12 hours. Treatment with kaolin and pectin failed. Paregoric caused the diarrhoea to abate somewhat, but the patient remained very weak and could not leave his bed. During the day he drank fluids, usually tea or ginger ale, and ate some cooked rice with apple sauce. The next day he felt stronger and, despite 5 soft bowel movements, could leave his room in the afternoon. On the third day he resumed his activities but at a reduced tempo; on the fourth day after the onset he was completely well.

The diarrhoea itself varies from a softening and general change in the consistency of the stool with a doubling or tripling of their daily number, to 40 bowel movements per day. Blood is almost never found in the stool in the diarrhoea of travellers. In addition to the diarrhoea, other symptoms that develop are:

General abdominal pain and cramps	71%
Nausea	65%
Vomiting	22%
Fever over 37°C	76%
Generalised body and joint aches	25%
Headache	21%
Weakness, dizziness and faintness	15%
Chills	52%

The temperature is rarely above 38°C and seldom lasts more than 2 days. The chills may be severe. Recovery may be delayed by exhaustion and lassitude that may persist for a fortnight.

DIAGNOSIS

Diagnosis is based almost exclusively on the history and clinical symptoms, the absence of protracted fever and the patient's spontaneous recovery (almost invariably on schedule) and, retrospectively, by the elimination of other causes following examination of the stool.

DIFFERENTIAL DIAGNOSIS

Shigellosis, salmonellosis, staphylococcal food poisoning, amoebic dysentery, are the most important diseases to be distinguished from the diarrhoea of travellers. At the onset of the illness, clinical differentiation may be impossible, and by the time laboratory studies are completed, the patient has recovered. Acute appendicitis, perforated peptic ulcer, diverticulitis and malaria are sometimes confused with the initial stages of the diarrhoea of travellers.

The absence of significant fever and the fact that blood and mucus are not present in the stool are important features in the differential diagnosis.

PROPHYLAXIS

General

Since the cause of traveller's diarrhoea is not known, intelligent prophylaxis must be based on general experience with the entity. The more practical preventive measures assume the faecal-oral route of transmission of an infectious agent. The use of boiled water or bottled beverages for drinking, ice cubes and toothbrushing is recommended. Food should be served in clean containers and dishes well protected from flies, vermin and rodents. All food handlers should be instructed in personal hygiene rules and in the art of sanitary food handling. Travellers should eat a hearty breakfast, a mild lunch and simple dinner, and should avoid exotic foods and over-indulgence in alcohol. Adequate rest is important.

Drugs

Half of all travellers to Mexico carried some nostrum with them—ranging from iodochlorhydroxyquin (Entero-Vioform) to Pepto-Bismol. Since Entero-Vioform has long been highly recommended, it was one of the drugs included in two controlled studies conducted in Mexico; 37 per cent of those who took this preparation developed turista, but so did 36 per cent of those who took a placebo.

The recent association of iodochlorhydroxyquin or clioquinol (Entero-Vioform) with the newly described syndrome of subacute myelo-optic neuropathy (SMON) supports the view that this drug should have no place in the prophylaxis or treatment of 'turista' (Kean, 1972).

Two antimicrobial agents were effective in preventing the diarrhoea of travellers among college students in Mexico; neomycin and phthalyl-sulphathiazole were efficient in reducing the attack rate of the more incapacitating degrees of diarrhoea by two thirds.

A recent study by Turner suggested that Streptotriad (each tablet containing streptomycin sulphate 65 mg, sulphadimidine 100 mg, sulphadiazine 100 mg, and sulphathiazole 100 mg) might be used prophylactically. A study of 1100 people showed that the preparation reduced the incidence of turista, the duration of attacks and the development of associated symptoms, but not significantly. A combination of neomycin and trisulphonamides reduced symptoms but not diarrhoea.

The British used this preparation (Streptotriad) during the 1968 Olympics in Mexico with dubious success. The Japanese used *Lactose bacillus acidophilus* for their athletes, obviously believing that bacterial flora were important. After extensive studies which indicated lack of toxicity and no adverse effect on performance, the United States team used sulphasuxidine with no dramatic effect.

It is recommended that drug prophylaxis should not be used except during brief visits (a week or 10 days) to the tropics; for patients who have a history of being prone to diarrhoea; for those who will find it impossible to follow hygienic strictures; and for those on missions of vital importance. If drug prophylaxis is employed, the use of either phthalylsulphathiazole or sulfasuxidine, 1 g twice a day, is advised. Used in this dosage for a brief period, the toxic reactions (rash, fever and haematologic abnormalities) associated with the sulphonamides will be negligible or non-existent. The nitrofurans e.g. (Furoxone) are not recommended; their toxicity is too great and their efficacy questionable. There is no vaccine that can be recommended.

TREATMENT

Treatment is directed toward control of symptoms and maintenance of hydration. A diet of tea, boiled rice and apple sauce (a small amount of each, consecutively, on the hour) is recommended during the acute phase. As the symptoms subside, small amounts of other simple foods can be added until a normal diet can be resumed. Nausea, if severe, may be controlled by anti-emetics such as Compazine (prochlorperazine).

Diarrhoea may be treated with paregoric or Lomotil (diphenoxylate hydrochloride with atropine sulphate).

If the vomiting and diarrhoea during the acute phase are so severe as to preclude the use of drugs by mouth or rectal suppository, it may be necessary to control the symptoms parenterally.

Modest fever needs no treatment, remaining a good index of the accuracy of the diagnosis. Antibiotics such as the tetracyclines and the sulphonamides are not indicated. If fever is high and persists for more than 2–3 days, the diagnosis probably is not the diarrhoea of travellers and antibiotics may then be considered.

PROGNOSIS

Prognosis is excellent except in the aged, the chronically sick, the very young, the diabetic—those who cannot tolerate 2–3 days of dehydration. If medical attention is directed more toward maintaining the fluid and electrolyte balance rather than toward the disease *per se*, recovery is prompt and complete.

Unhappily a very small percentage of patients who start with what appears to be a typical attack of traveller's diarrhoea continue to have symptoms for variable periods of time—up to a year or longer—despite many treatments of various sorts. These cases may represent other diseases or the establishment of an irritable bowel syndrome in the disposed.

FURTHER READING

DANDOY, SUZANNE (1966) The diarrhea of travelers. Incidence in foreign students in the United States. *Calif. Med.*, **104** (6), 458–462.

EDITORIAL (1971) The two faces of pathogenic *Escherichia coli. J. Amer. med Ass.*, **218**, 248.

HILL, J. A. (1961) Diarrhoea in Aden—A therapeutic trial. *Trans. roy. Soc. trop. Med. Hyg.*, **55**, (4), 355–360.

KEAN, B. H. (1963) The diarrhea of travelers to Mexico. Summary of a five-year study. *Ann. intern. Med.*, **59** (5), 605–614.

KEAN, B. H. (1969) Turista in Teheran. Travelers' diarrhea at the Eighth International Congresses of Tropical Medicine and Malaria. *Lancet*, **2**, 583–584.
——(1972) Subacute myelo-optic neuropathy. *J. Amer. med. Ass.*, **220**, 243.
ROWE, B., TAYLOR, J. and BETTELHEIM, K. A. (1970) An investigation of travellers' diarrhea. *Lancet*, **1**, 1.
THOMAS, CLAYTON L. (1968) Public health problems in the Olympic Games setting. *J. Amer. med. Ass.*, **205** (11), 754–756.
TURNER, A. C. (1967) Traveler's diarrhoea. A survey of symptoms, occurrence and possible prophylaxis. *Brit. med. J.*, **4**, 653–654.

17
Cholera

SYNONYMS. Cholera asiatica, cholerine, para-cholera, melon pulp epidemic, Olautha.

DEFINITION

Cholera is an acute endemic or epidemic enteric disease of varying severity caused by infection with *Vibrio cholerae* and characterised in a typical case by profuse painless evacuations, with vomiting, producing dehydration, metabolic acidosis and circulatory collapse which may be rapidly fatal if not treated.

AETIOLOGY

Koch in 1883 discovered *V. cholerae* in Egypt and confirmed it later in Calcutta (Koch, 1884). It is a Gram-negative curved rod-shaped bacterium, actively motile by a single terminal flagellum and is agglutinable by O-1 group antiserum. There are two biotypes, namely the non-haemolytic classical cholera vibrio and the haemolytic El Tor vibrio. The latter has now almost lost its haemolytic characteristic and is distinguished from the classical one by its resistance to phage IV and polymyxin B, and its ability to agglutinate chicken red blood cells. The two biotypes are separated antigenically into two main subtypes, Ogawa and Inaba, and rarely a third type, Hikojima.

The cholera vibrios appear in nature to be pathogenic only to man. A cholera-like condition can be produced in experimental animals, notably rabbit ileal loop, infant rabbit and dog (Sack and Carpenter, 1969), but the syndrome is not known to occur naturally in animals. Koch's view that cholera is a toxicosis was supported by production of cholera 'toxin' (De and Ghose, 1960; Seal, 1960; Panse and Dutta, 1961) later subjected to intensive studies.

The disease occurs in only a few of the susceptible individuals when vibrios are ingested. The size of the inoculum is important. Gastric acidity is a strong barrier (Napier and Gupta, 1942). It may be temporarily lowered, for example, by a drink of water on an empty stomach, which helps to carry the vibrios into the alkaline small intestine where they multiply in enormous numbers (to 10⁷/ml) but do not produce invasive infection. Disease results from vibrio colonisation if and when vibrios anchor themselves (Lankford and Legsomburana, 1965; Neogy and Sanyal, 1969) to the intact small bowel mucosa, so releasing during active multiplication an exotoxin (Feeley and Roberts, 1969) previously referred to as enterotoxin (De, 1959) and choleragen (Finkelstein and Lospalluto, 1969).

The exotoxin acts locally, altering the secretory function of the small intestine and causing a net flow of fluid by all segments (Leitch, Burrows and Stolle, 1967; Sack and Carpenter, 1969). Living vibrios need not be present, but sterile culture filtrates suffice (Sack and Carpenter, 1969), and there is no systemic toxaemia. In acute cholera, bidirectional flux of both water and sodium exists. An increased efflux, plasma to lumen, is the major factor responsible for fluid loss (Banwell *et al*, 1970). The exotoxin has been isolated and purified with the prospect of value in prevention and treatment.

The massive volume of fluid evacuated is almost isotonic with plasma but bicarbonate and potassium content is high, while plasma protein hardly escapes (Chaudhuri, 1954; Phillips, 1963). Adult cholera stool contains approximately (mean values ± standard deviation) sodium 126 ± 9 mEq/litre, potassium 19 ± 9 mEq/litre, bicarbonate 47 ± 10 mEq/litre, and chloride 95 ± 9 mEq/litre (Carpenter, 1970). The loss of sodium chloride, and bicarbonate is figuratively less and that of potassium more in paediatric cholera (Chaudhuri *et al*, 1971). Blood becomes concentrated and viscid and the plasma volume is reduced with increased protein content.

Other characteristic abnormalities causing hypovolaemic shock are elevated haematocrit, increased specific gravity of plasma and whole blood, increased red and white cell counts, decreased plasma bicarbonate, low arterial blood pH and slightly increased initial plasma potassium. The electrocardiographic changes after rehydration may resemble those of potassium deficiency (Kitamato *et al*, 1967). Blood calcium and sugar may be reduced (Rogers and Megaw, 1952). The appearance of the stools depends on the stage of

S

the disease and its severity. The characteristic rice-water appearance during the acute phase is attributed to the presence of mucus and massive numbers of vibrios. Isotonic diarrhoea is associated with isotonic dehydration.

EPIDEMIOLOGY

Cholera occurs in the lower socioeconomic groups under prevailing insanitary conditions, overcrowding and low standard of living, with poor basic health services, inadequate safe water supply and absent sewerage, promoting circulation of vibrio, and incidentally other entero-pathogens.

Since antiquity the worst endemic area has been the Ganges–Brahmaputra delta with epidemic outbreaks from time to time invading the adjacent areas. Six pandemics originated here between 1817 and 1923 and ravaged the world along the trade routes (Pollitzer, 1959). Thereafter, except for an outbreak in Egypt (1947–48) (Kamal, Messih and Kolta, 1948), cholera was not encountered until recently outside Asia other than as imported cases. Endemic areas exist in India, Nepal, Burma, Thailand, the Philippines and southern China. The recent (seventh) pandemic (1961–70) started from an endemic El Tor focus in Sulewesi spreading to nearby islands in Indonesia (Soemiatno, 1969). It then travelled to the western Pacific, and to South-east and Middle East countries, reaching Africa and eastern Europe. Some of these countries have been infected repeatedly after remaining free for some years, some have become truly endemic, while others have been free. Cholera was introduced into Japan, Australia, the United Kingdom and Czechoslovakia but did not gain a foothold there due to surveillance activities and good sanitation (Barua and Cvjetanovic, 1970).

The endemic foci represent a menace to adjoining areas, to neighbouring countries and, in these days of fast travel, to the rest of the world. El Tor vibrio had since its introduction into India in early 1964 (Barua *et al*, 1967), largely replaced the age-old classical vibrio (Mukherjee and Basu, 1967), until recently (Neogy *et al*, 1969). Both types of infection can cause severe cholera, but with the latter much milder and inapparent cases occur. El Tor vibrio is more resistant and survives longer in the environment.

Cholera patients or carriers are the only reservoirs and the mouth the only portal of entry of *V. cholerae*, the sources being liquid stool containing 10^7–10^9 vibrios per ml and formed stool containing 10^2–10^5 vibrios per 0.5 g, contamina-

ting water and food secondarily. Cholera is apparently maintained by a cycle of transmission from vibrio excretors to healthy subjects, a cycle in which water is most important (Mosley, 1970). The classical example of cholera as a water-borne disease was the explosive Broad Street Pump epidemic in London (Snow, 1955). An epidemic may, on the other hand, follow a protracted pattern; unconnected sporadic cases appear among susceptible hosts while occasional small outbreaks occur in groups having a common water or food supply. Besides this, there may be many inapparent infections (Mosley, 1970).

Thus cholera is a highly communicable disease of generally low attack rate depending on the susceptibility and habit of those concerned and the dose ingested. The protracted pattern may also be due to person-to-person spread (Sehgal and Pandit, 1968). The staff in the cholera wards usually do not suffer, but there have been victims among the relatives attending the last rites following deaths from cholera. Soiled moist clothes are contributory and flies may carry vibrios from faeces to food. Fomites are of minor significance. Neutral or alkaline food favour survival of vibrios, but they are readily killed by acid, heat, drying and disinfectants.

Seasonal prevalence differs in different countries. The climate or such factors as rains, monsoons and drought may increase or decrease the incidence according to conditions in a given area. Seasonal exacerbations, consisting sometimes of a yearly rise in two waves to epidemic proportions, may occur in an endemic area, and there may be sporadic cases and/or carriers throughout most of the year. Fairs, festivals and migration of population may lead to epidemic outbreaks and spread.

Both sexes and all age groups (rare under 1 year) are affected depending on the chances of infection. In endemic areas, cholera is largely a disease of children because of the development of immunity as they grow older. On the other hand, there is no difference between adult and paediatric morbidity in newly invaded non-endemic areas where the population has no basic immunity, although early in an epidemic there is higher incidence in male adults because of greater exposure (Mosley, 1970).

PATHOLOGY

Autopsy shows non-specific changes from depletion of fluids and electrolytes. The body is dehydrated with fluid accumulation in the intestine. The mucous surface of the small intestine is covered with a thick layer of tenacious, adherent mucus. Gut changes include congestion, oedema, hyperplasia of the lymphoid follicles and Peyer's patches, lymphocytic infiltration, dilatation of the intestinal crypts, and an increase in mucus-producing goblet cells (Rogers, 1913; De, 1961). Contrary to the former view, the small bowel mucosa is not destroyed or denuded, which may result from prolonged shock and post-mortem autolysis. Biopsy specimens at different levels during acute illness reveal no demonstrable damage to the epithelium (Gangarosa *et al*, 1960). Hence, cholera stool is virtually protein-free. Kidneys may show ischaemic tubular necrosis and hypokalaemic nephropathy (Benyajati *et al*, 1960; Hinman *et al*, 1963). Lungs may be oedematous and the liver shows centrilobular damage. The gall-bladder is distended with thick bile.

SYMPTOMATOLOGY

The incubation period is 1 to 5 days, at times a few hours to a week. The classical and El Tor vibrios can produce an identical syndrome (Wallace *et al*, 1966). Typical cholera occurs in a small proportion of infected and susceptible persons only.

It has a sudden onset. The lower bowel is rapidly emptied of faeces followed by large evacuations and disappearance of bile. Pints of pale fluid are painlessly poured out. The stools are clear or consist of opaque white watery fluid with floating mucus resembling rice-water in appearance. It is odourless or has a slightly fishy smell often emanated by patients with soiled clothes.

Vomiting starts after the diarrhoea, but may be absent in 20 per cent of cases. The patient is rapidly prostrated. Signs of dehydration appear when the fluid depletion corresponds to 6 per cent of the body weight. Profound loss may reduce it by 10 per cent within a few hours. The stool output varies, usually 5 to 10 litres, but may be much more during the course of the illness. The patient has a pinched face, sunken eyes and cheeks; he is apathetic, thirsty and speaks in a husky voice. The hands and fingers are shrivelled resembling washerwoman's hands. Striated muscle cramps are common particularly in the legs. Tetanic spasms may occur. The abdomen is soft and not tender with impaired skin elasticity, a pinched skin fold persisting longer than usual.

The patient passes into a stage of circulatory collapse with feeble or imperceptible pulse, fall of blood pressure and surface temperature. There may be cyanosis, and the urine flow stops. The patient is conscious, but may be drowsy and acidotic. The disease is self-limiting, the duration of illness being only a matter of hours or days. Recovery from rehydration is rapid and remarkable. Complications may arise from defective treatment. They are pyrogen reactions, persistent vomiting, recurring shock and renal failure. Pregnant women may have abortion or premature labour with high fetal mortality and retention of placenta.

Infection with cholera vibrio causes a high proportion of mild or subclinical cases. These have only one or two loose motions without rice-water character or dehydration. Many more inapparent infections may also be detected by bacteriological and serological surveys (Oseasohn *et al*, 1966). 'Carriers' are infected symptom-free persons in whom the organisms are multiplying and not just passive bearers of the organisms. Some may have occasional trivial diarrhoea. They may exist in endemic areas even in the absence of recognised cholera cases and move freely about in their community. The duration of the carrier state is relatively short, usually not more than a week or two, at times longer and rarely chronic. At the other extreme there is fulminant cholera sicca, a rare condition when death occurs within a few hours from shock before the appearance of diarrhoea and vomiting. The bowel is distended with rice-watery stool.

Cholera in children may have features which are rare in adults. These include tachypnoea, tympanitis, fever, stupor, convulsions, hypotonia and/or cardiac arrhythmia. There are problems of rapid dehydration, acidosis and hypokalaemia (Chaudhuri, 1966).

DIAGNOSIS

Cholera should be suspected in any acute case or outbreak of dehydrating diarrhoea, or 'gastroenteritis', occurring in an endemic or cholera-threatened area. Recognition of cholera gravis is easy. The initial diagnosis, upon which a patient's life may depend, must be made on clinical grounds with prompt treatment as an emergency measure. The final diagnosis remains primarily a bacteriological one. Dark-field microscopy has made possible a quick presumptive diagnosis (Benenson, Islam and Greenough, 1964). The fluorescent antibody technique has also been used with success directly and rapidly to identify vibrios in stool (Finkelstein and Gomez, 1963), however, the specialised microscope and reagents limit their usefulness.

Cultural isolation of vibrios is the mainstay in diagnosis. Different media, selective or non-selective, may be used for primary isolation.

TCBS agar (thiosulphate–citrate–bile salts–sucrose) (Kobayashi *et al*, 1963) has simplified the isolation and recognition of vibrios. Older media, such as bile salt agar and nutrient agar, continue to be widely used for vibrio isolation, particularly with the help of the oblique light technique. In addition to direct plating of cholera stool, liquid enrichment media are necessary for detection of small numbers of vibrios. Alkaline peptone water with pH of 9.2, as well as other modified liquid enrichment media, are adequate for this purpose.

Proper collection of stool is important. Before giving any antimicrobial drug, the liquid stool specimen is collected in a sterile screw-capped vial or test tube through a sterile rubber catheter passed into the rectum; or the specimen is collected on a sterile absorbent cotton swab inserted into the rectum and never from the bed or bed pan. One of the problems of diagnosing cholera in rural areas has been the difficulty of transporting specimens to distant laboratories. The time-honoured method of collecting stool in holding media, such as the sea-salt medium is still of great practical usefulness. An alternative is the use of blotting paper or a lump of cotton wool soaked with stool and transported in plastic bags or envelopes sealed air-tight (Barua and Gomez, 1967).

For patients who have taken antibiotics and for retrospective diagnosis, serological methods can be used because vibriocidal, agglutinating and toxin neutralising antibodies usually appear after infection (Sack *et al*, 1966). For detection of carriers of cholera vibrios, rectal swabbing and stool examinations alone may be partially satisfactory since vibrio excretion is scanty and intermittent. Purging with magnesium sulphate, duodenal intubation or the identification of Kappa phage (Takeya *et al*, 1965) in stools may be useful.

In the absence of vaccination serological follow-up is helpful. Serotype changes of vibrios may occur from time to time. Ogawa and Inaba organisms may show serological conversions from one to the other, in response to the selective presence of antibody. Also both smooth serotypes may undergo rough transformations with the loss of serological specificity, not only in the laboratory, but also in the long-term chronic carrier state.

DIFFERENTIAL DIAGNOSIS

Acute gastroenteritis due to salmonellosis or other food poisoning is usually associated with pain and fever, while vomiting precedes diarrhoea and there may be other cases among those who shared a particular meal. Acute bacillary dysentery rarely causes massive diarrhoea; tenesmus, griping, fever and mucus with blood are common features. Cholera patients may sometimes have mixed infection. Infantile diarrhoea due to *Escherichia coli* or virus, or 'parenteral diarrhoea' is excluded by clinical and stool examinations. In algid malaria stools and vomit contain bile and there may be a subicteric tinge of the conjunctiva. Such a patient should be given an antimalarial drug after taking blood smears for parasites.

The clinical picture of cholera can be produced by agents other than cholera vibrios, notably 'non-agglutinable' or 'non-cholera' vibrios (Carpenter *et al*, 1965), certain strains of *E. coli* (Sack, 1970) and *V. parahaemolyticus* (Chatterjee, Neogy and Gorbach, 1970). If *V. cholerae* is not isolated a special search for these organisms as well as for salmonellae and shigellae are made. There may however be cases in which no pathogens are isolated. Other conditions, like organic phosphorus and metallic poisoning and heat exhaustion, are excluded by history and local circumstances.

TREATMENT

Since all signs, symptoms and biochemical abnormalities in cholera result directly from the gut fluid and electrolyte loss, the principle is non-specific intravenous replacement of the losses supplemented by a specific antimicrobial drug given orally. Usually a litre of isotonic saline is followed by half a litre of isotonic alkali, namely, 1.3 per cent sodium bicarbonate (14 g per litre), or 1/6 molar sodium lactate (18.7 g per litre) and always repeated in the same 2 : 1 ratio. The solutions must be sterile and pyrogen free. This simple therapy (Chaudhuri and Carpenter, 1968) has proved uniformly successful in adult cholera and has replaced the traditional therapy with hypertonic saline and alkali. Ringer lactate (BP) or lactated Ringer solution (USP) is the intravenous fluid of choice for paediatric cases, and is also effective in adults. It is the most convenient single isotonic pyrogen-free solution available commercially and is useful for rehydration of cholera patients of all ages both for initial rehydration and maintenance (Chaudhuri, 1966; Carpenter, 1970; Chaudhuri *et al*, 1971).

Occasionally for direct puncture, a peripheral vein cannot be located in a pulseless patient. The 'cut down' method is avoided by starting infusion via the femoral vein and later changing to the antecubital or any other convenient vein. External jugular vein infusion has also been used in children. For initial rehydration of an adult, fluid is run in as rapidly as 1 litre every 15 minutes or less through a 17 or 18 gauge needle and then at a somewhat slower rate till the radial pulse volume is restored to normal along with improvement of the general condition. Vomiting invariably ceases also permitting oral fluid administration. The rehydrated state is then maintained by continuing the drip to replace subsequent losses as they occur, regulating the flow according to evacuations and giving to drink *ad libitum* additional water, which may be sweetened or flavoured with lemon juice.

The quality of the radial pulse is the single most reliable guide to fluid requirements as evaluated at 2-hourly intervals. The changing character of the stool—clear or whitish watery, yellowish watery and faecal—is also noted. The volume diminishes as the stool forms and the intervals between the bowel movements increase. A chart is maintained showing the amount of fluid intake orally and intravenously, and of output in the form of vomit, stool and urine. Overhydration is avoided. Urine flow is established soon after the patient is properly rehydrated. The infusion is terminated with cessation of watery diarrhoea while oral fluid is continued. Occasionally, purging recurs again necessitating infusion.

If the supply of intravenous fluid is limited as in rural areas, the majority of adult patients may be maintained, after initial intravenous rehydration, with oral glucose-electrolyte solution by mouth or nasogastric tube (Nalin *et al*, 1968). This may be prepared in the field by dissolving in 1 litre of water 4 g sodium chloride, 4 g sodium bicarbonate, 1 g potassium citrate and 20 g glucose. Potassium citrate improves the taste rather than potassium chloride (Chaudhuri, 1971). The solution is administered at the rate of 750 ml per hour for the first 4 hours. Following this the volume of oral solution for each 4-hour period should balance stool output with an additional 50 ml per hour for insensible loss. Close observation is essential with measurement of stool volume, and if the fluid is not retained or purging recurs resort must be had to intravenous management.

About 3 hours after the initiation of therapy when vomiting usually ceases, chloramphenicol, tetracycline or furazolidone is started. The minimal dosage of antibiotics is 500 mg 6-hourly for 48–72 hours, and that of furoxone 400 mg in single or divided doses for 72 hours. As a result, stools form early and become vibrio-negative in 24 to 48 hours, as compared with a week in the untreated patient, subject to adequate hydration.

Further, the duration of diarrhoea and consequently the intravenous fluid requirement are significantly reduced. The vibrios readily develop resistance to streptomycin. Sulphonamides are less effective while cholera phage therapy is of no therapeutic value.

If the infusion fluid contains no potassium, 1.75 g of a mixture containing potassium citrate 188 g, citric acid 84 g and potassium chloride 47g (4 : 2 : 1), or one containing 20, 10 and 5 grains respectively, is given with water 6-hourly. Alternatively, drinks of green coconut water containing 70 mEq/l potassium, if available locally, are given, 200 ml for every litre of stool. Fruit juice is allowed, and solid food is started early. Hospitalisation may not be necessary for more than 4 days if stools are vibrio negative.

Serious complications of cholera are prevented by proper therapy. Anuria due to renal tubular necrosis occurring in untreated or undertreated cases with prolonged hypovolaemic shock, usually responds to adequate fluid balance maintained by replacing the measured gastrointestinal fluid losses. Morphine or analgesics are avoided for muscular cramps which respond to rehydration, and the addition of calcium gluconate intravenously helps to relieve tetanic spasm. 'Stimulants' like adrenaline, noradrenaline, atropine, coramine, corticosteroids, or plasma substitutes for collapse, or oxygen for cyanosis and rapid breathing are unnecessary. These clinical features are corrected by adequate intravenous fluid therapy.

If pyrogen reactions occur the infusion rate is reduced, or better the fluid and tubing are replaced; an antihistaminic injection affords relief. Pregnant women with cholera should receive special care because of the risk of abortion or premature labour. There should be no maternal mortality. Retained placenta, if it occurs, is better left untreated for the time being. The organism may establish itself in the gall-bladder and treatment with vibriocides is not dependable.

In paediatric cholera, Ringer lactate is injected into a peripheral or scalp vein through a thin-walled 21 gauge needle. For initial rehydration 60 ml per kg is given in 4 hours. Half the amount is injected in the first hour and the rest in the next 3 hours. Thereafter, for maintenance, a slow drip is set up until watery diarrhoea stops. Glucose water, 5 per cent by mouth, is started early, at first in sips and later liberally. This makes an effective adjunct to intravenous fluid therapy. Excess in the rate or volume of infusion is strictly avoided, guarding against overhydration which is indicated by distended neck veins, pulmonary or peripheral oedema, disturbed sensorium and abnormal weight gain.

For maintenance, if intravenous therapy is difficult to continue under field conditions, Ringer lactate is given subcutaneously (Chaudhuri *et al*, 1971) or intraperitoneally, 500 ml being given in about 10 minutes through a No. 18 needle just below the umbilicus in the midline with aseptic cautions. Alternatively, oral maintenance therapy may be tried but it is less satisfactory than in adults.

Tetracycline, 50 mg/kg/day or furazolidone, 5 mg/kg/day in four divided doses is given for 3 days. The child is fed as soon as possible. Other measures include sponging for pyrexia and use of a flatus tube with administration of potassium for paralytic ileus. Potassium is also helpful in cardiac arrhythmia and muscular hypotonia. Glucose, 50 ml of 25 per cent solution, is given intravenously for prolonged stupor or convulsions with gardenal or paraldehyde injections for the latter. Hypoglycaemic convulsions respond remarkably. Cerebral oedema is another result of overhydration necessitating restriction of electrolytes. The passage of round worms is common, but antihelminthic treatment is postponed (Chaudhuri, 1971).

PROPHYLAXIS AND PREVENTION

Prophylactic vaccine consists of 8000 million killed smooth strains of prevalent cholera vibrios per ml of both Inaba and Ogawa serotypes in equal numbers. Each lot should pass appropriate potency and safety tests. The classical vibrio vaccine appears effective in both types of infection by stimulating an antibacterial but little or no antitoxic immune response; El Tor vaccine is also used. Individual immunisation is carried out in two doses, 0.5 and 1.0 ml (0.3 and 0.5 ml in children) given 1 to 4 weeks apart. A single dose of 1.0 ml in adults, and a proportionately lower dose in children, is given subcutaneously for mass immunisation in epidemic situations or in threatened areas, as an emergency measure. Mass vaccination as a routine seasonal measure is not necessary; it is much more expensive than modern treatment of cases.

Protection is effective a week after inoculation when the international certificate becomes valid. Immunisation of the exposed population is carried out in a concentric pattern around the infected area with priority to the population at risk. Cholera vaccination does not afford full protection; it can reduce the clinical case rate to 80 per cent for 2–3 months. It must not, however, be used as a substitute for public health measures. It does not modify the clinical severity nor reduce the fatality or carrier rate. Side reactions include malaise, headache, local tenderness and possibly some fever for 1–3 days. Vaccination is avoided in children under 1 year, advanced pregnancy and those with previous sensitivity reactions.

A suspected cholera case or an outbreak of 'gastroenteritis' should be notified as 'cholera' to the nearest health authority for prompt action including laboratory confirmation of the diagnosis. An essential step in prevention is early detection, isolation and treatment. Epidemiological enquiries are made about the possible source of infection and steps are taken for its removal. The infected house is cleaned and disinfected. Excreta are well mixed with bleaching powder or lime before disposal. In the absence of a sewerage system, as in rural areas, all excreta are buried at a safe distance. Dead bodies are wrapped in sheets soaked in 2 per cent lysol after plugging the orifices with cotton wool soaked in disinfectant. They must be disposed of properly—never thrown in a river or canal.

A single dose of furazolidone, 400 mg, is given to close household contacts for 3 days to prevent vibrio dissemination by infected persons. Acid drinks are encouraged. Health education is important with emphasis on food hygiene, handwashing after defaecation and before eating or serving food, and on the danger of unsafe water necessitating chlorination or boiling. Use of piped or tube well water is advised if available near by. Public gatherings and feasts are prohibited during an epidemic.

Final control of the disease will come only with improvement of environmental sanitation, water supply and personal hygiene. Treatment facilities should be made available in rural areas by trained field teams. Introduction of cholera into a country may not be prevented, but its spread can be limited by improving sanitation and by undertaking intensive surveillance. If surveillance is to be effective, the practising physicians in those countries must be fully informed about the nature of the disease, its optimal treatment and the trend of its spread. In addition, they should have the necessary supplies and means of sending suspected specimens to an appropriate laboratory for culture, even if it is far away. Experience has shown that even little improvement in sanitation and water supply markedly reduces the transmission of *V. cholerae*, a delicate organism (Barua, Burrows and Gallut, 1970)

PROGNOSIS

Modern therapy is simple and effective, making mortality from cholera at all ages unlikely. Prognosis depends on the degree of fluid and electrolyte loss and the length of time which elapses from the onset of illness to adequate therapy, but even a seemingly moribund patient may be saved. Prognosis is unfavourable in patients with renal failure. Extremes of age and pregnancy increase the risk.

Severity of the disease varies from epidemic to epidemic and with the individual patient. In remote areas there are logistic problems in initiating treatment when large numbers of cases occur. The fatality rate of untreated cholera gravis is about 60 per cent. A second attack of cholera may occur.

REFERENCES

BANWELL, J. G., NATHANIEL, F., PIERCE, R. C., MITRA, R. C., BRIGHAM, K. L., CARANASOS, G. J., KEIMOWITZ, R. I., FEDSON, D. S., THOMAS, J., GORBACH, S. L., SACK, R. B. and MONDAL, A. (1970) *J. clin. Invest.*, **49**, 183.

BARUA, D., BURROWS, W. and GALLUT, J. C. (1970) *Principles and Practice of Cholera Control*. World Health Organization, Public Health Series No. 40, Geneva.

BARUA, D. and CVJETANOVIC, B. (1970) In *Principles and Practice of Cholera Control*. World Health Organization, Public Health Series No. 40, Geneva.

BARUA, D. and GOMEZ, C. Z. (1967) *Bull. Wld Hlth Org.*, **37**, 798.

BARUA, D. *et al* (1967) *Bull. Wld Hlth Org.*, **37**, 804.

BENENSON, A. S., ISLAM, M. R. and GREENOUGH, W. B. (1964) *Bull. Wld Hlth Org.*, **30**, 827.

BENYAJATI, C., KEOPLUG, M., BEISEL, W. R., GANGAROSA, E. J., SPRINZ, H. and SITPRIYA, V. (1960) *Ann. intern. Med.*, **52**, 960.

CARPENTER, C. C. J. (1970) In *Principles and Practice of Cholera Control*. World Health Organization, Public Health Series No. 40, 53.

CARPENTER, C. C. J., BARUA, D., WALLACE, C. K., SACK, R. B. MITRA, P. P., WERNER, A. S., DUFFY, T. P., OLEINICK, A., KHANRA, S. R. and LEWIS, *Bull. Wld Hlth Org.*, **33**, 665.

CHATTERJEE, B. D., NEOGY, K. N. and GORBACH, S. L. (1970) *Indian J. med. Res.*, **58**, 234.

CHAUDHURI, R. N. (1954) *Brit. med. J.*, **22**, 423.

—— (1966) *Treatment of Cholera with Special Regard to Children*. WHO/Chol/WP. 66, 14.

—— (1971) *Tropical Doctor*, **1**, 5.

CHAUDHURI, R. N. and CARPENTER, C. C. J. (1968) *J. Indian med. Ass.*, **51**, 182.

CHAUDHURI, R. N. SHRIVASTAVA, D. L., MONDAL, A., SARKAR, B. K., GANGULY, ROMA, BHAKTI SAMANTA, B., DE, S. P. and DE, S. (1971) *Indian J. med. Res.*, **59**, 544.

DE, S. N. (1959) *Nature*, **183**, 1533.

—— (1961) *Cholera: Its Pathology and Pathogenesis*. Oliver and Boyd, Edinburgh.

DE, S. N. and GHOSE, M. L. (1960) *J. Path. Bact.*, **79**, 373.

FEELEY, J. C. and ROBERTS, C. P. (1969) *Tex. Rep. Biol. Med.*, **27**, 213.

FINKELSTEIN, R. A. and GOMEZ, C. Z. (1963) *Bull. Wld Hlth Org.*, **28**, 327.

FINKELSTEIN, R. A. and LOSPALLUTO, J. J. (1969) *J. exp. Med.*, **130**, 185.

GANGAROSA, E. J., BEISEL, W. R., BENYAJTI, C., SPRINZ, H. and PIYARATN, P. (1960) *Amer. J. trop. Med. Hyg.*, **9**, 125.

HINMAN, E. J., SAHA, T. K., WALKER, W. G. and CARPENTER, C. C. J. (1963) *Bull. Calcutta Sch. trop. Med.*, **11**, 154.

KAMAL, A. M., MESSIH, G. A. and KOLTA, Z. (1948) *J. Egypt. Publ. Hlth Ass.*, **31**, 185.

KITAMATO, O., HIRAISHI, K., TAKIGAMI, T., SAITO, M. and SHIMIZU, N. (1967) *Bull. Wld Hlth Org.*, **37**, 787.

KOBAYASHI, T., ENOMOTO, S., SAKAZAKI, R. *et al.* (1963) *Jap. J. Bact.*, **18**, 387.

KOCH, R. (1884) *Brit. med. J.*, **2**, 403, 453.

LANKFORD, C. E. and LEGSOMBURANA, U. (1965) *Proceedings of the Cholera Research Symposium*, p. 109. U.S. Public Health Services.

LEITCH, G. J., BURROWS, W. and STOLLE, L. C. (1967) *J. infect. Dis.*, **117**, 197.

MOSLEY, W. H. (1970) In *Principles and Practice of Cholera Control*. World Health Organization, Public Health Series No. 40, Geneva.

MUKHERJEE, S. and BASU, S. (1967) *Trop. geogr. Med.*, **19**, 138.

NALIN, D. R., CASH, R. A., ISLAM, R., MILLA, M. and PHILLIPS, R. A. (1968) *Lancet*, **2**, 370.

NAPIER, L. E. and GUPTA, S. K. (1942) *Indian med. Gaz.*, **77**, 717.

NEOGY, K. N. and SANYAL, S. N. (1959) *Bull. Wld Hlth Org.*, **40**, 329.

NEOGY, K. N., MUKHERJEE, M. K., SANYAL, S. N. and CHATTERJEE, B. D. (1969) *Bull. Calcutta Sch trop. Med.*, **17**, 39.

OSEASOHN, R., AHMAD, S., ISLAM, M. A. and RAHMAN, (1966) *Lancet*, **1**, 340.

PANSE, M. V. and DUTTA, N. K. (1961) *J. infect. Dis.*, **109**, 81.

PHILLIPS, R. A. (1963) *Bull. Wld Hlth Org.*, **28**, 297.

POLLITZER, E. (1959) *Cholera*. W.H.O. Memograph No. 43, World Health Organization, Geneva.

ROGERS, L. (1913) *Cholera and its Treatment*. London: Oxford University Press.

ROGERS, L. and MEGAW, J. W. D. (1952) *Tropical Medicine*. London: J. & A. Churchill.

SACK, R. B. (1970) Personal communication.

SACK, R. B. and CARPENTER, C. C. J. (1969) *J. infect. Dis.*, **119**, 138.

SACK, R. B., BARUA, D., SAXENA, R. and CARPENTER, C. C. J. (1966) *J. infect. Dis.*, **116**, 630.

SEAL, S. C. (1960) *Ann. Biochem. exp. Med.*, **20**, 205.

SEHGEL, P. N. and PANDIT, C. G. (1968) *Indian J. med. Res.*, **56**, 982.

SNOW, J. (1955) *On the Mode of Communication of Cholera*. New York: Oxford University Press.

SOEMIATNO (1969) *The Cholera Problem in Indonesia*. SEA/Cholera/sem. 2/4 Rev. 1.

TAKEYA, K., ZINNAKA, Y., SHIMODORI, S., NAKAYAMA, Y., AMAKO, K. and IIDA, K. (1965) *Proceedings of the Cholera Research Symposium*, p. 24. U.S. Department of Public Health.

WALLACE, C. K., CARPENTER, C. C. J., MITRA, P. P., SACK, R. B., KHANRA, S. R., WERNER, A. S., DUFFY, T. P., OLENICK, A. and LEWIS, G. W. (1966) *Brit. med. J.*, **2**, 447.

18
Typhoid Fever and Other Salmonella Infections

Typhoid fever has been known for many hundreds, if not thousands of years. Hippocrates described a fever which was probably typhoid, and it is said that Antonius Musa, a Roman physician, became famous by treating the Emperor Augustus with cold baths when he fell ill with typhoid.

Thomas Willis (1684), however, may be regarded as the pioneer in typhoid fever, and he was the first to separate this disease from the many which it mimics. Other important landmarks include Pierre Louis' description of Peyer's patches in 1829 and it was he who first used the word 'typhoid'. In 1837 Gerhard was the first to differentiate between typhoid and typhus.

Eberth's discovery in 1880 of 'B. typhus' and Gaffky's successful culture of *Salmonella typhi* in 1884 completed the diagnostic and prophylactic picture.

Achard and Bensaude in 1896 were the first to isolate *S. paratyphi B* and use the term 'paratyphoid fever'. Subsequently *S. paratyphi A* and *C* together with other members of the salmonella group were isolated.

Widal in 1896 described the Widal reaction, and the first prophylactic inoculation against typhoid was introduced by Pfeiffer and Kolle (1896) and Wright (1896). Two other great advances were Marriott's classical paper on salt and water depletion in 1947, and the first report on the use of chloromycetin synthesised as chloramphenicol in typhoid (Woodward *et al*, 1948). After 25 years no drug has yet been found to equal chloramphenicol in the treatment of typhoid fever.

AETIOLOGY

The salmonellae form a large group of pathogenic bacteria numbering 72 phage types, the typhoid bacillus itself having over 1000 species. All salmonellae are both irritative and invasive to some degree.

Those that are mainly of the invasive type give rise to an enteric type of disease, i.e. typhoid fever and paratyphoids A, B and C. These are on the whole the most serious types, and may lead to severe complications and death.

Those that are mainly of the irritative type tend to cause gastroenteritis, which is often mild and of short duration. This is not invariable, however, and occasionally a salmonella *other* than *S. typhi* and *S. paratyphi* A, B and C may give rise to a generalised disease difficult to distinguish from the true enteric fevers. The typhoid and paratyphoid bacilli on the other hand can occasionally cause an early gastroenteritis if ingested in massive doses.

The salmonellae are motile bacilli 1–3 $\mu\mu$ in length and 0.5–0.7 $\mu\mu$ in thickness. They are Gram-negative, have 8–12 flagellae, do not form spores, grow best at 37°C, and can survive freezing and drying for several weeks and sometimes longer. They are killed by a temperature of 60°C for 15 minutes and rapidly by boiling.

EPIDEMIOLOGY

Typhoid fever still occurs in epidemics in many of the tropical and subtropical parts of the world, and will continue to do so for many years to come. This is partly due to low standards of hygiene, but also to a lack of a completely effective prophylactic vaccine.

The number of notified cases each year in Britain has never fallen below a hundred, and the Aberdeen epidemic in 1964 with 507 cases showed that epidemics, especially those due to infection from other countries, is an ever increasing hazard. Switzerland also has had several epidemics, the worst of which was at Zermatt in 1963.

The number of notified cases from Italy alone in 1966 was 10 493 and over 2000 cases were notified each from France, Spain and Yugoslavia. Colombia had 7823, Mexico 6699, and Peru 6512 known cases in 1966 (*Epidem. vit. Statis. Rep.*, 1967) and the number of undiagnosed cases from these countries must be several times this number. In addition, unreported epidemics in India and

China probably number hundreds and thousands each year.

In many developing countries also, epidemics are getting larger, not smaller. Patnaik and Kapoor (1967), for instance, reported a rise in incidence in Delhi, India, from 245 in 1955 to 1076 in 1963 with a sevenfold increase in mortality rate.

Visitors to developing countries are by no means completely protected by TAB vaccine and Laverdant in 1966 showed that immunised soldiers still contracted severe typhoid in countries like North Africa with severe complications, relapses and death.

The paratyphoid fevers are usually, but not always, less serious than typhoid. They are common in Europe and North America, but unlike typhoid they are rare in most tropical countries. In Delhi, for instance, out of 5854 hospital admissions only 16 were paratyphoid and the rest typhoid (Patnaik and Kapoor, 1967).

The spread of infection in *typhoid* fever itself is usually from a carrier contaminating water or milk supplies. Other sources include ice cream, vegetables, salads, and classically but uncommonly oysters infected in polluted river estuaries. Occasionally flies and dust have also been incriminated, and recently infected meat from South America has caused several epidemics in Britain (Meers and Goode, 1955).

In salmonella enteritis, on the other hand, the sources of infection are usually different, and commonly include processed food, synthetic cream, pies, dried eggs and incompletely cooked meat and poultry. Animal reservoirs of infection both live and dead, tame and wild, can be considerable and are almost universal (Huckstep, 1967b). Imported meat from endemic countries is also an important source of infection (Payne, 1958).

The *paratyphoid* fevers are spread mainly by prepared foodstuffs, and contaminated milk and ice cream. They also have, as have the other salmonella infections, a very definite geographical distribution. Paratyphoid A is found mainly in eastern Europe, the United States, the Middle East and India. Paratyphoid B is common in Europe and forms 20 per cent of cases found in North America while paratyphoid C is found mainly in eastern Europe and Guyana.

The pathology, diagnosis and treatment of typhoid fever will now be discussed in detail, and this will be followed by sections on paratyphoid fevers and other salmonella infections. Many of the views expressed are based on a series of 1300 typhoid patients treated personally in East Africa

between 1954 and 1968 (see Huckstep, 1957, 1960, 1961, 1962, 1967a, 1968).

PATHOLOGY

The typhoid bacillus is ingested by the oral route and invades the body by way of the small intestine. A normal gastric acidity will probably kill small doses of bacteria. If this acid has been diluted by draughts of water or neutralised by milk, or if a massive dose of bacteria has been ingested, some live bacteria reach the duodenum where a high concentration of bile forms an ideal culture medium for salmonellae.

After invasion of the intestinal mucosa, bacilli first enter the mesenteric lymph glands by way of Peyer's patches. They probably multiply here, and to a lesser extent to the lymphoid follicles and Peyer's patches of the intestinal wall during the incubation period. They then pass into the blood stream and reach other organs, especially liver, spleen and reticulo-endothelial system. Some reach the gall-bladder and bile ducts, and a second and heavier invasion of the intestines takes place through the infected bile.

The typhoid bacillus exerts its main effect by an endotoxin produced after destruction of the bacilli. The constitutional upset is mainly due to this toxaemia, while local tissue changes are the result of both toxaemia and bacteraemia. Descriptions of the effects of this on individual organs apply to both typhoid and the paratyphoids A, B and C, although the latter are usually, but not always, milder.

Peyer's patches. Microscopically in the follicles there are numerous large mononuclear cells which phagocytose typhoid bacilli, red blood cells and lymphocytes. There are also numerous lymphocytes but very few polymorphs. In the stage of necrosis these lymphocytes are replaced by macrophages (Cater, 1953) and this necrosis may progress to ulceration. On the peritoneal surface of the bowel this may cause a considerable fibrous exudate, and where there are microscopic or macroscopic perforations the bowel may be necrotic and adherent. Ulceration may also lead to haemorrhage from the blood vessels exposed in the base.

Liver. The liver is hyperaemic, soft and enlarged, and microscopically may show the cloudy swelling of toxaemia. Abscesses, cholangitis and hepatitis may also occur.

Gall bladder. During the acute stage the bile may be a constant nidus of infection, as may the bile passages. This may progress to a chronic carrier state or to the formation of gallstones in some cases.

Spleen and mesenteric lymph glands. These are enlarged and hyperaemic, and the lymphoid follicles are packed with large clear mononuclear cells instead of lymphocytes.

Genito-urinary system. The kidneys show cloudy swelling due to toxaemia, and albuminuria is common. Typhoid bacilli are classically excreted in the urine during the third week, but pyelitis, pyelonephritis and cystitis are uncommon. Orchitis is rare, and usually occurs during convalescence.

Respiratory system. Mild bronchitis occurs in over half the cases and typhoid lobar pneumonia is not uncommon.

Cardiovascular system. Fatty change of the heart muscle is common in typhoid with severe toxaemia. Thrombosis of the veins may cause pul-

true typhoid abscesses, and the infecting organism is usually *Staphylococcus aureus*.

SYMPTOMATOLOGY

During an epidemic the diagnosis of typhoid fever is of course simplified. Many isolated cases however may be misdiagnosed, especially if atypical or mild. The severity of an attack depends not only on the dosage and virulence of the organism, but also on the resistance of the patient and the time that treatment is started.

Symptoms (Table 1)

These may vary from a completely asymptomatic patient only diagnosed on routine stool

TABLE 1. *Main symptoms on admission (975 typhoid patients)*

	Research (240 pts.)	Subsidiary (735 pts.)	Total (975 pts.)
Headache	179	552	731 (74.9%)
Abdominal discomfort	168	424	592 (60.7%)
Joint pains	105	422	527 (54.0%)
Diarrhoea *without* blood	88	201	289 (29.6%)
Vomiting	59		(24.6%)
Cough (mainly slight)	84	128	212 (21.7%)
Chest pain (mainly slight)	68	141	209 (20.4%)
Backache	17	94	111 (11.4%)
Severe sore throat	15	52	67 (6.9%)

monary embolism. There is usually a neutropenia but the presence of complications may give rise to a leucocytosis.

Nervous system. Meningitis may occur as may a mild peripheral neuritis.

Skeletal system. Typhoid osteomyelitis is uncommon as is typhoid infection of the spine and typhoid arthritis. Infection of bones and joints by other salmonellae, however, is not uncommon, especially in sickle cell anaemia (Hendrickse and Collard, 1960; Huckstep, 1968, 1970).

Zenker's degeneration of muscles may be associated with thrombosis as well as toxaemia. It may occur in other muscles besides the classical site of the rectus abdominis (Huckstep, 1962).

Other pathological changes. Rose spots are due to clumps of typhoid bacilli under the skin, with round cells and large vascular spaces. *Parotitis* is usually due to secondary pyogenic infection in a very toxic patient. *Typhoid abscesses* are often deep seated and are common in the back and buttocks. *Boils* are usually more superficial than

culture to an extremely virulent and rapid onset very much like that of severe gastroenteritis.

A good clinical history may be difficult to take if the patient is mentally dull or confused, as may occur in the later stages of the disease.

The incubation period of typhoid is usually 10–14 days but may be as short as 5 days or as long as 21. It is shorter in the paratyphoid fevers. A history of exposure may be helpful with the diagnosis in non-endemic communities.

The mode of onset is usually insidious except in children and in massive infections. General malaise, anorexia and early lassitude, together with headache are common, and last longer than in many other conditions.

Vague abdominal discomfort tends also to be early. Vomiting is usually mild. Constipation is commoner than diarrhoea and usually occurs *without* blood (cf. bacillary dysentery).

Mild joint pains and backache are common but the joints are not swollen. A dry cough is also common and epistaxis is a variable symptom.

Signs (Table 2)

TABLE 2. *Main signs on admission*
(240 research patients)

Abdominal tenderness (mainly slight)	61%
Bronchitis	56%
Toxicity	54%
Coated tongue	39%
Mental confusion	29%
Abdominal guarding (mainly slight)	25%
Palpable *and* tender spleen	14%
No definite signs in any system	9%
Rose spots (black skin)	5%

Superficially the patient has a dull lethargic expressionless face which is typical of very few other diseases except typhus. The mental state may vary through normal mentality to frank mental confusion.

In the early stages the cheeks are usually flushed and the eyes bright, but by the second and third weeks the expression becomes dull, the pupils dilated, and the skin and lips dry.

There tends to be a lack of marked coughing or sputum, an absence of herpes simplex (Wright *et al*, 1953) and a musty odour. The patient shows an indefinite state on admission best described as 'toxic', and slight deafness is common (Fig. 18.1).

Rose spots mainly on the abdomen and chest, slightly raised, fading on pressure and seldom more than twelve in number (though more numerous in paratyphoid fever, may occur. They may be seen on a black skin with the help of a drop of oil.

The classical pyrexia of the untreated typhoid patient is a step ladder rise during the first week with an evening increment of 2°F (1°C) and a morning fall of 1°F (0.5°C) until it has reached about 104°F (40°C). During the second week it is 101–102°F (39°C) in the morning and 103–104°F (40°C) in the evening, and during the third week in the uncomplicated case starts to fall in the same way as it rose.

There are many atypical cases, however, and a complication such as lobar pneumonia may cause a sudden rise while intestinal perforation or haemorrhage may cause a sudden fall.

The temperature after treatment with chloramphenicol usually shows a fall in about 4 days in the uncomplicated case with a lag of about 2 days in many cases before any effects on the pyrexia are noted.

The respiration rate is seldom over thirty in adults, and bronchitis is common, 56 per cent of the author's cases presenting with some degree of it. This, when correlated with the typical abdominal findings in typhoid, constitutes one of the most valuable diagnostic signs in the disease.

The pulse is classically described as slow and dicrotic. A better description is that the pulse rate is relatively slow compared with the temperature during the *first* week of illness and is seldom above 100. This may *not* be true in children and very ill patients.

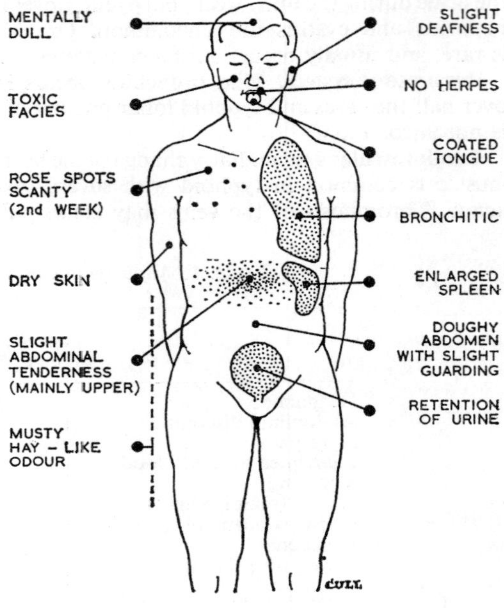

PULSE	RESPIRATION	TEMPERATURE
		REMITTENT
LESS THAN 100 (1st WEEK ONLY)	LESS THAN 30	MORNING 101–102
		EVENING 103–104

FIG. 18.1. *Signs on admission.* (From Huckstep, R.L., 1962.)

The tongue may be dry and coated, with brown fur on the dorsum and marked diminution of saliva during the second and third weeks.

The most valuable abdominal sign is slight tenderness in the liver and splenic regions. A tender palpable spleen may be a valuable positive finding in countries where hypersplenism is uncommon. There is often slight guarding and general tumidity of the abdomen similar to the doughiness of tuberculous peritonitis, and moderate abdominal distension is common in the second and third weeks of illness.

Meningism may be seen at an early stage of the

disease and may mimic true meningitis. There may be retention of urine but usually no other genito-urinary signs.

LABORATORY DIAGNOSIS

Ward tests. The classic 'pea soup' stool of typhoid fever is now less frequent as use of purgatives is uncommon. Albuminuria is very common and of little diagnostic value.

Simple laboratory tests. A blood slide for malarial parasites must always be examined in endemic areas. A low white blood count with a relative lymphocytosis is a useful test. An even more useful negative guide is a white blood count over 10 000 which is very much against a diagnosis of enteric fever except in children and when complications are present. A stool examination for ova and entamoebae may be useful in differentiating schistosomiasis and amoebiasis from the more chronic forms of typhoid in endemic areas.

Diazo test of urine. The urine of typhoid patients, especially between the fifth and fourteenth days of illness, when shaken with the diazo reagents, gives a red coloration to the froth. This test is easily performed in the ward and is useful especially during an epidemic. Eighty to 90 per cent of the author's patients gave a positive reaction at some stage of their illness, usually in the early pyrexial phase (Table 3). Only 5–7 per

TABLE 3. *Results of diazo test of urine*

	Positives
638 TYPHOID PATIENTS	
On admission	79.4%
Irrespective of when tested	82.9%
5th to 14th day of illness only	90.6%
2115 CONTROL PATIENTS (107 different medical and surgical conditions)	
Mainly *weakly* positive	5.7%

cent of a control series gave a positive reaction. Laboratory details of the test have been described elsewhere (Huckstep, 1962). The test was found very useful, especially when the blood had been sterilised by previous chloramphenicol and the Widal test invalidated by previous TAB inoculations.

Culture of typhoid bacillus. Blood culture may be positive at any stage of the clinical illness, particularly during the first week. Chloramphenicol usually sterilises the blood within 2 hours and it is therefore important to take a blood sample before chloramphenicol therapy is started. Blood clot culture is positive more often than the whole blood culture, and this may be so even some time after chloramphenicol administration.

Stool culture is not as often positive as blood culture. Several specimens should be cultured and contrary to the usual teaching it is *often* positive *before* the third week of illness and is a valuable diagnostic test.

Urine culture is not as frequently positive as stool culture and usually is positive only after the second week of illness.

Culture of pus from abscesses and post-mortem culture will occasionally yield a positive result when other results have been negative.

Agglutination tests. These are of limited value, especially when TAB inoculations have been given or where typhoid is endemic. In any un-immunised patient the test does not become positive until at least the seventh to tenth day of illness.

The H antibody can be raised by previous TAB inoculations, and is of little value. The O agglutination is of much more value, and a rising titre of 1 : 200 or over, with a clinical picture of typhoid, is very suggestive but not diagnostic of typhoid fever.

DIFFERENTIAL DIAGNOSIS (Table 4)

Typhoid fever may mimic or be mimicked by a large number of diseases. The following are the commoner ones.

Paratyphoid A, B and C. The geographical distribution of these diseases has already been mentioned, and the diagnostic criteria are discussed below. They are uncommon in many tropical countries and rarely cause difficulty in diagnosis. The laboratory is required as the final authority.

Salmonella infections and gastroenteritis. These usually cause a much more acute gastrointestinal type of illness of much shorter duration, and are also described later.

Malaria. This may be mistaken for typhoid in countries where both are endemic, but history of previous attacks, more rapid onset, shivering and sweating, high early pyrexia, relative infrequency of abdominal symptoms and signs, and a positive blood slide all point to a diagnosis of malaria.

Influenza. This is usually of much more rapid onset with a high temperature, severe sore throat and cough, and absence of a palpable spleen and rose spots.

Bacillary dysentery. The onset is usually acute. There is severe diarrhoea *with* blood, although in mild cases the blood may be absent. Diarrhoea *with* blood is rare early in typhoid. The signs and

TABLE 4. *Differential diagnosis of typhoid fever.* (From Huckstep, R. L., 1962)

Column groups: columns *Acute Onset* through *Vomiting* are under **History**; *Diagnostic Rash* through *Abdominal Signs* are under **Clinical Examination**; *Diazo Test Urine* through *Stool Culture* are under **Laboratory Investigations**.

Disease	Epidemic	Previous History	Acute Onset	Headache	Shivering	Cough	Abdominal Pain	Diarrhoea	Vomiting	Diagnostic Rash	Mental Confusion	Toxicity	High Initial Pyrexia	Chest Signs	Abdominal Signs	Diazo Test Urine	Leucocytosis	Blood Slide	Blood Culture	Agglutination Reaction	Stool Microscopy	Stool Culture
Typhoid	±	−	±	+	−	+	+	±	±	±	+	+	±	+	+	+	−	−	+	+	−	+
Paratyphoid	±	−	±	+	−	+	+	±	±	+	±	±	±	+	+	+	−	−	+	+	−	+
Other Salmonellae	+	−	+	±	−	±	+	+	+	−	±	±	±	−	+	±	−	−	±	±	−	+
Gastroenteritis	+	−	+	−	−	−	+	+	+	−	−	−	±	−	+	−	−	−	−	−	−	+
Abscesses	−	−	±	−	±	−	±	±	−	−	−	±	±	−	±	−	+	−	±	−	−	−
Acute Abdomen	−	−	+	−	−	−	+	±	+	−	−	±	±	−	+	−	+	−	−	−	−	−
Amoebiasis	−	±	−	−	−	−	±	±	−	−	−	±	−	−	±	−	±	−	−	−	+	−
Bacillary Dysentery	±	−	+	−	±	−	+	+	−	−	−	−	±	−	+	−	+	−	−	−	−	+
Bacterial Endocarditis	−	−	±	−	±	−	−	−	−	−	−	±	±	+	−	−	±	−	+	−	−	−
Brucellosis	±	±	±	+	±	−	±	−	−	−	−	−	±	−	±	−	−	−	+	+	−	−
Influenza	+	−	+	+	+	+	−	−	−	−	−	±	+	+	−	−	±	−	−	−	−	−
Malaria	±	+	+	+	+	−	−	−	−	−	±	+	+	−	−	−	−	+	−	−	−	−
Meningitis (TB)	−	−	±	+	−	±	−	−	±	−	±	−	±	±	−	±	−	−	−	−	−	−
Pneumonia	−	−	+	±	±	+	−	−	−	−	−	±	+	+	−	−	+	−	−	−	−	−
Pyelonephritis	−	±	+	−	+	−	+	−	±	−	−	±	+	−	+	−	+	−	−	−	−	−
Rheumatic Fever	−	±	±	−	±	−	−	−	−	−	−	±	±	+	−	−	±	−	±	−	−	−
Schistosomiasis	±	±	−	−	−	−	±	±	−	−	−	−	−	−	±	−	−	−	−	−	+	−
Septicaemia	−	−	+	±	+	−	−	−	−	−	−	−	+	−	±	−	+	−	+	−	−	−
Trypanosomiasis	±	±	+	±	−	−	−	−	−	+	±	−	±	−	−	−	−	+	−	−	−	−
Tuberculosis	−	±	−	−	−	+	±	−	−	−	−	−	−	+	±	+	−	−	−	−	−	−
Typhus and Rickettsial Diseases	±	−	+	+	+	+	±	−	−	+	+	+	+	+	±	+	±	−	−	+	−	−

symptoms of dysentery are usually abdominal and remain so, the mental state and chest being clear.

Typhus and other rickettsial infections. These are important in differential diagnosis, as both typhus and typhoid can cause a febrile illness with delirium, chest signs and abdominal discomfort. In typhus, however, the onset is acute and the temperature high at an early stage. Shivering attacks are common at the onset and prostration rapid. The rash is quite different, brownish-red in colour, much more profuse and does not fade on pressure like the rose spots in typhoid. There is a leucocytosis, and the Weil-Felix test becomes significantly positive at about the tenth day.

Tuberculosis. In economically poor countries, pulmonary tuberculosis and atypical abdominal tuberculosis are probably the most difficult diseases to differentiate from typhoid fever. The pyrexia and vague symptoms and signs may be very similar, and an X-ray of the chest or laboratory confirmation of typhoid may be the only sure method of diagnosis.

Other diseases. Brucellosis may cause difficulty, but tends to be more insidious, the patient is alert and a painful joint is frequently present. Trypanosomiasis in endemic areas should also be considered in the differential diagnosis.

The other diseases which enter the diagnostic field are much too numerous to mention individually. It should suffice to say that there are few conditions which cannot mimic, or be mimicked by typhoid fever.

Typhoid presenting with one of its complications. Typhoid itself may first present with one of its complications such as typhoid pneumonia, meningitis, orchitis, nephritis or as an abscess. An acute abdominal emergency also may prove to be a perforated ileum in an otherwise unsuspected case of typhoid fever.

TREATMENT

General (Fig. 18.2)

The general management of the typhoid patient is still of great importance even with specific chemotherapy. Barrier nursing plus care of the patients the various stages of a gastric diet such as soups, egg dishes and milk puddings should be given.

In economically poor countries a good standby is chocolate protein consisting of:

Skimmed milk	6 oz (170 g)
Cocoa	0.125 oz (7 g)
Sugar	2 oz (57 g)
Water	to 1 pint (568 ml)

Other local proprietary foods may be given, but they should be low in roughage, especially during the third week when the risk of haemorrhage and perforations is high.

Constipation should be left untreated unless of more than 3 days' duration, when nothing stronger than liquid paraffin or two suppositories should usually be given.

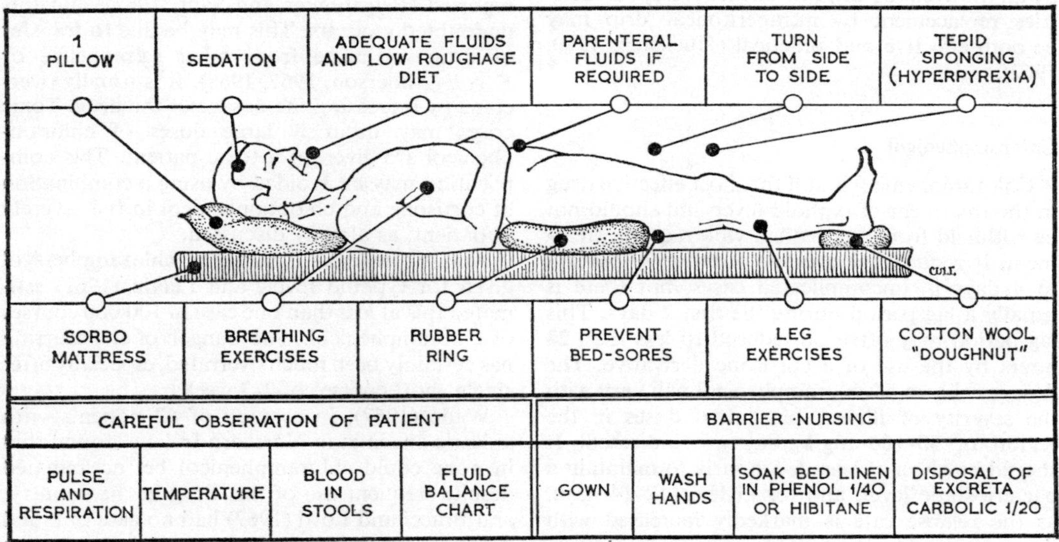

FIG. 18.2. *Nursing care and physiotherapy.* (From Huckstep, R. L., 1962.)

skin, eyes and mouth are important while physiotherapy will diminish chest complications and venous thrombosis of the legs.

Feeding of the patient must include adequate fluid and mineral intake and low roughage diet. Peptonised milk 2-hourly during the day and 4-hourly at night, plus orange or lemon drinks with added glucose are important. In very toxic cases parenteral fluids will be required plus half-strength milk or glucose by mouth.

In mild or moderate cases a high protein, high calorie diet with low residue and no roughage can be given, and milk can be fortified by milk protein such as Casilan, or by eggs. In convalescent

Retention of urine may be 'silent' in severe toxaemia and may require catheterisation. Carbachol should never be used.

Hyperpyrexia over 103–104°F (40°C) should be treated with tepid sponging and mental disturbances and insomnia may require phenobarbitone 30 mg t.d.s. or occasionally chloral and nepenthe 900 mg of each. Paraldehyde 5–10 ml intramuscularly or by mouth can be given in addition if necessary.

The general observation of the patient is important, and recording of the pulse half-hourly in seriously ill patients and 4-hourly in other patients is essential. The stools should be carefully observed for blood and the patient watched for severe toxaemia or evidence of intestinal haemorrhage or perforation.

Fluid and electrolyte balance

It is essential to keep the patient in adequate fluid and electrolyte balance, as loss by sweating, vomiting, diarrhoea or into a distended gut may be considerable. Five pints a day is the minimum fluid requirement of the ordinary adult patient, but allowance must be made not only for the extra losses already mentioned but also for the state of dehydration before admission, especially in tropical and subtropical countries.

Replacement should be by mouth where possible, but this may often have to be supplemented by an intravenous drip. In underdeveloped countries replacement by intraperitoneal drip may be both effective and practical (Huckstep, 1960, 1962).

Chloramphenicol

Chloramphenicol is still the most effective drug in the treatment of typhoid fever and should not be withheld from any patient who requires treatment. It reduces the average duration of pyrexia to 4 days in uncomplicated cases, but there is usually a lag period during the first 2 days. This lag period may often be reduced to less than 24 hours by the use of a cortisone derivative. The dosage scheme of chloramphenicol will vary with the severity of illness, but initial doses in the region of 50–100 mg/kg/day are indicated. It should be given at least 6–8 hourly to maintain a bacteriostatic level, and for at least 12–14 days, as the relapse rate is markedly increased with doses of shorter duration. In very toxic patients hydrocortisone and prednisone should be given in addition, but *not* in routine cases, due to the possible increased risks of intestinal haemorrhage and perforation.

Dosage. The following are average dosage schemes for adults.

In the acute fulminating or very toxic cases: 1 g chloramphenicol 6-hourly for 3 days, then 500 mg chloramphenicol 6-hourly for 12 days.

In marked toxaemia, cortisone should be given as well in the following doses: 200 mg hydrocortisone by intravenous or intramuscular injection immediately, then 15 mg prednisone t.d.s. on the first day, 10 mg prednisone t.d.s. on the second day, 5 mg prednisone t.d.s on the third day, 5 mg prednisone b.d. on the fourth day and 5 mg prednisone daily for the next 3 days. In very ill patients parenteral hydrocortisone should be continued instead of prednisone.

In the moderate or mild case: 500 mg chloramphenicol 6-hourly for 3 days, then 250–500 mg chloramphenicol 6-hourly for 12 days, depending on the severity of the illness.

Methods of administration. The oral route is still the best. 250 mg capsules of chloramphenicol are given to the adult patient and a suspension of chloromycetin palmitate to children. In the severely ill patients an attempt should still be made to administer the drug by the gastro-intestinal route through a Ryle's tube if necessary. Intramuscular or intravenous administration will also be required.

Disadvantages of chloramphenicol. Occasional cases of chloramphenicol resistance have been reported (Belgaumker and Sant, 1967), and this undoubtedly occurs. This may be due to transfer of drug resistance from other salmonellae or *E. coli* (Anderson, 1967, 1968). It is usually overcome by increasing the dosage of the drug. Toxic crises may occur if large doses of chloramphenicol are given to a toxic patient. This complication may be avoided by using a combination of cortisone and chloramphenicol in the severely ill patient, as already discussed.

Aplastic anaemia is rare after chloramphenicol given for typhoid fever, and Leikin (1961) estimated this at less than one case in 100 000 courses of chloramphenicol. The danger of it occurring has certainly been much overrated, especially after single short courses of 2–3 weeks.

Wade (1967), in a study of 42 patients with aplastic anaemia in Northern Ireland, found that in none could chloramphenicol be incriminated despite frequent use of this drug in the country, and Bracci and Lotti (1967) had no case of blood dyscrasia in 4000 patients treated with chloramphenicol over a 10-year period. Tolentino *et al* (1967) reported 2409 children treated over 15 years with no case of haematological toxicity, while Staudacher (1967) reported only 18 cases of allergic reaction out of 12 017 patients treated with chloramphenicol but no case of blood dyscrasia. Rondanelli and Magliulo (1967) made a comprehensive blood evaluation in patients with typhoid fever treated with chloramphenicol and confirmed the safety of chloramphenicol.

Fiaschi and Scuro (1967) point out that the use of chloramphenicol has increased over the years in all countries except the Anglo-Saxon, and that no less than 934 *tons* were manufactured in 1965 in countries other than the Soviet Union and China.

Other drugs

Cortisone and prednisone are not always effective alone, and should be restricted to the very toxic patient and always combined with chloramphenicol.

The only other drug of real value is ampicillin (Penbritin) but it is less effective than chloramphenicol in the acute case (Manriquez, 1965) and should be restricted to treatment of the carrier.

Relapse

Proof should be obtained by positive blood culture. Relapses may be of any severity, and are commoner in patients who have been treated with chloramphenicol for less than 14 days. The risk should be minimised by giving adequate doses of chloramphenicol. Treatment is the same as for the initial attack.

COMPLICATIONS

There are many complications in typhoid fever, and it may sometimes be difficult to differentiate between a complication and the natural course in so variable a disease. Complications are often associated with the gross toxaemia and prostration of the disease, and are especially common where nursing care is inadequate.

General

The general complications include typhoid abscesses, boils, bedsores, otitis media, Zenker's degeneration of muscle, severe mental confusion, deafness, severe dehydration and tonsillitis.

Typhoid abscesses are often missed, as they tend to be deep in the buttocks. They may, however, be superficial and present like boils. Treatment is by repeated aspiration under local anaesthetic and only rarely by incision.

Medical (Fig. 18.3)

Acute bronchitis is so common that it should be considered as a manifestation of the disease itself rather than as a complication.

Typhoid lobar pneumonia presents with the typical symptoms and signs of lobar pneumonia except that 'rusty' sputum is uncommon and the white blood count low. It responds well to chloramphenicol.

T

Myocarditis is extremely common in developing countries, particularly in the very toxic patient. The cardiac muscle is affected, even in convalescence. Pathania and Sachar (1965) also found that this complication was common in India and that it was responsible for most of their deaths.

Typhoid meningitis is rare and must not be confused with meningism, which is common. Chloramphenicol diffuses well into the cerebrospinal

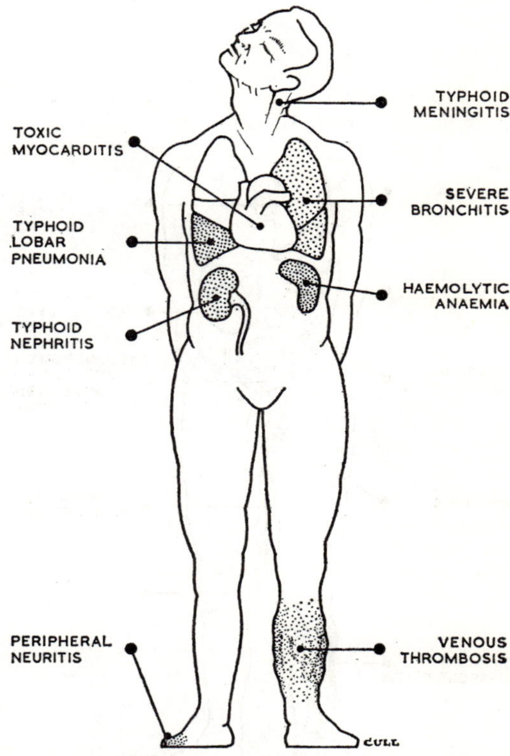

FIG. 18.3. *Medical complications.* (From Huckstep, R. L., 1962.)

fluid, and intrathecal chloramphenicol is only indicated in the severe case.

Mild haemolytic anaemia is fairly common in the very toxic typhoid patient. A marked degree is rare, and the mortality high. It should be treated with prednisone.

Other complications. Febrile albuminuria is common, but a true acute typhoid nephritis rare. Peripheral neuritis and 'tender toes' should be treated with large doses of vitamin B complex, and this vitamin should also be given routinely in typhoid fever as a prophylactic measure.

Surgical (Fig. 18.4)

Acute parotitis is a lethal complication and pus should be drained by transverse incision under local anaesthetic as early as possible.

Intestinal perforation. This is one of the most serious complications of typhoid. It occurs classically during the third week of illness but may occur before then. Diagnosis may be difficult and many of the usual symptoms may be masked by the general toxic state of the patient, and by local

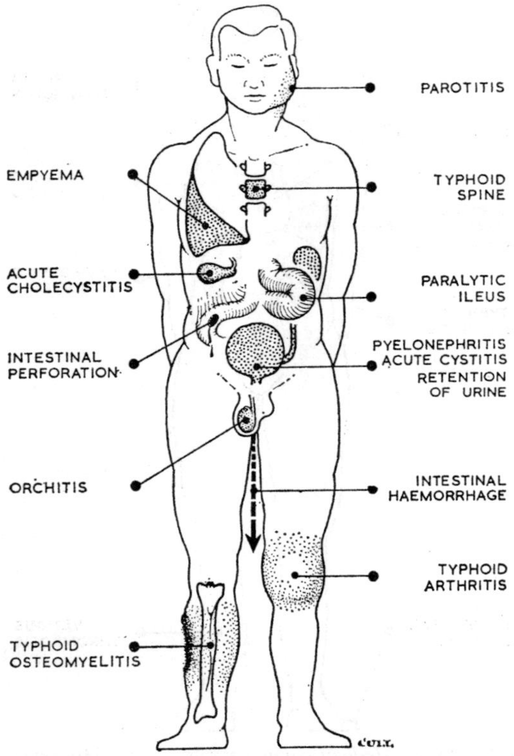

FIG. 18.4. *Major surgical complications.* (From Huckstep, R. L., 1962.)

adhesions around the leakage. In many cases, especially in the very toxic, the first indication of perforation may be the presence of free fluid, either generalised or localised, with deterioration of the condition of the patient, absent bowel sounds and vomiting. In the sudden perforation in the otherwise fairly well patient, the classical signs of perforation may be present with tenderness and guarding, but deterioration in the general condition is always rapid.

The gut is friable and often adherent, there may be more than one perforation (Dickson and Cole,

1964) and the patient tolerates general anaesthesia very badly. Sutures pull out and an adequate operation is often difficult. Most reported mortality rates after operation are very high, even with chloramphenicol.

An erroneous picture of the relative merits of operative versus conservative treatment is given by those surgeons who only report on patients presenting with the classical signs of perforation and who become relatively fit after a single perforation (Li, 1963). Badoe (1966) reported an operative mortality of only 30.4 per cent among his perforations. His *overall* mortality was no less than 57 per cent of all 241 patients, most of whom did not have perforations, and this mortality is probably the highest ever recorded, at least in this century. Dickson and Cole (1964) report an overall mortality of 50 per cent after operation for perforation with a mortality of 100 per cent in 4 patients who had a resection of the ileum for multiple perforations. Although their mortality after conservative treatment was high, they note, as do many other surgeons, that patients who have been treated conservatively are often those who have never been fit for surgery.

Many authors have found that patients often do better with conservative than with operative treatment. These include El Ramli (1950), Huckstep (1960) and White (1967).

The patient who is toxic and ill, and is already receiving chloramphenicol, often responds better to conservative treatment than to operative interference, and in a personal series of 23 perforations and peritonitis in typhoid treated conservatively, an overall mortality of 22 per cent was obtained.

Conservative measures, if instituted, must be adequate and should include large doses of chloramphenicol, both parenterally and by Ryle's tube and careful intravenous replacement of fluid, and an Oschner-Sherren regime. There are indications for operation, however, and these are as follows (Huckstep 1960, 1962, 1968a):

1. Sudden typhoid perforation in the otherwise fairly fit patient.

2. Complications caused by perforations, such as intestinal obstruction and localised abscess formation.

3. In addition to the above two absolute indications for operation, there is a third category in which in *certain* circumstances operation may be indicated. These include perforation in patients who have not had chloramphenicol, or in whom localisation and improvement on a conservative regime is not

occurring. Operation is also indicated where the diagnosis is in doubt.

It must be stressed that in all these cases the minimum possible must be done at operation and with the greatest speed possible, with the shortest and least toxic anaesthetic possible. Multiple perforations of gut must be treated by exteriorisation and not resection (Dickson and Cole, 1964). Simple closure, with care, of friable gut, with or without drainage, is all that is indicated in patients with less than three perforations. Even so, subsequent perforations may occur above or below the closure. If the bowel is very adherent or if an abscess is opened, simple drainage is probably the safest procedure.

Intestinal haemorrhage is a lethal complication which usually occurs 14–21 days after the onset of the illness, and is often 'silent'. The patient may have several small bleeds or there may be massive silent haemorrhage, and the first evidence may be a shocked patient with very pale conjunctivae.

It should be treated by early blood transfusion, nothing by mouth for 24 hours, adequate doses of morphia and very careful nursing and medical supervision. Thereafter a low roughage gastric diet is indicated.

Other surgical complications. *Typhoid cholecystitis*, like cholecystitis due to other organisms, occurs more frequently in women than in men. Diagnosis may be difficult because of the upper abdominal tenderness which is often present in typhoid fever.

Paralytic ileus may be secondary to a perforation, or to severe toxaemia. *Intestinal obstruction* may also be due to a localised abscess or adhesions.

Typhoid orchitis usually occurs in convalescence, while *acute pyelitis* is more common than generally recognised. *Typhoid arthritis* and *osteomyelitis* are uncommon and a true *typhoid spine* is rare. *Infection of bones* due to other salmonellae, however, such as *S. typhimurium*, is common, especially in sickle cell anaemia, where several bones may be involved (Huckstep, 1962, 1967a, 1968b).

All these complications should be treated along routine surgical lines with local rather than general anaesthesia if operation is required.

Concomitant diseases

In tropical countries concomitant diseases, such as bacillary dysentery, malaria, amoebiasis and worm infestations, are common. They should always be borne in mind, and treated with due regard to treatment already in progress and the side effects of drugs such as mepacrine and antihelminthics in the toxic patient.

TYPHOID FEVER IN CHILDREN

Typhoid fever in young children is uncommon and only 8 out of 507 patients in the Aberdeen outbreak were under 2 years (Galloway *et al*, 1966).

The incubation period in children is often shorter and the onset more acute than in adults, and may present as a gastroenteritis. The child often, but by no means invariably, has a less severe attack than the adult, and Patnaik and Kapoor (1967) found that infants in fact had the highest mortality. Complications tend to be less common, but when they do occur they usually progress more rapidly and are more severe. Dehydration and mineral loss may be particularly severe and need early treatment.

TYPHOID FEVER IN ECONOMICALLY POOR COUNTRIES

Despite the publicity given to Zermatt and Aberdeen, the outbreaks in these places and the problems associated with them are trivial compared with the world problem. Most cases occur in countries where hygiene is poor, equipment and trained medical and nursing staff extremely short, and transport to hospital sometimes non-existent.

Diagnosis must be mainly on clinical findings plus simple tests such as a low white count and the diazo test for urine. Confirmation is obtained from a single specimen of clotted blood which can be used for both culture and the Widal reaction, while a culture of faeces in glycerol will allow for delay in transport of the specimen. Finally, in doubtful cases it may be necessary as a matter of practical expediency to cover the possibility of malaria being present by giving chloroquine, if pneumonia is suspected, penicillin and for bacillary dysentery sulphaguanidine or tetracycline.

Treatment must be simple and dosage schemes of drugs realistic. Intraperitoneal fluid replacement may be necessary, and chloramphenicol can sometimes be given only three times a day, and for only 2 days after the temperature has dropped to normal, because of the expense involved.

The severity, morbidity and complication rate in developing countries is much higher than in Britain and the U.S.A.

THE CARRIER

The screening of all patients, suspects and contacts is essential in countries where adequate medical facilities exist. Three, and preferably six, negative stool and urine cultures and a negative Vi blood test should be the minimum before a proved case of typhoid is discharged from hospital.

The Vi test, although of value in Britain and North America, is of very limited use in countries where typhoid is endemic (Bokkenheuser and Smit, 1965; Forrest and Matthews, 1967).

The treatment of the chronic carrier is a difficult problem. Trials with ampicillin have met with some success (Christie, 1964; Troy, 1964; Simon and Miller, 1966) but even prolonged ampicillin administration in the convalescent stage does not prevent carriers (Russell *et al*, 1966). Treatment for the persistent carrier must be for at least a month and often much longer. Cholecystectomy (Perkins *et al*, 1967; Katz, 1967) and even nephrectomy, combined with ampicillin, may sometimes be necessary in the chronic carrier, and even these operations are not always successful. Vogelsang (1965), McFadzean and Ong (1966) think that this may be because an intrahepatic carrier state may occur with a recurrent pyogenic cholangitis. They reported 8 patients who had remained carriers for periods of 2–16 years despite both cholecystectomy and various antibiotics. They also pointed out the very real danger of such symptomless excreters working in Britain. In schistosomiasis urinary obstruction may be a further factor preventing the successful treatment of the carrier by conservative measures alone (Hathout *et al*, 1966).

PARATYPHOID FEVERS

The paratyphoid fevers A, B and C resemble typhoid fever and usually, but not always, run a milder course. *S. paratyphi*, however, requires a medium in which to multiply, and meat pies, synthetic cream and milk are the usual vehicles for this. Paratyphoid fever resembles other non-specific salmonella infections in this respect, and paratyphoid B may occasionally also have an onset similar to salmonella gastroenteritis. Despite this, paratyphoid fever is primarily an invasive type of disease like typhoid fever.

Partyphoid A, however, is less likely to cause complications than typhoid fever, but more likely to relapse. Paratyphoid B, which is common in Europe, is milder than typhoid, but is more likely to result in carriers and to cause jaundice, thrombosis and suppurative lesions. Paratyphoid C differs clinically from typhoid fever and the other paratyphoids in causing more septicaemic manifestations such as arthritis, cholecystitis and abscesses, with little in the way of gastrointestinal lesions.

Chloramphenicol is probably still the best drug in the treatment of paratyphoid fever, but the response may be poor (Anderson, 1962). In less severe cases neomycin or ampicillin are probably safer but are even less effective (Sharp *et al*, 1964; Sleet *et al*, 1964). Achromycin may also be worth a trial.

The paratyphoid carrier state is common after infection and may not respond to drugs like ampicillin and chloramphenicol (Parry, 1966). O'Toole and Jones (1964) reported success with the use of BRL 1060, a drug similar to, but more soluble than, ampicillin, in cases where ampicillin itself had failed to cure a carrier.

Many cases of paratyphoid fever, however, do not require specific chemotherapy, especially if mild (Christie, 1968).

OTHER SALMONELLA INFECTIONS

Salmonella infections are responsible for more attacks of food poisoning than all other bacterial infections and chemical poisons put together, and many thousands of new cases are reported each year in Britain alone. In Colombia over half the stool cultures showed a pathogenic salmonella (Fournelle *et al*, 1967). Salmonella infections are not always transitory and short-lived, and a single outbreak of food poisoning due to *S. typhimurium* in Sweden caused 7717 cases with no fewer than 90 deaths (Lundbeck *et al*, 1955).

There are over 1000 known species of salmonella at present, and more are continually coming to light. They may cause diseases not only in man but in cattle, pigs, dogs, cats, rats and many birds including ducks and chickens. Almost every animal (both tame and wild) may be infected; even the lion is not exempt, and the commonness of animal reservoirs of infection is often not appreciated (Huckstep, 1967b).

Salmonella infections in animals and birds are, therefore, potent sources of disease in man and infection is usually transmitted by ingested meat, milk products or eggs. Schothorst and Kampelmacher in 1967 isolated salmonellae from a sample of 34.7 per cent of the horse meat and 13.5 per cent of the frozen beef imported into Holland from South America.

In order to produce infection large doses of the

organism usually need to be ingested in comparison with the typhoid bacillus, and as a result food and milk products are much more often the source of infection than water which would have to be heavily contaminated. The salmonella organism grows in food products and produces an active endotoxin. The danger of this is that the food may show no evidence of infection, and also, although the bacteria are rapidly killed by heat, the toxin may survive 100°C for 30 minutes.

Diagnosis

The history of a salmonella infection is usually of an acute gastroenteritis following the ingestion of made-up food; often it occurs as an epidemic. The disease is confined to the gastrointestinal tract in most cases and is usually not severe. The incubation period is usually between 10 and 30 hours, but may be much shorter if the dosage of pathogenic bacilli is high.

The onset is abrupt with vomiting, diarrhoea *without* blood, headache and abdominal pain. The temperature is slightly raised, but seldom over 100°F (38°C). The symptoms gradually abate over 1–4 days, but occasional complications and even death may occur due to dehydration and electrolyte imbalance, and occasionally septicaemia and toxaemia.

The differential diagnosis as shown in Table 4 is straightforward when there is a typical history and a number of people are affected. The main differential diagnosis is from staphylococcal food poisoning due to a heat stable exotoxin, but here the vomiting is profuse and the incubation period much shorter.

Occasionally a generalised illness is caused as well with a bacteraemia and septicaemia (Neves and Martins, 1967) with complications similar to typhoid fever. Occasionally also, abdominal symptoms and a persistent carrier state may continue for several months.

Investigation should include stool culture, and occasionally blood culture, white blood count and a Widal test for non-specific salmonellae.

Treatment

The general treatment is important and includes adequate fluid and electrolyte replacement. The majority are mild cases and can be treated at home with bed rest, milk drinks and thin soup, and this is gradually increased to a normal diet.

The moderate and severe case is best treated in hospital, and in the case of severe fluid and electrolyte loss, intravenous replacement may be necessary. The value of non-specific treatment for diarrhoea, such as tincture of opium kaolin, chlorodyne and tincture of opium is in doubt.

There is no universally effective specific chemotherapy (Christie, 1968). Tetracycline at the present time is probably as effective as any drug, and can be tried in severe cases, and in those patients who do not respond rapidly to general measures. *In vitro* sensitivities unfortunately bear little relation to those *in vivo*, but may occasionally be helpful. Chloramphenicol should only be given in severe cases with septicaemia or toxaemia which do not respond to other drugs.

As with the paratyphoid fevers, salmonellae may be present in the faeces for weeks or months after the clinical recovery. Antibiotic therapy not only often fails to eradicate organisms from these symptomless excreters, but may prolong recovery (Dixon, 1965).

PROGNOSIS

The prognosis in both typhoid fever and other salmonella infections varies considerably from epidemic to epidemic and depends on many factors, including the resistance and health of the patient, the dose and type of organism, and the effectiveness and speed of treatment.

There seems to be such variation in mortality rates with different epidemics, especially in typhoid fever, that probably other factors such as differences in phage types and strains of bacteria are also important factors.

In non-specific salmonella infections the mortality rate is usually about 1 per cent, but it is higher in the very old and the very young.

In typhoid fever the mortality rate varies considerably from about 1 per cent in Britain and North America to 10–25 per cent in most developing countries, and Ikeme and Anan (1966) reported a mortality rate of 24 per cent from Nigeria. In large specialist hospitals in the tropics there will probably be a lower rate, and the mortality rate in Nairobi, Kenya was 5.4 per cent (Huckstep, 1962). In countries where only the very ill can be admitted to hospital, a huge mortality rate such as that reported from Ghana of 57 per cent out of 241 patients may occur (Baboe, 1966). The mortality rate in the paratyphoid fevers usually lies between that of typhoid fever and other salmonella infections; the prognosis appears to be worse in paratyphoid C, and best in paratyphoid A.

PROPHYLAXIS

In both typhoid fever and other salmonella infections, general prophylaxis is far more effective than specific vaccines. In typhoid fever prevention is mainly by ensuring pure water supplies and clean milk, raw vegetables and shellfish. In the paratyphoid fevers and other salmonella infections, on the other hand, the accent is much more on improvement of hygiene and prevention of contamination of prepared foods. Contamination by human carrier is an additional problem, especially as the carrier in both typhoid and other salmonella infections may be completely asymptomatic.

Prophylactic measures should be directed towards prevention and to the treatment of every suspected carrier as well as to improvement in hygienic standards of food handlers and the public generally. Water supplies must be pure, sewage disposal adequate, milk products supervised and shellfish purified. The manufacture of tinned meats, and also of prepared foods such as meat pies, sausages, puddings and cakes needs very careful supervision.

There are stringent regulations in Britain and North America and visitors from these countries to countries with lower standards must be warned of the dangers of drinking contaminated water and eating potentially infected food such as ice cream. Conversely, food prepared abroad such as tinned meat and dried eggs may introduce infection when imported, without adequate safeguards from endemic countries.

TAB is only of limited value, and the value of the paratyphoid components of the vaccine has never been proved. World Health Organization trials have confirmed this. In trials in Yugoslavia and British Guiana (W.H.O., 1962, 1964) it was shown that heat-phenol-inactivated vaccine and acetone-inactivated and dried vaccine gave partial protection, with the acetone vaccine being the more effective. Alcohol-killed and preserved vaccine on the other hand gave no protection.

In another trial by the World Health Organization in the Soviet Union, 181 cases of typhoid, 58 cases of paratyphoid A and 101 cases of paratyphoid B occurred (Hejfec *et al*, 1966). Every one of these cases of typhoid fever had had at least two doses of vaccine with the second dose at least 30 days before the onset of illness. It must however also be stressed that in these totals the incidence of typhoid fever was significantly less in the vaccinated than in the unvaccinated control groups.

Misleading information may be obtained from the laboratory on the value of TAB (Hejfec *et al*, 1966; Ashcroft *et al*, 1967). Felix in 1943, for instance, reported that an alcohol-killed and preserved vaccine appeared on the basis of laboratory tests to be superior to the previously used heat-killed and phenol-preserved vaccine. The vaccine was however subsequently found to have no apparent protective value in man (Huckstep, 1957, 1962; W.H.O., 1962).

It is important to note that there is *no* vaccine known at present which will give complete protection against typhoid and that even the best vaccines will probably only give *limited* protection against *small* doses of bacteria. In addition, these vaccines have little effect in altering the severity of the disease once typhoid has been contracted. In the Soviet Union, for instance, it was shown that the onset was more acute and relapses more *frequent* in the vaccinated than the unvaccinated, although serious complications appeared slightly less in the vaccinated (Shamov, 1966).

Intradermal vaccines appear to be more effective than vaccines given subcutaneously and constitutional upsets are much less, although the local reaction is still marked. 0.2 ml of phenolised-vaccine given intradermally in two doses at intervals of 4 weeks is recommended in England (Roodyn, 1968). Reinoculation is carried out once a year.

In North America typhoid immunisation is often given subcutaneously, as it is also in many other parts of the world. The dose recommended is 0.5 ml subcutaneously in two doses at 4-weekly intervals with 0.5 ml booster dose every 3 years. Children between 6 months and 10 years are given half this dose (*Ann. intern. Med.*, 1966). Routine immunisation, however, is not recommended for those *not* at risk in view of the constitutional upset. The addition of paratyphoid A and B is also not recommended by the U.S. Public Health Service Advisory Committee on Immunisation Practices. Ashcroft *et al* (1967) in their study found that one dose of vaccine gave better protection than two doses. If this finding is confirmed it will further confuse the controversy on the value of TAB.

The composition of phenolised vaccine for subcutaneous use is 1000 million *S. typhi* and 500 million each of *S. paratyphi* A and B, and if necessary *S. paratyphi* C, per ml. The intradermal vaccine has similar doses in 0.2 ml. It is important to note the composition and storage recommendations and dosage schemes supplied with each batch of vaccine as these may differ. The vaccine must be kept in a refrigerator when not in use. It is likely that this heat-killed phenol-preserved vaccine will be superseded by acetone-killed and dried vaccine in the near future.

Many other types of vaccine have been tried in the past. None has given more than partial protection, and the final answer may yet be a living attenuated vaccine of several phage types (Huckstep, 1957). Experimental work is, in fact, being carried out with an attenuated live vaccine (Singh, 1966). At present, however, our main weapon must be continued improvements in public health standards.

REFERENCES

ACHARD, D. and BENSAUDE, R. (1896) *Bull. Soc. med. Hop. Paris.*, 3s, **13**, 820.
ANDERSON, E. S. (1967) *Ann. Inst. Pasteur*, **112**, 547.
—— (1968) *Brit. med. J.*, **1**, 293.
ANDERSON, J. P. (1962) *Newc. med. J.*, **27**, 202.
Ann. intern. Med. (1966) **65**, 1300.
ASHCROFT, M. T., SINGH, B., NICHOLSON, C. C., RITCHIE, J. M., SOBRYAN, E. and WILLIAMS, F. (1967) *Lancet*, **2**, 1056.
BADOE, E. A. (1966) *Ghana med. J.*, **5**, 83.
BELGAUMKAR, P. H. and SANT, M. V. (1967) *Ind. J. med. R.*, **55**, 199.
BOKKENHEUSER, V. and SMIT, P. (1964) *Amer. J. pub. Hlth*, **54**, 1507.
BRACCI, U. and LOTTI, T. (1967). *Postgrad. med. J.*, *Suppl.*, **43**, 27.
Bull. Wld Hlth Org. (1962) **26**, 357.
—— (1964) **30**, 623.
CATER, D. B. (1953) *Basic Pathology and Morbid Histology*. Bristol: John Wright & Sons, Ltd.
CHRISTIE, A. B. (1964) *Brit. med. J.*, **1**, 1609.
—— (1968) *Medical News Magazine*, Feb. p. 5.
DICKSON, J. A. S. and COLE, G. J. (1964) *Brit. J. Surg.*, **51**, 893.
DIXON, J. M. S. (1965) *Brit. med. J.*, **2**, 1343.
EBERTH, C. J. (1880) *Virchows Arch.*, **81**, 58.
EL RAMLI, A. H. (1950) Wld Hlth Org. *Lancet*, **1**, 618.
Epidem. vit. Stat. Rep. (1967) **20**, 2.
FELIX, A. (1943) *Brit. med. J.*, **1**, 435.
FIASCHI, E. and SCURO, L. A. (1967) *Postgrad. med. J.*, *Suppl.*, **43**, 84.
FORREST, C. R., MATTHEWS, R. N., ROBERTSON, M. J. and HANLEY, W. P. (1967) *Brit. med. J.*, **2**, 472.
FOURNELLE, H. J., GRACIAN, M. and MEDINA, P. (1966) *Bol. Sanit. Pan-am.*, **61**, 408.
GAFFKY, G. (1884) *Mitt. GesundhAmt. Berl.*, **2**, 372.
GALLOWAY, H., CLARK, N. S. and BLACKHALL, M. (1966) *Arch. Dis. Child.*, **41**, 63.
GERHARD, W. W. (1837) *Amer. J. med. Sci.*, **20**, 289.
HATHOUT, S., EL-DIN., EL-GHAFFAR, Y. A., AWNY, A. Y. and HASSAN, K. (1966) *Amer. J. trop. Med. Hyg.*, **15**, 156.
HEJFEC, L. B. (1966) *Bull. Wld Hlth Org.*, **34**, 321.
HENDRICKSE, R. G. and COLLARD, P. (1960) *Lancet*, **1**, 80.
HUCKSTEP, R. L. (1957) MD Thesis, Cambridge, pp. 409.
—— (1960) *Ann. roy., Coll. Surg. Engl.*, **26**, 207.
—— (1961) *Nursing Mirror*, **112**, xiv–xvi.
—— (1962) *Typhoid Fever and Other Salmonella Infections*. Edinburgh: E. & S. Livingstone.
—— (1965) *Curr. Med. Drugs*, **5**, 19.
—— (1967a) *Brit. med. J.*, **3**, 739.
—— (1967b) *Brit. med. J.*, **4**, 681.
—— (1968a) *Companion of Surgery in Africa*, ed. Davey, W. W., p. 214. Edinburgh and London: E. & S. Livingstone.
—— (1968b) *E. Afr. Med. J.* **45**, 429.
—— 1970 *J. W. Pacific Ortho. Assoc.*, **VII**, 65.
IKEME, A. C. and ANAN, C. O. (1966) *J. trop. Med. Hyg.*, **61**, 15.
KATZ, M. (1967) *Clin. Paed.*, **6**, 137.
LAVERDANT, C. (1966) *Rev. int. Serv. Santé Armées*, **39**, 175.
LEIKIN, S. L., WELCH, H. and GUIN, G. H. (1961) *Clin. Proc. Chil. Hosp. Wash.*, **17**, 171.
LI, F. W. P. (1963) *Brit. J. Surg.*, **50**, 976.

LOUIS, P. C. A. (1829) *Recherches Anatomiques, Pathologiques et Therapeutiques sur la Maladie connue sous Les Noms de Gastro-enterite, Fievre, putride, ataxique, typhoide, etc.*, 2 volumes. Paris: Bailliere.

LUNDBECK, H., PLAZIKOWSKI, U. and SILVERSTOLPE, L. (1955) *J. Appl. Bact.*, **18**, 535.

McFADZEAN, A. J. S. and ONG, G. B. (1966) *Brit. med. J.*, **1**, 1567.

MANRIQUEZ, L., SALCEDO, M., BORGONO, J. M., MARZULLO, E., KRALJEVIC, R., PAREDES, L. and VALDIVIESO, R. (1965) *Brit. med. J.*, **2**, 152.

MARRIOTT, H. L. (1947) *Brit. med. J.*, **1**, 245, 285, 328.

MEERS, P. D. and GOODE, D. (1965) *Lancet*, **1**, 426.

NEVES, J. and LOBO MARTINS, N. R. L. (1967) *Trans. roy. Soc. trop. Med. Hyg.*, **61**, 541.

O'TOOLE, C. P. and JONES, D. E. (1964) *Lancet*, **1**, 1332.

PARRY, W. H., MORONEY, P. J. and KHAN, S. M. S. (1966) *Med. Officer*, **116**, 27.

PATHANIA, N. S. and SACHAR, R. S. (1965) *Amer. J. trop. Med. Hyg.*, **14**, 419.

PATNAIK, K. C. and KAPOOR, P. N. (1967) *Ind. J. med. Res.*, **55**, 228.

PAYNE, D. J. (1968) *Brit. med. J.*, **1**, 702.

PERKINS, J. C., DEVETSKI, R. L. and DOWLING, H. F. (1966) *Arch. intern. Med.*, **118**, 528.

PFEIFFER, R. and KOLLE, W. (1896) *Dtsch. med. Wschr.*, **22**, 735.

RONDANELLI, E. G. and MAGLIULO, E. (1967) *Postgrad. med. J.*, *Suppl.*, **43**, 32.

ROODYN, L. (1968) Personal Communication.

RUSSELL, E. M., SUTHERLAND, A. and WALKER, W. (1966) *Brit. med. J.*, **2**, 555.

SCHOTHORST, M. VAN. and KAMPELMACHER, E. H. (1967) *J. Hyg. Camb.*, **65**, 321.

SHAMOV, Yu. A. (1966) *Zh. Mikrobiol.*, **43**, 94.

SHARP, J. C. M., BROWN, P. P. and SANGSTER, G. (1964) *Brit. med. J.*, **1**, 1282.

SIMON, H. J. and MILLER, R. C. (1966) *New. Engl. J. Med.*, **274**, 807.

SINGH, R. B. (1966) *Med. J. Malaya*, **21**, 177.

SLEET, R. A., SANGSTER, G. and MURDOCH, J. McC. (1964) *Brit. med. J.*, **1**, 148.

STAUDACHER, V. (1967) *Postgrad. med. J.*, *Suppl.*, **43**, 49.

TOLENTINO, P. BRAITO, A. and CHIOSSI, F. M. (1967) *Postgrad. med. J.*, *Suppl.*, **43**, 61.

TROY, P. (1964) *Brit. med. J.*, **1**, 1252.

VOGELSANG, TH. M. (1964) *J. Hyg Camb.*, **62**, 443.

WADE, O. L. (1967) *Postgrad. med. J.*, *Suppl.*, **43**, 19.

WHITE, L. A. N. (1967) Hamilton Bailey's *Emergency Surgery*, 8th edn. Bristol: John Wright & Sons Ltd.

WIDAL, G. F. I. (1896) *Bull. Soc. med. Hop. Paris*, 3s, **13**, 561.

WILLIS, T. (1684) *Practice of Physick*, pp. 137, 234. London.

WOODWARD, T. E., SMADEL, J. E., LEY, H. L., GREEN, R. and MANKIKAR, D. S. (1948) *Ann intern. Med.*, **29**, 131.

WRIGHT, A. E. (1896) *Lancet*, **2**, 807.

WRIGHT, F. J., COOKE, E. R. N. and D'SOUZA, J. St. A. M. (1953) *Trans. roy. Soc. trop. Med. Hyg.*, **47**, 117.

19
Plague

Plague is an acute infectious disease of high mortality caused by *Pasteurella pestis*. Although primarily a disease of rodents, it may affect human beings. In the case of bubonic plague, infection is conveyed from rodent to man through their fleas, whereas in pneumonic plague transmission occurs from man to man by droplet infection.

Bubonic plague is characterised by inflammation of the regional lymph glands. Severe septicaemia occurring in bubonic plague without evidences of inflamed lymph glands is sometimes called septicaemic plague.

Primary pneumonic plague, in which the lungs are primarily involved through inhalation of infective material, is characterised by cough with bloodstained expectoration.

Plague occurring in wild rodents is known as sylvatic plague.

GEOGRAPHICAL DISTRIBUTION

Plague has been assumed to have originated from Central Asia. During historical times it was first recorded as occurring in North Africa, and the rest of the inhabited world when it was known as the Justinian pandemic, and later in Europe and Asia as the Black Death.

Areas where plague continues to exist are the coastal regions of China and Yunnan, Indo-China, Thailand, Central Burma, parts of India, Java, Madagascar, Central and South Africa, Brazil, Peru and Ecuador.

Plague epidemics have occurred in recent times in parts of Manchuria, India, the Middle East, North and Central Africa.

Sylvatic plague foci exist in western United States, Brazil, Argentina, Peru, Ecuador, parts of South Africa, South-east Russia, Mongolia and Manchuria.

AETIOLOGY

Plague is caused by *P. pestis*. The organism is a short, ovoid, Gram-negative bacillus with bipolar staining. It is an encapsulated organism and immotile.

The plague bacillus has feeble powers of resistance to adverse extrinsic influences. It is easily killed by sunlight, one hour's exposure to the sun being sufficient (Pollitzer, 1936). But if sheltered from light, it may remain virulent up to 54 days (Ori, 1933).

The plague bacillus is highly virulent and possesses a specific endotoxin (Petri 1929). It has two antigens, a *capsular* antigen which is of importance in conferring immunity against plague infection and is called the 'specific immunising fraction' and a *somatic* antigen which is water-soluble and does not provoke specific protective antibodies in man or monkey (Schutze, 1929).

Plague is essentially a disease of rats, or other rodents, and fleas are the vectors responsible for transmission of the infection from host to host. When a flea bites and sucks the blood of an infected rodent. the *P. pestis* present in the blood of the rodent are also imbibed and multiply rapidly in the lower end of the oesophagus and the stomach of the flea. Consequently the stomach of the flea becomes blocked with blood and plague bacilli, and the flea is called a 'blocked flea'. During subsequent feeds the flea ejects the bacilli in the process of biting and thus the infection is transmitted to the bitten victim.

Fleas tend to leave dead rats to seek living hosts, and if the usual rat hosts are not found, the rat flea readily attacks man, thereby transmitting the disease to man. This is the commonest method of transmission of bubonic plague. Occasionally the infection may be transmitted by the organisms present in the faeces of infected fleas being rubbed into the tissues through abrasions or flea bites. Rarely, entrance may be gained through the conjunctiva, tonsils of through abrasions in the skin during dissection or skinning of infected wild rodents.

Transmission by droplet infection

Patients whose lungs are involved, as in primary or secondary pneumonic plague, will have the organisms in their sputum, and may transmit the disease from man to man by droplet infection.

EPIDEMIOLOGY

Epidemiologically, there are two forms of plague—urban and sylvatic. The factors concerned with the prevalence and distribution of human plague are those that affect the rodent hosts and the insect vectors.

Rodent hosts

Wild rodents. In central Asia, wild rodents are believed to be the hosts of sylvatic plague infection. Species involved are marmots, sisels, *Tatera brantsi*, and ground squirrels.

Commensal rodents. Commensal rodents are those dependent upon man for their food supplies. The three species of commensal rodents implicated in plague outbreaks are *Rattus norvegieus*, *Rattus rattus* and *Mus musculus*. In India, wild and commensal rodents occur together extensively. There is interbreeding between them.

Insect vector

The common rat fleas are (a) *Xenopsylla cheopis* which is found in tropical and subtropical countries, and is commonly associated with outbreaks of plague; (b) *Xenopsylla brasilienses* and (c) *Xenopsylla astia*, both of which are less efficient vectors.

Fleas find more favourable conditions for survival on the specific hosts and still more in inhabited burrows or in other sheltered conditions than under artificial conditions. The optimum condition for *X. cheopis* is a temperature of 59–68°F (15–20°C) and relative humidity of 85 per cent. A favourable temperature leads to a rapid increase in the number of blocked fleas and a favourable humidity increases the length of survival of infected fleas. Climatic conditions which favour the survival of infected fleas would help the transmission of plague.

In the opinion of the plague research commission, plague epidemics are checked by temperatures above 80°F (27°C) and a dry atmosphere with relative humidity less than 80 per cent, as under such adverse conditions fleas fail to transmit infection. A large proportion of infected fleas become capable of transmitting the infection at a temperature of 68.8–76.8°F (20.5–24.9°C) and relative humidity of above 80 per cent, and such conditions therefore favour plague epidemics.

Spread of plague

Plague invasion of various countries was due mainly to importation by sea-routes. Establishment of the infection depends on local conditions. The infection fails to establish itself if the prevailing climate at the time of invasion or throughout the year is unsuitable. Inefficient vector fleas will also impede the spread of plague. After infection is brought into a port, the disease spreads to inland towns by railway or by other means of communications. Subsequently adjacent rural areas become involved and the wild rodents in these localities are infected. Sporadic cases keep on appearing so long as the disease remains in rodent reservoirs.

An epizootic develops when the conditions are suitable. There is a close relationship between *R. rattus* epizootic and bubonic plague epidemic in man. The average time interval between the epizootic and the appearance of the epidemic is 10–14 days (Wu Lien Teh, 1926). In the case of increasing rat fall in a locality, dissection of rats and demonstration of the *P. pestis* in organ smears should be done to confirm the plague epizootic. If necessary, further investigations such as culture and animal inoculation tests of the organ smears may be carried out.

In North China, the outbreaks start in late summer and autumn. In North India, the peak incidence is in March. In Burma, the usual plague season is between November and April, with a peak in February.

Urban plague. Plague becomes firmly established among rats of the affected towns, if the climate is suitable, if the rodent population is large and susceptible, and if a sufficient number of capable vectors is present. The disease may persist in the rodent population for some years. The disappearance of an epizootic may be due to the considerable reduction in number of susceptible rats.

Rural plague. Rural plague is due to importation of infection from plague-affected urban centres. Both commensal rodents and peridomestic wild rodents are infected. The transportation of grain after harvest facilitates the transportation of rats and fleas, and leads to increased numbers of village infections. Usually infection is transmitted from the affected to unaffected villages through the transport of infected fleas in rice cargoes. Rural plague may last for very long periods.

Sylvatic plague. Sylvatic plague may exist in extensive rural areas for many years among rodents such as squirrels, gerbils, chipmunks, fieldmice and marmots. When semi-domestic rats (*R. norvegieus*) which normally haunt human habitats, come into contact with infected field rodents through the use of common burrows, they become infected themselves, and pass on the infection to house rats (*R. rattus*), which in turn spread it to man, usually within a few days, through the bite of their fleas. A hunter who catches infected animals may contract the disease through their fleas.

Primary pneumonic plague (demic). Initially, primary pneumonic plague is contracted through contact with a bubonic plague patient who has secondary lung involvement. Transmission occurs through inhalation of infected sputum. Subsequent spread from man to man also takes place in a similar manner by droplet infection. Poor economic conditions leading to overcrowding, ill-ventilated houses and high relative humidity favour the spread of disease, whereas dry weather causes decline and eventual termination of an outbreak.

PATHOLOGY

Human plague may be classified into two main types:

1. Primary bubonic plague.
2. Primary pneumonic plague.

Bubonic plague. The regional lymph nodes draining the site of the bite become enlarged and appear as buboes. They are characterised by marked reaction in the surrounding tissues, haemorrhagic inflammation and coagulation necrosis. The individual nodes become matted to each other and to the surrounding tissues with eventual softening, suppuration and abscess formation.

When multiplication of the organism becomes too great, the lymph node filters are no longer capable of holding them back and allow the bacilli to enter the circulation, with resultant bacteraemia.

In bubonic plague, the lungs may be involved due to infection being carried by the blood stream. Toxic inflammation of the endothelial linings of lymphatics and blood vessels is common. There may be haemorrhagic pericardial effusion. The liver and spleen are enlarged and congested, with small haemorrhages below the capsule. Hyperaemia of gastric mucosa and congestion of intestines are usually found. Congestion and oedema of the brain and meninges have been seen in autopsies.

Primary pneumonic plague. The trachea and bronchi are congested and covered with a blood-stained exudate. Haemorrhages may be seen beneath the visceral pleura. In some cases acute congestion and oedema of the lungs is marked but without consolidation. In others, areas of pneumonic consolidation may be present. The bacilli multiply in enormous numbers in the lungs and cause severe bacteraemia and toxaemia. The bronchial lymph nodes may be enlarged and hyperaemic.

CLINICAL FEATURES

General

The incubation period of bubonic plague varies from 2 to 10 days, and is usually less than 6 days; that of pneumonic plague is 2 to 4 days.

The clinical picture is one of a severe septicaemia and is due to the action of *circulating plague* toxins (Pollitzer, 1936). The onset is sudden with a rapid rise of temperature accompanied by chills, shivering or rigors and an increase of pulse rate. The disease may become fully developed within a day. Prodromal symptoms such as malaise, headache, giddiness, mental apathy, restlessness, nausea and pain in the limbs or lumbar region may occur in some patients.

The general appearance of a severely affected plague patient is one of prostration and a greatly weakened condition. It may be characteristic enough to make the disease suspect when such a picture is seen during an outbreak. The face is flushed and the conjunctivae are almost invariably injected initially. The facial expression depicts anxiety and distress but later it becomes listless and apathetic. The eyes may be staring or show aimless movement if consciousness is impaired.

Fever may be continuously high, remittent or irregular. Temperatures of 103–104°F (40°C) are reached within hours or a day. In typical bubonic plague the temperature may show primary and secondary peaks with an interval of low temperature. It then subsides gradually, the whole pyrexial period lasting 6–7 days, or shorter if the disease is mild. Successful treatment will shorten the febrile period. Suppuration of the buboes will influence the course of the fever. Septicaemic and pneumonic forms have a high temperature, often with an irregular course.

The pulse is rapid, often dicrotic, and may in the later stages become so rapid and feeble as to be imperceptible and uncountable, denoting the presence of progressive heart failure. The heart is dilated and the heart sounds are feeble. Sudden death from heart failure may occur at any stage of the disease and may follow even slight exertion.

Polymorphonuclear leucocytosis is the rule in severely affected patients though severe septicaemic plague may give rise to leucopenia.

Initial bacteraemia usually occurs in bubonic plague patients and is transient in benign forms, but progressive in severely affected cases. Conspicuous bacteraemia therefore denotes a bad prognosis.

The respiratory system is almost invariably involved in severely affected patients suffering from any form of plague. Physical signs are usually inconspicuous, but in dying patients dyspnoea and cyanosis due to terminal lung oedema is almost always present.

The neurological manifestations due to toxic effects on the nervous system contribute to the characteristic clinical picture of plague and vary in intensity and form. Dulling of the senses and a degree of incoordination of the voluntary muscles occur in all; delirium or stupor and confusion may occur. The gait may be staggering and the speech hesitant, stuttering and indistinct. Convulsions may be seen in children.

Plague patients usually have no appetite and invariably have intense thirst. Nausea and vomiting is usually present. The tongue is thickly coated and the lips, teeth and gums are covered with sores. There is either constipation or diarrhoea.

The liver and spleen are moderately enlarged and occasionally there is abdominal tenderness and meteorism.

Epistaxis is not uncommon and submucous haemorrhages may occur in the gastrointestinal tract and bladder in severe cases.

If not treated specifically, pneumonic plague victims will usually die within 1 day and those with the 'septicaemic' form in 1 to 3 days. Patients surviving longer than 5 days have an increased chance of recovery. On the other hand, patients with the benign form of bubonic plague without bacteraemia will invariably recover even if left untreated. Occasionally meningeal complication may prolong convalescence. Sudden heart failure and other fatal complications may occur even at this stage.

The mortality rate was very high in the days before specific drugs were known. Nowadays, with the introduction of sulphonamides and antibiotics, the death rate has fallen spectacularly.

Bubonic plague

In mild cases, the general symptoms are inconspicuous, whereas in severe cases, invasion of the blood stream by organisms takes place so rapidly and so early that the clinical picture of septicaemia predominates before the appearance of inflamed regional lymph nodes.

Buboes. Groin buboes are most frequent, constituting from 55 to 70 per cent of cases, axillary buboes constituting 20 per cent and cervical buboes 10 per cent respectively. Primary invasion of tonsils by *P. pestis* may lead to the formation of tonsillar buboes.

As a rule the patient complains of discomfort or even some pain at the site of future buboes. These sites are tender on palpation. In the early stages the affected lymph nodes are slightly enlarged and of normal consistency. The enlargement of lymph nodes progresses and marked periadenitic changes take place with infiltration and oedema of surrounding tissue. These changes are manifested in the first 12 hours of illness.

Within 1 to 5 days after the onset of disease, well-marked buboes appear. The size of a well-developed bubo varies from a walnut to that of a hen's egg. At first they are movable, but later they become adherent to the surrounding tissues.

On palpation, a fully developed bubo reveals the presence of doughy or baggy consistency. The patient complains of dull or stabbing pain. During the acute stage of the disease, the buboes are invariably sensitive to touch, and even comatose patients react when the affected lymph nodes are palpated. This marked tenderness to touch in the early stage of the disease is an outstanding clinical sign of bubonic plague.

After a few days primary buboes subside along with improvement of the general condition of the patient. The affected lymph node remains enlarged and indurated. The skin over the lymph node may remain pigmented. Frequently suppuration commences in the centre of a bubo early in the second week of illness and an abscess is formed. The abscess may burst spontaneously and sloughing may take place. If there is secondary infection, healing may be delayed and sinuses may form. In such cases, a chronic ulcer may develop and the patient may die some weeks later of sepsis, exhaustion or amyloid disease.

The three cardinal signs of bubonic plague are (*a*) rapid rise of temperature, (*b*) congestion of conjunctiva bulbi, (*c*) painful swellings of peripheral lymph nodes.

Complications. In severe bubonic cases, bacteraemia and/or septicaemia may take place, leading to involvement of the lung as a complication. Lung lesions vary from simple catarrh to severe congestion and specific bronchopneumonia. As the physical signs are inconspicuous, secondary plague pneumonia is often difficult to recognise. The sputum may be bloodstained, but laboratory examination may not show *P. pestis*. Marasmus may develop after an attack of bubonic plague and lead to death.

Primary plague carbuncles may develop on any

part of the body as a result of metastatic infection through the blood stream.

Plague meningitis, arising with symptoms such as headache, painful stiff neck, Kernig's sign and coma, is a serious complication.

Benign forms. AMBULANT PLAGUE is characterised by the formation of a vesicle at the site of infection and slight local lymphangitis. Constitutional signs are absent. Such cases might be overlooked.

PESTIS MINOR. This type manifests the usual symptoms of bubonic plague without bacteraemia. The general condition is usually not serious. They may be overlooked.

Chronic forms. In this type, the disease runs a chronic course from the onset. The course is prolonged with the appearance successively of many buboes variously situated, alopecia, cachexia, followed by slow recuperation, prolonged convalescence or death.

Fulminant forms. In this type, the characteristic features are high fever, heart failure, pulmonary oedema, delirium and coma. Stool and urine may contain blood. Haemorrhages in skin and mucus membranes are conspicuous.

Primary pneumonic plague

The general clinical features are identical with those met within other severe forms of plague. In the early stages respiratory signs are inconspicuous. There may be little or no cough. Expectoration is scanty. Smear of the sputum will show only a few suspicious bacilli.

Pulmonary signs begin to appear about 24 hours after onset of disease. Cough becomes frequent and troublesome with expectoration at first of mucoid or mucopurulent sputum, but this soon shows streaks of bright red blood and is then followed by a considerable amount of uniformly pink or bright red coloured sputum. The sputum will now contain numerous *P. pestis*.

Dyspnoea is usually present and the patient may complain of pain and a restricted feeling in the chest. On auscultation, rales may be absent, but when present, they are of the fine variety. When oedema of the lungs occurs, numerous rales may be heard and breath sounds are feeble. There may be pleural rub or pleural effusion. Signs of progressive heart failure may follow. Patients with pneumonic plague rarely survive longer than 2-4 days.

DIAGNOSIS

The definitive diagnosis of plague depends upon the results of laboratory examinations. However, clinical diagnosis is important from the point of view of plague prevention and early treatment, especially in rural areas where laboratory facilities may be inadequate.

Bubonic plague

The diagnosis of typical bubonic plague is not difficult. During an outbreak of plague, patients who suddenly become very ill and have a high temperature, injected conjunctivae and painful buboes, are readily recognised as suffering from bubonic plague. Confirmation may be sought by puncture of the affected lymph node and demonstration of *P. pestis* in the stained smear. If the smear examination results are equivocal, culture or animal inoculation of the punctured material may be made.

Bubonic plague must be differentiated from other infections with enlarged lymph nodes, such as filarial or other forms of adenitis, glandular fever and lymphogranuloma venereum.

In acute severe septicaemia with enlarged regional lymph nodes, there is usually a septic wound in the affected region and the clinical picture of septicaemia is manifest. It would be very difficult to differentiate such septicaemia from bubonic plague. Gland puncture and demonstration of *P. pestis* will decide the diagnosis.

Mild cases of bubonic plague may have to be distinguished from lymphogranuloma venereum and filarial adenitis by appropriate laboratory tests.

Severe bubonic plague with septicaemia may be difficult to differentiate from other acute febrile illnesses such as typhus, pernicious malaria and acute haemorrhagic fever. In such cases, blood smear examinations, blood culture and serological tests are essential.

Bubonic plague must also be differentiated from infection caused by other members of the genus *Pasteurella*, especially *Pasteurella pseudotuberculosis*, which produces a typhoid-like syndrome with icterus. Guinea pig inoculation and other appropriate tests such as motility tests will distinguish *P. pestis* from *P. pseudotuberculosis*.

Primary pneumonic plague

There will be difficulty in the clinical diagnosis of this condition during the initial 24 hours of primary pneumonic plague when only general signs of serious illness are present and pulmonary localising signs are absent. Also, sputum examination is mostly inconclusive or negative during this stage. However, a history of recent contact with patients suffering from plague with lung involvement is highly significant and points towards a diagnosis of incipient pneumonic plague. X-ray demonstration of pneumonic foci serves as an additional diagnostic feature of importance.

During the later well-developed stage, the clinical features of a serious, rapidly progressive illness, insignificant lung signs, and expectoration of a bloodstained sputum, make the diagnosis of primary pneumonic plague easy. Sputum will show numerous plague bacilli on smear examination and this may be further confirmed by culture and/or animal inoculation.

Pneumonic plague may have to be differentiated from acute haemorrhagic fever. In the latter, haemorrhagic manifestations are usually generalised, starting from petechial haemorrhages and followed by haemorrhages in the mucosa, nose, mouth, stomach, intestines and kidneys. In addition, there is clinical evidence of renal involvement, whereas generally in cases of pneumonic plague bleeding is from the lungs only and the kidneys are not involved. Sputum examination will finally decide the diagnosis.

TREATMENT

In 1896, Yersin began to use therapeutic antiplague serum. More recently sulphonamides have been used on a large scale in the treatment of bubonic plague, and streptomycin and other antibiotics in the treatment of all forms of plague, all with consistently good results.

Rest in bed

The patient must be strictly confined to bed during the acute stage as well as in early convalescence, as there is the risk of acute heart failure, which may require special treatment and may cause sudden death.

Diet and fluid intake

Nourishing and adequate light diet with ample fluid intake is advised. The urine output is noted and the urine examined daily for albumin or blood.

Sulphonamide therapy

Sulphadiazine, sulphamerazine and sulphadimidine are effective in mild cases and are useful in prophylactic treatment of contacts and of those entering epidemic zones shortly after inoculation. As prophylaxis, 1 g three times a day for 6 days is adequate. For the treatment of bubonic plague, the recommended dosage is 4 g initially by mouth, followed by 2 g 4 hours later, and then 1 g 8-hourly till the temperature remains normal for 2 days.

Usually a total dosage of 50 g is required for a full course of about 7 days. To achieve the sufficiently high blood level of 100 mg per 100 ml, it is advisable to give the initial dose intravenously. It is essential to continue treatment during the first few days of convalescence to avoid relapse or complications.

As a rule, primary pneumonic plague is not amenable to sulphonamide therapy, which should be reserved in these cases for prophylaxis only.

Antibiotic therapy

PENICILLIN, even in high dose, has no action on *P. pestis*.

STREPTOMYCIN. In 1949 Meyer and Quan studied the effect of streptomycin on plague-infected animals and concluded that it has powerful bactericidal action on *P. pestis*. Streptomycin is effective both in bubonic and pneumonic plague. In 1947, Videla used streptomycin in the treatment of human plague.

For mild cases, treatment is started with an initial dose of 0.6 g intramuscularly, followed by 0.3 g 4-hourly until the temperature remains normal for 24 hours. In severe cases, 0.6 g is given 4-hourly until the temperature remains normal for 2 to 3 days.

Cases of primary pneumonic plague are treated with streptomycin 0.5 g intramuscularly every 3 hours for the first 2 days, 4-hourly on the third day, and 6-hourly for another 3 days. The same dosage is recommended for severe cases of bubonic plague with septicaemia.

Other antibiotics. Meyer (1950) stated that aureomycin, terramycin and chloramphenicol are good alternatives in plague therapy. But they are less bactericidal than streptomycin against the plague bacillus.

Chloramphenicol is given initially by intravenous injection, 0.5 g every 3 hours for three doses, along with 0.5 g by mouth 3-hourly for three doses. Subsequently three to four doses of 0.5 g are given orally every 3 hours, then 0.25 g 2-hourly until the temperature drops to 37°C; this is continued for a further 2–3 days. The total dosage amounts to 20–25 g.

In rural areas where funds are low it is advisable to start with sulphonamides alone. Antibiotics may be started if the patient fails to respond to sulphonamides.

Cases of plague must be detected as early as possible. Benign forms of bubonic plague, if detected early, should be treated with sulphonamides only. If the condition of patients treated with sulphonamides deteriorates, antibiotics must be used in addition to sulphonamides.

Patients suffering from primary pneumonic plague and from septicaemic plague, or severe cases of bubonic plague presenting for treatment at a late stage, or bubonic forms with serious complications like meningeal involvement, must all without exception be given antibiotic therapy, especially streptomycin.

Sulphonamides are the drugs of choice for abortive treatment. Known contacts, particularly those who are attending pneumonic plague patients, may be treated with specific serum and sulphonamides.

Treatment should be started immediately on clinical evidence, without waiting for the laboratory report.

CONTROL AND PREVENTION

The ultimate control and prevention of plague lies in controlling the rodent reservoir and insect vectors of the infection. Antirodent measures are aimed at commensal rodents and wild rodents respectively.

Commensal rodents

Control is effected by various methods of destruction and rat-proofing.

The methods employed to exterminate commensal rats include killing by mechanical means, the use of predators such as cats, trapping, poisoning and fumigation. The most suitable method will obviously depend on the circumstances in which it is to be used. In general, fumigation and poisoning appear to be more effective in permanently reducing the rodent population. Trapping is of supplemental value only, unless an intensive campaign can be launched. Other methods are ineffective in any large scale rat destruction campaign.

Poisoning. The various poisons that may be used are arsenic trioxide, barium carbonate, red squill, zinc phosphate, sodium fluoroacetate, and anticoagulants.

Whenever possible, poisoning compaigns should be conducted on a community-wide scale or should at least embrace blocks of buildings. A 'vertical' system of rodent control to include all foci such as infested buildings, outhouses and underlying sewers is of importance. Such a campaign, to be successful, should be accompanied also by public health propaganda campaigns.

Fumigation. The following chemicals may be used: carbon disulphide, carbon dioxide, carbon monoxide, chloropicim, hydrocyanic acid, calcium cyanide, methyl bromide and sulphur dioxide.

Some of these are effective not only against the rodents, but also against their fleas. They are used to destroy the rodents in their burrows or in closed spaces like warehouses, ships' holds, huts and houses.

Rat-proofing. This broadly aims at the separation of rat and man. Rodents may be denied ingress into houses by construction methods and other mechanical means. 'Internal' rat-proofing may be accomplished by the abolition of shelter and nesting facilities. Also measures to prevent access of commensal rats to food supplies should be instituted, together with general sanitary measures such as proper disposal of household refuse.

Wild rodents

Large-scale campaigns aimed at destruction of wild rodents are impractical. The main principle of control is to keep sylvatic foci under surveillance and prevent the infection from becoming established in commensal rodents in close proximity to man.

Vectors

Control is effected by the use of D.D.T., B.H.C. and to lesser extent by other insecticides and fumigants.

D.D.T. is used as a 5 per cent emulsion for indoor residual spraying, or as a 10 per cent dusting powder for insufflating rat burrows and harbourages and surface dusting of rat runs. It is of outstanding value in rodent flea control. B.H.C., whilst more rapidly lethal, has a shorter residual action. Fumigants such as calcium cyanide are mostly used for ridding grain supplies of fleas.

Control of bubonic plague

Hospitalisation, quarantine and evacuation. From the viewpoint of plague prevention it is not essential to isolate bubonic plague patients with lung complications. However, hospitalisation is desirable so that better nursing and treatment facilities may be utilised.

The patient should be in a rat-free room and medical attendants should wear masks and flea-proof garments.

There is no longer any need to quarantine contacts nor for mass evacuation of plague-infected areas.

Control of pneumonic plague

The aim is to prevent spread of infection from man to man. The methods used in dealing with primary pneumonic plague patients and those developing secondary lung involvement during the course of bubonic plague are similar and are dealt with together.

Rapid and early case detection is essential for effective suppression of pneumonic plague. The cooperation of the public is sought in reporting all suspicious cases. A system of house-to-house inspection may also have to be adopted.

Prompt isolation and hospitalisation of all pneumonic plague patients is essential. During an outbreak, those who show evidence of lung involvement should be treated with 1 g of streptomycin immediately, and thereafter 0.25 to 0.5 g 4-hourly.

Contacts should be quarantined for 6 to 10 days. If this is impossible, arrangements will have to be made for observation and abortive treatment within the house.

All persons attending the patient must wear masks, and hospital staff should wear masks, gown (with hood) and goggles. All objects contaminated with the patient's sputum should be disinfected. Boiling water may be used for disinfection of sputum.

The dead should be handled by burial squads provided with masks, protective garments, boots and gloves, and should be buried deep or cremated.

Vaccination, though of no direct value in preventing pneumonic plague in man, is of indirect value in reducing the frequency of bubonic manifestations.

Mass vaccination

This is of definite value in the prevention of plague and confers active immunity for at least 6 months from 5 to 7 days after vaccination. Killed vaccine has to be given in two doses with an interval of 7 days, while live avirulent vaccine is effective in single dose.

Immunoprophylaxis is useful in the control of sylvatic plague. Those who are staying in foci of sylvatic plague should be vaccinated 6-monthly.

Control of spread to distant areas

Careful medical examination must be made of intending travellers and their baggage should be de-flead with D.D.T. or calcium cyanide. Inoculation must be completed at least a week before their departure. Those who have had contact with pneumonic plague patients must be quarantined for 6–10 days before they are permitted to leave. Sea-going ships must be fumigated periodically. D.D.T. should be applied to railway carriages, buses and trucks to keep them free from fleas.

REFERENCES

MEYER, K. F. (1950) *J. Amer. med. Ass.*, **144**, 982.

MEYER, K. F. and QUAN, S. F. (1949) In *Streptomycin: Nature and Practical Applications*, ed. Wakesman, S. A., p. 394. Baltimore.

ORI, A. (1933) *Ann. Igiene*, **43**, 276.

PETRIC, G. F. (1929) In *A System of Bacteriology in Relation to Medicine*. Medical Research Council, London, **3**, 137.

POLLITZER, R. (1936) In *Plague: A Manual for Medical and Public Health Workers*, ed. Wu Lien-teh, Chun, J. W. H., Pollitzer, R. and Wu, C. Y. Shanghai.

SCHUTZE, H. (1929) In *A System of Bacteriology in Relation to Medicine*. Medical Research Council, London, **4**, 446, 474.

VIDELA, C. A. (1947) *Día méd.*, **19**, 1.

WU-LIEN-TEH (1926). *A Treatise on Pneumonic Plague*. Geneva: League of Nations Publication C.H. 474.

20
Brucellosis

Infections due to organisms of the genus *Brucella* occur primarily in mammals, birds and arthropods. They reach man almost exclusively from domestic animals. The varying reactions of the human host to these infections are included in the term brucellosis which, however, does not include tularaemia, the causative organism of which, sometimes classified as *Brucella tularensis*, is more commonly placed in the genus *Pasteurella* and produces a disease showing some affinities to plague.

Brucella melitensis, first described by Bruce in 1886 in Malta and called by him *Micrococcus melitensis*, infects goats and sheep. In the U.S.S.R. 10 strains have been isolated from 40 species of animals including rodents. Transovarian infection occurs in ticks which can act as vectors between animals. Three subtypes are recognised.

Brucella abortus is an infection of cattle and was first described by Bang in 1897 in Austria as the cause of contagious abortion in cows. Nine subtypes are now distinguished, type 5 resembling *Br. melitensis* in a number of laboratory tests. An attenuated strain, S.19, is used for vaccination of calves.

Brucella suis is acquired from infected pigs, as shown by Traum in the U.S.A. in 1914. Three subtypes occur. Type 2 has been found in hares in France and type 3 in rodents in Kenya.

EPIDEMIOLOGY

After the culture of the organisms from goats' milk in Malta by Horrocks in 1905, the importance of unheated goats' milk as a source of infection was quickly established.

Bevan, a veterinary surgeon in Rhodesia, in 1921 associated human disease in farmers with contagious abortion in cattle. Unpasteurised milk from infected cattle, including erroneously called 'safe milk' when tuberculin tested, conveys *Br. abortus*. As only a small proportion of those who drink infected untreated milk acquire overt brucellosis, the public has been slow to appreciate the danger.

These infections may also be acquired from unpasteurised derivatives of milk, such as cream and fresh cream cheeses. Mature cheeses are safe but the exact time or degree of maturity required to kill all the organisms has not been determined. Buffaloes, camels and reindeer have also been found commonly to be sources of infection.

Brucellosis may also be acquired by direct contact with goats, sheep and cattle. In highly endemic areas this commonly occurs in those tending animals or sharing accommodation with them, and *Br. abortus* infection is frequently acquired by veterinary surgeons, particularly after delivering retained placentas. The systemic disease is probably chiefly acquired by ingestion from unwashed hands but a dermatosis may result from contact of the forearms with infective discharges. Under dusty conditions, aerosols may convey the infection. Accidental inoculation of the vaccinator with the attenuated strain 19 may take place during the vaccination of calves.

Br. suis infections are usually acquired from handling infected carcases of pigs. The eating of inadequately cooked pork is also a possible method.

In bacteriological laboratories, if cultures of the organisms are not handled with great care, infections readily occur from aerosols being inspired or from the organisms entering through the conjunctiva.

In spite of brucellae being excreted at times in the urine, interhuman spread is exceedingly rare. In most cases of multiple infections in a family, a common external source can be postulated.

GEOGRAPHICAL DISTRIBUTION

Br. melitensis appears to have a somewhat patchy distribution but it is found in most tropical and subtropical countries as well as in some temperate zones of Europe and America.

Br. abortus infections are even more widespread but eradication programmes have met with considerable success in Scandinavia and elsewhere. It is the only form of brucellosis endemic in Britain.

Br. suis has been eradicated from Denmark but persists in some other European countries, the U.S.A. and the Far East.

Pathogenesis

Except for contact dermatosis, the pathological changes result from a bacteraemia and the spread of brucellae to many tissues. The organisms, presumably by endotoxins, cause fever of variable degree and duration. Bacteraemia may persist even when the patient is afebrile. In many cases, however, bacteraemia is intermittent and the organisms remain largely intracellular, making eradication difficult.

Morbid anatomy

The histological changes are due mainly to infiltration with cells producing characteristic small granulomas, which are not, however, pathognomonic of brucellosis. Brucellae may be cultured from such tissues but the organisms are not identifiable in the lesions. Usually the granulomas consist of epithelioid cells, lymphocytes and plasma cells, often with some multinuclear giant cells, varying in size from cells with a few nuclei to others with 50 nuclei (Hunt *et al*, 1967). Exceptionally, but particularly in *Br. suis* infections, caseation and eventually areas of calcification may develop. The spleen and liver enlarge, but not necessarily enough for the enlargement to be detected clinically. In chronic infections gross splenomegaly and considerable hepatomegaly may be present. Biopsies and necropsies have shown characteristic granulomas in the liver. Particularly at autopsy, cirrhosis of the liver may be found. In most cases this may well be coincidental, but rarely the clinical history and prior biopsies suggest that brucellosis may have caused the portal cirrhosis. The gall-bladder often shows evidence of inflammatory changes. In persistent infections, especially those due to *Br. melitensis*, osteomyelitis may occur, particularly in one or more vertebrae, and may lead to collapse and angulation, but only rarely is a paravertebral abscess formed. Osteophytes joining vertebrae together are a characteristic feature. Abscesses may occur in other bones, especially in ribs. The histological changes in joints and periarticular tissues are not well documented, but free fluid in a joint may be a feature.

Lymph nodes, when enlarged, show non-specific changes which may be erroneously attributed to sarcoidosis or Hodgkin's disease.

Cellular infiltration has been found in the testes, epididymis and heart muscle.

Pulmonary changes are not usually evident at autopsy, but caseous granulomas due to *Br. suis* are well known.

Suppurative foci in chronic infections may be found in the kidney, liver and elsewhere. Brucellae are sometimes the causative organisms in bacterial endocarditis and, in a case of long duration, calcification of a cusp margin has resulted, but brucellae do not tend to affect the endocardium of previously normal heart valves.

To avoid repetition, changes that may occur in the blood and in certain other tissues are described only in the following section.

Age and sex incidence

Although newborn calves are immune, human children are susceptible and the age and sex incidence is dependent upon exposure to infection.

Historical

Brucellosis is a disease of protean manifestations, but the occurrence of a fever differing from other prolonged fevers was for long recognised as occurring in the Mediterranean littoral. In 1863 Marston gave an excellent review of fever in Malta and gave the first convincing account of brucellosis under the names of Mediterranean remittent or gastric remittent fever in the following words:

'By this is meant a fever characterized by the following symptoms and course:—A preliminary stage of subacute dyspepsia, anorexia, nausea, headache, feeling of weakness, lassitude, and inaptitude for exertion, mental or physical, chills, muscular pains; lastly, a fever, having a very long course—three to five, or ten weeks—marked by irregular exacerbations and remissions, great derangement of the assimilative organs, tenderness in epigastric region, splenic enlargement, slight jaundice, without any exanthem. Neither bronchitis nor diarrhoea, as a rule. The patient is prone to relapses, and the disorder is followed by a protracted convalescence and a chloro-anaemic aspect; very frequently also by rheumatism of some form or other, but without any tendency to lesions of the peri- or endocardial membranes. Pathologically, it is marked by congestion or inflammation, with softening of the enteric mucous membrane, (particularly that of the stomach and duodenum) without any lesion of the Peyerian follicles, but with hypertrophies of the liver and spleen.'

This description can scarcely be bettered today except, as Marston said elsewhere, icterus of any degree is uncommon except in very toxic patients.

The disease thus became known as Malta fever.

Fever

Hughes, in 1897, after himself suffering from the disease in Malta, wrote a monograph in which he suggested the name 'undulant fever', as a variable fever is so characteristic. This has sometimes been misinterpreted as indicating that the temperature chart should show a regular rise and fall resembling the Pel-Ebstein fever of Hodgkin's disease. Hughes, however, was careful to point out that 'the term need not be held to mean a definite quantity or amount of intensity but as in nature undulations vary from gentle ripple or broader swell to chopping wave or overwhelming breaker, so may the expression be applied to the various pyrexial waves of this fever, however much they vary in length and magnitude'.

The onset of the disease is usually insidious and hence the incubation period indefinite. In those with more abrupt onset it varies from a few days to 3 weeks. Exceptionally, in virulent infections, the onset is relatively abrupt, the patient rapidly becomes toxic and comatose, sometimes with hyperpyrexia. More commonly, the patient, even though highly febrile, appears much less toxic than someone with a similar temperature from typhoid fever and he may remain ambulant. Fever is rapidly curtailed by antibiotic therapy. Untreated, the duration is unpredictable with remissions and exacerbations, and lasts not uncommonly for from 1 to 2 years, while an infection lasting 25 years has been reliably reported (Spink 1964). The patient may remain afebrile, or nearly so, for weeks or months only to relapse again. Particularly in temperate climates, in *Br. abortus* infections, profuse sweating is often a noticeable feature and sometimes in addition to sudamina indefinite erythematous rashes may appear. As with typhoid fever, but in contrast to many fevers, a crop of herpes labialis is rare.

Spleen

Less than half the patients when first examined are found to have a palpable spleen, but this proportion increases with the duration of the illness. Usually the spleen is only of moderate size and soft, but in chronic neglected infections, as may be seen in underdeveloped tropical countries, the spleen may extend to the right iliac fossa and become also very prominent and firm. A large spleen may be the site of infarcts accompanied by perisplenitis and severe pain.

Liver and gall-bladder

Appreciable enlargement of the liver is rather less frequent than splenomegaly, but particularly when the spleen is very big, the liver is usually considerably enlarged also. In endemic areas kala azar is closely mimicked. Occasionally the liver may be large and tender and the spleen not palpable. Severe pain in the region of the liver may be due to infarcts or cholecystitis. Hepatitis may be severe enough to cause jaundice (Wright *et al*, 1953).

Cholecystitis, sometimes associated with jaundice, may occur and brucellae have been cultured from a duodenal aspirate.

Lungs

In acute brucellosis areas of pneumonitis may develop, sometimes with haemoptysis and a positive sputum. A sterile pleural effusion or an empyema yielding brucellae on culture may occur. Chronic granulomatous foci in *Br. suis* infections may give radiographic appearances suggesting a carcinoma of the lung. A smouldering fever due to brucellosis accompanying inactive or healed pulmonary tuberculosis is liable to be incorrectly attributed to activity of the tuberculosis. Prior to the introduction of streptomycin, such patients sometimes lingered in sanatoria incorrectly diagnosed as suffering from active tuberculosis.

Locomotor system

Pain in the back, particularly in the lumbosacral region, is very frequent in prolonged infections. The pain may be localised and agonising or it may be felt throughout the spine. Sometimes it is of sudden onset, suggesting a slipped intervertebral disc. Untreated, the pain may continue to be distressing or may suddenly be relieved. It usually subsides rapidly with antibiotics, suggesting that it is due to inflammatory oedema of periarticular tissues. In certain infections, however, particularly when due to *Br. melitensis* or *Br. suis*, deformity of the spine may resemble Pott's disease and radiographic evidence of destruction of vertebral bodies may be evident. There is usually less evidence of disc destruction than in tuberculosis. Very rarely a paravertebral abscess gives rise to paraplegia.

When a cervical vertebra is affected, the stiff

neck and fever may simulate meningitis. Inflammation of the hip joint is common. When the knee, wrist or ankle are affected, the joints are obviously swollen. Usually only one or two joints are affected at the same time and the arthritis does not flit from joint to joint as is characteristic of untreated acute rheumatism.

A relatively painless swelling may develop at the site of inflammation in a rib, costochondral junction or the sternum. Fluid aspirated from a joint or local swelling is often sterile but sometimes is purulent and yields a brucella on culture.

There is no evidence to suggest that brucellosis is a factor in causing rheumatoid arthritis or a common cause of osteoarthritis but in endemic areas it is a significant cause of locomotor disability.

Lymph nodes

A slight degree of lymphadenopathy is frequently observed but its significance is often doubtful. Pronounced enlargement of multiple lymph nodes occurs in some 3 per cent of cases. In childhood this may be accompanied by a lymphocytosis simulating infectious mononucleosis.

Blood

A moderate iron deficiency anaemia is commonly present. Occasionally, particularly in malnourished children, very severe anaemia may develop. When this is combined with considerable splenomegaly, a dyshaemopoietic anaemia may be incorrectly suspected.

There is usually a slight leucopenia, in particular the number of granulocytes being below normal. The leucopenia is not as constantly profound as in developed kala azar, but when a low count is present as well as hepatosplenomegaly, the resemblance to this disease is increased. The ESR is often increased in febrile patients but nevertheless may be normal in the presence of a persistent infection.

Granulomas may be detected in smears from bone marrow and the organism may be successfully cultured from it, otherwise the changes are not diagnostic.

Central nervous system

Usually there is no evidence of central nervous system involvement. In highly virulent infections a comatose state may develop. On occasion, in patients who do not otherwise appear to be particularly ill, a mild meningitis develops. The cerebrospinal fluid then shows a moderate pleocytosis and may yield a brucella on culture. Cases resembling viral encephalomyelitis have also been described. Acute anterior poliomyelitis may be simulated (Debono, 1964). In long-continued infections evidence of peripheral neuritis may be found, but this is probably caused by concomitant malnutrition. Mental depression was a notable feature of this trying illness before antibiotics were available and if the underlying infection is not appreciated the patient may be incorrectly diagnosed as suffering from a psychoneurosis. A carefully controlled series of observations indicated that a neurosis did not tend to be produced by brucellosis unless the person was constitutionally unstable (Imboden *et al*, 1959).

Genitourinary system

In chronic infections an abscess may develop in the kidney or perinephric space and be associated with recurrent pyrexia over a period of years. Some cases present with pyelonephritis. Although abortion may occur during a bout of fever, unlike the infection in animals, abortion and infections of the female genital organs are not common. Orchitis and epididymitis, sometimes with a blood-stained seminal discharge, may be observed.

Eye

Some cases come to light by the investigation of keratitis or uveitis causing papilloedema.

Skin

Sudamina and evanescent rashes may occur during fever. Veterinary surgeons who do not protect their forearms from infected bovine vaginal discharges may develop a cutaneous hypersensitivity to contact with *Br. abortus* and develop a maculopapular eruption on the exposed areas after removing a retained placenta.

Other manifestations

Probably no organ is exempt from infection; thrombophlebitis causing pulmonary embolism, chronic miliary peritonitis and thyroiditis have all been attributed to brucellosis.

Indefinite ill health and hypersensitivity

Patients after treatment for brucellosis or after spontaneous recovery often remain somewhat below par for months. It is difficult to exclude a continuing infection in these circumstances, yet no benefit may follow from repeated chemotherapy. There is evidence that patients may remain hypersensitive, even to the injection of dead brucellae, and some bouts of symptoms may be due to such hypersensitivity.

Human disease due to the ingestion of milk containing viable *Br. abortus* strain 19 has not been recorded, but when this organism has accidentally entered through the conjunctiva or by subcutaneous injection, a typical febrile illness may result and the organism may be recovered by blood culture. The fever is usually only of short duration although antibodies and some minor ill health may persist.

DIAGNOSIS

As with many infections in the tropics the following questions have to be answered. Has the patient been infected? Is the disease still active? How much of the patient's illness is due to this particular infection?

Culture of organism

From blood. If a brucella is successfully isolated, a continuing infection is established. Even so, other diseases may be present. For example the disease may be coincident with kala azar, and in one patient both *S. typhi* and *Br. abortus* were cultured from the blood (Wright *et al*, 1953). Blood culture is of prime importance. It is helpful to use a double-phase medium as devised by Castañeda (1961). The culture should be carried out under normal atmospheric conditions and also, to facilitate the growth of the classical strain of *Br. abortus*, in a mixture of air with 10 per cent carbon dioxide. Cultures should be kept for 6 weeks before being discarded as negative. Attempted subcultures are made every few days by tilting the container and only when a growth is seen on the solid medium should the container be opened.

From other sites. Successful cultures may also be obtained from bone marrow or a liver biopsy, but not usually if the blood culture is negative. The organisms have also been isolated from urine, serous effusions, the cerebrospinal fluid, other tissues and abscesses.

Inoculation into guinea pigs is a valuable procedure for contaminated material, penicillin being added.

Results. *Br. melitensis* is readily recovered and may sometimes be cultured from the blood even while the patient is afebrile. The classical strain of *Br. abortus* may defy isolation, especially if preceding antibiotics have been taken. However, some strains of *Br. abortus* which do not require a reduced oxygen tension are grown as easily as *Br. melitensis*. Species differentiation is achieved by noting if hydrogen sulphide is produced, the inhibition of growth by dyes and the agglutination of a monospecific antiserum.

Serological tests

Delays or failures in culturing brucellae make serological tests of considerable importance.

A conventional agglutination test, using standard antigens (preferably expressing the results in International Units), is of considerable value. In established infections a high titre is usually found and is diagnostic of present or recent brucellosis. Only in the exceptional patient such as a laboratory worker, or in severe infections, are sera obtained early enough in the disease for rising titres, in successive specimens, to be observed. A rise in titre in a chronic infection may, however, indicate an exacerbation.

This test has certain shortcomings. In some patients there is not only a negative prozone in the lower dilutions, but no agglutination may take place at any dilution, yet on the addition of anti-human globulin (Coombs' test) antibodies associated with immunoglobulins (IgG) may be revealed. Inactivation of the serum with 2-mercapto-ethanol may be used to retain the 7S agglutinating antibodies associated with IgG and believed to indicate active disease.

False positive titres may be obtained by cross-agglutination with *Vibrio cholerae* or *Pasteurella tularensis* from cholera or tularaemia or from vaccination against these diseases.

A titre below 40 iu is of very doubtful significance although rarely negative sera are reported in culturally confirmed infections. Owing to cross-agglutination the causative *species* can only be deduced by absorption tests.

Complement fixation test. This test yields consistently positive results in active brucellosis and is comparable to the Coombs' test in detecting the disease. A falling titre suggests a favourable result to treatment but it is not yet clear whether a persistently positive result necessarily indicates a continuing infection (Kerr *et al*, 1966).

Intradermal tests

Sensitivity to the products of brucellae develop in those who have been in contact with these organisms, either by external contact (perhaps only if abrasions are present), by subclinical infections or overt disease. The carbohydrate fraction of brucellae induces an immediate cutaneous response; the nucleoprotein fraction contained in the commercial product Brucellergin produces a delayed tuberculin-like reaction. A negative test makes a diagnosis of brucellosis unlikely. Otherwise the test is of little value except as an epidemiological tool in indicating the degree of exposure of a population to infection. Some rise in seroagglutinins may follow the intradermal test and this does not, as has been claimed, necessarily indicate systemic infection.

Diagnosis in animals

Preliminary screening by means of the ring or ABR (Abortus Bang Ringprobe) test of milk or cream is a useful adjunct to the seroagglutination test and culture from milk (W.H.O., 1964).

DIFFERENTIAL DIAGNOSIS

As brucellosis is almost ubiquitous it should be considered as a possibility in any patient with an undiagnosed persistent or intermittent fever. In other patients hepatosplenomegaly, or enlargement of either viscus, will be the presenting problem. Arthritis, particularly spondylitis, is an alternative presentation. Less commonly brucellosis masquerades as severe anaemia, with lymphadenopathy, as meningoencephalitis or as an ocular disorder. Pulmonary lesions, especially in those possibly exposed to *Br. suis*, require differentiation. Smouldering ill health causing psychological stress should suggest the possibility of brucellosis in those whose occupations or habits render infection to be likely, namely veterinary surgeons, farmers, artificial inseminators, meat handlers and workers in bacteriological laboratories.

Coincidence of brucellosis and Hodgkin's disease may occur (Hunt *et al*, 1967), but the histology of the lymph nodes is similar.

TREATMENT

Before the introduction of antibiotics, brucellosis might consist of a subclinical infection, a short-term or more prolonged fever or a chronic febrile illness with complications including agonising pain in the back or hip. Spontaneous recovery ensued in the majority but its timing was unpredictable. The first combination frequently to produce a remission, and sometimes cure, was streptomycin and a sulphonamide. Tetracycline

alone is more successful and 2 g daily for 3 weeks is frequently curative. A more reliable therapeutic measure is a combination of streptomycin 1 g and tetracycline 2 g daily for 3 weeks. Although not fully substantiated by statistics, the dramatic relief of bone pain, formerly seen in patients treated with streptomycin and a sulphonamide, led the author to use a combination of streptomycin 1 g, tetracycline 2 g and sulphadimidine 4 g daily for 14 to 21 days, and in chronic infections this appeared to be the best combination followed by the fewest relapses. A combination of trimethoprim and sulphamethoxazole (Septrin, Bactrim) also appears to be effective and may be especially successful in reaching intracellular brucellae.

In the elderly it may be unwise to give streptomycin for fear of damage to the auditory nerve and in the malnourished, particularly, it may be wise to avoid precipitating an avitaminosis by administering also vitamin B complex. In children under 5 years of age the disease tends to be mild and tetracyclines less effective. If spontaneous recovery is delayed, a short course of oxytetracycline, which produces the least objectionable staining of children's teeth, is indicated (Rizzo-Naudi *et al*, 1967). For the exceptional highly febrile toxic adult patient it may be necessary to give, in addition, a corticosteroid for the first 24 to 72 hours only (Spink, 1960). In some exceptionally prolonged relapsing infections, cure has only been achieved after locating and draining or removing a brucellar abscess. Thus operations on bones, splenectomy, nephrectomy and the drainage of a perinephric abscess have been found to be necessary.

Experimental infections in mice have been found to persist after antibiotic therapy (Spink *et al*, 1960). Repeated courses of antibiotics may be necessary in human infections, but unless the organisms are still being recovered it is often difficult to decide if an infection is still present. The use of a vaccine in apparently chronic infections has its advocates, but there is little evidence that it is of any value.

PROGNOSIS

Exceptionally the untreated acutely ill patient may die of toxaemia. Prior to the introduction of antibiotics, a few others died of intercurrent infections or malnutrition after prolonged illness. The majority survived, many in a state of variable misery for months or years, some with permanent locomotor disabilities. With early treatment full recovery can now be expected, but when treatment is delayed, the illness or its sequelae may still be trying for many months.

PREVENTION

Br. abortus. All milk and milk products from infected herds should be pasteurised. Control of infection in cattle can be achieved by vaccination of calves with *Br. abortus* strain 19 and improved hygiene at parturition. A killed vaccine, strain 45/20, is used in adult cattle. Eradication programmes based on these methods, followed by the elimination of infected animals, has met with success and is financially rewarding. While cattle remain infected, those attending them are at risk.

Human protection of those at special risk by a living vaccine 19–BA has been widely employed in the U.S.S.R. (Vershilova, 1961) but because of undesirable reactions has not yet received universal acceptance.

Br. melitensis. The elimination of the infection in sheep and goats is difficult, but vaccines have been employed in the U.S.S.R. The relative importance of rodents as a reservoir of infection has not yet been established.

Br. suis. Elimination, by slaughter of pigs known to be infective, has been achieved in some countries. Personal hygiene amongst those handling pigs and pork products is highly essential to prevent human infections.

REFERENCES

CASTAÑEDA, M. RUIZ (1961) *Bull. Wld Hlth Org.*, **24**, 73.
DEBONO, J. E. (1964) *Lancet*, **1**, 1132.
HUGHES, M. L. (1897) *Mediterranean, Malta or Undulant Fever*. London.
HUNT, A. C. and BOTHWELL, P. W. (1967) *J. clin. Path.*, **20**, 267.
IMBODEN, J. B. *et al* (1959) *Arch. intern. Med.*, **103**, 406.
KERR, W. R. *et al* (1966) *Lancet*, **2**, 1181.
MARSTON, J. A. (1863) *Army Medical Department, Statistical, Sanitary and Medical Reports* (for 1861), p. 486. London.
RIZZO-NAUDI, J. *et al* (1967) *Postgrad. med. J.*, **43**, 520.
SPINK, W. W. (1960) *J. Amer. med. Ass.*, **172**, 697.
—— (1964) *Amer. J. med. Sci.*, **247**, 129.
SPINK, W. W. and BRADLEY, G. M. (1960) *J. Lab. clin. Med.*, **55**, 535.
VERSHILOVA, P. A. (1961) *Bull. Wld Hlth Org.*, **24**, 85.
WORLD HEALTH ORGANIZATION (1964) Techn. Rep. Ser., No. 289.
WRIGHT, F. J. *et al* (1953) *Trans. roy. Soc. trop. Med. Hyg.*, **47**, 117.

21

Leprosy

SYNONYMS. Hansen's disease, Hansen's infection, hansenaisis elephantiasis graecorum.

DEFINITION

Leprosy is a chronic disease of the peripheral nervous system of man, commonly involving the skin and less often involving the mucosa of the mouth and upper respiratory tract, the reticulo-endothelial system, eyes, bones and testes. The incubation period is usually between 2 and 7 years.

AETIOLOGY

The generally accepted, but as yet unproved, cause of the disease is *Mycobacterium leprae*, a bacterium discovered by Hansen in Norway in 1874. It is a rod-shaped organism similar in appearance to *M. tuberculosis* under the light microscope and, when stained by Ziehl-Neelsen method, it is less alcohol fast and acid-fast. It cannot be grown on artificial media, and all attempts to obtain bacillary multiplication in laboratory animals failed until Shepard (1960) successfully infected the footpads of mice. This work has been amply confirmed since then, and, using Shepard's technique, local multiplication of *M. leprae* has been obtained by different workers in the ears of mice, in the footpads and ears of hamsters, and in the footpads of rats. More recently it has been shown that systemic infections can be established in mice previously treated by thymectomy and whole-body irradiation (Rees *et al*, 1967).

EPIDEMIOLOGY AND DISTRIBUTION

The two important factors in the spread of leprosy are the proportion of susceptible persons in the population and the opportunities for contact with the disease. Observations on the incidence of leprosy in marriage partners, when one partner has the disease in an infectious form, show that only about 5 per cent of those at risk acquire the disease. The much higher incidence in children born into leprous families supports the view that children are more susceptible than adults. Transplacental infection does not occur.

The greatest endemicity of leprosy is in the tropics and subtropics, with a lower incidence in certain temperate zones such as the Mediterranean, Adriatic and Black Sea regions.

PATHOLOGY

The mode of infection in leprosy is unknown, and although it is generally believed to be via the skin during direct contact, transmission via the respiratory or gastrointestinal tracts, or by insect bite, is equally possible. The relatively few attempts to infect volunteers have failed. Whether the invading bacilli enter nerve twigs in the dermis near the point of entry in the skin (Khanolkar, 1952, 1955), or whether they enter the body by some other route and are carried to nerves by the blood stream (Weddell *et al*, 1963), the target organ is the Schwann cell. Once bacilli have been engulfed by Schwann cells their subsequent fate, and the type of disease which ensues, is decided by the resistance of the infected individual.

Tuberculoid leprosy (TT)

If the infected person has good resistance, the Schwann cells which engulf and destroy intraneural bacilli become fixed epithelioid cells, and these, by grouping together, become giant cells. In patients with a high degree of immunity the infection may not proceed further and pure neural tuberculoid leprosy results, but if resistance is inadequate to anchor the infection within nerves, one or two skin lesions develop. Histological examination of a skin lesion or of a damaged nerve reveals a tuberculoid granuloma. In the skin the cellular reaction tends to collect in foci surrounding neurovascular elements and to extend up to the epidermis without leaving the papillary zone clear (i.e. the zone immediately beneath the epidermis). Caseation is absent. Acid-fast bacilli are not seen, and cutaneous nerves within the granulomatous foci are unrecognisable because of the intense cellular reaction within and around them.

Lepromatous leprosy (LL)

If the infected person has a poor resistance the intraneural bacilli which are engulfed by Schwann cells become macrophages (Weddell *et al*, 1963) which carry their bacterial load throughout the peripheral nervous system eventually to rupture and liberate large numbers of bacilli. The whole process is then repeated. Intraneural bacilli may reach the posterior root ganglia and sympathetic ganglia but do not invade the spinal cord or brain. There is no structural damage to nerves at this stage and therefore pure neural lepromatous leprosy is not a clinical entity. Bacilli which enter the skin, either via the blood stream or by emerging from cutaneous nerves, are engulfed by histiocytes which fail to inhibit bacterial multiplication and, as wandering macrophages, carry their contents to other parts of the skin, or to other tissues, via tissue fluid, lymph and blood. These are known as lepra cells and, depending on the type of stain employed, appear as foamy cells or as globi in skin sections. Lepra cells eventually rupture and discharge their bacillary load, and the whole process is repeated by fresh histiocytes.

Thus there is, during the incubation period, an unimpeded build-up and distribution of bacilli throughout the body, and this process continues after the appearance of skin lesions. The factor which triggers the development of skin lesions is not known. Smears taken from skin lesions and from apparently normal skin of the same patient reveal the presence of leprosy bacilli at both sites, the only difference being the greater numbers in the actual lesions. Histological examination of skin lesions, stained by haematoxylin and eosin, shows thinning of the epidermis, flattening of rete ridges, a clear zone immediately beneath the epidermis, and in the remainder of the dermis the typical diffuse lepromatous granuloma consisting of large numbers of histiocytes and/or foamy-looking macrophages, and small numbers of lymphocytes and plasma cells. Sections stained by Fite-Faraco method show enormous numbers of acid-fast bacilli, some single, some in clumps, and others in globi of various sizes. The globi correspond with the foam cells seen in the H. and E. sections. Cutaneous nerves appear normal apart from the bacilli within them.

Examination of a skin section of a patient under treatment shows the granuloma to be breaking up into discrete foci with fibrocytes at their periphery; the bacilli are concentrated in these foci, and, as treatment continues, the proportion of granular bacilli increases and the foci become progressively smaller (Ridley and Wise, 1964). The term 'granular' implies that the bacilli are no longer solid-staining rods but are in the form of acid-fast granules. Electron microscopy has shown that these granules are dead (Rees and Valentine, 1962).

Borderline leprosy

This also goes by the name dimorphous and is the type of leprosy which is intermediate between the two polar types described above. Histological features vary according to the position in the borderline spectrum (Ridley and Jopling, 1967); those cases nearer the tuberculoid end of the spectrum (borderline tuberculoid or BT) have a similar epithelioid cell granuloma to that in tuberculoid leprosy but tending to be more diffuse. There is usually a free, although narrow, sub-epidermal zone. Lymphocytes are plentiful, giant cells are scanty or absent, cutaneous nerves are swollen and there is cellular infiltration within and around them. Acid-fast bacilli are scanty, either confined to cutaneous nerves or lying singly in the dermis as well.

Those cases nearer the lepromatous end of the borderline spectrum (borderline lepromatous or BL) have histological similarities to lepromatous leprosy but histiocytes are more numerous than macrophages (foam cells), lymphocytes are present in dense clumps, cutaneous nerves always contain bacilli as well as slight cellular infiltration, and acid-fast bacilli in the dermis are not only less numerous but are less likely to be contained within globi. Immunological instability is a feature of borderline leprosy and some cases may evolve, whether under treatment or not, into one or other of the polar types.

Indeterminate leprosy

This is an uncommon form of leprosy occurring as a transient phase which is either self-limiting or may evolve into one or other of the determinate types described above. Histological changes in the skin are slight and non-specific, and only rarely can an acid-fast bacillus be found within a cutaneous nerve.

HAEMATOLOGY

Blood changes in leprosy are confined to the lepromatous type (LL) and to some cases of the borderline lepromatous type (BL). They consist of anaemia which is normocytic and normochromic; reversal of the albumin-globulin ratio; false positive tests for syphilis; and positive tests for thyroglobulin antibodies, LE cells, antinuclear factor, rheumatoid factor, and cold precipitable protein (Bonomo *et al*, 1965; Matthews and Trautman, 1965).

SYMPTOMATOLOGY

Tuberculoid leprosy (TT)

The only tissues involved are nerves and skin. Symptoms may be purely neural with pain in the affected nerve followed by anaesthesia and/or paresis, the affected nerve being thickened on palpation (Jopling and Morgan-Hughes, 1965). Palpation for nerve thickening is simplified by the fact that peripheral nerves are thickened where they are most cool (Brand, 1959) and this coincides with where they are most superficial, e.g. the great auricular in the neck, the ulnar just above the elbow, the radial at the lateral border of the wrist, the lateral popliteal at the neck of the fibula, the superficial peroneal in front of the ankle, and the posterior tibial behind the medial malleolus. Cranial nerves which travel outside the skull may be damaged, principally the fifth and seventh. Facial nerve thickening cannot be palpated, but thickened branches of the trigeminal nerve can be felt on the forehead. Tendon reflexes are preserved.

More commonly the patient will present with dermal as well as neural symptoms and, on examination, there is usually only one skin lesion which begins as a macule and rapidly becomes a plaque which is erythematous, irrespective of the patient's skin colour, sometimes with a purple hue. It tends to be large, with a dry and rough surface, sometimes scaly, hairs are absent, sensation is impaired, and it has a raised and well-defined outer edge with a gradual slope from the raised periphery to the flattened centre. The nearest peripheral nerve is likely to be thickened, and there will be associated anaesthesia or muscle wasting depending on the type of nerve involved. Rarely a cold abscess of the nerve may develop and form a painless rubbery swelling attached to the nerve.

There are two characteristics of facial lesions which should be mentioned; firstly, anaesthesia may be difficult to demonstrate, and secondly, the lesion stops short at the hair-line and does not invade the scalp. Eye damage is secondary to corneal anaesthesia (fifth nerve) or to lagophthalmos (seventh nerve). An anaesthetic hand or foot is liable to be injured repeatedly and as abrasions or burns are neglected (because they are painless), chronic skin ulceration and bone infection may complicate them.

Lepromatous leprosy (LL)

Early manifestations are dermal, never neural, and consist of macules and papules. Macules are small, multiple, with vague edges and a shiny surface, are not anaesthetic, and are distributed bilaterally and symmetrically. They are faintly erythematous, whether on light or dark skins, but on dark skins may appear hypopigmented with a superadded erythema or copper tinge. Plaques and nodules appear as the disease advances, as well as fresh macules and papules, so that all four types of lesions may be seen in the same patient. Lesions (as in all types of leprosy) avoid the warmer parts of the skin such as the scalp, axillae, groins and perineum. Hair growth and sensation are not impaired over the lesions. Nodules on the mucosa of mouth and nasal septum sooner or later ulcerate, and in the nose cause epistaxis and nasal discharge. Leprous deposits in the eyes cause superficial punctate keratitis, iris atrophy, and recurrent attacks of iridocyclitis.

As the untreated disease advances, eyebrows and eyelashes become thinned and may disappear, chronic oedema of the legs leads to a waxy appearance and hard texture of the skin; sometimes chronic ulcers of the legs are superadded. Ichthyosis of the thighs and lower legs may develop (Schulz, 1965). The skin of the face and ears becomes thick and irregular, with deepened lines on the forehead (leonine facies). Narrowing of the glottis due to fibrosis causes stridor, and hoarse voice is caused by ulceration of the larynx or by paralysis of the vocal cords. Palpable enlargement of lymph glands is rare except during lepra reaction (q.v.). Testicular atrophy is a common late development, with consequent sterility, impotence and gynaecomastia. At this stage of the disease there is palpable thickening of peripheral nerves due to fibrosis, with associated regional anaesthesia and muscle wasting; as nerve fibrosis is bilateral, 'glove and stocking' anaesthesia is a usual sequel. Shortening of fingers and toes is due to a combination of factors, chief of which are repeated trauma (because of anaesthesia) and impaired blood supply secondary to leprous endarteritis of nutrient arterioles particularly during lepra reactions (q.v.).

Damage to motor nerves leads to wasting of intrinsic muscles of hands and feet, to foot drop or facial palsy, and X-rays of bones show characteristic changes. In the hands these consist of absorption of terminal phalanges and, less commonly, phalangeal cysts; changes in the feet consist of absorption of terminal phalanges and typical 'pencilling' of the heads of metatarsals due to concentric bone absorption at the site of maximal thrust when walking. Two radiological abnormalities in the skull have been described (Møller-Christensen, 1961), namely, atrophy of the anterior nasal spine and of the maxillary alveolar process; the former is associated with collapsed nose deformity and the latter with loss of upper central incisor teeth.

The commonest cause of death is pulmonary tuberculosis; renal failure from chronic nephritis or renal amyloidosis is a less usual cause, and rarer still is death during a lepra reaction either from severe necrotising reaction (Waters and Ridley, 1963) or from asphyxia secondary to oedema in an already narrowed glottis. These causes of death do not apply to tuberculoid or borderline leprosy, and in these the only form of tuberculosis likely to occur is glandular.

One particular variety of lepromatous leprosy requires special mention, namely, the diffuse type described by Lucio and Alvarado in Mexico in 1852 (Latapi *et al*, 1948). Until recently it was thought to be confined to Mexico, but it is now known to occur, albeit rarely, in other regions (Frenken, 1963). Patients first notice sensory impairment or paraesthesiae in hands and feet, followed by gradual loss of eyebrows, eyelashes and body hair. At the same time the skin of the whole body slowly becomes diffusely thickened, rendering it smooth and stiff as in scleroderma. There may be alopecia, nasal and laryngeal involvement, and widespread small telangiectases, but skin lesions such as nodules and plaques do not occur. The eyes have a shining appearance and escape leprous changes. Although *erythema nodosum* may occur in these patients, a more likely development is a unique form of reactional state known as Lucio's phenomenon (q.v.). Although skin biopsy is diagnostic even in the earliest stages, it is usual for skin changes to be well advanced by the time the diagnosis is suspected, and it may even require the development of Lucio's phenomenon to arouse the first suspicion of the underlying disease (Donner and Shively, 1967).

Borderline leprosy

As in tuberculoid leprosy, nerves and skin are the only tissues directly involved, and evidence of nerve damage often precedes the appearance of skin lesions, maybe for years (Jopling, 1956). Skin lesions vary in number and size, in definition of edges, in surface and sensory changes, according to the patient's position in the spectrum between tuberculoid and lepromatous, and their distribution is asymmetrical except in some BL cases. Macules are erythematous or hypopigmented, but plaques are always erythematous, sometimes with a purple or brown hue. Annular lesions are common and sometimes the band of raised tissue, instead of forming a ring, takes a bizarre shape. In some cases an oval area of hypopigmented skin is in the centre of a plaque which has a vague outer edge but a clear-cut inner edge giving a 'punched-out' appearance. In contrast, annular lesions are not a feature of tuberculoid leprosy, and tuberculoid plaques have well-defined *outer* borders with a gradual flattening towards the centre.

Nodules may occur in borderline leprosy but differ from lepromatous nodules in being less numerous and distributed asymmetrically. Cases in which borderline leprosy has evolved to lepromatous leprosy are distinguished by two findings; firstly, some older-standing borderline lesions will be present in addition to the newer lepromatous lesions, and, secondly, thickened nerves will be palpable from the very beginning.

Indeterminate leprosy

This is purely macular and can be very difficult to diagnose as the hypopigmented macules have no distinctive clinical features. Diagnosis is assisted by the family history, by absence of fungus in skin scrapings and by the histamine test (q.v.). Only rarely can any sensory impairment be demonstrated or any thickened nerve be palpated.

Reactional states.

The doctor treating leprosy must be on the lookout for reactional states for they occur all too commonly and can result in crippling deformity. From the clinician's viewpoint there are two distinct types of reaction. One type can occur early in the course of treatment of any of the three determinate types of leprosy, particularly borderline, and is manifested by a rapid swelling and erythema of skin lesions, painful swelling of peripheral nerves, and by oedema of feet, hands and face. Fever, if any, is slight and constitutional disturbance unusual. This is known as 'exacerbation reaction'.

The other type of reaction is confined to lepromatous leprosy and occurs late in the course of the disease when clinical improvement is well marked and the majority of acid-fast bacilli are granular. It is known as 'lepra reaction' and is characterised by one or more of a number of manifestations, the best known of which is *erythema nodosum leprosum* (ENL). Erythema nodosum in leprosy differs from that in other conditions by its evanescent nature and its distribution; the erythematous nodes and patches fade after 2–3 days and leave a blue stain in the skin. They may appear anywhere apart from those sites listed on page 303 as devoid of leprosy lesions, but are most commonly seen on arms and thighs. The leprosy lesions appear unchanged clinically.

When erythema nodosum leprosum lesions are few there may be no systemic disturbance, but if they are multiple there is likely to be fever, malaise and some of the following: nerve pain and swelling; tender swelling of lymph glands; swollen joints; acute iridocyclitis; pains in the bones of limbs, especially tibiae; oedema of feet, hands and face; acute epididymo-orchitis; insomnia; and mental depression. Any of the above may occur singly, or in combination, even in the absence of erythema nodosum leprosum.

The usual precipitating factor of a reactional state is effective treatment, especially with sulphone, but other factors include intercurrent infection, physical or mental stress, and iodides. Sulphonamides are potent factors and this is probably due to their antileprotic action. Blood examination during exacerbation reaction reveals little change, but during lepra reaction there is anaemia (normocytic and normochromic), a polymorphonuclear leucocytosis, increased globulin—particularly gamma globulin—and a raised erythrocyte sedimentation rate.

DIAGNOSIS

From the foregoing it will be readily appreciated that the clinician will not fail to make a diagnosis of leprosy if the possibility of this diagnosis is considered whenever he is confronted by a patient with an unusual skin disorder. The clinician in the tropics must not fail to think of leprosy because the patient has a white skin, and the clinician in Europe should not fail to ask patients the question: 'Where have you lived or travelled abroad?' A combination of skin lesions and nerve thickening is pathognomonic of leprosy, and systematic palpation of peripheral nerves is therefore essential. Again, a skin lesion which is anaesthetic is diagnostic. A skin lesion which is not anaesthetic will usually contain acid-fast bacilli, therefore a skin smear may be diagnostic.

Aids in diagnosis

Skin smear. The lesion is cleaned with ether and a fold is gripped firmly between thumb and forefinger of the left hand to render it avascular. With a small-bladed scalpel (size 15 Bard Parker blade) an incision is made 5 mm long and 3 mm deep; the blade is then turned at right angles to the cut and, without relaxing finger pressure, the wound is scraped several times in one direction. Fluid and pulp from the dermis collects on one side of the blade and is gently smeared on to a glass slide. The smear is then fixed by heat over a flame and stained by the Ziehl-Neelsen method. As *M. leprae* is less acid and alcohol-fast than *M. tuberculosis*, care must be taken to stop decolourising when the smear has a faint pink tinge and not to continue until all colour has been removed.

Skin biopsy. The important point is to carry the incision down to subcutaneous fat so that the whole depth of the dermis is included. The fixative devised by Ridley is recommended and consists of 10 ml 40 per cent formaldehyde; 2 g mercuric chloride; 3 ml glacial acetic acid; and tap water to 100 ml. After leaving the tissue in 3.5 ml of this fixative for 3 hours, it is transferred to 10 ml of 70 per cent alcohol in which it can remain indefinitely.

Nerve biopsy. This is essential to establish the diagnosis of pure neural leprosy, and a thickened nerve which is purely sensory can safely be biopsied, e.g. the great auricular in the neck, the radial at the wrist, or the superficial peroneal in front of the ankle.

Histamine test (Rodriguez and Plantilla, 1933). This test conveniently demonstrates damage to sympathetic nerves in the skin. A drop of 1 in 1000 histamine diphosphate is placed on the hypopigmented macule and another drop on a control area in the same region; a superficial pinprick is then made through each drop. A bright flare develops within 1–2 minutes if sympathetic nerves are intact, but is delayed, faint or absent, in a macule due to leprosy. This test can also be of value in a patient complaining of regional anaesthesia, for there will be depression of flare in peripheral neuritis from any cause (including leprosy). Thus anaesthesia such as that of hysteria or syringomyelia, and that due to psychological disturbances or to brain or cord dysfunction, can be differentiated.

Lepromin test. This is a non-specific test of value in classifying a case of leprosy; it is not a diagnostic test as the majority of adults who have never come in contact with leprosy give a positive reaction, the reason being unexplained (Shepard and Saitz, 1967). Once a diagnosis of leprosy has been made, however, the test gives valuable information as to classification and prognosis. It is strongly positive in the tuberculoid type, negative in the lepromatous, and ranges from moderately positive to negative in the border-line type, the reaction varying according to the position of the patient in the spectrum between BT and BL. The test is unpredictable in indeterminate leprosy. The early (Fernandez) reaction is similar to a tuberculin reaction and is read at 48 hours. The late (Mitsuda) reaction is read at 3–5 weeks: an erythematous-purple papule 3–5 mm in diameter is assessed as one-plus (+), one which is more than 5 mm as two-plus (+ +), and a papule of any size which ulcerates is three-plus (+ + +). The antigen for the test has not been standardised; it is therefore important to know if the lepromin is of the Fernandez-type or Mitsuda-type.

DIFFERENTIAL DIAGNOSIS

Pure neural leprosy

Regional anaesthesia with or without muscle wasting but with palpable nerve thickening.
1. *Primary amyloidosis* involving peripheral nerves begins insidiously in the second or third decades and usually affects the lower limbs with impairment of sensibility, foot drop, and amyotrophy; late effects are loss of tendon reflexes, trophic ulceration of the feet, and shortening of digits (Andrade, 1952). Evidence of amyloidosis can be found in other organs, especially kidneys.
2. *Familial progressive hypertrophic interstitial neuritis* commences in childhood and slowly progresses to produce flaccid muscular atrophy of the limbs commencing distally, with claw hand, dropped foot, loss of sensation and loss of tendon reflexes (Déjerine and Sottas, 1893).

Regional anaesthesia with or without muscle wasting but without palpable nerve thickening. The various forms of peripheral neuropathy need to be considered, but absence of nerve thickening in them and preservation of tendon reflexes in leprosy helps to exclude them. Difficulty may be experienced in cases of meralgia paraesthetica (Bernhardt's disease) due to compression or irritation of the lateral cutaneous nerve of the thigh at the inguinal ligament; this condition most often occurs in obese persons and during pregnancy (Annotation, 1961). The patient complains of paraesthesia and sensory loss over the antero-lateral aspect of the thigh, and, as in all other forms of peripheral neuropathy, including leprosy, the histamine flare (q.v.) is depressed. Compression palsy is another condition likely to cause difficulty; diabetes may predispose to it, and a familial tendency is well documented (Annotation, 1965). The histamine test is normal in cases

of regional anaesthesia due to changes in brain or spinal cord, thus the test can be helpful in differentiating syringomyelia from neural leprosy. In addition, sensory loss in syringomyelia is peculiar in that tactile sensation is retained while thermal and pain sensation is lost. The histamine test is also useful in excluding hysteria as a normal flare is obtained.

Dermal leprosy

Hypopigmented macules. Macules in leprosy tend to be oval in shape, are hypopigmented but never depigmented, the histamine flare is depressed, and there may or may not be anaesthesia of the macule and a thickened nerve in the vicinity.
1. In *vitiligo* (leucoderma) there is depigmentation (achromia) rather than hypopigmentation and hairs growing in the macule may be achromic. Lesions are multiple and of varying sizes and shapes, and the histamine test is normal.
2. In localised *scleroderma* (morphoea) there is a white macule which may be slightly raised in parts, the edge is often purple, hair growth and sweating are lost in the lesion, and when sclerosis is marked there is some degree of sensory loss.
3. Lesions of *pityriasis alba* occur in young Negroes and although their oval shape is suggestive of leprosy, the confinement of the macules to the face, together with their scaliness and positive histamine flare, help to differentiate them.
4. *Pityriasis rotunda* occurs on trunk or limbs, the macules being circular and scaly. Histamine flare is normal, and histology shows the changes of ichthyosis (Findlay, 1965).
5. *Pityriasis versicolor* in dark skins (tinea flava) can be differentiated by the scaliness of the lesions and the presence of *Malassezia furfur* in skin scrapings.
6. In *post-kala azar dermal leishmaniasis* hypopigmented macules appear on the trunk and limbs, rarely on the face. In addition there may be erythematous or orange-coloured papules and nodules on the face, less commonly on other parts of the skin, and there may be facial erythema with a 'butterfly' distribution over the nose and cheeks.
7. Depigmentation in *yaws* is mainly confined to hairless areas of the upper limbs and tends to be bilaterally symmetrical (Browne, 1962). It occurs chiefly in adults over the age of 30. Hyperkeratosis of palms and soles may be present, less commonly other signs such as juxta-articular nodes, gangosa, or sabre tibiae. Serological tests are positive as for syphilis.
8. Depigmentation in *onchocerciasis* is confined to the pretibial regions of both legs.

Pigmented lesions. Such lesions in leprosy can be diagnosed by two simple tests—pin-prick and smear. Either there is blunting of pin-prick or a smear is positive for acid-fast bacilli, and sometimes both tests are positive. Neither is positive in the conditions described below.

1. *Granuloma annulare.* Lesions consist of papules arranged in rings which are usually present on the extremities but occasionally occur elsewhere. They run a chronic course, disappear spontaneously, and may or may not reappear. Children and young adults are chiefly affected, and histology is characteristic.

2. *Granuloma multiforme* (Leiker *et al*, 1964). This is a chronic condition usually affecting those over 40. Lesions may be papulo-nodules, plaques, or circinate in appearance with slight hypopigmentation. They irritate, and sometimes new ones appear while old ones are subsiding. Histologically there is a tuberculoid infiltrate not arranged round neurovascular elements, and cutaneous nerves are undamaged.

3. *Sarcoidosis* (James and Jopling, 1961). Every kind of leprotic lesion can be mimicked by sarcoidosis, most commonly the plaque. Similarity will be heightened if there is evidence of peripheral neuritis (*Brit. med. J.*, 1965). but nerves are not thickened. The Kveim test is positive in sarcoidosis and negative in leprosy, and the tuberculin test is usually negative in sarcoidosis. The histology may be indistinguishable from tuberculoid leprosy apart from the fact that cutaneous nerves appear normal.

4. *Lupus vulgaris.* This commences as a papule which coalesces with neighbouring papules to form a plaque, yellowish-red in colour and irregular in shape. It chiefly affects those under 20, and the face is commonly involved; develops slowly and has a chronic course. The lesion becomes white when a glass slide is pressed on it, and the papules appear as brown apple-jelly spots. The tuberculin test is positive. Histological differentiation from tuberculoid leprosy is by the presence of caseation and by the normal appearance of cutaneous nerves.

5. *Lupus erythematosus.* The chronic localised or discoid form usually affects women in the age group 30–50 years. The round or oval plaques have a scaly surface and a predilection for the face, ears and scalp. A characteristic lesion is the 'butterfly' erythema of the face. Whitish patches with red margins may appear on the buccal mucosa, and lesions on the lips look like dried collodion. The histology is diagnostic.

6. *Cutaneous leishmaniasis.* Early nodular lesions, before becoming crusted, may simulate lepromatous leprosy, but should not cause confusion as they are too few in number, their distribution is asymmetrical, and there are no macules. Leishmaniae can be demonstrated in fluid which is extracted from them with a capillary pipette. The type of cutaneous leishmaniasis most likely to be confused with lepromatous leprosy is the disseminated anergic form (Convit and Kerdel-Vegas, 1965) which was previously thought to be peculiar to the New World but has recently been described in Ethiopia. Nodular lesions are numerous and closely simulate the nodules of lepromatous leprosy, but are teeming with L-D bodies and not with acid-fast bacilli.

7. *Atypical necrobiosis of the face* (Dowling and Wilson Jones, 1967). This occurs in adult females who are not diabetic. The annular lesions resemble lesions of borderline leprosy, but the scalp is commonly involved (compare leprosy) and histology is diagnostic.

8. *Tinea corporis* (tinea circinata). Ringworm infection of annular and plaque type may superficially resemble borderline or tuberculoid leprosy, but skin scales contain the causative fungus.

9. *Psoriasis.* The lesions may simulate scaly plaques of tuberculoid leprosy but tend to be too numerous and to involve regions such as the scalp and flexures which are spared in leprosy. The silvery scales are characteristic, and if they are scraped away a moist red surface is revealed through which dilated capillaries appear as red points which may bleed. Fingernails may be involved. Skin biopsy confirms the diagnosis.

10. *Kaposi's sarcoma.* Presentation is with nodules and oedema usually affecting the feet and lower legs. The legs feel firm or hard on palpation, as in lepromatous leprosy, and 50 per cent of the nodules ulcerate. Histology is diagnostic.

11. *Ichthyosis vulgaris.* An ichthyotic condition of the skin of arms and/or legs may develop in lepromatous leprosy, and the brown scales closely resemble those of the sex-linked type of ichthyosis vulgaris, but trunk, face and scalp are spared (Schulz, 1965).

Other conditions. 1. *Chronic ulceration* of the lower legs may occur in neglected lepromatous leprosy and may simulate conditions such as yaws, gummatous ulceration, tropical ulcer and sicklaemia, but anaesthesia below the knees will be present together with other signs of leprosy.

2. *Follicular mucinosis* (alopecia mucinosa). Skin-coloured plaques with scaling and hair loss, particularly affecting eyebrows, may be mistaken for leprosy (Fan *et al*, 1967), but histology is diagnostic.

Chemotherapy

Sulphones. In spite of the improved prospect of finding new antileprosy drugs opened up by Shepard's (1960) discovery that he could cultivate *M. leprae* in the footpads of mice, sulphones still hold pride of place in the treatment of leprosy. The sulphone in most common use is dapsone (DDS; 4,4-diaminodiphenyl sulphone) which is usually given orally. Until recently the usual adult dose was 600–700 mg/week, but such doses are now considered unnecessarily large. Until controlled trials have been carried out it will be impossible to say what is the optimum dose, but it is likely that a dosage of 100–200 mg/week will be found adequate. This can be given as 100 mg twice a week or as 25 mg daily. DDS for parenteral use is usually suspended in an oily medium, but at University College Hospital, London, DDS is dissolved in alcohol and propylene glycol. It is given by intramuscular injection, and the formula is:

Dapsone	5 g (100 mg in 2 ml)
Alcohol 95 per cent	40 ml
Benzyl alcohol	5 ml
Propylene glycol	to 100 ml

It is advisable to give small commencing doses, in the region of 5 mg twice a week, in order to reduce the likelihood of precipitating a reactional state (q.v.), and this is particularly important in borderline leprosy. It is to be hoped that pharmaceutical firms will produce a 5 mg tablet of dapsone as at present the usually available strengths are 50 mg and 100 mg. Already a step in the right direction has been taken by Arthur H. Cox and Co. Ltd of Brighton, England, in manufacturing small-dose tablets.

Side effects of DDS are rarely encountered with doses of 700 mg/week or less; they include haemolytic anaemia, methaemoglobinaemia, hepatitis, and various types of dermatitis and fixed drug eruption. One case of agranulocytosis has been described (McKenna and Chalmers, 1958), and one case of chronic nephritis in a patient treating himself with enormous doses of DDS on the mistaken assumption that he had leprosy (Browne, 1965). Psychosis is usually listed as a toxic effect but it is doubtful whether this should be accepted. Bacterial resistance to sulphone is rare and is confined to those who have been treated for many years in an irregular fashion. So far there have been no reports of infections with sulphone-resistant strains of leprosy bacilli.

Length of treatment depends on the type of leprosy. Tuberculoid and indeterminate patients require treatment for 5 years, or until all signs of activity have ceased, whichever is longer; borderline patients are treated for 5–15 years depending on their position in the borderline spectrum; lepromatous patients should be treated for life. 4,4-diacetyldiaminodiphenyl sulphone (DADDS) is under investigation; it is a repository preparation which is injected intramuscularly once every 75 days.

Thiourea compounds. Thiambutosine (Ciba 1906; SU 1906; DPT) is a disubstituted thiourea which is a useful alternative to DDS; it is virtually free from side effects, and its only disadvantage is that bacterial resistance is likely to develop after about 2 years. One tablet of 500 mg is given daily at first, slowly increasing to a maximum of four tablets daily. Maximal absorption occurs after a single dose of three tablets (1.5 g), therefore any daily dose larger than this must be divided. Recently a parenteral compound has been marketed and is administered by intramuscular injection once a week.

Thiacetazone (TBI; Conteben: Tibione; Amithiazone), a monosubstituted thiourea, is another alternative to DDS but has largely been displaced by the non-toxic thiambutosine. It is administered orally in a commencing dose of 25 mg/day, slowly increasing to a maximum of 150 mg/day, but bacterial resistance is likely to develop after 2 years. The commonest side effects are nausea and anorexia, but others are rare; they include headache, vertigo, proteinuria, skin rash, anaemia, agranulocytosis and hepatitis.

Long-acting sulphonamides. There is a growing literature on the use of these compounds in leprosy but they have not been proved more effective than DDS or less likely to precipitate reactional states.

Riminophenazine derivatives. Clofazimine (Lamprene; B663) is an aposafranine dye which has been undergoing trials in leprosy since the first report of successful treatment (Browne and Hogerzeil, 1962). It is a compound of very great interest to leprologists, for not only does it appear to have an initial activity against *M. leprae* equal to that of DDS but has an anti-inflammatory effect which reduces the incidence and severity of lepra reaction. Optimum dosage is one capsule of 100 mg twice a week but larger doses must be given to control lepra reaction. Side effects are few and include diarrhoea, skin irritation, red coloured urine and a red coloration of the skin which is most marked in the actual lesions. Later the lesions become slate grey in colour before becoming black. Pigmentation slowly disappears after stopping the dye.

Rifamycin. This antibiotic is proving very effective in a dosage of 600 mg daily for adults.

Other treatment

Burns and other injuries to anaesthetic hands require splinting until healed, otherwise the patient will continue to use the injured limb as pain is absent. Trophic ulceration of the anaesthetic foot usually responds to bed rest or to a below-knee walking-plaster maintained for about 4 weeks. After this it is necessary to supply specially made footwear to avoid pressure on the healed area; this problem has been well covered by Brand (1966). The use of insoles of Plastazote (expanded polyethylene) is a development of great effectiveness (Tuck, 1967).

Reconstructive surgery is required for clawing of the fingers, paralysis of the thumb, foot drop, and hammer toe, and plastic surgery can correct facial disfigurement caused by loss of eyebrows, facial palsy, saddle nose, ectropion, pendulous earlobes, and excessive folds of skin. Paralysed muscles must be supported by suitable forms of splinting, and this is combined with physiotherapy.

Dry skin can be relieved by daily soaking in water followed by the application of soft paraffin (Harris and Browne, 1966); daily washing of feet will prevent the formation of callosities over pressure points if combined with the use of pumice stone. The patient must learn to inspect his anaesthetic hands and feet daily for injuries so that he can have prompt treatment; the wearing of gloves at work or when cooking will help to prevent injuries, and the use of a cigarette holder will reduce the chances of burns to fingers. Nasal symptoms will be relieved if the nares are kept well greased with an ointment such as Ung. Hydrarg. Nit. Dil. (B.P.).

Treatment of reactional states

This is the most difficult aspect of treatment. A mild reactional state may respond to a reduction in dosage of antileprotic drug, but treatment should be temporarily suspended if the reaction is severe. Intramuscular injections of a trivalent antimonial such as Stibophen Injection (B.P,, U.S.P.) are often helpful and are given in a dosage of 2–3 ml of the solution containing 63 mg/ml daily or every other day for up to six injections. Corticosteroids are effective but should be reserved for acute epididymo-orchitis, acute iridocyclitis not responding to local treatment, and for threat-ened muscle paralysis. An initial dose of 30 mg prednisone daily is recommended and dosage can be reduced to the lowest which will relieve symptoms. Treatment with steroids should be given for the shortest possible time. The antileprotic drug can be given again when the reaction has been controlled, but very small doses should be used and these can be slowly increased. Some patients may require a prolonged course of steroid therapy, and in these cases antileprotic treatment should be given concurrently and the smallest effective dosage of steroid used. If available, clofazimine should be tried in these cases in place of standard antileprotic drugs.

Relief of nerve pain can be obtained by an intraneural injection consisting of 1500 units of hyaluronidase (Hyalase) dissolved in 1 ml of 1 per cent lignocaine solution and mixed with 1 ml of hydrocortisone suspension (25 mg/ml). A nerve abscess calls for surgical evacuation. Prompt local hourly instillation during the day of steroid eyedrops will usually relieve acute iridocyclitis; a steroid eye ointment can be used at night. Homatropine drops are required to keep the pupil dilated. Iridectomy must be considered if iridocyclitis is recurrent or chronic. Epistaxis, a common event in lepra reaction, is controlled by inserting into the nostril an absorbable gelatin sponge—Sterispon (Allen and Hanbury Ltd); size no. 3 is suitable. New prospects in the management of lepra reaction are being opened up by research into the nature of the reaction (Bonomo *et al*, 1965) and by the advances which are taking place in the development of new immunosuppressive drugs.

PROPHYLAXIS

Case finding and early treatment are very important in limiting the spread of leprosy. In addition, child contacts can be given BCG vaccination (Brown *et al*, 1968) and, in selected cases where medical supervision is possible, contacts can be given DDS for at least 2 years. Married women suffering from leprosy should be advised to avoid pregnancy until the disease is arrested. In the event of a baby being born to a mother suffering from 'open' leprosy, the infant should, if possible, be taken away immediately after birth and may be returned when treatment has rendered the mother non-infectious. The importance of improvement in living conditions, especially in housing, must not be overlooked in any campaign to eradicate leprosy.

REFERENCES

ANDRADE, C. (1952) *Brain*, **75**, 408.
ANNOTATION (1961) *Lancet*, **2**, 1133.
—— (1965) *Lancet*, **1**, 310.
BONOMO, L., TURSI, A., TRIMIGLIOZZI, G. and DOMMACCO, F. (1965) *Brit. med. J.*, **2**, 689.
BRAND, P. W. (1959) *Int. J. Lepr.*, **27**, 1.
—— (1966) *Insensitive Feet*. London: The Leprosy Mission.
Brit. med. J. (1965) **2**, 316.
BROWN, J. A. KINNEAR, STONE, M. M. and SUTHERLAND, I. (1968) *Brit. med. J.*, **1**, 24.
BROWNE, S. G. (1962) *Derm. trop.*, **1**, 148.
—— (1965) *Lepr. Rev.*, **36**, 55.
BROWNE, S. G. and HOGERZEIL, L. M. (1962) *Lepr. Rev.*, **33**, 6.
CONVIT, J. and KERDEL-VEGAS, F. (1965) *Arch. Derm.*, **91**, 439.
DÉJERINE, J. and SOTTAS, J. (1893) *C. R. Soc. Biol. (Paris)*, **45** (9me sér., **5**, pt. 2), 63.
DONNER, R. S. and SHIVELY, J. A. (1967) *Ann. intern. Med.*, **67**, 831.
DOWLING, G. B. and WILSON JONES, E. (1967) *Dermatologica*, **135**, 11.
FAN, J., CHANG, H-S. and MA, B. (1967) *Arch. Derm.*, **95**, 354.
FINDLAY, G. F. (1965) *Brit. J. Derm.*, **77**, 63.
FRENKEN, J. H. (1963) *Diffuse Leprosy of Lucio and Latapi*. Detroit, Michigan, U.S.A: Blaine Ethridge Books.
HARRIS, J. R. and BROWNE, S. G. (1966) *Lancet*, **1**, 1011.
JAMES, D. G. and JOPLING, W. H. (1961) *J. trop. Med. Hyg.*, **64**, 42.
JOPLING, W. H. (1965) *Trans. roy. Soc. trop. Med. Hyg.*, **50**, 478.
JOPLING, W. H. and MORGAN-HUGHES, J. A. (1965) *Brit. med. J.*, **2**, 799.
KHANOLKAR, V. R. (1952) *Lepr. India*, **24**, 62.
—— (1955) *Indian J. med. Sci.*, **9**, Suppl. 1.
LATAPI, F. and ZAMORA, A. C. (1948) *Int. J. Lepr.*, **16**, 421.
LEIKER, D. L., KOK, S. H. and SPAAS, J. A. J. (1964) *Int. J. Lepr.*, **32**, 368.
MATTHEWS, L. J. and TRAUTMAN, J. R. (1965) *Lancet*, **2**, 915.
McKENNA, W. B. and CHALMERS, A. C. (1958) *Brit. med. J.*, **1**, 324.
MØLLER-CHRISTENSEN, V. (1961) *Bone Changes in Leprosy*. Bristol: John Wright.
REES, R. J. W. and VALENTINE, R. C. (1962) *Int. J. Lepr.*, **30**, 1.
REES, R. J. W., WATERS, M. F. R., WEDDELL, A. G. M. and PALMER, E. (1967) *Nature (Lond.)*, **215**, 599.
RIDLEY, D. S. and JOPLING, W. H. (1966) *Int. J. Lepr.*, **34**, 255.
RIDLEY, D. S. and WISE, M. J. (1964) *Int. J. Lepr.*, **32**, 24.
RODRIGUEZ, J. N. and PLANTILLA, F. C. (1933) *Int. J. Lepr.*, **1**, 49.
SCHULZ, E. J. (1965) *Brit. J. Derm.*, **77**, 151.
SHEPARD, C. C. (1960) *J. exp. Med.*, **112**, 445.
SHEPARD, C. C. and SAITZ, E. W. (1967) *J. Immunol.*, **99**, 637.
TUCK, W. H. (1967) *Physiotherapy*, **53**, 368.
WATERS, M. F. R. and RIDLEY, D. S. (1963) *Int. J. Lepr.*, **31**, 418.
WEDDELL, A. G. M., PALMER, E., REES, R. J. W. and JAMISON, D. G. (1963) *The Pathogenesis of Leprosy*. Ciba Foundation Study Group No. 15. London: J. & A. Churchill.

Virus Diseases

Yaws

Leptospirosis

Fungal Diseases

Venereal Diseases

22
Virus Diseases

Probably all the virus infections of the temperate zones are common in the tropics but owing to the relatively undeveloped state of virus diagnostic services in the latter our detailed knowledge of their significance in the causation of disease—particularly mild disease—is very scanty. This chapter will therefore deal mainly with the virus infections peculiar to the tropics and subtropics (mainly arthropod-borne viruses) and mention briefly any peculiarities known about the behaviour of other virus infections in a tropical environment. These peculiarities are mainly epidemiological rather than clinical except where factors like malnutrition play a part. The virus infections which are of special importance in the tropics are mainly zoonoses: infections maintained in species other than man and of which man is only an incidental host. Most of these infections fall into the so-called arbovirus group (*arthropod-borne viruses*), which includes more than 200 (perhaps 250) viruses—a number which has been increasing regularly by about 20 per year over the last decade or so. As we shall see, by no means all of these are arthropod-borne but all, or nearly all, are zoonoses and this very heterogeneous but convenient grouping of viruses can perhaps best be described as the virus zoonoses, although certain other defining characteristics such as sensitivity to ether and bile salts are recognised, and certain virus zoonoses such as rabies, lymphocytic choriomeningitis and encephalomyocarditis virus are otherwise classified. Rabies will receive special attention because it is a much more prevalent problem in underdeveloped than developed areas.

ARBOVIRUSES

A recent W.H.O. Study Group (W.H.O., 1967) defined these viruses as follows:

'Arboviruses are viruses which are maintained in nature principally, or to an important extent, through biological transmission between susceptible vertebrate hosts by haematophagous arthropods; they multiply and produce viraemia in the vertebrates, multiply in the tissues of arthropods, and are passed on to new vertebrates by the bites of arthropods after a period of extrinsic incubation.'

One dissenter, however, proposed the following alternative:

'Arboviruses are zoonotic viral agents which, when circulating in natural foci of infection, are transmitted in a more or less regular manner by arthropods, but in certain cases may be transmitted in other ways than by arthropods.'

Arbovirus is clearly a heterogenous and ill-defined classification of convenience which will be subdivided and subclassified as our knowledge of the physical, chemical and biological properties of the constituent viruses accumulates. At present they are divided into antigenic groups and Tables 3–10 show those viruses so far known to cause human disease together with an indication of their probable mode of transmission to man. These tables are derived largely from information in the *Catalogue of Arthropod-borne Viruses of the World* (1968) which is based on the information available in February 1967. The W.H.O. Study Group report (W.H.O., 1967) differs from this in minor respects but these differences are of no clinical significance.

Epidemiology

As zoonoses, these viruses are, in general, maintained in nature by hosts other than man, and with certain exceptions are not normally or frequently transmitted from man to man. Disease in man is often the only overt indication of the presence of these viruses because the viruses and their maintenance hosts have normally evolved to a state of symbiosis in which no disease is caused in the hosts. From the point of view of the virus, disease in its host is no advantage unless it contributes to its onward transmission: for example, a respiratory infection may require coughs and sneezes to project it towards its next host, or rabies virus requires biting for its transmission. However, most zoonosis viruses are transmitted either by blood-sucking arthropods (in which case viraemia is the only important feature for the virus) or in secretions or excretions of vertebrates

313

(where the level of virus in the appropriate excretion is the important feature). Understanding of the virus zoonoses can be made clearer by distinguishing the types of host:

1. *Maintenance hosts* are vertebrates or arthropods which are responsible for the long-term maintenance of the infection in nature (for example, monkeys and the mosquito *Aedes africanus* in yellow fever).

2. *Amplifier or link hosts* are not always easily distinguished but represent very useful concepts. Amplifiers are vertebrate hosts which amplify the amount of infection in close juxtaposition to man and thus greatly increase the risk of infection to him; for example, Japanese encephalitis in Japan is fundamentally maintained through the summer months by birds and mosquitoes, but pigs (amplifier hosts) become infected, circulate virus, and infect large numbers of mosquitoes close to man, thus increasing the risk. Link hosts carry the infection from the maintenance complex of hosts into a complex which involves man. Thus in parts of Uganda *Ae. simpsoni* (a link host) can carry yellow fever virus from the forest canopy (monkeys and *Ae. africanus*) to the man-*Ae. aegypti* complex of the villages by biting both monkeys and man in the banana plantations in which it breeds.

3. *Incidental hosts* are vertebrates or arthropods which become infected but do not contribute to a significant degree to the continued existence of the virus. Man is an incidental host of most of the virus zoonoses although he has become a major maintenance host of a few infections (notably yellow fever and dengue) at least at times of epidemic. This is an important warning that he may well be capable of becoming a maintenance host of many other arboviruses (with consequent epidemic disease), particularly if he continues to interfere irresponsibly with the environment in which virus zoonoses dwell (see below). Although incidental hosts do not contribute directly to virus maintenance they are of considerable importance in at least two ways. Firstly they provide opportunities for evolution of the virus itself in a variety of ways and for the development of new complexes of maintenance hosts, particularly if exposed to severe pressure by human interference with the hosts or their environment. Secondly in an arthropod-borne zoonosis, an incidental host may be of critical importance in maintaining the arthropod maintenance (or link) hosts. Thus in Kyasanur Forest disease (q.v.) cattle do not contribute to maintenance of the virus but are very important hosts of the adult stage of the principal maintenance tick host (*Haemophysalis*

spinigera) since the disease became epidemic. It was probably increased human population pressure in the Kyasanur Forest area which led (during the 10 years or so before the disease appeared in epidemic form) in turn to an increase in the cattle population and to an increase in cattle grazing in the forest because of the unavailability of other land for grazing. The great increase in cattle in the forest then led to a great increase in the population of *H. spinigera* in the forest. The Kyasanur Forest disease virus was probably previously present but maintained by tick and vertebrate species (perhaps small ground-living mammals) without human involvement. *H. spinigera* in its various stages bites a wide range of hosts, thus it may be that an immature tick picked up the infection from a small mammal host.

There are major epidemiological differences between Diptera-transmitted (mosquito, *Phlebotomus, Culicoides*) and tick-transmitted infections. Because Diptera feed frequently and are quite short-lived, continued maintenance of the virus depends on the availability of a sufficient number of vertebrate hosts capable of exhibiting viraemia (i.e. which have not previously been infected). Such infections therefore tend to move as a wave through a population of susceptible vertebrates and it cannot readily reverse its direction of movement because the hosts behind the wave have been largely immunised. The best known example was provided by the yellow fever epizootic (which could be traced by monkey deaths) in Central America from 1949 to 1956. The epizootic started south of the Panama Canal, crossed it in 1949 then spread through the belt of forest on the Atlantic side of the mountains and continued, with one or two forays from the main line, until it reached southern Mexico in 1956 and eventually petered out because it had reached the limit of distribution of its maintenance hosts.

Ticks, on the other hand, feed relatively infrequently and live for longer periods. Furthermore, they often depend on animals such as rodents which have marked territorial behaviour. The tick-borne infections therefore characteristically exist for very long periods in fixed foci. For example, Smith (1956a) isolated the Langat virus in a small area of forest near Kuala Lumpur, Malaya, from the tick *Ixodes granulatus* in 1956. Since then the virus has been repeatedly isolated from the same tick species in precisely the same area—the last isolation attempt was from three ticks in 1966 and was successful.

There is a further important epidemiological difference between Diptera-borne and tick-borne virus infections in the temperate zones: ticks provide an excellent over-wintering mechanism for the infection, but as only the adult female stage of mosquitoes becomes infected, there are much greater difficulties in explaining the over-wintering of mosquito-borne viruses which nevertheless continue to exist and cause disease as far north as Finland and Saskatchewan. Although no complete explanation has yet been devised for any virus, a variety of mechanisms have been suggested: hibernating infected adult mosquitoes, hibernating vertebrates (including bats and snakes) which have been infected in late autumn and which with a very damped-down metabolism carry the infection through the winter and exhibit viraemia in the spring, annual re-introduction from tropical areas by migrating birds. Similar considerations and difficulties apply to understanding how mosquito-borne infections survive through long dry periods in tropical areas.

The factors affecting the frequency of transmission of virus infections (particularly zoonoses) are as follows:

1. The duration and degree of infectivity in the hosts, i.e. in vertebrates the duration and intensity of viraemia or virus excretion. Arthropods are infective for life after the end of the extrinsic incubation period.
2. The duration of the incubation period in the vertebrate and of the extrinsic incubation period (the time from infection to infectivity) in the arthropod.
3. The stability of the virus outside the host (viruses not transmitted by arthropods).
4. The population density of the hosts and the proportion of vertebrates susceptible to infection.
5. The frequency of contact between the hosts, i.e. their behaviour.
6. Climate, which influences the breeding and longevity of arthropod hosts and also the length of the extrinsic incubation period.
7. Vegetation which provides breeding places and also the microclimate for resting arthropods, thus influencing their longevity.

The factors which influence the risk of infection for man from the maintenance hosts of a zoonosis are:

1. Occupation, e.g. forest workers and yellow fever, veterinarians and Wesselsbron disease.
2. Leisure activities which cause man to intrude into the habitat of a zoonosis, e.g. hunting, picnicking.
3. Keeping domestic animals, e.g. pigs as amplifiers of Japanese encephalitis, dogs and rabies.
4. Standards of housing and hygiene, e.g. rodents and Bolivian haemorrhagic fever, *Ae. aegypti* and dengue.
5. Agriculture, particularly irrigation or desalinisation of surface water, e.g. virus encephalitis in southern California, West Nile fever in the Camargue.
6. Civil engineering—dams, road-building—by affecting mosquito breeding, etc.
7. Control measures, e.g. DDT poisoning of cats leading to increased rodent populations in and around houses (cf. Bolivian haemorrhagic fever).

Further details of the examples quoted will be found under the appropriate diseases. While intrusion into an area where a zoonosis constitutes an obvious risk of infection, human interference with the environment will be a much more important and larger scale factor in the future. With increasing efforts to increase food production by irrigation, desalinisation, deforestation, etc., very profound changes may occur in the frequency with which man is exposed to infection and new complexes of maintenance hosts may become involved with a greater risk of human infection and with possible changes in the virulence of the infection.

Pathogenesis

As with other virus diseases, the precise mechanisms which cause symptoms, signs or indeed death in arbovirus diseases are poorly understood. However, the broad picture can be drawn from observation of cases, from limited studies of experimental infections of man (Southam and Moore, 1951; Webb *et al*, 1966) and from a large amount of work on experimental infections of laboratory animals, especially monkeys and other larger animals (see reviews: Smith, 1968, 1970).

In general, arbovirus infections cause biphasic illnesses but in any particular infection only one phase (either the first or second) may predominate clinically. The first phase occurs during viraemia and is normally manifested clinically by a relatively undifferentiated febrile illness. In fully developed biphasic illnesses, such as Central European tick-borne encephalitis, there is then an afebrile interval followed by the second phase illness which involves the central nervous system; in dengue there is often a prodromal rash during the first phase but the characteristic rash is an expression of the second phase.

Available evidence suggests that the infective process proceeds as follows. After infection by the bite of a blood-sucking arthropod (or other route), the virus multiplies first in the regional lymph node where early antibody formation is initiated. From this primary site the virus reaches the general circulation through the lymph channels, then all parts of the body through the blood stream, infecting a variety of tissues and multiplying there—perhaps in the endothelium of capillary vessels although this is as yet by no means clear. Secondary release of virus from cells in these tissues then gives the detectable viraemia and the febrile first phase of illness. At this stage the circulating virus is probably already coated with antibody although without notably impairing its infectivity. Antibody cannot be detected at this time by classical methods because of their low sensitivity and because there is little or no free antibody which attaches, as soon as it goes into circulation, to the large amount of available virus and its antigens.

As the available antibody increases, single virus particles coated with antibody become bound together to form larger and larger aggregates which, in due course, are deposited on the walls of small vessels and engender an Arthus-type inflammatory reaction. This is the stage of onset of the second phase of illness. Although considerable cellular destruction must result from virus multiplication in cells throughout the body, the overlay of inflammatory damage with associated oedema, hypoxia, etc., is probably responsible for many of the more severe clinical manifestations of disease—especially in the central nervous system where, because of its rigid walls, oedema is of special importance. That this is so is well demonstrated by the often remarkable degree of recovery from paralytic disease in patients who survive the acute encephalitis—if the paralysis had been entirely due to viral destruction of neurones rather than inflammatory dysfunction, this recovery could not occur. Suppression of the antibody response might therefore ameliorate the clinical disease and cortisone given at the right moment appears to be beneficial although more critical studies are required.

In addition, deposition of virus-antibody complexes in vessels is probably the trigger mechanism of acute disseminated intravascular coagulation (McKay and Margaretten, 1967) in which a large number of small vessels are suddenly blocked by intravascular clotting which *inter alia* uses up platelets, leads to thrombocytopenia and haemorrhagic disease. This may be a major factor in the pathogenesis of the haemorrhagic fevers.

Laboratory diagnosis

Specific diagnosis of arbovirus infections is relatively expensive and requires well-developed virus laboratory facilities. Except for epidemiological research and for the investigation of major epidemics, facilities for routine diagnosis cannot at present be justified in underdeveloped countries, especially as the diagnosis can rarely be established before the patient is dead or better and there is no specific treatment for these infections. Only a brief account will therefore be given here of the complex laboratory procedures required: diagnosis depends either on isolation and identification of the causative virus or on the demonstration of a specific antibody response coincident with the course of the illness.

Virus isolation and identification. SPECIMENS. These are usually either blood taken during the first febrile phase or post-mortem tissue. Bone marrow has been successfully used in Venezuelan encephalitis. Cerebrospinal fluid has often been tried but seldom with success except in Kyasanur Forest disease, where there is an unusually intense vitraemia and contaminant blood is the probable source of virus in the CSF. Because much of the viraemia may be over before the patient is seen, blood for virus isolation must be taken as early as possible in the course of the illness: Table 1 shows why the success rate decreases as the disease proceeds. Isolation from the blood is very rare in

TABLE 1. *Viraemia and neutralising antibody in accidental human chikungunya infections* (Buescher, 1963)

Patient		\multicolumn{5}{c}{Day of disease}				
		1	2	3	4	5
1	Viraemia*	5.3	3.0	0.7	0	0
	Neut. index†		0	1.7		4.5
2	Viraemia	1.8	4.0	0	0	0
	Neut. index		0	2.1		4.7
3	Viraemia		2.5	0	0	0
	Neut. index		0	2.7		4.3

* Log LD50/0.03 ml blood.
† Log neutralising index.

encephalitis patients because the viraemia, which occurs during the often unrecognised first phase, is over by the time of onset of CNS symptoms. By special arrangement with the laboratory a finger-prick sample can be used but a specimen of venous blood is preferable, especially as it gives an opportunity for the collection of a first serum sample which is essential whether the diagnosis is to be established by virus isolation or serology. At least 10 ml of blood should therefore be withdrawn with sterile precautions, a small sample removed and either sent immediately to the virus laboratory or stored in a sealed container at low temperature on dry ice, in a $-65°C$ refrigerator, or in liquid nitrogen. Serum should be separated from the remainder of the blood and suitably stored until a later specimen is obtained 2–3 weeks later.

Post-mortem material should be obtained as soon as possible after death. In general, small representative pieces of as many tissues as possible should be placed in screw-cap containers and either sent immediately to the virus laboratory or stored as above. For relatively short periods of travel the virus may survive in tissue if it is sent in pH 7.4 buffered 50 per cent glycerol saline in a screw-cap container packed in ice in a thermos flask. The success rate in virus isolation from tissue depends very much on the duration of the illness. Buescher (1963), in a study of 27 fatal cases of Japanese encephalitis, isolated virus from the brains of seven of eight patients dying after 1–2 days' illness, from four of seven patients dying after 3–5 days' illness, but from only one of ten dying after more than 5 days of illness. This is mainly because of the increase of circulating antibody which neutralises the virus when the tissue is ground up.

As with many other infectious diseases, *post-mortem examinations must be made with great care wearing adequate protective clothing, gloves and preferably face-shields*, otherwise dangerous infections may be transmitted to the operators by contact, cuts on sharp bone edges, aerosols or splashing. Great care must also be taken in cleaning down the table, instruments, etc., with a suitable antiseptic (preferably 5 per cent hypochlorite) after the autopsy.

ISOLATION. The blood (usually defibrinated), or serum, or suspensions of the tissues in a buffered protein-containing saline diluent (usually with added antibiotics) are inoculated into baby mice, other laboratory animals, or into suitable cell cultures. Ninety-four per cent of the arboviruses were first isolated in baby mice (aged 1–4 days) which have been most commonly used. On primary isolation the incubation period in these animals is very variable, depending both on the dose of virus they receive and on the type of virus. Usually, however, some mice become sick or die within 14 days and often much sooner. The tissues of sick or dead mice are usually passaged in further groups of baby mice in which a shorter and more uniform incubation period is likely and antigens made from their tissues may enable a preliminary serological identification of the infecting virus to be made. Sometimes, however, several passages are required to achieve sufficient adaptation.

Cell cultures are being increasingly used but there is still no cell type so susceptible as baby mice to such very wide range of arboviruses on primary isolation. In local situations, however, a cell culture may be suitable for isolation of most of the likely viruses: for example chick embryo cell cultures are generally suitable for group A viruses, and the monkey kidney line LLC-MK2 is generally suitable for isolation of arboviruses in Bangkok. However, a range of cell cultures may have to be used and interference methods have sometimes been necessary with difficult viruses like those responsible for recent dengue epidemics in the Caribbean (Russell *et al*, 1966). In these, the presence of virus growing in a culture without evidence of cytopathic effect can be demonstrated by challenging the cultures with a virus of known cytopathic effect. If the cultures are infected, the challenge virus will fail to cause a cytopathic effect due to interference by the first virus.

IDENTIFICATION. Once a sufficient titre of virus has been attained either in an experimental animal or in a cell culture, an antigen can be prepared and tested in one or more of the serological tests (below) against antisera to known viruses. If the laboratory possesses the appropriate antisera, an identification can sometimes be achieved within 2–3 weeks of the collection of the specimen. If, however, the virus is an unfamiliar one, the identification will take much longer. In any case in certain virus groups (e.g. group B) where a number of viruses are very closely related antigenically, precise identification may be slow although a preliminary rough identification may be possible earlier. The virus isolated must also be confirmed as the cause of the disease. This can be done in two ways, the first of which is applicable particularly to post-mortem material, the second is much more rigorous:

1. Re-isolation of the same virus from the same material.
2. Testing of paired sera from the patient against the virus isolated so as to demonstrate a rise in antibody during the course of the illness.

Confirmation is essential lest the virus isolated is a contaminant from the laboratory or an adventitious infection of the patient.

Serology. Three main serological tests are used in diagnosis: the complement fixation (CF), the haemagglutinin-inhibition (HI) and the neutralisation tests. Other tests such as the agar gel precipitation (Clarke, 1964) and immunoelectrophoresis tests (Cuadrado and Casals, 1967) are used for special purposes and may come into more frequent use for rapid diagnosis. Fluorescent antibody methods are also likely to come into greater use: Emmons and Lennette (1966) found that they could make a diagnosis in Colorado tick fever within hours by testing for antigen in acute-phase blood clot. Standardisation of all these tests is important in order to achieve comparable results (Smith, 1967), but in any case paired sera from a patient should always be tested together in the same test. Whenever possible, a strain of virus locally isolated should be used in serological tests as minor antigenic differences may affect the success rate in diagnosis.

The complement fixation test can be carried out by a variety of techniques, the only special feature being the production of suitable antigens from the tissues of infected animals or cell cultures. The CF antibody response is usually later than that of HI or neutralising antibody. In a study of 84 proved cases of Japanese encephalitis, Buescher (1963) found that by 2 weeks after the onset of disease, CF antibody appeared in less than half the patients but HI antibody in over 90 per cent of them. The CF test is therefore sometimes able to demonstrate a significant increase in antibody (at least fourfold) when the initial serum sample has been taken so late as to already contain HI and neutralising antibody. The general problem of specificity is discussed below.

The haemagglutinin-inhibition test (Clarke and Casals, 1958) depends on the ability to prepare a haemagglutinin (HA) for the appropriate virus from the tissues of infected animals or from infected cell cultures. This has been successfully achieved with many but by no means all arboviruses. Some viruses have proved very difficult even with elaborate procedures (e.g. Ardoin and Clarke, 1967). The antigens are generally stable at high pH (9.0), but each virus agglutinates goose erythocytes at a specific acid pH. Sera are treated with kaolin or acetone-extracted to remove non-specific HA inhibitors, heat-inactivated (56°C) to prevent erythrocyte lysis, then goose-cell agglutinins are absorbed out. The sera are then diluted twofold in pH 9.0 buffered saline and a measured amount of HA (usually 8 units) added in a similar buffer. After incubation at pH 9.0, a goose erythrocyte suspension is added in an adjusting buffer which brings the mixture to the optimum pH for haemagglutination by the particular virus. HI tests can be carried out either by testing serum dilutions (usually twofold starting at 1 : 10) against 8 units of antigen (as above), or alternatively by testing serum (usually at 1 : 10) against a range of dilutions (usually twofold) of antigen. O'Reilly *et al* (1968) compared the two methods in sheep following infection and re-infection with louping ill virus. Both were suitable but the second procedure was more sensitive.

NEUTRALISATION TESTS. There are two parts to any neutralisation test:

1. A measured dose of virus is incubated with a measured amount of serum, or serum dilution in the presence of any necessary accessory factors. For maximum neutralisation of at least some arboviruses, a heat-labile factor present in normal serum is required. Sera are therefore usually heat-inactivated (56°C) before testing and a measured amount of normal serum added to provide the same amount of accessory factor in all the reaction mixtures.
2. After incubation, the serum-virus mixtures are tested for the presence of virus which has not been neutralised, by inoculation into susceptible animals (usually mice) or into cell cultures.

These tests can be done in one of two ways:

(*a*) Dilutions of virus, usually tenfold (or $\sqrt{10}$-fold), are incubated with standard amounts of undiluted serum. The residual log virus titre can then be calculated and compared with a control. The difference is the log *neutralising index* of the serum. A log difference between the neutralising indices of two sera of 1.7 (fiftyfold) is regarded as significant, although in well-controlled tests, differences of 1.1 or 1.2 (thirteen- or sixteenfold) may be significant.

(*b*) Dilutions (usually twofold) of serum are incubated with a standard amount of virus (usually 100 LD50 or TCD50) and scored as either neutralising or failing to neutralise this amount of virus. Differences of fourfold or greater are usually significant.

O'Reilly *et al* compared the two methods following infection and re-infection with louping ill virus in sheep. They found that procedure (*a*) was best for antibody surveys but (*b*) for diagnosis. Tests done in tissue culture tubes and judged by cytopathic effects are of about the same accuracy as those done in comparable numbers of animals although generally cheaper. However, there must be available a cell culture which gives a clear-cut cytopathic effect when infected by the relevant virus and there are therefore still some viruses which have to be tested in mice. Cell culture methods in which the remaining virus is enumerated by plaque counts are considerably more accurate and therefore enable smaller differences in antibody titres to be established as significant.

In all these tests the timing and spacing of the paired sera in relation to the course of the illness are critical for successful diagnosis. Table 2 shows

TABLE 2. *The influence of time of initial serum upon serological diagnosis of Japanese encephalitis using paired sera* (Buescher, 1963)

Day of illness of initial serum	No. of patients	% showing significant increase in indicated antibody	
		CF	HI
1–4	35	86	92
5–8	35	83	60
9–16	13	93	62
17–27	1	100	0

the relative degrees of success probable with the CF and HI test for various combinations of times of collection. The picture for neutralisation tests would be broadly similar to that for the HI test. In diseases which are seen mainly in the second phase, notably encephalitis, the CF test is often more successful in diagnosis because CF antibody increases occur later than HI or neutralising antibody increases. No reliable serological diagnosis can be made on the basis of a single serum specimen because, as will become apparent, subclinical infections with arboviruses are common. Thus only a *significant increase in antibody coincident with the course of the illness* can be a basis for serological diagnosis.

In areas where a number of antigenically related viruses coexist, the problem of diagnosis is greatly aggravated; this is particularly true of group B viruses of which several are found in most tropical areas. When a person is first infected with a group B virus, his antibody response is reasonably specific for the infecting virus although some antibody cross-reacting with other group B viruses is likely to be formed. When, however, he is later infected with a second group B virus he will probably have a very broadly cross-reacting antibody response in which it may be difficult or even impossible by normally available methods to make a precise diagnosis. Sometimes it may be possible to say only that the infecting virus was a member of group B.

Theiler and Casals (1958) attempted serological diagnosis of patients with yellow fever in Trini-

dad from which yellow fever virus had actually been isolated and the diagnosis was therefore not in doubt. In those not previously infected with a group B virus, the CF test gave a clear-cut diagnosis, and the HI (though less specific) generally gave higher titres against yellow fever than related viruses, especially in earlier convalescent sera. In those with previous group B infections, however, very broad cross-reactions were found by both tests and the only diagnosis generally possible was of a group B infection. The neutralisation test is usually most specific but it is difficult to predict the relative specificity of the CF and HI tests as this varies with the reagents used, the history of previous infections and the timing and spacing of the paired sera available for test.

Disease patterns in man

In general, arbovirus diseases are biphasic, the first phase being an undifferentiable febrile illness which often goes unrecognised. The second phase, which may follow an afebrile remission, is most characteristically encephalitic, but well-developed rashes and haemorrhagic disease are probably also features of the second phase. Recognisable clinical manifestations are absent following the majority of infections with many arboviruses although the ratio of inapparent infections to disease varies widely between viruses and probably between situations with epidemic or sporadic infections. Our knowledge of the geographical distribution of mild disease or sporadic severe disease due to arboviruses is very incomplete and mostly exists in the vicinity of the few well-equipped research laboratories which have studied them. The types of illness have been categorised (Catalogue, 1968) into:

1. Febrile illness
2. Febrile illness with a rash
3. Haemorrhagic fever
4. Encephalitis

However, only a few cases of disease due to many of the viruses have been recognised so that there is insufficient information to categorise them; and many viruses which predominantly cause one category of disease also cause one or more of the other categories in a variable proportion of cases. Thus Venezuelan encephalitis virus causes a febrile illness in the vast majority of cases and encephalitis only in a small proportion; dengue viruses cause a febrile illness with a rash in some situations but haemorrhagic fever in a considerable proportion of cases in others; Kyasanur Forest disease and Machupo viruses (both categorised as causing haemorrhagic fevers) cause encephalitis in a significant proportion of cases. This deceptively attractive subdivision of the viruses on disease category has not therefore been used here and the infections are arranged alphabetically within the serological groups of the causative viruses.

There is no specific treatment for any of these infections and supportive therapy will be mentioned only when some special feature merits attention. The methods for laboratory diagnosis are similar for all these infections and have been

epidemics in Indian cities. Infections with this virus have also been common in cities of Southeast Asia in association with the dengue haemorrhagic fever epidemics (q.v.). The first known chikungunya epidemic occurred in Tanzania in 1952–53 and involved some 40 per cent of the inhabitants of the affected area. Outbreaks have also occurred in Rhodesia and eastern Transvaal. In Africa, clinical disease has also been reported in Zambia and the Congo, and the virus has been isolated from man and mosquitoes in Uganda and South Africa. In Asia it was isolated from man in

TABLE 3. *Group A arboviruses which are known to cause human disease and occur in the tropics and subtropics*

Virus	*Probable transmission to man*	*Geographical distribution of viruses*	*Other features*
Chikungunya	Mosquito	E. and W. Africa, S. and S.E. Asia	
Eastern encephalitis	Mosquito	N. and Central America, Trinidad, Guyana, Brazil, Argentina	? present in S.E. Asia and Philippines
Mayaro	Mosquito	Trinidad, Brazil	
Mucambo	Mosquito	Brazil	
O'nyongnyong	Mosquito	E. and W. Africa, Rhodesia	Epidemics E. Africa and Rhodesia only
? Ross River	Mosquito	Australasia	Possibly a related virus responsible for disease
Sindbis	Mosquito	Africa, E. Mediterranean, S. and S.E. Asia	Disease recognised only in Africa
Uruma	Mosquito	Upper Amazon	
Venezuelan encephalitis	Mosquito	Venezuela, Colombia, S. and Central America	
Western encephalitis	Mosquito	N. America, Mexico, Guyana, Brazil, Argentina	

discussed above. Only special features will therefore be mentioned under the individual diseases. Pathological studies have largely been confined to those arbovirus diseases which have caused epidemics with a considerable proportion of fatal cases—often in temperate areas. Where the pathology is not mentioned, little or nothing has been recorded in the literature. The Catalogue (1968) is freely referred to but contains much additional information and many references to the literature about the viruses.

Group A (Table 3)

Chikungunya virus has caused several epidemics in Africa and more recently a series of large

Thailand in 1958 during a dengue haemorrhagic fever epidemic and infections are probably fairly common there and in neighbouring countries. In India since 1963, chikungunya has caused large epidemics in Calcutta, Vellore, Madras, Pondicherry and also in Colombo in Ceylon. In Calcutta, the chikungunya epidemic immediately followed an epidemic of dengue haemorrhagic fever. In Asia, the main mosquito transmitting the disease to man in urban epidemics has been *Ae. aegypti*, but the virus has also been isolated from a number of *Culex* species. In Africa the vertebrate maintenance hosts of this virus may be wild primates, and the virus has been repeatedly isolated from *Ae. africanus*, but there seems little doubt that in time of epidemic (particularly in association with dense urban *Ae. aegypti* populations) man himself must be acting as a temporary maintenance host.

Clinical features. The incubation period is estimated as 3–12 days. As seen in Africa (Robinson, 1955) there is a sudden onset of severe joint pains which very rapidly (within minutes or hours) cripple the patient. With a rapid rise in temperature the patient soon becomes doubled up and immobile. There is frighteningly severe pain in the spine and limbs which may require morphine for relief, but the headache is not severe and retro-orbital pain is not mentioned. The fever is often biphasic with an afebrile interval of 1–3 days occurring 1–6 days after onset. During the second phase, about 80 per cent of patients have an irritating maculopapular rash on the trunk and extensor surface of limbs.

The acute illness lasts 6–10 days but recurrences of the joint pains, sometimes severe, occur for up to 4 months without fever. Otherwise recovery is uniform and no sequelae have been recorded other than oedema of the ankles in a few cases. In Asia, the disease seems to have been more dengue-like, but with some severe complications and some deaths. The bone and joint pains seem to have been less spectacular but there was fever (3–4 days), headache, backache, general aches and pains, lymphadenopathy, vomiting in some, cough in 50–60 per cent, a rash in 50 per cent, haemorrhages in 5–7 per cent and neurological symptoms in a small number. These estimates of the prevalence of severe complications may well be exaggerated as, during such large epidemics, the recording of mild cases must be greatly underestimated. Myocarditis and peripheral circulatory failure were recorded.

Halstead (1966) states that 'the most severe form of chikungunya infection observed in Thailand has been a febrile illness with minor haemorrhagic manifestations (haemorrhagic fever without shock) and not a life-threatening disease'. Deller and Russell (1968) have described 10 cases in American soldiers in Vietnam. There was a brief illness with an acute onset of fever, chills, headache, arthralgia, and signs of arthritis with or without a macular rash. In Calcutta, Sarkar *et al* (1965) described nine cases with haematemesis or melaena, four with skin petechiae or purpura, and 2 who died of shock (peripheral circulatory failure): the death rate was estimated at 0.4 per cent, but 2.8 per cent in children under 1 year of age and 1.6 per cent in persons over 50.

No vaccine is yet available for prophylaxis, but experimental vaccines are under development. A formalinised vaccine grown in green monkey kidney cultures has given good protection against experimental infections in mice and monkeys (Harrison *et al*, 1967).

Eastern encephalitis virus is distributed along the east of the New World from the north-eastern United States to Argentina. Small outbreaks have occurred in the United States, the Dominican Republic (1948–49) and Jamaica (1962). Epidemics of encephalitis in horses have occurred in these and other areas, sometimes with no recognised human cases. The virus has also been isolated in Panama, Trinidad, Guyana, Brazil and Argentina. Isolations have been reported in the Philippines, Thailand, Poland and the U.S.S.R., but their significance is still uncertain. The rate of inapparent infections with eastern encephalitis is rather low compared with other encephalitis arboviruses. This virus is probably maintained by wild birds and mosquitoes: many mosquito species have been found infected, but the maintenance species in tropical areas have not been clearly determined. *Culiseta melanura* seems to be the main mosquito infecting birds in North America; in Brazil and Trinidad the virus has been isolated from *Ae. taeniorhynchus*, *Culex taeniopus* and *C. nigripalpus*. Outbreaks of disease occur among pheasants in the United States, probably transmitted between them by pecking and feather picking.

Clinical features. Little is known about the disease in many tropical areas where it is at most sporadic and has seldom been recognised. In the United States (Farber *et al*, 1940) encephalitis occurs mainly in infants and children. A mild febrile first phase may or may not be apparent, but usually there is an abrupt onset of high fever (102–106°F; 38.9–41.1°C), headache and vomiting, followed by drowsiness, coma, twitching and severe convulsions within 48 hours of onset. Control of convulsions is often an important aspect of the treatment. On examination there is usually neck stiffness, spasticity, bulging fontanelles in infants, and loss of abdominal reflexes. There may be oedema of the legs and face, and cyanosis. The CSF is under pressure and may contain increased protein and up to 1000 cells/mm³, mostly polymorphs in the acute stage. Death usually occurs within 3–5 days but some die later, often of complications. Mental retardation, convulsions and paralyses are common and severe sequelae in surviving young children, while older individuals usually recover much more completely.

At autopsy gross examination reveals only generalised congestion and oedema of the viscera and central nervous system (Farber *et al*, 1940). Histologically there is marked and diffuse meningoencephalitis with widespread neuronal damage of varying severity. There is neuronophagia and marked perivascular cuffing. In venules and arterioles there is cellular infiltration of the walls, thrombi and fibrin deposits. The basal nuclei and brainstem are most severely affected and there is notable involvement of the cortex in the frontal and occipital lobes and in the hippocampus. No vaccine is available for use in man although a formalinised chick embryo vaccine is used in horses and is apparently effective.

Mayaro virus has been isolated from man in Trinidad (Anderson *et al*, 1957) and has caused a febrile outbreak of 50 cases in Para, Brazil (Causey and Maroja, 1957). The infection is probably fairly widespread in American tropical forest habitats. The virus has been isolated from *Mansonia venezuelensis* in Trinidad where the infection was commonest in forest workers; and from a wide variety of mosquito species (especially *Haemagogus* spp.) in Brazil where antibody was found in a wide range of wild forest mammals and marsupials.

Clinically there was fever lasting 2–6 days with headache, prostration, conjunctivitis, aches and pains in muscles and joints, and a rash. In some patients there was severe frontal headache, vomiting and/or jaundice. The five Trinidad cases were very mild: apart from fever, aches and pains and headache, one patient had a loose stool and one a swollen finger joint. No rash was observed. Virus was isolated from the blood of all five on the first or second day of illness. There has been one accidental laboratory infection with overt illness (Catalogue, 1968).

Mucambo virus, closely related to Venezuelan encephalitis virus, has been responsible for at least eight cases of naturally occurring febrile illness in Brazil, and serological surveys suggest that it is distributed in Amazonas and Para, Brazil and in French Guiana. It has been isolated from a variety of species of mosquitoes and from rodents and marsupials. Clinically there was fever, headache, prostration and muscle pains (Catalogue, 1968). De Mucha-Macias and Sanchez-Spindola (1965) have described two accidental laboratory cases in persons previously vaccinated against Venezuelan encephalitis: they had fever, severe headache, and severe pharyngitis together with symptoms suggestive of CNS involvement. No deaths or sequelae are known to have occurred and there is no vaccine.

O'nyong-nyong virus has caused one very major epidemic which started in Uganda in 1959 and spread to Kenya, Tanzania and Malawi involving an estimated 2 million people. Small outbreaks were still active in 1962. In the worst affected areas 70 per cent of all age groups were affected within a short time. There appears to have been little or no pre-existing immunity, suggesting that it was a new disease the origin of which is still obscure. The virus is closely related to chikungunya and Semliki Forest viruses, both previously isolated in East Africa, and O'nyong-nyong may have been a variant of one of them. O'nyong-nyong fever was transmitted to man by two man-biting *Anopheles* mosquitoes (*An. gambiae, An. funestus*) from which the virus was repeatedly isolated during the epidemic. The incubation period is estimated at 8 days or less. There was a sudden onset, sometimes with rigors and epistaxis, followed by aches and stiffness in the back and joints (often severe), headache, pain in the eyes, an irritating rash which usually began on the face and spread to the trunk and limbs, and marked lymphadenitis especially of the cervical nodes, the swelling of which was obvious (Shore, 1951). About a third of the cases were considered to be afebrile and marked fever was relatively infrequent. Fever when present lasted about 5 days, the rash 4–7 days, but aches, pains and malaise often considerably longer. There were no sequelae or deaths due directly to the disease.

Ross River or a closely related group A virus has caused epidemics of febrile illness with rash and polyarthritis in Australia (Shope and Anderson, 1960). Ross River virus has been isolated from the mosquito *Ae. vigilax* and residual antibody found in various parts of Australia and New Guinea. The epidemics involved thousands of cases in the Murray Valley. Similar epidemics have occurred on islands in the South-west Pacific and in troops in North-east Australia. The rash, which in many cases covered the whole body, began as discrete macules, progressed to papules and in a few cases to small vesicles. Petechiae and an enanthem were also recorded. Joint pains preceded the rash (in one case by as long as 10 days) and mainly affected the small joints of the hands and feet. Joint swelling was rare. The arthritis lasted 2–28 days (8 months in one case). Few cases complained of fever. Tenderness of the palms and soles was notable in six of 36 cases and five had paraesthesiae.

Sindbis virus has been isolated in Egypt, Uganda, South Africa, India, Malaya, Sarawak, Philippines and northern Australia from a variety of *Culex* mosquitoes (*C. univittatus, C. tritaeniorhynchus, C. pseudovishnui*) and from wild birds and man. Although the presence of antibody indicates the occurrence of infections of man in these areas, little disease has been attributed to Sindbis virus. In 1961, five cases were seen in Uganda with fever, headache, aches and pains, and slight jaundice in two (E.A.V.R.I., 1962). In South Africa there has been rather more severe illness; fever, severe headache, soreness of tendons and joints (especially of the hands or feet), a rash and painful vesicles on the toes, from the fluid of which the virus was isolated (Malherbe *et al*, 1963).

Uruma virus is very closely related to, and perhaps identical with, Mayaro virus and was responsible for an undetermined proportion of cases in an epidemic in the eastern Bolivian rain forest. Although deaths occurred during the epidemic there is no evidence that they were attributable to Uruma virus. Antibody surveys show that infections of man are fairly common in the upper Amazon basin in Bolivia and Peru. The small number of diagnosed cases had fever, headache and prostration only (Schaeffer *et al*, 1959).

Venezuelan encephalitis virus derives its name from the large epizootics of encephalitis which it causes in horses, mules and donkeys. In man, encephalitis occurs in a small proportion of cases but the majority have only a non-fatal febrile illness. Evidence of infections with this virus (or very closely related viruses) has been found in Venezuela, Guyana, Colombia, Brazil, Ecuador, Argentina, Panama, Trinidad, Mexico and Florida, and it is probably present in neighbouring countries. Human disease has definitely occurred in Venezuela, Colombia, Trinidad and most of Central America. The virus has been frequently isolated from wild-caught mosquitoes—most often from *Ae. serratus* or *Ae taeniorhynchus* but also from a wide range of other species, and from wild rodents (*Heteromys*, *Sygodontomys* and *Oryzomys* spp.). Its maintenance in nature is poorly understood but may depend on mosquitoes and rodents. Transmission to man and horses is by mosquito although, as the virus can readily be isolated from throat swabs from patients and 'contact' transmission between horses has been described, the possibility of occasional aerosol or mouth-to-mouth transmission between cases cannot be excluded. There have certainly been many accidental laboratory infections with Venezuelan encephalitis virus, most of them due to aerosol infection.

In a large epidemic which occurred in 1962–63 in Venezuela and Colombia involving both man and horses, there were estimated to have been more than 30 000 human cases with only about 200 deaths. Two-thirds of the patients were children under 15. This epidemic followed very heavy rainfall in Venezuela in 1962 with flooding which led both to intense mosquito breeding and to the crowding of animals on small areas not flooded. More recently there has been a very large epidemic affecting both man and horses over several countries in central America and spreading to affect the southern United States. Vaccination provided successful protection where it was used.

Clinically there is a short febrile illness with a sudden onset and malaise, nausea or vomiting, headache which may be severe, and aches and pains in bones and muscles (Sanmartin-Barberi *et al*, 1954). The fever lasts up to 4 days. Convalescence may take up to 3 weeks, during which there is general asthenia. Following the febrile illness, a small proportion of patients (0.5–6 per cent in different estimates) develop encephalitis which may be severe or fatal. This is a typical virus encephalitis with no obvious special clinical or pathological features. Briceno-Rossi (1964a) reported successful isolations from blood during the first 3 days of illness in 64 per cent of 145 cases, and from nine throat swabs. Virus was isolated from nine of 20 brain samples.

The first significant mortality in man due to Venezuelan encephalitis occurred in the large epidemic in Venezuela and Colombia. There were no recorded deaths in those with the acute febrile illness, but of 397 encephalitis patients, 42 died. The usual sequelae of encephalitis may be expected in a few cases but recovery from laboratory infections appear to have been complete with one possible exception.

Vaccines. There is an effective and safe live attenuated vaccine which has been widely used in laboratory workers. It causes a low viraemia in 10 per cent of recipients and a significant antibody response in all. Some degree of non-specific reaction occurs in 37.5 per cent but it has been significant only in 10 per cent of recipients (Alevizatos *et al*, 1967). The very slight degree of viraemia found has allayed some of the concern felt about the administration of this vaccine to people likely to be bitten by susceptible mosquitoes which might transmit the infection perhaps with increased virulence. This possibility should however be borne in mind and vaccine given outside the mosquito season, or vaccinated individuals protected from mosquito bites whenever possible for a few days after inoculation.

Western encephalitis virus has been isolated in the United States, Canada, Guyana, Brazil and Argentina, but human disease has been recognised only in North America and Brazil. Large epidemics have occurred in North America, where it also causes encephalitis in horses. Recent epidemics and the circumstances leading to them were reviewed by Hess and Hayes (1967). Residual antibody has also been found in man in Mexico. Reeves *et al* (1962) have estimated the relationship between infections and cases as 58 : 1 in infants and children under 5, increasing with age to 1150 : 1 in people over 15 years of age. The virus has been isolated from many species of wild birds and from many mosquito species (mainly *Culex tarsalis* in western United States and *Culiseta melanura* in the east) and there is little doubt that these are the maintenance hosts of this virus at least in North America. Little is known about its maintenance in tropical areas although it is probably basically similar.

Clinically (Kokernot *et al*, 1953) the disease varies somewhat with age, but fever and drowsiness are common at all ages. Convulsions occur in 90 per cent of affected infants, in 40 per cent of children aged 1–4 years, but rarely in adults. There is fever (usually 102–104°F or higher), headache, vomiting and stiffness of the neck and back. In children, there is notable restlessness and irritability. Drowsiness and severe occipital headache, often with mental confusion, and coma occur in 35–40 per cent of adults. Pleocytosis and increased protein are found in the CSF, the levels and type of cell depending on the stage of the illness. In less severe cases, recovery occurs in 3–5 days and even in severe cases within 5–10 days, although complete return to strength may take several weeks. Severe and permanent sequelae are rare in adults but are increasingly common and severe with reducing age. In infants under a month of age, more than half are left with convulsions, motor or mental changes; in children over 1 year, convulsions are the commonest residual problem. The mortality rate varies between outbreaks from 2 to 15 per cent.

Vaccines. There is no vaccine for human use. A formalinised chick embryo vaccine has been effectively used in horses and suggested for use in man (Robinson *et al*, 1966). Recently an attenuated live vaccine has been developed and used in horses (Binn *et al*, 1966).

Group B (Table 4)

Banzi virus (syn. H336, and probably Uganda S, Makonde) has been isolated from mosquitoes in Uganda and South Africa and from the blood of a febrile child in Natal (Smithburn *et al*, 1959). Antibody in man suggests that infection is distributed very widely in Africa and possibly in South and South-east Asia although interpretation of

Group B antibody surveys is very difficult due to cross-reactions.

Dengue viruses of which at least four serological types (and perhaps six) exist have been responsible both for classical dengue and for dengue haemorrhagic fever. The various types (dengue-1, dengue-2, dengue-3, dengue-4) are closely related and no significant biological differences are known between them. Many of the largest epidemics have been caused by dengue-1, but a recent Caribbean epidemic was due to dengue-3. However, in many situations several types coexist and successive epidemics may be due to different types; in North Queensland dengue-2 caused an epidemic in 1942-44, and dengue-1 in 1953-55. A significant number of people were affected in both epidemics and Sabin (1952) has shown that cross-protection between dengue types in man lasts only a short time.

CLASSICAL DENGUE. Epidemics of 'dengue' have been reported since the late eighteenth century and there was a great wave of urban epidemics in tropical and subtropical regions during the nineteenth and early twentieth centuries (Smith, 1956d). These epidemics seem to have followed the migration of *Ae. aegypti* along trade routes from Africa, particularly round the coast of Asia from southern India to Hong Kong and across the Pacific to Hawaii, and probably occurred when towns became large enough and urban *Ae. aegypti* populations sufficiently dense. Dengue was probably previously a rural infection in tropical Asia transmitted by indigenous *Stegomyia* such as *Ae. albopictus*. However, no virological diagnosis was possible in these epidemics and 'dengue' is a symptom complex which can be caused by quite a number of arboviruses and can be closely mimicked by other infections.

The disease is endemic over wide areas of Asia, the Pacific and Australasia wherever *Stegomyia* species are active throughout the year. The boundaries are about the winter isotherms for 64°F (17.8°C). Outside these areas large urban epidemics occur from time to time such as those in Brisbane (1906), in Durban (1927) and in Athens (1928). Since 1920, epidemics each of ½ to 2 million cases have occurred in the United States, Greece, Japan and Australia. Within the endemic regions the presence of the disease may be almost unrecognised among the undifferentiated mild fevers, and epidemics are usually small and restricted to immigrant groups such as military forces or to institutions such as schools (Smith, 1956bc, 1957). However, in 1963 a large epidemic started explosively in Puerto Rico and Curacao and swept through the Caribbean area wherever

TABLE 4. *Group B arboviruses which are known to cause human disease and occur in the tropics and subtropics*

Virus	Probable transmission to man	Geographical distribution of viruses	Other features
Banzi	Mosquito	S. Africa and neighbours	
Dengue types 1–4	Mosquito	S., S.E. and E. coast Asia, Pacific Is., New Guinea, Caribbean area	Tropics and subtropics wherever the virus and a *Stegomyia* vector exist
Ilheus	Mosquito	Central America, Trinidad, Colombia, Brazil	
Japanese encephalitis	Mosquito	E., S.E. and S. Asia, W. Pacific	
Kyasanur Forest	Ixodid tick	Mysore, India	
Langat	Ixodid tick	Malaya	
Murray Valley encephalitis	Mosquito	Australia, New Guinea	
Rio Bravo	? Bat saliva	U.S.A., Mexico	Lab. cases more severe
St Louis encephalitis	Mosquito	N. America, Panama, Jamaica, Trinidad, Brazil, Argentina	
Spondweni	Mosquito	E., W. and S. Africa	
Wesselbron	Mosquito	S. Africa and neighbours	
West Nile	Mosquito	E. and W. Africa, S. and S.E. Asia, Mediterranean area	Disease recognised mainly in Israel and S. France
Yellow fever	Mosquito	W. and Central Africa, S. and Central America	Periodical epidemics in neighbouring areas, e.g. Ethiopia.
Zika	Mosquito	E. and W. Africa, S. and S.E. Asia, Philippines	One case in Uganda

Ae. aegypti was prevalent, to Venezuela where an epidemic of more than 10 000 cases occurred. In 1971–72 there has been a very large epidemic in Colombia. The high susceptibility of the populations in these areas was probably attributable to the gap in transmission of dengue there following *Ae. aegypti* eradication over most of the area (which had previously had endemic dengue) followed by recrudescence of the species in a number of areas in recent years. There were considerable fears of epidemic spread to the United States, especially from Puerto Rico, but this did not occur. In Asia and the Pacific other *Stegomyia* such as *Ae. albopictus*, *Ae. polynesiensis* and *Ae. scutellaris* play a role in transmission, particularly in rural areas, but *Ae. aegypti* is more important in urban transmission. Although evidence of infection has been found in monkeys and some other mammal species, there is as yet no convincing evidence of a vertebrate maintenance host other than man.

Sabin (1952) studied the disease in volunteers. Skin biopsies showed endothelial swelling, perivascular oedema and mononuclear infiltration. In petechial lesions there was blood extravasation but little inflammatory reaction.

The *clinical picture* of classical dengue was well described by Siler *et al* (1926) and Simmons *et al* (1931). The incubation period is estimated as 5–8 days. The onset of fever may be sudden or preceded by malaise. The illness starts with headache, retro-orbital pain, backache, and pains in the muscles and joints, all of which may be severe. During this stage a transient mottled erythematous rash (sometimes scarlatiniform) may be seen (although seldom observed on darker skins). The fever may be continuous or biphasic ('saddleback'). During the second phase or second half

Y

of the fever there is marked loss of appetite and often considerable malaise and weakness, relative bradycardia and, around the third to fifth day of the illness, frequently a rash first on the trunk then spreading to the face and limbs. The rash is usually maculopapular but may be scarlatiniform or even petechial. In the larger and more severe epidemics in non-endemic areas (e.g. Durban, 1927; Athens, 1928) epistaxis, haematemesis, intestinal and skin haemorrhages, and a positive tourniquet test were mentioned. These epidemics were retrospectively confirmed as due to dengue viruses. There were thus earlier indications that dengue viruses were capable of causing illness resembling dengue haemorrhagic fever. In classical dengue, recovery is complete but convalescence may be prolonged with weakness and depression lasting several weeks.

DENGUE HAEMORRHAGIC FEVER. This severe disease, caused by infection with one of the dengue viruses in children under 15 (mainly aged 3–6 years) first appeared in epidemic form in Bangkok in 1953 and has since involved cities and later rural areas in Thailand (from 1958), and cities in North (1958) and South Vietnam (1963), Malaysia (from 1960) and India (from 1963). Halstead (1966) wrote an excellent review of the disease in South-east Asia and Symposia are to be found in *Bull. Wld Hlth Org.* (1966) and in *Ind. J. med. Res.* (1965). The precise epidemiological picture is confused by the concurrence in most epidemics of large numbers of chikungunya infections transmitted by the same mosquito, *Ae. aegypti*. Both viruses cause diseases of a wide range of severity and Halstead estimated that in Bangkok in 1962, while there were over 8000 cases of dengue haemorrhagic fever with or without shock, there were probably between 150 000 and 300 000 cases of less severe febrile illness (mild fevers and classical dengue) in the population at risk— about 870 000 under 15 years of age. In Thailand, at least, all but 25 of 10 367 cases with 694 deaths were in children under 14 years of age. Because of multiple group B virus infections, serological diagnosis of the precise type of dengue virus responsible for individual cases has been very difficult. However, by virus isolation from the blood all four types of virus have been incriminated. Types 3 and 4 appeared to be mainly responsible for the first Philippine epidemic, and dengue-2 has been recovered most frequently from fatal cases in Bangkok. *Ae. aegypti* is undoubtedly the main (and probably the only important) arthropod maintenance host and the disease has occurred only in areas with exceptionally dense *aegypti* populations because of an abundance of breeding places provided by water containers in and around houses. Epidemics have occurred annually in Bangkok and have tended to be more severe in alternate years. In Calcutta the epidemic coincided with the wet season and hence peak *aegypti* population. Apart from Singapore and Penang, where the number of cases was relatively small, most of the epidemics have been large with thousands of cases.

Clinically the onset is often slow with fever, upper respiratory symptoms, headache, anorexia, abdominal pain and vomiting. This stage lasts 2–4 days and the majority of children then recover. In a proportion, however, there is an abrupt onset of collapse with hypotension, peripheral vascular congestion, which may give the skin a diffuse purplish appearance, a maculopapular rash, petechiae and ecchymoses. A positive tourniquet test is usual even in milder cases. Other haemorrhagic manifestations also occur: epistaxis, haematemesis, melaena. Commonly there is abdominal pain and tenderness, and hepatomegaly has been common in Bangkok cases. Some patients progress to a state of shock which has a bad prognosis: the patient is restless, sweating, with cold clammy limbs and a hot trunk—various CNS symptoms and signs including convulsions may occur at this stage. Pleural effusions and pneumonitis have been demonstrated by X-ray (Nelson, 1960) and myocardial damage by electrocardiogram. Apart from death in shock, recovery is usual and fairly rapid. Laboratory investigations demonstrate haemoconcentration, prolongation of the bleeding time, thrombocytopenia, and other deficiencies of the blood clotting mechanisms (Weiss and Halstead, 1965). Both leukopenia and leukocytosis have been reported. The bone marrow may show maturation arrest of megakaryocytes and phagocytic activity by reticulum cells. Liver function tests show changes paralleling the severity of the disease. Hypoproteinaemia is frequent and important in relation to shock. In immunoelectrophoretic studies of serum protein, disappearance of the $\beta 1C$ line at the onset of shock has been reported suggesting that this is an immunological phenomenon—a massive antigen-antibody reaction. The very rapid rise in group B antibody commonly found during the early stages of the disease suggests that patients may have been previously sensitised to the infecting virus by earlier infection with a closely related virus and perhaps another type of dengue virus.

At autopsy vascular changes are dominant: vasodilatation with congestion, oedema and haemorrhages. Pleural and peritoneal effusions are found and haemorrhages in the stomach and intestines. Petechial haemorrhages are widespread, including interventricular and subendocardial haemorrhages in the heart. There is marked proliferation of large mononuclear cells in the spleen, lymph nodes and elsewhere in the reticulo-endothelial system. Some Thailand cases have shown hyaline necrosis in both parenchymal and Kupffer cells in the liver.

Diagnosis depends on the epidemiological situation and on virus isolation from the blood during the first 3 days of illness. Serological diagnosis is unusually difficult because of the broad group B antibody response which is usual: the first serum specimen should be obtained before the fourth day of illness to provide a reasonable chance of success.

Treatment is symptomatic except where haemorrhage or, more important, shock supervenes. Intravenous fluids or blood should be used as in shock due to other causes, with careful attention to blood electrolytic levels and balances. Nelson (1960) found that cortisone given sufficiently early could be a life-saving measure. This would be consistent with an immunological aetiology for the shock. Phentolanime (an adrenergic blocking agent) appears to be beneficial in shock (Chundermpadetsuk, 1966). Transfusions of concentrates of fresh platelets or of packed cells may be necessary in the treatment of haemorrhage. On the basis that the pathogenesis of this disease may be fundamentally acute disseminated intravascular coagulation (McKay and Margaretten, 1967), anticoagulants given before the onset of haemorrhage and shock might theoretically be of benefit but would have to be used with caution and only in situations where full facilities for treatment and its laboratory control were available.

A poor *prognosis* is associated with shock, gastrointestinal haemorrhage, haematuria or cerebral haemorrhage. A high level of dengue HI antibody during the first 3 days of illness was of good prognosis.

Control of either type of dengue depends mainly on control of urban populations of *Ae. aegypti* which has been eradicated in many areas of America. Much can be done by eliminating water containers such as jars, flower pots, old tyres and tin cans from the environment of houses, and by the intelligent use of insecticides although many resistant strains are known. Where *Ae. aegypti* also breeds in tree holes, eradication can probably not be achieved, and for similar reasons control of the other *Stegomyia* species is difficult. No vaccine is yet available but live attenuated strains have been shown to be protective and Wisseman

et al (1963) have developed an experimental dengue-1 vaccine which causes completely inapparent infections in man. Probably a vaccine containing all four antigenic types will be required to give complete protection. Such a vaccine would be of particular value for military forces operating in endemic areas: dengue epidemics were a militarily serious cause of disease in the Pacific area during the Second World War.

Ilheus virus has been isolated in Brazil, Colombia, Trinidad, Panama, Guatemala and Honduras. Serology suggests that it also occurs in forest areas of Surinam, Guyana and Venezuela. It is probably maintained by a forest complex of wild birds and mosquitoes: it has been isolated repeatedly from wild birds, antibodies have been found in rodents; numerous isolations have been made from mosquitoes of six genera (mostly commonly *Psorophora*). Knowledge of the disease in man is limited to five naturally occurring cases in Trinidad and Brazil and nine cancer patients infected experimentally by Southam and Moore (1951). There were no detectable symptoms in half of these infections, three had undifferentiated mild febrile illnesses and four had more marked illness with involvement of the CNS. The fully developed disease probably comprises fever, headache, aches and pains, which may be severe and disabling, photophobia and signs of encephalitis. Diplopia and mental changes were reported in one case, followed by tachycardia and circulatory collapse. The CSF has an increase in cells and protein. No deaths or sequelae were reported.

Japanese encephalitis virus occurs over the whole of the eastern seaboard of Asia and its offshore islands, from the maritime province of the Soviet Union to Singapore, in Borneo, Indonesia and South India; also probably in Burma, Bangladesh and Ceylon. Epidemics have been recognised in Japan possibly since 1871 but almost certainly since 1924, and have occurred annually since, varying in size from a few to over 8000 cases. Epidemics have also occurred in the maritime province, Korea, China, Guam, Okinawa and Taiwan. Epidemics usually occur in late summer, but further south the disease is sporadic and enzootic throughout the year. Japanese encephalitis virus also causes encephalitis in horses and abortion in pigs.

The main mosquito hosts throughout its distribution are rice-field breeding mosquitoes: the *Culex vishnui* complex, especially *tritaeniorhynchus*, and probably *C. annulirostris* in Guam. In tropical Asia, Borneo and Indonesia, *C. gelidus*, which breeds particularly in association with pigs and cattle, is also involved. In Japan, extensive studies by Scherer *et al* (1959) showed that in the spring there is intense virus transmission among young herons by *C. tritaeniorhynchus*. These mosquitoes then infect pigs which appear to act as amplifier hosts to infect *C. tritaeniorhynchus* populations in close juxtaposition to man. Human cases can be predicted in time and place in any year by surveillance of abattoir pigs for evidence of infection (antibody conversion, especially IgM) which precedes outbreaks of human disease by 2–3 weeks. The mechanisms of over-wintering are obscure, although hibernating *C. tritaeniorhynchus* have been found in substantial numbers in the U.S.S.R. and evidence of frequent infections in bats suggests that virus may hibernate in them. In tropical Asia, the vertebrate maintenance hosts are not yet defined—evidence of infection in wild birds has been scanty. Studies in Sarawak (Macdonald *et al*, 1965, 1967) suggest that there the main maintenance hosts throughout the year may be pigs and *C. gelidus* and that during the monsoon, when *C. tritaeniorhynchus* is numerous, the risk to man is increased in association with rice fields. Southam (1956) estimated that, in Japanese children, 500–1000 were infected for each case of encephalitis, however Halstead and Grosz (1962) found a very much lower rate (25 : 1) among American soldiers in Korea during an epidemic. The risk may therefore be higher to immigrants into endemic areas than to residents.

Clinical description. Reports of large numbers of cases come from the epidemic areas (e.g. Edgren *et al*, 1958; Green *et al*, 1963) but the sporadic cases of tropical areas are broadly similar (e.g. Phoon and Lim, 1963). The disease may start with a mild febrile illness but the first phase is usually absent or unnoticed and there is a sudden onset of fever, headache and vomiting. The fever, usually with relative bradycardia, is commonly continuous, reaching a peak and subsiding after 2–4 days. Lethargy may be predominant with expressionless facies, and motor and sensory disturbances affecting speech, the eyes and limbs; or there may be confusion and delirium. Either state may progress to coma. In children, convulsions may be the first indication. Weakness or paralysis may affect any part of the body and the lesions are usually upper motor neurone in character. Lesions of the extrapyramidal tracts are common. There is usually neck rigidity, a positive Kernig's sign, and the reflexes are disordered. There may be an initial leukocytosis followed by leukopenia. The CSF is usually clear and under pressure with up to about 400 cells/mm³ (occasionally more) and a moderately raised protein. The duration of the illness is very variable: sudden improvement may occur after a few days, or with modern intensive care the patient may remain largely unconscious for months and then show a reasonable and often surprising degree of recovery; fatal cases usually die within 10 days but death due to complications may occur much later in patients under intensive care.

Convalescence is often prolonged and sequelae are fairly common (Weaver *et al*, 1958) especially in children under 10 years and particularly severe in infants. There may be incoordination, tremors, nervousness, mental impairment, emotional or personality changes. There may be residual paralysis (either upper or lower motor neurone) and less frequently aphasia, cerebellar ataxia, psychoses and even decerebrate rigidity. Over a period of time with adequate care, skilled physiotherapy and occupational therapy, considerable slow improvement is usually possible in all but the most severely affected. In Singapore children (mainly under 5) the mortality was low (7 per cent) but there was a high incidence of sequelae (Phoon and Lim, 1963); while in Taiwan the death rate under 3 years of age was 37 per cent, in ages 3–15 19 per cent and in people over 15, 17.5 per cent (Green *et al*, 1963).

Post-mortem examination shows only oedema and congestion of the central nervous system. Histologically, neuronal degeneration and necrosis with marked neuronophagia is widespread—including the cerebral cortex, the cerebellum and the cord. Perivascular cuffing is general and adjacent tissue is infiltrated with round cells. There is striking damage to the Purkinje cells of the cerebellum and often severe involvement of the spinal cord (Zimmerman, 1946).

Treatment. There is no specific treatment, but much can be done by intensive care procedures. Hiraki *et al* (1958) suggested that ACTH was of benefit in severely ill cases, and a large dose of intravenous cortisone is probably worth trying. Control of convulsions may be necessary.

No really satisfactory and available vaccine yet exists but a formalinised mouse-brain vaccine appeared to give some protection to Japanese school children (Tigertt and Berge, 1957; Matsuda, 1962) although no properly controlled trial has been conducted. More recently a formalinised vaccine made from an attenuated strain of virus grown in hamster kidney cultures shows considerable promise (Darwish *et al*, 1967). Vaccination of the amplifier hosts, pigs, is worthy of consideration as a means of breaking the infection link to man; mosquito control in large rice-field areas appears to be impracticable at present.

Kyasanur Forest disease broke out suddenly in 1956 as an epidemic associated with an epizootic and deaths in monkeys in the Kyasanur Forest in the western Ghats (Mysore, India). First impressions were that it might be the first outbreak of yellow fever in India but the virus was soon isolated and found to be closely related to the tick-borne complex of group B viruses, e.g. tick-borne encephalitis, louping ill, Omsk haemorrhagic fever, Langat (Work, 1958). In 1957 there were probably about 500 cases in an area of about 70 square miles. The infection rate in man during this period may have been as high as 33 per cent, with disease in at least 55 per cent of those infected. The death rate was about 10 per cent. Although residual antibodies suggestive of Kyasanur Forest disease infection have been found in Saurashtra, the disease itself has not been recognised outside the area of the Kyasanur Forest. The disease is acquired in the forest mainly in the dry season: March to June. The virus has been isolated from several tick species but most from *H. spinigera* and *H. turturis*. Monkeys suffer from the disease and many die; they may be amplifier hosts but are obviously not the long-term vertebrate hosts of the virus, which are probably ground-living rodents and/or birds. The virus has been isolated from two *Rattus* species and the shrew *Suncus murinus*. Cattle are incidental hosts of the virus but important hosts of the adult stages of the ticks and the increase in cattle population prior to the epidemic may have permitted *H. spinigera* to have become infected initially as an incidental arthropod host and have triggered off a new cycle of infection involving monkeys and man. Laboratory infections with this virus have been common but generally with relatively mild disease.

Clinically (Webb and Rao, 1961) the disease has a sudden onset of fever, headache, severe muscle pains (chiefly in the lower back and calves), severe general prostration, bradycardia (usually from about the ninth day) and hypotension (especially between the fifth and twelfth days). There is commonly cough (sometimes with haemoptysis), conjunctival injection (sometimes with photophobia), lymphadenopathy (most marked in neck and axillae), maculopapular haemorrhagic spots on the palate, vomiting, diarrhoea and marked dehydration. In a minority of cases there are also haemorrhagic complications which begin as early as the third day: bleeding from nose, gums, stomach or intestines. This first phase of illness lasts 6–11 days. Mental confusion and drowsiness have been seen. A small proportion have a second febrile illness after an interval of 9–21 days. In this there is severe headache and central nervous system abnormalities including pleocytosis and increased globulin in the cerebrospinal fluid. During the first phase the CSF was normal but virus has several times been isolated from it—probably due to blood contamination. The laboratory findings (Chatterjea *et al*, 1963) included leukopenia during the first phase and a slight leukocytosis during the second. There was a fall in the haematocrit and phagocytosis of erythrocytes, leukocytes and platelets was seen in the peripheral blood between the twelfth and twentieth days. Albuminuria appears about the third or fourth day with granular casts and pus cells.

At autopsy (Iyer *et al*, 1959) general congestion is found with, in haemorrhagic cases, haemorrhage and consolidation in the lungs and haemorrhage in the gastrointestinal tract. The liver shows patchy and variable but generally slight histological damage; phagocytosis of erythrocytes was seen in Kuppfer cells. The kidneys show some swelling of the glomeruli and degenerative changes in the convoluted and collecting tubules. The lungs have patchy consolidation, sometimes a haemorrhagic alveolar exudate, and bronchiolitis. Moderate pleurisy has been seen in one case.

Vaccines. No satisfactory vaccine is yet available. A formalinised Russian spring-summer encephalitis vaccine has been tried without very noticeable effect. Recently Mansharamani *et al* (1967) have produced an inactivated vaccine in chick embryo cultures.

Langat virus is known to occur only in Malaya where it is probably maintained in forest by the tick *I. granulatus* and ground-living rodents. There is little evidence of infection in man in Malaya and no evidence of natural disease, probably because *I. granulatus* rarely bites man. The only evidence that it can cause human disease results from experimental infections of cancer patients by Webb *et al* (1966). Two of some 27 patients infected developed encephalitis and one of them appears to have died of it.

Langat virus is of some general interest as a possible live virus vaccine either alone or in series with yellow fever vaccine and attenuated West Nile virus (Price *et al*, 1963) against group B viruses, especially the tick-borne complex. Various experiments have been made, and except for some doubts about safety (although the above encephalitis cases were at special risk because they had leukaemia) the vaccine might well come into use. Smorodintsev *et al* (1967) have given a suitable strain to over 1000 people with satisfactory results. An exceptionally promising avirulent strain of the virus has been developed and can be grown in chick embryo (Thind and Price, 1966).

Murray Valley encephalitis has caused epidemics of encephalitis (originally called Australian X disease) in south-eastern Australia and the southern half of Queensland and sporadic cases in New Guinea where antibody has been found in man and chickens. It is very closely related to Japanese encephalitis virus. Evidence of infection has been found in every state of Australia, and epidemics (confined so far to the above areas) occur in late summer (February to April). *C. annulirostris* appears to be the main arthropod concerned in epidemics but the virus has been isolated also from other species (*Ae. normanensis, C. bitaeniorhynchus*) in the enzootic tropical and subtropical areas. The virus is probably maintained by birds and mosquitoes in the Australasian tropics (Miles, 1960). Inapparent infections are common. Anderson *et al* (1952) estimate the ratio of infections to disease as between 500 : 1 and 1000 : 1.

Clinically and pathologically the disease (Robertson and McLorinan, 1952) very closely resembles Japanese encephalitis. There is no vaccine available.

Rio Bravo virus (syn. U.S. bat salivary gland virus) has been isolated from the salivary glands of bats (*Tadarida, Eptesicus*) in Texas and California. It does not appear to cause disease in bats and is probably transmitted from bat to bat by bite and not by arthropods. Knowledge of the human disease it causes is limited to five accidental laboratory cases. One naturally occurring case with fever only is mentioned in the Catalogue (1968). Although not a tropical virus, it is mentioned here to illustrate the wide range of types of disease that arboviruses can cause. The general picture was febrile illness with pharyngitis, cough and lymphadenitis. Three of the cases were fairly severe and complicated by aseptic meningitis, orchitis or oophoritis.

St Louis encephalitis virus is widespread in the United States where it is the most important mosquito-borne disease. It has also caused cases of encephalitis in Jamaica and there is evidence of its presence in Argentina, Brazil, Colombia, Trinidad, Panama and Mexico, where sporadic cases may be occurring unrecognised. In the western United States the important mosquito host is *C. tarsalis*, in the central states *C. pipiens* and *C. quinquefasciatus*, and in Florida and Jamaica probably *C. nigripalpus*. These mosquitoes transmit to man but, apart from *C. tarsalis* in the west, may not be the true maintenance hosts. In Trinidad and Panama, the virus

has been isolated from *Culex, Psorophora* and *Sabethes* species. The vertebrate maintenance hosts appear to be wild birds and the virus is probably maintained in a woodland or forest habitat. Inapparent infections are common: in Texas the ratio of infections to disease was estimated as 64 : 1 (Brody *et al*, 1959); in Florida as 39 : 1 (Quick *et al*, 1965a).

Clinical descriptions of the disease are based on the large epidemics (Kunin and Chin, 1957; Quick *et al*, 1965b). The majority of patients have a febrile illness with severe headache lasting a few days followed by complete recovery. A variable proportion progress to aseptic meningitis or encephalitis. There is a sudden onset of fever with lassitude and nausea, the headache becomes severe, and confusion and drowsiness develop. Vomiting is common and there may be convulsions which have a poor prognosis. The fever normally lasts 3–10 days, falling slowly. A stiff neck with positive Kernig and Brudzinski signs are common. The CSF shows increased pressure and moderate increases in cells and protein. Muscular weakness and pains, tremors or spasticity, dysphasia, photophobia and visual disturbances may all occur. Coma or delirium may lead to death or persist for some time. On the other hand, really dramatic recovery can occur even in very ill patients. In the aged there is a higher incidence of disease, greater severity, greater mortality and more severe sequelae: in an epidemic at Tampa Bay, Florida, which affected a population with a very high proportion of old people, 22 per cent had an uncomplicated febrile illness, 12 per cent aseptic meningitis and 66 per cent encephalitis with or without paralysis. There were 43 deaths (42 over 50 years of age) in 222 cases (Quick *et al*, 1965b). People with debilitating diseases seem to be unduly susceptible; of 67 cases at Houston, Texas in 1964, eight had preexisting brain damage, nine hypertension, nine chronic alcoholism, three diabetes, two pulmonary tuberculosis and three other chronic illness. The disease also tends to be severe in children (Barrett *et al*, 1965); 11 of 26 affected in Houston, in 1964, had severe disease and more than half had neurological abnormalities. Although convalescence may be prolonged, permanent sequelae are relatively uncommon but include mental and personality changes, weakness or paralysis.

At autopsy, congestion and a few small haemorrhages are found in the CNS. Histologically there is perivascular cuffing and small perivascular haemorrhages. Neuronal damage tends to occur in clusters and changes are most marked in the midbrain and brainstem, but the cerebral cortex, the cerebellum and the anterior horns of the cord are also affected.

Vaccines. No vaccine is yet available but Darwish and Hammon (1966) have prepared an experimental formalinised vaccine in hamster kidney cultures.

Spondweni virus has been isolated from the blood of a febrile child in Nigeria, has caused two accidental laboratory infections and a volunteer has been infected. Clinically there was brief fever with headache and malaise. It has been repeatedly isolated from mosquitoes in South Africa and antibody surveys suggest that it is widely distributed in Africa.

Wesselbron virus appears to be widely distributed in South Africa, Botswana, Mozambique and probably neighbouring countries. It has been isolated from several mosquito species and causes epizootics in sheep with abortion and death in pregnant ewes, and death in newborn lambs. A few human cases have been described (both naturally occurring and laboratory infections): the disease is moderately severe, influenza-like with severe headache, a feeling of pressure behind the eyes, and aching and stiffness of joints and muscles. Convalescence may be prolonged. Splenomegaly and hepatomegaly with liver tenderness were found in one case. One patient had disturbances of vision.

West Nile virus has been isolated in Egypt, Uganda, Congo, South Africa, India, Borneo, Israel and France. Disease due to it has been clearly recognisable only in Israel, where it has been epidemic, and France where, in the Camargue, it has caused febrile illnesses in man and encephalitis in horses. In Egypt the disease appears to be a mild febrile illness mainly of young children. The virus has been isolated from a number of species of *Culex* mosquitoes, from *Mansonia metallica* and from *Argas* ticks. There have also been isolations from wild birds in Egypt, in South Africa and in Borneo. This virus is probably maintained by bird-biting *Culex* mosquitoes and wild birds, and in the case of birds which live in colonies perhaps by *Argas* ticks and birds. The epidemiology has been well studied only in Egypt (Taylor *et al*, 1956) and in Israel where sharp epidemics occur between May and October (Klingberg *et al*, 1959) in the north and central parts of the country. The epidemics start and end rather suddenly and, in one of the early epidemics, illness occurred in 60 per cent of the population in the affected area. West Nile virus (especially in low passage) has caused many laboratory infections—mainly by aerosol.

Clinical features. The incubation period is estimated as 3–6 days. In areas where disease has been readily recognisable there is a sudden onset of fever (sometimes biphasic), severe headache, pains in the muscles, rash and lymphadenopathy. The rash is maculopapular and mainly on the trunk. Most cases recover uneventfully. However, the disease is more severe in the elderly: 12 of 49 such patients in one outbreak were severely ill with neurological signs and four of them died (Spigland *et al*, 1958). Myocarditis has also been reported. Viraemia may last 6 days, probably 2 days of it before the onset of symptoms. Goldblum *et al* (1957) isolated virus from acute phase blood in 38 per cent of cases and from 77 per cent when the blood was taken on the first day of illness.

Vaccines. No vaccine exists although Price *et al* (1961) have experimentally used an attenuated strain of virus which had markedly reduced encephalitogenic properties in monkeys but has remained immunogenic.

Yellow fever. In Africa yellow fever (a disease with a vast literature including a comprehensive book by Strode, 1951) has probably always been enzootic in forest monkeys (who do not suffer recognisable disease), endemic and periodically epidemic in man by spread from the forest maintenance hosts. Whether the virus existed in America before the advent of *Ae. aegypti*, or, perhaps more probably, was imported with the mosquito, is not clear. However, yellow fever is now enzootic in forest monkeys in tropical America. Some American monkey species develop disease and die of yellow fever. Epidemics have been known in the Americas since the seventeenth century and the great urban American epidemics in the seventeenth, eighteenth and nineteenth centuries almost certainly followed the importation of *Ae. aegypti* from Africa and its subsequent establishment and spread. With the great propensity of *Ae. aegypti* for travel along trade routes, the infection spread widely in tropical and subtropical America and is said even to have reached Spain, France, England and Italy. As late as 1905 there was an epidemic of 5000 cases with 1000 deaths in parts of the southern United States, and in 1928 there was an epidemic in Rio de Janeiro. Eradication of *Ae. aegypti* has all but eliminated urban yellow fever from America, although it remains enzootic in its forest hosts.

Epidemiology. In Africa, the main maintenance hosts are monkeys and *Ae. africanus* which maintain the infection in the forest canopy. *Ae. simpsoni* which breeds in plant axils (particularly those of the false banana) has been mainly responsible for the Ethiopian epidemic (1959–66) which was associated mainly with riverine forest with an abundant monkey population and in which *Ae. africanus* is present. In some areas of Africa *Ae simpsoni* seldom bites man. In the severe Nuba Mountains (Sudan) epidemic of 1940, one or more of *Ae. vittatus*, *Ae metallicus* and *Ae. taylori* were thought to be responsible. Urban yellow fever in West Africa is transmitted by *Ae. aegypti* and, in epidemic circumstances, man is the temporary vertebrate maintenance host.

In tropical America where yellow fever is now essentially a disease of forest workers, the infection is maintained in monkeys and mosquitoes of which several species are involved. Most important is *Haemagogus spegazzini*, but also other *Haemagogus* species, *Sabethes chloropterus* (which may be responsible for maintaining the infection over dry periods in Central America), and *Ae. leucocalaenus*. Between 1948 and 1957, 1600 cases were reported from Guatemala in the north to Argentina in the south (Kerr, 1959). Many yellow fever infections both in Africa and America are mild or inapparent.

There has long been speculation as to why yellow fever has never reached Asia although *Ae. aegypti* was highly successful in doing so (see *Dengue*). The probable reasons are (*a*) that yellow fever has not been prevalent in East Africa—indeed the danger would be greater than ever before if yellow fever persists in Ethiopia, spread further up the Rift Valley and reached the Awash Valley which leads down to the Red Sea; and (*b*) that there may be a limit (say six or seven) to the number of group B viruses which can successfully establish themselves in a given area and most receptive areas in Asia already have a considerable complement of such viruses: the mechanism is probably vertebrate immunity where increasing antibody cross-reactions following multiple infections are likely to reduce viraemia in titre and duration and thus the chances of infecting mosquitoes.

The infection is permanently enzootic in the Congo and Amazon basins, the only areas now large enough for the infection to travel continuously as a wave through the monkey population without meeting an area where too high a proportion have been eliminated by death or immunity by a previous infection wave before the population has regenerated. From these permanent areas of maintenance the infection periodically spreads to cause epidemics where suitable arthropods exist in sufficient numbers, where mosquito control is inadequate, and where vaccination has been insufficient. Thus in recent years

there have been outbreaks in Nigeria (1951–54), Trinidad (1954), Central America (1948–57), Congo (1958), Sudan and Ethiopia (1959–66) and Senegal (1965). The largest of these by far was in Ethiopia, an area where the disease was not known previously, where the total number of cases is unknown but there were at least 15 000 deaths in 1960–62 (Serié *et al*, 1964). There were between 2000 and 20 000 cases in Senegal in 1965 (Chambon *et al*, 1967).

The danger of abandoning *Ae. aegypti* control was well illustrated by the narrow escape from urban yellow fever in Trinidad in 1954 (Downs, 1957), and the danger of abandoning systematic vaccination and mosquito control was demonstrated by the Senegal epidemic—some degree of complacency had been induced by a long period of freedom from epidemics due to previous systematic control measures. Yellow fever is almost certainly ineradicable from its maintenance cycles and those who live within reach of the Congo and Amazon basins must maintain constant vigilance and control measures.

Clinically the illness ranges from inapparent infection to the fully developed and fatal classical syndrome. Downs (1957) estimated that hundreds of unrecognised cases of yellow fever occurred in Trinidad in 1954. The incubation period is estimated as 3–6 days. The onset is usually sudden. Mild cases last about 1 week with fever, headache, aches and pains and perhaps nausea. Classical yellow fever often has a biphasic course. The first phase closely resembles a mild case although it may be more severe with vomiting. Following a brief remission of fever, the second phase develops with bradycardia, jaundice and haemorrhages. The jaundice is usually not severe (despite the name). There is bleeding of the gums, epistaxis, haematemesis (often 'coffee-ground' in character), melaena and internal haemorrhage. Oliguria and albuminuria are common but anuria uncommon. The blood pressure falls and coma and delirium may supervene. Death may follow either of these or profuse coffee-ground vomiting. Sometimes the disease is fulminating with earlier death and cases have been described with an atypical encephalomyelitis but without jaundice, albuminuria or haemorrhages. Increased serum bilirubin, a prolonged prothrombin time and a raised blood urea are common but tend to be more severe and to occur earlier in cases which subsequently die. A more detailed account of the clinical picture is given by Strode (1951).

At autopsy there is moderate jaundice and haemorrhages in many organs; the stomach and intestines may contain partly digested blood. The liver shows characteristic microscopic changes; there is midzonal cloudy and fatty degeneration of the parenchymal cells, necrotic cells coalesce and become markedly acidophilic to form the Councilman bodies. In severe cases almost the entire liver lobule may have been destroyed. There is a marked lack of inflammatory reaction. Severe changes may be found in the kidney tubules with debris and casts in their lumina. Petechial haemorrhages may be found in the brain and myocardium. Strode (1951) has given a detailed account of the pathology.

Diagnosis. Classical yellow fever is relatively easily diagnosed in areas where clinicians expect to encounter it. When, however, it occurs in a new area or in one where it has been absent for a number of years it is often misdiagnosed. The existence of yellow fever in Trinidad in 1954 was accidentally discovered by isolation of the virus from the blood of a patient with a mild febrile illness. Retrospectively three fatal cases were found to have occurred in one hospital and to have been diagnosed as 'typhoid with jaundice', 'malaria with jaundice'; and in Panama in 1948, after a long period of absence, four fatal cases were diagnosed by a pathologist as 'acute yellow atrophy'.

Virus can usually be isolated from the blood during the first 4 days of illness and has been isolated as late as the twelfth day. It can sometimes be isolated from the liver at autopsy. A serological diagnosis on paired sera is relatively easy if the patient has not previously been infected with a group B virus but can be difficult or impossible if there have been multiple group B infections (Theiler and Casals, 1958). Fatal yellow fever can also be diagnosed with a fair degree of certainty by histological examination of the liver provided that the epidemiological background is consonant. The viscerotome was designed so that non-medical personnel could collect suitable samples from cadavers and this method has been the basis for surveillance of jungle yellow fever in the Americas. The fixed tissue can be sent long distances without trouble so the method is particularly appropriate wherever there is no nearby expert staff or where communications are difficult.

Treatment is symptomatic except where fluid and electrolyte balances require intravenous infusions or where haemorrhage requires transfusion.

Because mild cases are seldom recognised in sufficient numbers during times of epidemic and because some infections are subclinical, mortality rates are difficult to establish and estimates are very varied. There are no notable sequelae to yellow fever.

Two live attenuated virus vaccines are available: the 17D strain which was attenuated in tissue culture and is prepared in chick embryos; and the French neurotropic strain which was attenuated and is produced in mouse brain. The French vaccine is administered by scarification and 17D vaccine by subcutaneous injection although it has been successfully used by scarification (e.g. Cannon and Dewhurst, 1953; Roever-Bonnet and Hoekstra, 1958). This method offers very considerable economy in effort and vaccine but is less suitable than injection in populations which already have a high incidence of antibody to other group B viruses (Smith *et al*, 1962). Meers (1960) produced a 17D vaccine by one passage in mouse brain and by scarification successfully vaccinated 60 000 Nigerian children without ill effects. 17D vaccine has been very widely used and is one of the most innocuous vaccines. The only serious complications have been non-fatal encephalitis in a very small proportion of children vaccinated under 1 year of age (Stuart, 1956). Macnamara (1953) described the reactions following French vaccine: mild febrile reactions were common, viscerotropic reactions were rare but included albuminuria and jaundice, neurotropic reactions were characterised by encephalitis with a high mortality rate. During the Senegal epidemic in 1965, about 1.9 million received French vaccine and about 120 000 17D. Of the former, at least 246 subsequently developed encephalitis with 23 deaths; about 90 per cent were children under 12 and the risk in this age group was between 1 and 2 per 1000. Only two children developed encephalitis following 17D vaccine (1 : 10 000) and both survived (Chambon *et al*, 1967). Immunity following yellow fever vaccination is long-lasting and an International Vaccination Certificate is valid for 6 years. Because 17D vaccine is labile once suspended in saline, and because of the importance of the validity of International Certificates, vaccination for this purpose can be obtained only at specially designated centres.

Control. Apart from vaccination, control of yellow fever depends on control of *Ae. aegypti* in any infected area. The disease is internationally notifiable and especially careful precautions are taken about vaccination of travellers to and from infected areas and against importation of infected mosquitoes to receptive areas (where it is thought the disease might be spread) such as tropical Asia.

Zika virus has been isolated only in Uganda from man and repeatedly from the mosquito *Ae.*

africanus. It is probably maintained in forest by these mosquitoes and monkeys. Residual antibodies to Zika virus have been reported in many parts of Africa and tropical Asia. These findings, however, must be treated with caution because of difficulties in interpretation of group B serology due to cross-reactions. Knowledge of the disease caused is limited to one accidental laboratory infection which resulted in a brief illness with fever, headache and a rash (Catalogue, 1968).

Group C (Table 5)

Of this group of 13 viruses, nine have each caused small numbers of cases of human disease: Apeu, Caraparu, Itaqui, Madrid, Marituba, Murutucu, Oriboca, Ossa and Restan. They appear to be widely distributed in tropical South and Central America and one has been isolated in Florida. Various members have been isolated from rodents, marsupials and a sloth and from a range of mosquito species. Disease has been mainly among forest workers although a laboratory case due to Apeu virus has been described.

TABLE 5. *Group C arboviruses known to cause human disease*

Virus	Probable transmission to man	Geographical distribution of viruses
Apeu	Mosquito	Brazil
Caruparu	Mosquito	Brazil (Trinidad, Panama)
Itaqui	Mosquito	Brazil
Madrid	Mosquito	Panama
Marituba	Mosquito	Brazil
Murutucu	Mosquito	Brazil
Oriboca	Mosquito	Panama
Ossa	Mosquito	Brazil
Restan	Mosquito	Trinidad, Surinam

The diseases are similar, with fever lasting 2–6 days, headache, backache and general aches and pains. Photophobia, conjunctivitis, vertigo, nausea, pain or tenderness in the right upper quadrant of the abdomen or lymphadenopathy may occur and the fever may be biphasic. Recovery has been complete although convalescence may be protracted. These viruses are probably quite common causes of mild febrile illness in forest workers in tropical South and Central America and their prevalence can be guessed at from the fact that in 1960 in the Belem area of Brazil, 406 isolations were made mainly from sentinel mice (Shope and Causey, 1962).

Bunyamwera group (Table 6)

Members of this group have been found in almost all parts of the inhabited world except Australasia. They have been isolated from a very wide range of mosquito species but their vertebrate maintenance hosts remain obscure. The group contains 14 viruses but only four (probably five) have definitely been incriminated as causes of human disease.

TABLE 6. *Bunyamwera Group arboviruses which are known to cause human disease and occur in the tropics and subtropics*

Virus	Probable transmission to man	Geographical distribution of viruses
Bunyamwera	Mosquito	Africa
Ilesha	Mosquito	E. and W. Africa
Germiston	Mosquito	S. Africa and neighbours
Guaroa	Mosquito	S. and Central America

Bunyamwera virus has caused mild disease in South Africa, Nigeria, Uganda and Zanzibar (Catalogue, 1968), but the total number of cases recorded is eight (five of them probably laboratory infections). In addition to fever, the symptoms included headache, backache, joint pain, a macular rash and abdominal pain. All recovered without incident (E.A.V.R.I., 1962). Southam and Moore (1951) infected four cancer patients, one of which developed severe but non-fatal encephalitis. The virus has been isolated repeatedly from *Ae. circumluteolus* and *Ae. pembaensis* mosquitoes in South Africa and once in Uganda. Antibody surveys suggest that infection is widely distributed in Africa.

Ilesha virus has been recorded as the cause of three mild febrile illnesses in Nigeria and antibody provides evidence of human infection in Ghana and possibly Uganda.

Germiston virus has caused one natural and one laboratory infection in South Africa. Antibody in man has been found in Angola and Botswana and in man and cattle in Kenya. The illnesses were mild with headache and aches and pains.

Chittoor virus has been isolated from *Anopheles* mosquitoes in India, *Batai virus* from *Culex* mosquitoes in Malaya and a closely similar virus from *Aedes* mosquitoes in Sarawak: mild febrile illnesses have been attributed by serological diagnosis to the latter and a very similar virus (*Calovo*) has caused fever and headache in Czechoslovakia.

Guaroa virus has been repeatedly isolated from

man in Colombia and Brazil, both from healthy people and from people with a mild illness: fever, headache, pains in muscles and joints. One patient had alopecia and paresis but the aetiology of these is uncertain (Catalogue, 1968). In Brazil, the virus has been isolated from a liver biopsy from a febrile patient. Residual antibody shows that human infection is common in tropical America, especially Venezuela and Colombia. The virus has been isolated from *Anopheles* mosquitoes in Colombia and Panama.

Phlebotomus group (Table 7)

The Phlebotomus group of viruses has at least 10 members, two of which (Chagres and Candiru) are mentioned below. However, only the Naples and Sicilian viruses are known to be regularly transmitted by *Phlebotomus* flies and to cause sandfly (or *Phlebotomus*) fever.

TABLE 7. *Phlebotomus group arboviruses known to cause human disease*

Virus	Probable transmission to man	Geographical distribution of viruses
Candiru	?	Brazil
Chagres	?	Panama
Naples sandfly fever	Phlebotomus	Mediterranean area
Sicilian sandfly fever	Phlebotomus	Middle East, W. Pakistan, ? India
Punta Toro	?	Panama

Phlebotomus fever. The disease had been recognised and described in the Mediterranean area by 1886, and by 1905 *Phlebotomus papatasi* had been suspected as the vector. Doerr *et al* (1909) successfully proved that *P. papatasi* would transmit the disease from man to man. The disease is broadly distributed throughout the Old World between 20° and 45°N wherever there is a dry climate and suitable breeding places for *P. papatasi*: it has been reported in Malta, Italy, Greece, Cyprus, North Africa including Egypt, Israel, Jordan, Iraq, Sudan, Pakistan, India and in the southern U.S.S.R. Where it is endemic the disease occurs from April to October, is mild, mainly affects children and goes unrecognised unless virological investigations reveal it. However, in such areas it may be rapidly revealed by an epidemic when a new population (usually military) is introduced. Outside the endemic areas, large epidemics occur from time to time. Between

1946 and 1951 large epidemics affected Yugoslavia and surrounding territories: in 1948 in northern Serbia, 75 per cent of a population of 1.2 million were affected (Guelmino and Jevtic, 1955). Epidemics were reported in the Sudan in 1847.

The extrinsic incubation period in *P. papatasi* is 7–10 days. The Sicilian virus has been successfully transmitted from man to man and the virus has been isolated from wild-caught flies. Barnett and Suyemoto (1961) have isolated strains (some of them close to Naples virus) from *Sergentomyia* sandflies. Both Naples and Sicilian virus have been isolated in Italy, Egypt, Iran and Pakistan. No vertebrate maintenance host other than man is known for these viruses, nor is their overwintering mechanism known although there is suggestive evidence that transovarial infection occurs in both *Phlebotomus* and *Sergentomyia* flies.

Clinical descriptions of natural (Fleming *et al*, 1947) and experimentally induced disease (Sabin *et al*, 1944) are similar. The incubation period is usually 3–4 days (2½–6 days). There are occasional prodromal symptoms (constipation, abdominal discomfort, dizziness and malaise) but the onset is usually sudden with severe frontal headache, pain behind the eyes especially on movement, photophobia, backache, joint pains, stiffness of the neck and back, anorexia, nausea, often vomiting, and constipation followed by diarrhoea. There may be slight sore throat, shivering followed by profuse sweating, dizziness and fatigue. The fever lasts about 3 days (limits 1–9 days), is usually highest on the first day, and may fall slowly or be irregular. There is a relative and sometimes a true bradycardia. Marked flushing (which may amount to an erythematous rash) of the face and neck is common and there is congestion of the conjunctiva, fauces and soft palate, tenderness of the eyeballs and a hot skin.

Convalescence is variable: some feel well even before the fever has completely subsided while others have weakness and depression for some time after. Recovery has invariably been complete. Second or even third attacks have been reported, probably due to different viruses in the group, but possibly due to some of the many other infections which can cause a similar symptom complex. Differential diagnosis on clinical grounds between sandfly fever and these other infections is very difficult. Perhaps the question most often asked is whether an epidemic is dengue or sandfly fever —on the basis of many cases they can be distinguished because lymphadenitis is usual in dengue but absent in sandfly fever, and a true rash is common in dengue but uncommon in sandfly fever.

Control depends on control of sandflies usually by insecticide spraying. The malaria eradication programme in Yugoslavia seems virtually to have eliminated sandfly fever. Insect repellents may be helpful under some circumstances. No vaccine is available.

Three other members of the Phlebotomus group, *Candiru, Chagres* (Catalogue, 1968) and *Punta Toro* (personal communication Dr G. E. Sather), have each caused a single natural case of human disease. In Brazil, Candiru virus caused fever, headache, coryza, and aches and pains in muscles and joints. In Panama, Chagres virus caused fever, headache, retro-orbital pain and vomiting; and Punta Toro virus fever, headache, muscle pains, hepatomegaly, splenomegaly and an increased CSF protein (66 mg/100 ml) without an increase of cells. Their modes of transmission or of natural maintenance are unknown.

Arenoviruses (Table 8)

Junin virus: Argentinian haemorrhagic fever. This disease appears to have been known in the north-west of the Buenos Aires province since the early 1940s, but epidemics have occurred annually in the area since 1958 and it seems to have spread further north-west. Between 300 and 1000 cases have been reported annually. The death rate seems

TABLE 8. *Arenoviruses known to cause human disease in the Tropics*

Virus	*Probable transmission to man*	*Geographical distribution of viruses*
Junin	Rodent urine	Argentina
Machupo	Rodent urine	Upper Amazon
Lassa	?	Nigeria

to have been falling: from 20 per cent in 1958, to 3 per cent in 1963 (PAHO, 1963). The disease occurs in autumn and early winter: March to August with the peak in May. Males make up 80–85 per cent of cases and two-thirds were aged 16–55 years, probably because infection is acquired in the maize fields at harvest time. The virus has been isolated from rodents in endemic areas (*Mus musculus* (repeatedly), *Hesperomys laucha, Akodon arenicola*) and they are possibly (even probably) the maintenance hosts. The infection is probably transmitted (as is the closely related

Machupo virus) in their excreta, especially urine. The virus has been isolated from mites but they may be incidental hosts.

Clinical features. The incubation period is estimated as 7–16 days (usually 10–12 days). There is a slow onset of fever, malaise, drowsiness, general weakness, headache, back and muscle pains, anorexia, nausea and vomiting. There is general pallor but facial erythema associated with conjunctival injection and palpebral oedema. After 3–5 days an enanthem in the mouth, which may be visible earlier, becomes pronounced: the gum margins are red and bleed easily; characteristic vesicles with a red-violet background are seen on the soft palate and fauces. About the same time a petechial rash appears, most marked in the axillae and on the chest. There is no detectable splenomegaly or hepatomegaly. About half the cases have a dry cough but no changes in chest X-rays. Signs of dehydration including a dry tongue, foul breath and oliguria often occur between the third and sixth days. Anuria or haematuria are uncommon. Most patients also have hypotension (both systolic and diastolic), relative bradycardia and often ECG changes, mainly in the ST segment. Lymphadenopathy, mainly axillary, is slow to subside. Two-thirds of patients have loss of equilibrium and half of them ataxia. More severe cases may have haemorrhages from mucous membranes, epistaxis, haematemesis, haematuria or melaena.

Death may occur in uraemic coma or in profound hypotension and shock. In non-fatal cases the fever lasts about 8 days and falls by lysis. There is a marked diuresis and fairly rapid recovery although convalescence may be prolonged. There are no known sequelae. A temperature over 104°F (40°C), haematemesis or melaena are of bad prognosis. About 20 per cent of cases had only a mild febrile illness while between 3 and 7 per cent were gravely ill. This account is based on an account of 1700 cases in several papers by Rugiero *et al* (1964).

Laboratory findings include marked leukopenia for 6–8 days, absence of eosinophils, almost constant and sometimes severe thrombocytopenia, increased blood urea which may reach 200 mg/ml, moderate to severe albuminuria, and large numbers of cellular and granular casts in the urine together with characteristic round cells with cytoplasmic inclusions. The ESR increases only when the patient begins to improve. There is marked reduction in serum albumin and an increase in beta globulin which return to normal levels in convalescence. Gamma globulin increases markedly during recovery and convalescence.

At autopsy there is general congestion of the viscera, especially the liver and kidney which are also oedematous. Histologically there is moderate granular degeneration of parenchymal cells and central veins in the liver. In the kidney there is granular degeneration of the epithelium of the glomeruli and convoluted tubules; haemorrhage, hyaline and blood casts can be seen in the tubules.

Diagnosis. Virus has been isolated from blood 3 to 8 days after onset and from liver, spleen, kidney and brain. Guinea pigs have been most commonly used: they die usually 11–15 days after inoculation and show fever, weight loss and viraemia. At post-mortem there are subcutaneous petechial or larger haemorrhages in tissues, abdominal lymph nodes, adrenals and intestinal walls. Newborn mice are susceptible to intra-cerebral inoculation. There is no vaccine and only supportive therapy.

Machupo virus: Bolivian haemorrhagic fever. Machupo virus is closely related to Junin virus and causes a rather similar disease. Bolivian haemorrhagic fever was formerly an occasional disease of rural workers, but was first recognised when epidemics occurred between 1959 and 1962 during the dry season in two separate areas of the Beni Department of North-east Bolivia. The disease was of exceptionally high incidence (an attack rate of up to 10 per cent) and of such severity that in some places the people fled their homes. It was twice as common in males over 15 than in females and commoner in those aged over 15 than in children under 10.

The best studied outbreak was in San Joachim, where there were 650 cases and 115 deaths in a population of only 2500. The town was found to have a large population of a rodent *Calomys callosus* (normally a grassland species but found in peridomestic and domestic habitats) which was found to be infected with the virus, to excrete it in the urine for at least 100 days, and to have viraemia for at least 42 days. The infection was probably transmitted to man by urinary contamination from the rodents and the epidemic was brought to an end by eradication of *Calomys* from the town. There is a strong suggestion that the establishment of a dense population of *Calomys* was facilitated by previous DDT spraying (in a malaria eradication campaign) which caused a high mortality in cats in the town.

In rural situations the disease is associated with areas of riverine forest where the spiny rat, *Proechimys cayannensis* and *C. callosus* live together. Although there was no evidence of infection from man to man in Bolivia, one of the scientists studying the disease acquired it and was evacuated to Panama, where he infected his wife. Kissing was suggested as the mode of transmission because virus could be recovered from throat swabs.

Clinically (MacKenzie *et al*, 1964) there is an acute febrile onset with headache, pains in the limbs and back, intention tremor of the tongue and hands, and haemorrhagic manifestations such as petechiae in the mouth and on the skin (especially in the axillae), epistaxis, haematemesis and melaena. Vomiting, diarrhoea, conjunctivitis and respiratory symptoms may occur. After 7–10 days there may be marked hypotension and the onset of central nervous symptoms (in about 25 per cent): death usually occurs during this stage. The death rate in frank cases is estimated at 30 per cent. Temporary alopecia is common during convalescence but there are no other notable sequelae.

The *pathology* of eight fatal cases has been described (Child *et al*, 1967). Congestion and interstitial haemorrhages especially in the gastrointestinal tract and CNS were the most striking features. Eosinophil inclusions were seen in Kupffer cells in the liver and local coagulative necrosis in some cases. There was widespread proliferation of the reticuloendothelial system in liver, spleen and lymph nodes. Interstitial pneumonitis was common.

Lassa fever was first recognised in January 1969 when a missionary nurse become ill in Lassa, North-Eastern State, Nigeria. She was flown to hospital in Jos, where two other nurses were affected—the first case and one of these died. The other was flown for treatment to the United States, where two laboratory workers were affected. In January and February 1970, a short sharp outbreak of 28 cases occurred in Jos. Serological studies indicate that Lassa virus infection is widespread in Nigeria and occurs at least as far west as Guinea. Although no host other than man has yet been identified for this virus, its classification as an arenovirus suggests that its maintenance hosts are rodents (Carey *et al*, 1972; Henderson *et al*, 1972). Transmission can clearly occur between patients and from them to staff in hospitals although the mode is unknown.

Clinically the disease presents with high fever, toxicity, headache, vomiting, diarrhoea, severe pharyngitis with white patches on the pharynx, soft palate and tonsillar pillars, cough, epigastric pain and tenderness, and a bleeding tendency. Symptoms and signs of both gastrointestinal and respiratory involvement were present in all cases. About half the patients had renal changes—albuminuria, granular casts, raised blood urea.

Cardiac failure occurred in about a quarter and was probably the cause of death in them. Confusion and delirium were recorded and several patients (mostly those in shock) were unconscious for varying periods before death. Abnormal bleeding (injection and cut-down sites, haemophilia, haematemesis, haematuria, espistaxis) occurred in about a third of the patients and constitutes a risk of infection to others. The clinical and laboratory data are described by White (1972).

Edington and White (1972) have described the pathology of two cases as somewhat similar to mosquito-borne and monkeys may be its vertebrate maintenance host. Antibody surveys show infection of man to be widespread in Africa and a closely related virus (*Pongola*) is found in South Africa (Catalogue, 1968).

Changuinola virus, isolated in Panama from *Phlebotomus* sandflies has caused a natural mild febrile illness in a mosquito catcher. He had fever, headache and joint pains (Catalogue, 1968).

Guama and **Catu** are related viruses known only from Trinidad and Brazil. They have been isolated from *Culex* and *Mansonia* mosquitoes, rodents

TABLE 9. *Smaller arbovirus groups of which members are known to cause human disease*

Virus	Antigenic group	Probable transmission to man	Geographical distribution of viruses	Other features
Bwamba	Bwamba	Mosquito	E. and W. Africa	Cases only in Uganda
Changuinola	Changuinola	Phlebotomus	Panama	
Guama	Guama	Mosquito	Brazil, Trinidad	
Catu	Guama	Mosquito	Brazil, Trinidad	
Chandipura	Piry	?	India	
Piry	Piry	?	Brazil	Lab. cases only
Oropouche	Simbu	Mosquito	Trinidad, Brazil, Colombia	
Quaranfil	Quaranfil	Argas tick	Egypt, S. Africa	
Vesicular stomatitis	Vesicular stomatitis	Contact, ? Phlebotomus	U.S.A., S. and Central America	Most human cases from contact with infected domestic animals

that of dengue and Bolivian haemorrhagic fevers. There is generalised capillary damage with increased permeability which accounts for the serous effusions. Haemorrhages are widespread and there is severe liver damage with eosiniphil necrosis of liver cells and eosinophilic bodies in the sinusoids resembling those in yellow fever. There were focal pneumonitis, gross oedema of the intestine with haemorrhages, oedema and haemorrhages in the myocardium. Kidney changes were less severe than the clinical findings suggested.

Other groups (Tables 9 and 10)

Bwamba virus was isolated in western Uganda in 1937 from the blood of nine patients with an acute febrile illness of sudden onset, together with headache, backache, and sometimes conjunctivitis, lasting 5–7 days. It is probably and marsupials. Three cases of febrile illness have been reported due to each virus in forest workers in the Belem area. The illness lasted 4–6 days with headache, aches and pains, and sometimes dizziness, photophobia and nausea. All recovered completely (Causey *et al*, 1961).

Piry virus has caused five cases of febrile illness in laboratory workers with headache, aches and pains in muscles and joints, anorexia and tenderness in the right upper abdominal quadrant. It was isolated in Brazil from an opossum but its mode of transmission is unknown.

Chandipura, a related virus, was isolated in India from two patients with fever, and aches and pains in muscles and joints during an outbreak of febrile disease in Nagpur in the presence of infections with chikungunya and dengue viruses (Catalogue, 1968).

Oropouche virus was first isolated in Trinidad from the blood of a patient with fever, backache and cough. More recently, there was an outbreak involving more than 7000 people in the suburbs of Belem, Brazil (Theiler and Downs, 1963). The illness lasted 2–7 days with fever, headache, backache, general aches and pains. Some cases had conjunctival injection, photophobia and delirium, but there were no deaths, notable complications or sequelae. There were also inapparent infections. The virus has been isolated from *Ae. serratus* and *Mansonia* mosquitoes and there is evidence of human infections but not, so far, of disease in Colombia, Brazil and Trinidad.

TABLE 10. *Ungrouped arboviruses known to cause human disease*

Virus	Probable transmission to man	Geographical distribution of viruses	Other features
Congo	? Tick	Tropical Africa ? Pakistan	*syn.* Crimean haemorrhagic fever
Nairobi sheep disease	Ixodid tick	E. and Central Africa	
Rift Valley fever	Mosquito, Contact	E., S. and Central Africa	Most human cases from contact with infected domestic animals

Quaranfil virus is probably transmitted to man by *Argas* ticks in heron colonies and has caused febrile illnesses in two children in Egypt. The virus has been isolated from birds and *Argas* ticks in Egypt and South Africa (Catalogue, 1968).

Vesicular stomatitis is a disease of cattle, horses and pigs but can affect man. It is endemic in the United States, Mexico, Panama, Colombia, Ecuador and Peru. There are two serotypes (New Jersey and Indiana) and the Indiana type has been repeatedly isolated from *Phlebotomus* sandflies in Panama, where there is also evidence of fairly frequent human infections particularly in forest areas. Knowledge of the disease in man is limited to cases due to laboratory infections or to contact with diseased domestic animals. However, *Phlebotomus*-transmitted infection in Central and South America must be regarded as possible. Residual antibody shows that infections of man are common in Panama.

The disease in laboratory workers has a sudden onset of fever with shivering and profuse perspiration, generalised aching, pain in the eyes, headache and dizziness. Anorexia is common but few have nausea. Sore throat occurs in 30 per cent and respiratory distress and coryza in 10 per cent. 'Fever blisters' on the buccal surface of the lips are common and raised vesicles are also seen. These may be due to reactivation of latent herpes simplex. Cervical and submaxillary lymphadenopathy is common. Conjunctivitis occurs in 20 per cent but may be due partially to sand from the tissue-grinding process. The disease lasts 2–3 days but a second phase starting about the fourth day occurs in 10 per cent. Recovery has been complete. However, if it occurs, the disease may differ in several respects when the infection is arthropod-transmitted.

Congo viruses (Simpson *et al*, 1967) seem to be widely distributed in tropical Africa and a related virus has been isolated in Pakistan. A Congo virus is responsible for Crimean haemorrhagic fever (Casals, 1969). Twelve strains have been isolated from the blood of patients in East Africa and elsewhere from cattle and ticks.

Clinically it causes fever, prostration, severe headache and backache, and photophobia. Anorexia, nausea and vomiting occurred in several patients. The illness lasts 5–10 days and is followed by gradual recovery. One patient died when he was about to be discharged from hospital following a sudden severe haematemesis.

Nairobi sheep disease virus which causes acute gastroenteritis in sheep, with a high mortality, has caused mild disease with fever and aches and pains in a laboratory worker, and antibody to this virus is common in East Africans. Three subclinical human infections have been detected serologically. The infection is transmitted by the tick *Rhipicephalus appendiculatus* and is distributed in a broad belt of Africa south of a line from Nairobi (Kenya) to Kisenyi (Congo), as far south as the Kalahari, Botswana, Zululand and Mozambique (Catalogue, 1968).

Rift Valley fever is an important disease of sheep, cattle and goats in Africa and is probably transmitted to them by mosquitoes. Some human cases have been due to mosquito transmission but most appear to have been due to contact with infected animal tissues and have thus affected farmers, veterinarians, butchers and laboratory workers. In 1950–51 a great epizootic with 100 000 deaths in sheep and cattle occurred in South Africa and an estimated 20 000 people were infected. In man, the onset of disease is sudden with fever, malaise, aches and pains; vertigo and discomfort over the liver are common. Epistaxis or retinopathy may occur. Only one fatal case has been recorded and recovery is usually uneventful although sometimes slow. A formalinised vaccine prepared in monkey kidney cell cultures exists and has given good antibody responses without notable adverse reactions in over 1000 people. It has been successful in preventing illness following laboratory infections and immunity lasts about 18 months (Randall *et al*, 1963).

ADENOVIRUSES

This group of viruses seems to be worldwide in distribution. Three types of human disease are recorded:

1. An acute non-fatal respiratory disease mainly studied in epidemics among military recruit populations in U.S.A.
2. Pharyngitis sometimes associated with conjunctivitis.
3. Follicular conjunctivitis and keratoconjunctivitis.

Large outbreaks of keratoconjunctivitis have occurred in the Far East and in Hawaii as well as in North America and Europe. Spread may be partly due to poor aseptic technique in dispensaries.

ENTEROVIRUSES

In conditions of poor hygiene, which are common in most tropical countries, the opportunities for transmission of enteroviruses are abundant and the general epidemiological pattern is of universal infection with a variety of enteroviruses in early infancy. This pattern existed in many temperate countries where the population was sufficiently dense until the advent of modern hygiene—particularly water-borne sanitation and its educated use. In any community there was probably a limited number of enteroviruses in some sort of equilibrium with the human and perhaps to some extent the animal population of the area. This situation probably still exists in relatively isolated rural communities, but with the growth of towns and cities, with major population movements particularly in recent wars, and with the great increase of travel, new strains of virus must often be introduced into communities. There are no known substantial differences between the enterovirus diseases whether they occur in tropical or temperate areas; the differences are epidemiological and therefore may affect different age groups. The diseases are well described in standard medical texts. The milder enterovirus diseases are of course seldom recognised in underdeveloped areas. Special attention is directed to the risks of exposure to infection when people from a country with a high level of hygiene (and possibly little or no previous infec-

tion with enteroviruses) go to an area where enteroviruses are highly prevalent.

Poliomyelitis. Until recent years the picture in tropical areas has been of 'infantile paralysis': very high rates of infection but only sporadic cases almost entirely in children under 5. Small outbreaks occurred (mainly in Europeans), notably epidemics among allied troops in Africa during the Second World War. More recently epidemics have begun to appear in cities such as Colombo without any very noticeable improvement in the general standards of hygiene. Factors in the change include increasing overcrowding, changes in behaviour and falling neonatal and infantile mortality rates. In contrast to the seasonal occurrence of poliomyelitis in temperate regions, infections occur throughout the year in the tropics with perhaps the highest rate at the hottest period of the year.

The remedy lies in vaccination, and live virus vaccines taken orally have in large measure taken over from inactivated vaccines because of their relative cheapness and ease of administration. The three types of poliovirus can be given one at a time or in a triple vaccine and the appropriate procedure is usually determined by logistic considerations. In general, three doses of triple vaccine are advisable. The vaccines are usually administered as a few drops on a sugar lump or in a syrup. Highly potent inactivated vaccines also exist and are preferred by some authorities for vaccination of individuals as opposed to large numbers, especially where cost is a minor factor.

Everyone travelling to the tropics should be vaccinated against the polioviruses. It is more difficult to decide whether and when to advise mass vaccination in underdeveloped areas. If such vaccination is contemplated it must cover as high a proportion as possible of the children and young adults and must be accomplished as quickly as possible. The cost in effort and money is substantial and must be balanced against other medical and public health needs. Each situation must be judged on its merits, but at the stage where endemic sporadic cases change to small outbreaks, there is an indication for vaccination, because larger epidemics are likely to follow. Once mass vaccination has been done, it is essential to set up a long-term, well-designed and adequately financed scheme to vaccinate all children born subsequently. Usually each type is given separately some time after 3 months of age and a fourth dose of triple vaccine given soon after the first birthday.

In the face of an actual epidemic, mass vaccination with live vaccine given very quickly can arrest it. Usually a monovalent vaccine of the type of virus causing the epidemic is used and followed later by measures to vaccinate against the remaining types.

Coxsackievirus. These viruses fall into groups A and B largely on the basis of the type of lesions they cause in newborn mice and hamsters. They are common enteric infections throughout the world. The following types of illness have been attributed to them: aseptic meningitis, occasionally paralysis, rash, hepatitis, pneumonitis. In addition, group A viruses have caused herpangina and coryza; and group B pleurodynia, meningoencephalitis and myocarditis in infants. A full account of diseases due to Coxsackieviruses has been given by Dalldorf and Melnick (1965).

Echovirus. These viruses, which can be isolated only in cell cultures, are commonly found in the intestinal tract in all parts of the world. They can cause febrile illnesses with or without rash, and are common causes of aseptic meningitis. A wide range of other lesions have been attributed to them (Melnick, 1965). German *et al* (1968) recently described an outbreak of febrile illness with a wide range of signs and symptoms due to echovirus-5 in a maternity unit in Singapore.

ENCEPHALOMYOCARDITIS VIRUS

Strains are widely distributed in the world and probably have rodents as their maintenance hosts. The virus has been isolated from cases clinically diagnosed as paralytic poliomyelitis, aseptic meningitis and encephalomyelitis. No fatal cases have been recorded. Myocarditis does not seem to be a feature of the human disease although it occurs in experimental animals. Fourteen cases of mild CNS disease were reported by Gadjusek (1955). An epidemic of '3 day fever' among American troops in Manila in 1945–46 appears to have been due to encephalomyocarditis virus (Smadel and Warren, 1947). There was a sudden onset of severe headache and fever lasting 2–3 days with pharyngitis, stiff neck, positive Kernig's sign, increased reflexes, and coma in a few. The CSF contained 50–500 cells/mm³, mainly lymphocytes. All recovered. For diagnosis, both virus isolation from the blood and demonstration of an increase in circulating antibody are desirable as these viruses may be present in the experimental animal colonies used for isolation.

HEPATITIS VIRUS

Infectious hepatitis and serum hepatitis. The viruses of these diseases are not yet well defined,

Z

but they appear to be of worldwide distribution. They seem to be highly prevalent in the Mediterranean area, the Middle East, parts of Africa, the East, and Central and South America. Epidemics have occurred in immigrant military populations in many of these areas, but no accurate estimates can be made of the prevalence in their indigenous populations because the diseases are not notifiable and laboratory diagnostic procedures are not available. The infectious hepatitis virus (or viruses) is probably excreted mainly in the faeces and contamination of water or food is the most likely vehicle of transmission. Thus wherever water or food hygiene is of low standard, transmission of infectious hepatitis is likely to be frequent. Inapparent infections and a carrier state are probably common in endemic areas especially among infants and young children. Shellfish from infected water can be infected. Outbreaks of infectious hepatitis are often preceded by a wave of gastroenteric illness.

Serum hepatitis is spread mainly by contamination of syringes with blood from symptomless carriers or cases, or similarly by blood transfusion, renal dialysis, tattooing, etc. Diagnosis in carriers or cases is by demonstration of hepatitis-associated (Australia) antigen in serum (Zuckerman, 1970). The incubation period of serum hepatitis is often much longer than that of infectious hepatitis.

Control depends on good food and water hygiene, on careful use of syringes and needles, and on careful control of donors of blood and blood-products for transfusion. All injections (including dental injections) should be given with a separate syringe and needle for each patient—much easier now with disposable equipment. Mass vaccinations should be carried out with a well-designed jet injector which does not carry over blood contamination from one recipient to the next. Needles for vaccination by scarification must be carefully sterilised, usually by flame, between use. No really satisfactory method has been found for sterilisation of blood or blood-products although storage of plasma at 90°F for 6 months (a hardly practical procedure) has sharply reduced incidence of hepatitis in recipients (Allen, 1960). However, serum albumin can be made safe by heating at 60°F and the cold ethanol process for gamma globulin preparation also seems to be effective.

There is no vaccine. Contacts (e.g. family contacts) can be partially protected by the administration of gamma globulin. Passive partial protection lasts from 3–6 months depending on dose. There is some evidence that natural infection during passive protection may confer active immunity with little or no disease and a dose of

0.05 ml/pound body weight every 6 months has been advised for immigrants to heavily infected areas. This regime has been used to a considerable extent in the American forces in Vietnam. However, there must be some doubt about the advisability of more than a very small number of doses of gamma globulin which may be slightly altered by processing and lead to possible long term autoimmunity problems.

Although serum hepatitis is probably transmitted *in utero* to result in symptomless carriers and all possible infective donors cannot be excluded, no blood donors should be accepted (except in extreme urgency) who have a history of hepatitis or of close contact with cases of hepatitis during the previous 6 months, or who have received a transfusion of blood or plasma within 6 months. Plasma should be made from the blood of not more than two donors to avoid contamination of large pools and transmission to large numbers of patients from a single source (W.H.O., 1953).

HERPESVIRUSES

Known human infections comprise herpes simplex virus (Herpesvirus hominis), the B virus of rhesus monkeys (Herpesvirus simiae) and chickenpox virus (Herpesvirus varicellae). Primary infections with herpes simplex can cause herpetic dermatitis which may present as an infection of pre-existing eczema, traumatic herpes, herpetic gingivostomatitis, herpetic rhinitis, herpes of the genitalia, herpes keratoconjunctivitis or keratitis, herpes meningoencephalitis—all of these usually in infants or children. Neonatal herpes which often includes severe hepatitis is usually fatal. Recurrent herpes results from reactivation of a latent infection; 'cold sores' are its commonest form but more severe lesions can occur, particularly ophthalmic herpes. Primary infections are common in conditions of poor hygiene and particularly under primitive conditions and are most prevalent between 1 and 3 years of age. There are no control measures other than good hygiene and no effective specific treatment exists except for ophthalmic herpes where 5-iodo-2'-deoxyuridine and related compounds appear to be effective (Kaufman and Heidelberger, 1964).

B virus usually causes an ulcerative stomatitis in rhesus monkeys from which the infection can be transmitted to man by bite or by salivary contamination of scratches. Monkey kidney tissue cultures may also present a hazard for laboratory workers. In man there is an acute and frequently fatal encephalomyelitis. A history of monkey bite should always be sought in cases of encephalitis where recent contact with rhesus monkeys is possible. Other monkey species have now been shown to harbour herpesviruses and each primate species probably has a herpesvirus. The pathogenicity for man of simian herpesviruses (other than B virus) is unknown but any monkey bite should be regarded as potentially dangerous and avoided. There is no vaccine available and no specific treatment for B virus infection.

Chickenpox and its recurrent form, herpes zoster, are worldwide and have no known special tropical features.

MYXOVIRUSES

Influenza, para-influenza and mumps virus infections have a worldwide distribution and no notable differences are known between their characteristics in tropical and non-tropical areas.

Measles. Now a relatively mild disease in most parts of the world, measles is a severe one in Central and South America and in West Africa and therefore deserves special mention. Mortality from measles is 10 times as high in South America and 20 times as high in Central America as in North America. However, it is a mild disease in the Caribbean area. In West Africa a doctor is likely to encounter 250 deaths in a measles epidemic for every death he would encounter in a similar epidemic in England.

Clinical features. In West Africa the disease is common in the first year of life and most children have been infected by the age of 3 years. Epidemics are commonest in the dry season but may occur at any time. The degree of confluence of the rash seems to have little bearing on the outcome of the disease but there is a progressively increasing mortality with the degree of darkening of the rash and with the size of the desquamation plaques. There is a higher mortality in children with purulent discharge from the eyes as opposed to injected conjunctivas. 4.5 per cent have a purulent discharge from the ears. Children with 'thrush' or ulceration in the mouth (reflected in impairment of sucking) have a notably higher mortality. Laryngeal obstruction causes a very high mortality. Half the children have dyspnoea or other evidence of pneumonia and bronchopneumonia is a common cause of death. Associated diarrhoea is an outstanding feature: mucus and blood in the stool have a poor prognosis and prolapse of the anus may occur. Mortality increases with the degree of dehydration. Symptoms of malnutrition (oedema or the skin changes of kwashiorkor) tend to be aggravated by the disease and the prognosis is impaired by malnutrition. Convulsions and other manifestations of CNS involvement are not uncommon. The body weights of children admitted to hospital with measles are well below the average for the area either because they have lost weight before admission or because underweight children are at higher risk. The mortality is about 14 per cent of admissions to hospital in children up to 3 years of age and about 7 per cent in older children although higher rates have been reported in Africa.

Vaccines. In recent years a number of measles vaccines have become available and have been widely used. Extension campaigns have been carried out in Latin America and in West Africa in recent years (Foege, 1971). The inactivated vaccines made from whole virus preparations are now generally discarded because of the poor immunity they induce and because there is evidence that they can aggravate disease due to subsequent natural infection (Fulginiti *et al*, 1967; Scott and Bonnano, 1967). Newer inactivated vaccines prepared by fractionation and purification of the whole virus material are however showing promise and may take over again where cost is not a major factor. A number of live vaccines are now available (Morley, 1967), and have been accepted for general use in Britain and elsewhere. There is no doubt about their efficiency and the desirability of their use in areas where measles is a severe illness. With the newest vaccines the reaction and complication rates are very low although the earlier live vaccines caused mild clinical measles.

Morley (1967) recommends that in situations such as West Africa, children should be vaccinated at the age of 6–7 months and again at 9–10 months of age because some of the earlier vaccinations will have failed due to persistent maternal antibody. He also discusses the costs and procedures such as the use of jet injectors for mass vaccination against measles. Cooper *et al* (1966) have described the use of the dermojet.

A comparison has been made in Hong Kong children between two live attenuated vaccines. One gave a higher complication rate and higher antibody responses than the other. Both were satisfactory (over 96 per cent antibody conversions) given intramuscularly but neither gave acceptably high conversion rates (at the dose given) by intradermal inoculation (75–86 per cent conversion) (Hong Kong Measles Vaccine Committee, 1967). In infants at special risk, e.g. with chronic illnesses, gamma globulin may be used (10 iu/kg body weight) and if given within 5–6

days of exposure will usually prevent overt disease. A smaller dose (2 iu/kg) given in the same way will often make the disease mild without preventing the development of subsequent lasting immunity (Katz and Enders, 1965).

RABIES

All warm blooded animals are susceptible to infection with rabies virus which causes fatal disease of the central nervous system in most of them, and because it is frequently excreted in the saliva it is usually transmitted by bite. Most human infections are derived from dogs, but the disease exists in wild life from the Arctic to the tropics in both the Old and the New Worlds. Wild-life rabies is often unrecognised except when wild animals attack and infect man or his domestic animals. The true maintenance hosts may be the Mustelidae and Viverridae, but this account will concentrate on important sources of infection in the tropics. In India, jackals and mongooses are most important, in Asia Minor wolves have caused serious outbreaks in man. In Africa, a variety of animals have been incriminated, notably meerkats in South Africa. In Central and South America and in the Caribbean, the vampire bat (*Desmodus rotundus*) is an important source of infection, especially for cattle, and is able to act as a symptomless carrier for up to 5 months. A few human cases have occurred in America and elsewhere, due to bites by insectivorous or frugivorous bats, but this appears to be a relatively unimportant source of infection except perhaps in limited areas of western North America. Introduced Indian mongooses have been responsible for human rabies in Puerto Rico and Grenada. With wild-life rabies, the most important lesson to be learned is that the disease often causes a change in behaviour: a 'friendly' wild animal which children can play with is quite likely to have rabies and should be avoided at all costs. Similarly, a sick wild animal must be regarded as dangerous and not handled.

Dog rabies is however by far the most important source of human disease, and anyone who lives in an area where rabies occurs should be able to recognise the early signs of the disease. The incubation period is very variable, but usually 10–12 weeks. The infecting bite often goes unnoticed and has usually healed when rabies occurs. The first sign is a sudden change in disposition: an affectionate dog becomes snappy and uncertain or a reserved and uncertain dog becomes affectionate and seeks human companionship. It is of the greatest importance to recognise this stage, which lasts 2–3 days. It is followed by 'furious' or 'dumb' rabies and one or other of these forms tends to predominate in particular outbreaks. In the furious form the dog is first restless, has a watchful, puzzled or apprehensive look and may snap at imaginary objects. There is a characteristic 'howl'. The dog then acquires more than normal energy and strength and an insensitivity to pain: it will run aimlessly for long distances biting anything in its path, or if restrained will attack bars, chains or wire netting to such an extent as to reduce its teeth to stumps with gross laceration of the mouth. The furious stage lasts 1–4 days and is followed by ataxia, paralysis and death. In the dumb form, the dog bites only when disturbed but develops paralysis, coma and dies. In either form death occurs 3–7 days after onset but virus may be present in the saliva for as long as 3 days before onset of signs of disease.

Rabies in man

The disease in man follows a rather similar course. The incubation period varies from 10 days to about 7 months but is usually about 6 weeks and incubation periods longer than 3 months are uncommon. Bites with deep and large lacerations, bites in children and particularly bites of the head, neck or upper limbs are all associated with a short incubation period and prophylactic treatment of these should be especially urgent and vigorous.

During the premonitory stage of the disease, lasting 1–4 days, there is usually low fever, malaise, anorexia, nausea and headache. Respiration is often so shallow that the patient has to stop speaking and take long sighing breath. Changes in personality and nervousness are common and there may be attacks of acute anxiety. In more than three-quarters of cases there is some form of abnormal sensation around the causative wound (itching, aching, stabbing pains, etc.) and there may be mild local inflammation due to scratching or the application of counter-irritants. The patient may be hypersensitive to stimuli such as cold, draughts, bright lights, noises. He may complain of pain in the back, epigastrium or elsewhere. Vomiting may occur, often associated with severe headache.

In most patients, a stage of excitement follows and may last until death which occurs within 1–3 days. Aimless wandering about the room is common and speech is often incoherent. Periods of acute mania may alternate with depression and acute morbid anxiety. Convulsions which may

be fatal often occur during these maniacal attacks. Pyrexia is usual and may reach 103°F. The classical, although not constant, symptom of hydrophobia is very characteristic: when the patient tries to drink, or even sometimes thinks of drinking, the muscles of the pharynx go into sudden acute spasm so that any fluid taken is violently ejected and the head is thrown back. Cases with typical hydrophobia yet able to swallow solids have been described. The respiratory muscles may be affected causing apnoea followed by cyanosis and severe dyspnoea.

In the late stages Cheyne-Stokes breathing is not uncommon. The patient is unable to swallow his saliva and becomes dehydrated due to lack of fluid intake. The saliva, which may be infective, becomes very ropy and tenacious. Tremors and weakness especially of the ocular and facial muscles may be observed. The reflexes may be increased in the early stages but are usually absent later. There may be some stiffness of the neck but Kernig's sign cannot be elicited. Babinski's sign may be positive. Patients who survive the stage of excitement pass quickly into apathy, paralysis and coma which occasionally lasts as long as 10 days but is usually brief and most patients retain consciousness until near the end. Rare cases are paralytic from the onset and show little of the stage of excitement. Recently a small number of cases of recovery from rabies has been reported following prolonged very intensive medical care with particular attention to controlling respiratory function. This should obviously be followed up wherever suitable intensive care facilities are available.

Diagnosis. There may be a relative or absolute polymorphonuclear leukocytosis. The CSF is usually normal, seldom under pressure, the protein may be slightly increased and the cell count rarely exceeds 100 lymphocytes/mm³. There is usually marked albuminuria and there may be glycosuria.

There is no treatment other than symptomatic for the disease. *Medical and nursing staff should exercise care and recognise that the patient's saliva and other secretions may be infective.*

Diagnosis depends on the history of bite, sensory symptoms at the site of the bite and the clinical picture. Virus has occasionally been isolated from the saliva and is probably often present in it. Definitive diagnosis usually depends on the isolation of virus from the CNS at post-mortem and on the demonstration of Negri bodies in the brain. Fluorescent antibody tests on fresh brain are now commonly used. *Great care must be exercised in removing the brains from the skulls:*

protective clothing, heavy gloves and eye shields are essential. Infected tissues stored in neutral glycerol retain infectivity for several weeks at room temperature and for months at 4°C. Part of the brain can thus be sent to the laboratory in 50 per cent glycerol in buffered saline for virus isolation and part in an appropriate fixative for histology. Virus isolation attempts are made by intracerebral inoculation of mice, in the brains of which Negri bodies can usually be demonstrated when they are moribund.

Autopsy. Gross examination of the brain reveals meningeal congestion and some cerebral oedema. When the bite is in a limb, the cut surface of the cord frequently shows unilateral pinkish-grey discoloration most marked in the posterior horn. Microscopically there is general congestion and maybe perivascular haemorrhages, especially in the thalamus and beneath the ependyma. Severe damage to nerve cells is widespread—usually most marked in the medulla and midbrain but also in the cortex of cerebrum and cerebellum and in the spinal cord. When changes are present in the spinal cord they are found also in the corresponding posterior root ganglia. No lesions can be found in the root ganglia in neuroparalytic accidents, a helpful feature in distinguishing them from paralytic rabies. A variable degree of demyelination is common. Interstitial round cell infiltration and perivascular cuffing vary in degree with the duration of the disease. There may be infiltration of the meninges.

Negri bodies are the only characteristic findings and are diagnostic when seen. They vary greatly in numbers however and cannot always be found. About 10 per cent of suspect brains in which Negri bodies cannot be demonstrated can be shown to contain rabies virus by animal inoculation. Negri bodies are round or oval eosinophil inclusions found in the cytoplasm of nerve cells. There may be several in one cell and they vary in size. The characteristic internal structure which confirms their nature can be seen in the larger bodies and consists of a central granule or a ring of granules which show as vacuoles by some staining methods. When present, Negri bodies are usually most numerous in the hippocampal gyrus but common also in the pyramid cells of the cortex and in the Purkinje cells of the cerebellum. They are also found in the basal ganglia, cranial nerve nuclei and in the spinal cord.

Prophylactic treatment for bitten persons. When treatment is sought for any animal bite, the responsible animal should, if at all possible, be identified, caught and placed under veterinary observation. Biting dogs should not be killed immediately as this makes diagnosis difficult. If the biting animal is dead, its brain should be examined for Negri bodies as soon as possible and virus isolation attempted from it. If the dog is known to have been effectively vaccinated against rabies sufficiently recently, it is unlikely that its bite would be infective.

The bite wound should be washed out as soon as possible with plenty of water and 20 per cent soap solution, a quaternary ammonium compound, or other suitable antiseptic. Soap must be washed from the wound before a quaternary ammonium compound is used, because soap neutralises the activity of these compounds. Vigorous scrubbing or interference with the wound should however be avoided. Cauterisation with nitric acid is of doubtful value and should, if used, be reserved for deep puncture wounds inaccessible to washing. Surgical debridement or repair should be avoided whenever possible.

The following compounds are known to have a lethal effect on rabies virus *in vitro* (W.H.O., 1966): 0.1 per cent benzalkonium chloride, 0.1 per cent cetrimonium bromide, 1 per cent Hyamine 2389, 1 per cent methyl-benzethonium chloride, 1 per cent benzethonium chloride, 1 per cent SKF 11831, 43-70 per cent ethanol, tincture of thiomersal, tincture of iodine, 0.01 per cent aqueous iodine solution and 1–2 per cent soap solution.

VACCINE AND HYPERIMMUNE SERUM. The recommendations of the W.H.O. Expert Committee (W.H.O., 1966) are shown in Table 11. Hyperimmune serum (or better, hyperimmune globulin) should be given whenever possible in all cases of severe bite and especially bites of the head and neck. It should be given as soon as possible (after a small intradermal test dose) and certainly within 72 hours of the bite. It is probably of little value after 72 hours. The dose is large: 40 iu of serum per kg body weight given by intramuscular injection. Local infiltration of the tissues around the bite or topical application of serum or powdered globulin to the wound are also of value. Allergic reactions to the serum occur in about 15–20 per cent of patients, some of whom may be severely affected. Reactions have been less common with hyperimmune horse or rabbit serum than with sheep serum. When purified hyperimmune globulin is used, reactions are much less common. All patients must be given a small dose of serum intradermally to test for hypersensitivity before the whole dose is administered. If the patient is hypersensitive, he should be desensitised with small doses perhaps under cover of prophylactic ephedrine and/or antihistamines. Whenever serum

TABLE 11. *Recommendations on prophylactic treatment by the World Health Organization Expert Committee on Rabies (W.H.O. 1956)*

Nature of exposure	Status of biting animal (irrespective of whether vaccinated or not)		Recommended treatment
	At time of exposure	During observation period of 10 days	
I. No lesions; indirect contact	Rabid	—	None
II. Licks: (1) unabraded skin (2) abraded skin, scratches and un-abraded or abraded mucosa	Rabid (a) healthy (b) signs suggestive of rabies (c) rabid, escaped, killed or unknown	— Clinical signs of rabies or proven rabid (laboratory) Healthy —	None Start vaccine[1] at first signs of rabies in the biting animal Start vaccine[1] immediately; stop treatment if animal is normal on fifth day after exposure Start vaccine[1] immediately
III. Bites: (1) mild exposure	(a) healthy (b) signs suggestive of rabies (c) rabid, escaped, killed or unknown (d) wild (wolf, jackal, fox, bat, etc.)	Clinical signs of rabies or proven rabid (laboratory) Healthy — —	Start vaccine[1,2] at first sign of rabies in the biting animal Start vaccine[1] immediately; stop treatment if animal is normal on fifth day after exposure Start vaccine[1,2] immediately Serum[2] immediately, followed by a course of vaccine[1]
(2) severe exposure (multiple, or face, head, finger or neck bites)	(a) healthy (b) signs suggestive of rabies (c) rabid, escaped, killed or unknown (d) wild (wolf, jackal, pariah dog, fox, bat, etc.)	Clinical signs of rabies or proven rabid (laboratory) Healthy —	Serum[2] immediately; start vaccine[1] at first sign of rabies in the biting animal Serum[2] immediately, followed by vaccine; vaccine may be stopped if animal is normal on fifth day after exposure Serum[2] immediately, followed by vaccine[1]

[1] Practice varies concerning the volume of vaccine per dose and the number of doses recommended in a given situation. In general, the equivalent of at least 2 ml of a 5 per cent tissue emulsion should be given subcutaneously daily for 14 consecutive days. Many laboratories use 20 to 30 doses in severe exposures. To ensure the production and maintenance of high levels of serum-neutralising antibodies, booster doses should be given at 10 days and at 20 or more days following the last daily dose of vaccine in *all* cases. This is especially important if antirabies serum has been used, in order to overcome the interference effect.

[2] In all severe exposures and in all cases of unprovoked wild animal bites, antirabies serum or its globulin fractions together with vaccine should be employed. This is considered by the Committee as the *best* specific treatment available for the post-exposure prophylaxis of rabies in man. Although experience indicates that vaccine alone is sufficient for mild exposures, there is no doubt that here also the combined serum-vaccine treatment will give the best protection. However, both the serum and the vaccine can cause deleterious reactions. Moreover, the combined therapy is more expensive; its use in mild exposures is therefore considered optional. As with vaccine alone, it is important to start combined serum and vaccine treatment as early as possible after exposure, but serum should still be used no matter what the time interval. Serum should be given in a single dose (40 IU per kg of body weight) and the first dose of vaccine inoculated at the same time. Sensitivity to the serum must be determined before its administration.

is administered, adrenaline etc. should be at hand so that serum sickness can be promptly dealt with. When hyperimmune serum is not available a blood transfusion from someone of compatible blood group who has recently received a course of rabies vaccine treatment may be of value.

When serum or globulin is given, vaccine treatment is started 24 hours later, and the usual course of 12–14 daily doses given. Booster doses are also required 10 and 20 days after the end of the vaccine course because the hyperimmune serum may interfere with full antibody production. The serum provides passive immunity for about 14 days and a sufficient immune response must have been built up by then to continue protection of the patient.

The vaccines used are mainly either the β-propiolactone-inactivated duck embryo vaccine of phenolised brain tissue vaccine (Semple vaccine). The latter may be more antigenic but carries a risk of neuroparalytic accident (q.v.). In either case, 14 daily doses are given and local or general vaccine reactions, usually allergic in type, may be experienced. If the biting animal is under observation and shows no signs of rabies up to 7 days after the bite, treatment may be terminated. If brain tissue vaccine is to be used, it should be given only when there is a clear risk (even though a small one) of rabies infection. Treatment is often demanded by patients who have had no physical contact with the animal but are activated by fear.

Neuroparalytic accidents. These usually occur about the end of the 14-day courses of treatment or soon after. They are classified by McFadzean and Choa (1953) as follows:

Group	Pathology	Clinical syndrome
1	Perivascular myelinoclasis	(*a*) Dorsolumbar myelitis which may be ascending (Landry). (*b*) Encephalomyelitis. (*c*) Encephalitis without paralysis.
2	Polyradiculo-neuronitis	Neuritis varying from isolated cranial nerve palsies (often seventh) to extensive paralyses of the Guillain-Barré type which may be fatal.

About two–thirds of their cases were of the dorsolumbar myelitis group. The ascending (Landry) type have a 30 per cent mortality, but only about 5 per cent of the myelitis cases die. Approximately 25 per cent of cases have facial paralysis usually bilateral. The other syndromes are less common but encephalomyelitis carries a very high mortality. McFadzean and Choa reported polymorphonuclear leucocytosis in group 1 accidents but not in group 2. Variable increases were found in cells and protein in the cerebrospinal fluid in group 1, while in group 2 is found a great excess of protein with either a normal cell count or at most only a moderate number of mononuclear cells as is characteristic of the Guillain-Barré syndrome. Constitutional disturbances were present and sometimes severe group 1; these might precede the nervous system symptoms by 24–48 hours. Systemic symptoms were trivial in group 2.

ACTH and cortisone seem to be of definite value and may give dramatic relief. Vaccine should normally be discontinued if nervous system signs appear, but McFadzean and Choa suggest that the course of vaccine may be completed if essential, under cover of cortisone or ACTH. Antihistamine drugs may be of value although there is little evidence of this. The occurrence of any constitutional symptoms during vaccine treatment should be regarded as possibly the onset of neuroparalytic accident and cortisone or ACTH should probably be started immediately. Stoppage of vaccine treatment should also be considered unless the risk of rabies is considered to be high. An account of the experimental evidence of the value of the hyperimmune serum was given by Habel (1954).

Prophylactic vaccination for non-bitten persons. Recently a number of vaccines made from virus grown in chick or duck embryos have been developed and there is now even a hope of a practicable tissue culture vaccine. These avian embryo vaccines are free of brain tissue and thus of the risk of inducing neuroparalytic accident. The HEP (high egg passage Flury) vaccine made in the same way as the Flury canine (low egg passage) vaccine, has been widely used for prophylactic vaccination. Although HEP is a live virus vaccine, the virus does not multiply in man and the response depends only on the antigen mass administered. A duck embryo vaccine inactivated with β-propiolactone has also been used for prophylaxis. The effectiveness of all these vaccines depends on the amount of virus antigen they contain.

Prophylactic vaccinations are usually confined to occupations at special risk, e.g. veterinarians and their assistants in enzootic areas. Even with the best schedule of doses, HEP vaccine produces antibody in only 80–90 per cent of recipients. Atanasiu *et al* (1961) showed that antibody responses were best when there was an interval of 20 days between two of the doses. Anderson *et al* (1960) using duck embryo vaccine found that at least 75 per cent of the recipients of three doses had developed significant antibody but that a later booster dose gave an antibody response in 96 per cent. It is usually recommended that three intradermal doses of HEP or duck embryo vaccine are given 5–7 days apart, followed by a fourth dose 2–6 months later. Booster doses are required every 2–3 years to maintain protection.

As antibody responses do not always result from prophylactic vaccination, it is essential that a serum sample be tested for antibody 1–2 months after the last dose of vaccine. If antibody is not present, further vaccine doses should be given until antibody is demonstrated.

When a successfully immunised person is exposed to rabies infection, one booster dose of vaccine is recommended for a mild exposure; for a severe exposure five daily doses of vaccine followed by a booster 20 days later (W.H.O., 1966).

SMALLPOX

Smallpox is still endemic in large areas of the world, especially in India, Pakistan, Indonesia, parts of Africa and some South American countries. During and immediately after the Second World War there was increased spread of the disease especially in Africa and Asia, but since then the prevalence has fallen in many countries. In South America smallpox has been predominantly of the minor type (alastrim), but in Asia and in epidemics introduced to other countries from Asia, smallpox major has been more common. In tropical areas where the disease is prevalent, smallpox has a higher incidence and is most fatal in the first year of life (D. Morley, personal communication). W.H.O. commenced a smallpox campaign in 1967 and great strides have been made. The number of cases reported in the world fell by about a third annually between 1967 and 1970 (Henderson, 1971). Until, if ever, smallpox is eradicated from the world, the risk of introduction and spread exists everywhere where the prevalence of immunity due to vaccination is inadequate. For this reason smallpox is internationally notifiable and vaccination of travellers prescribed by the International Health Regulations. Eradication and control is discussed by W.H.O. (1964) and the requirements for smallpox vaccine in W.H.O. (1959).

Vaccination of contacts should be done as soon as possible, but if they have previously been vaccinated, revaccination is much more effective in preventing disease. Although there is no specific treatment for smallpox, the thiosemicarbazones have been shown to have considerable prophylactic value particularly when the contact is first seen rather too late for vaccination to be effective. Bauer (1965) reported a trial of N-methylisatin β-thiosemicarbazone in Madras: in 2297 close contacts who received both vaccine and the drug in various dosages (some too low) there were six cases and two deaths, while in 2842 similar controls who received vaccine only there were 114 cases and 20 deaths. This was confirmed by do Valle *et al* (1965) in alastrim contacts who had not been vaccinated and received no vaccine in São Paulo, Brazil: of 187 contacts given 3–6 g of thiosemicarbazone, seven developed alastrim, compared with 38 of 219 control contacts. Nausea and vomiting are the only important side effects and occurred in two-thirds of the São Paulo contacts treated.

BEDSONIA INFECTIONS

The *Bedsonias* or psittacosis-lymphogranuloma-trachoma group of agents are obligate intracellular parasites which are really small bacteria rather than viruses but have been habitually called viruses. Unlike viruses, they are susceptible to treatment with tetracyclines and certain other antimicrobial drugs. Ornithosis (transmitted from birds) and psittacosis (from psittacine birds) are of world-wide distribution and the diseases are largely occupational among those concerned with pet birds or poultry. Man-to-man infection can, however, occur and small outbreaks, particularly among nurses, have occurred. However, there are no features applying specially to the tropics. Lymphogranuloma venereum is also probably of world-wide distribution but little information of prevalence exists in most countries. It appears to be particularly prevalent in some tropical countries, in the Mediterranean area and in southern and eastern ports of the United States, but this is almost certainly more because of poor socioeconomic and hygienic conditions than because of climate. Transmission is normally venereal but has occurred from infected clothing, and surgeons and other hospital staff have been infected from patients. Sulphadiazine or tetracycline appear to be effective in controlling infection and a course of sulphadiazine followed by a course of tetracycline is probably even more effective (Erskine, 1958).

Trachoma and inclusion conjunctivitis. These are also caused by agents of this group—the

TRIC agents. Agents isolated from inclusion conjunctivitis of the newborn and the adult, and from the cervices of mothers of babies with ophthalmia neonatorum are indistinguishable in the laboratory from agents isolated from patients with trachoma. Inclusion conjunctivitis is found mainly in temperate countries but trachoma is world-wide and flourishes wherever there is poverty and poor hygiene. Trachoma is believed to affect 400–500 million people and is the greatest single cause of blindness and impaired vision. The worst affected areas are North Africa, the Middle East, the northern parts of the Indian subcontinent and large areas of the Far East such as Vietnam and China. The disease is moderately prevalent in large areas of Africa, southern India, the Far East and Australasia. Transmission is probably mainly by direct contact, or through fomites such as clothing, towels and bedclothes. Flies are often blamed, but the disease flourishes in areas which are comparatively free of such insects.

Clinical features. The earliest detectable lesion is subepithelial infiltration especially of the upper tarsal and bulbar conjunctiva. Papillae are formed in the palpebral conjunctiva in response to any prolonged infection or irritation. In trachoma they become so numerous that the lid looks velvety and gross hypertrophy may occur at the upper tarsal border and fornix. Retention cysts may form. Follicles are seen mainly in the palpebral conjunctiva, frequently at the limbus. At first they are small pale areas among the red papillae, later they enlarge to form pale elevations. When they regress they leave pigmented depressions (Herbert's pits) which are virtually pathognomic of trachoma. In the early stage of keratitis there may be generalised avascular superficial punctate lesions of the epithelial layers: small discrete greyish-white opacities are seen mainly in the upper half of the cornea. In pannus there is vascular and cellular infiltration of the cornea characteristically most marked in the upper half. The cornea becomes hazy, greyish-white foci appear between the vessels and may on resolution leave permanent small opacities. Cicatrisation occurs during the slow healing of the disease; small white stellate scars replace follicles on the palpebral conjunctiva, and characteristically horizontal streaks of fibrous tissue appear on the tarsal conjunctiva. Sequelae include contraction of the fornices, entropion, trichiasis, ectropion or xerosis (Sowa *et al*, 1965).

Diagnosis. Apart from ophthalmological examination, diagnosis depends on demonstration of the characteristic inclusion bodies in conjunctival scrapings either by an iodine stain or Giemsa/May-Grunwald stain. By the iodine stain the intracytoplasmic inclusions stain a deep copper-brown in contrast to the pale yellow of the epithelial cells. By the Giemsa/May-Grunwald method the inclusions can be seen to consist of a mass of elementary bodies. Isolation of the agent by inoculation of the yolk sac of embryonated eggs is a more sensitive but more expensive and elaborate method of diagnosis (Sowa *et al*, 1965).

Treatment of the stages varies according to whether it is done on an individual or a community basis. For individual adults a soluble sulphonamide can be used by mouth; 40 g given in divided doses over a period of 10 days is usually adequate. Alternatively, tetracycline 2 g daily for 3–5 days may be used. These dosages are reduced appropriately for children. Oral therapy may with advantage be supplemented by twice daily applications of 1 per cent tetracycline eye ointment. For mass treatment reliance must usually be placed on twice daily topical applications of 1 per cent tetracycline ointment extending over a period of several months. Long-acting sulphonamides (e.g. sulphor-methoxine 20 mg/kg body weight every 12–15 days for 3 months) may also be used for community treatment provided that adequate supervision can be maintained. There is usually rapid clinical improvement but keratitis and necrotic follicles may persist for 3–6 months after the infection has been eliminated. Surgical repair may be necessary for cicatricial sequelae.

No effective vaccine for trachoma is yet available. The requirements and problems of manufacture are discussed by Collier (1966) who also reviews progress.

VERVET MONKEY DISEASE

This disease, also called Marburg/Frankfurt disease, occurred in about 30 laboratory workers in Germany and Yugoslavia during the summer of 1967. All had had contact with the blood or tissues of vervet monkeys (*Cercopithecus aethiops*) from Uganda, or with tissue cultures from them, or with the blood of patients suffering from the disease. Those who fed and watered intact monkeys were not affected. There is no known record of this disease in Africa (or elsewhere) and there is a possibility that the monkeys were infected in transit by other animals they were housed with at London Airport. The disease appears to be uniformly fatal in vervet monkeys and is also highly lethal to guinea pigs, hamsters and rhesus monkeys. As its maintenance host and geographical distribution are uncertain, this disease may reappear in a quite different situation although its present importance is mainly to those who work with monkeys and their tissues, and for those responsible for ensuring that it does not get into vaccines made from monkey tissue. However, it can be transmitted from man to man by blood contamination when blood samples are taken from patients (a risk aggravated by their bleeding tendency) and venereal transmission has also occurred (see below). The agent has been found in the throat and urine of both patients and infected monkeys. The causative agent is a large rod-shaped RNA-virus, but it has so far defied classification and no specific treatment has been found. No vaccine has yet been developed.

Clinical features. Twenty-three cases occurred in Marburg and six cases in Frankfurt. Estimates of the incubation period lie between 4 and 9 days. There was a sudden onset of marked nausea, severe headache (mainly frontal or temporal) and tenderness of the eyeballs. During the first few days there was increasing fever, relative bradycardia, pain and a feeling of tension in the trunk muscles and around the hips, and vomiting was common. After 1–2 days there was often watery diarrhoea with up to 10 motions a day. As the fever subsided from about the seventh day of illness, the vomiting decreased but the diarrhoea continued for several more days. In some patients there was a second febrile phase from the twelfth to the fourteenth days associated with myocarditis and orchitis. The severity of the diarrhoea in general paralleled the severity of the disease although a few patients showed constipation at least for a time. Dryness of the mouth was a common complaint, even before onset of diarrhoea and vomiting.

Between the fifth and seventh day of illness, a rash appeared, most marked on the buttocks, trunk and the outer aspects of the upper arms. At first there were red 'pinhead' spots around the hair follicles; after about 24 hours the rash became maculopapular, then confluent. In severe cases there was a diffuse livid erythema on the face, trunk and limbs, sometimes associated with marked cyanosis of the lips. Some cases had dermatitis of the scrotum or labia. In a few there were vesicles (on lips, abdomen or thumb) some or all of which may have been due to recrudescent herpes simplex. After about the sixteenth day, there was fine desquamation of the rash, especially on the palms, soles, forearms and legs, lasting about 2 weeks. About half the patients

had conjunctivitis at one time or another. There was also an enanthem which appeared a day before the rash in some patients: deep red discolouration and 'sago-like' vesicles on the soft palate sometimes spreading to the hard palate. Some had inflamed tonsils with yellowish pinhead areas of exudate. Lymph nodes were small and not tender, but palpable, sometimes before the onset of the rash, in the neck and axilla.

Two patients had signs of meningeal irritation but the cerebrospinal fluid was essentially normal. Most patients were peevish and uncooperative at the height of the illness but some had confusion, depression or anxiety, and in some of the fatal cases, restlessness and confusion were succeeded by coma and death. Some had loss of memory for the acute stage of the illness. There were also changes in peripheral sensation: hypersensitivity to pain and touch, 'pins and needles' or a feeling of 'lying on crumbs'. Myelitis was recorded in one patient after the end of the acute stage of illness.

There was a marked bleeding tendency, notably from the gums and from needle punctures. Haematemesis and melaena occurred but the rash was never haemorrhagic. There was marked thrombocytopenia (less than 10 000/mm³ in two fatal cases) but no other changes in blood clotting factors sufficient to account for the bleeding. Transaminase levels (especially SGOT) were raised and atypical lymphocytes and plasma cells were seen in association with leukopenia. Serum proteins (all components) declined in all cases but significant proteinuria was not seen.

Seven patients died and the remainder had a slow convalescence. Three patients relapsed: one had a marked rise in serum transaminase 31 days after recovery; a second had a similar rise after 73 days associated with an acute psychosis and the agent was isolated from a liver biopsy; the third appears to have infected his wife by sexual intercourse 11 weeks after recovery, and the agent was detected in his semen.

At autopsy necrotic changes appeared first to affect the liver and lymphatic system, then the pancreas, gonads, adrenals, hypophysis, thyroid, kidneys and skin. There was evidence, supported by liver biopsy findings, that the liver damage was quickly repaired by regeneration after the acute stage. Basophilic bodies were seen in cells in and around necrotic lesions. In lymphoid tissue there was a notable transformation to plasma cells and monocyte-like cells. There was diffuse infiltration with similar cells of the mucosa of stomach, small intestine and less of the large intestine. Evidence was seen of the haemorrhagic tendency. All cases had severe parenchymal damage and evidence of tubular failure in the kidneys, associated with cerebral oedema. In patients who died in coma, there was either some evidence of encephalitis (glial nodules) or a haemorrhagic state in the central nervous system.

Diagnosis depends on the inoculation of blood or tissue suspensions into experimental animals—guinea pigs are most suitable. Alternatively paired sera can be tested—most conveniently in a complement fixation test.

The literature on Marburg disease was reviewed by Smith (1971).

REFERENCES

ALEZIVATOS, A. C., MCKINNEY, R. W. and FEIGIN, R. D. (1967) *Amer. J. trop. Med. Hyg.*, **16**, 762.

ALLEN, J. G. (1960) *Stanford med. Bull.*, **18**, 40.

ANDERSON, C. R., DOWNS, W. G., WATTLEY, G. H., AHIN, N. W. and REESE, A. A. (1957) *Amer. J. trop. Med. Hyg.*, **6**, 1012.

ANDERSON, C. R., SCHNURRERBERGER, P. R., MASTERSON, R. A. and WENTWORTH, F. H. (1960) *Amer. J. Hyg.*, **71**, 158.

ANDERSON, S. G., DONNELLEY, M., STEVENSON, W. J., CALDWELL, N. J. and EAGLE, M. (1952) *Med. J. Aust.*, **1**, 110.

ARDOIN, P. and CLARKE, D. H. (1967) *Amer. J. trop. Med. Hyg.*, **16**, 357.

ATANASIU, P., CANNON, D. A., DEAN, D. J., FOX, J. P., HABEL, K., KAPLAN, M. M., KISSLING, R. E., KPOROWSKI, H., LEPINE, P. and GALLARDO, F. P. (1961) *Bull. Wld Hlth Org.*, **25**, 103.

BARNETT, H. C. and SUYEMOTO, W. (1961) *N.Y. Acad. Sci.*, Ser. II, **23**, 609.

BARRETT, F. F., YOW, M. D. and PHILLIPS, C. A. (1965) *J. Amer. med. Ass.*, **193**, 381.

BAUER, D. J. (1965) *Ann. N.Y. Acad. Sci.*, **130**, 110.

BINN, L. N., SPONSELLER, M. L., WOODING, W. L., MCCONNELL, S. J., SPERRZEL, R. O. and YAGER, R. H. (1966) *Amer. J. vet. Res.*, **27**, 1599.

BRICENO-ROSSI, A. L. (1964a) *Rev. Venez. San. Asist. Soc.*, **29**, 354.

BRODY, J. A., BURNS, K. F., BROWNING, G. and SCHATTNER, J. D. (1959) *New Eng. J. med.*, **261**, 644.

BUESCHER, E. L. (1963) Paper presented at *7th Int. Cong. trop. Med. Malar.*, Rio de Janeiro.

CANNON, D. A. and DEWHURST, F. (1953) *Ann. trop. Med. Parasit.*, **47**, 381.

CAREY, D. E., KEMP, G. E., WHITE, H. A., PINNEO, L., ADDY, R. F., FOM, A.L.M.D., STROH, G., CASALS, J., HENDERSON, B. E. (1972) *Trans. R. Soc. trop. Med. Hyg.*, **66**, 402.

CASALS, J. (1969) *Proc. Soc. exp. Biol. Med.*, **131**, 233.

CATALOGUE (1968) *Catalogue of the Arthropod-borne Viruses of the World.* U.S. Govt. Printing Office.

CAUSEY, O. R., CAUSEY, C. E., MAROJA, O. M. and MACEDO, D. G. (1961) *Amer. J. trop. Med. Hyg.*, **10**, 227.

CAUSEY, O. R. and MAROJA, O. M. (1957) *Amer. J. trop. Med. Hyg.*, **6**, 1017.

CHAMBON, L., WONE, I., BRES, P., CORNET, M., LY, C., MICHEL, A., LACAN, A., ROBIN, Y., HENDERSON, B. E., WILLIAMS, K. H., CAMAIN, R., LAMBERT, D., REY, M., DIOPMAR, I., OUDART, J. L., CAUSSE, G., BA, H., MARTIN, M. and ARTUS, J. C. (1967) *Bull. Wld Hlth Org.*, **36**, 113.

CHATTERJEA, J. B., SWARUP, S., PAIN, S. K. and RAO, R. L. (1963) *Ind. J. med. Res.*, **51**, 419.

CHILD, P. L., MACKENZIE, R. B., VALVERDE, L. R. and JOHNSON, K. M. (1967) *Arch. Path.*, **83**, 434.

CHUNDERMPADETSUK, S. (1966) *Bull. Wld Hlth Org.*, **35**, 76.

CLARKE, D. H. (1964) *Bull. Wld Hlth Org.*, **31**, 45.

CLARKE, D. H. and CASALS, J. (1958) *Amer. J. trop. Med. Hyg.*, **7**, 561.

COLLIER, L. H. (1966) *Bull. Wld Hlth Org.*, **34**, 233.

—— (1971) In *Management and Treatment of Tropical Disease.* ed MAEGRAITH, B. G. and GILLES, H. M. S. Oxford: Blackwell Publications.

COOPER, C., MORLEY, D. C., WEEKS, M. C. and BEALE, A. J. (1966) *Lancet*, **1**, 1076.

CUADRADO, R. R. and CASALS, J. (1967) *J. Immunol.*, **98**, 314.

DALLDORF, G. and MALNICK, J. L. (1965) In *Viral and Rickettsial Infections of Man*, 4th Edit., ed. HORSFALL, F. L. and TAMM, I., p. 474. London, Philadelphia: Pitman, Lippincott.

DARWISH, M. A. and HAMMON, W. M. (1966) *Proc. Soc. exp. Biol. N.Y.*, **123**, 242.

DARWISH, M. A., HAMMON, W. M. and SATHER, G. E. (1967) *Amer. J. trop. Med. Hyg.*, **16**, 364.

DELLER, J. J. and RUSSELL, P. K. (1968) *Amer. J. trop. Med. Hyg.*, **17**, 107.

DE MUCHA-MACIAS, J. and SANCHEZ-SPINDOLA, I. (1965) *Amer. J. trop. Med. Hyg.*, **14**, 475.

DOERR, R., FRANZ, K. and TAUSSIG, S. (1909) *Das Pappa tacifieber*, Deuticke, Liepzig.

Do Valle, L. A. R., De Melo, P. R., De Salles Gomes, L. F. and Proenca, L. M. (1965) *Lancet*, **2**, 976.

Downs, W. G. (1957) In *Yellow Fever*, Symposium in commemoration of Carlos Juan Finley, p. 71. Philadelphia: Jefferson Med. College.

Eavri (1962) *Ann. Rep. E. Afr. Res. Inst.*, No. 12, Entebbe.

Edgren, D. C., Palladino, V. S. and Arnold, A. (1958) *Amer. J. trop. Med. Hyg.*, **7**, 471.

Edington, G. M. and White, H. A. (1972) *Trans. R. Soc. trop. Med. Hyg.*, **66**, 381.

Emmons, R. N. and Zennette, E. H. (1966) *J. lab. clin. Med.*, **68**, 923.

Erskine, D. (1958) *Brit. J. ven. Dis.*, **34**, 163.

Farber, S., Hill, A., Connerly, M. L. and Dingle, J. H. (1940) *J. Amer. med. Ass.*, **114**, 1725.

Fleming, J., Bignall, J. R. and Blades, A. N. (1947) *Lancet*, **1**, 443.

Foege, W. H. (1971) *Int. Conf. on applic. of Vaccines against viral, rickettsial diseases of man.* PAHO, W.H.O. 14-18 Dec. 1970, Washington DC, p. 207.

Fulginiti, V. A., Eller, J. J., Downie, A. W. and Kempe, C. H. (1967) *J. Amer. med. Ass.*, **202**, 1075.

Gajdusek, C. (1955) *Pediatrics*, **16**, 819.

German, L. J., McCracken, A. W. and Wilkie, K. M. (1968) *Brit. med. J.*, **1**, 742.

Goldblum, N., Sterk, V. V. and Jasinska-Klingberg, W. (1957) *Amer. J. Hyg.*, **66**, 363.

Green, I. J., Want, S-P., Yen, C-H., Hung, S-C. (1963) *Amer. J. trop. Med. Hyg.*, **12**, 668.

Guelmino, D. J. and Jevtic, M. (1955) *Acta trop.*, **12**, 179.

Habel, K. (1954) *Bull. Wld Hlth Org.*, **10**, 781.

Halstead, S. B. (1965) *Ind. J. med. Res.* **53**, No. 8.

—— (1966) *Bull. Wld Hlth Org.*, **35**, 1.

Halstead, S. B. and Grosz, C. R. (1962) *Amer. J. Hyg.*, **75**, 190.

Harrison, V. R., Binn, L. N. and Randall, R. (1967) *Amer. J. trop. Med. Hyg.*, **16**, 786-791.

Henderson, B. E., Gary, G. W., Kissling, R. E., Frame, J. D. and Carey, D. E. (1972) *Trans. R. Soc. trop. Med. Hyg.*, **66**, 409.

Henderson, D. E. (1971) *Int. Conf. on applic. of Vaccines against viral, rickettsial diseases of man.* P.A.H.O., W.H.O., 14-18 Dec. 1970, Washington DC, p. 139.

Hess, A. D. and Hayes, R. O. (1967) *Amer. J. med. Sci.*, **253**, 333.

Hiraki, K., Demiya, Y., Kageyama, H. and Kiyama, A. (1958) *Acta med. Yokohama*, **12**, 51. (*Bull. Hyg.*, **34**, 115, 1959).

Hong Kong Measles Vaccine Committee (1967) *Bull. Wld Hlth Org.*, **36**, 375.

Iyer, C. G. S., Rao, R. L., Work, T. H. and Murthy, D. P. N. (1959) *Ind. J. med. Sci.*, **13**, 1011.

Johnson, K. M., Webenga, N. H., Mackenzie, R. B., Kuns, M. L., Tauraso, N. M., Shelokov, A., Webb, P. A., Justines, G. and Beye, H. K. (1965) *Proc. Soc. exp. Biol. N.Y.*, **118**, 113.

Katz, S. L. and Enders, J. F. (1965) In *Viral and Rickettsial Infections of Man*, 4th Edit., ed. Horsfall, F. L. and Tamm, I., p. 784. London, Philadelphia: Pitman, Lippincott.

Kaufman, H. E. and Heidelberger, C. (1964) *Science*, **145**, 585.

Kerr, J. A. (1951) In Strode (1951) *Yellow Fever*, p. 385.

—— (1959) *Proc. 6th int. Cong. trop. Med. Malar.*, **5**, 219.

Klingberg, M. A., Jasinska-Klingberg, W. and Goldblum, N. (1959) *Proc. 6th int. Cong. trop. Med. Malar.*, **5**, 132.

Kokernot, R. H., Shinefield, H. R. and Longshore, W. A. (1953) *Calif. Med.*, **79**, 73.

Kunin, C. M. and Chin, C. D. Y. (1957) *Publ. Hlth Rep.*, **72**, 519.

Macdonald, W. W., Smith, C. E. G., Dawson, P. S., Ganapathipillai, A. and Mahadevan, S. (1967) *J. med. Ent.*, **4**, 146.

Macdonald, W. W., Smith, C. E. G. and Webb, H. E. (1965) *J. med. Ent.*, **1**, 335.

Mackenzie, R. B., Beye, H. K., Valverde, C. L. and Garron, H. (1964) *Amer. J. trop. Med. Hyg.*, **13**, 620.

Macnamara, F. N. (1953) *Trans. R. Soc. trop. Med. Hyg.*, **47**, 199.

Malherbe, H., Strickland-Cholmley, M. and Jackson, A. L. (1963) *S. Afr. med. J.*, **37**, 547.

Mansharamani, H. J., Dandawate, C. N. and Krishnamurthy, B. G. (1967) *Ind. J. Path. Bact.*, **10**, 9.

Matsuda, S. (1962) *Bull. Instr. publ. Hlth, Tokyo*, **11**, 173.

McFadzean, A. J. S. and Choa, G. H. (1953) *Trans. R. Soc. trop. Med. Hyg.*, **47**, 372.

McKay, D. G. and Margaretten, W. (1967) *Arch. intern. Med.*, **120**, 129.

Meers, P. D. (1960) *Trans. R. Soc. trop. Med. Hyg.*, **54**, 493.

Melnick, J. L. (1965) In *Viral and Rickettsial Infections of Man*, 4th Edit., ed. Horsfall, F. L. and Tamm, I. p. 513. London, Philadelphia: Pitman, Lippincott.

Miles, J. A. R. (1960) *Bull. Wld Hlth Org.*, **22**, 339.

Morley, D. C. (1967) In *Modern Trends in Medical Virology*, ed. Heath, R. B. and Waterson, A. P., p. 141. London: Butterworth.

O'Reilly, K. J., Smith, C. E. G., McMahon, D. A., Bowen, E. T. W. and White, G. (1968) *J. Hyg. Camb.*, **66**, 217.

PAHO (1963) *Panamer Hlth Org. Report* RES 63.1, Rio de Janeiro.
PHOON, W. O. and LIM, K. A. (1963) *Singapore med. J.*, **4**, 11.
PRICE, W. H., LEE, R. W., GUNKEL, W. F. and O'LEARY, W. (1961) *Amer. J. trop. Med. Hyg.*, **10**, 403.
PRICE, W. H., PARKS, J., GANAWAY, J., LEE, R. and O'LEARY, W. (1963) *Amer. J. trop. Med. Hyg.*, **12**, 624.
QUICK, D. T., THOMPSON, J. M. and BOND, J. O. (1965b) *Amer. J. Epid.*, **81**, 415.
QUICK, D. T., SERFLING, R. E., SHERMAN, I. L. and CASEY, H. L. (1965a) *Amer. J. Epid.*, **81**, 405.
RANDALL, R., BINN, L. N. and HARRISON, V. R. (1963) *Amer. J. trop. Med. Hyg.*, **12**, 611.
REEVES, W. C., HAMMON, W. M., LONGSHORE, W. A., McCLURE, H. E. and BEIB, A. F. (1962) *Univ. Calif. Publicn. Publ. Hlth*, **4**, 1.
ROBERTSON, E. G. and McLORINAN, H. (1952) *Med. J. Aust.*, **1**, 103.
ROBINSON, D. M., BERMAN, S., LOWENTHAL, J. P. and HETRICK, F. M. (1966) *Appl. Microbiol.*, **14**, 1011.
ROBINSON, M. C. (1955) *Trans. R. Soc. trop. Med. Hyg.*, **49**, 28.
ROEVER-BONNET, H. DE and HOEKSTRA, J. (1958) *Trop. geog. Med. (Amst.)*, **10**, 289.
RUGIERO, H. R. *et al* (1964) *Rev. Asoc. med. Argentina*, **78**, 221, 281, 500, 611; **79**, 153.
RUSSELL, P. K., BUESCHER, E. L., McCOWAN, J. M. and ORDONES, J. (1966) *Amer. J. trop. Med. Hyg.*, **15**, 573.
SABIN, A. B. (1952) *Amer. J. trop. Med. Hyg.*, **1**, 30.
SABIN, A. B., PHILIP, C. B. and PAUL, J. R. (1944) *J. Amer. med. Ass.*, **125**, 603, 693.
SANMARTIN-BARBERI, C., GROOT, H. and OSBORNO-MESA, E. (1954) *Amer. J. trop. Med. Hyg.*, **3**, 283.
SARKAR, J. K., CHATTERJEE, S. N., CHAKRAVARTI, S. K. and MITRA, A. C. (1965) *Ind. J. med. Res.*, **53**, 921.
SCHAEFFER, M., GAJDUSER, D. C., LEMA, A. B. and EICHENWALD, H. (1959) *Amer. J. trop. Med. Hyg.*, **8**, 372.
SCHERER, W. F. *et al.* (1959) *Amer. J. trop. Med. Hyg.*, **8**, 644.
SCOTT, T. F. McN. and BONANNO, D. E. (1967) *New Eng. J. Med.*, **277**, 248.
SERIE, C., ANDRAL, L., LINDREC, A. and NERI, P. (1964) *Bull. Wld Hlth Org.*, **30**, 299.
SHOPE, R. E. and ANDERSON, S. G. (1960) *Med. J. Aust.*, **1**, 156.
SHOPE, R. E. and CAUSEY, O. R. (1962) *Amer. J. trop. Med. Hyg.*, **11**, 283.
SHORE, H. (1951) *Trans. R. Soc. trop. Med. Hyg.*, **55**, 361.
SILER, J. F., HALL, M. W. and HITCHENS, A. P. (1926) *Manila Bur. Sci. Monogr.* No. 20, 62, 170.
SIMMONS, J. S., ST JOHN, J. H. and REYNOLDS, F. H. K. (1931) *Manila Bur. Sci. Monogr.* No. 29, 19, 112, 189.
SIMPSON, D. I. H., KNIGHT, E. M., COURTOIS, G., WILLIAMS, M. C., WIENBREN, M. P. and KIBUKAMASOKE, J. W. (1967) *E. Afr. med. J.*, **44**, 87.
SMADEL, J. E. and WARREN, J. (1947) *J. clin. Invest.*, **26**, 1197.
SMITH, C. E. G. (1956a) *Nature*, **178**, 581.
—— (1956b) *Med. J. Malaya*, **10**, 289.
—— (1956c) *J. Hyg., Camb.*, **54**, 569.
—— (1956d) *J. trop. Med. Hyg.*, **59**, 243.
—— (1957) *J. Hyg. Camb.*, **55**, 207.
—— (1967) *Int. Symp. Immunobiol. Methods of Biol. Standardization Symp. Series Immunobiol. Standard*, **4**, 263.
—— (1968) *Abstr. Hyg.*, **43**, 1397.
—— (1970) *J. R. Coll. Phycns, Lond.*, **5**, 31.
—— (1971) *Sci. Basis of Med. Ann. Reviews* 1971, p. 58.
SMITH, C. E. G., TURNER, L. H. and ARMITAGE, P. (1962) *Bull. Wld Hlth Org.*, **27**, 717.
SMITHBURN, K. C., PATERSON, H. E., HEYMANN, C. S. and WINTER, P. A. D. (1959) *S. Afr. med. J.*, **33**, 959.
SMORODINTSEV, A. A., ILYENKO, V. I. and PLATONOV, V. G. (1967) *Jap. J. med. Sci. Biol.*, **20**, 132.
SOUTHAM, C. M. (1956) *J. inf. Dis.*, **99**, 155, 163.
SOUTHAM, C. M. and MOORE, A. E. (1951) *Amer. J. trop. Med.*, **31**, 724.
SOWA, S., SOWA, J., COLLIER, L. H. and BLYTH, W. (1965) *Med. Res. Council spec. Rep. Ser.*, No. 308. London: H.M.S.O.
SPIGLAND, J., JASINSKA-KLINGBERG, W., HOFSHI, E. and GOLDBLUM, N. (1958) *Harefuah*, **54**, 275.
STRODE, G. K. (ed.) (1951) *Yellow Fever*. New York, Toronto, London: McGraw-Hill.
STUART, G. (1956) *Wld Hlth Org. Monogr.*, No. 3, 143.
TAYLOR, R. M., WORK, T. H., HURLBUT, H. S. and RIZK, F. (1956) *Amer. J. trop. Med. Hyg.*, **5**, 579.
THEILER, M. and CASALS, J. (1958) *Amer. J. trop. Med. Hyg.*, **7**, 585.
THEILER, M. and DOWNS, W. G. (1963) *Yale Scient. Mag.*, **37**, 10, 26.
THIND, I. S. and PRICE, W. H. (1966) *Amer. J. Epid.*, **84**, 193, 214, 225.
TIGERTT, W. D. and BERGE, T. O. (1957) *Amer. J. publ. Hlth*, **47**, 713.
WEAVER, O. M., HAYMAKER, W., PIEPER, S. and KURLAND, R. (1958) *Neurol.*, **8**, 887.
WEBB, H. E. and RAO, R. L. (1961) *Trans. R. Soc. trop. Med. Hyg.*, **55**, 284.
WEBB, H. E., WETHERLEY-MEIN, G., SMITH, C. E. G. and McMAHON, D. (1966) *Brit. med. J.*, **1**, 258.
WEISS, H. J. and HALSTEAD, S. B. (1965) *J. Pediat.*, **66**, 918.
WHITE, H. A. (1972) *Trans. R. Soc. trop. Med. Hyg.*, **66**, 390.
WISSEMAN, C. L., SWEET, B. H., ROSENZWEIG, E. C. and EYLAR, O. R. (1963) *Amer. J. trop. Med. Hyg.*, **12**, 620.

WORLD HEALTH ORGANIZATION (1953) *Wld Hlth Org. tech. Rep. Ser.* No. 62.
—— (1959) *Wld Hlth Org. tech. Rep. Ser.* No. 180.
—— (1964) *Wld Hlth Org. tech. Rep. Ser.* No. 283.
—— (1966) *Wld Hlth Org. tech. Rep. Ser.* No. 321.
—— (1967) *Wld Hlth Org. tech. Rep. Ser.* No. 369.
WORK, T. H. (1958) *Progr. med. Virol.*, 1, 248.
ZIMMERMAN, H. M. (1946) *Amer. J. Path.*, 22, 965.
ZUCKERMAN, A. (1970) *Bull. Wld Health Org.*, 42, 957.

23

Yaws

SYNONYMS. Framboesia (German, Dutch), pian (French), buba (Spanish), bouba (Portuguese). Populations in which the disease is endemic have either their own language names for yaws or for some of its lesions, or use a word from another language meaning 'foreigner', such as 'parangi' (Ceylon) which suggests that the disease has been introduced during the past few centuries.

DEFINITION

Yaws is a communicable disease, often of high prevalence, among rural populations in humid tropical countries. Its course is characterised by latency interrupted by early infectious lesions and after some years by late destructive lesions. Some relapses probably occur in all patients. Only the skin and bones are affected. The causal organism is *Treponema pertenue* which is transmitted non-venereally usually before puberty. It is a crippling, not a killing disease.

HISTORICAL

The earliest record of yaws is probably in bone lesions from the Mariana Islands, West Pacific, which Stewart and Spoehr (1952) dated by carbon–14 estimation of an associated tridacna shell at A.D. 854±145. In many early written accounts the destructive lesions of yaws are confused with venereal syphilis (Hackett, 1936). Yaws was probably carried to the Carribbean Islands and Americas with African slaves from the sixteenth century onwards and there it has largely remained restricted to populations of African stock (Hackett, 1963). There is a possibility that yaws was in Indonesia at least a thousand years ago (Hackett, 1970).

It was not until the end of the nineteenth century that the late destructive lesions were recognised as the late stage of the infection. The causal organism, *T. pertenue*, was discovered by Castellani in 1905 in Ceylon.

In many parts of the world during the 1920s neoarsphenamine, following Ehrlich's discovery

in 1910, established the power of modern medicine among indigenous populations by the relief it brought to afflicted communities. Bismuth came into use in the next decade following its introduction by Levaditi in the treatment of syphilis. The efficacy of penicillin in yaws was demonstrated by F. N. Guimarães in Brazil, and Findlay and co-workers in the Gold Coast in 1943.

The relapsing and latent characters of yaws were recognised by Harding (1949) in Sierra Leone and the frequency of latency was demonstrated by serological studies by Li and Soebekti (1955) in Indonesia in the 1950s: this knowledge made possible the full use of the great efficacy of long-acting penicillin in mass treatment which is rapidly hastening the eradication of yaws.

The first rapidly effective mass treatment campaign against yaws using single injections of PAM started in Haiti in 1950 and was estimated at the time to have increased national production by 5 million U.S. dollars anually.

AETIOLOGY

The causal organism is *T. pertenue* of the pallidum/pertenue group of morphologically identical spiral organisms that are also associated with pinta treponarid* (endemic syphilis) and venereal syphilis. It is 8–16 μm long and 0.2 μm wide, has about 8–16 regular spirals and divides according to estimates based upon animal experiments about every 30–33 hours (Turner and Hollander, 1957).

T. pertenue readily infects monkeys, rabbits and hamsters and causes subclinical infections in rats, mice and guinea pigs. *T. carateum* of pinta has recently been passed to chimpanzees. None of these treponemes has been cultivated.

Turner and Hollander (1957) found that the inoculation of yaws treponemes into the testes of rabbits produced granular periorchitis with little induration; on intracutaneous inoculation there was no induration and but few generalised lesions. Treponemes from venereal syphilis produced

* To avoid confusion the term 'treponarid' will be used in this chapter as a synonym for 'endemic syphilis' or 'bejel'. This was recently suggested by Dr Calvin Wells.

The text of this chapter is based upon that published in DEMIS, D. J., CROUNSE, R. G., DOBSON, R. L. and MACGUIRE, J. eds (1972), *Clinical Dermatology*. New York: Harper and Row.

contrary results. In hamsters yaws treponemes produced extensive skin lesions and skin metastases and few treponemes were found in the lymph glands; the opposite was found after inoculation of treponemes from venereal syphilis. Those from treponarid gave intermediate results. Occasional yaws treponemes in experimentally infected animals tended to change character towards treponemes from venereal syphilis. The induration in venereal syphilis infections in animals was found to be due to accumulation of a mucopolysaccharide, hyaluronic acid, apparently produced by the treponemes.

No differences have been found in the serological response of patients with any of the treponematoses to any serological test for syphilis, nor in their response to antibiotics (Turner and Hollander, 1957).

The treponemes in nature have little resistance outside the body although they retain their virulence for some years in 15 per cent glycerol at $-70°C$. Transmission through inanimate objects such as floors is thus most unlikely.

In experimental infections in rabbits resistance to reinfection had usually developed by the third month. It continued as long as infection was present and in some cases persisted after therapy, especially if the infection had lasted some months (Turner and Hollander, 1957). The persistence of treponemes in lymph glands in syphilitic patients and in experimental rabbit infections with reactive sera after adequate antibiotic therapy late in the infection needs to be taken into account in these studies (Collart et al, 1964), and may indicate the foci from which treponemes come to initiate relapses.

There was some reciprocal immunity between all pathogenic treponemes due apparently to common antigenic components (Turner and Hollander, 1957). The extent of cross-protection between different treponemes varied. Most strains of venereal syphilis treponemes gave fairly good cross-immunity in rabbits. The same was found in yaws. There did not, however, appear to be a general cross-immunity between treponemes from venereal syphilis and yaws but it was often good. There was no cross-immunity between non-pathogenic cultivated treponemes and pathogenic ones, but the naturally occurring T. caniculi of the rabbit possessed some cross-immunity with the human pathogenic treponemes. A few cross-infections of yaws with syphilis in man, especially when only a month or two has separated the two infections, have been reported, but most field workers are agreed that there is considerable protection against syphilis from childhood yaws.

Turner and Hollander (1957) called attention to the inherent capabilities of treponemes for adaptation and the possibility of future changes in the present balance in favour of the host. They also called for constant vigilance concerning the mutational capabilities of the treponemes.

EPIDEMIOLOGY AND DISTRIBUTION

In early lesions many treponemes are present and serum exuding from the papillomata teems with them. In the late destructive lesions, treponemes are very scanty, rather than absent, as F. N. Guimarães of Brazil has demonstrated. Probably infection occurs through some breach of skin surface, minor though it may be. Because most initial lesions are on an exposed part of the body and especially below the knee, trauma is probably important. In experimental syphilis as few as 10 treponemes have produced infection. Insects such as flies play only a small part in transmission (Barnard, 1952). Although the widespread application of residual insecticides for the destruction of mosquito vectors of human disease has greatly reduced other domestic diptera such as flies, no reduction in yaws transmission directly due to it has been recognised. The transmission of yaws by contaminated fingers needs further consideration.

Hudson (1965) and some others maintain that there is only one treponeme, T. pallidum, which produced different clinical patterns under different environmental conditions.

Yaws is a disease of rural populations in many tropical countries. Prevalence rates of active disease of over 10 per cent, and reactor rates in adults to the older serological tests for syphilis of 80 per cent or higher were probably not uncommon in the past. For every patient with active yaws there were two to five infected persons with no lesions; many of these latent infections, especially in young adolescents and children, could be expected to relapse with infectious lesions within a year. The sexes are equally infected. There are at present a few million people infected with yaws in a total population of about 50 million living in endemic areas, but the prevalence of active yaws in many such areas might be only a few per thousand.

In many endemic populations until 20 years ago, infectious yaws in children and destructive lesions in adults were to be seen in any gatherings of people, e.g. markets. After a few years of national mass treatment campaigns, surveillance resurveys have often failed to reveal any active lesions. Mass treatment campaigns have been carried out or are now in progress in most countries where yaws is or has been recently present. Thus, a map of the probable distribution of yaws (and the other treponematoses) about the beginning of this century (Hackett, 1963) is useful to show where it should still be considered in differential diagnosis.

In some countries, however, sero-immunological surveys (*Guthe et al*, 1972) have shown, some years after mass treatment campaigns, an unexpected presence of sero-reactors in children with no active yaws. The numbers depend upon the original prevalence and the thoroughness of the campaigns. These findings suggest modified treponemes and subclinical infections.

During the first quarter of this century yaws was more prevalent in Africa than in other continents where its recession had already started. In parts of Africa at that time yaws was thought to have been a bigger burden on the infected community than all other communicable diseases. Recent improvements of standards of living, however, have greatly reduced the transmission, the luxuriance and prevalence of early yaws, and the prevalence and destructiveness of late lesions. This recession of the disease in many countries, especially in South-east Asia, had commenced before the effective use of mass treatment with penicillin which has so greatly hastened these trends. The hazard is now the exposure to venereal syphilis of a rising generation reaching sexual maturity unprotected by childhood yaws.

Figures for the prevalence of active yaws of over 20 per cent sometimes result from including persons with 'yaws scars', the diagnosis of which is uncertain and which indicates past, not present, active disease, or erroneous diagnosis of non-yaws plantar and palmar lesions.

In some West African coastal cities in the mid-1950s the sero-reactor rates of primiparae was about 20 per cent, but congenital syphilis did not occur in their children. These young women had probably had childhood infections with yaws in rural areas and had recently come into the cities.

Yaws is restricted to humid tropical countries. Notable is its coastal distribution in South America because of its limitation to populations of African stock, its limited distribution in India to certain previously isolated aboriginal tribes, and its presence until recently in Taiwan.

The infection, under naturally endemic conditions, is usually contracted from about the age of 2–3 years when children's movements start to extend beyond the family. By the age of 15 years most of the population is infected. Susceptible children are infected by contact with infected children from other households rather than from their own brothers and sisters. In many countries its prevalence is not uniform throughout the yaws endemic area, but high and low prevalence may be found adjacent. In some African countries active yaws is more prevalent in the wet season than in the dry, hotter one (Harding, 1949). The 'last cases' towards the end of an eradication campaign are often difficult to account for, but perhaps arise from exceptionally delayed infectious relapses.

Yaws is not transmitted in cities or towns by sexual contact, nor to the unborn child, probably because infection occurs long before sexual maturity so that the mother is no longer infectious. In syphilis, intrauterine transmission to the fetus after 5 years of the mother's infection is unusual. Until recently natural infection of wild animals in yaws endemic foci was unknown. Fribourg-Blanc and co-workers (1963) however, found that the sera of 65 per cent of 111 baboons (*Papio cynocephalus*) from Guinea gave a positive reaction to the fluorescent treponemal antibody (FTA) test for Nichol's strain of *T. pallidum*, and recently treponeme-containing skin lesions have been reported in these animals.

This test reacts positively with sera from syphilis, yaws and pinta patients. The same monkey sera also reacted to the treponemal immobilisation (TPI) test. No search was made for treponemes at that time, but the monkeys came from a highly endemic area for human yaws. Because these two tests are specific and do not give false positive reactions, nor reactions with non-pathogenic treponemes, the authors concluded that a treponematosis is present in these monkeys. Their suggestion that these animals might thus serve as a reservoir for human infection has direct relevance to yaws eradication although it may not be important.

In subsequent studies of 24 apparently healthy *P. cynocephalus* with no cutaneous or genital scars, within a month of their departure from Guinea, the same workers (Fribourg-Blanc *et al*, 1966) found that 22 gave positive reactions with the FTA test. In autopsies on 18 no microscopical abnormality was found. Treponemes of the pallidum/pertenue type, however, were found in seven of these 18 animals but only in the popliteal lymph nodes. Usually the treponemes were numerous and readily and constantly found in smears. Twenty-eight hamsters were then inoculated with popliteal lymph node tissue from 12 sero-positive baboons. Positive TPI and FTA tests were obtained after 3–6 months and four hamsters developed treponeme-rich skin

2 A

lesions. The lesions resembled those of *T. pertenue* inoculation in the hamster but their evolution was slower, more restricted and they healed more rapidly. Reactions to the fluorescent antibody treponemal test were not found among 1236 cynomolgus from Cambodia and 106 *P. cyno-cephalus* from Kenya.

PATHOLOGY

Treponemes can penetrate the skin in a few minutes (animal experiments) and are presumably soon carried to the related lymph nodes and throughout the body. Multiplication continues in the early skin lesions and lymph nodes until the rising immunity processes overtake it. Lesions only arise in the skin and bones. Pathological changes in the central nervous and cardio-vascular systems have not been substantiated. Latent infection probably resides in the skin and lymph nodes.

The pathological basis of the early lesions (Ferris and Turner, 1937) is epithelial hyperplasia with prolongation of the epithelial papillae into the dermis, and oedema (Plate 7). There are exudation of leucocytes into the epidermis and foci of lymphocytes and plasma cells, sometimes perivascular, in the dermis. Turner and Hollander (1957) in experimental animal infections found that leucocytes were more frequent when the surface of the skin had been destroyed. Treponemes are present in the hypertrophied epidermis and in the cellular foci in the dermis where they multiply. Because much epithelial tissue is present without much destruction, little scarring remains on healing.

The changes of the late skin lesions resemble those in syphilis and histological criteria for their differentiation are unsatisfactory. Vascular changes are reported to be absent or at most not more frequent than in other inflammations although endarteritis may be more frequent in late syphilis than in late yaws. At present differences between the late pathological changes in syphilis and yaws appear to be quantitative rather than qualitative. Treponemes are scanty rather than absent. Opportunities for adequate pathological study of yaws in man may now have passed.

SYMPTOMATOLOGY

Yaws is characterised by latency interrupted by relapsing lesions of two kinds: early (secondary) multiple, non-destructive lesions, and the late (tertiary) less abundant destructive ones. Only the skin and bones are involved in yaws. Lesions in other tissues or organs, such as the cardio-vascular or central nervous systems, have not been confirmed. Increased cells in the cerebro-spinal fluid have been reported in yaws patients in the absence of organic nervous symptoms.

Initial lesion (Plate 8)

In many patients, an initial lesion develops at the site of infection after an incubation period of 3–5 weeks or longer. Powell (1923) failed to find initial lesions in only 20 per cent of 205 closely observed patients who had developed generalised early yaws lesions. The interval between initial lesions and the generalised lesions was 25–121 days.

The lesion resembles a large papilloma and is usually on an exposed part of the body; three-quarters are on the lower part of the leg and foot. The initial lesion is round or oval and 2–5 cm in diameter. It heals after several months unless it develops into a chronic ulcer which may remain to give a false impression of an initial lesion developing into a late yaws ulcer. Scars may at first be depigmented but may darken later when they may be difficult to detect.

Early lesions (Plates 9–16)

Some weeks or months after the appearance of the initial lesion, before or after it has healed, the generalised early eruption of papillomata commences often as a widely dispersed fine papular rash. At this time there may be lymph node enlargement and malaise, but these are often not recognised among other causes of ill health. Within a week or so many of these papules disappear and the others develop into the characteristic papillomata. There may be hundreds of them from a few millimetres up to 1–2 cm in diameter. In patients where yaws is in recession, however, there may be only a few large papillomata.

The round papillomata have a raised convex or flat granular surface. Their surface is reddish-yellow with an arabesque pattern caused by the paler hypertrophic epithelial tissue. They exude a clear yellowish serum which dries to form a yellowish-brown or black scab. The scab may be shed frequently or remain for some time and become thick. The first generalised eruption heals after a few months to leave little or no scarring. Bone pain with or without radiographically demonstrable lesions is often present.

During the early stage of infection, which is roughly the first 5 years or so, several relapses of the early lesions may occur. With each relapse there are fewer lesions. The palms and soles may be involved in painful papillomata or 'crab yaws' in later relapses and these may exceptionally arise years later when the prevalence of active yaws has fallen below 1 in 1000. Then, because they may be missed, they may cause some of the 'unaccountable' new infections or 'last cases'. Towards the end of the early stage too, and in cooler areas such as mountains, papillomata may be more frequent in the anogenital region than elsewhere; they may also be circinate.

Other early lesions are patches of acuminate and squamous macules. On the palms and soles squamous and hyperkeratotic macules may also occur. Early bone lesions such as periostitis, osteitis and osteomyelitis, involving at times most of the shaft of several long bones, are frequent. These are painful but not destructive and on healing leave little bony alteration (Hackett, 1951). Polydactylitis is frequent. Bony swellings, usually bilateral, of the frontal processes of the maxillae, goundou, have occurred in all yaws endemic populations in Africa; at times their prevalence in patients with papillomata has been 15 per cent. Its absence or extreme rarity from all other continents has not been explained.

Papillomatous buccal mucous membrane lesions were seen in Lango district of Uganda in a few children with yaws papillomata and biopsies were taken (Hackett, 1946). This is most unusual in all other yaws populations. Lango is not far from the southern Sudan where treponarid is present; in this infection mucous membrane lesions are characteristically frequent.

After a few years infectious relapses cease but the infection continues as a symptomless latency for usually at least 3 years before late lesions appear. In a few patients the passage into the late stage may be delayed for some years during which exceptional papillomatous relapses may appear, usually on the hands and feet. Early lesions and late lesions are due to different tissue responses and do not occur at the same time.

Late lesions (Plates 17–21)

These are characteristically destructive and thus on healing leave scars which may be thin and at first depigmented. Later they may contract or become keloid. They are often solitary and are most frequent in older adolescents and adults, though they may occasionally occur in children of about 10 years of age after early lesions have healed and within 3–5 years of their infection. In a yaws population fewer patients have late yaws ulcers and bone lesions than early lesions, but late palmar and plantar hyperkeratoses are often frequent.

Frequent late lesions are cutaneous and subcutaneous inflammatory nodules which break down and ulcerate to form either superficial sergipinous ulcers healing in the centre in some parts and extending widely in others, or round, deeper, less active ones. The margins are raised and the bases are coarsely granular or even nodular. Scars always remain on healing and may be extensive in area. Contractures may develop.

Hyperkeratotic palmar and plantar lesions are frequent in older patients and may accompany or result in depigmentation and atrophy. These lesions may be confused with mycotic infections or other conditions not at present well understood (Hackett and Lowenthal, 1960). Well-defined squamous erythematous plaques, especially about the hands and feet, are also seen. In highly endemic yaws areas in the past other skin diseases were often mistaken for yaws.

Late bone lesions consist of hypertrophic periostitis, gummatous periostitis, osteitis and osteomyelitis with nodular or general enlargement of the bones of the limbs, hands and feet and calvaria. These lesions are usually single and frequently ulcerate through the skin when pyogenic infection might rarely be added. On healing bony thickening usually remains. In some series bone lesions have been found in 10–15 per cent of patients with active yaws. Arthritis, bone necrosis and spontaneous fractures are not frequent in yaws but may perhaps be associated with added pyogenic infections. Destructive ulceration of the nose and mouth, gangosa ('rhinopharyngitis mutilans') occurs in all highly endemic yaws populations and can result in extensive destruction of the nose and palate. Its active stage is rarely seen now.

Painless firm fibrous nodes up to about 2 cm in diameter over bony prominences (juxta-articular nodules), pre-patellar bursal enlargement and ganglia of tendon sheaths may occur. The last are seen in both stages of the disease and usually resolve spontaneously.

Late yaws lesions relapse as do the early ones, but less frequently and at longer intervals. The last lesions to appear are those of the palms and soles. With increasing age the active disease becomes less frequent and ceases, but crippling contracture of the scars of late lesions may remain. The course of yaws may be perhaps comparable with that of untreated syphilis as found in the Oslo study (Gjestland, 1955). Spontaneous cure with sero-reversal may perhaps occur at any stage of the infection, although its frequency is unknown.

Several other lesions have been attributed to

yaws, such as sabre tibias, flexor contractures of the fingers resembling Dupuytren's contracture, in the absence of plantar skin changes, and depigmentation elsewhere than on the hands and feet: there is no general agreement about their yaws origin. An international nomenclature of the lesions of yaws has been drawn up in a World Health Organization monograph (Hackett, 1957).

With the progress of national treatment campaigns, the usually more florid and abundant yaws lesions become less frequent, and less typical manifestations attract more attention. The specific effect of arsenical preparations in the treponematoses at one time provided a practical therapeutic diagnostic test which is not available with the more widely effective penicillin.

The disabling sequelae of yaws are those of the late stage. They consist of contractures following late ulcers about joints, gangosa, contractures of the fingers accompanying palmar hyperkeratosis and discharging sinuses from pyogenic infection of ulcerated late yaws bone lesions.

In non-yaws countries the most frequent clinical manifestations in adult visitors and immigrants from yaws endemic areas are bone pain and bone swellings. Occasionally in the children of such migrants infectious early yaws may relapse but transmission would not be expected.

DIAGNOSIS

Where facilities are available the diagnosis of early yaws lesions would depend upon their appearance and the demonstration by darkground microscopy of characteristic treponemes in their exudates. Serological tests for syphilis become positive in yaws within the first few weeks of the infection. Thus there is no serological test that will distinguish yaws from other treponemal infections. Differentiation from syphilis remains a problem, especially in adults in towns; in doubtful cases if a patient comes from a rural area where yaws has recently occurred the infection is probably yaws, but if from a city or town it is more likely to be venereal syphilis.

In the rural areas of tropical countries serological tests are rarely employed. They may have little practical value in field work except in exploratory surveys of persons under 15 years of age in populations with very low prevalence of active yaws but thought to be at special risk. Such serological surveys would indicate the prevalence of infection in what is usually the most susceptible age group but, of course, the longer extensive active transmission has ceased, the higher the age of the susceptibles. Recent field studies in tropical countries where yaws is in recession have shown that lipoidal serological tests for syphilis, in persons with active yaws, and especially in children may give up to 30 per cent false reactions when compared with the TPI test. These are often transient and are probably due to infections with other communicable diseases (W.H.O., 1964). A specific test is needed in endemic areas and it is hoped that the fluorescent treponemal antibody test will provide this. In field work, past and present, diagnosis is based on clinical observation and considerable accuracy may be soon acquired.

In late yaws the clinical appearance and reactive serological tests are of some value. Judgement will, however, be needed in assessing the value in any particular patient of a reactive test to a syphilitic antigen. In an adult population with over 80 per cent serological reactives, although a treponemal infection may be present, symptoms may arise from one or more additional diseases.

DIFFERENTIAL DIAGNOSIS

In mass treatment of yaws, accuracy of diagnosis is most needed towards the end of the campaign to indicate the amount of active yaws remaining. Upon this the immediate operations must depend. Accuracy is less essential, though it is desirable, at the start when often all persons are treated. Initial prevalence figures for few yaws campaigns are reliable. Exaggerated prevalences of clinically active yaws in field work may arise from attributing to yaws certain conditions resembling yaws such as impetigo, tropical ulcer, ecthyma, tungiasis, occupational hyperkeratoses, the effects of vitamin deficiencies, mycoses, certain palmar and plantar lesions that are not due to yaws, and also by regarding 'yaws scars' as a yaws lesion.

A tropical ulcer commences as an inflammatory oedema and vesicle which soon gives way to extensive necrosis: this on separating leaves a chronic granulating ulcer. It reponds to penicillin therapy. Impetigo is most often seen about the face. Its thin-walled vesicles become pustular and result in scabs covering non-elevated inflammatory areas. Ecthyma may accompany impetigo or be present alone; on removing the scab a depressed loss of dermis is seen which is very different from the raised more granular yaws papillomata.

Tungiasis is likely to be confused with plantar papillomata. It is frequent on parts of the sole not in direct contact with the ground. The posterior extremity of the parasite may be found extruding reddish-brown pellets of faeces, or ova. *Tunga penetrans* may parasitise the buttocks. Certain vitamin deficiencies may result in papular lesions especially at the angles of the lips which may resemble early yaws lesions: other signs of the deficiencies should be sought. Mycoses of the soles have less induration than yaws lesions.

Macular leprosy lesions may resemble early yaws macules or maculo-papules. Acid-fast bacilli and other manifestations of leprosy, especially loss of sensation, should be sought. Plantar perforating ulcers may be mistaken for papillomata, but the ulcers are always painless. Gangosa has been confused with leprosy or syphilitic lesions and also with American dermal leishmaniasis and blastomycoses. Bone lesions of sickle cell anaemia and the dactylitis of tuberculosis may also need to be excluded from early yaws bone lesions. Pyogenic osteomyelitis and periostitis are usually more painful and of more rapid development than yaws bone lesions, but when they are added to an ulcerated late yaws bone lesion their recognition may be difficult without radiography, except that they are likely to be more painful.

A number of palmar and plantar lesions are not well understood nor are their causes known. They are characterised by thickening and fissuring of the epithelium and by pitting of the surface. They are usually worse in the wet season. These and other conditions to be differentated from yaws lesions have been dealt with in a World Health Organization monograph (Hackett and Lowenthal, 1960).

Depigmentation may occur in any of the treponematoses, but in patients with pinta there will also be the earlier stage dyspigmented areas in which treponemes should be sought in expressed serum. Depigmentation alone should not be attributed to yaws.

The differentiation of yaws from syphilitic lesions, especially late lesions in adults, may be very difficult. Often the only help to be obtained is from the rural or urban origin of the patient.

Corns and callosities due to ill-fitting shoes, warts and even rat gnawing of the soles while the victim sleeps may all be mistaken for yaws plantar lesions.

TREATMENT

The treatment of the occasional yaws patient in medically advanced countries is that of the corresponding stage of syphilis with antibiotics. Because lesions of the central nervous and cardiovascular system do not occur in yaws, single dose mass treatment can be used. Hume and Facio (1956) showed in Haiti that a single injection of 0.6 mega-units of procaine penicillin with 2 per cent aluminium monostearate (PAM) gave satisfactory results in active early yaws as judged by the absence of infectious relapses during the first year after treatment. This finding was of great importance in the eradication of yaws and hastened the abandonment of arsenical preparations of yaws.

Penicillin aluminium monostearate is in general use in mass treatment campaigns because of its effectiveness and low cost although some other antibiotics are also effective. It is usually given in single intramuscular doses of 1.2 mega-units for adults and 0.6 mega-units for patients under 15 years of age; half doses are given to latent cases (Hackett and Guthe, 1956). When this policy was generally applied in 1954, after the demonstration of its effectiveness in the Haitian national mass campaign, the population group treated as latent cases depended upon the prevalence of active yaws. If this prevalence was over 10 per cent all persons without active lesions were given half doses; if it was 5–10 per cent all children under puberty; and if it was under 5 per cent only household contacts of infectious patients received half doses.

So great has been the effect of the first of the above schemes, total mass treatment, that perhaps now, with the low cost of penicillin aluminium monostearate, many workers would recommend its use in all areas of yaws prevalence. Only a small part of the cost of the treatment surveys is for the drug and total mass treatment is simpler to carry out and is better received by most populations than other schemes; penicillin is known by many populations to be effective in a number of prevalent infections.

The response to these small doses of penicillin aluminium monostearate is excellent. Early lesions become non-infectious within a few days and are healed in 7–10 days. Subsequent relapses of infectious lesions are few and are delayed for a year or longer. Late lesions also heal, but a little more slowly. A prevalence of active lesions of 10 per cent at the first survey will probably be less than 2 per cent at a re-survey a year later and may mostly be among persons not previously seen; a further single injection to patients with active lesions and to their immediate contacts is followed by a further fall the following year.

Intense individual treatment in the early stage may result in sero-reversal but in the late stage this change is slower and less frequent. Following single injection mass treatment, sero-reversal is less rapid and less frequent, but the suppression of infectious relapses is of great public health importance.

Early treatment will rapidly heal all early lesions and limit the destruction of late ones. Early slight goundou will reduce and disappear with treatment, but late severe lesions may need surgical removal.

The prevention of yaws and the maintenance of its eradication depends upon the continued improvement of standards of living. In this are inextricably mingled adequate water supplies, adequate nutrition and road communications, all of which depend upon economic development. The factors favouring the transmission of yaws seem to be so unstable as to be readily displaced by such simple measures and the use of soap and water if these are not, indeed, mere indicators of improved standards of living. Recession of the infection has been noticeable everywhere since the 1920s, though when properly carried out, modern mass treatment is able to reduce a generation of time to a few years.

The development of adequate rural health services is essential—after mass treatment has reduced the prevalence of active yaws to under 2 per cent and infectious cases to 0.5 per cent— to maintain the necessary surveillance to bring to immediate treatment all infectious patients. This will ensure eradication at low cost. Yaws mass treatment teams, after the first or second resurvey, usually extend their activities to include other communicable diseases and other public health measures. Especially suitable for this purpose are operations, such as nation-wide smallpox vaccinations, which need only a brief single annual contact with each individual in the population.

It must be stressed again that the proper use of penicillin aluminium monostearate in mass treatment of yaws depends upon taking into account the high prevalences of latent infections. Treatment of these will take care of contacts which are usually impossible to recognise accurately. Examinations of over 80 per cent of the population in surveys at intervals of not more than 1 year are important for success.

Eradication is defined by the World Health Organization (W.H.O., 1960) as being achieved when no indigenous active case of yaws has appeared in the population for 3 years and no sero-reactor is found in persons under 5 years of age.

In the Nigerian national mass treatment campaigns, a team of 10 trained auxiliaries with an experienced field supervisor and under medical direction examined and treated 1500 people daily as long as sufficient persons were available (Zahra, 1956). After a few days 2–3 of the staff remained while the others moved to the next community where preparations had already been made.

In the Haiti campaign the surveys were made by house-to-house visits because of the scattered population; this has not been used so successfully elsewhere (Petrus et al, 1953).

In Indonesia mass treatment has been carried out by careful and frequent surveys and resurveys with the treatment of active cases only. The long-established village health administration in Java has made this successful but it may not be so successful in other countries lacking this important service (Soetopo et al, 1956).

In national yaws eradication campaigns, assisted by W.H.O. and U.N.I.C.E.F., up to 1970, over 160 million persons had been examined in initial treatment surveys and several times that number in all surveys and resurveys of whom 60 million had received penicillin (PAM) injections. Active yaws in most of these populations is now well below 0.5 per cent (Guthe et al, 1972)

In Indonesian mass treatment campaigns, after several annual surveillances the prevalence of infectious yaws has fallen below 0.5 per cent. In a number of such districts where disturbed conditions stopped annual surveillances for some years no active yaws in any age group was seen.

There may still be some millions of infected persons with a low prevalence of active yaws. For this reason governments may not regard the problem as justifying very active measures while there are so many more urgent calls on limited national finances; however, some reliable system of surveillance of the rural child population should be maintained. The success of yaws eradication campaigns by mass treatment surveys depends upon the recognition of the latency of yaws, the efficacy and proper use of long-acting penicillin, and the rising standards of living.

PROGNOSIS

Without treatment many grave disabilities may result from scarring, particularly about joints and from gross nasopalatine destruction. After single intramuscular injections of penicillin aluminium monostearate, the burden of the disease rapidly disappears, transmission of infection will cease and thus the present gradual recession of the disease will be hurried to eradication.

REFERENCES

BARNARD, C. C. (1952) *J. trop. Med. Hyg.*, **55**, 100, 135.
BOTREAU-ROUSSEL, J. N. (1922) *Osteitis Pianiques 'Goudou'*. Paris: Masson.
COLLART, P., BOREL, L-J. and DUREL, P. (1964) *Brit. J. vener. Dis.*, **40**, 81.
FERRIS, H. W. and TURNER, T. B. (1937) *Arch. Path. (Chicago)*, **24**, 703.
FRIBOURG-BLANC, A., NIEL, G. and MOLLARET, H. H. (1963) *Bull Soc. Path. exot.*, **56**, 474.
—— (1966) *Bull Soc. Path. exot.*, **59**, 54.
GJESTLAND, T. (1955) *Acta derm.-venereol. (Stockh.)*, **35**, Suppl.
GRIN, E. (1961) *Bull. Wld Hlth Org.*, **24**, 229.
GUTHE, T., RIGET, J., VORST, J., D'COSTA, J. and GRAB, B. (1972) *Bull. Wld Hlth Org.*, **46**, 1.
HACKETT, C. J. (1936) *Med. J. Aust.*, **1**, 733.
—— (1946) *Trans. roy. Soc. trop. Med. Hyg.*, **40**, 206.
—— (1951) *Bone Lesions of Yaws in Uganda*. Oxford: Blackwell.
—— (1957) *Wld Hlth Org Monogr Ser.*, No. 36.
—— (1963) *Bull Wld Hlth Org.*, **29**, 7.
—— (1970) *Trans. roy. Soc. trop. Med. Hyg.*, **64**, 615.
HACKETT, C. J. and GUTHE, T. (1956) *Bull. Wld Hlth Org.*, **15**, 869.
HACKETT, C. J. and LOEWENTHAL, L. J. A. (1960) *Wld Hlth Org. Monogr. Ser.*, No. 45.
HARDING, R. D. (1949) *Trans. roy. Soc. trop. Med. Hyg.*, **42**, 347.
HUDSON, E. H. (1958) *Non-Venereal Syphilis—a sociological and medical study of Bejel*. Edinburgh and London: Livingstone.
—— (1965) *Bull. Wld Hlth Org.*, **32**, 735.
HUME, J. C. and FACIO, G. (1956) *Bull. Wld Hlth Org.*, **15**, 1057.
LI, H-Y. and SOEBEKTI, R. (1955) *Bull. Wld Hlth Org.*, **12**, 905.
MAGNUSON, H. J., THOMAS, B. W., OLANSKY, S., KAPLAN, B. J. and CUTLER, J. C. (1956) *Medicine (Baltimore)*, **35**, 33.
NITSON, R. VAN (1944) *Mem. Inst. colon. Belge Soi. nat.*, **13**, No. 7.
PETRUS, E., LEVITAN, S., PAOLIELLO, A. and NICOL, R. (1953) *Bull. Wld Hlth Org.*, **8**, 261.
POWELL, A. (1923) *Proc. roy. Soc. Med.*, **16**, (3), 15.
SCHOEBL, O. (1928) *Philipp. J. Sci.*, **35**, 209.
SOETOPO, M. and WASITO, R. (1953) *Bull. Wld Hlth Org.*, **8**, 273.
SOETOPO, M., WASITO, R., SOEDARSONO, H. and TICKRODIPO, D. (1956) *Bull. Wld Hlth Org.*, **15**, 937.
STEWART, T. D. and SPOEHR, A. (1952) *Bull. Hist. Med.*, **26**, 538.
TURNER, T. B. and HOLLANDER, D. H. (1957) *Wld Hlth Org. Monogr. Ser.*, No. 35.
WORLD HEALTH ORGANIZATION (1960) *Wld Hlth Org. Tech. Rep. Ser.*, No. 129, 29.
—— (1964) *W.H.O. Chronicle*, **18**, 403.
ZAHRA, A. (1956) *Bull. Wld Hlth Org.*, **15**, 911.

24
Leptospirosis

SYNONYMS. There are no synonyms for leptospirosis. Numerous terms, used in the past, have stressed clinical and epidemiological features of some of these infections.

The notion, still prevalent, that 'leptospirosis' equals 'Weil's disease' equals 'spirochaetosis icterohaemorrhagica' is untenable. A patient may be suffering from leptospirosis even though he is not jaundiced, bleeding at various sites, in the throes of renal failure, and surrounded by *Rattus norvegicus*. Moreover, the syndrome described by Weil and others may be caused by agents other than *Leptospira* as well as by serotypes of *Leptospira* other than those which belong to the Icterohaemorrhagiae serogroup.

DEFINITION

Leptospirosis is infection of a vertebrate host with a strain of *Leptospira*, a genus of aerobic Gram-negative spirochaetes.

AETIOLOGY

Pending the collection of sufficient valid taxonomic data, strains of the genus *Leptospira* are tentatively arranged under one species—*Leptospira interrogans*. Within this mono-specific genus two 'complexes' are recognised. The parasitic and pathogenic strains—which comprise the interrogans complex—can be distinguished by biological and serological reactions from the saprophytic and non-pathogenic strains, which seem to exist without passage through any host; these comprise the biflexa complex. Preliminary studies of a few strains have already revealed four genetic groups of *Leptospira*. Within each complex the strains are arranged into serogroups and serotypes on the basis of cross-agglutination and agglutinin-absorption studies with antisera prepared in rabbits. In *Leptospira*, as in *Salmonella*, each strain possesses numerous agglutinogenic factors; but the analysis is not yet completed.

Some idea of the number of pathogenic serogroups and serotypes is provided in the latest published list of 16 serogroups and 120 serotypes (*W.H.O. Technical Report Series*, No. 380, 1967).

The serogroups, and the number of serotypes in each, are: Icterohaemorrhagiae 13, Javanica 5, Celledoni 2, Canicola 10, Ballum 3, Pyrogenes 9, Cynopteri 3, Autumnalis 13, Australis 10, Pomona 6, Grippotyphosa 2, Hebdomadis 25, Bataviae 7, Tarrasovi (syn, Hyos) 10, Panama 1, and Shermani. 1. This total of serotypes contrasts with the 11 which were recognised in 1939.

The reference laboratories do not agree unanimously with the status of some of these serotypes and of others reported more recently. The techniques of preparing suitable antisera in rabbits and of the agglutinin-absorption procedures have still to be standardised.

DISTRIBUTION

It has been stated that leptospirosis is probably the world's most widespread zoonosis; it probably occurs everywhere except in regions of permanent ice, tundra and desert. The extent of our knowledge has been, and will be, determined by the quality and quantity of laboratory investigations of materials from animals and man. During the last 30 years infections of man, his pets and livestock, and of a wide range of wild animals have been disclosed in many countries where they had been unsuspected. In some parts of the world leptospirosis presents a veterinary and economic problem to the livestock industry which rivals brucellosis in importance. Where an occupational risk of infection has been established, this has been countered by improvements in hygiene or by prophylactic vaccination.

EPIDEMIOLOGY

The natural history of leptospirosis can be considered under three headings: survival of leptospires outside their hosts, the modes of transmission, and the reservoir or maintenance hosts.

Survival outside host

Environmental conditions—the microclimate of a locality—affect the duration of survival of pathogenic and parasitic strains after they have been shed from the host. Optimal conditions are moisture, warmth (about 25°C), and pH values of surface waters and soil around neutrality. Adverse factors include desiccation, excessive sunlight (ultraviolet irradiation), pH values outside the range 6.2 to 8.0, salinity, chemical and bacterial pollution, and certain properties of soil (e.g. the adsorptive capacity of clays). Under favourable conditions leptospires can survive in water or damp soil for 3 weeks or more.

Modes of transmission

The commonest mode is indirect contact with an environment such as surface water (ponds, streams), mud, soil, foodstuffs or bedding which is contaminated with urine shed from a carrier host. Direct contact may occur: venereal transmission is common in some rodents (and leptospires may be present in the semen); transplacental infection of the fetus is common in livestock; and both modes have been reported in man. Bites by animals may provide a portal of entry, but leptospires are not excreted in the saliva. Blood-sucking arthropods—ticks, bedbugs, mosquitoes—may harbour leptospires, and passive transfer by flies is possible; but transmission by insects is not important in practice. In theory predatory animals might be infected by eating a recently killed animal carrier. Carrion eaters are less at risk because leptospires may survive for only a short time after death of the host—until the onset of post-mortem autolytic processes in the tissues and of bacterial contamination.

Reservoir or maintaining hosts

The natural reservoirs of *Leptospira* are wild animals, mainly mammals; but birds, reptiles, amphibians and fish can harbour the organisms in the cloaca. The order *Rodentia* is the most important: this includes mice, voles, gerbils and coypu, as well as rats. Any of these may be important in a particular locality; and many rats other than *Rattus norvegicus* are implicated. Orders other than *Rodentia* are also involved: *Insectivora* —hedgehogs, shrews: *Carnivora*—jackals, foxes, mongoose, skunks, racoons, civets, as well as dogs; *Marsupialia*—bandicoots, opossums; *Artiodactyla* —deer; and *Chiroptera*—bats.

Domesticated animals—livestock and hounds —are important; they can be affected by an outbreak of infection (epizootic) and they can maintain enzootic infection in the herd, flock, or pack.

Pets and laboratory animals may become infected—often without any sign of ill health. This applies particularly to rats and mice, as well as to dogs, guinea pigs and hamsters. The owners or laboratory staff may become infected and are liable to be seriously ill.

The interrelationships of the principal epidemiological categories of reservoir and incidental hosts are summarised in Fig. 24.1.

The reservoir state is not fully understood. A biological equilibrium is established between a strain of *Leptospira* and a host in which the organisms are able to survive and multiply in the convoluted tubules of the host's kidneys without any evident effect on the tissues. From here they are shed intermittently in the urine.

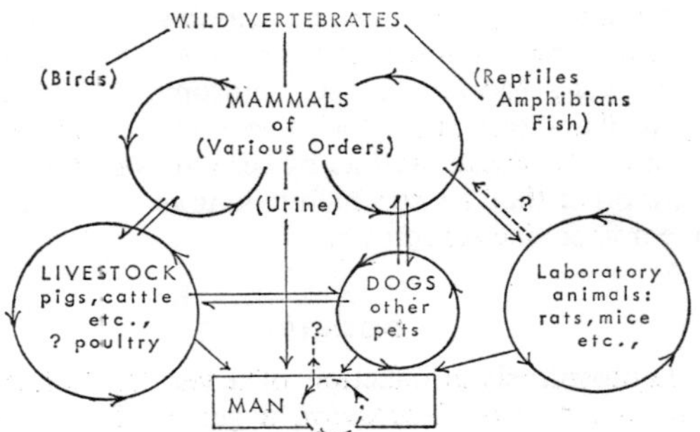

FIG. 24.1. *Relationships of the principal reservoir hosts of* Leptospiro.

A host species may act as a reservoir for various serotypes of *Leptospira*, sometimes for more than one in an individual animal. The same species of host may be infected by and become a temporary or convalescent carrier and urinary-shedder of other serotypes.

The extent of enzootic infections in animals varies from time to time and from place to place. The proportion of infected animals is affected by variations in the local microclimate, the availability of common water supplies and of food, the population densities of the various species, and the proportion of young to old animals.

The overall situation is dynamic. Interference by the works of man can also affect the situation —by altering the environment and therefore the ecological niches of the local fauna. The fauna must then adapt themselves to the new conditions or migrate in search of food or a more suitable habitat; they may thereby come closer to man and in increased numbers. Perennial operations such as harvesting may cause significant but temporary changes. More permanent effects result from the clearing of forest or scrub and by drainage or irrigation works.

Such changes are liable to affect the overall incidence of leptospirosis in man as well as the incidence of infections with various serotypes of *Leptospira*. The incidence of various syndromes may be affected by the prevalence of various serotypes—in the particular locality and at that time.

Thus the overall pattern of leptospirosis—the medical, veterinary, public health and bacteriological aspects—varies from region to region and from time to time. Such variations may be gradual,

The course in any vertebrate host is of two overlapping phases: *leptospiraemia* followed by increasing concentrations of antibodies with localisation of the organisms in the kidney and shedding resulting in *leptospiruria*.

Leptospires enter the blood stream within an hour or two of penetrating the host's epithelium. The usual incubation period is 7–14 days (range, 3–20 days or more). Meanwhile the organisms in the blood can reach, and may affect, any tissue or organ. The range of clinical manifestations is therefore wide.

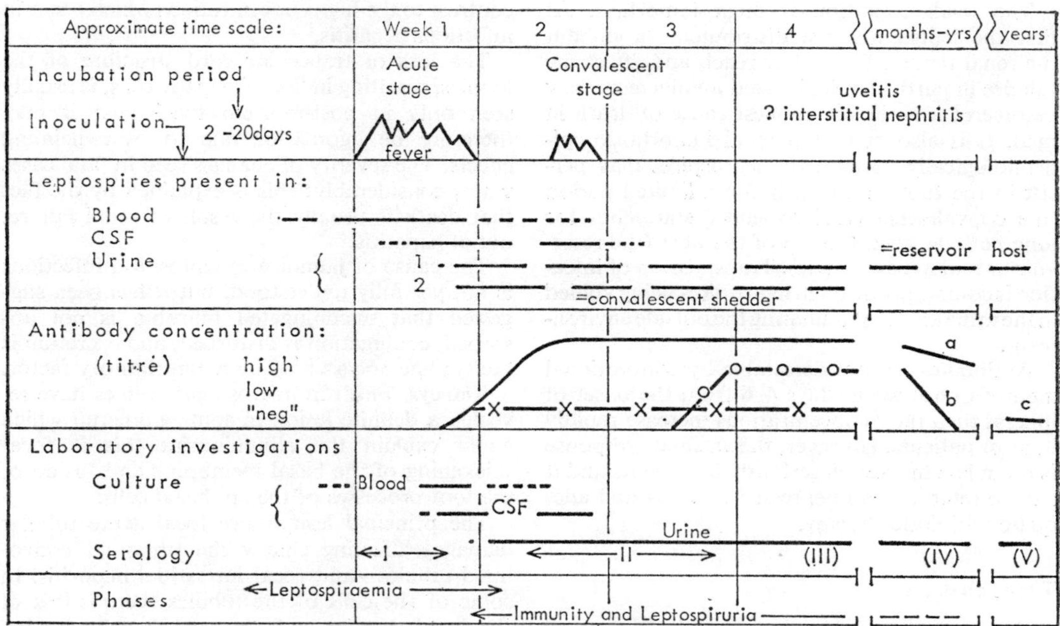

FIG. 24.2. *Leptospirosis: phases and relevant diagnostic procedures.*

or they may be more sudden, even dramatic. Surveillance of the situation is desirable and, for this to be effective, adequate laboratory facilities are essential.

PATHOLOGY

Course of infection

Some knowledge of the course of these infections is required for an understanding of the various clinical features which may occur, of the epidemiological and enzootiological aspects, of some preventive measures, and for the selection of appropriate specimens for laboratory investigations (see Fig. 24.2).

Infection in man usually results in fever with one of various clinical syndromes (see under *Differential diagnosis*), or with no localising signs (pyrexia of unknown origin, PUO), or with unusual features (e.g. Fort Bragg or 'pre-tibial' fever). Among pets and livestock, clinically mild infections seem to be common judging by the proportion of seroreactors to animals which have shown overt clinical signs. Severe infections are associated with jaundice, haemoglobinuria or haematuria, and raised concentrations of urea in the blood; they may be fatal. The flaccid mastitis syndrome occurs in cattle. The fetus may be affected leading to abortion, stillbirth, premature births, or weakly offspring. Recurrent iridocyclitis (periodic ophthalmia, moon blindness) has been associated with leptospirosis in horses; and uveitis may complicate infection in other animals. Interstitial nephritis has been associated with *canicola* infections in dogs, but the acute syndrome (Stuttgart disease) with ulcerative stomatitis is now rarely seen.

Leptospires are removed from most tissues by non-specific defence mechanisms, assisted later by increasing concentrations of specific antibodies. There are, however, two notable exceptions—the interior of the eye and the convoluted tubules of the kidneys—in which sites the leptospires are seemingly not affected by antibodies.

The renal condition is most important. At first the leptospires are distributed throughout the renal tissues. Later they reach and affect the tubules in particular. This renal involvement may be severe; it is the commonest cause of death in man. It is also of fundamental importance epidemiologically because the leptospires may persist in the tubules not only for a limited period (the convalescent carrier-shedder state) but for long periods, even the life of the host (the reservoir or maintenance state). Transmission of infection is commonly through leptospires being voided in the urine and contaminating the outside environment.

Antibodies are not detectable by conventional methods until about days 4–6 from the onset of illness; then their concentrations increase rapidly in most patients. However, the antibody response is often less marked in seriously ill patients and it can be retarded and depressed by early and adequate antibiotic therapy.

Tissue changes

Recent studies of biopsy material of liver and kidney by electron microscopy as well as by conventional histological methods have extended our knowledge. Most of the patients were moderately or severely ill with Icterohaemorrhagiae infection.

The lesions are focal. At lower magnifications seemingly normal tissue, foci of degenerated tissue and foci of regenerating tissue may all be observed in the same microscopic field. In electron micrographs, normal cells are seen next to abnormal cells. The abnormalities so observed suggest the action of some locally produced toxic substances. No endotoxin or exotoxins have yet been demonstrated, but certain strains of leptospires (e.g. of *pomona*) are associated with haemolysis and haemoglobinuria in some animals.

Capillaries. Localised swelling of the endothelium may be associated with interstitial oedema and haemorrhages.

Liver. In biopsy material, the lobular structure is maintained. Pathological effects are mainly restricted to the central zone of the lobule— enlarged liver cells, some multinucleate, with clear cytoplasm containing granules of bile pigments; and occasional acidophilic bodies resembling Councilman bodies. Küppfer's cells show hypertrophy and hyperplasia and may contain granules of bile pigments and haemosiderin. Biliary canaliculi often contain bile thrombi. Actual necrosis of liver cells is not a marked feature: this is also evident from the slight increase in concentration of serum transaminases which is usual, in marked contrast to the high concentrations which occur in infectious hepatitis.

The loss of trabecular cord structure of the lobules, resulting in 'loose' hepatic cells, is usually seen only in post-mortem specimens; it may therefore be agonal or due to overwhelming effects. The severity of changes seen in fatal cases varies considerably: this is explained by the fact that death is usually the result of renal failure, not of hepatitis.

The cause of jaundice in leptospiral infections is not yet fully understood, but it has been suggested that unconjugated bilirubin is not absorbed, conjugation is disturbed, and excretion is faulty; haemolysis may be a contributory factor.

Kidneys. Electron microscopic studies have revealed a definite lesion in some glomeruli which could explain the albuminuria: this is focal thickening of the basal membrane and fusion of the foot processes of the epithelial cells.

The principal lesions are focal acute tubular damage—affecting chiefly the proximal convoluted tubules—and focal interstitial nephritis. In some of the cells of the tubules there is loss of the brush border and areas of detachment between cells; in some there is depletion of mitochondria and diffuse rarefaction; in others, dense bodies (which may be altered mitochondria, or lysosomes) are seen. Casts and dilatation of the tubules may be prominent features. The precise mechanism of renal failure has still to be explained though it would seem to depend on the lesions of the tubules.

Voluntary muscle. Focal lesions may affect single muscle fibres or groups of fibres; they are not confined to the muscles of the leg. The gross appearance of the muscle is normal except, perhaps, for punctate haemorrhages. The microscopic changes include loss of cross-striation of the fibres, swelling and hyalinisation. There is seldom any permanent scarring or fibrosis. The presence of leptospiral antigen in such foci has been revealed by immunofluorescence.

Other organs and tissues. Focal infiltrations and haemorrhages, slight to severe, may occur in the skin, lungs, brain, spleen, lymph nodes, gastro-intestinal tract and in the adrenal glands.

CLINICAL FEATURES

The dissemination of leptospires during the phase of leptospiraemia would account for the wide variety of symptoms and signs—in various combinations—which can occur.

The clinical effects—severity of illness, symptoms and signs—are determined by an interplay of factors: the strains of *Leptospira* and the condition of the hosts. The factors which determine the virulence and pathogenicity of strains of *Leptospira* are not known. The agglutinogenic characters are not an essential factor: thus, for example, oriental strains of serotype *bataviae* tend to cause severe illness in man (e.g. Weil's syndrome), whereas European strains produce only a mild or moderately severe illness. Other examples of such geographical differences are known; more may remain to be reported.

The condition of the host may affect the clinical manifestations. Thus, in patients with a poor general condition the illness tends to be more severe. If there is pre-existing derangement, even subclinical in degree, of any particular system or organ this may seem to be most seriously involved, and to dominate the syndrome. If such conditions are prevalent among the population, the incidence of these leptospiral syndromes will tend to be higher than in other, healthier, populations.

The clinical manifestations in one region (country or part of a country) tend to be fairly constant at any particular time; but they may seem to be atypical to the inexperienced (see *Differential diagnosis*). Occasionally some bizarre feature may dominate the clinical pattern. An example was the skin rash localised to the front of the legs in 'pretibial' or Fort Bragg fever which was eventually proved to be caused by strains of an unknown serotype, *fort-bragg*, which belongs to the Autumnalis serogroup.

The fallacy of regarding leptospirosis as synonymous with Weil's syndrome cannot be over-emphasised. In some parts of the world this hepatorenal syndrome is common; elsewhere it is not. The clinical manifestations of leptospirosis are varied. Clinical diagnosis is therefore unreliable until astute physicians have seen more than a few patients in whom the diagnosis has been established by laboratory investigations.

The commoner symptoms and signs are indicated below; they occur in various combinations and permutations.

Onset: often sudden, with or without rigors. Fever is usual and may be biphasic in untreated patients.

Malaise: prostration is often more severe than the signs seem to warrant; sore throat; joint pains.

Gastrointestinal tract: nausea, vomiting; diarrhoea or constipation.

Muscles: pain; tenderness, often acute; weakness. The calves are often affected; but other groups may be involved—pectorals, back, and abdomen (which may lead to a presumptive diagnosis of acute abdominal emergency, laparotomy, and a baffled surgeon). Pseudo-paralysis may be due to reluctance to use affected muscles.

Meninges: headache is often severe and intractable; analgesics may be of no avail but lumbar puncture relieves the pain. Meningism and stiff neck are quite common and often dominate the clinical picture during the febrile relapse, if not from the onset.

Cerebrospinal fluid: increased pressure; pleocytosis; increased protein but normal concentrations of sugar and chloride. Routine cultures are 'sterile', but leptospires may be isolated.

Eyes: conjunctival injection is common. The small blood vessels which radiate over the bulbar conjunctiva appear distended, but signs of acute inflammation are lacking. There may be sub-conjunctival haemorrhages. Later, uveitis or optic neuritis are uncommon sequelae.

Central nervous system: altered reflexes; Babinski's and Kernig's signs may be elicited. Rarely the spinal cord is affected or transverse myelitis occurs.

Skin: rashes are not common; petechiae, ecchymoses; occasionally macular (morbilliform, etc.); may be localised (e.g. to the front of the leg).

Lymph nodes: enlargement of superficial groups is not uncommon; may be a prominent feature.

Lungs: basal rales are common; sputum may be blood-tinged. Actual pneumonitis, with radiological signs, may be the dominant feature.

Vascular system: haemorrhages may be slight or gross (even fatal), affecting the skin, muscles, kidneys (may only be evident from increased red cells in centrifuged deposit of urine), lungs, stomach, intestines; epistaxis (at onset; should be part of the questionnaire in taking the patient's history).

Heart: arrhythmias, defects of conduction, hypotension.

Blood: the ESR is usually raised. The total white cell count is often within normal limits for the population; sometimes raised, occasionally below normal limits. In all cases there is a tendency to neutrophilia (leptospirosis must always be considered when there is leucopenia with normal or increased numbers of neutrophil cells).

Kidneys: albuminuria is very common, but may be transient in the early stage; casts (commonly granular), red cells and leucocytes may be detected in centrifuged deposits of urine. The blood urea concentration may be increased without signs of renal failure. Renal failure is the commonest cause of death.

Liver: jaundice is common in some territories, rare in others. Jaundice supervenes after a few days of fever and when the patient's condition is deteriorating; associated commonly with evidence of renal involvement. Liver function tests suggest hepatocellular derangement. Serum transaminase concentrations are usually not very much increased, in marked contrast to the findings in infectious hepatitis.

DIFFERENTIAL DIAGNOSIS

The symptoms and signs in leptospiral infections often occur in combinations which may mimic, to a greater or lesser extent, those of various well-known febrile syndromes many of which are more often presumed, by clinicians, to be caused by viral infections. Leptospirosis should therefore be considered in the differential diagnosis of the following kinds of febrile illnesses, particularly if the original presumptive diagnosis is not confirmed by serological or other laboratory investigations.

Influenza-like illness, especially in sporadic cases.

Aseptic meningitis.

Other febrile illnesses associated with involvement of the nervous system (e.g. encephalitis, non-paralytic poliomyelitis).

'*Dengue*' and the other '*-algias*' which often constitute a high proportion of so-called diagnoses in the monthly returns of diseases.

Rickettsioses (Q fever, tropical typhuses).

'*Enteric.*'

'*Glandular fever.*'

Brucellosis and other fevers with recurrences or relapses of fever.

Jaundice with fever, especially if associated with signs of renal involvement or haemorrhages (e.g. yellow fever, etc.).

'*Atypical*' *pneumonias.*

Nephritis for which no obvious cause is evident.

Pyrexia of unknown origin (PUO) in which the duration of fever is less than 14 days and whatever the clinical symptoms and signs may be.

DIAGNOSIS

Clinical diagnosis of leptospiral infections is unreliable because they may seem to mimic so many syndromes or to evoke no pathognomonic symptoms or signs. However, physicians who are served with adequate laboratory facilities and who see more than a few patients with leptospirosis soon become adept in suspecting the correct diagnosis. Cynics regard the conditions listed above (*Differential diagnosis*) as comprising a diagnostic rubbish dump. However, laboratory investigations if properly used will supply some, if not many, of the answers. Fortunately, a definitive diagnosis of 'leptospirosis' can be established in a very high proportion of leptospiral infections by means of various serological tests, some of which can be carried out in any general-duty laboratory.

Serological tests for leptospirosis are of two sorts: first the so-called 'genus-specific' tests which differentiate leptospiral infections from those caused by other aetiological agents and second, agglutination tests which will often indicate the serogroup to which the infecting strain belongs, though they should not be regarded as 'serotype-specific'.

The 'genus-specific' tests can be carried out in any laboratory where serological procedures are performed. Four kinds of 'genus-specific' tests are available: complement fixation (using any reliable technique), the sensitised erythrocyte lysis or hemolytic (SEL or HL) test, indirect immunofluorescence, and the biflexa agglutination test. Each of these tests requires only one antigen preparation. The complement fixation test is preferred because the leptospiral antigen can be included with a battery of viral antigens in screening tests of sera from patients with febrile illnesses. The other 'genus-specific' tests require a separate procedure.

Agglutination tests are of two kinds—microscopic and macroscopic. The standard microscopic agglutination test requires a battery of antigen suspensions prepared from cultures of various strains; it is likely to be restricted to few laboratories. Antigens for the macroscopic test are available commercially; but if appropriate positive and negative controls are not included these may give misleading results.

In the serology of leptospirosis, as in other infections, the time at which specimens of sera are taken is important but, regrettably, is very often ignored. A serum obtained in the early days of illness may be 'negative', but it may contain residual antibodies from some previous infection. However, this is a very important specimen for comparison with those obtained later in the course of illness. The duration of the illness should always be stated to the serologist to whom the date of admission to hospital (quite often divulged) is meaningless. Serum specimens should also be adequate in volume: few patients will suffer adverse effects from being deprived of 10 ml of blood!

The infecting strain may be isolated, from patients who have not received antibiotics, from the blood during the first 6–7 days from onset of illness, from the CSF, and from the urine (day 7 onwards). Isolation may be achieved by direct inoculation of suitable culture media, or by inoculation of laboratory animals.

TREATMENT

The methods of treatment are not influenced by the identity of the infecting strain of *Leptospira*. Patients with mild or moderately severe illness recover without any special treatment, antibiotics or other methods.

Antibiotics, other than chloramphenicol which seems to be the least effective, are useful. If administered in adequate dosage during the first 3–4 days from onset of illness, they will relieve the symptoms and prevent the onset of complications (jaundice, renal failure) and sequelae (e.g. uveitis). They may cause a transient exacerbation of symptoms with a Herxheimer type of reaction which may be dealt with by conventional supportive measures. Military physicians in Malaya came to regard this reaction as a confirmation of their presumptive diagnosis of leptospirosis. As judged by agglutination tests, early and adequate antibiotic therapy may also retard and depress the antibody response. The later antibiotic therapy is begun, the less effective it will be.

Penicillin is the antibiotic of choice because it is least likely to affect the patient adversely; but tetracyclines, erythromycin and others are effective. The dosage of penicillin depends on the severity of illness. A minimum of 2.4 mega-units in 24 hours is advisable, but the dosage may be greatly increased, and be administered with intravenous fluids, unless contraindicated. The course of antibiotics should continue for 6–7 days, or for 2 days after the temperature has reverted to normal.

Other treatment is supportive: analgesics for pain; lumbar puncture for intractable headache; dietary restriction and correction of electrolyte imbalance for hepatic and renal dysfunction. The state of renal function should be carefully monitored; when evidence of renal failure is obtained, recourse to peritoneal dialysis or the artificial kidney should not be delayed. Renal failure is the commonest cause of death and these measures have saved lives.

PROPHYLAXIS AND PREVENTION

Vaccines have been used successfully in occupational groups exposed to risk of infection (e.g. miners in Japan and Poland; rice-field workers in Italy and Spain). The vaccine should be prepared from local strains of the predominant serotypes. No so-called wide-spectrum vaccine is yet available.

When a person has been exposed to great risk of infection (e.g. laboratory accidents with known virulent strains) a course of antibiotic treatment will abort the infection. With less urgent exposure the alternative to prophylactic treatment is for any fever which may occur within the subsequent 5 weeks to be regarded as possibly leptospiral in origin. This incident should be reported at once; blood is taken for attempts to isolate the strain; then treatment is begun.

Personal and communal hygienic measures to counter contamination by infected urine from carrier hosts are advised.

Control of reservoir hosts is, in practice, seldom effective except in restricted environments.

PROGNOSIS

Prognosis is good. Many patients recover without specific treatment (and without correct diagnosis of their illness). The more severely affected will recover provided renal and hepatic function is supported. There is no evidence that significant permanent renal or hepatic dysfunction results from leptospiral infections in man.

FURTHER READING

Current problems in leptospirosis research
WORLD HEALTH ORGANIZATION (1967) *Wld Hlth Org. techn. Rep. Ser.*, No. 380. (This contains the latest list of serotypes and serogroups.)

Serology (discussion of methods and interpretation of results)
TURNER, L. H. (1968) *Trans. roy. Soc. trop. Med. Hyg.*, **62**, 880.

Isolation and maintenance of strains
TURNER, L. H. (1970) *Trans. roy. Soc. trop. Med. Hyg.*, **64**, 623.

Laboratory techniques
GALTON, MILDRED M., MENGES, R. W., SHOTTS, E. B., NAHMIAS, A. J. and HEATH, C. W. (1962) *Leptospirosis: Epidemiology, Clinical Manifestations in Man and Animals, and Methods in Laboratory Diagnosis.* U.S.P.H.S. Publication No. 951. Washington, D.C.: U.S. Government Printing Office.
ALEXANDER, A. D., GOCHENOUR, W. S. Jr., REINHARD, K. R., WARD, M. K. and YAGER, R. H. (1970) Leptospirosis. In *Diagnostic Procedures and Reagents*, 5th edn., pp. 382-421. New York: American Public Health Association.

25
Fungal Diseases

Clinical mycology is such a wide subject that only the manifestations of greatest importance to medicine in the tropics can be discussed in a work of this nature.

The *Thallophytae* form one of the four main subdivisions of the plant kingdom. They are divided into *algae* and *fungi* or *mycetes*. Algae are differentiated from the fungi in that they contain chlorophyll and can synthesise their food from carbon and water with the aid of sunlight. Fungi cannot do this.

Fungi reproduce through the agency of spores. Reproduction starts with the spore enlarging lengthwise to form a tube-like process called the germ spore. This elongates into a filament known as a hypha. In some fungi septa form transversely dividing the filament into chains of cells known as septate hyphae. Others remain essentially unicellular throughout. The hyphae branch and rebranch eventually forming a complicated network called the mycelium. The mycelium is divided into two functionally distinct units. The vegetative mycelium constitutes the main bulk of the fungus and is concerned with obtaining nutrition. The aerial mycelium has long fine particles projecting above the vegetative mycelium. It is from the aerial mycelium that the spores are formed.

Many fungi are dimorphic, existing in two separate forms. When dimorphic fungi invade the body they do so in the shape of unicellular parasitic yeast-like organisms. On the other hand, under natural conditions, in the soil for example, fungi exist as filamentous saprophytes. The form the organisms assume depends largely on temperature. Many dimorphic fungi can be grown on acid-dextrose-peptone agar (Sabouraud's medium). If they are cultured at 37°C (body temperature) they take the form of unicellular yeast-like organisms similar to their appearance when invading human tissue. If grown at 22°C (room temperature) they form filamentous growths similar to their appearance under natural conditions.

The diseases caused by fungi may conveniently and simply be classified into two groups:

1. *Dermatomycoses*: fungus diseases affecting the skin only.

2. *Systemic mycoses*: diseases caused by fungi which affect the skin but which under certain circumstances can invade the internal tissues of the body.

DERMATOMYCOSES

The classification of the dermatomycoses is more conveniently based upon the part of the body affected rather than the type of fungus responsible because different species of fungi can produce identical clinical results.

Tinea pedis

Fungus infection of the feet is extremely common in tropical countries especially in European residents. Less sophisticated indigenous people, who do not wear socks or shoes, are seldom affected. Reinfection is extremely common so that the disease assumes the aspect of a chronic affection.

The infecting fungus is usually *Epidermophyton floccosum* though species of *Microsporum* or *Candida albicans* may be responsible.

Clinically the first indication is usually irritation of varying severity between the toes, frequently between the fourth and fifth toes. A small red linear fissure may be present in this area which may spread to the areas between other toes. Ultimately a chronic intertrigo is produced. The skin in the affected areas becomes thickened, white and sodden. Flakes of epithelium may peel of exposing areas of pink erythematous skin. A more acute form may be present with vesicles or pustules which may spread to the sole of the foot. An unpleasant odour is frequent. Secondary infection with pyogenic organisms is not unusual, perhaps leading to lymphadenitis of the groin. A more chronic form is encountered chiefly affecting the heel and sole of the foot. The skin is flaky and thickened with hyperkeratosis. Scales can be scraped off revealing a background of erythematous skin.

Diagnosis is made by digesting a snippet of skin in 10 per cent potassium hydroxide solution when the appropriate fungus may be revealed under the microscope.

2B

Treatment consists in immobilising the patient in bed if much inflammation is present and frequent bathing of the affected parts in a 1 : 400 solution of potassium permanganate until the acute stage has subsided. Then Castellani's paint or half-strength Whitfield's ointment should be applied twice daily and continued for a week after all traces of the infection have disappeared. For the average patient with a chronic indolent infection an ointment containing merthiolate or one of the undecylenate compounds is less messy and generally more acceptable. Griseofulvin given orally, 0.5 to 1 g daily in divided doses for 3 to 4 weeks, is effective for obstinate infection of the soles of the feet, but fails to clear toe-web infection.

Prophylaxis is important as reinfection is so common. This implies frequent washing of the feet, which should be thoroughly dried, especially between the toes. A thymol iodide salicylic acid dusting powder should be employed. Cotton socks should be used and changed daily. If circumstances permit sandals rather than shoes should be worn. Frequently, infection arises from communal showers, bath mats and the sodden surrounds of swimming baths and these should be avoided.

Tinea cruris (eczema marginatum, Dhobie's itch)

This extremely frequent infection is usually due to *E. floccosum*. It usually causes a bilateral affection of the groins though it may appear in the axillae. It takes the form of a raised area of erythematous skin in the upper and inner aspect of the groin from which it may spread to the scrotum or posteriorly towards the perineum. A diagnostic feature is the abrupt margin between affected and normal skin. The periphery is the spreading margin of the lesion and in this area the inflammation is more intense, perhaps resulting in small closely set vesicles or pustules. Occasionally the surface of the lesion shows more acute inflammation with weeping exudate and an offensive odour. In long-standing cases the skin is dry, thickened and lichenified.

Diagnosis is effected from skin scrapings. Treatment consists in bathing with a dilute solution of potassium permanganate if inflammation is acute and the subsequent application of half-strength Whitfield's ointment or Castellani's paint.

Tinea corporis

This is not so common as fungus of the feet or groins. It is the result of infection with various species of *Trichophyton* or *Microsporum*. Any portion of the body may be affected. A single lesion or many may be present. The individual lesions are usually round or annular in shape. They may coalesce to form larger plaques. The centre of the lesion is usually scaly but the more active periphery is erythematous often with vesicles or pustules.

Diagnosis is made by demonstrating the presence of the fungus in skin scrapings. The lesions readily resolve after the application of 5 per cent ammoniated mercury ointment or a 3 per cent sulphur and salicylic acid preparation.

Tinea versicolor (Plate 22)

Tinea versicolor has a world-wide distribution being encountered with great frequency in the tropics. The fungus responsible for the infection is *Malassezia furfur*. It particularly affects young adults. It causes a superficial discoloration of the affected skin forming brownish sheets with rather indistinct margins. Extensive areas of skin, usually on the trunk, may be involved. Although usually asymptomatic slight irritation may result. Long-standing cases may exhibit pseudoachromia in which case the colour of the skin becomes paler than normal.

The condition is important to recognise because in dark-skinned individuals the pale areas of skin not infrequently cause a suspicion of leprosy. Scrapings of skin will demonstrate the thick-walled round fungus and budding forms may be encountered. Treatment involves frequent hot baths with vigorous rubbing of the affected areas. Half-strength Whitfield's ointment or 3 per cent sulphuric and salicylic acid are then applied. Reinfection should be prevented by boiling bed linen and underclothes.

Tinea imbricata

This is the result of infection from *Trichophyton concentricum*. It is encountered in the Pacific Islands, China, Ceylon and in South-east Asia. It does not occur in Africa or the Middle East. The disease often affects broad sheets of skin on the trunk but rarely attacks the nails or the hair. The lesions consist of brown maculo-papules which undergo scaling. It is characteristic of the scaling that the free borders of the scale face inwards towards the centre of the lesion. There is often a brown or erythematous colour at the active spreading periphery. The lesions are concentric and may be very profuse. The treatment consists in the application of 5 per cent sulphur and salicylic acid or full-strength Whitfield's ointment.

Trichomycosis axillaris

This disease has a ubiquitous distribution. It affects the hair of the axillary or occasionally the pubic region. The responsible fungus is *Nocardia tenuis*. It is apt to affect individuals who sweat excessively in the axillae. The hairs contain yellow, black or red concretions which form around the shaft of the hairs sometimes surrounding them in a sheath-like tube. The concretions are firmly cemented on to the hairs, rendering them lustreless and brittle and altering their colour. The various colours are said to be formed by pigment-producing cocci. The roots of the hairs and the adjacent skin are not involved. The treatment is to shave the hairs from the affected parts and to apply 2 per cent formalin in alcohol or a 1 per cent solution of bichloride of mercury.

Rhinosporidiosis

Although this truly horrible disease is usually classed among the dermatomycoses it is not strictly a skin disease. It confines its attention mainly to the mucous membranes.

It is due to infection with *Rhinosporidium seeberi*. It occurs in the tropics generally and is especially common in India and Ceylon. It is suggested that the fungus primarily attacks fish and that man is only accidentally infected. The fungus is commonly acquired through contact with water, particularly stagnant water. Males are almost exclusively affected.

Clinically the nose is the most frequent site of the lesion, being involved in 72 per cent of 280 patients. The first symptom is nasal irritation which is accompanied by a mucoid discharge from the nares. Small sessile papillomata form in the nasal mucous membrane. They enlarge and become pedunculated. Eventually polypoidal tumours protrude from the nares and hang in festoons over the upper lip. The tumours extend posteriorly and overhang the pharynx. In the conjunctivae granulomatous masses form and may eventually evert the eyelids, or they may block the lacrimal duct and cause infection. Lesions in the ear resemble aural polyps. The rectum or vagina may be involved and in these situations the tumours may be confused with piles or condylomata. The disease is exceedingly chronic and cases persisting for 35 years have been described. The general health of the patient is little affected.

Treatment consists in removal of the growths by means of a snare. The bases of the tumours are then touched with the electrocautery. Tartar emetic injections intravenously have been reported to disperse the lesions. Neostibosan 0.2 g daily given intravenously for a total dose of 3 g has also been advised.

Chromoblastomycosis (Plate 23)
(verrucous dermatitis, 'mossy foot')

The various fungi causing chromoblastomycosis exist in soil and woodpulp and are introduced into the skin by trauma. The disease does not occur in Asia but is found in most tropical and subtropical countries especially in males of the labouring classes in Central, South and North Africa.

Clinical. Chromoblastomycosis commonly commences on an exposed area of skin, frequently on the foot, as a small irritating papule. It gradually enlarges extending from the periphery to resemble a tinea infection. The margins of the lesion are sharp and often of a violaceous hue. With the passage of time, often several months, crops of new lesions appear along the areas of superficial lymphatic drainage. These gradually become elevated and the surface of the lesion assumes a papular and wart-like appearance. These growths extend so gradually that it may take anything between 4 and 15 years before the greater part of the leg or arm is affected. Islands of normal skin are left unmolested. Extensive fibrosis occurs so that the lymphatic drainage is blocked and elephantoid oedema appears. The general health remains good and the disease is localised to the skin and subcutaneous tissues.

Diagnosis is affected by finding the fungus, which has typical gondispores, in the lesion.

Treatment by potassium iodide is sometimes effective. The drug is given by mouth and gradually increased until a daily dose of 3 g is reached and maintained for long periods. Amphotericin B is to be preferred. If the lesions are superficial and not too extensive, surgery is indicated.

Tinea favosa

Favus is prevalent in countries in the Middle East, especially in Iran, Iraq and Israel. It is one of the commonest fungus infections of Egypt. According to a World Health Organization newsletter there are villages in northern Syria where every child is affected. The disease also occurs in Eastern Europe. It tends to favour conditions of poverty, dirt and squalor.

The fungi responsible are *Trichophyton schoenleini*, *T. violaceum* and *Microsporum gypseum*. The disease affects children and adolescents in the main but may also attack adults.

Clinically, the first sign appears on the scalp as a minute yellowish red puncture area. This soon becomes covered with concave cup-shaped crusts. Soon the condition spreads and in a relatively short period of time a large area of scalp becomes covered with crusts or scutula. Hairs frequently protrude through the scutula. Removal of the crusts reveals depressed ulcers with weeping red bases. The hair loses its sheen and drops out. The whole scalp may be affected and crusted over. The disease has serious consequences because as the infection reaches the deeper layers of the skin it may result in much scarring and baldness. The scalp often exudes a peculiar mousy odour. Sometimes the eruption resembles seborrhoeic eczema. The glabrous skin may be affected and rarely the nails.

Diagnosis is revealed by the typical concave scales. The lesion fluoresces under Wood's light. Microscopical examination of the scales will reveal the fungus.

Treatment. To affect a cure depilation is required. This is usually achieved by X-rays which should be administered by an expert. The remaining hairs should be removed manually. Afterwards 3–5 per cent ammoniated mercury ointment should be applied and well rubbed in. Half-strength Whitfield's ointment may also be used. Griseofulvin produces excellent results orally in doses of 0.5–1 g daily. Treatment must continue until the infection has completely resolved.

SYSTEMIC MYCOSES

The diseases caused by pathological fungi when they invade the body have certain features in common. They tend to produce chronic lesions which often take the form of granulomata. These may form pus which reaches the surface and discharges through indolent sinuses. The fungi causing systemic infection are mostly of the dimorphic type, the fungi assuming a yeast-like form in the body. There are exceptions to this, for example actinomycosis and aspergillosis.

Infection by fungi may be acquired in a variety of ways. Inoculation may take place of a fungus deep to the skin, for example through an open wound or on the point of a thorn as in mycetoma. There is seldom any general dissemination from this type of lesion. The fungus may be inhaled, as in histoplasmosis or aspergillosis. When this occurs infection of the lungs takes place. Blood-borne dissemination from the lungs may then result. If this happens the favourite target organs are the brain, bones and the suprarenal cortex, though the liver, spleen and heart may also be involved.

Diagnosis is usually achieved by finding the fungus in pus, sputum or biopsy material. Cultural methods are frequently successful using Sabouraud's medium. Cultures should always be set up at room temperature and at body heat. Skin tests for hypersensitivity to a particular fungus are widely used but their specificity is limited.

Mycetoma

Mycetoma is the term employed to describe a clinical condition which can be caused by a number of different fungi. It commonly affects the foot when it is usually referred to as Madura foot or maduramycosis.

Mycology. The fungi responsible for the infection exist as saprophytes in the soil or plants. The organisms commonly belong to the genera *Nocardia*, *Streptomyces* or *Madurella*. In the body the fungi produce characteristic granules of

TABLE 1. *Characteristics of the main species of fungi causing mycetoma*

Species	Colour of granules	Habitat
Nocardia asteroides	Yellow, white	America, Asia, Europe, Africa
Nocardia braziliensis	Yellow	South America, Central America
Streptomyces madurae	Yellow, white or red	India (Madura), Asia, Africa, Europe, America
Streptomyces pelletieri	Red	Africa, America, India, Sudan
Streptomyces somaliensis	Yellow	Somaliland, Sudan, Ethiopia, Nigeria
Madurella mycetomi	Black	India, South America

various colours, yellow, white, red or black. The fungi are sometimes identified by the colour of the granules but the accuracy of this procedure is doubtful owing to unpredictable variations. The commonest fungi causing mycetoma are given in Table 1 together with the usual colour of the granules and the countries in which they occur.

Clinical. The disease occurs in India, Sudan, the Somalilands, Ethiopia, West Africa and in Central and South America. The male sex is affected ten times more frequently than the female. The infection commonly attacks young adults though it is not unknown in teenagers. Nearly all the patients are farm workers or engaged in agriculture. The source of infection is exogenous and there is frequently a history of trauma such as a wound from an agricultural implement or a scratch from a thorn. The foot is involved in 80 per cent of cases, the leg in 10 per cent and the hand in 7 per cent.

The first manifestation is a small nodule in or beneath the skin which soon becomes attached to deeper structures. Occasionally a vesicle is first encountered. A chronic granulomatous process occurs which is accompanied by pus formation and which spreads deeply into the tissues involving fascia, muscles, tendons, ligaments and bones and joints. A chronic osteomyelitis, essentially destructive with little formation of new bone, is set up. The disease progresses slowly, but in spite of remissions at first, proceeds in a remorseless manner. The skin and subcutaneous nodules become multiple. They rupture and discharge an oily looking fluid which contains the coloured granules. Sinuses form which lead deep into the affected tissues. As many as eight abscesses or sinuses may be present on the foot. The skin of the foot becomes indurated and discoloured. Areas of fibrous tissue representing attempts at healing and forming depressed scars are encountered. The foot undergoes considerable elephantoid enlargement and becomes clubbed.

The disease runs a very chronic course and may persist for 15 or more years. X-rays reveal the osteomyelitis with much erosion of bone and destruction of joint surfaces. The condition is not usually painful and locomotion is usually well maintained. There are no constitutional symptoms unless secondary infection is present.

Treatment. Medical treatment may well be effective though it has to be continued for long periods. It should always be tried before resort to surgical measures. A wide-spectrum antibiotic should be given for 1 week to remove any secondary infection. After this diamino-diphenylsulphone (dapsone) is given in doses of 100 mg by mouth twice daily and continued for 2 years. Initially the patient should be under close observation as toxic effects, such as exfoliative dermatitis or haemolytic anaemia, may occasionally occur with large doses of dapsone. Not all fungi respond to this treatment. The result is usually good if the infection is caused by the genus *Nocardia* or by *Madurella mycetomi*.

In early cases in which the disease has not been arrested by medical treatment excision must be undertaken. It must be appreciated that involvement of deeper structures is always more extensive than it appears and that the excised area should include a wide zone of apparently healthy tissue. In very advanced cases if medical treatment is of no avail amputation of the limb may be required.

Sporotrichosis (Plate 25)

Sporotrichosis usually presents as a chronic granulomatous disease affecting the skin and superficial lymphatics, though occasionally the disease is encountered in disseminated form. It occurs in all continents particularly affecting North America and France. It mainly affects agricultural workers. It has been described in South Africa as an epidemic affecting gold miners, the fungus being found saprophytic in mine timbers.

The fungus, *Sporotrichium schenkii*, is found in soil, wood and plants. It affects many animals and man has been infected from animal sources though as a rule the fungus is acquired from inoculation into the skin from an abrasion. The disease attacks all ages being most frequent in adult males.

Clinical. Between 1 and 3 months after inoculation a small nodule forms at the site. This extends in size becoming pink in colour. It is known as a sporotrichotic chancre. Its colour gradually deepens to purple eventually becoming necrotic and ulcerated. The ulcer may persist for many months. After several weeks or months spread through the superficial lymphatics occurs. Nodules appear in the lymph drainage of the area. They become pink and may ulcerate and discharge thin pus from which the fungus may be recovered. The lymph vessels connecting the nodules become thickened and can be palpated as firm cords. The disease is remarkably chronic. It may become arrested or spread to involve a major group of glands such as those in the axillae or groins.

The disseminated form is rare. The disease may attack the lungs or invade extensive areas of skin where a varying picture is produced with the formation of plaques, crusted, weeping, fungating or verrucose lesions. Multiple subcutaneous nodules represent one of the commonest of disseminated forms but the mucous membranes or bone may be involved. Very rarely the viscera are affected. Pyelonephritis, orchitis, epididymitis and mastitis have been described.

Treatment. Fortunately sporotrichosis responds to potassium iodide by mouth. The commencing dose is 0.3 g given in solution. The dose is gradually increased until a daily dose 2 g is reached. This is maintained for 6 weeks after the clinical cure. Surgery is contraindicated. Sodium iodide has been used intravenously with good results.

Cryptococcosis (torulosis, European blastomycosis)

This infection may be regarded as a true blastomycosis in that the fungus appears in the tissues as a budding organism. It is a chronic ailment appearing as a primary infection of the lungs and disseminating to the skin, lymph nodes, bone and particularly the central nervous system. It occurs in all parts of the world especially in America and Australia.

The fungus, *Cryptococcus neoformans*, affects many animals and causes mastitis in cows. The fungus has been found in cow's milk and in milking utensils. Man is probably not infected from animals. The fungus has also been found in soil and it is likely that human infection is the result of aspiration of the fungus into the lungs. Individuals with a pre-existing reticulosis seem specially liable to attack and cryptococcosis is not infrequently found in association with Hodgkin's disease, leukaemia or lymphosarcoma.

Clinical. The *pulmonary form* appears as a subacute disease, but may be almost symptomless, the first indication being dissemination into the central nervous system. There are usually mild constitutional symptoms with a variable degree of cough and sputum. The condition is usually bilateral. The X-rays may show dense massive opacities or a miliary appearance resembling that of tuberculosis.

The *central nervous system form* is the variety most commonly encountered. Clinically the picture is that of a chronic meningitis with fever, headache and the signs of meningeal irritation. Lumbar puncture reveals a fluid which may be xanthochromic and which contains up to 1000 lymphocytes per mm³. The protein and globulin are much increased whilst the chlorides and sugar are reduced. These changes closely resemble those produced by tuberculous meningitis.

Dissemination may occur from the pulmonary focus into other organs such as bone, the kidney, skin, spleen and lymph glands.

Treatment has been revolutionised by the introduction of amphotericin B which is derived from a soil *Streptomyces*. This drug is given intravenously in a saline drip which should last 6–12 hours. The dose is 0.25 mg per kg gradually increasing to 1 mg. The drip is set up on alternate days and must be continued for several weeks. Fever and rigors are common, as are nausea and vomiting. These symptoms do not call for cessation of treatment and can be controlled by simultaneous administration of prednisolone.

North American blastomycosis (Gilchrist's disease)

This disease occurs as a chronic granulomatous primary skin affection with a strong tendency to pus formation and also a systemic form which results in wide dissemination. It is practically confined to the United States and Canada.

It is not known how the fungus, *Blastomyces dermatitidis*, reaches man but presumably it is acquired from exogenous sources. It attacks people of all ages but half of those affected are between 20 and 40 years of age. Males are attacked nine times more frequently than females.

Clinical. The *cutaneous form* affects exposed areas of skin, especially the face. The earliest indication is a papule or vesicle which soon proceeds to point and discharge pus. The lesion then extends towards its edges and tends to heal in the central areas forming light scars. There are two characteristic features. The extending periphery is raised and thrown up into fine wart-like processes which have a violaceous hue. There are also many small pointing abscesses. These special features make for ready diagnosis.

The *systemic form* of the disease results from a pulmonary focus from which dissemination occurs. The onset is usually insidious with moderate fever, cough, chest pains and variable sputum. Sooner or later the sputum becomes blood stained. The severity of the disease gradually increases so that after some weeks or months the general condition has declined and sweats and wasting occur whilst the fever increases. X-rays often show widening of the mediastinum from glandular enlargement with the projection of wedge-shaped opacities from the hilum. There may be parenchymatous shadowing or miliary lesions evenly scattered throughout the lung fields.

Dissemination is usual, the symptoms depending on the affected tissue. Bone is involved in 60 per cent of cases. Backache or chest pains may indicate the spread to the vertebrae or ribs which are the commonest bones to be attacked. The brain is affected in 30 per cent of cases. The symptoms are often those of brain abscess. Abscesses may form in the subcutaneous tissues or ulcers may develop in the skin. Other organs affected are the liver, spleen, kidneys or prostate. The disease has a poor prognosis in its disseminated form. Without treatment over 90 per cent of the patients die within 2 years.

Treatment consists in the intravenous administration of the aromatic amide hydroxystilbamitine isethionate. This is given in infusions of 300 ml of 5 per cent dextrose solution. The commencing dose is 50 mg and during the course of fifteen infusions the dose is gradually worked up to 250 mg. If required a second course may be given after an interval of several weeks. Amphotericin B is also effective. (See Plate 24*a* and *b*.)

South American blastomycosis (Almeida's disease)

This disease, caused by infection with *Blastomyces braziliensis*, is confined to South America and shows a special predilection to affect the lymph nodes. It is encountered most frequently in Brazil but also occurs in the Argentine, Venezuela, Bolivia, Peru and a few other South American states. It is not yet ascertained how the infection is acquired. It occurs predominantly in young males. Several forms of the disease are recognised.

Clinical. The *mucocutaneous form* is presumably acquired from exogenous sources and its onset not uncommonly follows a dental extraction. Primary lesions of the skin show hyperkeratosis of a small circular area which may be papilliferous. Central necrosis of the primary lesion takes the form of an ulcerating papule situated on the lips, palate, cheek or tongue. The ulcer extends deeply and spreads at the periphery. Adjacent nodules soon become visible and extend. Considerable destruction of tissue occurs and as the disease extends erosion of the hard palate, epiglottis, uvula and vocal cords may lead to complete destruction of these organs. The lymph nodes of the neck become involved and undergo necrosis with rupture of their contents and persistent sinuses. Blood stream infection may lead to involvement of the skin or the more remote lymph nodes (Plate 26).

The *lymphangitic form* is attributed to infection acquired through the nasopharynx. Often no trace of the portal of entry can be discovered. It gives rise to massive cervical glandular enlargements which proceed to soften and rupture.

In the *visceral form* the infection is thought to enter through the gastrointestinal tract and leads to ulceration of the large bowel particularly in the appendicular regions. This gives rise to anorexia, nausea, vomiting and diarrhoea. Spread to other organs takes place. The lungs are affected in 80 per cent of cases and the liver and spleen may be enlarged. There is moderate fever.

Diagnosis in all forms is achieved by direct microscopy of the lesions.

Treatment consists in the administration of nystatin, 2-hydroxystilbamidine or amphotericin B.

The latter drug has produced the most promising results. The drug should be given for 4–6 weeks as described under the treatment for cryptococcosis. The aromatic amide, 2-hydroxystilbamidine, is given daily by slow intravenous infusion working up to a dose of 225 mg which is maintained for 40–50 days.

Histoplasmosis (Plate 27)

Epidemiology. Histoplasmosis is due to infection with *Histoplasma capsulatum* and is a common disease in certain parts of the United States particularly the Mississippi Valley and the Ohio Valley regions. It also occurs sporadically in Central and South America, Australia and Europe. Cases have been described in the United Kingdom.

In certain parts of tropical Africa, notably Ghana, Nigeria, the Congo and the Sudan, there is a variant of the fungus, *H. duboisi*. This is distinguished by the large size of the intracellular form. Clinically, although the skin may be affected the organism specially selects the viscera causing a much higher mortality than *H. capsulatum*. The lymphatic glands, the liver and the spleen may be affected but infection of the lungs has not been reported. In the bones rounded cyst-like lesions result.

H. capsulatum affects man by causing either a pulmonary infection which is often symptomless or by producing a generalised disease. It is probable that man's natural immunity to infection is high. Histoplasmin skin test surveys have shown that in some areas of the United States as many as 80 per cent of the population show evidence of a past infection. It is considered that 85 per cent of all infections are symptomless.

The fungus commonly attacks animals but infection from animals to man has not been proven. The saprophytic form of the fungus has been found in soil, especially if contaminated by animal droppings. Infection probably arises through the inhalation of dust contaminated with spores.

Recently the close association between histoplasmosis and exposure to infection in caves has been recognised. Indeed it is sometimes known as 'cave disease'. Infection from caves has been reported from Venezuela, East and South Africa. In East Africa the caves at Matapos are regarded as 'm'tagate' or bewitched. The floor of many of these caves is covered with bat guano, in some cases eight feet deep. The substance is sought commercially and people who go into the caves in search of it run a high risk of infection. Wearing a respirator is a protection. The fungus has been demonstrated in the filters of respirators.

Infection has also been reported from enclosed areas such as pigeon lofts and hen-houses.

Clinical. Histoplasmosis can present in either a primary pulmonary form or as a disseminated progressive form.

Primary histoplasmosis is a relatively benign infection of the lungs. In some instances following exposure there may be a short illness with mild fever, cough and sputum with rales at the lung bases. In most cases infection is symptomless. In areas where the disease is endemic routine chest radiology reveals the extent of past infection. The radiological changes in the lungs usually reveal multiple bilateral fluffy opacities with hilar glandular enlargement. These resolve slowly over the years eventually undergoing fibrosis and calcification. In other cases very many small round opacities are found dotted about both lung fields causing a strong resemblance to miliary tuberculosis. The rare solitary opacity may cause difficulty in diagnosis. The sputum seldom shows evidence of the fungus though attempts to culture it should be made. Infrequently the gastric contents or lung biopsy may yield positive results.

Progressive histoplasmosis is a rare and frequently fatal sequel which occurs in less than 1 per cent of all primary infections. The primary lesion is not infrequently extrapulmonary being situated in the mucous membrane of the lips, tongue, nasopharynx or larynx. The ear or even the penis may afford entry to the fungus. The disease has a special tendency to affect children in whom it produces a chronic wasting disease somewhat resembling kala azar. Fever is prolonged. The affinity to affect the reticuloendothelial system is shown in enlargement of the spleen, liver and lymph nodes. There may be intestinal ulceration giving rise to abdominal symptoms. Bone may be affected, the osteitis being revealed radiologically. It may be possible to obtain the fungus from bone marrow aspiration.

Treatment with amphotericin B has been shown to be effective. The dosage and method of administration is described under the treatment for cryptococcosis.

Coccidioidomycosis

This infection, caused by *Coccidioides immitis*, has many resemblances to histoplasmosis. It is encountered in the dry south-western states of America attaining a high endemicity in the San Joaquin Valley of California. It also occurs in Texas, Arizona, New Mexico and Utah. The disease also occurs in South America where the coccidioidin skin test shows that infection is frequent though clinical manifestations are not common. Infection is acquired through inhalation of the spores in dust. People of any age may be affected. Males are predominantly attacked. About 60 per cent of all primary infections are symptomless as judged by the coccidioidin skin test.

Clinical. Symptoms, when they occur, take place about 14 days after inhalation of the fungus and consist of those of a mild upper respiratory tract infection with low-grade fever and cough. Dry pleurisy may be a prominent feature. About 80 per cent of patients have abnormal radiological findings which are less specific than those encountered in histoplasmosis. Soft hilar flares, patchy pneumonic consolidation persisting for several days, hilar adenopathy, isolated and well circumscribed nodular lesions and small pleural effusions indicate the wide variety of pulmonary pathology. A sequel to the primary lung lesion is the occurrence of allergic skin manifestations closely resembling erythema nodosum or erythema multiforme which may occur anywhere in the body.

In about 1 per cent of primary lung infections a progressive form of coccidioidomycosis develops. The lung lesions extend, fever becomes high, wasting commences and the patient enters a decline which frequently terminates fatally with involvement of bones, joints, skin and meninges.

Occasionally the primary infection is on some exposed area of skin. This may result in a chronic spreading granulomatous and ulcerative lesion which, if the face is affected, may lead to considerable disfigurement.

Treatment has been attempted with various drugs but as experience accumulates it seems probable that the best results are to be attained with amphotericin B.

Aspergillosis

This disease is of importance because it affects the bronchi and lungs but it can also cause inflammatory granulomatous lesions in the skin, nasal sinuses or external ear.

Man may be infected with several species of *Aspergillus* but *A. fumigatus* is most frequently involved. This fungus is widely distributed in nature and infections occur in all parts of the world. Cases are reported with increasing frequency in Europe and America. Aspergillosis is a common disease of birds. Pigeon fanciers are said to become infected from allowing birds to pick up grains of corn from their lips. Dust from threshers may contain spores and infect agricultural workers. Fur cleaners who use contaminated rye flour are at risk.

Clinical. *Pulmonary aspergillosis* can occur as a more or less innocent saprophyte in lungs which are already attacked with pre-existing disease. It has frequently been found in association with pulmonary infarcts and also invades the damaged lungs of miners. It has been found complicating sarcoidosis. In individuals who develop a sensitivity to the fungus more serious effects result. The fungus may settle down in the alveoli. In this case asthmatic symptoms are frequent. There may be cough, tightness and wheeziness of the chest and perhaps low-grade fever. The sputum may exhibit tough plugs which contain the fungus. Eosinophilia is present in the blood and in the sputum. The bronchi may be affected and bronchiectasis may be demonstrated by opaque oil. The radiograms may show opacities in the lung fields.

Occasionally the case presents as a mycetoma (aspergilloma) with a pre-existing cavity in the lung containing masses of mycelium. Multiple, repeated small haemoptyses may indicate this situation. Radiographically there is a rounded body surrounded by a halo of air. Calcification may follow death of the fungus. The ear is occasionally affected. The auditory canal becomes oedematous and eythematous and there are numerous crusts. Itching is intense. The epithelium is exfoliated and may cause obstruction and secondary infection may result. The tympanic membrane is seldom involved. Rarely the orbit, nasal sinuses or the vulva are the sites of infection.

Diagnosis depends upon finding the fungus in the lesion. In pulmonary aspergillosis the frequency of the fungus as a contamination during culture requires repeated examinations of the sputum.

Treatment is somewhat unsatisfactory. If sensitisation to the fungus is present desensitisation with aspergillin and administration of steroids should be tried. Nystatin is too toxic for parental use. Good results have been reported from giving it in tablets of 500 000 units by mouth thrice daily for 3 weeks. Amphotericin B is usually employed. Older treatments, still used, are potassium iodide by mouth or sodium iodide intravenously.

An aspergilloma causing haemoptysis should be resected if this is practicable. Instillations of thick suspensions of amphotericin B or nystatin into aspergilloma cavities have been used as an alternative to surgery in patients with respiratory insufficiency.

FURTHER READING

CONANT, N. F., SMITH, T. S., BAKER, R. D. and CALLAWAY, L. C. (1971) *Manual of Clinical Mycology*, 3rd ed. Philadelphia: Saunders.

WOLSTENOLME G. E. W. and PORTER, R. (Eds) (1968) *Systematic Mycoses, a Ciba Foundation Symposium*. London: Churchill.

26
Venereal Diseases

SYNONYMS. Climatic bubo, lymphopathia venereum, esthiomene, inguinal poradenitis.

Definition

A generalised virus infection usually transmitted by venereal infection and associated with a self-healing primary sore and changes in the lymph nodes draining the area where the sore is situated. In addition there may be a genito-anorectal syndrome with inflammatory stricture of the rectum, or more rarely meningoencephalitis and eye lesions.

Aetiology

The causative agent, first isolated in 1930 by Hellerstrom and Wassen, was formerly described as a large virus but is more closely related to bacteria and is a typical member of the psittacosis, trachoma, inclusion conjunctivitis, enzootic hepatitis of sheep group of organisms called *Bedsonia* (Meyer, 1953) or *Chlamydia* (Andrewes, 1967).

Morphological and cultural characteristics. The organism is an obligatory intracellular parasite which is found in leucocytes and consists of minute particles which can be stained by Victoria blue, Giemsa (bluish purple) or Castaneda's stain (reddish purple). Both large and small forms of the parasite can be demonstrated outside the cells lying close to cell debris in compact colony-like masses which may attain considerable size forming cyst-like spaces, and later the cyst wall may rupture. These resemble similar bodies found in psittacosis in which large morula-like particles break up to form the small virus or elementary bodies. When they are within cells the elementary bodies may be found in the cytoplasm of either mononuclear or polymorphonuclear leucocytes.

The most reliable methods of isolation are by inoculation into the yolk sac of eggs and the intracerebral inoculation of white mice (Wassen test). The organism can also be cultured in tissue culture or on chick chorioallantoic membranes. In inoculated mice after 5 to 70 days weakness, paresis, opisthotonos, and convulsions occur.

Dilutions greater than 1 : 10 000 fail to give positive results.

Transmission. In every instance infection is acquired by sexual intercourse either normal or abnormal.

Immunology

Antigenically lymphogranuloma venereum virus closely resembles the psittacosis trachoma group of viruses, but tests with viricidal antibodies have shown that these viruses are not antigenically identical.

There is a marked increase in the serum globulin and the total protein content of the serum lies between 8.1 and 10.3 g per cent. The total globulin varies between 3.9 and 5.6 g per cent so that a positive formol gel test may be found. Combes and his co-workers (1945) found that 38 out of 42 cases gave a positive formol gel reaction and concluded that hyperglobulinaemia is of value in diagnosis and in delineating the activity of the disease since it reverts to negative with cure.

There is a well-marked delayed hypersensitivity which can be demonstrated by the Frei Hoffmann test (Frei and Hoffmann, 1928).

Frei Hoffmann test. Frei originally prepared antigen from the pus withdrawn from a suppurating bubo which had not burst. At present antigen is prepared from the virus grown in the yolk sac of developing chick embryos (Rake *et al*, 1940) which is commercially available under the proprietary name of Lygranum.

0.1 ml of antigen is injected intradermally into the skin of the forearm and 0.1 ml of control material made from egg yolk into the other. The test is read at 48 to 72 hours. In positive reactions a red raised papule of at least 6 mm appears at the site of the injection and some induration may persist for a few days.

The test becomes positive at varying intervals after infection from 1 week to 6 months, but usually within 2–3 weeks, and remains positive for many years, perhaps for life. False-positive reactions may arise and cross-reactions occur with trachoma.

Complement fixation test. A complement fixation test is available using the same antigen,

Lygranum. The test becomes positive early in the course of the infection and becomes negative following successful treatment. A positive titre of 1 : 16 or above means recent or active infection in a patient with clinical manifestations of the disease when acute and convalescent sera are available, and a titre of 1 : 40 is diagnostic (Annamunthodo, 1962). Low titres persist for a long time in past infections. Cross-reactions occur with psittacosis and an antigen made from this organism gives equally satisfactory results.

Mouse protection test. Test serum diluted 1 in 5 with normal saline is mixed with virus-infected mouse brain and kept overnight at 4.0°C. 0.5 ml of the suspension is inoculated intracerebrally into another mouse and sera containing viricidal antibodies will protect the second mouse against encephalitis.

Epidemiology and geographical distribution

Lymphogranuloma inguinale is world-wide in distribution and has been called the 'sixth venereal disease'. It occurs especially among Negroes of both sexes in West Africa, North and South America and in seaports throughout the world. More recently it has been described in Europe and there are numerous reports of its occurrence in France, England, Italy, Rumania, Scandinavia and the whole of Europe.

Sex incidence

Lymphogranuloma inguinale is commonest in the male but it is now recognised that this infection does occur in women although inguinal buboes are comparatively rare on account of the different anatomical disposition of the lymphatic system in the female. Typical inguinal buboes have been found in prostitutes in Singapore and inguinal buboes with a positive intradermal reaction have been reported by French writers. Definite evidence of infection of the wife by her husband has been obtained in an English case.

Inguinal syndrome (climatic bubo)

Pathology. The *primary lesion* consists of an ulcer surrounded by plasma cells and histiocytes containing the cone or dumb-bell shaped basophilic inclusion bodies which can be found in Giemsa-stained smears of pus. Occasionally eosinophils are prominent.

The *secondary lesions* are found in the lymph nodes where there is a proliferation of monocytes and plasma cells with a few neutrophil polymorphonuclear leucocytes and eosinophils present.

There is a granulomatous reaction with a proliferation of macrophages and epithelioid cells and sometimes central necrosis with giant cells which may simulate tuberculosis. These granulomata are scattered in a pin-point manner all through the node and a Giemsa-stained preparation may show intracytoplasmic inclusion bodies. In the late stages a central area of necrosis is surrounded by a palisade of epithelioid cells merging with a wall of acellular hyaline material which may be of diagnostic significance.

Pathological changes in the spleen, liver, heart and central nervous system have been described and generalised lymphadenopathy may occur.

Clinical features. The incubation period is short, perhaps less than 1 week but periods of 3–5 weeks and longer have been reported.

Symptoms and signs. PRIMARY SORE. Hanschell (1926) described a small herpetiform ulcer on the prepuce which usually heals in a few days although it may ulcerate. The adenitis proper does not commence until after the primary lesion has healed.

Hanschell (1926) believed that the disease does not usually occur in the circumcised. The primary lesion is an erosion with clean edges and is surrounded by a reddened zone but with only slight infiltration and induration. The base of the ulcer is usually whitish-grey.

ADENITIS. The incubation period of the adenitis is 3–4 weeks after coitus, but it may be as long as 6 weeks to 2 months. The disease generally commences with remittent pyrexia which may precede the actual localising signs and may be mistaken for typhoid. Soon subacute inflammatory swellings of the groin nodes are noted. The inflammation may be unilateral or bilateral. While the oblique nodes are most frequently affected, at times the crural nodes are attacked.

Sometimes one groin is affected after the other. In well-marked cases the internal iliac nodes and sometimes the lumbar nodes also can be felt enlarged and tender on deep palpation. Signs of intoxication from absorption may be widespread producing prolonged or intermittent fever, sometimes up to 40°C. Rigors, vomiting and slight jaundice have been noted. Rheumatic-like pains in the joints and painful effusions into joint cavities may also occur.

The affected nodes slowly enlarge to the size of a hen's egg or even larger and after several weeks or months gradually subside. Usually the periglandular connective tissues inflame and become adherent until suppuration ceases. Fistulous tracks may form, continuously exuding a clear sticky fluid.

The most striking clinical feature in the male is the extensive inflammation of the periglandular tissues with comparatively little pain and suppuration.

Four stages of adenopathy are recognised:

1. A firm solitary node with no apparent causative lesion other than a recently healed ulcer on the genitalia.

2. A firm solitary node adherent to overlying skin and deeper tissues. Adjacent nodes are enlarged including external iliac nodes which are palpable as a mass above Poupart's ligament. The affected nodes tend to coalesce.

3. The nodes in the groin soften and fluctuate. If incised a cavity is disclosed trabeculated by coarse fibrous strands.

4. The softened node mass ulcerates through the skin and spontaneous fistulation occurs. Secondary infection follows.

Genital syndrome (Genital elephantiasis, esthiomene)

Pathology. Esthiomene is an ulceration of the vulva associated with elephantiasis of the labia and is the counterpart of lymphogranuloma in the male.

The primary lesion is probably hidden in the posterior wall of the vagina and the anorectal lymph node is the first to be attacked. The infiltration of this node extends via the lymph flow to the anterior part of the vulva and posteriorly to the rectum, resulting in the genito-anorectal syndrome which is much more common in women than in men.

Clinical features. There is swelling due to chronic lymphatic oedema of the vulva. The male genitalia may be affected by the same process but less commonly.

Vegetations and polypoid growths develop on the skin surface and fistulae may form and break down to destructive ulceration.

The oedema may extend from the clitoris to the anus and elephantiasis in the male involves the penis and scrotum.

Urethral syndrome

Involvement of the urethra with infiltrative lesions in the posterior part, followed by stricture and fistula formation, may present as nongonococcal urethritis.

Anorectal syndrome

Pathology. The virus spreads from the initial site of implantation by the lymphatics to the inguinal and pelvic nodes. Later in the female the lymphatics of the anus and rectum become involved, producing at first proctitis and later stricture of the rectum. In the male stricture of the rectum follows the occurrence of a primary lesion in the rectum.

Clinical features. The earliest symptom is bleeding from the anus followed by purulent anal discharge. Proctoscopy may reveal proctitis, rectal ulceration or rectal stricture.

RECTAL STRICTURE. Several varieties of rectal stricture are recognised:

1. Anal stricture, in women associated with esthiomene, annular rectal stricture, or tubular rectal stricture which may extend to the sigmoid or even the descending colon and may cause 'skip lesions' on radioscopy (Middlemiss, 1962).

2. Rectal communicating strictures from ulceration between the rectum, bladder, vagina, prostate and seminal vesicles.

3. Associated with carcinoma of the rectum and in some cases causing a tender, fixed and palpable ileum resembling Crohn's disease.

Extragenital infections

Extragenital infections have been recorded on the tongue with node enlargement in the neck and axilla, and on the foot. A few cases of meningo-encephalitis due to the virus of lymphogranuloma venereum have now been recorded.

Ocular lymphogranuloma

This was described by Macnie (1941). The whole globe may be covered with granulation tissue and washings of the conjunctival sac will infect monkeys.

A number of cases of uveitis and keratoconjunctivitis have given positive intradermal tests and fundus changes have been reported with peripapillary oedema and dilatation and tortuosity of the veins.

Complications

If too much lymphatic tissue is removed by excision of the nodes, elephantiasis of the scrotum and leg on the affected side may develop and secondary sepsis may ensue. Rupture of lymphogranulomatous suppuration into the bladder has been recorded.

Malignant changes have been described as a sequel to genital elephantiasis and the anorectal syndrome (Levin *et al*, 1964), and Rainey (1954) found that out of 220 cases diagnosed as rectal stricture, after a period of 14 years the Frei test became negative in 5 and carcinoma became apparent.

Blood changes. There is usually a leucocytosis accompanying the suppuration and the leucocyte count varies between 8000 and 27 000 per mm³.

Diagnosis

The disease must be differentiated from soft sore, filarial adenitis, ambulant plague (pestis minor), tularaemia and femoral hernia.

The diagnosis is made by isolation of the virus, Frei skin test, complement fixation test and node biopsy.

The virus may be demonstrated in a smear of the lesion and stained with Giemsa showing intracytoplasmic inclusion bodies, and may be isolated by the inoculation of pus from buboes intracerebrally into the yolk sac of an embryonated hen's egg. The Frei skin test and complement fixation reaction are described under *Immunology*. Node biopsy will show the characteristic histological changes described under *Pathology*.

The formol gel test is positive in active cases and will return to negative following successful treatment.

Treatment

ANTIMONY DRUGS have been used in the past and are now largely superseded. Anthiomaline 2 ml on alternate days intramuscularly for four to five doses has been recommended (Willcox, 1952).

SULPHONAMIDES give good results in early cases. Sulphathiazole, sulphadiazine or sulphadimidine may be given in a dose of 5 g daily in divided doses for 7 days (Willcox, 1952). Sometimes it is necessary to prolong the course for as long as 2–3 weeks or give another course of the same or another sulphonamide drug. Long-acting sulphonamides, sulphamethoxypyridazine 1.5 g initially followed by 500 mg daily, may be of use. Genital elephantiasis and the anorectal syndrome should be treated first with sulphonamides, but the results are disappointing.

ANTIBIOTICS. Penicillin and streptomycin are ineffective (Greenblatt *et al*, 1950). Tetracycline, chlortetracycline, and oxytetracycline should be used when sulphonamides have failed. The main effect is possibly on the secondary infection. Greenblatt and associates (1950) gave 75 to 100 g of chlortetracycline (Aureomycin) over 37 to 60 days, and sinuses, proctitis and inflammatory strictures showed marked improvement, but ulcers responded poorly. Oxytetracycline (Terramycin) has been given successfully in doses of 15 to 36 g over a period of 15 to 30 days.

Surgical treatment should only be undertaken after adequate antibiotic therapy has been given. Fluctuant abscesses in the groins should be repeatedly aspirated and incision avoided. The lymph nodes should not be removed. Treatment of rectal stricture is difficult. Palliative measures consist in dilating by graduated bougies. Operative measures depend on the type of stricture present. Various alternatives are internal proctotomy, complete proctotomy, excision of the stricture and rectum and colostomy. Local vulvectomy may be indicated for genital elephantiasis.

GRANULOMA INGUINALE

SYNONYMS. Ulcerating granuloma of the pudenda, donovanosis.

Definition

An infective and granulomatous condition of the pudenda, widespread in some parts of the tropics, conveyed by sexual contact and auto-inoculation.

Aetiology

The cause of the granuloma inguinale is a bacterium *Donovania granulomatis* (*Calymmatobacterium granulomatis*) which can be seen in mononuclear cells of the lesion as a small Gram-negative pleomorphic bacillus (1–2 μm in length). It may show bipolar staining and appears to be capsulate. Extracellular forms may also be observed.

Cultural characteristics. It is difficult to cultivate on ordinary media but it may be grown readily at 37°C in the yolk sac of chick embryos when after adaptation growth can be obtained on enriched artificial media. Laboratory animals are not susceptible to inoculation but the disease has been reproduced in man by inoculation with yolk sac cultures.

Transmission. Transmission is by sexual intercourse and autoinoculation.

Immunology

The organism has morphological resemblances to *Klebsiella* and cross-reacts serologically with *Klebsiella rhinoscleromatis*.

Sterilised cultures will give an allergic skin reaction in infected persons and a positive complement fixation with the serum. The capsular material also fixes complement in patients' serum, but intradermal and complement fixation tests are of little use in diagnosis because of frequent false-positive reactions.

Epidemiology and geographical distribution

Granuloma inguinale is widely spread in India, Guyana, Brazil, West Indies, Puerto Rico, Pacific Islands and northern Australia. It occurs sporadically in the southern United States, on the west coast of Africa and in southern China. One case has been described from Scotland (Ferguson and Roberts, 1953).

It is extremely common in New Guinea, where in 1925 one quarter of a population of 20 000 were affected and in 1946, 422 cases were found in 8761 persons examined (Maddocks, 1967).

Ulcerating granuloma has only been found after the age of 13 or 14 and up to 40 to 50. It occurs in both sexes but more often in women, especially where polyandry is practised.

Pathology

Histologically this disease is allied to rhinoscleroma and a close association between these two diseases has been found in Sumatra. It is a reticuloendotheliosis and on microscopical examination the new growth at the margins of the sores is found to be made up of nodules or masses of nodules consisting of round cells with large badly staining nuclei, embedded in a delicate fibrous reticulum. The predominant cells are plasma and endothelial cells forming small polymorphonuclear abscesses. An important feature is the presence of a peculiar pathognomic cell. It is a large mononuclear varying from 25 to 90 μm in diameter, probably derived from a plasma cell. This specific cell laden with Donovan bodies can best be shown by the *Dieterle silver impregnation* method in which these bodies appear as dark brown or black elongated ovoid masses with intense bipolar staining. The nodular masses are for the most part covered by epithelium, their under surfaces merging gradually into a thick dense fibrous stroma in which small clusters of similar round cells are here and there embedded.

The growths, though very vascular, contain no haemorrhages and there are no signs of suppuration caseation or giant cells and no tubercle bacilli.

In vertical section of the small nodules, the round cell mass will be found to be wedge-shaped, the base of the wedge being towards the surface; the deep-lying apex is usually pierced by a hair or two. The growth is found around sebaceous follicles, blood vessels, lymphatics and sweat glands, but is especially abundant and most deeply situated around hair follicles.

Clinical features

The incubation period is comparatively short, from 2 to 8 days after sexual contact, but it may be as long as 12 weeks. The disease commences in the great majority of cases somewhere on the genitals, usually on the penis or labia minora, the pubes or groin as an insignificant circumscribed nodular thickening and elevation of the skin. The affected area is elevated above the surrounding skin and is covered with a very delicate pinkish, easily rubbed off epithelium which excoriates, readily exposing a surface which tends to bleed and break down although it rarely ulcerates deeply.

The disease advances in two ways: by continuous eccentric peripheral extension and by autoinfection of an opposing surface. It exhibits a distinct predilection for warm moist surfaces, particularly the folds between the scrotum and thighs, the labia and the flexures of the thighs. Its extension is very slow, years elapsing before it covers a large area. Concurrently with peripheral extension a dense contracting uneven, readily breaking down scar forms on the surface traversed by the coarsely or finely elevated new growth which constitutes the peripheral part of the diseased area. Occasionally islands of active disease spring up in this scar tissue; but it is at the margin of the implicated patch that the special features are best observed. In long-standing cases the partially healed areas are covered with thin depigmented skin and thus show up as white patches.

In the female the disease primarily attacks the crura of the clitoris and extends into the vagina over the labia and along the flexures of the thighs. The women thus affected are rendered sterile. In the male the disease may spread over the penis and involve the glans scrotum and upper part of the thighs. Occasionally the glans penis is not involved. In either sex it may spread over the course of years into the pubes, over the perineum and into the rectum, the rectovaginal septum in the female ultimately breaking down.

At times a profuse watery discharge exudes or drips from the surface of the new growth, soiling the clothes, soddening the skin and emitting a peculiarly offensive odour. The general health is not materially affected.

In neither sex do the lymph nodes become involved, but in the process of cicatrisation the lymph channels may become blocked and pseudo-elephantiasis of the genitals may occur. Impassable strictures of the urethra may result and rectovaginal fistulae are common. Invasion of the bladder with septic cystitis may result.

Constitutional symptoms occur when there is gross secondary infection and phagedenic ulceration with tissue destruction.

General dissemination has been described in which there were metastases in the bones and Donovan bodies were cultured from the blood (Packer *et al*, 1948).

Carcinoma may be associated with the disease in India, and pseudocarcinomatous proliferation in association with the disease in the rectum has been described.

Diagnosis

The differential diagnosis must be made from malignant and syphilitic ulceration of the groin and lupus vulgaris. Ulcerating granuloma is characterised by extreme chronicity of 10 or more years and absence of cachexia or any mortality, and by non-involvement of the lymphatic system.

It differs from lupus vulgaris since it is confined to the pudendal region and is not associated with any tuberculous histology. Unless complicated by syphilis, the Kahn and WR are negative and the characteristic mode of spread distinguishes it from epithelioma and carcinoma. A fungating form affecting the cervix uteri greatly resembles the ulcerative and vegetative type of carcinoma of the cervix, and in New Guinea where genital amoebiasis occurs this must be excluded. The characteristic Donovan bodies may be demonstrated on biopsy.

Treatment

STREPTOMYCIN is specific in most cases (Greenblatt *et al*, 1947).

The optimum dosage is 4 g a day in divided doses. Healing commences in 2–3 days and is complete in 1–2 weeks. Resistance can develop and 10 per cent of cases relapse, half of which fail to respond to a second course.

ACHROMYCIN can be combined with streptomycin with good results (Greenblatt *et al*, 1948). The maximum curative dose is 20 g given in doses of 500 mg 6-hourly for 10 days.

CHLOROMYCETIN in the same dosage cured 32 out of 34 cases (Greenblatt *et al*, 1948).

TRIACETOLEANDOMYCIN was successful in one case (Kerdel Vegas *et al*, 1961).

REFERENCES

ANDREWES, G. H. (1967) *Viruses of Vertebrates*, 2nd edn., p. 365. London: Baillière Tindall and Cassell.
ANNAMUNTHODO, H. (1962) *W. Indian med. J.*, **11**, 73.
COMBES, F. C., CANIZARES, O. and LANDY, S. (1945) *Amer. J. Syph.*, **29**, 611.
FERGUSON, A. G. and ROBERTS, G. B. S. (1953) *Brit. med. J.*, **1**, 1257.
FREI, W. and HOFFMANN, H. (1928) *Arch. Dermat. Syph. (Berl.)*, **153**, 179.
GREENBLATT, R. P., DIENST, R. R., KUPPERMAN, H. S. and REINSTEIN, C. R. (1947) *J. vener. Dis. Inform.*, **28**, 183.
GREENBLATT, R. P., DIENST, R. R., CHEN, C. and WEST, R. M. (1948) *S. med. J.*, **41**, 1121.
GREENBLATT, R. P., WAMMOCK, V. S., CHEN, C. H., DIENST, R. R. and WEST, R. M. (1950) *J. vener. Dis. Inform.*, **31**, 41.
HANSCHELL, H. D. (1926) *Lancet*, **2**, 276.
HELLERSTROM, S. and WASSEN, E. (1930) *VIIIe Congres Internationale de Dermatologie et de Sypholographie*. Copenhagen.
KERDEL VEGAS, E., CONVIT, J. and SOTO, J. (1961) *Arch. Dermat.*, **84**, 248.
LEVIN, I., ROMANO, S., STEINBERG, M. and WELSH, R. A. (1964) *Dis. Colon. Rect.*, **7**, 129.
MACNIE, J. P. (1941) *Arch. Ophthalm.*, **25**, 255.
MADDOCKS, I. (1967) *Papua N. Guinea med. J.*, **10**, 49.
MEYER, K. F. (1953) *Acad. Sci.*, **56**, 545.
MIDDLEMISS, H. (1961) *Tropical Radiology*, p. 229. London: William Heinemann Ltd.
PACKER, H., TURNER, H. B. and DULANEY, A. D. (1948) *J. Amer. med. Ass.*, **136**, 327.
RAKE, G., MCKEE, S. M. and SHAFFER, M. E. (1940) *Proc. Soc. exp. Biol. (N.Y.)*, **43**, 332.
WILLCOX, R. R. (1952) *Trans. roy. Soc. trop. Med. Hyg.*, **46**, 658.

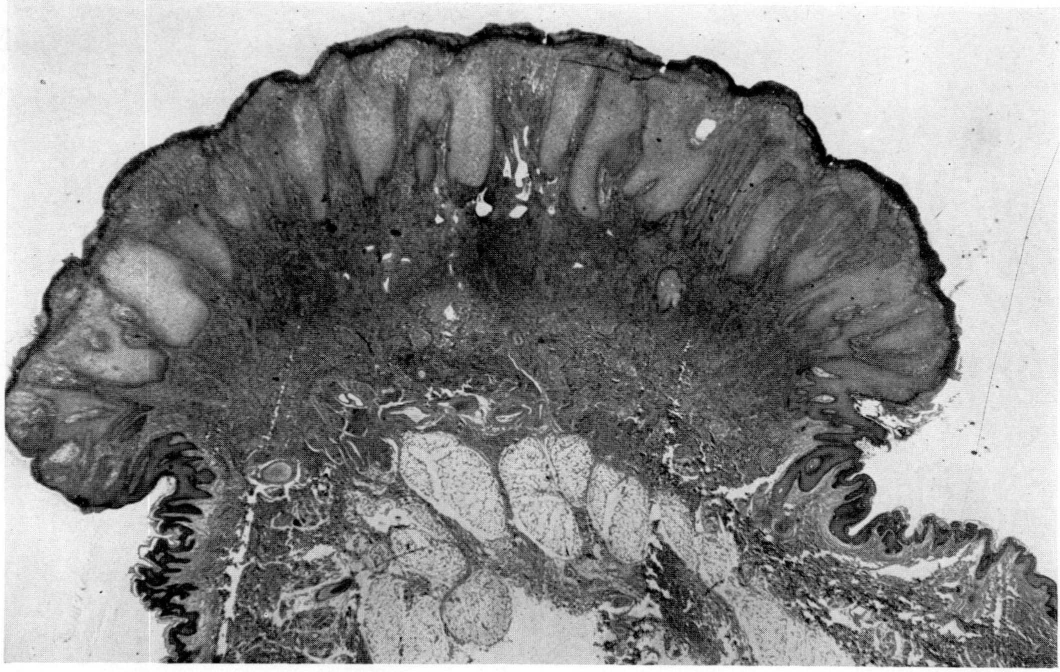

PLATE 7 *Papilloma of early yaws. Marked epithelial hyperplasia with prolongation of epithelial papillae into dermis. There is considerable cellular infiltration which may be perivascular in the dermis. Treponemes are numerous in the hypertrophic epidermis.*

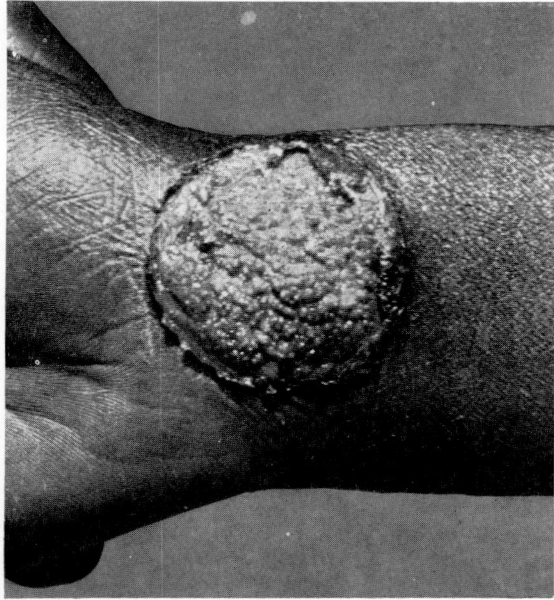

PLATE 8 *Initial lesion on child's wrist; closely resembles the papilloma of the early generalised early eruption* (Plate 10).

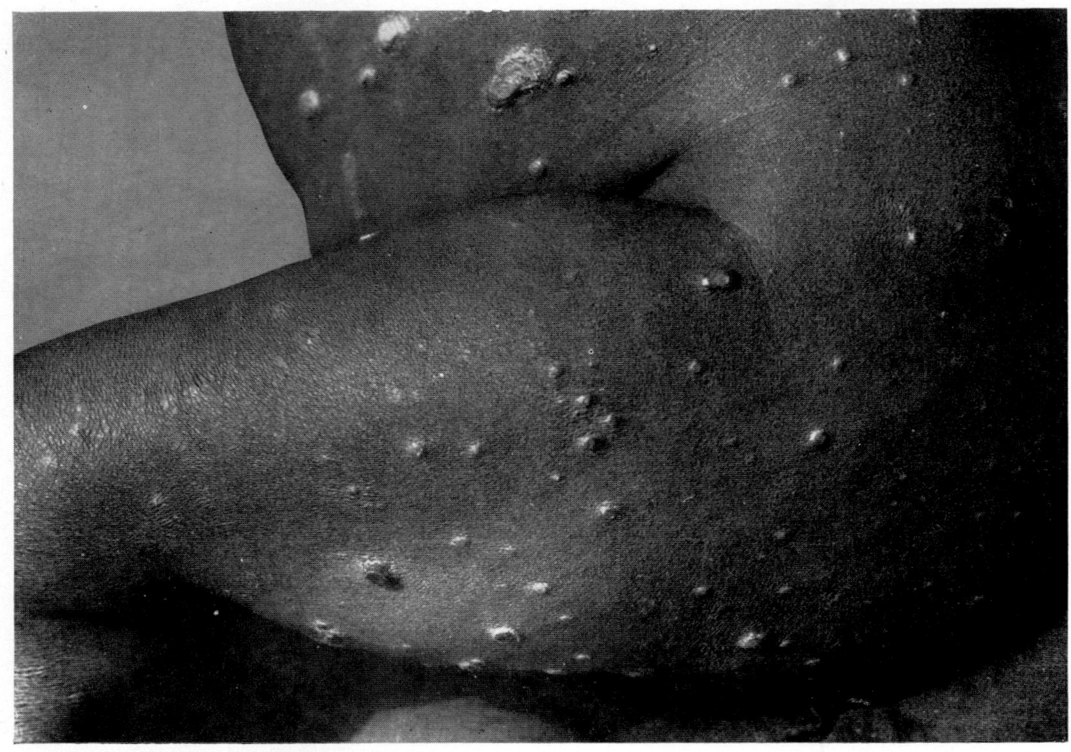

PLATE 9   *Papules and early papillomata. Some of these will develop into the larger characteristic papillomata while others will recede.*

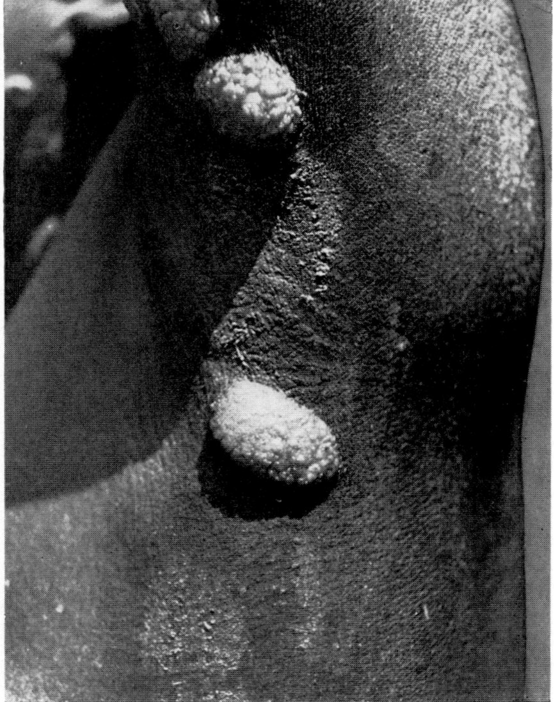

PLATE 10   *Characteristic yaws papillomata in left axilla. The pale, reddish yellow, coarsely granular surface arises from the hypertrophic epithelial papillae. Healing leaves little or no scar because destruction is slight or absent. The secretion from these lesions contains many treponemes; scaling from drying of such secretion is seen below the upper lesion.*

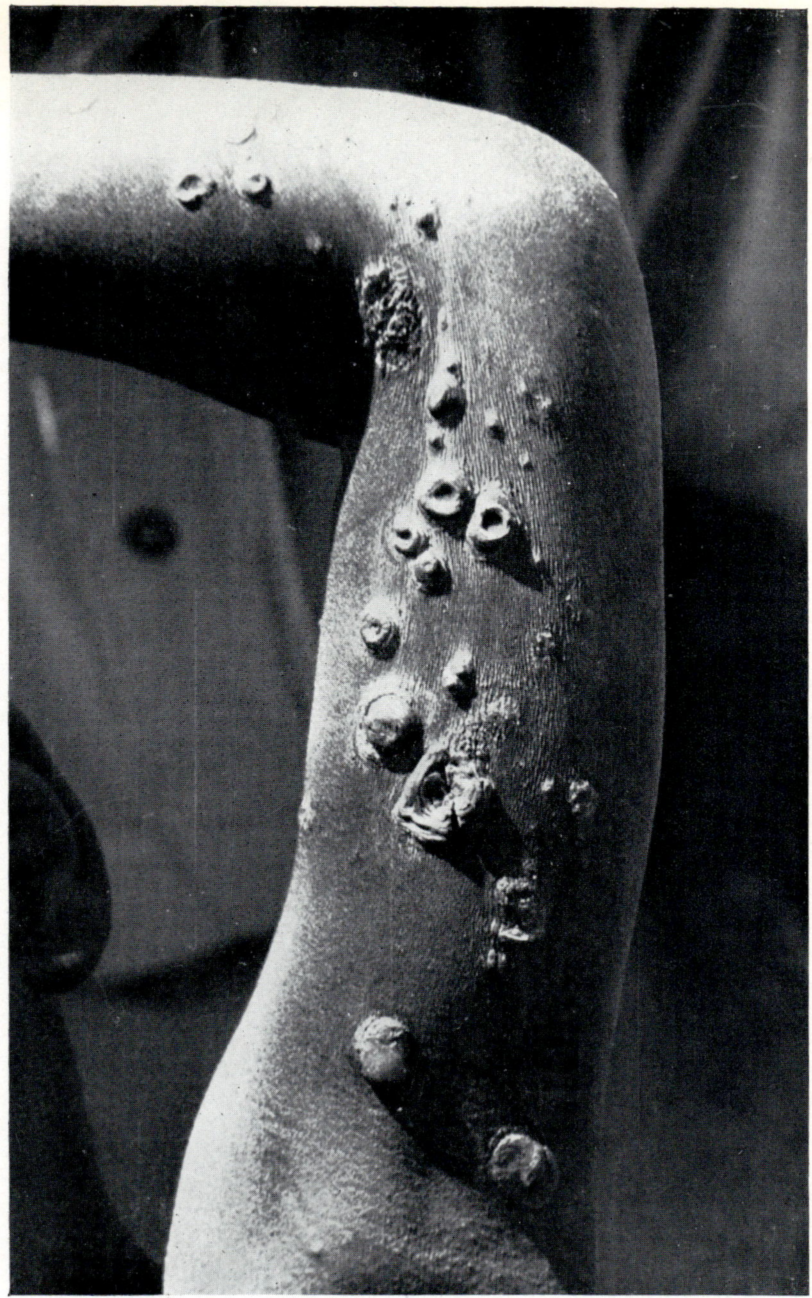

PLATE 11 *Papillomatous early lesions of less activity so that the secretion has dried to form scabs.*

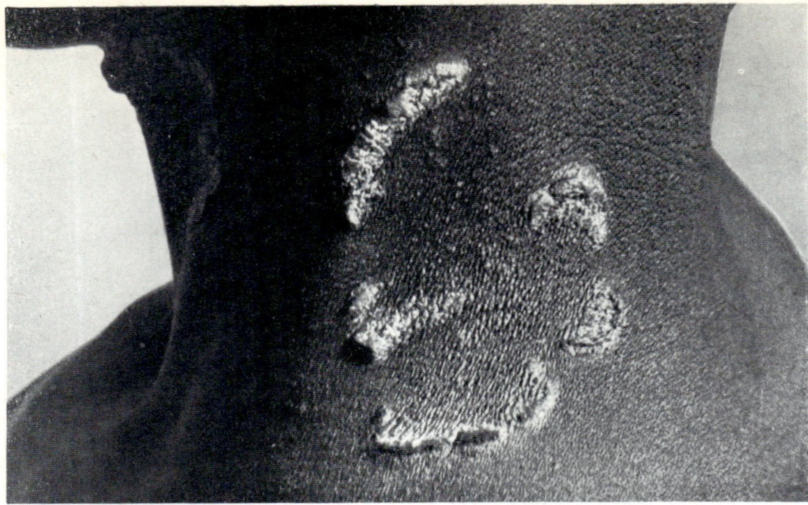

PLATE 12   *Circinate papillomata resulting from peripheral extension and central healing of large papillomata. The healed centre is free of scars. This lesion occurs towards the end of the early stage of the disease.*

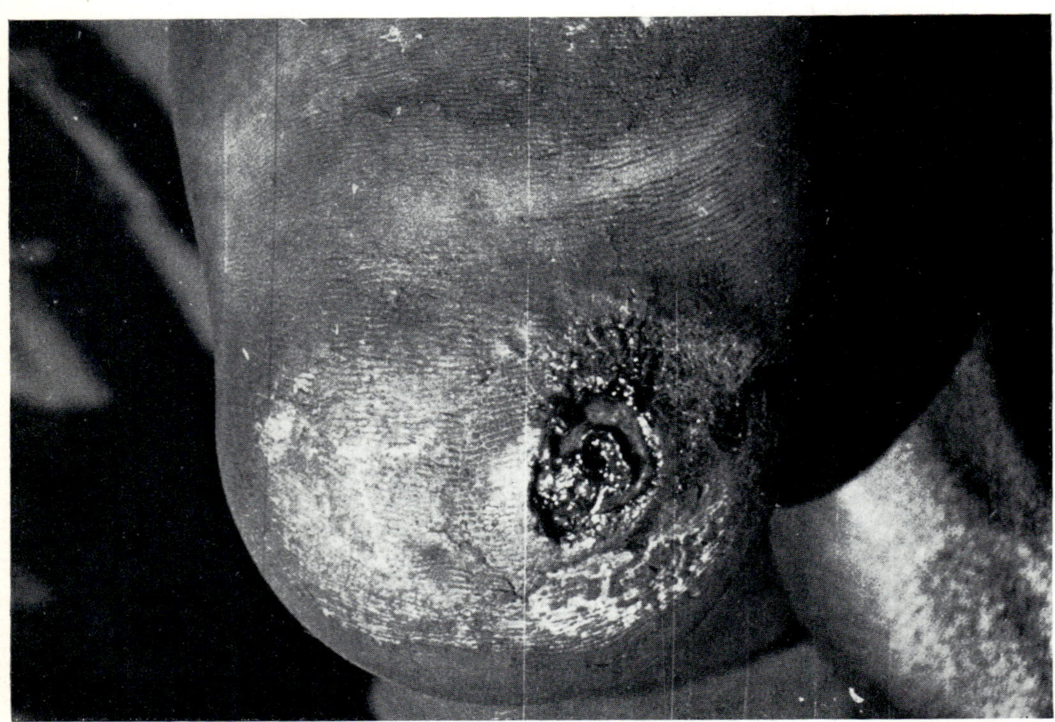

PLATE 13   *Papilloma of the heel, so-called crab yaw. The moist surface is seen in the perforation through the thick epithelium. These lesions are very painful, especially before the epithelium is perforated. As long-delayed relapses they may give rise to new infections of which the originating patient may be missed.*

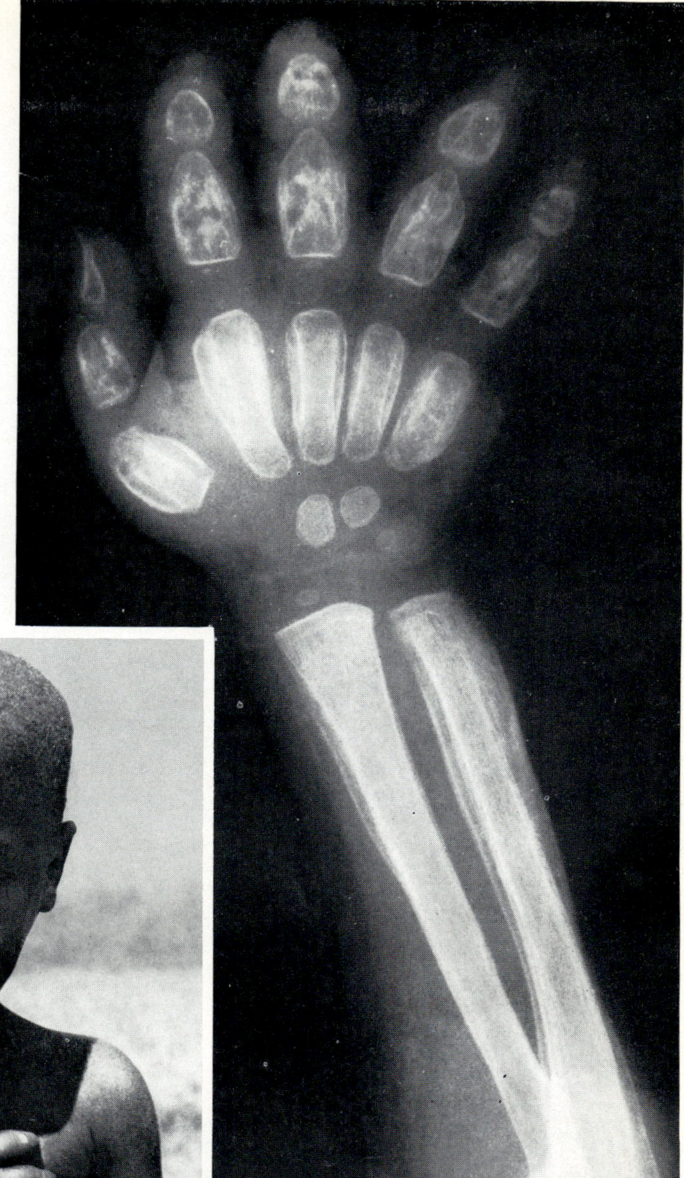

PLATE 14 *Bone lesions of early yaws are hypertrophic, extensive and not destructive. Goundou may be present. Early bone lesions may accompany or follow early skin lesions.*

PLATE 15 *Extensive periosteal deposits and some focal cortical rarefaction in early yaws. On healing there is little or no bony change.*

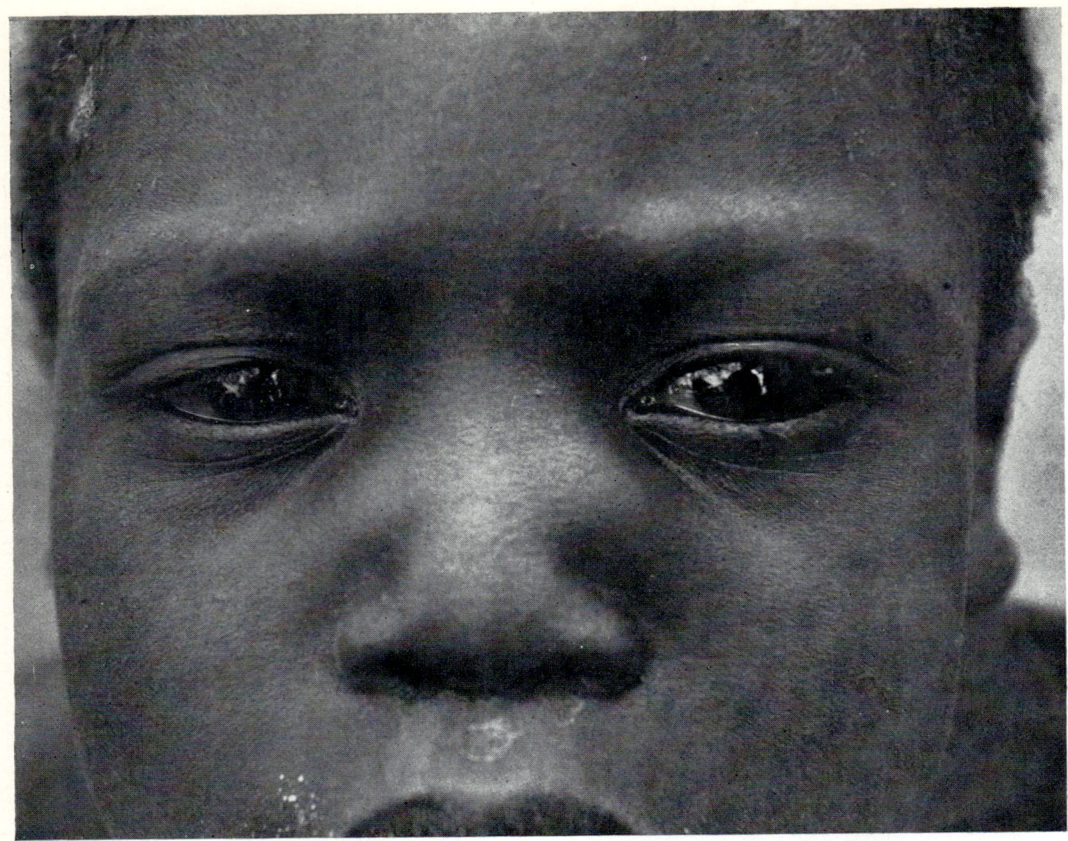

PLATE 16   *Goundou; an early yaws lesion frequent in Africa but rarely seen elsewhere. In its early stage the bony swelling will disappear with chemotherapy, but not in long-standing lesions.*

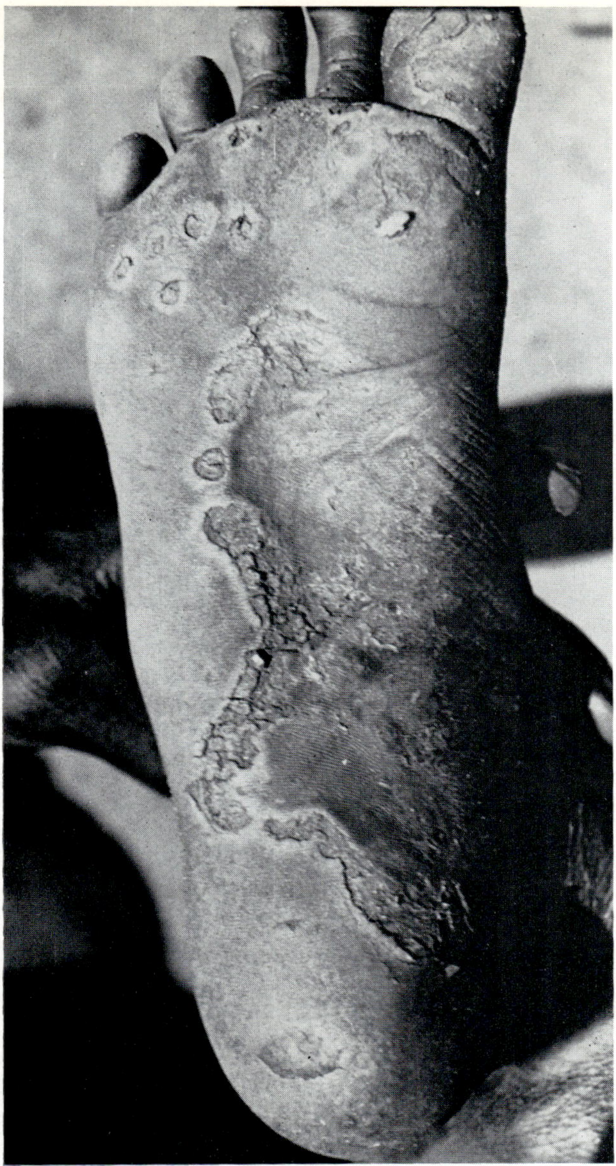

PLATE 17 *Plantar lesions of the early stage. Their relation to the papillomata is seen in the anterior changes. The circinate ribbon-like pattern in the instep is typical. Palmar and plantar lesions of the late stage are less characteristic. (From* Trans. R. Soc. trop. Med. Hyg., **40**.)

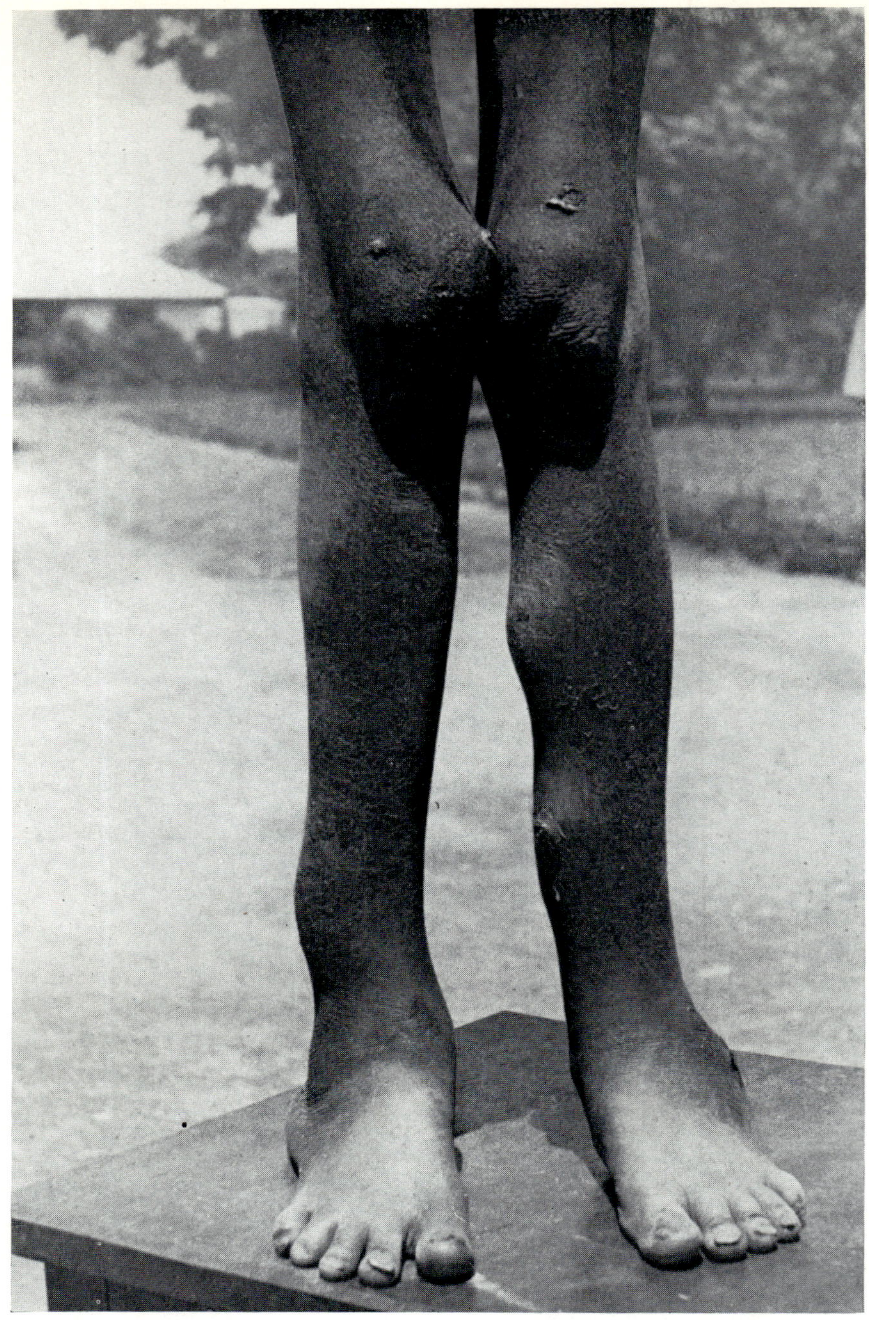

PLATE 18 *Late yaws bone lesions are more often nodes than general expansions as in early stage lesions. They are destructive and often open by small sinuses on to the skin (left tibia).*

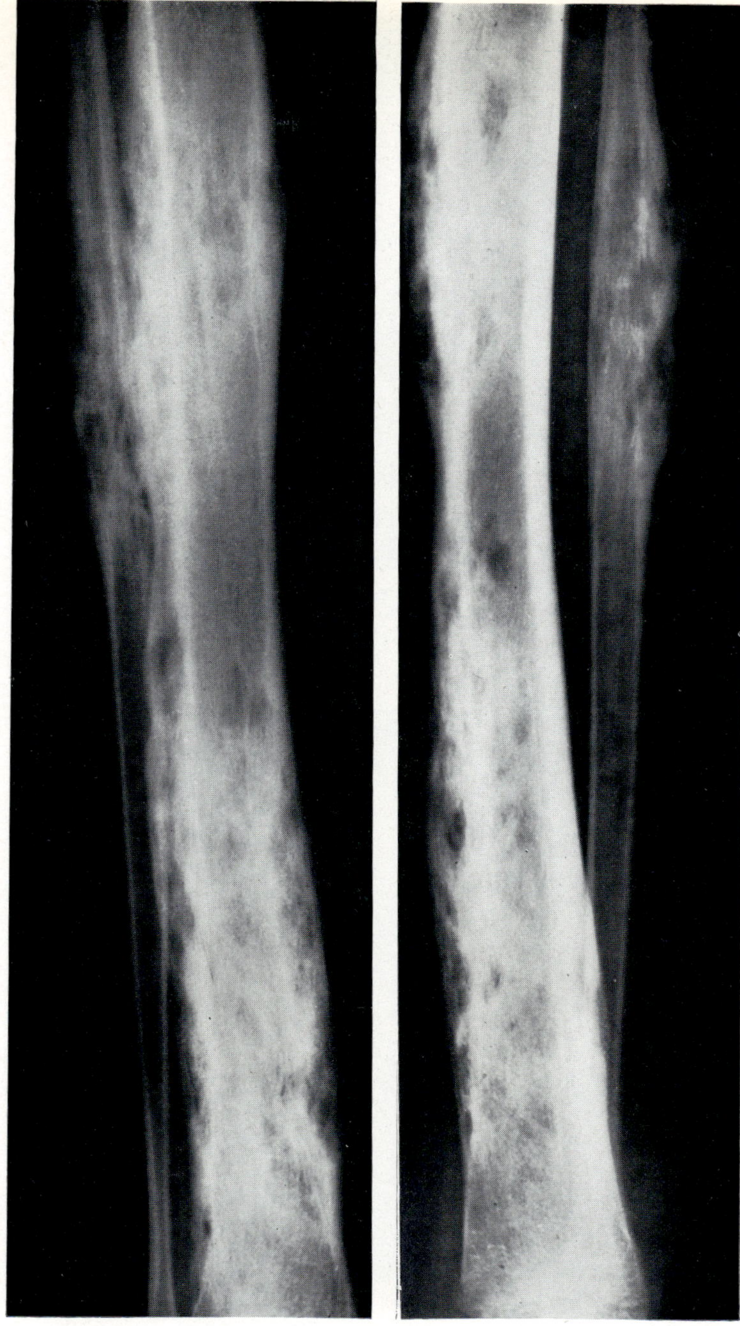

PLATE 19 *Late bony nodes with superficial small cavities in tibia and fibula. Healing always leaves bony thickening. This is a characteristic treponemal bone lesion.*

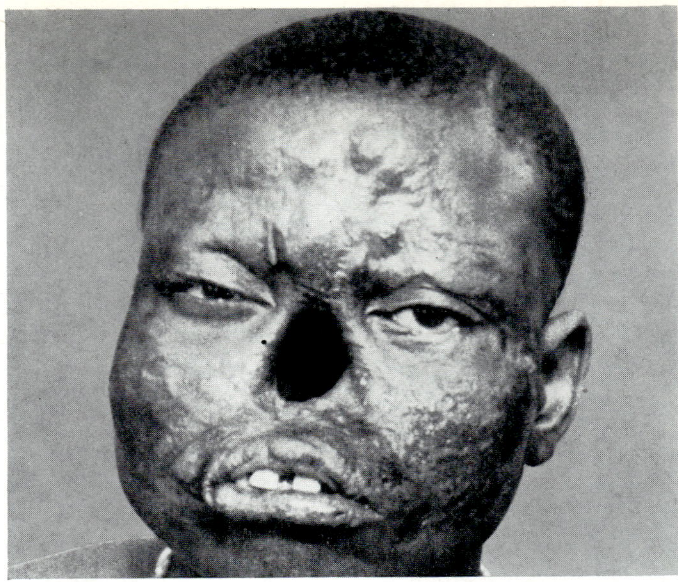

PLATE 20 *Destruction and scarring of late yaws lesions. Nasopalatine destruction is known as gangosa. (Courtesy of Dr A. Zahra.)*

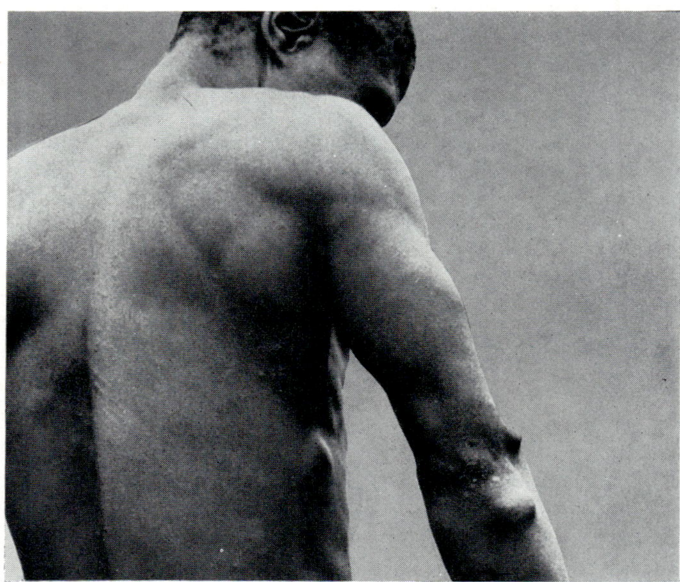

PLATE 21 *Juxta-articular nodules occur under the skin over bony prominences and are painless, firm and movable. They appear many years after infection. (Courtesy of Dr A. Zahra.)*

Plates 7–21 have appeared in the *W.H.O. Monograph Series*, No. 36 (1957) 'An international nomenclature of yaws lesions'.

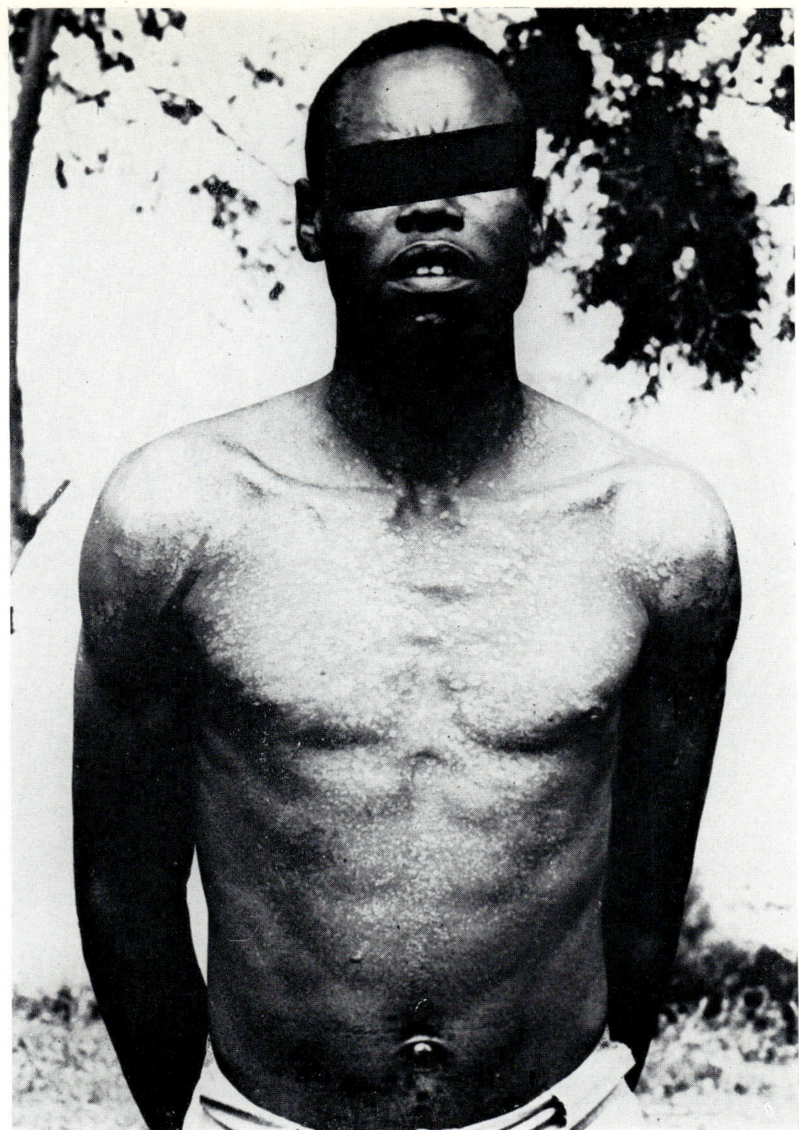

PLATE 22 *Pityriasis versicolor*. (Courtesy of Dr P. Hutton.)

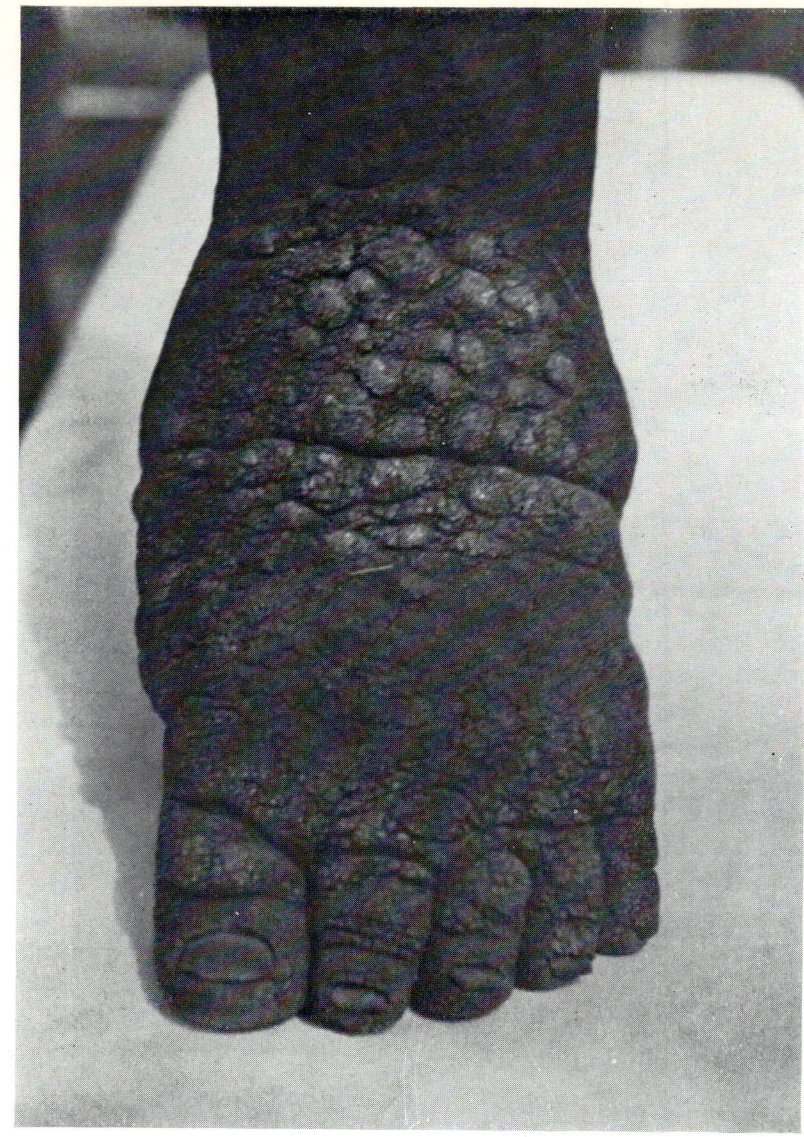

PLATE 23 *Chromoblastomycosis, showing the typical wart-like appearance.* (Courtesy of Dr J. Densfield.)

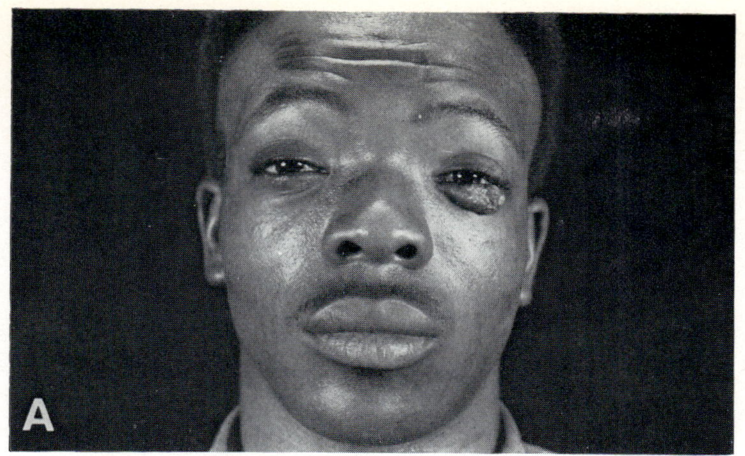

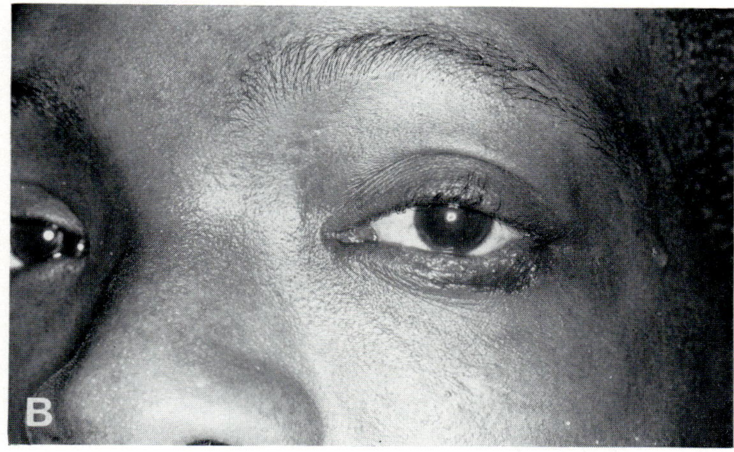

PLATE 24 *North American blastomycosis.* A *Granuloma of eyelid.* B *Same patient after treatment.* (Courtesy of Armed Forces Institute of Pathology, Washington, D.C.)

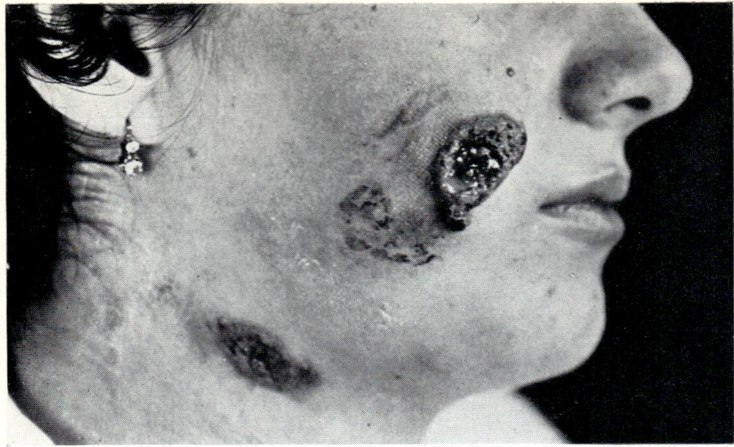

PLATE 25 *Sporotrichotic chancre of the face with lymph node involvement.* (Courtesy of Professor C. S. Lacaz and Professor Pupo.)

PLATE 26 *South American blastomycosis. Widespread papules involving the face and neck.* (Courtesy of Professor C. S. Lacaz and Professor Pupo.)

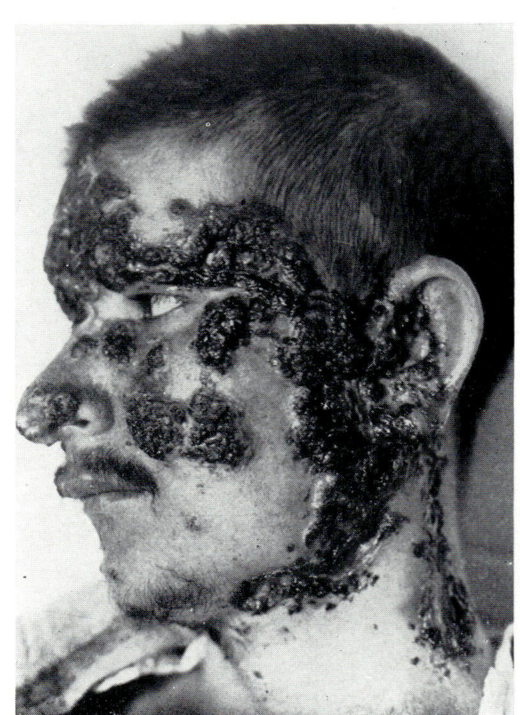

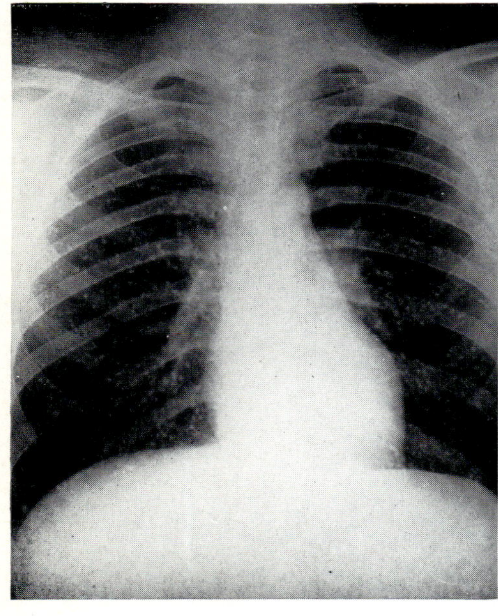

PLATE 27 *Histoplasmosis. X-ray showing fine miliary areas of calcification.* (Courtesy of Wellcome Museum of Medical Science.)

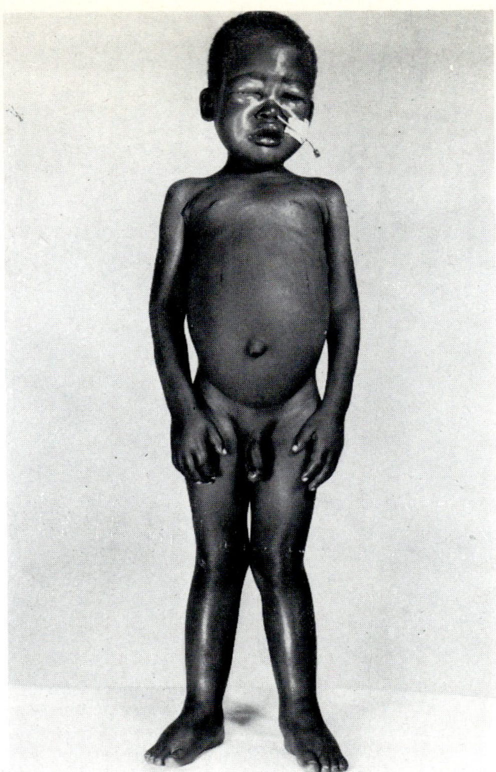

PLATE 28   *Kwashiorkor in Uganda, pre-school child showing oedema, wasted muscles, misery and growth failure.*

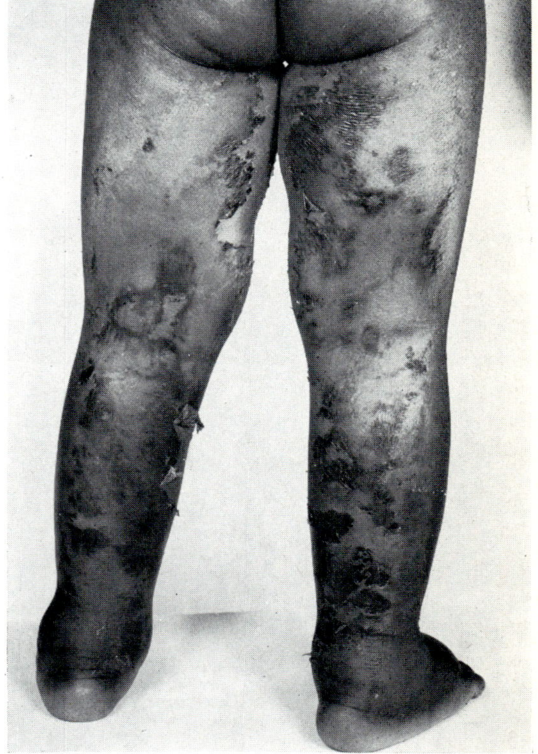

PLATE 29   *'Flaky paint' rash, pathognomonic of kwashiorkor, on backs of legs, made up of hyperpigmented patches peeling off to leave very light, thin skin beneath.*

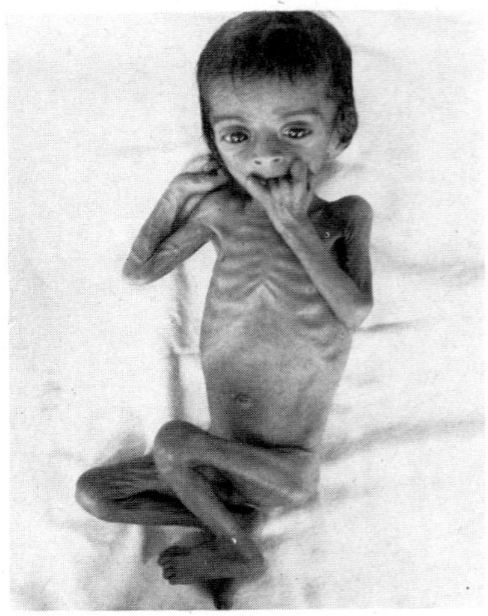

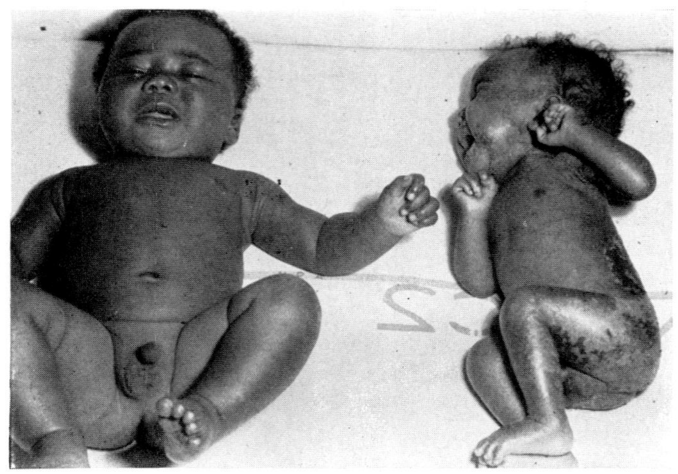

Plate 30 *Nutritional marasmus in 3-month-old Trinidadian infant, following bottle feeding with diluted contaminated cow's milk formula.*

Plate 31 *Twins—one normal (left) following breast-feeding and adequate supplementary foods, contrasted with the other (right) with kwashiorkor, following artificial feeding and largely carbohydrate gruels as weaning foods.*

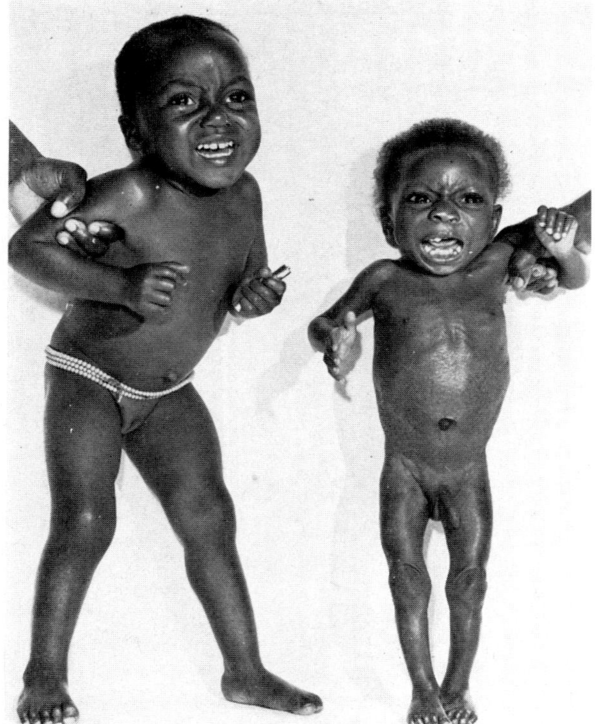

Plate 32 *Twins—one normal growth, and one with late nutritional marasmus resulting from severe untreated cleft-palate.*

Nutritional Diseases

Protein-Calorie Malnutrition of Early Childhood

Vitamin Deficiencies

Nutritional Anaemias and Small Intestinal Diseases in the Tropics

Haemoglobinopathies

Heat Disorders

Occupational Diseases

Venomous Bites and Stings

Hazards from Plants and Aquatic Organisms

Cardiovascular Diseases

27

Protein-Calorie Malnutrition of Early Childhood

The group of conditions known collectively as 'protein-calorie malnutrition of early childhood' (PCM) or 'protein-calorie deficiency diseases', constitute the most widespread and serious nutritional public health problem in the world, involving tens of millions of young children.

The term 'protein-calorie malnutrition of early childhood' was introduced (Jelliffe, 1959) to cover all categories from the severe syndromes of kwashiorkor and nutritional marasmus, to the much more numerous mild-moderate cases. This group label also has the advantage of emphasising the importance of calories, both in infant feeding designed to prevent protein-calorie malnutrition, and in the therapeutic regimens for the cure of established cases. In addition, the time-span covered by 'early childhood' is designedly imprecise, covering both infancy and the 1–4 year so-called 'pre-school' period, as the age-prevalence of the various forms of protein-calorie malnutrition is not the same in different regions of the world.

It can, in fact, occur in all forms, including kwashiorkor, in older children and in adults, especially in multiparous women, as a form of maternal depletion syndrome. Severe degrees are, however, rare outside early childhood, except in famine conditions.

Biological stages

The nutritional dangers of the early years of life can best be understood in relation to the concept of the 'extrauterine fetus' (Bostock, 1962), which postulates that the newborn is essentially fetal until the achievement of quadrupedal locomotion, or, in other words, that the human fetal period lasts for 18 months.

Nutritionally, three interrelated biological stages of early life can be differentiated—the *intrauterine fetus*, the *extrauterine fetus*, and the *transitional* (Jelliffe, 1968a). They are helpful in understanding the aetiology of protein-calorie malnutrition of early childhood and, conversely, in planning a rational preventive programme, including infant feeding.

The *intrauterine fetus* is plainly directly dependent on the nutrients acquired transplacentally from the mother. The *exterogestate fetus*, covering approximately the first 9 months of life in traditional circumstances, is dependent nutritionally on stores laid down *in utero*, and on mother's milk. During this period, the breast has the function of an external placenta and umbilical cord. The *transitional* is the young child subsisting on an increasing range of foods together with breast milk. This is a period of multiple stresses—nutritional, dietary, immunological and psychological. The period of transition commences at a variable age in different cultures, and is tending to occur earlier (page 394). In traditional circumstances, the second year of life is the most dangerous for the transitional, and the process is completed when the young child is on the full adult diet and has acquired immunity to the local microbial and parasitic infections.

Statistical stages

Early childhood is usually considered statistically in two stages—'infancy' (0–11 months) and 'pre-school period' (12–59 months). Both are arbitrary chronological categories, and the pre-school span covers much too wide a range of rapidly changing years with differing problems and risks, and has a 'fill-in' connotation. Also, the term pre-school child is incorrect for large areas of the world where a high percentage of the child population may never have the opportunity of attending school.

Statistically, there is a need to analyse 'pre-school child' data by 1-year age groups. The second year is a time of special risk, even in technically advanced countries, when more than one third of the pre-school deaths occur. In pre-industrialised less technically developed regions, as much as three quarters of the pre-school deaths occur in this year, as a result of a combined burden of malnutrition and infection (Gordon *et al*, 1967), and to emphasise this neglected year the neologism 'secotrant' has been suggested for the second year transitional (Jelliffe, 1969a).

The present account of protein-calorie malnutrition is intended to have a practical, rather than a metabolic, orientation, with major emphasis on preventive approaches in the community. The severe syndromes—kwashiorkor, marasmus and intermediate forms—are described first, followed by mild-moderate forms, and by general considerations concerning prevention.

KWASHIORKOR

SYNONYMS. The word 'kwashiorkor' was introduced to scientific medical literature by Cicely Williams (1933). It is from the Ga language of Ghana and implied the 'disease that the young child developed when displaced from his mother by another child or pregnancy'.

A wide variety of synonyms have been used in the past, although by general agreement kwashiorkor is the term most usually employed at the moment. Other names for the condition can be grouped as follows Jelliffe, 1966):

> *Appearance:* culebrilla ('snakeskin'—from the rash), nutritional oedema, enfants rouges (from the light skin and hair).
>
> *Outcome:* malignant malnutrition.
>
> *Pathological change:* fatty liver disease.
>
> *Diet:* mehlnährschaden (flour-feeding disease), sugar baby, syndrome pluricarencial (multiple deficiency syndrome).
>
> *Social:* kwashiorkor, obwosi (Luganda) and numerous other African terms, with similar meanings to 'displaced child'.

Definition

Kwashiorkor is one of the severe syndromes of protein-calorie malnutrition of early childhood. Most characteristically it has its main incidence in the second year of life. It is due to an imbalanced diet, which is very low in protein but contains carbohydrate calories, associated with a variable burden of microbial and parasitic infections and psychosocial factors. The four main clinical features—the tetrad of kwashiorkor—comprise *oedema, growth failure, psychomotor change* and *wasted muscles, with retention of some subcutaneous fat.*

Aetiology

As with all forms of protein-calorie malnutrition, the precise aetiology of kwashiorkor varies from region to region. It is, however, always due to the cumulative effect of multiple factors— dietary, infective and psychosocial.

Diet. The primary cause of kwashiorkor is always an imbalanced diet, low in protein but containing some carbohydrate calories, in the early years of life, when protein needs for growth are relatively much higher than in later childhood

or adult life (Table 1). Kwashiorkor can be produced experimentally in young animals with such diets.

TABLE 1. *Protein and calorie requirements*

Age	Weight (kg)	Total calories	Total protein (g)	
			Reference	Practical
Birth	3.5	420	8	10
3 mths	5.7	680	13	16
6 mths	7.6	840	14	17.5
1 year	10.0	1000	12	17.5
1½ yrs	11.4	1300	12	17.5
2 yrs	12.6	1300	13.5	19
3 yrs	14.6	1300	15.5	22

Notes

1. Weights = Harvard standard, 50th percentile, boys. If subjects are underweight for their age, they should still have the proper amount for their age.
2. Calorie requirements taken from F.A.O. Nutritional Studies (1957) No. 15, page 27.
3. Protein requirements from W.H.O. (1965) Tech. Rep. Ser. No. 301, Fig. 2.
4. 'Reference' protein = protein which is 100 per cent utilised (ideal). 'Practical' = assuming that the birth to 6/12 months protein = milk with utilization of 80 per cent. From 6/12 months onwards, protein = mixed protein with utilization of 70 per cent.

In many traditional communities, kwashiorkor is mainly a disease of the secotrant—that is the child in the second year of life. The background to this can best be understood by the four-stage weight curves commonly seen in these circumstances (Fig. 27.1). For the first 6 months or so (Stage 1), the breast-fed infant usually gains weight well and is protected from infections by maternal antibodies acquired transplacentally. In the second semester of the first year of life (Stage 2), growth is often less good, as the diet frequently comprises decreasing quantities of breast milk, together with small amounts of carbohydrate gruels or pastes. This inadequate and imbalanced nutrient intake is associated with waning passive immunity to infections.

The third stage of growth is usually a feature of the second year of life. Breast feeding may have been stopped, or if lactation is continuing, the quantity of mother's milk received is inadequate for the child's needs, and other foods will often consist of low protein, mainly carbohydrate foods. At the same time, the non-immune child is exposed to a wide and cumulative burden of bacterial, viral and parasitic infections of nutritional consequence. During this dangerous phase, the

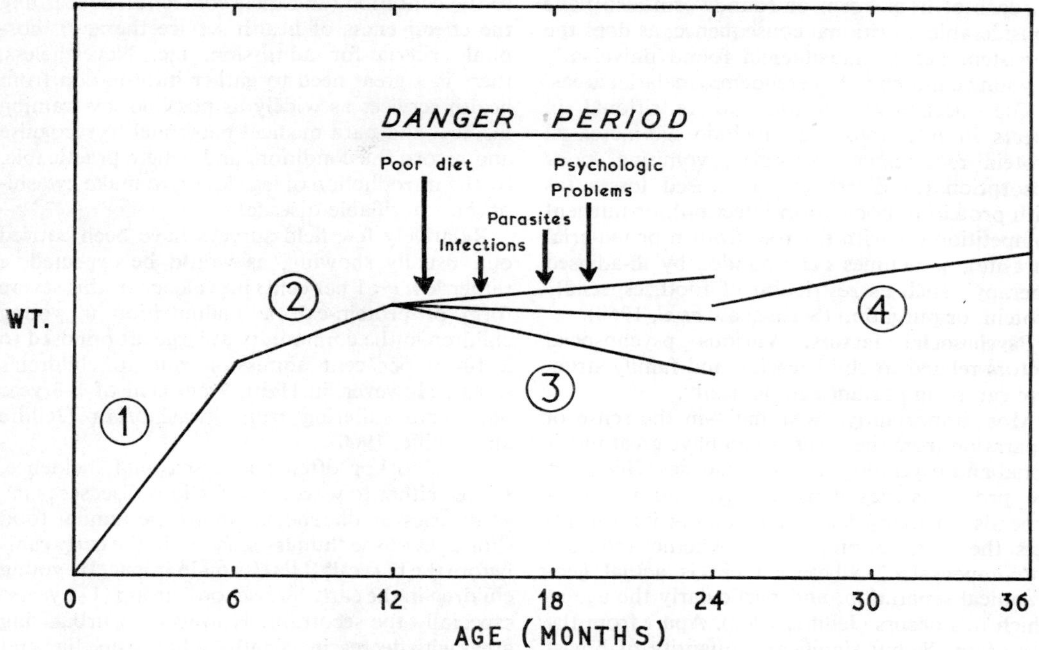

FIG. 27.1. *Typical weight curve in early childhood in tropical regions.*

weight curve may remain flat, or decline, and, in severe instances, kwashiorkor develops.

Subsequently (Stage 4), the child's weight gradually starts to increase in the third or fourth years of life, although the curve usually remains below standard levels.

The main defect of this type of diet is in protein, although recent work has shown that some deficiency in calorie intake also occurs, especially if the child's main food is a high bulk staple, such as the plantain, with a considerable content of water and cellulose and with a consequent low calorie density. In addition, associated defective intakes of various vitamins and minerals may be present in different combinations.

An inadequate diet of the type outlined may be fed to a child by his parents for one or more of the following reasons:

POVERTY. Protein-rich foods, especially those of animal origin, are the most costly items in the diet all over the world.

LACK OF AVAILABILITY. For geographico-climatic and agricultural reasons, including preservation and marketing, the appropriate foods for young children may be unavailable locally.

LACK OF KNOWLEDGE. Parents usually do not appreciate the need for protein-rich foods for young children, in fact a highly sophisticated concept.

'INCORRECT KNOWLEDGE'. Numerous food attitudes may act as 'cultural blocks' (Jelliffe, 1957) between available protein foods and physiologically vulnerable groups, especially young children. More important of these include the overvaluation of the local 'cultural super-food'—usually a mainly carbohydrate staple—for feeding young children, physiological group foods which are considered to be suitable or harmful for young children, the reserving of prestige foods (usually protein) for adult males, and the classification of foods in relation to non-scientific concepts of body physiology, e.g. into 'hot' and 'cold' (Jelliffe, 1967).

Infections. With waning transplacentally acquired immunity, the young child is continuously involved with a procession of infections—major and minor, simple and additive.

Important as conditioning infections are measles, whooping cough, diarrhoeal disease* and tuberculosis. Parasitic infections with heavy

* The useful term 'weanling diarrhoea' has been introduced by Gordon *et al* (1963) to describe an epidemiological entity, due to a variable mixture of alimentary infection (including organisms that are not classical enteropathogens), malnutrition and poorly digestible ill-cooked diet.

burdens of hookworm or roundworm also have considerable nutritional consequence, as does the persistent heavy parasitaemia found universally in young children in hyperendemic malarial areas.

The mechanisms leading to nutritional ill effects in infections may include an increased protein requirement, anorexia, vomiting, poor absorption (in diarrhoea), increased losses (as with protein in hookworm infection), or nutrient competition (as with the roundworm or malarial parasite), sometimes compounded by ill-advised 'therapy', such as restriction of food, especially protein, or purgation (Scrimshaw *et al*, 1968).

Psychosocial factors. Various psychosocial factors related to child rearing and family structure can be important aetiologically.

Most importantly, 'weaning'—in the sense of separation from the breast—can have great nutritional and psychological consequences. However, the process varies considerably, and its effect depends on many factors, including its abruptness, the degree of preparation, whether the child is 'compensated', whether there is actual geographical separation, and particularly the age at which this occurs (Jelliffe, 1962). Apart from the loss of small, but significant, quantity of breast milk, the psychological trauma of the process may lead to a form of 'maternal deprivation syndrome', characterised, among other features, by poor appetite, apathy and vomiting.

Family instability has much nutritional relevance. In particular, illegitimacy and paternal irresponsibility may lead to protein-calorie malnutrition directly by lack of finance to purchase protein foods, and indirectly as a result of lack of child care when mothers leave to go out to work to support their family.

Epidemiology and distribution

Kwashiorkor has been seen in most parts of the world, including the U.S.A. and the U.K. In the early years of the century, it was a common problem in Europe (mehlnährschaden). However, as with all syndromes of protein-caloric malnutrition, kwashiorkor is related to poverty, defective education, poor sanitation, insufficient food production and inadequate health services, so that currently it is principally a public health problem in less technically developed regions of the world, mostly situated in the tropics.

Factual information on its incidence or prevalence is very incomplete. Most statistics are derived from hospitals or health centres, and are therefore biased by many circumstances, including local transport problems, the attitude of the population to the condition (and their conviction concerning the effectiveness of health service therapy), hospital criteria for admission, etc. Nevertheless, there is a great need to gather information from health services as widely as possible, by training medical and para-medical personnel to recognise and record the condition, and, where practicable, by the introduction of legislation to make kwashiorkor a notifiable disease.

Relatively few field surveys have been carried out, usually showing, as would be expected, a rather low (< 1 per cent) prevalence of this severe form of protein-calorie malnutrition in young children in the community at large, as opposed to a 10–20 per cent admission rate to children's wards. However, in Haiti, 7 per cent of 1–3 year olds were suffering from kwashiorkor (Jelliffe and Jelliffe, 1960).

Kwashiorkor often has a seasonal incidence, related either to waves of infectious diseases (such as measles or diarrhoea), or to the annual food shortages of the 'hungry season', in the early rains before the harvest. It has its main impact on young children in the early 'pre-school' group (1–4 years) especially the secotrant. However, in urbanising areas with decreasing lengths of breast-feeding and with use of carbohydrate gruels, infantile kwashiorkor is seen increasingly, as in Trinidad where the peak incidence was between 5 and 7 months (Jelliffe *et al*, 1960). Also, in disasters, such as the Congo civil disturbances of the mid-1960s, the age emphasis widened to include late pre-school children, school children and even adults.

The question as to whether kwashiorkor is mainly a disease of urban or rural areas is uncertain, and may vary from place to place. Likewise, no real knowledge exists as to whether kwashiorkor occurred in traditional communities before contact with outside cultures, as, for example, in Africa prior to European penetration. Again, this may have varied, but it seems likely that various practices, such as prolonged lactation (associated with a cultural proscription on sexual intercourse) and polygamy, may have resulted in child spacing at longer, more nutritionally physiological intervals.

Pathology (Vitale *et al*, 1964)

The main pathological ill-consequences of kwashiorkor are on the organs with the highest turnover rate of protein. However, even here, the body adapts in a way most likely to spare the more essential tissues and organs responsible for vital life functions (Waterlow, 1968).

Firstly, the slowing in growth is itself an

adaptive function, while the primary tissue to show depletion is the musculature, which can be regarded as the body's labile and relatively expendable reserves of protein. The pale, pinkish-grey wasted muscles are characteristically contrasted with a layer of subcutaneous fat, paralleling the less defective calorie intake. Protein-rich compact bone is also much thinned (Garn, 1966).

The liver is often, but not always, enlarged, but is invariably yellow in colour, due to extreme periportal fatty infiltration. Hepatic dysfunction is indicated by defective synthesis of serum albumin. The pancreas is atrophic, with loss of secreting granules. The small intestines are very thin-walled, almost transparent, and distended; microscopic examination shows villous fusion, broadening, atrophy and flattening. Some degree of steatorrhoea is common.

Haematopoiesis is interfered with, because of lack of protein and often other associated factors needed for red cell formation, such as iron or folic acid, and concurrent secondary infections.

Enzyme systems throughout the body are affected, and their output usually decreased, including, for example, serum cholinesterase and alkaline phosphatase. Particularly important is the diminished output of pancreatic and small intestinal secretions.

Mineral metabolism is much affected and body stores of potassium (Garrow *et al*, 1968) and magnesium (Caddell, 1967) are greatly depleted.

Symptomatology

The clinical features of kwashiorkor vary from one region of the world to another, depending upon the genetic characteristics, the age of onset, the rapidity of development, the chronicity, the dietary defects and the types of conditioning infections present.

Kwashiorkor is a variable syndrome and it is unwise to generalise too widely from the picture seen in one area. Nevertheless, it is possible to divide the clinical features into three groups: constant, usual, and occasional.

Constant. The basic four features are oedema, growth failure, psychomotor change and wasted muscles with overlying subcutaneous fat. This 'kwashiorkor tetrad' is all that is required for a clinical diagnosis in early childhood in areas where protein-calorie malnutrition is a public health problem (Plate 28).

Pitting oedema is *the* cardinal feature. It is first present over the feet, ankles, lower legs and sacrum, but in severe cases may be generalised involving the hands, forearms and face. Strangely, the pathophysiology of this oedema is not fully understood. The impaired osmotic pressure associated with low serum albumin is only partly responsible, and probably the oedema results in part from metabolic effects on the endocrine system, particularly the adrenals.

Growth failure is best detected by a failure to gain or a loss of weight on serial measurements, or by a low body weight for age if only a single measurement is available (usually below 80 per cent of standard). However, the degree of underweight varies in different kwashiorkor syndromes seen in various parts of the world, depending, for example, on the amount of subcutaneous fat present. Also, the full extent of the depleted body weight is masked by the associated oedema, and is only revealed in early therapy when the oedema subsides.

Psychomotor change is characteristic, but impossible to measure objectively. It is characterised by a whining apathetic lethargy, or by a dull withdrawal. Psychomotor change is of complex aetiology, partly a direct effect of protein depletion on brain metabolism (as suggested by an abnormal EEG), partly psychological change due to maternal deprivation, and partly the result of decreased movement due to the wasted muscles and oedematous limbs.

The last feature of the kwashiorkor tetrad is *muscle wasting with some overlying subcutaneous fat*. In the severely oedematous child, muscle wasting is most obvious in the neck muscles, especially the trapezii, and the upper arms, where the much diminished belly of the biceps can be easily seen and palpated.

Usual. In addition to the basic four features, various characteristics are usually present in varying degrees. *Hair changes* are very common, although neither universal nor necessary for diagnosis. The hair may, for example, be quite normal in kwashiorkor of acute onset in the first year of life. *Dyspigmentation of the hair* can be striking. Various shades may occur, including light-brown, red-brown, blonde and grey. These represent an abnormal melaninisation, probably associated with deficiency of sulphur-containing amino acids. Bouts of protein-calorie malnutrition followed by recovery may unusually lead to the striped hair, termed the 'flag sign' (signa de bandera). Dyspigmentation of the hair is *not* necessary for the diagnosis of kwashiorkor, and conversely occurs widely in children with mild-moderate protein-calorie malnutrition in some areas of the world. The hair in kwashiorkor is also often *sparse, easily pluckable, silky* and *straight* (in groups with naturally curly hair). Paralleling the dyspigmentation of the hair, there is often a *lightening in colour of the skin*, especially of the face.

Anaemia of some degree is usual in kwashiorkor (*Brit. med. J.*, 1967). Aetiologically, this is basically due to protein lack (Woodruff, 1968), together with associated deficiency of other different haematinics, such as iron or folic acid. The haemolytic effects of malaria, or the blood loss from such intestinal helminths as the hookworm (which may lead to severe anaemia) or the whipworm, or the general effect of any bacterial infection may also be contributory.

The degree of deficiency in total erythrocyte mass is not accurately indicated by haemoglobin concentration estimations. In kwashiorkor, the haemoglobin level falls during therapy initially, as a result of haemodilution. Likewise, secondary deficiencies of haemopoietic substances may result during later therapy when rapid growth in red cell mass occurs, unless these are supplied in the diet.

Diarrhoea of some degree is usually present. Its aetiology is often mixed. Classical enteropathogenic organisms, such as shigella and salmonella, may be responsible from an antecedent diarrhoeal conditioning infection, but, in addition, the protein deficiency itself leads to loose stools from decreased secretion of intestinal and pancreatic enzymes, from altered microbial flora and possibly from changes in gut motility. Recently, attention has been given to the diminished lactase production seen, leading in some cases to diarrhoea during milk-based treatment, as a result of lactose intolerance.

Moon-face is commonly seen. It is partly due to subcutaneous fat, but it is similar to the Cushingoid facies seen in steroid therapy.

Occasional. *Hepatomegaly* is an occasional clinical sign in kwashiorkor, especially in the infantile cases seen in some parts of the Caribbean. As extreme fatty infiltration is a constant pathological finding, it is uncertain why hepatomegaly is only a variable feature. Splenic enlargement is not a sign of kwashiorkor, although often found coincidentally in areas where malaria is hyperendemic. Likewise, the hepatomegaly seen in some children with kwashiorkor is also due in part to malarial infection. Also, an enlarged liver may be present because of heart failure which can occur as a complication of kwashiorkor, especially during treatment (page 400).

Skin lesions are occasionally present, including small *indolent sores*, *groin rash* and the pathognomonic *flaky-paint rash* (Plate 29), which characteristically presents as dark, hyperpigmented patches on the buttocks, backs of legs and arms, later flaking off to reveal thin light-coloured skin or superficial ulceration underneath. The flaky-paint rash is the main reason that kwashiorkor was once mistakenly labelled 'infantile pellagra'. The dermatosis differs from that of pellagra in that it is not related to exposure to sunlight, but rather to pressure areas.

Signs of *associated infections* may also be present, such as tuberculosis. However, more usually associated infections are cryptic and difficult to detect clinically because of the malnourished child's lack of characteristic response —for example, bronchopneumonia with no fever, tachypnoea or rales. Dehydration should be sought for even in oedematous children, but, in view of the abnormal skin elasticity found in severe protein-calorie malnutrition, the primary signs to look for are dry mouth, sunken eyeballs, the state of the anterior fontanelle, and the pulse rate.

Associated vitamin deficiencies may influence the clinical picture and therapy, especially the 'quiet destruction' of the eye due to the keratomalacia of severe vitamin A deficiency, or the cherry-red sore mouth of ariboflavinosis. Other vitamin deficiencies may become apparent during the course of therapy, including avitaminoses A and D, and infantile scurvy.

INFANTILE KWASHIORKOR. The clinical picture in infantile kwashiorkor seems to vary somewhat from that seen in the classical 1–3 year age period. Hair changes are often minimal, and the flaky-paint rash is unusual. Conversely, liver enlargement tends to be considerable, often reaching below the level of the umbilicus.

Diagnosis

Kwashiorkor is usually diagnosed clinically by the presence of the tetrad of oedema, growth failure (as judged by weight), psychomotor change and muscle wasting with overlying subcutaneous fat, in a young child in an areas of the world where the diet is such that protein-calorie malnutrition is likely to occur. The aim in any community nutrition programme is, of course, to diagnose protein-calorie malnutrition long before the kwashiorkor stage.

No laboratory tests are required for diagnosis, but the level of serum albumin will give an index of the severity of the kwashiorkor (usually below 2 g per 100 ml). Also, interference with amino acid metabolism is indicated by an abnormal amino acid imbalance test (Whitehead and Dean,

1964), while growth failure is mirrored by a low hydroxyproline excretion (Whitehead, 1965).

Various routine tests should be carried out to assist in the detailed diagnosis of the aetiological factors responsible for the particular case and as a guide to treatment. These may include: a haemoglobin estimation, a sickling test, a thick blood film for malaria parasites, stool examinations for ova and occult blood, urine for microscopy, and a chest X-ray. A tuberculin test, usually a Heaf test, should be undertaken, but it should be realised that in malnutrition children infected with tuberculosis may give negative results.

Differential diagnosis

Other causes of oedema may need to be excluded. The nephrotic syndrome will show no other signs of kwashiorkor and the urine will be

Therapy has to be routinised, but with opportunities for intelligent flexibility. Details of standard treatment will plainly vary from one region to another, depending on staff and hospital facilities, on prevalent conditioning infections and associated mineral and vitamin deficiencies, and on available indigenous foods. A major role of a nutrition or paediatric centre in a region should be to devise a locally appropriate therapeutic regimen, bearing in mind overall cost-effectiveness as judged by simplicity of administration, length of hospitalisation, lack of side effects, and mortality rate, as well as expenditure on items included in treatment.

At the same time, it must be admitted that the details of current methods of treatment vary considerably in different centres, and this may be due in part to dogma rather than factual evidence (Wharton, Jelliffe and Stanfield, 1968).

TABLE 2. *Standard routine calorie reinforced dried skimmed milk mixture* (King, 1966)

| | 2 Pint, 1100 ml quantity | | | Bulk | |
	Rounded dessert spoonfuls	Imperial fl oz oz	Metric ml g	Weight % parts	Volume % parts
Dried skimmed milk	9	7 $4\frac{1}{4}$	194 120	65 4	72 19
Sugar	2	$1\frac{1}{4}$ 1	36 30	16 1	13 $3\frac{1}{2}$
Vegetable oil	5	$1\frac{1}{2}$ $1\frac{1}{4}$	39 35	19 1	15 4

loaded with albumin. Hookworm infection may lead to severe anaemia, in which case the child will show very pale conjunctivae, tachycardia, a haemoglobin below 5 g per cent and no signs of kwashiorkor, apart from oedema. The situation is, however, complicated by the fact that, in some regions of the world, hookworm infection may be a precipitating feature in kwashiorkor, as a result of the protein drain of continuous blood loss.

The dyspigmentation of the hair seen in some cases of kwashiorkor is not pathognomonic, and care must be taken to consider other causes of lightening of the hair, including genetic factors, and the influence of such environmental circumstances as sunlight, salt spray, hair-dye or oiling.

Treatment

Therapy can be divided into initial and subsequent, and the two basic principles of all forms of standard initial treatment are to supply adequate quantities of a high protein, high calorie diet, and to treat overt (or locally prevalent) infections.

Diet. The diet in the initial therapy of severe kwashiorkor should be liquid or semi-solid, and high in protein and calories.

Although cure can be obtained with vegetable protein mixtures or even balanced mixtures of essential amino acids, therapeutic diets have been (and still are) characteristically based on a formula of dried skimmed milk (DSM) with added calories in the form of sugar and/or vegetable oil. Various mixtures can be used, with the aim of administering about 4 g/kg of protein, about 100 cal/kg and adequate potassium and magnesium. Details of a suitable routine formula are given in Table 2, together with a chart for calculating feeds of 125 ml/kg/day (2 fl oz/lb/day) (Fig. 27.2).

Additional to the basic diet, it is desirable to administer potassium and magnesium by mouth, as in modified PCM Mixture containing 1.6 g of potassium chloride, and 0.15 g of magnesium hydroxide in 15 ml (0.5 fl oz), mixed with each pint of milk formula given (King, 1966).

Alternatively, if facilities exist, the IMRU (1968)

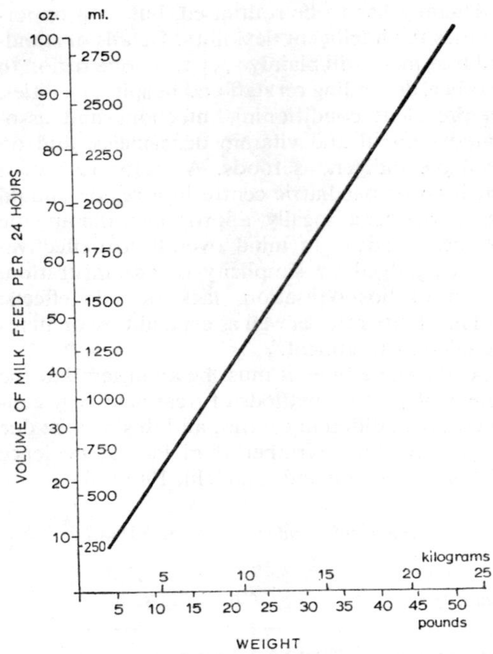

FIG. 27.2. *Chart for administration of milk diets in the therapy of protein-calorie malnutrition of early childhood* (from King, 1966).

CaDSu diet (with added minerals) may be premixed and used (Table 3).

With the present decreasing world supplies of available dried skimmed milk and with the occasional diarrhoea seen in the therapy of protein-calorie malnutrition from lactose intolerance, it is becoming increasingly necessary to investigate other forms of diet therapy; for example, CSM (processed gelatinised corn (maize) flour, 68 per cent, defatted roasted soya flour, 25 per cent, dried skimmed milk, 5 per cent, vitamin and mineral pre-mix). Reliance will probably have to be increasingly on vegetable proteins, including the soya bean and other legumes, and on new genetic varieties of cereals, such as high lysine corn, or on animal-vegetable protein mixtures.

Anorexia is a major hazard, especially in the usual understaffed tropical children's ward. In less severe cases, a ward help, or, preferably, the mother, can feed the child with small quantities of formula at frequent intervals. Alternatively, feedings may be given by a transnasal intragastric polythene tube (1–2 mm diameter), which can be left *in situ* for a week. Through it may be given either intermittent syringe feeds at 2–3 hourly intervals or continuous drip feeds throughout the 24 hours.

The routine administration of vitamins in early therapy is controversial, largely because the use of proprietary vitamin preparations would increase the cost of therapy greatly. Ideally, a non-proprietary vitamin mixture covering recognised daily requirements should be added to the feeds. If a particular deficiency is well recognised in the local dietary, this nutrient should be given routinely in larger amounts to all cases. For

TABLE 3. *Ingredients and nutritional value of routine Casilan (casein)— dried skimmed milk—sucrose diet (CaDSu) (I.M.R.U., 1968)*

Ingredients of the 'dry' mixture g		Nutritional value per 100 g of reconstituted diet	
Casilan	33	Protein g	4.0
Dried skimmed milk	30	Fat g	6.1
Sucrose	30	Carbohydrate g	4.6
Cottonseed oil	60	Calories	90
Potassium chloride	2.7	Potassium mEq	4.7
Magnesium hydroxide	0.3	Magnesium mEq	1.3
Sodium chloride	None	Sodium mEq	0.9

Notes

1. The diet devised by Dean and Swanne (1963), previously used, contained 5.9 mEq of sodium per 100 g of the reconstituted diet.
2. The mixture of 'dry' ingredients is prepared for use by taking 174 g of this mixture and making it into a paste with a little cold boiled water, in scalded equipment, and then adding, gradually, enough cold sterile water to make a total of 1000 g.
3. The reconstituted diet is fed at the rate of 100 g per kg of bodyweight per day.
4. At present the cost of this diet is 105 E.A. cents for a 10 kg child per day.

example, in areas where keratomalacia is a problem, 10 000 iu of water-dispersible vitamin A should be given daily by mouth for 7 days; while if megaloblastic anaemia is prevalent, all cases should receive 5 mg folic acid daily. Ferrous sulphate (300 mg/day) should be given to all patients.

Less severe kwashiorkor may have to be treated at home, using a protein supplement or additive, as will be described in the therapy of mild-moderate protein-calorie malnutrition (page 410).

After 1–2 weeks, the dietary will be widened. This will usually consist of continuing milk feeds, together with an increasing quantity and range of low-cost, soft, easily digestible local dishes that are suitable for young children and are rich in protein, calories, vitamins and minerals. These can be based on the principles of 'multimixes' (page 414) and should be an important tangible form of nutrition education for attendant mothers. Group discussion-demonstrations should be carried out on the wards, with, if possible, the mothers assisting in preparing and cooking the dishes, in feeding their children with them on the spot, and in using the changing appearance of the improving child as a 'visual teaching aid' for the group.

Less severe kwashiorkor (or, if health facilities are very inadequate, all cases) may have to be treated outside hospital. The best local mechanism will vary from home treatment by parents, which will not often be successful, to domiciliary treatment reinforced by home visits from public health nurses (Cook, 1971), or even from educated village volunteers, to the use of some form of day feeding centre, such as a 'nutrition rehabilitation centre' (Bengoa, 1967).

Infections. There is much disagreement between authorities as to the routine use of antibiotics in kwashiorkor, and, if employed, which to select. A decision has to be made for the particular local area or, if the situation permits, for the individual case, but in view of the extreme commonness at autopsy of clinically undetectable bronchopneumonia at least a 5-day course of inexpensive procaine penicillin (200 000 units intramuscularly daily), or of oral tetracycline (25 mg/kg/day) may be logical.

Other overt or highly probable infections also require immediate therapy, that is commenced in the first few days. For example, in a hyperendemic malarial area, a 5-day course of oral chloroquine should be given, or if heavy roundworm infections are known to be widespread, single dose piperazine can be instituted at once, or if enlarged

cervical glands suggest the possibility of tuberculosis, appropriate therapy should be commenced immediately.

Infections discovered in the course of hospital investigation should be dealt with as soon as possible. In particular, severe hookworm infection, with large numbers of ova and a strongly positive occult blood in the stools, can be treated with tetrachlorethylene (0.1 ml/kg/dose) for 3 consecutive days, combined with a slow transfusion of sedimented red cells (3 ml/kg), if anaemia is severe with a haemoglobin below 5 g per 100 ml.

Special features. PSYCHOLOGICAL. The speed and effectiveness of cure is increased by TLC (tender loving care)—that is by attention, affection and cuddling by the mother, if admitted, or by nursing staff.

DIARRHOEA is a usual feature of kwashiorkor, and it may be due to a variety of causes, singly or in combination. Moderate loose stools are best ignored initially and will usually settle with a high protein diet. If facilities exist, severe diarrhoea should be investigated microscopically and bacteriologically, and if enteropathogens are present and/or if naked eye or microscopic blood cells, pus and mucus occur, it should be treated with a 5-day course of oral tetracycline. If the stools increase in frequency with a milk-based diet, and if they are acid (with a pH below 6, using Universal indicator paper) and with a high sugar content (more than 0.5 per cent reducing substance as shown by Clinitest tablets), the child should be treated on a lactose-free diet, based either on soya or casein (Table 4), given together with vitamin supplements.

DEHYDRATION can occur even in the presence of oedema. Its clinical detection poses problems, and can best be carried out by inspection of the mouth and of the eyes, palpation of the fontanelle, and auscultation of the heart rate. Rehydration must be undertaken *cautiously*, preferably by intragastric tube, and the intravenous route is rarely warranted, as there is a considerable risk precipitating pulmonary oedema. Even if dehydration is diagnosed, not more than 150 ml/kg (70 ml/lb) should be administered as the *total* fluid, including feeds, for the first 24 hours. A hypotonic electrolyte solution, such as half-strength Darrow's solution in 5 per cent glucose water should be employed.

ANAEMIA requires appropriate therapy in addition to the high protein diet, depending upon the aetiology. Infection with malaria (page 27) and hookworm (page 161) may need treatment; while megaloblastic anaemia should be given folic

TABLE 4. *Ingredients and nutritional value of the Casilan (casein)—sucrose (CaSu) and Casilan (casein)—fructose (CaFru) diets (I.M.R.U., 1968)*

Ingredients of the 'dry' mixture g		Nutritional value per 100 g of the reconstituted diet	
Casilan	45	Protein g	4.0
Sucrose or fructose	40	Fat g	6.1
Cottonseed oil	60	Carbohydrate g	4.0
Potassium chloride	2.7	Calories	88
Potassium dihydrogen orthophosphate	1.4	Potassium mEq	4.7
Magnesium hydroxide	0.4	Magnesium mEq	1.3
Sodium chloride	0.5	Sodium mEq	1.1

Notes

1. If a very low sodium diet is required the sodium chloride may be omitted from the ingredients. The sodium content of the prepared diet is then 0.2 mEq per 100 g.
2. The mixture of 'dry' ingredients is prepared for use by taking 150 g of this mixture and mixing as for CaDSu.
3. The reconstituted diet is fed at the rate of 100 g per kg bodyweight per day.
4. At present the cost of a CaSu diet is 124 E.A. cents and that of the CaFru 759 E.A. cents for a 10 kg child per day.

acid (10 mg/day) and hypochromic anaemia, oral or intramuscular iron (Imferon).

HYPOTHERMIA may develop in kwashiorkor, but the problem becomes marked in regions of the world with low ambient temperatures at night or during the rainy season. It is important to ensure that kwashiorkor patients are kept warm in the ward, away from drafts and well covered, and, if necessary with special arrangements, such as electric heaters and carefully guarded hot-water bottles.

CONVULSIONS or SUDDEN COLLAPSE may occur shortly after admission or later in the first week or so of treatment. Some of these cases are produced by hypoglycaemia, and in an attempt to prevent, feeds, preferably via intragastric polythene tube, should be commenced as soon as possible; while all children with convulsions or sudden collapse should receive 10 ml of 50 per cent glucose intravenously, followed by a continuous intravenous infusion of 10 per cent glucose (100 ml/kg/day). It is possible that some may be related to low body magnesium, and 1–2 ml 50 per cent magnesium sulphate solution should be administered intramuscularly at once and repeated daily for 4 more days. The usual routine procedures for resuscitation should be carried out, including clearing the airway and mouth-to-mouth respiration.

CARDIAC FAILURE may occur in the course of therapy of kwashiorkor as a result of anaemia, circulatory overload, hypernatraemia and hypomagnesaemia. Appropriate therapy will be indicated, together with digitalisation and oxygen.

Various forms of 'recovery syndrome' have been observed in the course of therapy in different parts of the world, including a syndrome of tremors (Kahn, 1957), and hepatomegaly and signs suggestive of portal hypertension (Gomez *et al*, 1955). Both are transient and disappear with continued treatment.

Response to therapy

The two main clinical gauges of improvement are the body weight and the child's demeanour. In uncomplicated cases, the weight falls during the first 1–2 weeks as the oedema disappears, and thereafter rises slowly as resynthesis of muscle occurs and growth resumes. The importance of accurate weighing on a checked balance cannot be overestimated. It is *the* basic test in paediatric malnutrition, but is rarely appreciated as such and more usually carried out so carelessly on an unchecked scale that its value is slight.

Psychomotor improvement is also characteristic. The first indication is when the child's eyes become bright and alert, following activities in the ward with interest, while cure is virtually assured when the child commences sitting up and, ultimately, smiling.

Biochemical tests of different degrees of complexity may be carried out, but with the exception of rising serum albumin and haemoglobin, are not needed for the assessment of response to treatment.

Follow-up treatment

Pressure on hospital paediatric beds* is usually such in developing countries that children, including those with kwashiorkor, often have to be discharged too early, often after only a few weeks of treatment. Ideally, this should be further consolidated by a further period in a simple nutrition rehabilitation centre (page 416) either residential or day-care in type, capable of feeding the children and educating the parents.

If this is not practicable, children should be discharged only after their parents are fully and practically conversant with how they should be fed on returning home, and where they should attend for follow-up (e.g. at health centre, hospital out-patients, or special nutrition clinic). Usually, they will be issued with protein supplement or additive (page 410) for use at home, together with weekly chloroquine in hyperendemic malarial areas. This consolidation of cure should last for at least 3 months, during which time opportunity should be sought to immunise the child against outstanding infections.

Prophylaxis and prevention

The prevention of kwashiorkor can best be considered in relation to the whole problem of protein-calorie malnutrition (page 411).

Prognosis

In the community, presumably almost all patients with kwashiorkor die. It is difficult to compare the hospital mortality rates for kwashiorkor, as the syndrome varies in different parts of the world (e.g. age of onset, conditioning infections, etc.), admission policies concerning less severe kwashiorkor vary with numbers of cots available, and the local population has different views on the effectiveness of health service therapy.

Mortality probably ranges from 10 to 30 per cent in well-equipped, adequately staffed centres, to as much as 60 per cent in less favoured places. A high percentage of the total mortality in hospitalised children with kwashiorkor occurs in the first 24–48 hours, so that the early institution of treatment, with intragastric feeds, antibiotics, warmth and cautious rehydration (if needed) is most important. If staff and accommodation permits, it may be feasible to institute a modified 'intensive care' approach to children with kwashiorkor for the dangerous first two days.

From a long-term viewpoint, limited evidence suggests that children recovered from kwashiorkor show a diminished physique 5–8 years later, but often not more so than children from the same socioeconomic background, who have not suffered from kwashiorkor. However, these studies are extremely difficult as young children in this socioeconomic background are difficult to trace and have a high mortality from many causes, particularly infections.

Likewise, there is at present no evidence that these children show evidence of severe liver pathology, especially cirrhosis. The association between kwashiorkor in childhood and the development of calcification of the pancreas in adult life has been suggested, but lacks proof.

The question of permanent mental retardation after kwashiorkor is also unproven, but will be discussed further in relation to other forms of protein-calorie malnutrition (page 418).

NUTRITIONAL MARASMUS

SYNONYMS. In the older Continental European classification of malnutrition, marasmus was sometimes termed athrepsia or decomposition. The word 'marasmus' itself is derived from the Greek *marasmos*, meaning severe wasting.

Definition

Nutritional marasmus is a syndrome of severe protein-calorie malnutrition characterised by *growth failure* (notably a weight of 60 per cent or less of that expected for age), and *very wasted muscles and subcutaneous fat*. It is due to a diet that is extremely low in *both* protein and calories.

Aetiology

There are two aetiological forms of marasmus —early and late. Early marasmus (Plate 30) occurs in the first year of life, and is usually due to failure of lactation and attempts to artificially rear the infant with dilute, contaminated bottle feeds. It is the result of a downward spiral of starvation and infective diarrhoea.

---

* Recent studies indicate the inherent dangers of hospital treatment, and suggest that methods of extra-hospital therapy need further investigation (Cook, 1971)

Late marasmus is seen characteristically in the secotrant, or less commonly in the later 'pre-school' child. It is due to a low protein, low calorie diet composed of inadequate quantities of local foods together, in some cases, with a small amount of breast milk. Diarrhoea may also be present, as may tuberculosis.

Epidemiology and distribution

Marasmus has always been common, but, until recently, has received inadequate attention compared with the more striking syndrome of kwashiorkor.

the imitation of socioeconomic 'superiors' and the persuasive ill effects of advertising of costly and locally inappropriate commercial foods for young children (Jelliffe, 1962; McLaren, 1966).

The main determinant of successful lactation is the psychosomatic 'let-down' or 'milk-ejection' reflex. Anxiety, uncertainty or lack of interest inhibit this reflex, leading to a dissatisfied hungry baby and breast engorgement, and the likelihood of a vicious circle resulting in lactation failure (Fig. 27.3).

Breast feeding has the universal advantages of species-specific composition and proved protection against at least some enterovirus infections,

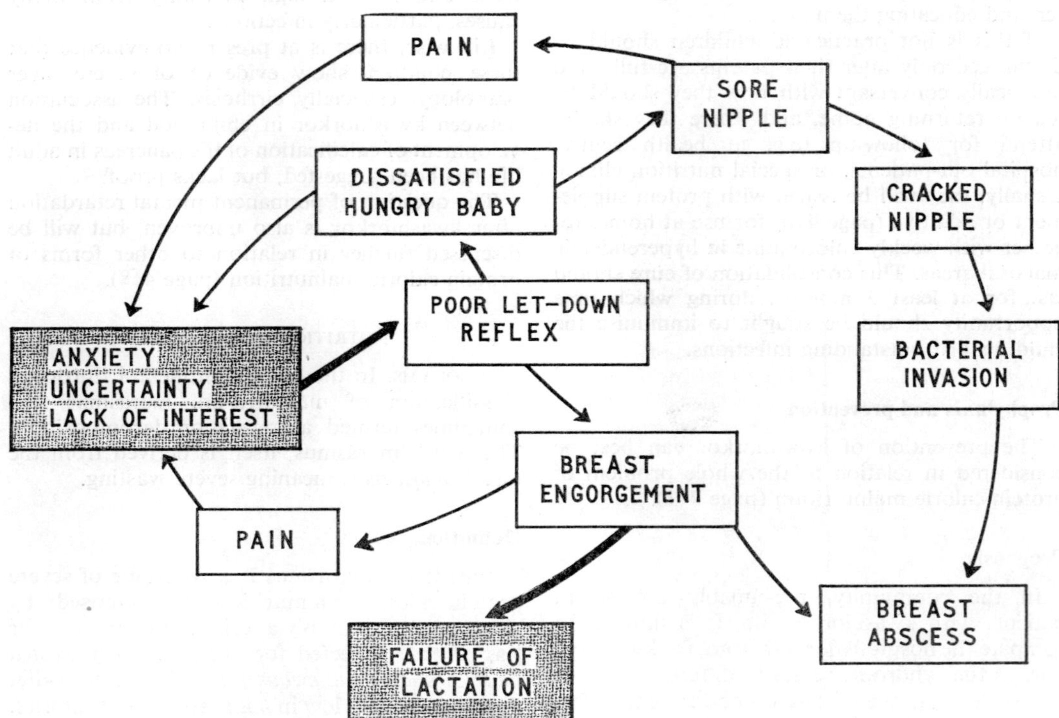

FIG. 27.3. *Failure of lactation from interference with the let-down reflex.*

It is of world-wide distribution, and, according to numerous observers, marasmus is now increasing in many urbanising areas, paralleling a decline in breast feeding resulting from women going out of the home to work, and from various complex social and cultural pressures, especially

as well as economy, ease of preparation of feeds, and a close initial mother-child emotional relationship (Jelliffe and Jelliffe, 1971).

However, for infants in less developed regions, breast feeding is not only desirable,* but virtually necessary for health or, indeed, for survival.

* From a wider viewpoint, breast milk needs to be considered among a nation's protein resources. In India, some 25 million litres are produced daily. The economic and food production consequences of widespread lactation failure need consideration, especially in relation to the current world 'protein gap' (Jelliffe, 1968b).

Artificial feeding with cow's milk preparations is beyond the parents' resources, while the environment, especially the kitchen and storage facilities, is such that a clean feed is almost impossible to prepare. Bottle-fed infants under these circumstances receive a homeopathic dose of milk and a high concentration of bacteria, with resultant mutually reinforcing marasmus and infective diarrhoea.

Pathology

The main brunt of the pathological changes seen is on the muscles and fat—both of which are very markedly wasted. The liver shows only minimal fatty infiltration, and the serum albumin and enzymes are less affected than in kwashiorkor. Recent studies have shown that the brain is decreased in size.

Symptomatology

There are two *constant clinical features* in nutritional marasmus: *extreme growth retardation*, as judged particularly by a weight of 60 per cent (or less) of that expected for age, and *severe wasting of both muscle and fat*. Numerous features may occasionally be present, including *anaemia, associated signs of avitaminoses* (especially keratomalacia or ariboflavinosis), *slight hair changes* (light colour, sparseness, straightness), and *associated signs of infection*, such as diarrhoea, dehydration, thrush and skin sepsis.

The overall physical appearance of the child is characteristic—that is a very wasted, long-seeming infant, with spidery-thin limbs and a large-looking head. The face is wizened and has been compared to a monkey or a little old man. The infant is often more alert and the appetite better than in kwashiorkor. The skin is loose, dry and inherently inelastic, even in the absence of dehydration.

Diagnosis

This is made on clinical grounds, largely on the basis of the appearance already described, backed by the extremely low bodyweight for age, and associated with a history of a very low intake of protein and calories.

Differential diagnosis

The clinical picture is diagnostic, although it will be necessary to differentiate the aetiological factors responsible in the individual case. In addition to a grossly inadequate diet, the presence of tuberculosis, infective diarrhoea and other infections need exclusion.

Tuberculosis may be suggested by a close relative with pulmonary disease, or by enlarged glands in the child's neck or elsewhere. Proof may be difficult as the tuberculin test may be falsely negative. A chest X-ray is desirable, if facilities exist.

The diarrhoea commonly seen in marasmic children is often difficult to diagnose aetiologically. Alimentary infection with classical enteropathogenic organisms, such as shigella, salmonella and *Escherichia coli*, or probably with other bacteria ingested from dirty feeding utensils and a generally contaminated environment, can lead to diarrhoea initially thereby contributing to the onset of marasmus as a result of poor intestinal absorption due to 'intestinal hurry', and often because of sometimes unduly prolonged dietary restriction as part of either indigenous or allegedly 'scientific' therapy. Additionally, enteral infection tends to be more chronic in marasmic infants, as, for example, with salmonella organisms, and leads to decreased intestinal enzyme production and defective absorption. Lastly, as with kwashiorkor, the pathological and biochemical changes of marasmus itself, especially the decreased output of lactase and other intestinal enzymes, may be in part responsible.

If available facilities exist, the stools should be cultured on three occasions for pathogenic organisms, or at least examined microscopically for the red and white cells suggestive of intestinal infection, as well as for parasites, especially *Giardia lamblia* and *Entamoeba histolytica*. Chemical examination of the stools for excess sugar and low pH (page 399) may be helpful in suggesting lactase deficiency.

Evaluation of the degree of dehydration presents special problems in marasmus. The skin is inherently inelastic, so that the classical decrease in skin turgor is difficult to interpret. Likewise depletion of body fat and muscle make the anterior fontanelle appear more prominent and the eyeballs seem sunken. If prior recordings are available, a *sudden* drop in weight can give an index of fluid loss. However, this is rarely the case and usually the state of the oral mucous membrane and the heart rate may be the best approximate clues to the degree of dehydration.

In industrialised parts of the world, 'failure to thrive'—leading in advanced severe instances to marasmus—is relatively uncommon and is usually due to one of a wide range of rare inherited metabolic anomalies, such as defects of sugar absorption or fibrocystic disease, or to congenital abnormalities, such as urogenital tract deformities with associated chronic infection. The incidence of these conditions in children in tropical regions is unknown. Probably they are occurring, but are currently 'buried' within the overwhelming mass of 'environmental' marasmus, due to an inadequate diet and associated infections.

Treatment

Marasmus is treated along similar lines to kwashiorkor (page 397). However, although the

portance of 'compact calories' in dietary management.

Despite the absence of clinical oedema, marasmic children have cellular overhydration, so that rehydration must be as cautious as in kwashiorkor (page 399).

Prophylaxis and prevention

Again this parallels the prevention of kwashiorkor, and is plainly based on breast feeding, the provision of high protein, high calorie transitional foods, and the avoidance of unnecessary dietary restriction in illness, especially in diarrhoeal disease. Details will be considered later (page 416).

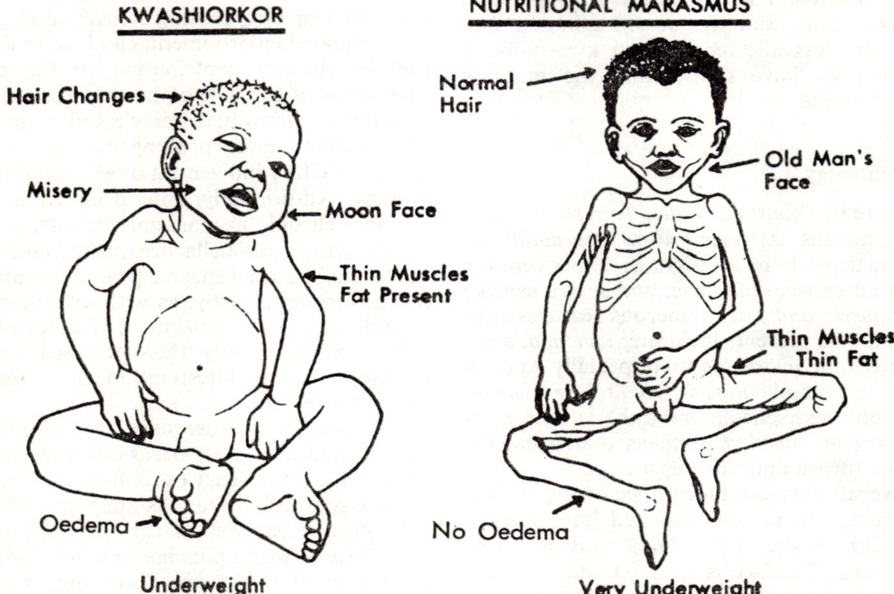

FIG. 27.4. *Clinical features of two main severe forms of protein-calorie malnutrition—kwashiorkor and nutritional marasmus—contrasted diagrammatically* (*Jelliffe* 1968c).

marasmic baby usually has a better appetite and is less apathetic than is the case in kwashiorkor, the patient is often infantile and so unable to assist in feeding himself.

The problem of the so-called 'stuck' marasmus also needs mention—that is the infant who, despite dietary therapy and control of infections, fails to gain weight. Some of these children may be suffering from undiagnosed infections or inherited metabolic defects, but many are due to an inadequate intake of calories. The aim should be to give the calorie requirements for the *expected* weight for the age. A difficulty here is the infant's stomach capacity, emphasising the im-

Prognosis

The prognosis in marasmus depends on the age and on the aetiology. 'Late' marasmus in the preschool age period is relatively easy to cure.

'Early' marasmus, in the first year of life, is notoriously slow to respond to therapy, often leading mothers to remove their infants from hospital. With adequate calorie intakes, the mortality rate is over 25 per cent in uncomplicated cases, while the death rate is still higher if single or multiple infections, or dehydration are present.

In addition, recent research has shown that different species have varying times of maximal growth and development for specific tissues and organs during which they may be damaged permanently by malnutrition or other adverse conditions. Modern studies have suggested that both brain development, and hence potential for intellectual development in later life, may be permanently interfered with by protein-calorie malnutrition in the early months of infancy. It is, then, possible that 'early' marasmus, which is tending to become more common, may have long-term irreparable effects of greater social magnitude than kwashiorkor (Scrimshaw and Gordon, 1968).

INTERMEDIATE-SEVERE PROTEIN-CALORIE MALNUTRITION

In all parts of the world, malnourished young children are seen who fall clinically between the two polar extremes of kwashiorkor and marasmus

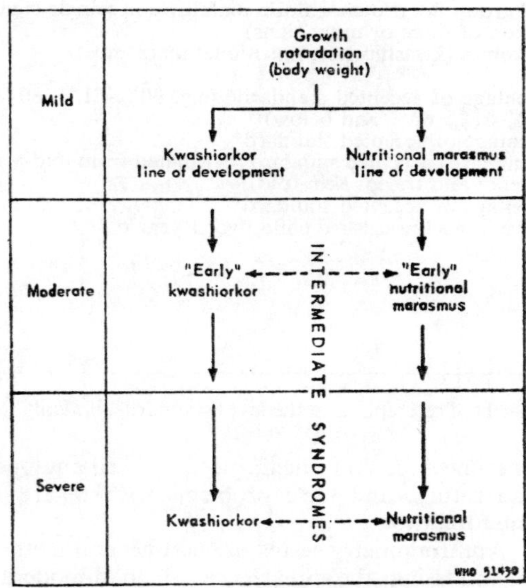

FIG. 27.5. *Lines of development in protein-calorie malnutrition of early childhood* (Jelliffe and Welbourn, 1963).

(Fig. 27.4, Plates 31 and 32). Cases may present with many of the features of kwashiorkor, but with only slight subcutaneous fat ('marasmic kwashiorkor'). In addition, inter-relationships between the two major syndromes are such that changing circumstances can result in the conversion of one clinical picture to another (Fig. 27.5). Thus, a child with early kwashiorkor can be forced into nutritional marasmus by severe infective diarrhoea and ill-advised, prolonged 'therapeutic' starvation or an infant with 'late marasmus' due to prolonged over-reliance on breast feeding alone may become ill with kwashiorkor during the second year of life, when mainly carbohydrate foods are introduced.

Provided the impossibility of categorising all severe cases of protein-calorie malnutrition into either marasmus or kwashiorkor is appreciated, the situation is somewhat academic. The aetiology, treatment and prevention follows similar lines in all instances.

MILD-MODERATE PROTEIN-CALORIE MALNUTRITION

Lesser degrees of protein-calorie malnutrition are far more common in the community than are the severe syndromes of kwashiorkor and marasmus. In addition, the inter-relationships between different degrees and forms of mild-moderate protein-calorie malnutrition are shown in the 'lines of development' diagram (Fig. 27.5).

SYNONYMS. Mild protein-calorie malnutrition may be termed growth failure. Moderate protein-calorie malnutrition in the kwashiorkor 'line-of-development' has been referred to as 'latent kwashiorkor', 'pre-kwashiorkor', 'mild kwashiorkor' or 'marginal malnutrition'. In the marasmus 'line-of-development', moderate cases have been called 'pre-marasmus' or 'mild marasmus'.

Definition

Mild-moderate protein-calorie malnutrition is difficult to define with objectivity. It is probably best to base the diagnosis on growth failure, as detailed later, as judged by a flattening weight curve, or, in community surveys, by a low weight for age (90–81 per cent standard: mild protein-calorie malnutrition; 80–61 per cent standard: moderate protein-calorie malnutrition).

Aetiology

This is identical with the aetiology of severe protein-calorie. In fact, children with mild-moderate protein-calorie malnutrition represent those who are passing through the transitional period with least immediate consequences.

Epidemiology and distribution

Inadequate information is available as most data on the incidence of protein-calorie malnutrition are derived from hospital or health centre

2 D

figures, and therefore mostly concerned with severe syndromes.

The improved collection of facts concerning severe cases of protein-calorie malnutrition attending health services is much required, while the incidence of lesser degrees of malnutrition can be estimated by analysing charts from Young Child Clinics for children demonstrating growth failure. In hospitals, *all* illnesses should be recorded for each child's admission and on death certificates (McKenzie *et al*, 1967).

Community assessment also needs to be undertaken by either *longitudinal surveys*, which are complicated to organise, expensive and time-consuming, but give detailed insight into the dynamic interplay of the different factors opera-

Tentative methods of direct assessment of protein-calorie malnutrition in the community are given in Tables 5 and 6, for areas where children's ages are known and unknown.

In community surveys, 11 clinical signs suggestive of protein-calorie malnutrition should be recorded (Table 7). They are useful in giving a general picture of the local nutritional pattern, but are too variable and subjective to give precise information. Two biochemical tests have been employed. The amino acid imbalance test (Whitehead and Dean, 1964), carried out on a small sample of serum, and the hydroxyproline excretion test, carried out on a random sample of urine (Whitehead, 1965). As with clinical signs, they are independent of exact age, but require the taking of

TABLE 5. *Tentative methods of direct assessment of protein-calorie malnutrition of early childhood as a community problem, where ages are known* (Jelliffe, 1966)

Method of assessment	*Remarks*
Clinical signs	'Suggestive' group for protein-calorie malnutrition (single signs, combination of three or more signs) Major syndromes (kwashiorkor, nutritional marasmus)
Anthropometry: Weight for age	Using percentage of accepted standard* (e.g. 90%–81%, 80%–71%, 70%–61%, 60% and below)
Height for age	Using percentage of accepted standard*
Mid-arm-muscle circumference for age	Using percentage of accepted standard (calculated from mid-arm circumference and triceps skin-fold)
Mid-arm circumference for age	Using percentage of accepted standard*
Chest/head circumference ratio	One or above in well-nourished child over 1 year old

Biochemical:
  Amino acid imbalance test
  Hydroxyproline excretion test	

Cytological: Buccal mucosa smear	

* Comparison should be made with both the general standards of reference and the local standards, if available.

tive, or by *cross-sectional point-prevalence surveys*, which are relatively economical of time, staff and money, but only give a picture of the situation at the particular season.

Data for the assessment of the status of protein-calorie malnutrition in the community may be obtained from the following approaches (Jelliffe, 1966):

> *Direct assessment of human groups:* clinical signs, biochemical tests, anthropometry.
> *Indirect assessment of human groups:* mortality and morbidity data.
> *Assessment of ecological factors:* conditioning infections, food consumption, cultural influences, socioeconomic features; food production, medical and educational services.

specimens in the field, need a well-equipped laboratory, and have problems with regard to interpretation.

Anthropometry seems the best general method of assessing the prevalence of mild-moderate protein-calorie malnutrition. Measurements most frequently used include the weight, the length, the circumference of the mid-upper arm, the chest and the head, and the triceps skinfold.

Pathology

The pathology of mild-moderate protein-calorie malnutrition is uncertain, as they have been but little investigated. Moderate wasting of muscle and fat is characteristic, and, at least in moderate cases in the kwashiorkor 'line-of-

TABLE 6. *Methods of direct assessment of protein-calorie malnutrition of early childhood as a community problem (where ages are unknown)* (Jelliffe, 1966)

Method of assessment	Remarks
Clinical signs	'Suggestive' group for protein-calorie malnutrition (single signs; combination of three or more signs)
	Major syndromes (kwashiorkor, nutritional marasmus)
Anthropometry:	
Weight for length*	Using percentage of accepted standard†
Weight for head circumference*	Using percentage of accepted standard†
Mid-arm circumference*	Using percentage of 16 cm (for 1–2 year old children)
Chest/head circumference ratio	One or above in well-nourished child over 1 year old
Biochemical:	
Amino-acid imbalance test	
Hydroxyproline excretion test	
Cytological:	
Buccal mucosa smear	

* Probably most valuable at age 1–2 years.
† Comparison should be made with both the general standards of reference and the local standards, if available.

development', some degree of fatty infiltration of the liver occurs.

Symptomatology

Growth failure and resultant body disproportion are the main features of mild-moderate protein-calorie malnutrition. Eleven clinical signs *suggestive* of protein-calorie malnutrition have been listed by World Health Organization (1962) (Table 7), but these vary in incidence in different communities and are, in any case, difficult to define objectively. In general, most will be more common in regions where the kwashiorkor 'line of development' is in evidence.

From the anthropometric point of view, mild-to moderate cases show abnormal measurements that might be expected from findings in the advanced syndromes of kwashiorkor and nutritional marasmus.

The principal anthropometric abnormality is a

TABLE 7. *Protein-calorie malnutrition in young children* (W.H.O., 1962)

The signs *suggestive* of protein-calorie malnutrition in young children are:

    oedema
    dyspigmentation of hair
    easy pluckability of hair
    thin sparse hair
    straight hair
    muscle wasting
    diffuse depigmentation of skin
    psychomotor change
    moon-face
    hepatomegaly
    flaky-paint dermatosis

low weight for age, *approximately* paralleling the severity of the malnutrition. Despite early interference with bone metabolism, there is much less interference with linear growth, as indicated by measurements of body length unless mild-to-moderate protein-calorie malnutrition is prolonged when stunting, or 'nutritional dwarfing', can result, with children both undersized as well as underweight.

The head circumference, though affected, is less so than the weight, especially if malnutrition occurs in the second year of life. This is because most of extrauterine skull growth occurs in the first year of life. The apparent largeness of the head is due to the contrast between a relatively normal-sized skull with the thin limbs, the wasted face—in children in the marasmus 'line of development'—and especially with the small chest, which is due in large part to wasted or poorly developed pectoral muscles, a finding which can be confirmed by a below-standard chest circumference. Muscle wasting is clinically evident and can be assessed approximately by the measurement of arm circumference *alone* (Jelliffe and Jelliffe, 1969).

In general terms, the clinical picture of mild-moderate protein-calorie malnutrition is of an underweight, disproportionate child, with a long-seeming body, thin limbs, a head that appears too large and feet that seem unduly elongated. The buttocks are flattened and the scapulae appear 'winged'. The chest is small, especially in contrast with the abdomen, which is often somewhat distended because of thin abdominal muscles, a bulky, fermentable, largely carbohydrate diet, sometimes associated with heavy burdens of roundworms and enlargement of the liver and spleen, often on a malarial basis.

Other signs in the grouping suggestive of protein-calorie malnutrition will be present in varying combinations, depending, among other things, on whether the child is in the kwashiorkor or marasmus 'line of development'.

In the kwashiorkor 'line of development', hair changes, including dyspigmentation, straightness, sparseness and easy pluckability, moon-face,

prevalence of kwashiorkor can be presented as shown in Table 8.

If ages of young children are not known accurately with documentary proof, children in their 'dental second year' (6–18 teeth) (Jelliffe and Jelliffe, 1968) can be examined for measurements which are relatively 'year constant' (especially the arm circumference, and for various ratios, especially the chest-head ratio (Table 6).

For children under surveillance (e.g. attending

TABLE 8. *Method of reporting percentages positive with (a) moderate and (b) severe calorie malnutrition of early childhood from data collected on a prevalence survey* (Jelliffe, 1966)

Age (months)	Number examined	Moderate* protein-calorie malnutrition (%)	Severe† protein-calorie malnutrition (%)
0–3			
4–6			
7–11			
Total 0–11			
12–13			
24–35			
36–47			
48–59			
Total 12–59			
Total 0–59			

* Total of children under 3rd percentile (80% of standard weight-for-age).
† Total of children with kwashiorkor (oedema) and below 60% of standard weight, for age.

psychomotor change and other signs in the suggestive grouping will be found in different combinations, together with a clinically obvious layer of subcutaneous fat. These cases—when marked have been termed 'pre-kwashiorkor', 'early kwashiorkor', 'subclinical kwashiorkor' or 'latent kwashiorkor'.

By contrast, in the marasmus 'line of development' the principal clinical signs will be low weight and diminished subcutaneous fat and muscle, sometimes with minor hair changes.

In community surveys, measurements of the weight, length, and arm circumference compared with standards (Jelliffe, 1966) give the best profile of the PCM status of the young children in the area. A combination weight measurements and

Young Child or Child Welfare Clinics), serial recording of weight graphically is the best method of early detection of lesser degrees of protein-calorie malnutrition, using a weight card such as that devised by Morley (1968) (Fig. 27.6), and also is excellent practical nutrition education for mothers.

Diagnosis (see above)

Differential diagnosis

Growth failure may be the result of acute or chronic infection or various long-standing metabolic or congenital abnormalities (e.g. cyanotic heart disease). Likewise, small anthropometric

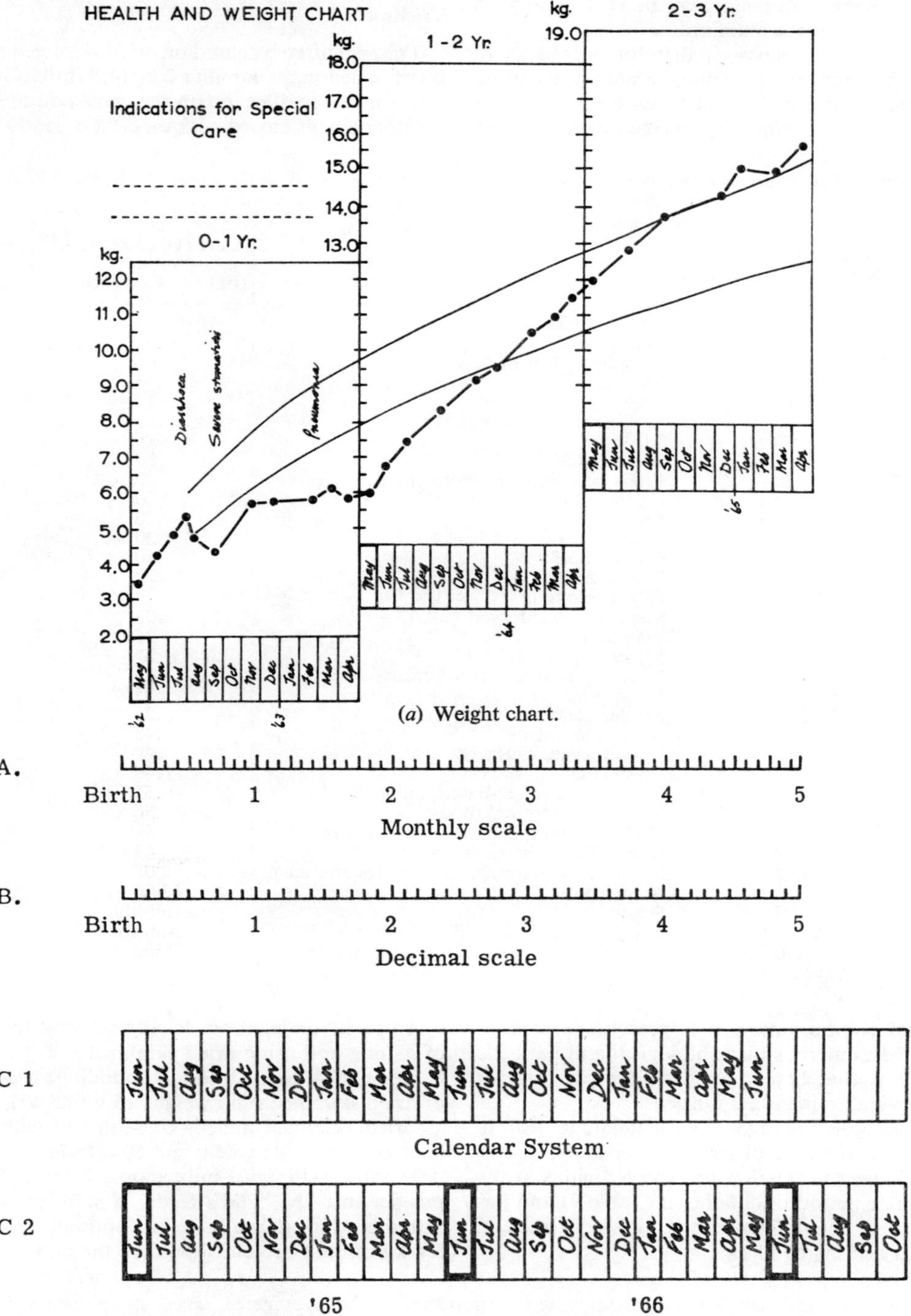

(b) Calendar system with birth month emphasised.

FIG. 27.6. *Child's health and weight record over first 5 years.* (Courtesy of Dr. D. Morley.)

measurements in a child may be due to genetic variation below the standard.

In community surveys, therefore, statistically adequate numbers of young children must be examined and due account taken for the normal variation of distribution of measurements. In

Treatment

This will often be based on dried skimmed milk, often issued in the familiar 2 kg (4.5 lb) UNICEF box, or in smaller quantities repackaged into polythene bags closed with an elastic band.

TABLE 9. *Average cost of foods in the West Indies as sources of protein and calories* (McKigney, 1968)

Cost per 1000 calories (Eastern Caribbean $)		Cost per 20 grams of protein (Eastern Caribbean $)
.25	Dry skimmed milk	.05
.22	Pulses	.06
.10	Cornmeal—wheat flour	.08
1.20	Salt fish	.10
.13	Rice	.12
.25	Macaroni—rolled oats	.15
.60	Sardines	.18
.55	Fresh milk	.20
.60	Fresh beef, goat, mutton, cheddar cheese	.20
1.80	Fresh fish	.20
.25	Bread	.20
1.10	Chicken necks and backs	.20
1.20	Corned beef	.20
.47	Peanut butter	.22
.55	Dry whole milk	.23
.25	Sweetened condensed milk	.23
.55	Evaporated milk	.25
.90	Minced (ground) beef	.25
.25	Ground provisions (root crops)	.28
.40	Fresh pork	.35
2.20	Broiler meat	.35
.60	Irish potatoes	.40
1.10	Frankfurters, sausages	.40
1.60	Fresh eggs	.40
.80	Milk-based, cereal-based, infant foods	.51
.80	'Health promoting' foods	.56
.29	Plantain, green bananas, ripe bananas	.59
4.87	Infant foods—strained meats	.69
4.58	Infant foods—strained vegetables and meat	2.08
.55	Arrowroot	13.00
.09	Sugar	Infinity
.15	Margarine, cooking oil	Infinity
.80	Glucose	Infinity

tropical circumstances, it is reasonable to consider the numerous microbiological and parasitic infections that beset young children as part of their overall nutritional burden.

On an individual basis, an 'inadequate' gain in weight can best be observed graphically, or has to be judged in relation to expected gains at the particular period of childhood (Table 9) and has to bear in mind fluctuations in weight seen in normal healthy children.

An easily understood, locally relevant method of issuing and using dried skimmed milk* has to be devised. A heaped dessert (pudding) spoonful of dried skimmed milk weighs 15 g (0.5 oz), and, as dried skimmed milk is one-third protein, this contains 5 g milk protein and 50 calories.

The dried skimmed milk should be mixed as a powder into the child's feeds. If sufficient dried skimmed milk is available, an optimal 'dose' of 3 g/kg of milk protein should be the aim, so that

* The size of usually employed local domestic measures needs to be investigated, especially spoons. A dessert (pudding) spoon usually has a volume of 12 ml, and a village teaspoon, 5–6 ml. A heaped dessert-spoonful = 3 level teaspoonfuls = 2 heaped teaspoonfuls. In addition, a wide variety of indigenous spoons, or similar utensils, may be available and more appropriate.

a 10 kg (20 lb) child would be given 30 g protein/day, which can be supplied by 2 heaped dessertspoonfuls three times daily, mixed into soft, digestible, locally acceptable cereal porridge. A 2 kg (4.5 lb) package will then last about 21 days.

However, as dried skimmed milk is often in limited supply (and is likely to be more so in the future), it may be more economically employed as the animal protein ingredient of a triple mix or quadrimix (page 414), including vegetable protein foods in the form of a cereal and a legume. In this case, 1–1½ heaped dessertspoonfuls of dried skimmed milk may be added to a multimix three times daily.

Alternatively, already processed mixtures may be available, as with the triple mix, CSM, i.e.

the health services, an appreciation of the wider approaches to the community forces responsible for childhood malnutrition is essential.

Community nutrition equation. As an oversimplification and as a rough guide to thinking, the level of nutrition in a community, especially of its highly vulnerable young child population, may be considered as being the end-result of numerous complex interacting ecological moulding forces, expressed diagrammatically in Fig. 27.7.

Each of the components affects the community nutrition level directly, and via the other factors. The educational level operates through numerous channels, such as the number, quality and relevance of technical training establishments and the existence of schools and their use for nutri-

Community level of nutrition ⟶	Educational level	Economic level	Food availability	Aspects of health	{ Conditioning infections { Preventive services

Population size

FIG. 27.7. Community nutrition equation.

corn (maize)–soya–dried skimmed milk, or with the triple mix, Laubina, i.e. *burghul* (parboiled wheat)–chick pea–dried skimmed milk (McLaren *et al*, 1966), or with the double mix, AK–1000 (King *et al*, 1966).

CSM has been quite widely used. It has a protein content of about 20 per cent, and, as it is partially pre-cooked, it can be rapidly and safely reconstructed by mixing with boiled water. In addition, its relatively high viscosity means that it cannot be bottle-fed and so will not be used in competition with human milk. Different preparations can be made as follows:

Parts of water (by volume)	Preparation	Cal/100 g	Protein g/100 g
2	Porridge	80	4.5
3	Thick gruel	57	3.25
4	Thin gruel	45	2.5
5	Drink	36	2.0

Moderate protein-calorie malnutrition is best treated at a nutrition rehabilitation centre (page 416), but may have to be undertaken at home, when special attempts should be made to supervise the parents by home visiting.

Prophylaxis and prevention

It is with the prevention of all degrees of protein-calorie malnutrition that the main concern of the health worker should centre, and, while his opportunities will be mainly in relation to activities in

tion education. End-results include the supply of technically trained personnel and the numbers of literates likely to be exposed to modern knowledge concerning food, nutrition and related matters.

The economic level operates on a country basis, when an increased national income can make more governmental budget available for social services, such as schools and health services, as well as for specific nutrition programmes directed at major problems. At the family level, improved earning capacity means that increased money will be available, which can be used for the purchase of a greater range of foods, especially higher cost, much needed protein items.

The vague expression 'food availability' covers a wide spectrum of circumstances and activities. Basically, this may be restricted by geographical realities of soil, water and climate. In particular, it refers to the quantity and, most importantly, the nutritional quality of foods currently produced (at village level or on a large scale) or imported, and how these are stored, processed, marketed, prepared and distributed within the family.

Also, certain 'aspects of health' particularly influence the community nutrition level, especially the widespreadness of 'conditioning infections', and the health services concerned with the prevention or early rehabilitation of child malnutrition, by nutrition education and growth supervision at young child clinics, by the issue of food supplements, and by measures designed to control relevant infectious diseases, as with immunisation or the chemoprophylaxis of malaria.

It is becoming increasingly apparent that the level of nutrition in a community is related to the number of mouths to be fed—that, in fact, population size is the 'universal denominator' for all other components of the equation.

The present serious world food situation is due in large measure to the disproportionate, and currently geometrical, increase in population size, constantly outstripping not only economic and educational development, but also *per capita* availability of food. As is well known, this trend particularly affects pre-industrial, largely tropical countries, where food supplies are often already inadequate and is most marked with regard to protein-rich foods, resulting in the grave and widening world 'protein gap', with its major impact on vulnerable young children.

effective National Food and Nutrition Committee or Council, leading to a rational food and nutrition policy, related to all components of the equation, including appropriate, relevant and economical maternal and child health services, and a co-ordinated programme of nutrition education directed through all extension channels.

Health service activities. Apart from general public health measures of indirect nutritional consequence, such as improved water supply and environmental sanitation, and malaria control, various more specific activities may be undertaken by health personnel to prevent protein-calorie malnutrition, including:

1. Improved feeding of young children.
2. Early recognition of less severe malnutrition (mild-moderate) and its correction by supplementary feeding.

TABLE 10. *Approximate protein content and amino acid deficiency of main categories of vegetable foods used in multimixes* (Jelliffe, 1968c)

Type of food	Protein (approx. %)	Amino acid deficiency
Cereal grain	± 10	Lacking in lysine
Legumes*	± 20	Lacking in methionine
Dark green leafy vegetable†	4–10	Lacking in methionine

* Soya Beans < 40 %   † Dried: 30 %

Lastly, and impossible to include as a single item in the equation, is the culture patterns of the community. The system of values, attitudes, beliefs and customs is interwoven into every aspect of life and affects each component of the equation.

Approaches to solutions. If the community level of nutrition is the end-result of numerous interlocking forces, it seems unlikely that a solution can often be reached by attention to one component of the equation alone.

A planned programme to improve the nutritional status of any community can logically, therefore, only be based on a simultaneous, co-ordinated approach designed to raise educational and economic levels, to supply inexpensive realistic health services, to increase the availability of protein foods, to improve family eating patterns, and to develop a locally acceptable family planning service.

In many parts of the world, a prime nutritional need is organisational—the development of an

3. Prevention and management of nutritional conditioning infections.
4. Improved treatment of severe protein calorie malnutrition.
5. Child spacing programmes.

IMPROVED FEEDING OF YOUNG CHILDREN. Methods recommended will have to be based on knowledge of local circumstances, such as current indigenous practices with regard to child feeding, the pattern of malnutrition and of childhood infections, the range of foods available and their cost in relation to nutrient value (Table 9), the status and activity of women, and such practical aspects of home economics as the type of stove and available cooking utensils.

Breast feeding should be the mainstay *alone* for 4–6 months, depending upon the local lactation performance. There is usually no need for other foods, including fruit juices during this period as the baby is receiving sufficient nutrients from mother's milk and fetal stores. Conversely, the

TABLE 11. *Village-level multimixes* (Jelliffe, 1968c)

	Ingredients
Double mix	Staple*+legume *or* Staple+animal protein† *or* Staple+dark green leafy vegetable (DGLV)
Triple mix	Staple+legume+animal protein *or* Staple+legume+DGLV *or* Staple+DGLV+animal protein
Quadrimix	Staple+legume+DGLV+animal protein

* Preferably a cereal.
† Mixtures with animal protein preferable in all mixes.

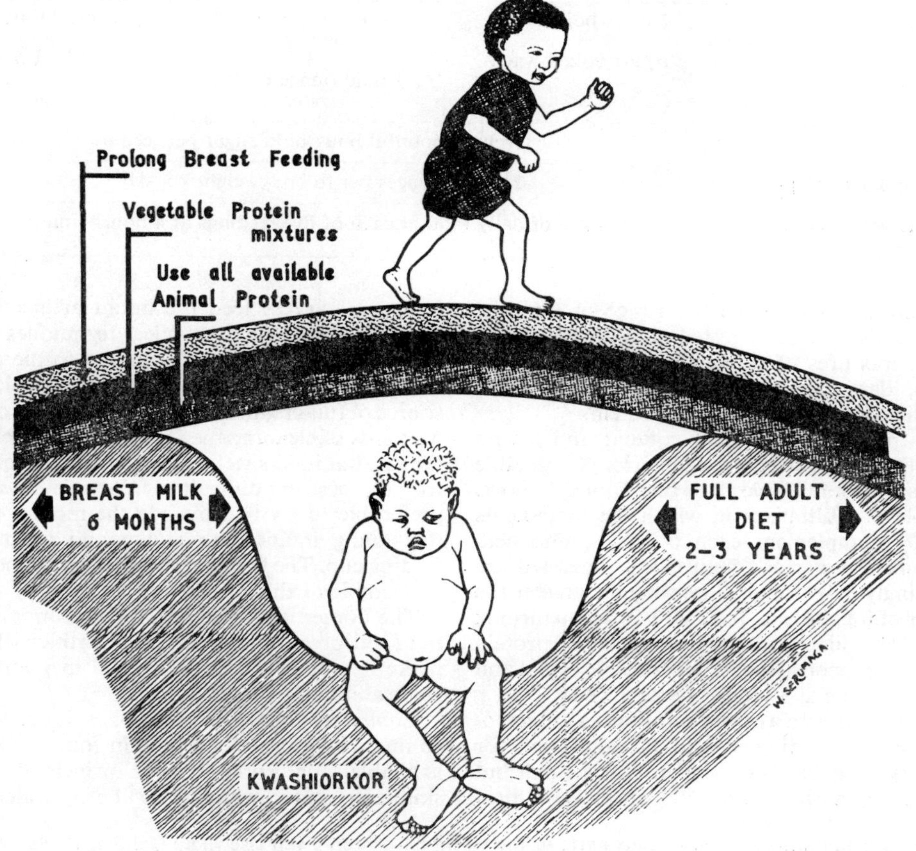

FIG. 27.8. *Three plank protein bridge.*

ingestion of other foods is accompanied by grave risk of infective diarrhoea.

The dependence of the young child on maternal nutrition, both via fetal stores and breast milk, emphasises the need to ensure as full a diet as possible, with special reference to locally available vegetable protein foods, for the mother during pregnancy and lactation.

From 4 to 6 months on, semi-solids should be gradually introduced, but in increasing quantity and range. The first food is often the indigenous carbohydrate gruel or paste, which, however, should be very soon combined with other items. Often a simple, economical *combination* of foods ('multimix') may be nutritionally desirable and

duced in late lactation, even in poorly nourished women.

As protein is the critical need in feeding in young children in developing tropical countries, the concept of the Three Plank Protein Bridge (Fig. 27.8) emphasises the need to use *all available protein sources*. The bridge is made up of the 'three planks' of *breast feeding* and mixtures of *animal and vegetable protein foods*, all of which assist the child in crossing the nutritional transition between 6 months and 2–3 years.

The dangers of artificial feeding, using cow's milk formulas and feeding bottles, has been stressed. The risk of marasmus and infective diarrhoea are very great (page 403). If, however,

TABLE 12. *Simplified use of cow's milk and its preparations in the feeding of babies up to 3 months of age* (Jelliffe, 1968c)

	Fresh cow's milk	Full cream powdered milk	Evaporated milk
Dilution	2 parts boiled milk + 1 part boiled water	1 level teaspoon milk powder + 1 fluid ounce boiled water	1 part evaporated milk + 2 parts boiled water
Add sugar	1 level teaspoonful household sugar per feeding		
Calculate daily volume	$2\frac{1}{2}$ fluid ounces per lb bodyweight per day		
Calculate volume per feed	One-fifth of daily total at each of five feedings at 4-hourly intervals		

practicable, in which the full range of essential amino acids can be ingested simultaneously by suitable mixtures of staple (preferably a cereal), legume, dark-green leafy vegetables and *small* quantities of expensive animal protein.

The approximate protein content and amino acid deficiency of the main categories of vegetable foods is shown in Table 10; while Table 11 shows village-level multimixes in which the ingredients mutually complement each others' amino acid spectrum. The various multimixes suggested are increasingly nutritionally desirable the greater the number of ingredients. In other words, quadrimix recipes are ideal, although vegetable protein double mixes, consisting of local staple cereal and legume, may be all that can be achieved.*

At the same time as these multimixes are introduced, breast feeding should be continued for 1–2 years, as it has been shown that a small but significant quantity (about 500 ml daily) is pro-

it is necessary to feed the infant artificially, the simplest and most economical techniques should be employed, and carefully taught to the mother or other relative. The cheapest, reliable local source of full-cream milk should be recommended. Methods of cleaning the feeding bottle need to be taught, but in less well-to-do circumstances in the tropics, these are difficult to follow, and it may be preferable to try to persuade the mother to feed the young infant with a cup and spoon or a feeding cup. The formula suggested must be basically simple (Tables 12 and 13).

The domestic mathematics, the economics and the food preparation aspects of artificial feeding make it unlikely to be successful in poorer, less well sanitated tropical homes.

Commercially processed protein foods. Various commercially processed protein foods have been available for some years, principally dried skimmed milk which has been widely dis-

* Recipes for multimixes from various parts of the world have been given elsewhere (Jelliffe, 1968c; W.H.O., 1968; Jelliffe, 1971).

TABLE 13. *Simplified use of cow's milk and its preparations in the feeding of infants over 3 months of age* (Jelliffe, 1968c)

	Fresh cow's milk	Full cream powdered milk	Evaporated milk
Dilution	Undiluted boiled milk	1 rounded teaspoonful milk + 1 fluid ounce boiled water	1 part evaporated milk + 1 part boiled water
Add sugar	1 level teaspoonful household sugar per feeding		
Calculate daily volume	$2\frac{1}{2}$ fluid ounces per lb bodyweight per day		
Calculate volume per feed	One-fifth of daily total at each of five feedings at 4-hourly intervals		

tributed by UNICEF for supplementary infant feeding.

The usefulness of commercially processed protein foods in combating protein-calorie malnutrition depends on various factors, including the availability of money to purchase foods and whether the community is dependent on a subsistence or a cash economy. In some parts of the world, mothers are already buying imported canned foods for their young children, although these are often highly expensive and nutritionally inappropriate.

Numerous attempts have been made in various parts of the world to produce economical, acceptable protein processed foods mainly from local resources, especially those not currently fully utilised for human feeding (e.g. soya, groundnut, cottonseed). The various foods have, in fact, been based on the same principles as discussed already for village-level multimixes (page 414). In some instances they have been entirely vegetable protein mixtures, as with AK-1000 (King *et al*, 1966) and Incaparina,* but more often are mixtures of vegetable protein together with *small* quantities of animal protein, such as CSM or Laubina (McLaren *et al*, 1966).

Their usefulness varies, but they may be expected to play an increasing role in urban areas. It is now appreciated that while they need governmental support and subsidy, their continued survival depends on their becoming commercially viable—that is, capable of making a reasonable, but continuing, profit as a status food on the open market.

EARLY RECOGNITION OF LESS SEVERE MALNUTRITION. Growth failure is the earliest sign of protein-calorie malnutrition, so that mild-moderate cases can be detected by serial weighing of children at Child Welfare Clinics, or, as they are more correctly known nowadays, Young Child Clinics or Under-Fives Clinics (Morley, 1963).

Serial weighings can best be recorded graphically and Morley (1968) has demonstrated the value of such cards in Africa and elsewhere (Fig. 27.6). If suitable cards are not available, inadequate weight may be judged by comparison with approximate standard figures (Table 14).

Too often weighing in Young Child Clinics is

TABLE 14. *Inadequate weight gains during the first 2 years of life* (Jelliffe, 1968c)

Age *(months)*	Minimum length of observation *(months)*	Inadequate weight gain
0–6	1	$\frac{3}{4}$ lb (226 g) per month
7–12	2	1 lb (453 g) per 2 months
12–24	4	1 lb (453 g) per 4 months

* Incaparina is a plant protein mixture containing corn (maize) flour 29 per cent, sorghum flour 29 per cent, cottonseed flour 38 per cent, torula yeast 3 per cent, calcium carbonate 1 per cent and vitamin A 4500 iu. (Behar and Bressani, 1966).

a farce. The scale is never tested, the weighing is carried out purposelessly by an uninterested, uninstructed junior staff member, and the weights obtained are not interpreted or made use of. It is necessary to lay down guidelines for action for the particular area. For example, children with early growth failure (mild protein-calorie malnutrition) should receive particular attention with regard to nutrition education, and should attend more frequently; children with more severe growth retardation (moderate protein-calorie malnutrition) should also be issued with supplementary protein food and, if feasible, some form of home visiting should be instituted.

The staff must be thoroughly familiar with the use of whatever supplementary protein food is being issued (e.g. dried skimmed milk). It should be pre-packaged and instructions given to mothers to use it as a powder added to local food mixtures. It should not be reconstituted as a liquid. Similarly, various newer protein-rich supplementary foods are becoming available, often also containing added calories. Thus CSM, i.e. corn (maize)–soya–dried skimmed milk, has been used widely.

PREVENTION AND MANAGEMENT OF CONDITIONING INFECTIONS. As noted earlier (page 411) protein-calorie malnutrition is the result of an interaction between dietary inadequacy and multiple infections, so that the prevention of conditioning infections is also an important method of combating malnutrition. Local priorities will vary, but often immunisation against whooping cough and tuberculosis are very important. Much attention is currently being given to the simplest, most economical 'compressed' immunisation schedules adapted to tropical circumstances (Stanfield, 1967).

Chemoprophylaxis against malaria may be considered advisable in hyperendemic areas, during the nutritionally vulnerable period of from 6 months to 2 years.

The control of diarrhoeal disease needs special emphasis, both by prevention (breast feeding, boiled water, clean feeding utensils, improved environmental hygiene), and by early attention to dehydration, especially by means of simple rehydration centres, often attached to health centres or hospitals (Jelliffe, 1969b).

Likewise, the *early* treatment of other nutritionally relevant infections is of importance preventively, including the avoidance of dietary restriction and, indeed, the use of supplementary protein when possible (e.g. in the therapy of measles).

IMPROVED TREATMENT OF SEVERE PROTEIN-CALORIE MALNUTRITION. The therapy of severe protein-calorie malnutrition has already been outlined (page 397). However, its preventive function needs stressing. Briefly, it seems more likely that parents will listen to advice on infant feeding, if they are convinced that the health staff are able to cure children with severe protein-calorie malnutrition.

In addition to hospital treatment, Bengoa (1967) has introduced the concept of the 'nutrition rehabilitation centre'. This has different forms according to the differing circumstances in various parts of the world, but basically it is a simple unit in which children with moderate (or even severe) protein-calorie malnutrition may be treated by a suitably prepared diet of local foods. It may be residential or for day-care only. Mothers are responsible for preparing the foods and for feeding the children under supervision. The unit has a double function—to rehabilitate the children economically and to educate (and convince) the mothers of the need to feed their children on nutritious, locally available foods.

CHILD SPACING. Many cultures seem to have recognised empirically the relationship between child spacing and the health and nutrition of both the mother and her children. Limitation of family size is related nutritionally not only to population pressure in a country in relation to limited food supplies, but also to family resources and to the nutritional effect on a mother and her children. Too frequently, yearly children lead to various forms of cumulative 'maternal depletion syndromes' and to inadequate breast feeding and defective feeding of the deposed young child. There is no doubt that family planning forms an integral part of MCH services of nutritional significance on a family basis as well as from a national viewpoint.

MCH programmes and child nutrition. A basic health approach to improving child nutrition is to develop a country-wide, locally appropriate MCH programme geared to the reality of the situation, especially finance and potentially available staff. The nutritional components of such a programme have been illustrated by Bengoa (1966) (Fig. 27.9).

This programme should include activities ranging from hospitals to health centres to, staff permitting, home visiting, for children at special risk (e.g. following measles, with moderate protein-calorie malnutrition etc.).

The major component of such a programme will be Young Child Clinics, with preventive, curative and promotive functions. Their activities will include weighing, practical health and nutrition education, examination and counselling, immunisation, and the issue of food supplements and/or simple medicines (if required).

The structure and functions of the MCH programme will have to be based on local priorities, on adaptation of methods, and on realistic training of suitable cadres, including non-traditional para-auxiliaries and volunteers.

For all activities and in all types of training, nutrition education will be a major theme. A main function of all health personnel in the prevention of protein-calorie malnutrition is as an needs. Non-nutritional motivation, including status, must be incorporated.

Major dietary topics for nutrition education will include diet for pregnant and lactating mothers, value of breast feeding, dangers of bottle feeding, types of foods, multimixes, harmful foods, and use of available processed protein foods.

A major goal is to ensure the evaluation of a coordinated flow of relatively uniform nutrition education through all responsible in the health

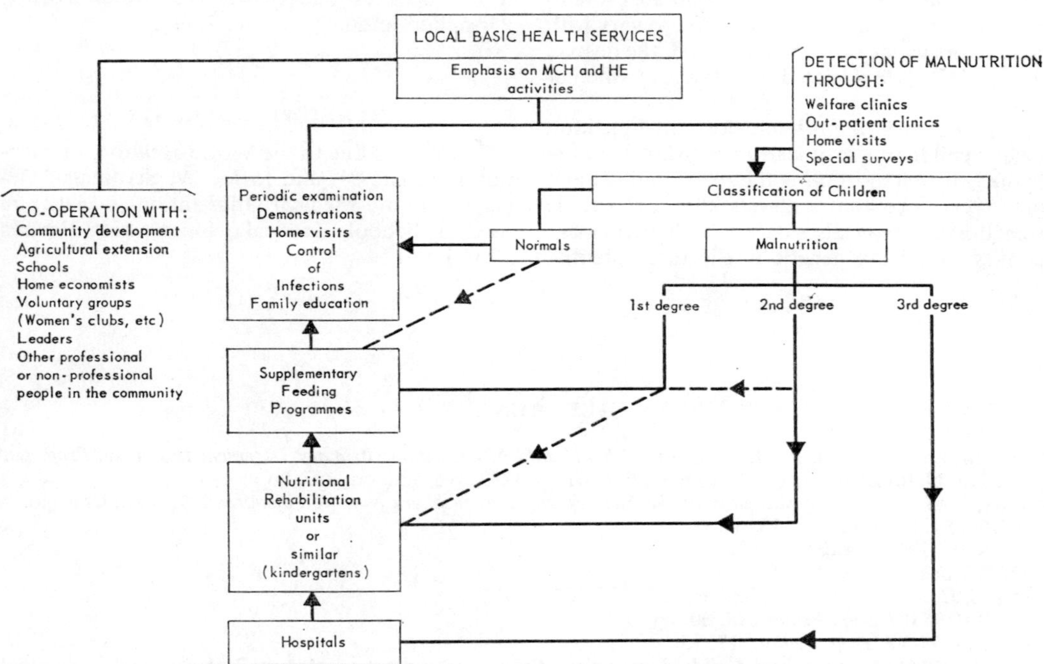

FIG. 27.9. *Organisation of a programme at a local level for the protection of young children from malnutrition* (Bengoa, 1966).

educator, and they should therefore receive instruction concerning methods, media and approaches to nutrition education and realise that this has to be incorporated into all their activities both with individual families, with small groups (as with parents' clubs) and, when feasible, via mass media. Certain groups should also be mentioned as targets for nutritional education, including politicians and administrators and parents of the near future, that is school children.

Nutrition education should include more than the supplying of information. Preferably it should be by means of lively, entertaining and convincing demonstration with involvement of mothers themselves and taking into account local felt-services and through those in other extension agencies, such as agriculture and community development (W.H.O., 1966).

Prognosis

Mild-moderate protein-calorie malnutrition involves from one third to three quarters of the young child population in most developing tropical countries. It is responsible for millions of deaths—not directly, but in combination with multiple infections. This is illustrated by the fact that, while the infant mortality rate in developing regions may be ten times as high as in Europe or North America, the 1–4 year mortality rate may be thirty to fifty times as great, with the secotrant showing a particularly high death rate (Gordon *et al*, 1967).

The relationship of many of these deaths to malnutrition is unappreciated. Tropical children at this early age usually have several illnesses at one time, and, if the cause of death is recorded, it is most often the terminal pathological burden, often bronchopneumonia or diarrhoeal disease. When feasible, death certificates should show all illnesses present.

The long-term effects of mild-moderate protein-caloric malnutrition may be expected to vary with such factors as the age when involved, the degree, the duration, associated infections, whether treated, etc.

Lesser degrees of protein-calorie malnutrition in early childhood may lead to physical stunting for life. More important is the recent animal and human evidence that suggests that irreparable brain damage may also occur, with permanent inability to achieve genetic intellectual potential

(Stock and Smythe, 1963; Scrimshaw and Gordon, 1968).

The economic prognosis in countries where protein-calorie malnutrition is rife needs stress. In addition to the costs of child wastage and of permanent mental impairment in regions attempting to develop technically, the actual expenditure on a programme to treat and rehabilitate under-nourished children may be formidable in relation to resources. In the Commonwealth Caribbean, with a population of between 4 and 5 million, it has been estimated that the overall cost is £4 million annually (Cook, 1968).

ACKNOWLEDGEMENTS

Thanks are due to the World Health Organization for Plate 31, and to Mr W. Serumaga, Department of Medical Illustrations, Makerere Medical School, Kampala, for drawing Figures 27.1, 3 and 5.

REFERENCES

BEHAR, M. and BRESSANI, R. (1966) In *Pre-School Child Malnutrition: Primary Deterrent to Human Progress*, p. 213. National Academy of Sciences, Publication 1282, Washington D.C.

BENGOA, J. M. (1966) In *Proceedings of the First Western Hemisphere Nutrition Congress*, A.M.A., Chicago.

—— (1967) *J. Trop. Pediat.*, **13**, 67.

BOSTOCK, J. (1962) *Lancet*, **1**, 1033.

British Medical Journal (1967) **2**, 446.

CADDELL, J. L. (1967) *New England Med. J.*, **276**, 535.

COOK, R. (1968) *J. trop. Pediat.*, **14**, 60.

COOK, R. (1971) *J. trop. Pediat.*, **17**, 15.

GARN, S. (1966) In *Pre-School Child Malnutrition: Primary Deterrent to Human Progress*, p. 43. National Academy of Sciences, Publication No. 1282, Washington, D.C.

GARROW, J. S., SMITH, R. and WARD, E. E. (1968) *Electrolyte Metabolism in severe Infantile Malnutrition*.

GOMEZ, F., GALVAN, R. R. CRAVIOTO, J. and FRENK, S. (1955) In *Advances in Pediatrics*, Vol. 27, p. 131. Chicago: Year Book Publishers.

GORDON, J. E., CHITKARA, I. D. and WYON, J. B. (1963) *Amer. J. med. Sci.*, **245**, 129.

GORDON, J. E., WYON, J. B. and ASCOLI, W. (1967) *Amer. J. med. Sci.*, **254**, 357.

JELLIFFE, D. B. (1957) *Pediatrics*, **20**, 128.

—— (1959) *J. Pediat.*, **54**, 227.

—— (1962) *Amer. J. clin. Nutr.*, **10**, 19.

—— (1966) *The Assessment of the Nutritional Status of the Community*. W.H.O. Monograph No. 53, Geneva.

—— (1967) *Amer. clin. Nutr.*, **20**, 279.

—— (1968a) *J. trop. Pediat.*, **14**, 217.

—— (1968b) *Clin. Pediat.*, **7**, 96.

—— (1968c) *Child Nutrition in Developing Countries*. U.S. Department of Health, Education and Welfare, Washington, D.C.

—— (1969a) *J. Pediat.*, **14**, 808.

—— (1969b) In *Alimentary Diseases in the Tropics*, Woodruff, A. London: Edward Arnold.

JELLIFFE, D. B. and JELLIFFE, E. F. P. (1960) *Amer. J. pub. Hlth*, **50**, 1355.

JELLIFFE, D. B. and JELLIFFE, E. F. P. (eds.) (1971) *Amer. J. Clin. Nutr.*, **24**, 968

JELLIFFE, D. B. and JELLIFFE, E. F. P. (eds.) (1972) *Amer. J. Clin. Nutr.*, **25**, 595.

JELLIFFE, D. B., SYMONDS, B. E. R. and JELLIFFE, E. F. P. (1960) *J. Pediat.*, **57**, 922.
JELLIFFE, E. F. P. and JELLIFFE, D. B. (eds.) (1969) *J. trop. Pediat.*, **15**, 177.
JELLIFFE, E. F. P. (1971) *J. trop. Pediat.*, **17**, 124
JELLIFFE, E. F. P. and JELLIFFE, D. B. (1968) *J. trop. Pediat.*, **14**, 71.
KAHN, E. (1957) *Centr. Afr. med. J.*, **3**, 398.
KING, K. W., FOUGÈRE, W. and BEGHIN, I. (1966) *Ann. Soc. belge Méd. trop.*, **6**, 741.
KING, M. (ed.) (1966) *Medical Care in Developing Regions*. Nairobi: Oxford University Press.
MCKENZIE, H. I., LOVELL, H. G., STANDARD, K. L. and MIALL, W. E. (1967) *Milbank Memorial Fund Quarterly*, **45**, 303.
MCKIGNEY, J. I. (1968) *J. trop. Pediat.*, **14**, 55.
MCLAREN, D. S. (1966) *Lancet*, **2**, 485.
MCLAREN, D. S., ASFOUR, R. Y., COWAN, J. W., PELLETT, P. L. and TANNOUS, R. I. (1966) *Proc. Seventh International Congress of Nutrition*, Vol. III, Braunshweig, W. Germany.
MORLEY, D. (1963) *Trans. roy. Soc. trop. Med. Hyg.*, **57**, 79.
—— (1968) *Trans. roy. Soc. trop. Med. Hyg.*, **62**, 200.
SCRIMSHAW, N. S. and GORDON, J. E. (ed) (1968) Malnutrition, Learning and Behaviour. Boston: M.I.T. Press.
SCRIMSHAW, N. S., TAYLOR, C. E. and GORDON, J. E. (1968) *Inter-actions of Nutrition and Infections*. W.H.O. Monograph No. 57, Geneva.
STANFIELD, J. P. (1967) *J. trop. Pediat.*, **13**, 102.
STOCK, M. B. and SMYTHE, P. M. (1963) *Arch. Dis. Childh.*, **38**, 546.
VITALE, F., BEHAR, M. and ARROYAVE, G. (1964) In *Mammalian Protein Metabolism*, Vol. 2. New York and London: Academic Press.
WATERLOW, J. C. (1968) *Lancet*, **2**, 1091.
WHARTON, B. A., JELLIFFE, D. B. and STANFIELD, J. P. (1968) *J. Pediat.*, **72**, 721.
WHITEHEAD, R. G. (1965) *Lancet*, **2**, 567.
WHITEHEAD, R. G. and DEAN, R. F. A. (1964) *Amer. J. clin. Nutr.*, **14**, 320.
WILLIAMS, C. D. (1933) *Arch. Dis. Childh.*, **8**, 423.
WORLD HEALTH ORGANIZATION (1962) *Expert Committee on Medical Assessment of Nutritional Status*. Tech. Rep. Ser. No. 258.
—— (1966) Joint F.A.O./W.H.O. Technical Meeting on *Methods of Planning and Evaluating in Applied Nutrition Programmes* Rech. Rep. Ser. No. 340.
—— (1968) *J. trop. Pediat.*, **14**, 149.
WOODRUFF, A. W. (1968) In *Calorie Deficiencies and Protein Deficiencies*, ed McCance, R. A. and Widdowson, E. M. London: J. & A. Churchill Ltd.

28
Vitamin Deficiencies

A vitamin may be defined as an *organic substance, soluble in fat or water, ordinarily needed only in minute quantities to maintain the biochemical and structural integrity of many cells and tissues*. Most vitamins are integral parts of certain organic molecules which are called coenzymes. Deficiency of vitamins may lead to functional or biochemical changes in the first instance, to be followed later by clinical manifestations.

Vitamin deficiencies arise usually from dietary inadequacy. Vitamin deficiencies may also be conditioned by factors interfering with the intake, absorption or utilisation of nutrients. Conditioning factors also include various stress factors that increase vitamin requirements like pyrexia, hyperthyroidism, diabetes and pregnancy and lactation.

While some clinical syndromes are attributable specifically to some vitamin deficiencies, generally vitamin deficiencies do not occur singly. They often coexist with other nutritional deficiencies.

In the following pages some major disorders arising from vitamin deficiencies are briefly described.

HYPOVITAMINOSIS A
SYNONYMS. Xerophthalmia, keratomalacia.

Definition

Vitamin A deficiency is due to inadequate intake of the vitamin in diet and produces severe eye lesions, which lead to blindness in many children. It is one of the major pediatric nutritional problems in many developing countries.

The ocular manifestations of vitamin A deficiency are xerophthalmia and keratomalacia which are the most important causes of preventable blindness.

Aetiology

Dietary intake. Inadequate dietary intake of vitamin A is the most important cause of the wide prevalence of the deficiency of this vitamin among the poor communities. Several important additional factors appear to have a contributory role.

Surveys carried out in South India revealed that the daily intake of vitamin A is about 70 μg while the recommended allowance for children is 300 μg (Gopalan *et al*, 1960). Vitamin A (as distinct from its carotenoid precursors) is limited to the animal kingdom. However, the sources of vitamin A like α and β carotene are important in human nutrition, β carotene being the most important. The β carotene content of the diet itself in many instances is very low and may fully explain the widespread prevalence of vitamin A deficiency in the poor communities.

Mother's nutritional status. SERUM LEVELS. There is a close relationship between vitamin A nutritional status of the mother and the infant. The concentration of carotene and vitamin A in the serum of expectant mothers is low. There is a progressive fall in the serum levels with the advance of pregnancy. Supplementation (Venkatachalam *et al*, 1962) of vitamin A in the diets of mothers during the last trimester can increase the vitamin A level of the cord blood significantly.

BREAST MILK CONTENT. Vitamin A concentration in breast milk is also considerably low in the poor communities. During the first 6 months of life of the infant, its vitamin A requirement must be completely met through maternal milk. Low levels, therefore, result in a deficiency. Infant feeding habits may have some bearing on this problem. If supplementary feeding is started at an early age, vitamin A may be obtained from other sources, whereas in places where the children are weaned at a later date, they may have to depend on breast milk alone, which may lead to a deficiency state (Gopalan *et al*, 1960). However, vitamin A content of milk can be increased considerably by providing vitamin A supplements (Venkatachalam *et al*, 1962).

HEPATIC STORES. Vitamin A is known to be transferred across the placenta to the fetus. Therefore, another important factor in conditioning vitamin A deficiency is hepatic storage of the vitamin during fetal life. Hepatic stores of vitamin A in fetuses born to mothers of poor income groups are considerably lower than the stores in fetuses born to well-nourished mothers (Iyengar and Apte, 1972). Infants born to undernourished mothers, therefore, are prone to develop vitamin A deficiency.

Infection. Infections in general affect nutritional status. Pyrexias, diarrhoeas and respiratory infections always precede nutritional deficiency disorders. Malnourished children particularly are prone to develop gastrointestinal disturbances. The results of recent studies have provided clear evidence that during infections, the intestinal absorption of both β carotene and vitamin A are seriously interfered with (Sivakumar and Reddy, 1971).

Therefore, in undernourished populations, a number of factors like inadequate dietary intake, poor vitamin A nutritional status of the mother, low hepatic stores in the infant and low concentration of vitamin A in milk lead to the widespread prevalence of vitamin A deficiency.

Epidemiology

Vitamin A deficiency is a major public health problem in several Asian countries like Burma, Ceylon, India, Indonesia, Malaysia, Pakistan, the Philippines and Thailand, in the Middle East, in many African countries, and in certain parts of Central America and in South American countries.

Age incidence

It is well recognised that age plays an important role in determining the incidence of vitamin A deficiency. It is rarely seen in infants below the age of 6 months. In infants between the ages of 6 and 12 months signs of vitamin A deficiency do occur. Children between the ages of 1 and 5 years are particularly vulnerable to the development of vitamin A deficiency. Recent surveys carried out in rural areas around Hyderabad revealed that nearly 8 per cent of children below 6 years had clinical signs of vitamin A deficiency (Prahlad Rao *et al*, 1969). Adults are rarely affected. It is more common in expectant women and nursing mothers.

Sex incidence

It is more common in males than in females. The reasons for this sex difference are not known.

Clinical features

Clinical manifestations are characterised by ocular signs. Formation of urinary stones and existence of nervous lesions have been demonstrated in experimental animals but this does not seem to have any significance in human beings. It has long been held that follicular hyperkeratosis (phrynoderma) is a manifestation of hypovitaminosis A. Clinical, therapeutic and biochemical studies have indicated that phrynoderma is due to the deficiency of essential fatty acids and not of vitamin A (Srikantia and Balavady, 1961; Bhatt and Belavady, 1967).

Ocular signs. NIGHT BLINDNESS. Inability to see in dim light is called night blindness or hemeralopia. This is the earliest clinical manifestation of the disease. Among adults it has been reported to occur in epidemic form during wars and famines. The diagnosis of nutritional night blindness depends upon a proper appraisal of the diet. The presence of other signs of vitamin A deficiency is not necessary. It must, however, be recognised that not all cases of night blindness are due to vitamin A deficiency and that all cases of vitamin A deficiency do not suffer from night blindness. If response to adequate treatment with vitamin A does not occur within a few days, vitamin A deficiency is an unlikely diagnosis.

XEROPHTHALMIA. Dryness of the cornea and of the conjunctiva has long been recognised in association with malnutrition. It is a manifestation of severe deficiency of vitamin A. The conjunctiva is involved earlier and more frequently than the cornea. The earliest sign is drying, roughness and wrinkling of the conjunctiva. This is followed by swelling and redness of lids, pain and photophobia. If the lids are held open, dry lustreless patches with muddy discolouration may be observed. The cornea also shows lack of lustre, dryness and haziness in the earlier stages. These changes are entirely reversible with prompt therapy.

BITOT'S SPOTS. At the canthi, particularly on the temporal side, triangular, whitish and foamy patches are frequently encountered. These are called Bitot's spots. In general, particularly in pre-school children, these disappear rapidly after therapy with vitamin A. However, in adults Bitot's spot do not respond to vitamin A administration.

KERATOMALACIA. Infants and young children are far more liable than are older children and adults to keratomalacia and permanent blindness due to lack of vitamin A. The first sign is a spreading opaque white spot in the cornea. The cornea appears dull, hazy and lustreless. Corneal sensibility, tested by touching the cornea with a wisp of cotton wool, is impaired. Infiltration of the stroma of the cornea occurs and this adds to the haziness already produced by keratinisation. The distinctive feature of the terminal stage is the dissolution of the corneal substance, known as colliquative necrosis. If the cornea gives way, there is perforation with subsequent prolapse of the iris. At the same time secondary infection may lead to ulceration and may end in pthisis bulbi.

Other features. Bladder stone formation, neurological manifestation and dermal lesions have been described as signs of vitamin A deficiency on the basis of studies in experimental animals. There appears to be, however, little evidence to suggest that these may be so in the humans.

Protein-calorie malnutrition. Vitamin A deficiency is frequently seen in association with signs of protein-calorie malnutrition in children. Levels of serum vitamin A are low in most children suffering from kwashiorkor whether or not they have ocular signs of vitamin A deficiency and tend to increase after therapy with protein alone (Gopalan *et al*, 1960; Arroyave *et al*, 1961). The intestinal absorption of vitamin A in children suffering from kwashiorkor is reported to be defective. This has, however, not been confirmed. Since vitamin A is transported in plasma bound to specific proteins, in kwashiorkor retinol-binding proteins may be low. Though there may be a relationship between protein nutritional status and vitamin A deficiency, administration of vitamin A definitely improves the ocular signs.

Pathology

The corneal epithelium shows characteristic metaplasia and vascularisation of the substantia propria. Metaplastic keratinisation follows atrophy of the epithelium. In experimental animals, changes in the epithelium lining the gastrointestinal tract, respiratory tract, urinary tract and olfactory tract have been described.

Diagnosis

Diagnosis of keratomalacia offers no difficulty. Conjunctival and corneal xerosis should be diagnosed earlier, since at this stage, the condition is completely reversible. Dark adaptation test may be helpful in cases of night blindness.

Levels of vitamin A in serum have been extensively used as indicators of vitamin A nutritional status. It has been found that levels of plasma vitamin A in children with corneal involvement are invariably much lower than levels in children exhibiting the milder conjunctival lesions. However, plasma levels of vitamin A need not necessarily reflect the tissue vitamin A status. Levels above 20 μg/100 ml are considered as being acceptable levels, whereas below 10 μg/100 ml are clearly indicative of a deficiency state.

Treatment

Signs like xerosis, Bitot's spots and night blindness respond quickly and satisfactorily to small amounts of vitamin A administered orally. Fish liver oils are excellent sources of vitamin A and can cure the condition. Synthetic vitamin A in doses of 5000 to 10 000 iu per day for a few days can bring about complete cure.

Corneal involvement is more serious and requires immediate attention. Vitamin A in doses of 100 000 iu has been employed. Even advanced cases of corneal xerosis are known to clear up satisfactorily.

Routes of administration. Parenteral administration is in vogue in many parts and this has been giving satisfactory responses. However, results of investigation indicate that oral administration of vitamin A is more efficient than intramuscular injection (Reddy and Srikantia, 1966). If the damage to the cornea has not become irreversible, obvious improvement becomes evident in as short a period as 12 to 24 hours and the cornea clears up completely in 48 to 72 hours. In the diet there must be enough fat to ensure proper absorption. Water-miscible preparations have been shown to raise readily the serum levels and liver concentrations of the vitamin, unlike the oily preparations. In protein deficient states, the absorption of parenterally administered vitamin A perhaps is ineffective due to defective absorption of the carrier fat base since a water-miscible preparation is absorbed better than the oily vitamin A.

Children showing vitamin A deficiency signs invariably have associated protein-calorie malnutrition. For treatment of such cases, if an oily preparation is used, the oral is preferable to the parenteral route. If the vitamin has to be given parenterally as in cases with severe diarrhoea, a water-miscible vitamin must be used. However, this should be followed by oral supplementation of oily vitamin A to improve the liver stores.

Supportive therapy. Attention to local sepsis is essential. Local treatment of the eye should be confined to saline irrigations when there is discharge. Secondary infection may be prevented by using antibiotic ointments.

Prognosis

Early diagnosis and prompt treatment are essential to cure hypovitaminosis A completely. However, if therapy is started late, various degrees of residual scarring like nebulae, maculae, leucomata or total blindness may ensue.

Prevention and prophylaxis

Dietary intake. Since inadequate dietary intake of vitamin A is the major aetiological factor, the most rational approach for control and prevention of the condition would be improvement in the diet so as to ensure adequate intake of the vitamin. Foods containing preformed vitamin A are expensive. However, there are less expensive sources of provitamin A. Green leafy vegetables are rich sources of β carotene. Results of recent study indicate that by encouraging the consumption of green leafy vegetables among people in poor communities, the incidence of vitamin A deficiency can be lowered considerably (Lala and Reddy, 1970). This, however, involves nutrition education and at present may be considered as a long-term approach.

Supplement of vitamin A concentrates. Periodic administration of vitamin A concentrates to infants and children is a useful short-term measure. For this adequate health services are essential. These supplements can be given from MCH centres, hospitals or through Health Units and personnel. However, even this has a limited application.

Single dose prophylaxis. Since vitamin A can be stored in the body for long periods of time in the liver, a single massive dose of vitamin A, preferably twice a year, can be given to ensure adequate stores, which will be made available to meet needs as they arise. The main objective of the use of a single dose is to prevent blindness arising out of vitamin A deficiency.

The results of such a study have recently been reported from India (Swaminathan *et al*, 1970). A single oral dose of 300 000 iu once a year (vitamin A palmitate) given orally not only increased serum vitamin A levels but also decreased the incidence of both conjunctival xerosis and Bitot's spots. Satisfactory levels of serum vitamin A were maintained for about 6 months. It is, therefore, now suggested that instead of one single annual dose, two doses of 200 000 iu may be given at intervals of 6 months so as to afford a better degree of protection.

RICKETS

Definition

Rickets is a disorder of phosphorus and calcium metabolism in which there is a failure of the orderly process of calcium and phosphorus deposition in the bones. This is a condition caused by deficiency of vitamin D, especially in infancy and childhood, with disturbance of normal ossification. The disease is marked by bending and distortion of bones under muscular action, by the formation of nodular enlargements on the ends and sides of bones, and by delayed closure of the fontanelles which result in various deformities.

Aetiology

Nutritional rickets, caused by lack of vitamin D, is still a common disease in many countries. Vitamin D in the body is derived from two sources—photosynthesis in the skin and absorption of ingested vitamin from the upper part of the small intestine.

The natural sources of dietary vitamin D are foods of animal origin, especially dairy products and eggs. Such food sources are expensive and hence the intake of this vitamin is inadequate. The intake of calcium among such children is also low.

Human skin contains 7-dehydrocholesterol, a provitamin D. Under natural living conditions this provitamin is activated by the ultra-violet rays of sunlight and converted into vitamin D_3 or cholecalciferol. The amount of cholecalciferol produced in the skin by exposure to sunlight is not known, but varies with such factors as the duration of exposure, the skin area exposed, the geographical location and the season of the year. In some countries, due to social customs, exposure to sunlight is prevented or reduced, particularly in the case of women and infants, and rickets is common in these places. It is, however, not known to what extent environmental factors influence the dietary requirement of vitamin D.

Though it has been claimed that the entire requirement of vitamin D can be obtained through this source, the incidence of vitamin D responsive rickets in the tropics, known to be adequately exposed to sunlight, raises doubts about this claim. Since the natural diets of infants contain very small amounts of vitamin D, rickets is still common in many underdeveloped countries, constituting an important cause of illness and deformity in childhood.

Deficiency of vitamin D may be caused by other factors like failure of absorption from the intestine, as in malabsorption syndromes and steatorrhea. Vitamin D resistant rickets has also been described. This is due to genetically determined metabolic abnormality.

Epidemiology

It is prevalent in South African countries, in the Philippines, India, Pakistan and Singapore.

Recently rickets has been found to be common among the immigrant population of Britain. In some European countries, nutritional rickets is still a common disease.

Age incidence

Congenital rickets occurs only under rare conditions and is caused by deficient maternal diet. Mild rickets is frequent in the first few months of infancy when no preventive measures are taken. Well-developed rickets occurs towards the end of the first and during the second year of life.

Osteomalacia is a disease which occurs in adults, particularly in women during the childbearing age.

Sex incidence

Children of both sexes are affected. In adults, however, only women suffer from this disease.

Clinical features

The principal manifestation of vitamin D deficiency in infants is rickets and in pregnant and lactating women it is called osteomalacia.

Early rickets. The early recognition of rickets is important, but the early signs are difficult to detect. Craniotabes manifests as softening of the occiput or the posterior parts of the parietal bones. This is an early sign and may be seen in the first few months of life when the rachitic process begins. Premature infants are particularly prone to it. Enlargement of the costochondral junctions and slight thickening of the wrist and ankles are suggestive of early rickets.

Advanced rickets. SKULL. Craniotabes may disappear, but the rachitic process continues. The softness of the skull results in asymmetry. The skull assumes a peculiar shape with protruding forehead and cruciform depressions along the sutures. The sutures are soft and remain separated. Frontal and parietal prominences give a box-like appearance (box headed or caput quadratum). The anterior fontanelle remains wide open even after 18 months. The head appears larger and may remain so throughout life.

THORAX. A line of enlargement at the costochondral junction of the rib gives rise to what is called the 'rickety rosary'. In many cases the beading of the ribs is not only palpable, but also visible. The costochondral junctions as well as the osseous part of the rib gradually soften. The softened ribs cave in from muscular action and cause 'pigeon chest' with broad grooves running antero-laterally on either side of the chest. This is called 'Harrison's sulcus'. The chest may show a variety of other deformities and the bones of the shoulder girdle may also be involved.

LIMBS. As the rachitic process continues, the epiphyseal enlargements at the wrist and ankles become more noticeable. Long bones like femur, tibia and fibula curve forwards, resulting in bowlegs and knock knees. Greenstick fractures occur in the long bones, but seldom cause clinical symptoms.

SPINE. Kyphosis and scoliosis are commonly encountered. Lordosis of the lumbar region may be seen in the erect position.

PELVIS. In children with lordosis there is a concomitant deformity of the pelvis. The rachitic pelvis is not only small but also continues to be small throughout life.

Teeth. Delayed eruption of primary teeth is characteristic. There may be defects of the enamel and extensive caries. The permanent teeth which are calcifying may be affected; usually the permanent incisors, canines and first molars show defects of the enamel.

Ligaments and muscles. Ligaments are loose and lax, especially of the spine and the larger joints and aid in producing deformities. The muscles are poorly developed and lack tone. The 'pot belly' is due to weakness of the abdominal muscles. This weakness delays the milestones like standing and walking in infants.

Radiological changes. The diagnosis of active and healing rickets is usually based on evidence obtained from X-rays of the joints. In active rickets, the distal ends of the long bones appear widened, concave or cupped and frayed. The distance between the distal ends of the ulna and radius and the metacarpal bones is increased. The shafts show decreased density and the trabeculae are prominent. Healing is indicated by the appearance of the line of preparatory calcification.

Other features. The rachitic infant is a tired, restless and unhappy creature. Gastrointestinal disturbances or respiratory infections are frequently encountered in these children. Deformities result in the reduction in height of the body producing a 'rachitic dwarf'. Clonic or tetanic spasms may be occasionally observed.

Osteomalacia in adults. In adults the epiphyseal line is already closed and endochondral calcification has ceased; consequently in osteomalacia disturbances in endochrondral and periosteal calcification do not occur. Osteomalacia is characterised by diffuse skeletal pain and tenderness, particularly involving the pelvis and lower extremities. This is aggravated by weight bearing. There is hip girdle muscular weakness with a waddling gait.

Pathology

Defective bone growth is observed. There is retardation or suppression of normal growth of epiphyseal cartilage and of normal calcification. The cartilage cells fail to complete their normal cycle of proliferation and degeneration along the epiphyseal-metaphyseal line. This results in a frayed, irregular epiphyseal line at the end of the shaft. The width of the epiphyseal cartilage continues to increase, but the columns are irregularly arranged.

In addition there is failure of normal mineralisation of osseous and cartilaginous matrix. The zone of preparatory calcification fails to mineralise and newly formed uncalcified osteoid is deposited. This is responsible for many of the skeletal deformities. Mineralisation is lacking in the subperiosteal bone and a shell of osteoid tissue is formed which surrounds the shaft. Cortical bone is reabsorbed and is replaced by osteoid tissue. This results in rarefied cortical bone which is prone to be deformed by mild stresses.

Pathogenesis of rickets. When there is a deficiency of vitamin D, absorption of calcium from the intestine diminishes. There is increased mobilisation of calcium and phosphorus from the skeleton and excretion of both in the urine is increased. The cumulative effect of these changes is to prevent calcification of cartilage to form bone. The fall in plasma calcium may stimulate parathyroid activity with resultant outpouring of calcium and phosphate from the bone to redress the balance. Parathyroid hormone also causes a reduction in renal tubular reabsorption of phosphate, and the net result is a lowering of plasma phosphate level.

Biochemical pathology. Unless the deficiency is very severe, the plasma calcium level usually remains at or near normal level, presumably maintained by parathyroid activity. The serum levels of phosphorus are invariably low. Serum alkaline phosphatase levels are high due to the stimulation of osteoblasts.

Diagnosis

Diagnosis is based on a history of inadequate vitamin D intake, on clinical observation and on radiological examinations. Biochemical indices may aid in diagnosing active rickets.

Treatment

Oral administration of vitamin D is quite effective. The daily administration of 1500 to 5000 iu will produce healing demonstrable on X-ray within 2 to 4 weeks. Parenteral administration is indicated in cases of malabsorption syndromes. Rickets can also be treated by massive doses of vitamin D (600 000 units) in two or three doses at fortnightly intervals.

Prognosis

Rickets is usually a self-limiting disease. Spontaneous healing occurs from exposure to sunshine. Deformities may be permanent in advanced cases. Rickets in itself is not a fatal disease, but complications and intercurrent infections are likely to cause death.

Prevention and prophylaxis

The daily requirement of vitamin D is estimated to be 400 iu. Improving dietary standards is an important measure to prevent rickets. Oral administration of vitamin D is the practical means for the prevention and treatment of rickets. Such preparations can be obtained in fish oils and in water-miscible vehicles. Fortification of milk with vitamin D has been successful in many countries. Rickets can be prevented by exposure to sunlight. Vitamin D should be administered to pregnant and lactating women.

BERI-BERI

SYNONYMS. Kakke, barbiers, polyneuritis endemica, linchavon, loempe, inchaco, perneiras, asjike.

Definition

Beri-beri is defined as a disease caused by aneurine or thiamine deficiency, occurring in population groups who subsist mainly on highly milled or polished rice. Beri-beri is a syndrome complex rather than a single clinical entity. Its most conspicuous features are gastrointestinal derangements followed by muscular weakness and polyneuritis. Cardiovascular symptoms and/ or neurological symptoms may dominate the clinical picture.

Aetiology

In the early twentieth century, Takaki (1906) reported the problem of beri-beri in Japanese sailors. The chief component of the Japanese sailor's diet was polished rice. Eijkman in his investigations in chickens, which were fed only on boiled polished rice, found a paralytic disease which he named as polyneuritis gallinarium. Later work on this field revealed that thiamine deficiency was the causative factor.

Thiamine is widely distributed in raw foodstuffs, the richest sources being whole cereals, especially the pericarp. During milling much of the vitamin is lost and hence people consuming polished rice develop the disease. Several enzymes capable of destroying thiamine have been found in food. These are known as thiaminases. These are present in raw tissues of many fishes, chiefly freshwater fishes, clams, shrimps and in mussels. However, on cooking, these thiamines are destroyed. It seems unlikely that these can play a significant role in the pathogenesis of beri-beri.

Conditioned thiamine deficiency may be associated with cases of chronic diarrhoea, trophic disorders of small intestine, chronic and severe diuresis as in diabetes mellitus and diabetes insipidus, thyrotoxicosis and degenerative arteriosclerosis. It is usually encountered in chronic alcoholics.

Epidemiology

This disease is common in rice-eating areas like Japan, Malaya, China, Indonesia, India, the Philippines and Sumatra. Epidemics have been reported in Australian aborigines, Ceylon and other Eastern countries. Epidemics of wet beri-beri were very common in coastal Andhra districts in India. But due to some unknown reasons, the acute form of this disease has completely disappeared though chronic cases are still encountered in these areas.

Age incidence

Commonly it affects adults between 20 and 60 years of age. It is not uncommon in the breast-fed infants of mothers with beri-beri. This form, called infantile beri-beri, may declare itself in varying ways.

Sex incidence

It attacks both sexes though it is more common in males than in females.

Clinical features

A striking feature of the disease is that it may assume a great variety of forms. The course of development of beri-beri is so variable that it is difficult to describe a common sequence of symptoms. It is insidious in onset, but it may occasionally be ushered in by acute symptoms, in which case it is fatal. For purposes of convenience the following clinical types may be considered separately.

1. Wet beri-beri or acute beri-beri or cardiac beri-beri.
2. Chronic, dry, atrophic type or polyneuritis.
3. Acute fulminating type or pernicious type of beri-beri.
4. Infantile beri-beri.
5. Wernicke's encephalopathy and Korsakoff's psychosis.

Gastrointestinal manifestations. In the earlier stages there is a feeling of heaviness in the epigastrium accompanied by nausea and vomiting. Anorexia which may progress to nausea is a common feature. These symptoms appear to be associated with gastroduodenal irritation. Vomiting often indicates the onset of an acute phase of the disease. Constipation is more common than diarrhoea.

Cardiac beri-beri. Cardiac symptoms occur at some stage of the disease in most patients. The subjects usually complain of weakness, shortness of breath, palpitations, dizziness and giddiness, particularly on arising from a recumbent posture. Swelling of the feet accompanied by oliguria is seen in the majority. There is marked variability in oedema formation. It may be great or minimal and gross oedema appears to have no relation to the severity of the case. Platt (1958) has observed that it occurs particularly in warmer weather because the temperature favours vasodilatation and congestion of the venous circulation.

Clinically, one can detect an enlarged heart with a rapid pulse which is full and bounding. Visible pulsations may be seen in the neck. Pallor and cold extremities are often encountered. Peripheral cyanosis is not uncommon. The systolic blood pressure increases with a fall in the diastolic element giving rise to a wide pulse pressure. The heart sounds are often loud, particularly the pulmonic second sound. The liver is enlarged and tender and epigastric pulsations are seen. As in all hyperkinetic circulatory states associated with a lowered peripheral vascular resistance, retention of sodium and water by the kidneys occurs, which increases the blood volume, raises the venous pressure and so further increases the cardiac output. The heart is enlarged on both sides but more markedly on the right resulting in congestive cardiac failure.

Atrophic or dry beri-beri or paraplegic beri-beri. In general the first symptom of beri-beri is a sensation of numbness of the feet. There is tingling in the extremities and the patient walks as little as possible. Paraesthesiae-like sensations of pins and needles, burning and cramps are common features. There is gradually increasing weakness in the limbs which ultimately results in flaccid paralysis. The clinical picture is one of ascending, symmetrical, bilateral peripheral neuritis.

Initially hyperaesthesia may be encountered but later anaesthesia predominates. This has a peculiar distribution in the sense that the longest nerve fibres are the first to be affected and so the loss of sensation is in the peripheral parts of the limbs. This is called 'the glove and stocking' type of anaesthesia. Calf muscles and other muscles become extremely tender and this is a useful diagnostic sign. Sensory disturbances involve the inner surface of the legs below the knees. Anaesthesia over the tibia is a very frequent finding. A delayed pain response is common. Anaesthesia may extend to involve both legs, arms, trunk and neck also. Superficial sensations are all lost in the later stages of the disease accompanied by loss of vibratory and position sense.

Motor disturbances usually follow the sensory abnormalities. The distal muscles like dorsiflexors of the foot, extensors and flexors of leg, etc., are affected. Foot drop and wrist drop are often encountered. Weakness gradually spreads upwards and finally there is a flaccid paralysis. There is profound atrophy of the musculature.

Alteration of the reflexes occurs fairly early. At first there is exaggeration of the knee and ankle reflex but in the later stages they disappear. Ataxic gait is commonly seen in these patients.

Involvement of cranial nerves. Lesions of the optic nerve have been described. They include loss of visual acuity, bilateral central scotomata, concentric contraction of the field of vision, temporal pallor of the optic disc and signs of retrobulbar neuritis. Involvement of the eighth nerve has also been described. These, however, may be due to a multiple deficiency of the B complex group vitamins.

Wernicke's encephalopathy and Korsakoff's psychosis. This is a syndrome that develops with very severe restriction of thiamine intake. It is seen usually in association with chronic alcoholism. It may be precipitated by overloading with glucose without adequate thiamine coverage. Denny Brown (1958) emphasised that the neurological manifestations of thiamine deficiency depend on the severity of dietary restriction. Mental symptoms and paralysis of cranial nerves dominate the picture. During early stages there are symptoms of disturbances of higher nervous centres, manifested as irritability, forgetfulness, disturbing dreams, vague fears and development of ideas of persecution. This progresses to a stage of apathy, confusion and delirium. Patients often complain of photophobia and diplopia. There is ophthalmoplegia associated with nystagmus and pupillary abnormalities. There is ptosis and ocular palsies, especially of the external rectus muscle. Papilloedema and haemorrhages have also been described. Ataxia and ophthalmoplegia are transitory and may disappear soon.

Korsakoff's psychosis is part of the psychic picture of Wernicke's encephalopathy and occurs after the subsidence of the original confusional state. Cardinal features of Korsakoff's psychosis are lack of retentive memory and confabulation. There is also extensive retrograde amnesia which may cover a period of months or even years.

Infantile beri-beri. This was first recognised in Japan and accounted for many infant deaths. It usually affects breast-fed infants of mothers who are either themselves victims of beri-beri or subsist on a diet poor in vitamins. It affects infants between 1 and 3 months of age. The frank condition develops rapidly and ends fatally. The syndrome may be of several types with acute or cardiac form predominating. The disease begins with vomiting, restlessness, pallor and insomnia. It may progress to dyspnoea, cyanosis, thready pulse and cardiac failure, or it may be a pseudo-meningitic type, with aphonia, neck retraction and opisthotonus. It may go into a convulsive stage. Vomiting is very common and is an important sign in the development of infantile beri-beri.

Acute pernicious type of beri-beri. The acute fulminating form of beri-beri has been called 'shoshin'. The whole picture is dominated by insufficiency of the heart and vessels. In addition, patients may have aphonia. Respirations are affected and there are widespread pulsations and vascular dilatation. Oedema develops due to acute failure and it may be associated with peripheral neuropathy. It usually runs a fatal course.

Pathology

Hypertrophy of the heart is a constant finding, usually associated with dilatation of the right side. Hydropericardium, hydrothorax and ascites are frequently encountered. Oedema of cardiac muscle has been reported. There is oedema of the lungs with pressure congestion of the liver (nutmeg liver).

In Wernicke's encephalopathy the histological changes are chiefly in the nature of capillary damage in the mammillary bodies, the related walls of the third ventricles, the aqueduct and in the tegmentum of the medulla. Pinpoint haemorrhages are seen. In the medulla, the nuclear region of the vagus is affected. The cerebral cortex may appear oedematous. It is only in the more chronic states that nerve cell damage occurs. They take the form of partial chromatolysis with displacement of the nucleus to one side.

In the peripheral nerves, Wallerian degeneration is seen beginning in the most peripheral part of the longest nerve fibres. Segmental thinning of the myelin has been observed. This is the early and reversible stage of the disease. In the peripheral nerves, in chronic cases, beading, distortion of axis cylinders and paucity of myelin are striking.

Diagnosis

Multiple symptoms like involvement of heart, brain and peripheral nerves are easy to detect, particularly when they occur as an epidemic. Sporadic cases may be difficult to diagnose. However, the dietary history associated with calf muscle tenderness is diagnostic. In cardiac beri-beri, therapeutic response itself is a valuable aid in diagnosing the heart condition.

Differential diagnosis

The cardiac condition must be distinguished from other states of hyperdynamic heart failure like anaemia, thyrotoxicosis and arteriovenous fistulae.

Neuropathy must not be mistaken for diseases like tabes dorsalis, progressive muscular atrophy, ascending spinal paralysis and arsenical neuritis.

Determination of thiamine excretion in the urine, load test of thiamine and transketolase assay may all be valuable aids to diagnose thiamine deficient status (Sauberlich, 1967; Bamji, 1970).

Treatment

The treatment of beri-beri consists in the administration of thiamine and the institution of a good diet. In adults 5 to 10 mg of the vitamin three times a day will be adequate. In severe acute forms, parenteral treatment is indicated.

Prognosis

The severity of the disease varies within wide limits. If the patient is properly treated at an early stage, most of the symptoms, particularly the cardiac and acute neurological symptoms, can be brought under control. In the chronic dry form of the disease, if serious damage has already been done to the nerves, recovery is slow and may never be complete. Acute pernicious type and infantile beri-beri are fatal unless promptly treated.

Prevention and prophylaxis

Measures must be devised to increase the intake of thiamine. The thiamine content of the diet may be increased by affecting a change from the use of highly milled rice to rice containing more thiamine, such as undermilled, parboiled or enriched rice. The use of home-pounded rice can be encouraged. Parboiling causes a change in the location of thiamine in the grain so that it is not removed in the milling process. Improved methods of cooking, like discouraging the process of washing rice before cooking or to cook rice in just enough water, helps to retain the vitamin.

In the Philippines rice was enriched with the vitamin and clinical surveys (Salcedo *et al*, 1949) indicated that in the experimental area the incidence of beri-beri was much less. However, in areas where there are large numbers of small rice mills, the organisation of enrichment is difficult.

Extensive production and distribution of synthetic vitamin may eradicate beri-beri completely.

ARIBOFLAVINOSIS

SYNONYMS. Shibi-gatchaki in Japan.

Definition

This disease is due to deficiency of riboflavin in the diet and is characteristised by lesions at the angles of the mouth, on lips, around the nose and eyes and by seborrheic dermatitis.

Aetiology

Riboflavin deficiency in man is due to an inadequate dietary intake of riboflavin or to some conditioning factor which causes impairment of absorption or utilisation of the vitamin as in diabetes, hyperthyroidism and malabsorption syndromes. Signs of deficiency often appear during periods of physiological stress such as pregnancy or childhood. It is frequently seen in association with pellagra.

Epidemiology

Ariboflavinosis is frequently encountered in the low socioeconomic groups in all developing countries. A comprehensive survey carried out in Hyderabad among pre-school children revealed that nutritional deficiency signs, particularly angular stomatitis, was prevalent in 19 per cent of the children (Pralhad Rao *et al*, 1969). The incidence of oral lesions is also high in pregnant women.

Clinical features

The clinical picture is characterised by orolingual and dermal lesions. The eye lesions of ariboflavinosis have been the subject of considerable controversy.

Orolingual lesions. A lesion at the angles of the mouth is known as angular stomatitis. It begins as small fissures and later extends outwards from the buccal mucous membrane. These fissures are often covered with yellowish crusts.

The tongue in ariboflavinosis is characteristically purplish or magenta-red in colour. The papillae may be swollen or mushroom-shaped giving a pebbled appearance. In chronic deficiency, the papillae may become atrophic. Lesions of the lips begin with redness and denudation along the lines of closure. The lips appear dry and chapped and shallow ulcerations or crusting may occur in severe deficiency. This is termed cheilosis.

The triad of angular stomatitis, glossitis and cheilosis has been associated so far only with riboflavin deficiency. However, there is evidence to indicate that deficiency of other vitamins like pyridoxine may play an important role in the causation of these orolingual lesions (Vilter *et al*, 1958; Krishnaswamy, 1971b).

Dermal lesions. An eczematous scrotal dermatitis is common in riboflavin deficiency. A seborrheic type of dermatitis is also found in the nasolabial and nasomalar folds, alae nasi, vestibule of the nose and around the eyes. The mouths of the sebaceous glands are plugged with inspissated sebum, giving the skin a roughened appearance. These hard sebaceous plugs or filiform comidones may be seen over the bridge of the nose, on the malar prominences and the chin.

Eye lesions. Sydenstricker and his colleagues (1939) in a study of riboflavin deficiency observed conjunctivitis and photophobia. The conjunctiva may be diffusely inflamed. Corneal vascularisation has also been described as a manifestation of vitamin B_2 deficiency. But a number of subsequent studies have indicated no correlation between corneal vascularisation and the dietary intake of riboflavin.

Anaemia. A normochromic and normocytic anaemia has been reported in patients fed on a synthetic diet severely deficient in riboflavin. This anaemia was accentuated by galactoflavin, a riboflavin antagonist (Lane and Alfrey, 1965). However, anaemia is not a regularly described component of the naturally occurring form of human riboflavin deficiency.

Pathology

Very little information is available about the histological changes in tissues, in riboflavin deficiency particularly in human subjects. The first tissue to suffer from riboflavin deficiency is the endothelium of the capillary system. The lesions are due to capillary congestion with impaired nutrition of skin and mucous membrane.

Diagnosis

Dietary history is very important. When the dietary history indicates an intake of less than 0.6 mg of riboflavin, deficiency is a likely possibility. However, it has been observed that sometimes there is lack of correlation between the dietary intake and oral lesions. Other vitamin deficiencies, particularly pyridoxine, have to be considered. It is a common observation that the oral manifestations sometimes fail to respond to riboflavin alone. The glossitis may be confused with that of deficiency of niacin, folic acid or vitamin B_{12}. Oral lesions in iron deficiency anaemia are commonly encountered. The Plummer-Vinson syndrome is a well known clinical entity with severe oral lesions, anaemia and dysphagia. Riboflavin deficiency may contribute towards the causation of orolingual lesions in this syndrome also.

Biochemical tests like the urinary excretion of vitamin B_2, load tests, red cell riboflavin and glutothione reductase activity (Bamji, 1969) may be useful parameters to diagnose ariboflavinosis.

Treatment

Riboflavin in doses of 5 and 10 mg has been found to be effective in curing the oral lesions and nasolabial dyssebacia. Oral administration is usually satisfactory. Cases of malabsorption require parenteral therapy. Symptoms disappear in a few days and the lesions resolve in a matter of a few days to a few weeks.

Prognosis

Ariboflavinosis is a condition which responds to therapy and does not leave any sequelae.

Prevention

General improvement in the diet is essential. The diet should include foods that are rich sources of riboflavin like milk, liver, meat, eggs, pulses and green leafy vegetables.

PELLAGRA

SYNONYMS. Mal de la rosa, mal rosso, Alpine scurvy, Austrian rose.

Definition

The name pellagra is a combination of two Italian words: *pelle* meaning skin, and *agra* meaning rough. Pellagra is a deficiency disease due to an insufficient dietary supply of niacin and its precursor tryptophan. It is characterised by a complexity of nervous, alimentary and cutaneous symptoms, which are relieved by the administration of niacin or tryptophan. In the past, pellagra was considered to be the result of a multiple deficiency of the vitamins of the B group. It is however, now realised that other B complex deficiencies often accompany pellagra and complicate the clinical picture.

Aetiology

Pellagra occurs most frequently in population groups in which corn or maize is the staple cereal. In 1680–1700, the disease was first described in Spain, where pellagra was believed to have made its appearance shortly after the introduction of maize as an article of food. In 1762, Gasper Casal, a Spanish physician, wrote the first satisfactory account of the disease.

Endemic pellagra has long been associated with maize consumption. Numerous studies indicate that the pellagragenic effect of corn diets may be due to their low tryptophan content. Also, the niacin in corn has been claimed to be present in bound form, which is unavailable to the body. Goldsmith (1956) has shown that essentially all the manifestations of endemic pellagra can be cured by either niacin or tryptophan. Gopalan and Srikantia (1960) reported the occurrence of pellagra in an endemic form among population groups in Hyderabad, India, whose staple diet is jowar (sorghum vulgare).

Unlike maize, jowar is not a poor source of tryptophan and its nicotinic acid is in an available form. But like maize, jowar has a high leucine content. The results of several studies have shown that dietary excess of leucine, leading to high leucine concentration, influences the metabolism of tryptophan and niacin and is concerned with the pathogenesis of pellagra (Belavady, 1963; Raghuramulu *et al*, 1965a; Raghuramulu *et al*,

1965b; Belavady and Gopalan, 1965; Belvady *et al*, 1967; Srikantia *et al*, 1968a; Madhaven *et al*, 1968).

Dietary inadequacy may precipitate niacin deficiency in situations where the food intake is restricted or when there is interference with the absorption or utilisation of nutrients. This is called 'secondary pellagra' and occurs in association with chronic alcoholism, cirrhosis of the liver, chronic diarrhoeal diseases, diabetes and neoplasia. Niacin deficiency may develop in patients with malignant carcinoid tumours (Bridges *et al*, 1957). Pellagra has occasionally been observed during therapy with isoniazid. In these instances, pyridoxine deficiency may have resulted in decrease in conversion of tryptophan to niacin.

Epidemiology

Pellagra has been reported to occur in European countries like Portugal, Spain, Italy, Bulgaria, Rumania and Germany. It is prevalent in Algeria, Tunis, Egypt, Sudan, Kenya and Tanganyika. Among Asian countries, it has been reported from Armenia, Syria, North Bihar and Deccan in India, the Malaya States and the Philippine islands. Cases are also reported from Canada, the southern states of U.S.A., Mexico, Central America, Brazil and Jamaica. The disease invariably appears in manifest and epidemic form during winter months.

Age incidence

Pellagra is a disease of middle age, the majority of cases occurring between twenty and fifty. Cases of 'infantile pellagra' that had been described in West and East Africa were found to be not due to deficiency of nicotinic acid. They were cases of kwashiorkor, a disease known to be due to protein-calorie malnutrition. Pellagra is rarely encountered below 15 years of age.

Sex incidence

Both sexes are liable, though in some countries, males are more affected than females. This may be particularly due to the fact that men are more exposed to sunlight than women and many women may be in a subclinal state of deficiency.

Predisposing factors

Infections and infestations may precipitate the disease, e.g. tuberculosis, diabetes and bacterial diseases. These may operate by interfering with the appetite or the absorption of food or by increasing the general metabolism and requirement of the vitamin, niacin.

Clinical features

The early signs of pellagra are non-specific and include lassitude, anorexia, nausea, weakness, digestive troubles and psychic and emotional changes such as insomnia, anxiety, irritability and depression. The prodromal period of ill health lasts for a few months and gradually the symptoms progress and culminate in the characteristic manifestation of pellagra, namely, the well-known diagnostic triad—diarrhoea, dermatitis and dementia.

Dermal lesions. The dermatitis of pellagra varies with the acuteness and severity of the deficiency state. It has a characteristic appearance and is distributed in those parts of the body which are exposed to sunlight. The lesions are precipitated by exposure to sunlight, fires and radiant heat. The dermatitis in the early stage resembles sunburn and is usually found on the extensor surfaces of the hands and forearms, and on the anterior surfaces of the feet and lower legs. It rarely extends to the thigh or upper limb, though in labourers, who are constantly working in the fields, it may be found also in these regions, if they happen to be frequently exposed to sunlight. Lesions also occur on the face and neck. In the latter area, they are so distributed that they often appear as a necklace, the so-called Casal's necklace. They are usually bilaterally symmetrical and sharply demarcated from the adjacent healthy skin.

These erythematous skin lesions change to a reddish-brown colour and later coarse desquamation sets in and the underlying skin is thickened. As the disease continues, the involved areas become darkly pigmented. Sometimes, the affected area is swollen and tense and blebs and bullae may be seen occasionally. Secondary infection may occur with formation of pus. Hyperkeratosis and callous formation is characteristic in chronic cases. The hyperkeratotic patch is seen over the elbows and knees and the dorsum of forearms and legs. Ichthyotic changes may also accompany these skin changes. It is on account of this roughness of the skin that the disease was originally called 'pellagra' (rough skin). The relationship of sunlight to pellagra has never been elucidated satisfactorily. Recent studies (Vasantha, 1970) indicate that perhaps it is related to urocanic acid in the skin. These skin changes heal completely with adequate therapy, without scarring or pigmentation.

Gastrointestinal symptoms. These precede the other symptoms and lesions and are usually the presenting ones. In acute cases, severe inflammation of the entire gastrointestinal tract is observed. Loss of appetite, nausea, indigestion, abdominal cramps and constipation alternating with diarrhoea are the early symptoms in many. Diarrhoea is not an invariable feature of pellagra as is generally believed. Constipation is not uncommon. Chronic diarrhoea, when it does occur, is distressing and sometimes the motions may be bloodstained, profuse and foul smelling.

The mucous membrane of the gastrointestinal tract is inflamed resulting in glossitis, stomatitis, oesophagitis, gastritis and, occasionally, proctitis. The tongue is inflamed and fiery red in the initial stages. Patients often complain of sore mouth and dysphagia. As the disease progresses desquamation of the superficial epithelium leaves a scarlet, smooth bald tongue. The desquamation may be irregular giving the appearance of 'geographical tongue'. This process extends to the buccal mucosa, producing stomatitis, to the pharynx and oesophagus producing oesophagitis, with reddening and superficial ulceration. The lips are also red and inflamed producing cheilosis, and fissures at the angles of the mouth may also be seen.

The majority of pellagrins have achlorhydria even after histamine stimulation. The acid reappears in the stomach after treatment with nicotinic acid.

Mental function. Mental symptoms of pellagra are numerous and varied. It has been found that when pellagra was rife, 4 to 6 per cent of pellagrins were admitted to mental hospitals in Italy. The initial nervous syndrome consists of hyperaesthesia to all forms of sensation, increased psychomotor drive and emotional instability with a definite trend towards depression and apathy. Jolliffe *et al* (1940) described an acute encephalopathy characterised by clouding of consciousness, cogwheel rigidity and uncontrollable grasping and sucking reflexes which responded to therapy with niacin. However, such violent reactions are rare in endemic pellagra and these manifestations may have been due to deficiency of other vitamins as well.

Insomnia, irritability, apprehension, lethargy, fatigue, loss of memory, confusion, hallucinations and delirium are frequently seen in pellagrins. Disorientation with regard to time and space is also encountered and a few cases may go into a violent maniacal stage. Often the personality is changed and paranoid condition may be observed. Mental symptoms may precede other symptoms, and a potential pellagrin may be diagnosed as neurasthenic. Electroencephalographic changes have also been reported to occur in pellagra (Srikantia *et al*, 1968b).

Neurological manifestations. These accompany or follow the other lesions of pellagra. Symptoms like tingling and numbness in extremities, burning sensation in the limbs and inability to walk are often encountered in pellagrins. Incoordination, tremors, ataxia, spastic paralysis, sensory abnormalities and subacute combined degeneration of the cord have all been reported to occur. However, such lesions may not be due to deficiency of niacin alone and those subjects may be deficient in thiamine, vitamin B_{12} and pyridoxine. Visual acuity and hearing capacity is decreased in pellagrins. Often there is some element of peripheral neuritis and the subjects' response is much better to a combination of B vitamins, rather than niacin alone.

Other features. Anaemia is a common finding. It is usually hypochromic and microcytic and is usually a manifestation of deficiency of iron. However, in some patients niacin administration itself is beneficial.

Nasolabial dyssebacia is frequently encountered in pellagrins. Facial lesions consisting of filiform, seborrhoeic excrescences (dyssebacia) are found in the nasolabial and nasomalar folds. Fissures and maceration at the angles of the mouth are also seen. These signs are attributed to concomitant riboflavin deficiency.

Pathology

Pathologically, the disease is characterised by changes in the skin, tongue, buccal cavity, mucous membrane of the gastrointestinal tract and nervous tissues.

Skin. In the initial stages there is rarefaction in the superficial portion of the corium with dilatation of blood vessels. This corresponds to the erythema observed clinically. Hyperkeratinisation and parakeratosis are prominent. The sebaceous glands may become atrophic. The dermis is spongy and there is disruption of elastic and collagen fibres. These changes in the corium lead to separation of the epidermis from the dermis over extensive areas. The pigment melanin is distributed through all layers of the epidermis and is almost absent in the basal layer.

Gastrointestinal tract. The mucous membrane is considerably inflamed and frequently ulcerated, particularly in the small intestine, colon and rectum. The epithelium becomes atrophic and cysts are filled with mucus and polymorphonuclear leucocytes in the colon.

Nervous system. Alterations in the nervous tissue in pellagra are much less clearly understood. Chromatolysis of ganglion cells in the brain and myelin degeneration in the cord have been reported. These changes may have been due to severe niacin deficiency. In recent times, all the mental symptoms are quickly reversed by niacin administration, suggesting that there may not be any permanent damage to the nervous system.

Pathogenesis

It has been observed that excess leucine in the diet is involved in the pathogenesis of pellagra. Administration of leucine results in increased excretion of quinolinic acid in the urine both in normals and pellagrins (Balavady *et al*, 1963). There is an increase in the urinary excretion of n-methyl nicotinamide also. Studies were next directed to elucidate the precise biochemical mechanisms underlying the effect of leucine on nicotinic acid metabolism. It has been shown that nicotinamide nucleotide synthesis is altered in pellagrins. It is significantly low when compared to normal subjects (Raghuramulu *et al*, 1965a). Also oral administration of leucine depresses the synthesising ability of erythrocytes both in normal subjects and pellagrins. Recent studies indicate that leucine inhibits the enzyme concerned in the conversion of quinolinic acid to nicotinic acid mononucleotide (Gafoorunissa and Narasinga Rao, 1971).

Experimental evidence also indicates that leucine can produce black tongue in dogs (Belavady *et al*, 1968; Madhavan *et al*, 1968). Leucine can also precipitate mental changes and alter the electroencephalograph (Srikantia *et al*, 1968b). The effect of leucine can be counteracted by isoleucine supplementation (Krishnaswamy and Gopalan, 1971).

Diagnosis

The diagnosis is made on the dietary history, the dermal lesions with orolingual lesions and mental and gastrointestinal disturbances. It is difficult to diagnose pellagra in the preclinical stages, as it may resemble other B vitamin deficiency diseases or may be mistaken for mental ailment.

Differential diagnosis

Pellagra must be differentiated from congenital icthyosis wherein the skin involvement is complete and there is no predilection for the extensor surfaces. It is present from a very young age, though exacerbations are frequent in winter months. It does not respond to niacin therapy. Protein deficiency also produces a crazy pavement dermatosis. In this condition, there is no clear demarcation between normal and abnormal skin. The skin lesions in the initial stages have to be differentiated from erythema multiforme and certain toxic dermatitoses.

Treatment

Nicotinic acid has been found to have a striking curative action, even in advanced cases, and therefore should be given in full doses. Patients with mild pellagra recover rapidly on a good diet containing adequate amounts of protein (tryptophan), nicotinic acid and other members of B group vitamins. Milk, meat, eggs and fresh vegetables must be incorporated into the diet. Exposure to sunlight should be minimised.

A moderately severe case is confined to bed and nicotinic acid or its amide is given in doses of 100–300 mg daily after food. Oral treatment is effective in all cases. Patients with mental depression are often given parenteral nicotinamide. Mental symptoms are cured within 24 to 48 hours of niacin administration, though the dermal lesions require 3–4 weeks of therapy.

Oral lesions are cured by niacin in a few cases. However, riboflavin in doses of 5–10 mg has to be supplemented in the majority, particularly in patients with severe nasolabial dyssebacia. Anaemia is cured by supplements of iron and folic acid. Preparations of B complex vitamins are given for neurological complaints.

Prognosis

Prognosis is excellent in cases where there are no complications. The patient recovers completely though recurrences are common. Mental condition and dermal lesions heal completely without producing any scars. Oral lesions also disappear quickly. Neurological manifestations, if any, require prolonged therapy.

Prophylaxis and prevention

Prophylaxis and prevention consists in supplying a suitable diet rich in all vitamins and a good diet rich in proteins. The use of maize and sorghum rich in leucine should be restricted. Among population groups in which pellagra is common, this is not an easy matter. Enrichment of corn with niacin is feasible in areas in which corn is milled in a few large plants. Since the leucine content of the cereal varies considerably, it may be possible to identify low-leucine strains of jowar and maize and selectively propagate them.

PERIPHERAL NEUROPATHY

SYNONYMS. Polyneuritis, polyneuropathy, multiple neuritis, parenchymatous neuritis.

Definition

This is a peripheral nerve disorder characterised by degeneration of peripheral nerves. Its aetiology is varied and may be produced by a variety of causes like toxic, degenerative, metabolic and deficiency disorders. The term peripheral neuritis is often a misnomer since the condition is rarely inflammatory.

Aetiology

In tropics, peripheral neuropathy is mainly due to dietary deficiencies of vitamins like thiamine, vitamin B_{12}, pantothenic acid and niacin. Neuritis has been described in association with beri-beri, megaloblastic anaemias and pellagra. The causation of neuropathy may be multifactorial, and may operate in several different ways and even at different points of the peripheral nerves. The syndrome may be associated with certain gastrointestinal disturbances like steatorrhea, metabolic diseases like diabetes and chronic alcoholism. The nerve cell and its axonal process are the most important parts of the peripheral nerve and damage to these structures due to vitamin deficiency results in axonal and cellular degeneration.

Epidemiology

The incidence of peripheral neuropathy due to various causes is not yet well documented. However, it is a common observation that patients with vitamin B deficiency signs frequently complain of tingling and numbness in the extremities. Nursing women frequently complain of paraesthesiae in the limbs.

Clinical features

Patients with neuropathy describe their symptoms by characteristic expressions—for instance, they use such words as tingling, numbness, prickling, burning, searing and jabbing pain in the extremities. Typically the symptoms are worse when the affected part bears weight, as in walking.

Peripheral neuropathy due to thiamine deficiency. This has already been described in beri-beri. This is one of the most commonly encountered polyneuropathies in temperate climates. The outstanding clinical findings in advanced thiamine deficiency are peripheral neuritis (dry beri-beri) and heart disease with oedema (wet beri-beri). The peripheral neuropathy of chronic alcoholism is often due to thiamine deficiency. It is mostly attributed to the poor dietary intake of thiamine in alcoholism. Alcohol actually requires less thiamine for its utilisation than does glucose.

The mechanism by which thiamine deficiency causes neurological lesions is not clearly understood. The action of pyrithiamine *in vivo* mimics the thiamine deficiency state, particularly with respect to the development of polyneuritis. Experiments by Cooper and Pincus (1967) indicate that the role of thiamine in conduction is independent of its function as a coenzyme and is perhaps mediated through ion transport.

Peripheral neuropathy due to vitamin B_{12} deficiency. Subacute combined degeneration of the cord is a disease usually associated with megaloblastic anaemia. It is characterised pathologically by degeneration of the white matter of the spinal cord—most evident in the posterior and lateral columns—and of the peripheral nerves and brain. Clinically it is manifested by paraesthesiae, sensory loss, especially impairment of deep sensibility, ataxia and paraplegia.

It is a popular misconception that subacute combined degeneration of the cord occurs only in cases of classical pernicious anaemia. It is, in fact, a manifestation associated with severe vitamin B_{12} deficiency and may occur in any condition leading to such deficiency. Thus it has been described in patients with dietary vitamin B_{12} deficiency (Badenoch, 1954; Wells, 1958). Nevertheless, it appears that subacute combined degeneration of the cord is much less common in cases of dietary deficiency seen in India and the tropics than it is amongst a group of pernicious anaemia patients in the West. This may be so because dietary deficiency of vitamin B_{12} is often not as marked as in cases of pernicious anaemia.

There is no relationship between the severity of the anaemia and the incidence of neurological changes.

The clinical picture is a mixture of posterior column, pyramidal tract and peripheral nerve degeneration. The onset of symptoms is gradual. The paraesthesiae begin in the periphery of the lower limbs and tend to spread slowly upwards; a sense of constriction around the chest or abdomen is common. Motor symptoms consisting of weakness and ataxia develop at variable intervals. Objective sensory changes are constantly present, and the forms of sensation mediated by the posterior column, such as postural sensibility and appreciation of passive movement and of vibration, are impaired. Cutaneous sensation to light touch, pin prick, heat and cold is impaired. Incoordination in the lower limbs is evident in the ataxic gait and by the presence of Romberg's sign. Moderate muscular wasting is usually present in the later stages in the extremities. The reflexes are variable. Usually, the ankle jerk is lost and the knee jerk is affected less frequently. The plantar response is extensor and depending on the column affected, either ataxia or spastic paraplegia is dominant.

Other associated clinical symptoms. Bilateral primary optic atrophy with some visual impairment is observed in many cases. Gastric achlorhydria and anaemia are invariably encountered. Glossitis is common and may in fact be the presenting symptom.

Neuritis associated with pellagra. Symptoms of peripheral neuritis are commonly seen in association with pellagra. But deficiency of riboflavin, thiamine and other B complex vitamins may complicate the clinical picture of endemic pellagra. Therefore, it is difficult to ascribe these symptoms to niacin deficiency alone.

Pyridoxine deficiency and neuritis. The role of vitamin B_6 in metabolism of the central nervous system is well established. Convulsions occurring in infants are cured by pyridoxine supplements (Scriver 1960). However, so far there is no evidence to implicate dietary deficiency of pyridoxine in any reported disorders of the peripheral nervous system. Large amounts of pyridoxine have been shown to prevent or alleviate the peripheral neuropathy which may develop during therapy with isoniazid (Vilter, 1955). Vilter *et al* (1953) demonstrated that patients receiving desoxypyridoxine develop peripheral neuropathy.

It is a common observation that patients with neuropathy often respond to a combination of B vitamins rather than to a single B vitamin. Biochemical parameters like transketolase activity do not always correlate with clinical signs (Bamji, 1970). These observations suggest that patients with neuropathy may also be deficient in other vitamins such as vitamin B_6. Pyridoxine deficiency does exist in population groups, particularly in pregnant women and in adults with severe oral lesions (Krishnaswamy, 1971a and b). Therefore, the possibility of pyridoxine deficiency contributing to peripheral neuropathy cannot be ruled out.

Pantothenic acid: burning feet syndrome. Outbreaks of 'burning feet' have been reported among malnourished populations and have often occurred in jails. This syndrome has been described as a separate clinical entity by Gopalan (1946).

This disease is usually encountered in rice-eating zones. The rice consumed is, in most cases, of the parboiled type, which contains enough thiamine. Females are more commonly affected, particularly after delivery. A burning sensation in the extremities is the characteristic feature. This is confined to the soles of the feet. Sometimes, the palms of the hands are also involved. The burning starts in the soles of the feet around the ball of the great toe and spreads upwards. This sensation is often mild but sometimes excruciating pain may incapacitate the patient. Paroxysms of burning may occur. Patients may also complain of 'pins and needles' in the distal parts of the limbs. Though the subjective symptoms are predominant, objective signs are often lacking. There is no wasting, no weakness, no sensory loss, no calf muscle tenderness and there are no alterations in reflexes. This is quite opposite to what is seen in peripheral neuropathy due to thiamine deficiency. Hyperidrosis is a common accompaniment and visible beads of perspiration may stand out. The hyperidrosis is limited to the areas of burning and follows paroxysms of burning sensation. The response to treatment with pantothenic acid is dramatic.

It is possible that the burning sensation may be due to abnormal and excessive stimulation of the peripheral sensory nerve endings by certain intermediate metabolites accumulating as a result of disturbances in cellular metabolism caused by the vitamin deficiency.

Pathology

Segmental myelin thinning, followed by demyelination and axonal degeneration are characteristic features of neuropathy due to vitamin deficiencies.

Diagnosis

Since peripheral neuropathy can be caused by multiple factors, several lines of enquiry should be followed in every case of polyneuropathy.

Differential diagnosis

Metabolic disturbances like porphyria, diabetes and collagen diseases can produce neuritis. Infections, for instance infectious mononucleosis, can result in neuritis. Toxic substances like arsenic and thalium should be considered. Certain hereditary neurological syndromes like peroneal muscular atrophy, sensory radicular neuropathy and hypertrophic interstitial neuropathy have to be differentiated.

Treatment

Vitamins of the B group have to be administered for complete clinical cure. Subacute combined degeneration requires large doses of vitamin B_{12} (50–100 μg) daily. Burning feet syndrome requires calcium pantothenate in doses of 50 and 100 mg. In addition, patients should be treated for associated conditions, like diabetes and chronic alcoholism.

Prognosis

Early diagnosis and prompt treatment are indicated. In advanced cases, where the axons and spinal cord are involved, reversal of symptoms may not be possible, though subjective sensations may disappear.

Prevention and prophylaxis

Dietary deficiencies can be overcome only by improving the standards of living. Distribution of synthetic vitamin preparations may solve the problem to a certain extent.

SCURVY

SYNONYMS. Haemorrhagic scurvy, infantile scurvy or Barlow's disease, Cheadle's disease, Moeller's disease.

Definition

This is a condition due to the deficiency of ascorbic acid in the diet and is marked by weakness, anaemia, spongy gums and a tendency to mucocutaneous haemorrhages.

Aetiology

This disease is due to a dietary deficiency of ascorbic acid which is present in all fresh vegetables and fruits. The vitamin is very sensitive to heating and drying and therefore is almost absent in tinned fruits and dried vegetables. Among the richest dietary sources of ascorbic acid are oranges, lemons, tomatoes, fresh strawberries and raw cabbage.

The instability of ascorbic acid during cooking

is a major cause of loss of this nutrient. As much as 25 to 60 per cent of this vitamin is lost during cooking. An enzyme, ascorbic acid oxidase, which slowly oxidises ascorbic acid, is liberated as soon as fruits or vegetables are bruised or macerated. Other important factors leading to the loss of the vitamin are cooking in iron, copper or badly tinned vessels and chopping the vegetables with a steel or metal knife. These procedures cause a loss of the vitamin even before the food is cooked. Deficiency of this vitamin is, therefore, not uncommon. However, clinical scurvy in adults has become a rare disease.

Epidemiology

In the past, the disease frequently occurred in sailors who received a diet devoid of vitamin C. Many epidemics have been observed during military campaigns and in prisons. While adult scurvy is rare, infantile scurvy is still encountered in many tropical countries.

Age incidence

Scurvy may occur at any age, but is extremely rare in the newborn infant. The majority of cases are seen in the latter half of the first and during the second year of life. This is the period of rapid growth. In a well-nourished population, the amount of ascorbic acid required from the mother is apparently sufficient to prevent scurvy for about 5 months. Scurvy is a disease of artificially fed infants past the age of breast feeding. In the United States, infantile scurvy became a major problem after the introduction of pasteurisation of milk.

Scurvy is occasionally seen in adults, when the diet is severely restricted because of disease, and in neurotics and faddists with self-imposed dietary restrictions.

Sex incidence

The incidence of scurvy in both male and female infants is similar.

Clinical features

All febrile episodes, particularly infections and diarrhoeal diseases, increase the need for vitamin C; they are therefore predisposing factors in the aetiology of scurvy.

The onset of infantile scurvy is insidious, with the child being fretful and refusing its food. The majority of patients present the triad of irritability, tenderness of the legs and pseudoparalysis

2 F

involving the lower extremities. The infant in the early stages resents handling, and within a day or two refuses to move his legs in anticipation of pain. Haemorrhagic manifestations may occur particularly around the erupting central incisors.

The infant assumes the characteristic 'pithed-frog' position. Costochondral beading is found in all patients. This scorbutic beading is produced by subluxation of the sternal plate at the costochondral junction. It is sharp with 'caving in' of the cartilaginous anterior chest wall. The limbs are tender and extremely painful.

The gums bleed easily. The subperiosteal haemorrhages around the shafts of the long bones are frequently palpable. Petechial haemorrhages occur in the skin, the mucous membrane and the soft tissues, as in the scalp. Extensive haemorrhages may occur behind and around the eyeball. Blood may be vomited or passed by the bowels and there may be haematuria. Subdural haemorrhage is an occasional manifestation, whereas intra-cerebral haemorrhages rarely occur.

Anaemia is very frequent in scorbutic infants. It may be hypochromic due to iron deficiency and sometimes it is megaloblastic. Specific haematological response to ascorbic acid alone is not seen.

Radiological findings. The diagnosis is usually based on radiological changes in the long bones, especially of their distal ends. These appear earliest at the sites of the most active bone growth such as the sternal ends of the ribs, the distal end of the femur, the proximal end of the humerus, both ends of the tibia and fibula and the distal ends of the radius and ulna.

The cortical atrophy or diminution of the ratio between the thickness of the cortex and the thickness of the shaft is an early alteration. Atrophy of the trabecular structure with increased transparency and blurring gives rise to a 'ground glass' appearance. The cortex is reduced in thickness and the epiphyseal ends are sharply outlined. The 'white line of Fraenkel', which represents the zone of well-calcified cartilage, can be clearly discerned.

A zone of rarefaction near the cortex, in conjunction with the thinning of the cortex, constitutes the 'corner sign'. As the scorbutic process proceeds, this area of rarefaction may extend completely across the cartilage shaft junction. The trauma of normal movement and weight bearing may produce fractures. Spur formation may also occur.

Scurvy in adults. The early symptoms are nonspecific like weakness, fatigue and listlessness. The appetite is reduced. The specific manifestations are perifollicular hyperkeratotic papules. These are found on the thighs and buttocks and later spread to the arms and the trunk. As the disease progresses, haemorrhages occur deep in the calf, thigh and forearm muscles, causing hard indurations. Phlebothrombosis may occur. Haemorrhages may occur in joints, particularly the knee. Haemorrhagic involvement of the gums is frequent. The gums are swollen, blue-red, spongy and very friable. Secondary infection, infarction and gangrene may occur. Low-grade fever is usually present. Wound healing is delayed in vitamin C deficiency. Repeated infections are common in vitamin C deficient subjects.

Pathology

Deficiency of vitamin C results in the defective formation and maintenance of intercellular substances in the supporting tissues of mesenchymal origin; these substances are collagen of fibrous tissues, the matrices of bone and the intercellular cement of vascular endothelium. Endochondral bone formation ceases in the absence of vitamin C, since osteoblasts are not capable of forming the matrix, osteoid.

Diagnosis

The tenderness of tissues and the pain are often mistaken for rheumatic arthritis. The age of the patient aids in identifying scurvy. Pseudo-paralysis of syphilis usually occurs at an earlier age and is accompanied by other signs of congenital syphilis. Diseases of the blood mimic the haemorrhagic tendencies of scurvy. However, X-rays are diagnostic. Vitamin C levels, particularly in white cells, go down in severe cases.

Treatment

Scurvy should be treated by both administration of adequate amounts of ascorbic acid and correction of the dietary pattern that led to its development. Adult scurvy will respond to as little as 10 mg of ascorbic acid daily, with healing of skin lesions in 10 days to 2 weeks. In infants 100 to 200 mg daily in divided doses will produce clinical response with cessation of pain and disappearance of pseudo-paralysis, in about 3 days. The oral route of administration gives satisfactory results.

Prognosis

Recovery occurs rapidly in cases correctly treated. Pain ceases in a few days, but the swelling caused by subperiosteal haemorrhages may require months to disappear. Permanent deformities are uncommon.

Prevention

Scurvy can be prevented by the administration of a diet adequate in vitamin C. All infants should receive fruit juices beginning at 2–4 weeks of age.

The optimal amount of ascorbic acid necessary for the maintenance of health in man is still a matter of controversy. The recommendations made by various national bodies range from 30 to 75 mg/day. The results of a study indicate that maximal leucocyte concentration can be maintained by the intake of as little as 10–22 mg/day (Srikantia *et al*, 1970).

REFERENCES

ARROYAVE, G., WILSON, D., MENDEZ, J., BEHAN, M. and SCRIMSHAW, N. S. (1961) *Amer. J. clin. Nutr.*, **9**, 180.
BADENOCH, J. (1954) *Proc. roy. Soc. Med.*, **47**, 426.
BAMJI, M. S. (1969) *Clin. chim. acta*, **26**, 263.
—— (1970) *Amer. J. clin. Nutr.*, **23**, 52.
BELAVADY, B. and GOPALAN, C. (1965) *Lancet*, **2**, 1220.
BELAVADY, B., MADHAVAN, T. V. and GOPALAN, C. (1967) *Gastroenterology*, **53**, 749.
BELAVADY, B., SRIKANTIA, S. G. and GOPALAN, C. (1963) *Biochem, J.*, **87**, 652.
BHAT, K. S. and BELAVADY, B. (1967) *Amer. J. clin. Nutr.*, **20**, 386.
BRIDGES, J. M., GIBSON, J. B., LOUGHRIDGE, L. W. and MONTGOMERY, D. A. D. (1957) *Brit. J. Surg.*, **45**, 117.
COOPER, J. R. and PINCUS, J. H. (1967) In *Thiamin Deficiency: Biochemical Lesions and their Clinical Significance.* Ciba Foundation Study Group No. 28, ed Wolstenholme, G. E. W. and O'Connor, M., p. 112. London: J. & A. Churchill.
DENNY-BROWN, D. (1958) *Fed. Proc.*, **17**, 35.
EIJKMAN, C. (1961) Quoted by Williams, R. R. in *Towards the Conquest of Beri-Beri*, p. 36. Cambridge: Harvard Univ. Press.

GAFOORUNISSA and NARASINGA RAO, B. S. (1972) In press.
GOLDSMITH, G. A. (1956) *J. Amer. diet. Ass.*, **32**, 312.
GOPALAN, C. (1946) *Ind. med. Gaz.*, **81**, 22.
—— (1969) *Lancet*, 197.
GOPALAN, C. and SRIKANTIA, S. G. (1960) *Lancet*, 954.
GOPALAN, C., VENKATACHALAM, P. S. and BELAVADY, B. (1960) *Amer. J. clin. Nutr.*, **8**, 833.
IYENGAN, L. and APTE, S. V. (1972) *Brit. J. Nutr.* **27**, 313.
JOLLIFFEE, N., BOWMAN, K. M., ROSEMBLUM, L. A. and FEIN, H. D. (1940) *J. Amer. med. Ass.*, **114**, 307.
KRISHNASWAMY, K. (1971a) *Int. J. Vit. Nutr. Res.*, **41**, 240.
—— (1971b) *Int. J. Vit. Nutr. Res.*, **41**, 247.
KRISHNASWAMY, K. and GOPALAN, C. (1971) *Lancet*, 1167.
LALA, V. R. and REDDY, V. (1970) *Amer. J. clin. Nutr.*, **23**, 110.
LANE, M. and ALFREY, C. P. Jr. (1965) *Blood*, **25**, 432.
MADHAVAN, T. V., BELAVADY, B. and GOPALAN, C. (1968) *J. Path. Bact.*, **95**, 259.
PLATT, B. S. (1958) *Fed. Proc.*, **17**, 8.
PRAHLAD RAO, SINGH, D. and SWAMINATHAN, M. C. (1969) *Ind. J. med. Res.*, **57**, 2132.
RAGHURAMULU, N., NARASINGA RAO, B. S. and GOPALAN, C. (1965a) *J. Nutr.*, **86**, 100.
RAGHURAMULU, N., SRIKANTIA, S. G., NARASINGA RAO, B. S. and GOPALAN, C. (1965b) *Biochem. J.*, **96**, 837.
REDDY, V. and SRIKANTIA, S. G. (1966) *Amer. J. clin. Nutr.*, **18**, 105.
SALCEDO, Jr., J., BAMBA, M. D., CARRASCO, E. O., JOSE, F. R. and VALENZUELA, R. C. (1949) *J. Philipp. med. Ass.*, **24**, 519.
SAUBERLICH, H. E. (1967) *Amer. J. clin. Nutr.*, **20**, 528.
SCRIVER, C. R. (1960) *Pediatrics*, **26**, 62.
SIVAKUMAR, B. and REDDY, V. (1972) *Brit. J. Nutr.*, **27**, 299.
SRIKANTIA, S. G. and BELAVADY, B. (1961) *Ind. J. med. Res.*, **49**, 109.
SRIKANTIA, S. G., MOHANRAM, M. and KRISHNASWAMY, K. (1970) *Amer. J. clin. Nutr.*, **23**, 59.
SRIKANTIA, S. G., NARASINGA RAO, B. S., RAGHURAMULU, N. and GOPALAN, C. (1968a) *Amer. J. clin. Nutr.* **21**, 1306.
SRIKANTIA, S. G., REDDY, M. V. R. and KRISHNASWAMY, K. (1968b) *Electroenceph. clin. Neurophysiol.*, **25**, 386.
SWAMINATHAN, M. C., SUSHEELA, T. P. and THIMMAYAMMA, B. V. S. (1970) *Amer. J. clin. Nutr.*, **23**, 119.
SYDENSTRICKER, V. P., GEESLIN, L. E., TEMPLETON, C. M. and WEAVER, J. W. (1939) *J. Amer. med. Ass.*, **113**, 1698.
TAKAKI, K. (1906) *Lancet*, 1369, 1520.
VASANTHA, L. (1970) *Ind. J. med. Res.*, **58**, 1079.
VENKATACHALAM, P. S., BELAVADY, B. and GOPALAN, C. (1962) *J. Pediat.* **61**, 262.
VILTER, R. W. (1955) *J. Amer. med. Ass.*, **159**, 1210.
VILTER, R. W., MUELLER, J. F., GLAZER, H. S., JARROLD, T., ABRAHAM, J., THOMPSON, C. and HOWKINS, V. R. (1953) *J. Lab. clin. Med.*, **42**, 335.
WELLS, R. (1958) *J. trop. Med. Hyg.*, **61**, 81.

29

Nutritional Anaemias and Small Intestinal Diseases in the Tropics

Those who work in tropical regions will not be surprised to find discussion of both the nutritional anaemias and disorders of the small bowel in the same chapter of a textbook. So interrelated are these that such an arrangement leads to clarity rather than confusion.

In tropical countries where nutritional deficiencies, infections and infestations are rife, it is sometimes difficult to know which of a multiplicity of abnormalities is afflicting the patient. In Fig. 29.1 there are shown some of the factors that may lead to anaemia in an inhabitant of a tropical country.

Iron deficiency due to hookworm infection is very widespread and may be severe, but although many inhabitants of tropical regions have an adequate supply of iron in the diet (and in some regions, excess), there are areas where dietetic habits and poverty result in primary iron undernutrition.

The factors leading to megaloblastic anaemia are particularly complex, and may vary considerably even in different areas of the same country. Primary malnutrition is an important cause that may result in deficiency of folic acid or vitamin B_{12} or both. In general, however, depletion of folate is the more usual, and it may occur even in vegetarians whose articles of diet contain adequate quantities of the vitamin. This is because they have destroyed it first by cooking for prolonged periods and then by throwing away the boiling water in which folate has accumulated. The patient may continue in a poorly nourished condition without overt anaemia, but the balance may be tipped by pregnancy, chronic infection, tropical sprue, diarrhoea, or haemolysis. Malaria does not by itself cause megaloblastic anaemia, but may lead to it in a patient with inadequate stores of vitamin B_{12} or folate. In certain of the haemoglobinopathies too, megaloblastic change may occur because of haemolysis in one who is poorly nourished and depleted of folate.

The content of this chapter is restricted to diseased states in the adult.

IRON DEFICIENCY ANAEMIA

Aetiology

Throughout the world, iron deficiency anaemia is an affliction of mankind that saps efficiency and leads to much ill health and misery. Even in the developed countries it is a significant problem amongst women of the childbearing age because so often the iron in the diet is insufficient in quantity to balance the monthly loss. Repeated pregnancies add to the negative balance.

Iron is widely distributed in many foodstuffs, there being a relatively high content in pulses. Vegetarians also obtain a good intake from green vegetables. Whole rice contains about 5 mg per 100 g, whereas the iron content of polished rice after cooking is only about 0.2 mg per 100 g. Initially the infant receives its iron stores from the mother, but thereafter additional supplies of the mineral must come from foodstuffs. In the adult, about 20 mg are liberated daily from the breakdown of red cells, but nearly all this is utilised again. In the male in temperate climates the output in the faeces, sweat and hair is less than 1 mg per day, but it has been claimed that in the tropics the loss from sweating may be considerably more than this. Indeed, figures from India have suggested a loss on occasion of as much as 6.5 mg daily in the sweat. It should, however, be added that no correlation has been shown between the incidence of iron deficiency in various countries and the environmental temperature, and that most investigators have tended to minimise the importance of the sweating of iron as a significant factor.

The menstrual loss varies considerably amongst women, but an output at a period of about 30 mg is probably not unusual. During a normal pregnancy a mother may lose about 3 mg a day if haemorrhage at delivery is included in the calculation, and during lactation there may be a loss of about 1 mg daily in the milk. Thus a man may need to absorb about 1 mg daily, a woman during the reproductive age about 2 mg and a pregnant female up to 3 mg. The iron intake varies considerably in different tropical countries, but the Western diet supplies about 15–20 mg of iron daily, and of this about 10 per cent is absorbed, the amount entering the blood stream being controlled to a certain extent by the ferritin mechanism of the small intestinal mucosa. It is now considered that this acts as a mechanism of excretion

Africa, the tendency throughout the tropics is for iron deficiency to be a scourge.

Clinical features

The patient with severe anaemia is tired and weak, but he may have become relatively well acclimatised to existing with an abnormally low

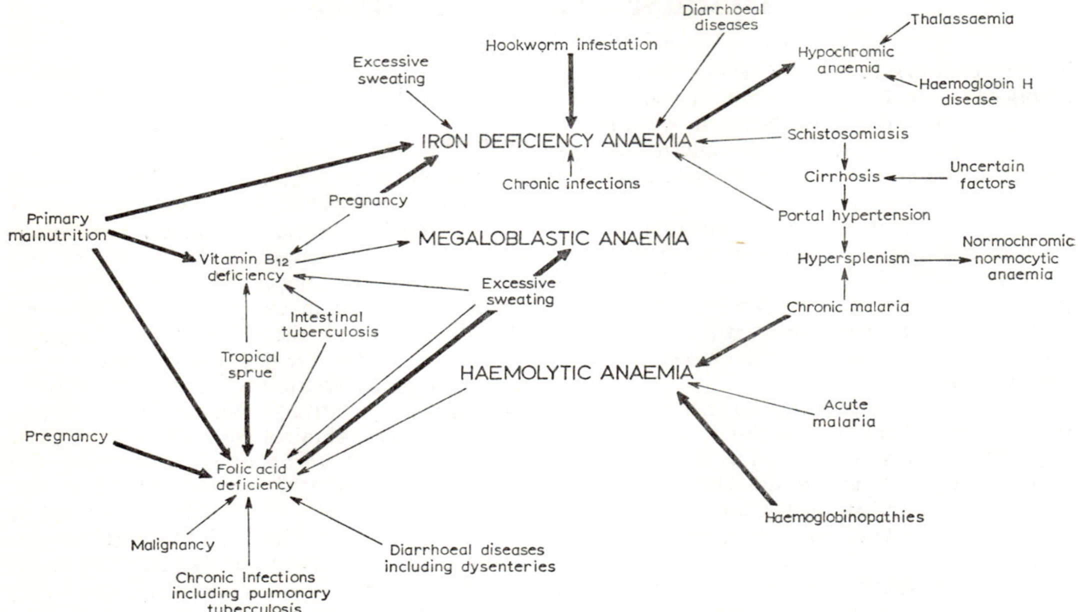

Fig. 29.1. *Factors causing anaemia in the tropics.*

in that cells loaded with ferritin iron will carry it back with them into the alimentary canal at the end of their life span. Where, however, there is a need for more iron to be absorbed, less ferritin is formed.

This barrier mechanism is not entirely successful and it is possibly for this reason that the Bantus in South Africa develop tissue siderosis. They obtain a considerable amount of iron from the utensils used for cooking and for the preparation of fermented alcoholic beverages. Indeed, some studies have suggested that the average Bantu male consumes from 50 to 100 mg of iron daily in beer alone. The controlling mechanism for iron absorption in the intestinal wall seems to be unable to deal with intakes of this magnitude, and hence iron is absorbed in excess and deposited in the tissues.

Nevertheless, although this condition of excessive absorption of iron is well known in South

level of haemoglobin. He is likely to be breathless on exertion and to suffer from dizziness and palpitations. The appetite may be poor, and glossitis may occur. Particularly if there is coronary atheroma, the patient may suffer from anginal symptoms.

On examination, oedema of the ankles is likely to be present, and if anaemia is severe this may also occur in the upper limbs and even the face. There is likely to be a rapid pulse, and systolic heart murmurs will be heard. The jugular veins may be prominent and the liver enlarged. There may also be splenic enlargement, but in tropical regions the causes of this are, of course, numerous, and the degree of enlargement in simple iron deficiency is relatively slight.

In hypochromic anaemia the nails of the fingers or toes may be flat or spoon-shaped, and parotid gland enlargement may be found; the reason for this is unknown. If the retinae are examined there may be found to be pallor of the optic discs, venous engorgement, and retinal exudates or haemorrhages.

Laboratory findings

In tropical countries an extreme degree of iron deficiency anaemia is not uncommon, and the haemoglobin level may even be as low as 1.5 g per 100 ml. Red cell counts are notoriously unreliable if they are not carried out with an electronic counter, but they will show that the colour index, MCH and MCV are very low. The MCHC will be considerably reduced, perhaps down to 22 per cent. The blood film shows hypochromia, microcytosis and anisocytosis. The reticulocyte count may be increased if there is active bleeding, but reticulocytosis may also be due to coincidental malaria or some other cause of haemolysis. If there is bleeding the thrombocyte count may be increased. With hookworm infestation, eosinophilia may be a feature. If the serum iron level is measured, it will be found to be reduced. The bone marrow will be normoblastic, the late normoblasts being hypochromic.

Diagnosis

Investigators in the tropics are well accustomed to seeing many anaemic patients, and the aim is to determine the type of anaemia and, if possible, find and treat the cause. Frequently there is a dual deficiency of folic acid (or, less commonly, vitamin B_{12}) and iron, but if iron deficiency is severe it may be difficult to determine this merely by studying the peripheral blood or bone marrow. A dimorphic picture in the peripheral blood suggests a dual deficiency, and the presence in the marrow of red cell precursors with an open chromatin pattern in the nucleus (the thrush breast appearance) indicates megaloblastic change.

Anaemia in the tropics is frequently due to a haemoglobinopathy (page 465) or to thalassaemia (page 495). The basic defect in thalassaemia is a failure to produce red cells with a normal adult haemoglobin content. There is hypochromic anaemia because of a deficiency of globin, there being defective production of the protein moiety. This results in a variation in the size of the red cells, and some are very thin and pale. Target cells and poikilocytes may be a feature, and basophilic stippling may occur in β-thalassaemia major or minor. The MCHC is not as low as is frequently found in iron deficiency in the tropics, and the serum iron level is increased if iron deficiency is not a complicating factor. Investigation

for fetal haemoglobin will show it to consist of 15 to 90 per cent of the total in β-thalassaemia major, but the increase is much less in β-thalassaemia minor. There is also usually an increase of haemoglobin A_2 compared with A. This type of anaemia does not respond to iron therapy.

Another genetically determined form of anaemia that gives a peripheral blood picture that may be mistaken for iron deficiency anaemia is haemoglobin H disease (page 498), and any coexisting iron deficiency has to be treated before it can be diagnosed. It should, of course, be remembered that a patient with iron deficiency may have a haemoglobinopathy such as sickle cell anaemia (page 487).

Other causes of anaemia that may be hypochromic include chronic infection and renal failure.

Treatment

Where possible the cause must be eliminated and this may include the treatment of ancylostomiasis (page 165). If anaemia is severe it should be treated with iron before an anthelminthic is given.

If oedema is marked or anaemia so severe that transfusion is considered necessary, it should be realised that this procedure may cause cardiac failure. Packed cells rather than whole blood should be administered and given very slowly. Digitalisation may first be carried out or 40 mg of frusemide can be given intravenously. An alternative method that is still under investigation for the treatment of severe anaemia is to use exchange transfusion. This is most easily done by removing blood from the veins of one arm and giving concentrated red cells into a vein in the other.

It should always be remembered that the dangers of transfusion include serum hepatitis, bacterial contamination, allergic and pyrogenic reactions, circulatory overloading and possibly citrate intoxication with a lowering of the blood level of ionised calcium.

ABO incompatibility can largely be avoided by careful blood grouping and cross matching, but there is no such thing as a universal donor, and plasma from group O donors may contain sufficient antibodies to antigens of groups A and B to give reactions. If a patient has received blood previously there may be reactions to rhesus and other blood group antigens or to white cells.

When iron is given, the inexpensive ferrous sulphate is as satisfactory as any preparation and should be given in a dosage of 200 mg thrice daily. Alternative preparations are ferrous fumarate (200 mg t.i.d.) or ferrous gluconate (300 mg b.i.d.). In a patient with iron deficiency, the absorption of iron from such preparations is satisfactory and in most instances it is unnecessary to give it by injection.

Iron preparations are available for intravenous or intramuscular use, but it should not be assumed that they give a more rapid rise in the haemoglobin level except when blood loss is occurring more rapidly than is iron absorption. It is reasonable to give iron by injection if it is believed that the patient will not take treatment by mouth, and certainly a few patients require it because they are unable to tolerate iron given orally. There may be a place for it in late pregnancy although in that event blood transfusion may be needed.

When iron is given by injection there is always a possibility of reactions. Accordingly, a test dose should be given and the maker's recommendations carefully followed. If a general reaction occurs, the treatment should be discontinued and 100 mg of hydrocortisone sodium succinate given intravenously. If this is not available, 0.5 ml of 1 in 1000 adrenaline tartarate should be given subcutaneously.

The preparations that are available vary in different countries and hence it would be unwise to give detailed instructions here. The form for intravenous use most commonly used in the United Kingdom for some years was saccharated iron oxide, but it is no longer listed as being obtainable there. Dextriferron is an iron dextrin complex for intravenous use, marketed as Astrafer I.V. (Astra Chemicals Ltd.). The dose is 1.5 to 5 ml (the equivalent of 30 to 100 mg of Fe) daily intravenously. It should not be used if there is liver damage.

The iron sorbitol preparation sold by Astra Chemicals Ltd. as Jectofer contains 50 mg per ml and each ampoule contains 2 ml. This latter amount will raise the haemoglobin level by about 0.6 per 100 ml. Iron sorbitol has to be given intramuscularly, and iron should not be given orally simultaneously because headache, dizziness nausea and vomiting may occur. It is said by some that the giving of the preparation may lead to exacerbations of pyelonephritis, but by others that it merely causes an output of white cells in the urine of patients prone to pyelitis. Even in the normal person the urine may turn black on standing when iron sorbitol has been given.

Iron dextran is marketed as Imferon (Fisons Pharmaceuticals). It contains 50 mg of iron per ml and was originally intended for intramuscular use. It can also be given intravenously as a 'total dose infusion'. The total dose is calculated and the iron dextran given in a drip diluted 1 in 20 with isotonic sterile saline (not dextrose). It has to be given slowly and should not be used if there is cardiac failure. Thromboses and reactions have been reported.

MEGALOBLASTIC ANAEMIA

Aetiology

Megaloblastic anaemia is very commonly encountered in developing countries, and is more frequently due to deficiency of folic acid than of vitamin B_{12}, but there may be depletion of both. The daily requirements of folate are believed to be about 50 to 200 μg per day and folate in a conjugate form occurs in liver and other organs and in meats. It is present in high concentration in vegetables, particularly of the leafy variety. It may be lost if foodstuffs are overcooked, especially if the water is thrown away. The body stores will prevent megaloblastic anaemia for about 8–12 weeks if a folate-free diet is given, but such a diet is difficult to prepare. Most tables purporting to give the folate content of foodstuffs are inaccurate because satisfactory methods of assay were not available when the tables were constructed. Some folate is lost in the sweat. Vitamin B_{12} does not occur in vegetable matter, but is present in large amounts in liver and kidney and is found in meats. The daily requirements are uncertain, but the figures given have ranged from 2 to 5 μg. There is enough stored in the body to last about 3 years if the source of vitamin B_{12} is cut off. Bacteria in the small or large intestine can synthesise folate under certain experimental conditions and vitamin B_{12} and related substances occur in the faeces, but there is no evidence to suggest that this is a significant factor in human metabolism.

In the absence of vitamin B_{12} or folate, a clinical feature which attracts particular attention is the development of abnormal red cell precursors, viz. megaloblasts in the bone marrow. This results in normochromic macrocytic anaemia if iron deficiency is not a complicating feature, but it should be realised that this anaemia is only one facet of an abnormal cellular metabolism that is generalised. The factors that are operative in the causation of megaloblastic anaemia in the tropics have already been referred to, but, in brief, they may include primary malnutrition, pregnancy, malabsorption, diarrhoea, chronic infection, and haemolysis, this last necessitating an increase in red cell turnover. In this way malaria or a haemoglobinopathy may aggravate the deficiency.

Clinical features

The general clinical features are similar to those of iron deficiency anaemia. There may be painful glossitis and the tongue is frequently red and angry. Diarrhoea may be a feature. If thrombocytopenia is marked, purpuric haemorrhages sometimes occur. Marked splenomegaly is not a feature of megaloblastic anaemia in itself.

Laboratory findings

Whether megaloblastic anaemia is due to deficiency of folate or of vitamin B_{12}, the anaemia is macrocytic and normochromic so that the colour index and MCV are raised and the MCHC is normal. There is likely to be leucopenia and thrombocytopenia, and the neutrophil polymorphs have an increased number of lobes. In tropical countries the anaemia is commonly dimorphic because of complicating iron deficiency, but if this is not so the serum iron level is normal. The bone marrow shows megaloblastic change, but this does not mean that no normoblasts are to be found in the marrow, and if there is severe iron deficiency the megaloblasts are more difficult to identify. Giant metamyelocytes in the marrow are a feature of megaloblastic anaemia. Sometimes megaloblasts are seen in the peripheral blood or in the buffy coat after the blood sample has been centrifuged.

Where facilities are available for further investigation, it will be found useful to measure the serum vitamin B_{12} level using *L. leichmannii* or *Euglena gracilis* as the test organism. The normal range varies slightly in different laboratories, but it is of the order of 150 to 1000 pg per ml. If vitamin B_{12} deficiency is the cause of megaloblastic anaemia the serum level is usually below 70 pg per ml. The serum folate level may also be measured, using *L. casei* as the test organism, but again the range of normal varies in different laboratories. It is of the order of 2.5 to 18 ng per ml, but it is possible to have megaloblastic anaemia due to folate deficiency with the serum folate level in this lower range of normal. Perhaps the red cell folate level is a better measure of established folate depletion, but the true value of this index has not yet been established. The normal range is from 150 to 650 ng per ml of packed red cells.

In vitamin B_{12} deficiency the serum folate level may be low, normal or raised, and in folate deficiency there may be some reduction of the serum vitamin B_{12} level, but not to the level found in megaloblastic anaemia from vitamin B_{12} depletion.

The amino acid histidine is normally metabolised to glutamic acid, but where there is folate depletion the metabolism proceeds only to the stage of formiminoglutamic acid (FIGLU), and this appears in the urine. Accordingly, a test that has been developed to demonstrate folate depletion is to give 20 g of histidine by mouth and show by electrophoresis using cellulose acetate paper that FIGLU is present in the urine. Unfortunately, a positive test may also occur in vitamin B_{12} depletion and, moreover, it is possible to have megaloblastic anaemia of pregnancy from folate depletion without finding FIGLU in the urine.

When there is doubt as to whether a patient is depleted of folate or of vitamin B_{12}, a therapeutic test involving the use of folic acid will not be helpful because there will be a response to this no matter which deficiency is present. If, however, the patient is depleted only of folic acid, he will not respond significantly to treatment with vitamin B_{12}.

Diagnosis

Reference has already been made to the differential diagnosis of various types of anaemia (page 443) and mention has been made above of laboratory tests that may help in differentiating between depletion of folic acid and of vitamin B_{12}.

Deficiency of either of these vitamins may lead to anaemia, weight loss, painful glossitis, diarrhoea, or confusion. Where there is diarrhoea, it may be difficult to be certain whether this is incidental or causative, or whether it is part of a syndrome of general malnutrition or possibly tropical sprue. The problem is simple in Africa since tropical sprue is not found there, whereas in many other tropical regions it may occur on an epidemic scale (page 448). In the South African Bantu there is little malaria, virtually no haemoglobinopathy and no tropical sprue, so that in this group nutritional megaloblastic anaemia is found in a relatively pure form, and occurs particularly in pregnancy and the puerperium. It is obvious, therefore, that in certain areas of the world the differentiation of factors causing megaloblastic anaemia is more easily done than in others. Methods for investigating malabsorption are referred to on page 446.

When splenomegaly is a marked feature, conditions that require consideration include malaria, hepatic cirrhosis, a haemoglobinopathy or bilharziasis. It seems likely that at least in some areas the condition known as idiopathic splenomegaly or big spleen disease does not differ from the syndrome formerly believed to be due to chronic malaria, and it may be that this is in fact the cause. The anaemia is normochromic and there may be leucopenia or thrombocytopenia. As has already been indicated, megaloblastic change may occur if the patient is, in addition, malnourished.

It has to be remembered that certain drugs, including pyrimethamine or anticonvulsants may give rise to megaloblastic anaemia.

Prevention and treatment

It is not possible to give a detailed account of methods of preventing nutritional megaloblastic anaemia since this will depend largely upon dietetic habits and the likelihood of altering these. Certainly avoidance of the overcooking of vegetables and throwing away of water in which they have been boiled will be helpful in a population suffering from folate depletion, but it is realised that it is difficult to persuade people to alter their cooking and eating habits. Where it is feasible, the administration of folic acid in a dosage of 5 mg daily will be more than sufficient to prevent folate deficiency, and where there is evidence that a population suffers from deficiency of vitamin B_{12}, this is one of the few indications for administering vitamin B_{12} orally. It is available in tablets containing 50 μg, and one may be given daily. In some regions a treble depletion of folic acid, vitamin B_{12} and iron may occur, and other deficiencies may also be found. A particular need for folic acid is likely to arise in pregnancy and where possible it is wise to give 5 mg of folic acid daily to all inhabitants of tropical countries who become pregnant. Apart from Europeans and Americans, or their descendants, there is little theoretical risk of encountering a woman with unsuspected pernicious anaemia. Even in countries where this disease is common, it is unlikely to be encountered in a pregnant woman.

The immediate treatment of severe megaloblastic anaemia may involve giving transfusions of packed cells or using exchange transfusion and taking all possible precautions to avoid reactions and not to overload the circulation (page 443). The patient is given 15 mg of folic acid daily, the first dose being injected, and if vitamin B_{12} depletion is suspected or shown to be present, there should also be given hydroxocobalamin or cyanocobalamin. The former preparation is preferable because vitamin B_{12} in this form is better retained in the body. It should be given in a dosage of 1000 μg intramuscularly for a few weeks. Naturally, however, if true Addisonian pernicious anaemia is encountered, treatment must continue

for life, a suitable dose of hydroxocobalamin being 1000 μg every 6 to 8 weeks. When a patient with megaloblastic anaemia responds to folic acid or hydroxocobalamin therapy, iron deficiency may supervene and require treatment.

DISEASES OF SMALL INTESTINE

Methods of investigation

Investigations that are commonly employed include radiography, examination of the stools for occult blood and tests for bacterial infection or parasitic infestation. Other laboratory investigations that may be required if malabsorption is suspected include the following.

Fat absorption tests. It is convenient to estimate the amount of fat in the faeces over two periods of 5 days, and if more than 6 g are passed per day this is considered to indicate malabsorption. This conclusion is based on invstigations carried out on subjects taking a normal European or American diet, and there is a dearth of reports from areas where the diet differs appreciably from this. More complex tests of fat absorption using iodine-labelled triolein and oleic acid have not proved to be particularly helpful.

Other tests of absorption that are commonly used involve the giving of glucose, xylose, or folic acid, or of vitamin B_{12} labelled with radioactive cobalt.

Xylose tolerance test. Many normal subjects have a 'flat' glucose curve in the blood after a 50 g dose, hence the xylose tolerance test is more useful. The patient is given 25 g of d-xylose in 250 ml of water while fasting and the urine collected for 5 hours. An output of more than 4 g occurs normally. An alternative method is to give 5 g of xylose, and the expected output is then not less than 1.2 g. The larger dose is more likely to cause nausea.

Folic acid absorption. Patients with tropical sprue or gluten enteropathy usually have malabsorption of folic acid and this can be demonstrated by one of a variety of methods provided there is available a laboratory in which microbiological assay for folic acid can be performed. One method that is reasonably satisfactory consists of giving 5 mg of folic acid by subcutaneous injection and collecting the urine for 24 hours, then administering 5 mg by mouth and again collecting the urine for 24 hours. The folic acid content of each 24-hour collection is estimated microbiologically. The amount of folic acid must be measured exactly, say with a tuberculin syringe, and in tropical climates the urine should be collected under toluene, put in a refrigerator, and tested as soon as possible. Normally the output after each dose is similar and exceeds 1.5 mg. If the patient is considerably depleted the output of folic acid in each collection is likely to be low. Hence it is better to 'saturate' the body by giving 15 mg of folic acid daily intramuscularly for 4 days before performing the test, and allowing 2 days to elapse thereafter before carrying it out. Under these conditions, if the output of folic acid in the urine after the oral dose is less than 1.5 mg and it is also less than 75 per cent of that after the subcutaneous dose, this is good evidence of malabsorption. The cause may be one of the sprue group of diseases or an organic lesion of the small intestine.

Reference has already been made to estimation of the serum or red cell folate level (page 445) and to the FIGLU test (page 445) in the assessment of folate depletion. In malabsorptive states of the sprue type the serum and red cell folate levels are usually low, and the FIGLU test is usually positive. It appears that histidine is well absorbed even in malabsorptive disorders.

Vitamin B_{12} absorption. Tests for the absorption of vitamin B_{12} necessitate the use of cyanocobalamin labelled with radioactive cobalt, the isotope that gives least radiation to the patient being ^{57}Cobalt. Probably the most satisfactory method involves the use of a whole body counter, but the necessary apparatus is not generally available and the simplest method is to give labelled cyanocobalamin by mouth and flush it out into the urine with an injected dose of 1000 μg of non-labelled cyanocobalamin (Schilling test). The test has not been standardised, but if 0.5 μg of labelled material is given by mouth, the output of radioactivity in the urine will normally exceed 12 per cent of that administered. If there is evidence of malabsorption of vitamin B_{12}, this may indicate lack of intrinsic factor, a disease of the sprue type, organic disease of the lower ileum or its resection, or the presence of blind or stagnant loops in the small intestine. In such areas bacteria may be deviating vitamin B_{12} from the host. If there is doubt about the mechanism, the test may be extended by repeating it, but with the addition of intrinsic factor by mouth: this should correct the malabsorption if lack of intrinsic factor is the problem. If, however, there are bacteria depriving the patient of vitamin B_{12}, the malabsorption should be temporarily corrected by a 4-day course of 250 mg of tetracycline q.i.d., and hence a Schilling test then repeated will probably give normal results. In the sprue group of diseases or where there is organic disease or resection of the terminal ileum, neither intrinsic factor nor tetracycline will correct the malabsorption.

Jejunal biopsy. This has now become a standard method of investigation. It is particularly valuable to have an instrument that will permit multiple biopsies by the oral route, such as the hydraulic tubes developed by Flick, Quinton and Rubin and by Baker and Hughes, but a satisfactory instrument for single biopsies is the capsule devised by Crosby and Kugler. When suction is applied by a syringe to a tube connected to the capsule, a piece of mucosa is first pulled into an aperture in it, and then cut by a small knife edge. The capsule is next withdrawn and it may be possible to examine a portion rapidly with a dissecting microscope. The remainder is prepared for examination under the ordinary light microscope.

The mucosa viewed with the dissecting microscope normally shows finger-like or leaf-shaped processes. In sprue-like disorders they may look like the convolutions of the brain, or the mucosa may have a mosaic-like appearance or even be granular with no evidence of true villi. In normal histological sections, the villi are clearly seen, but in various sprue-like conditions they are broadened and infiltrated with lymphocytes (abnormal villi or partial villous atrophy). Particularly in gluten enteropathy the abnormality may be more profound, no villi being visible. Here the mucosa is flat, but with prominent crypts and marked infiltration with lymphocytes. To this appearance the term 'flat mucosal pattern' is commonly applied. For satisfactory histological examination, serial sectioning is necessary.

Jejunal biopsy should be carried out under fluoroscopic control, and complications are few, but there have been some reports of perforation or of haemorrhage. Occasionally the Crosby capsule knife fails to sever completely a mucosal fragment and the capsule cannot then be withdrawn until the tissue has sloughed. Fortunately, this occurs within a day or two.

ACUTE INFECTIONS OF SMALL INTESTINE

Detailed consideration of such infections will be found in other chapters, and it is sufficient to state here that the conditions affecting the small intestine include typhoid and paratyphoid fever, in which lesions occur in the wall of the small bowel, and salmonella food poisoning in which there may be not only enteritis, but also septicaemia and, particularly in those suffering from a haemoglobinopathy, possible localisation in bones with resulting osteomyelitis.

It should be realised, too, that enteritis can be

caused by *Streptococcus faecalis*, *Staphylococcus aureus* and, occasionally, *Escherichia coli* infection, especially in infants. Such infections may have a high mortality rate.

Infections of the small intestine with protozoa or helminths are considered in earlier sections of this book.

TROPICAL SPRUE

SYNONYMS. The name military sprue is sometimes given by American authors to this disease.

Definition

When diarrhoea with glossitis and megaloblastic anaemia occurs in tropical countries other than Africa, it is commonly considered that the patient is suffering from tropical sprue, but in many instances the symptoms may be due to a combination of infective diarrhoea and nutritional anaemia. Differentiation between this and tropical sprue will be discussed later, but it may be beyond the capabilities of hospitals with small laboratories. Whether true tropical sprue is one condition or a group of disorders is uncertain, occurring as it does either sporadically or on an epidemic scale. It is essentially a disease of malabsorption occurring in the tropics, the causative factors being unknown.

Aetiology

It is true that a sprue-like disorder associated with flattening of the jejunal mucosal cells may occur in monkeys subjected to nutritional deficiency, but most authorities consider that primary malnutrition is not the cause of tropical sprue, and certainly it may occur in persons eating a satisfactory diet. Tropical sprue is similar to gluten enteropathy in its clinical features, but although gluten enteropathy may occur occasionally in dwellers in tropical climates or in those travelling in such areas, it is certain that tropical sprue is not due to or associated with gluten sensitivity and no other article of food has been shown to cause the disease. It has been said that those whose diet is lacking in fat are not likely to have the steatorrhoea of tropical sprue, but, on the other hand, it is possible to have tropical sprue without steatorrhoea. Bacillary dysentery and infections leading to gastroenteritis may precipitate sprue, and epidemics of the former may be followed by apparent epidemics of the latter. However, most infections of the small intestine are short-lived, and tropical sprue is frequently persistent.

No organism has been shown to be causative and yet there may be improvement from antibiotic therapy, particularly with the tetracyclines. Investigations to demonstrate viral agents by tissue culture preparations and suckling mice inoculations from rectal and throat swab material have given negative results. Serum antibody studies have also been negative. It has been suggested that the virus of infective hepatitis or an adenovirus (type 4) may cause changes in the small intestinal mucosal structure and impaired absorptive capacity, but these viruses do not cause tropical sprue.

It seems clear that although tropical sprue occurs sporadically it may also occur on a wide scale in a population, and there are some very odd features about its occurrence. It was seen amongst Indian and British troops in the areas east of the Brahmaputra river during World War II, but African troops in the same area were not affected. In more recent times there have been reports by Baker of a major outbreak of the disease amongst Indians living near Madras, and there is a report from the same area of a family unit in which 16 out of 27 members were affected. In this family, as in many others, the housing conditions were satisfactory, and there had been no known change in the diet or of the source of food or water before the onset of the disease.

In brief, therefore, the cause of tropical sprue is not known, but the fact that it may occur in epidemic form suggests that infection may be responsible in such outbreaks. Since no causative organism has been isolated, a viral agent is suspected, but none has been demonstrated. Although tropical sprue occurs widely in the tropics, this does not apply to Africa, and its virtual non-occurrence in the peoples of that continent may indicate a genetically determined difference in response to the hypothetical infection. The fact that African troops in Burma were not affected during World War II lends support to this view. This, however, is merely supplementing one hypothesis by another one, and it is hoped that before long a more satisfactory solution to the mystery of the causation of tropical sprue will emerge.

Pathology

If a patient has had sprue for any length of time, there will be generalised wasting and atrophic changes throughout the tissues. The bone marrow will show megaloblastic change to have occurred in the red cell precursors if malabsorption of folic acid has continued for more than a few weeks (page 444). Reference has already been made to the value of jejunal biopsy as an aid to diagnosis (page 447), but it should be said that there is evidence to suggest that variation in the normal villous architecture and cell content of the lamina propria occurs in different areas of the world. It has been claimed that in the Far East there may be more round cells in the lamina propria and greater blunting and branching of the normal villi than in Europe or North America. In tropical sprue the flat mucosal pattern is rare, and the abnormality is that of partial villous atrophy. Since, however, there is a range of normality, the appearances of the mucosa in tropical sprue may shade into those of the normal person.

It has been claimed that in malabsorptive states with folic acid deficiency, the jejunal epithelial cells may be enlarged, with foamy nuclei and enlarged nucleoli. This is in accord with similar changes in the epithelial cells of the mouth and stomach, and is due to folate deficiency in cells with a high rate of mitosis.

To complicate the picture, the gut of a patient dying of tropical sprue may be thin and transparent as a result of malnutrition.

Symptomatology

In the full blown picture of tropical sprue the patient has fatty diarrhoea, glossitis, megaloblastic anaemia and loss of weight, the stools being pale, frothy and bulky. He may develop deficiency of potassium, sodium and chloride and there may be evidence of deficiency of riboflavin, giving angular stomatitis and of nicotinic acid, leading to pellagra, with dermatitis, and mental disturbance. Oedema may be a feature and death may ensue from inanition, electrolyte loss or cardiac failure. Some authors consider that there are three stages of the disease, an initial diarrhoeic phase being followed by evidence of a deficiency state and then by anaemia.

Frequently, however, the condition is less clearcut and there may be watery diarrhoea, glossitis or megaloblastic anaemia as the main feature. Colicky abdominal pain may occur. Sometimes the condition supervenes upon infective diarrhoea or bacillary dysentery, making diagnosis particularly difficult. In an epidemic, tropical sprue makes its way from house to house along a street, but in due course, with or without treatment, the condition no longer troubles the area. Numerous deaths may occur before the disease ceases to spread.

The traveller from Europe, North America or elsewhere may develop sprue soon after arriving in a tropical country, and in wartime whole battalions may be severely affected. The condition may clear up spontaneously as soon as the affected individual leaves the tropics, but it may be very persistent or may even develop for the first time some years after the person has returned home. It is probable that at least some of the patients who appeared in the past to be affected in this way were, in fact, suffering from gluten enteropathy unrelated to their tropical experience.

Diagnosis

When a patient in the tropics develops a diarrhoeal disease, it is likely to be because of an infection, but even if the stools are not bulky, the possibility of sprue may require consideration. Diagnosis may be extremely difficult if malnutrition is rife, but the combination of steatorrhoea, glossitis and megaloblastic anaemia makes it likely that the patient suffers from sprue. Jejunal biopsy will be helpful in many instances, and if there is obviously partial villous atrophy, this serves as confirmatory evidence. If there is a flat mucosal pattern the possibility that the condition is gluten enteropathy should be considered.

It should be realised that partial villous atrophy may occur in other disorders, particularly dermatitis herpetiformis. Changes have also been reported in the villi in hookworm infection.

A barium follow-through examination may show small intestinal dilatation, prominent mucosal folds and perhaps flocculation of barium, but an abnormality is not always demonstrable. If laboratory tests can be done it is useful to estimate the fat in the stools and to measure the absorption of xylose, folic acid, and labelled vitamin B_{12}.

Differential diagnosis

The conditions to exclude first are primary malnutrition and an alimentary infection. A large number of diseases may be associated with malabsorption and the more important ones are listed in Table 1. Reference is made to a number of them later.

Treatment

The patient may be acutely ill and require immediate blood transfusion and replacement of electrolytes (see below). If anaemia is severe, exchange transfusion is the safest method of giving blood, since the weakened myocardium may be unable to withstand a sudden increase in blood volume. Alternatively, packed red cells should be given very slowly, 0.5 litres of cells being given in not less than 6 hours, together with 40 mg of frusemide intravenously (page 443).

It is most important to give folic acid, injecting 15 mg daily intramuscularly at first, and thereafter giving it by mouth. This not only improves the blood picture, but also diminishes diarrhoea and improves the general well-being of the patient. It has been shown, too, that folic acid therapy can lead to a rapid improvement in the abnormalities of the jejunal mucosa and lead to improved absorption of various substances.

TABLE 1. *Diseases that may be associated with malabsorption*

Sprue-like disorders	Tropical sprue
	Gluten enteropathy
	Idiopathic steatorrhoea
Organic change in intestinal mucosa of wall of small bowel	Tuberculosis
	Regional enteritis
	Eosinophilic granuloma
	Scleroderma
	Reticuloses
	Carcinoma
	Amyloid disease
	Radiation injury
	Radiomimetic drugs
	Neomycin
Lymphatic obstruction	Whipple's disease
	Intestinal lymphangiectasia
Inadequate absorptive area	Intestinal resection
	Intestinal bypass
Inadequate digestion	Gastric resection
	Pancreatic disease
	Disease of liver or bile ducts
	Intestinal hurry
Altered motility	Vagotomy
Altered flora	Blind or stagnant loops
	Jejunal diverticulosis
	Acute enteritis
	Parasitic infestation
Hormonal	Adrenal insufficiency
	Diabetes mellitus
	Zollinger-Ellison syndrome
Vascular	Mesenteric artery insufficiency
Biochemical disorders	Disaccharidase deficiency
	Cystinuria
	Hypogammaglobulinaemia

Since vitamin B_{12} depletion may also be a feature, it is wise to give injections of 1000 μg of hydroxocobalamin (or cyanocobalamin) intramuscularly weekly in the early stages of treatment. If there is osteomalacia, calciferol (vitamin D) should be injected, 100 000 units being given daily for 2 weeks and then weekly for 2 months, and a calcium preparation given by mouth (e.g. five tablets of calcium Sandoz effervescent daily). Thereafter the serum calcium level should be checked and further X-rays of the bones obtained. Excessive treatment with calciferol may give vitamin D intoxication and lead to deposition of calcium in the kidneys and elsewhere. Ferrous sulphate and multivitamin preparations may have to be given orally.

A method of treatment of tropical sprue that has had some success despite our ignorance of its mode of action is the administration of sulphonamides or wide-spectrum antibiotics by mouth for a period of about 3 weeks. For example, tetracycline may be given in a dose of 250 mg q.i.d., and this may cause haematological improvement, cessation of gastrointestinal symptoms, gain in weight, improvement in the jejunal mucosal appearances and increased absorption of various substances. Whether this is due to the tetracycline acting as an antibiotic on unidentified organisms or whether it makes available folic acid in conjugate form in the food or acts in some entirely different way is uncertain. In any case, folic acid should be given in addition.

When the nutritional state is extremely bad, it may be possible to save life by giving intravenously a hydrolysed casein or amino acid preparation (e.g. Aminosol, Vitrum Ltd., Paines and Byrne, Ltd; Vamin, Paines and Byrne, Ltd.). or administering a fat emulsion in this way (Intralipid, Vitrum Ltd., Paines and Byrne, Ltd.). The instructions given by the makers must be followed carefully.

If the patient is not responding to treatment, it is possible that the diagnosis is incorrect (gluten enteropathy being a possibility), but if deterioration continues, adrenocorticosteroids may give dramatic results. A suitable dose is 60 mg of prednisone daily by mouth for 2 weeks, the dose then being tailed off. Potassium depletion should be prevented during this form of therapy.

If the patient is acutely ill it may be necessary to give potassium salts orally or in an intravenous infusion. Although it is possible to give 10 grams or more of potassium chloride intravenously this is a very dangerous procedure if the serum potassium level cannot be measured, and if there is mixed sodium and potassium depletion at least part of the volume of extracellular fluid should first be restored with sodium containing fluids. If potassium chloride is then given intravenously, 1.5 grams may be given in a litre of isotonic saline over a period of four hours, this being repeated if hypokalaemia persists. Sometimes an ECG pattern is helpful.

Complications that may require treatment include multiple deficiency states, pneumonia and abdominal distension. Sometimes this last is associated with potassium depletion. Bacillary dysentery may complicate tropical sprue, and the patient may also have amoebiasis.

Visitors to the tropics who have been successfully treated for tropical sprue may be able to continue to reside there without suffering a relapse. It has been said that restoration of the normal absorption of vitamin B_{12} should be demonstrated before complete correction of the intestinal lesion can be accepted.

GLUTEN ENTEROPATHY AND IDIOPATHIC STEATORRHOEA

Since these conditions are but rarely seen in the tropics, they will not be considered in detail here.

The condition in infants and children that was formerly named coeliac disease is now known in most instances to be associated with sensitivity to the gluten fraction of wheat protein, and hence the condition in the infant or child is now commonly referred to as gluten enteropathy. Although gluten sensitivity is a major feature, this does not exclude with certainty the possibility that there is an underlying enzyme deficiency in the mucosal cells of the small intestine, but the important feature is that treatment with a gluten-free diet will cause remarkable improvement in absorption and in development of the child. In the disorder there is commonly a flat mucosal pattern, but the rigid exclusion of gluten from the diet will result in the mucosal cells reverting to their normal appearance. A puzzling feature is that although some patients will have to remain on a gluten-free diet indefinitely, this is not always the case.

A similar condition in the adult has had given to it many names, including idiopathic steatorrhoea, non-tropical sprue, primary malabsorptive disease and gluten enteropathy of the adult.

Some patients give a clear history of gluten enteropathy in childhood, but this is by no means invariable, and on occasion the sensitivity is to some other article of food such as milk. The mucosal appearance may be that of partial villous atrophy as in tropical sprue or there may be a flat mucosal pattern. If a rigid gluten-free diet is given there will, in most instances, be recovery with a return of the mucosal appearance to normal. The diagnosis is made by absorption tests, jejunal biopsy and trial of a gluten-free diet. If there is still doubt, a gluten challenge should then be given to see whether deterioration occurs.

In gluten enteropathy of the adult it may be necessary for the diet to be continued indefinitely, but in some instances reversion to normal eating may be possible, and the reason for this is unknown. Apart from the diet and the lack of value of antibiotic therapy, treatment is as for tropical sprue. A patient with gluten enteropathy should avoid travelling in tropical countries because of the difficulty of obtaining the necessary diet and because of the danger of exposure to alimentary infections.

ABDOMINAL TUBERCULOSIS

Of the granulomatous diseases of the small intestine, tuberculosis is the most important. It is rarely seen in many Western countries, but is still common in tropical areas.

Pathology

Tuberculosis of the small intestine may be ulcerative or hyperplastic. The ulcerative form is usually secondary to pulmonary tuberculosis, whereas the hyperplastic type appears to be a primary infection. Each tends to appear first in the ileocaecal region but may become widespread and accompanied by adhesions, exudation into the peritoneal cavity and enlargement of regional lymph glands. In the ulcerative form perforation into the peritoneal cavity may occur, but this may be localised by adhesions. A rectal fistula or perianal abscess sometimes is a complication of abdominal tuberculosis.

In the hyperplastic form of the disease the bowel is thickened and narrowed, so that a mass may form or intestinal obstruction occur.

Clinical features

The ulcerative form of the disease is found particularly in young adults who may or may not have the symptoms and signs of pulmonary tuberculosis. The usual features of tuberculous enteritis are abdominal pain, fever and weight loss. Diarrhoea is frequent, but this may occur in pulmonary tuberculosis without evidence of intestinal involvement. The pain is particularly in the lower abdomen and may be cramp-like in character. Sometimes there is constipation rather than diarrhoea, and intestinal obstruction may occur. Night sweats and amenorrhoea are a common feature and anaemia is likely to develop. A mass may be felt, particularly in the right iliac fossa, but if there has been considerable exudation, the abdomen will be protuberant.

In the hypertrophic form of the disease any of these features may occur, but the finding of a tender mass is more likely, and intestinal obstruction is particularly prone to occur.

If a barium meal with follow-through is done there may be narrowing, dilatation and delay in the emptying of loops, distortion of the caecum or evidence of fistulae between loops. Similar changes may occur in hypertrophic tuberculous enteritis. It is difficult to differentiate between the two on clinical grounds or radiographic appearances, and a chest X-ray should always be taken.

Diagnosis

Reference has already been made to the importance of radiographic studies of the small bowel and chest. The faeces and sputum should be cultured for tubercle bacilli or animal inoculation carried out. If sputum cannot be obtained, gastric washings may be used. It is important to remember that in the tropics where multiple pathology is so common, the finding of tubercle bacilli does not exclude the possibility that abdominal symptoms or signs are due to an unrelated disease such as amoebiasis. A negative tuberculin test suggests that the diagnosis of abdominal tuberculosis is incorrect.

Differential diagnosis

If a patient has features of ulcerative enterocolitis in association with pulmonary tuberculosis, diagnosis may not be difficult, particularly if tubercle bacilli are found in the faeces, but it should be remembered that he may also have amoebic or bacillary dysentery or both. If there is intestinal obstruction and a mass in the right iliac fossa, this may also be due to regional enteritis, an appendix abscess, chronic intussusception, amoebiasis, malignancy of the small bowel or caecum, or actinomycosis.

Treatment

It is important to diagnose and treat pulmonary tuberculosis at an early stage. In the tropics there may be particular problems about persuading patients to undergo full and adequate treatment for pulmonary or abdominal tuberculosis, and if both are present the treatment of the former must take priority.

In the treatment of tuberculous enteritis or peritonitis, chemotherapy should be continued for at least a year. In adults under the age of 40 years, streptomycin 1 g daily, together with sodium PAS 5 g thrice daily and isoniazid 100 mg twice daily should be given. If organisms are obtained and shown to be fully sensitive to all three drugs, one of these may be withdrawn, and if the patient is in hospital it is better to continue

with streptomycin and isoniazid. If he is not in hospital, the streptomycin may be withdrawn. Because of its effects on the vestibule, the dosage of streptomycin should not exceed 0.5 to 0.75 g daily in those over the age of 40. Where it is considered unlikely that the patient will take his treatment an attempt may be made to give twice weekly therapy with streptomycin 1 gram intramuscularly and 15 mg of isoniazid per kg of body weight by mouth.

Where, because of inadequate treatment, the organisms are resistant to these drugs, or if the patient suffers from sensitivity to them, other agents with a certain degree of antituberculous efficiency are cycloserine, 500 mg twice daily by mouth; ethionamide, 500 mg twice daily by mouth; thioacetazone 75 mg twice daily by mouth; pyrazinamide 40 mg/kg/day by mouth with a maximum of 1.5 g twice a day; ethambutol 25 mg per kg daily, this being reduced to 15 mg per kg after 60 days; rifampicin 600 mg daily. The possible adverse reactions to these drugs should be known before they are employed and any contraindications should be noted from the literature that accompanies each drug.

Treatment with one drug alone is unsatisfactory and a variety of regimes have been tried. For example, isoniazid 300 mg daily may be given with thioacetazone 150 mg daily, but it is better to give in addition streptomycin 1 g daily by injection in the first two months. Little is known about possible impairment of absorption of drugs given by mouth to patients with abdominal tuberculosis.

REGIONAL ENTERITIS

SYNONYMS. This is a condition which occurs particularly in the ileum, hence it is frequently referred to as regional ileitis, and as it was first described by Crohn, Ginzburg and Oppenheimer, it is sometimes called Crohn's disease.

Definition

It is a cicatrising inflammatory disease of unknown aetiology which usually commences in the terminal ileum, but may affect the jejunum or colon.

Epidemiology and distribution

The condition occurs both in temperate and tropical regions, but because of confusion with abdominal tuberculosis its true incidence and distribution is uncertain.

Pathology

The terminal ileum is thickened and rigid, and its serosal surface may be obscured by an extension of mesenteric fat and by exudate. The mesentery of the involved area is thickened and oedematous, and contains enlarged lymph glands. There may be fistulae between loops of bowel, or evidence of localised perforation into the mesentery, and the appendix may be buried in the latter.

There is great thickening of all coats of the small intestinal wall, considerable narrowing of the lumen and evidence of mucosal ulceration. This last may also occur proximal to the stenosed area. The extent of involvement of the small intestine is very variable and there may be segmented areas of disease with normal bowel in between. Extension may occur up into the jejunum or beyond the ileocaecal junction into the large intestine, where, again, segmented areas of involvement may be found.

The microscopic appearance is of thickening, particularly of the submucosa, with hyperplasia of lymphatic tissue and oedema from lymphatic obstruction. There may be well defined giant cell systems without caseation and these may occur not only in the submucous and subserous regions, but also in regional lymph glands. Acid-fast bacilli are not to be found. Ulceration of the mucosa is seen and this extends into the submucosa and may give lymphadenitis.

Clinical features

The original description referred to diarrhoea, lower abdominal pain, fever, loss of weight and anaemia. The symptoms depend upon the site of the lesion and its severity and are usually insidious but may be acute. The patient may be troubled only by a bloated feeling with borborygmus and flatulence. Diarrhoea or bouts of pain may eventually lead him to obtain medical advice. The condition may occur at any age, even in childhood, but is commoner in young men or women, being found slightly more often in males.

Intermittent abdominal pain is the commonest feature, and it may be very slight or cramping in nature. The pain may be experienced around the umbilicus or in the lower abdomen and may simulate appendicitis. In time the features may be those of intermittent obstruction with severe cramps and abdominal distension. Sometimes intestinal obstruction is the first evidence of the disease. In some patients there is a steady ache which is commonly felt in the right iliac fossa,

but may occur elsewhere in the abdomen, depending upon the site of the lesion. Back pain can be a feature, particularly if there is extensive mesenteric involvement.

Diarrhoea is usually less severe than in ulcerative colitis, and the stools are soft rather than liquid. Blood and pus are not a feature unless there is enterocolitis, but steatorrhoea may occur because of malabsorption. In some instances there is neither pain nor diarrhoea.

Sometimes these features are followed by the occurrence of perianal or perirectal fistulae, and this may be the first evidence of the disease. A rectovaginal fistula or an ischiorectal abscess may rarely develop, or there may be fistulae between loops of bowel. If operation is performed for suspected appendicitis or for treatment of regional enteritis, the patient may be very much troubled by the development of one or more fistulae opening through the abdominal wall.

Other manifestations that are found include melaena, fever, polyarthritis, iritis or iridocyclitis, electrolyte disturbances, hypoproteinaemia, amyloidosis, retardation of growth, amenorrhoea and anaemia. There may be deficiency of iron, folic acid or vitamin B_{12}. This last is to be expected if the terminal ileum is unable to absorb vitamin B_{12} for a period of many months or years.

On examination of the abdomen the abnormality that is most likely to be encountered is a mass that is relatively fixed and tender and is usually located in the right iliac fossa. Rectal examination may reveal a mass or merely an area of tenderness.

In most tropical countries abdominal tuberculosis is common and regional enteritis is rare. Differentiation between the two is difficult and unless the evidence to the contrary is very good, treatment for tuberculosis should be given.

Diagnosis

The first consideration in diagnosing regional enteritis is to think of the possibility and to avoid laparotomy if possible. A barium meal and follow-through examination should be done, and classically this will give the 'string sign' of incomplete filling in the lower ileum. It should, however, be realised that in the early stages there may be no X-ray abnormality other than rigidity of the ileal wall, and this is difficult to demonstrate. Unexpected fistulae between loops of bowel may be found in some instances. The disease may extend into the caecum and ascending colon, or beyond it.

2 G

Differential diagnosis

If there is a mass in the right iliac fossa this may be due to amoebiasis, tuberculosis, carcinoma, a reticulosis, an appendix abscess, chronic intussusception, or even actinomycosis.

The radiologist may be unable to differentiate between regional enteritis and other causes of narrowing of the small intestine such as tuberculosis, lymphosarcoma, lymphadenoma or carcinoma. On occasion, amoebiasis of the small bowel may be confused with regional ileitis. It may be impossible to differentiate on X-ray evidence between regional enteritis and tuberculosis. The latter tends to affect the colon to a greater extent, the mucosal markings are coarser because of greater ulceration, and the contours are more irregular.

If, when a barium enema is carried out, the caecum is deformed and the terminal ileum cannot be filled because of irritability and spasm, regional enteritis should be considered.

In tropical regions the occurrence of diarrhoea amongst the population is so common and the causes so numerous that it would be unrealistic to suggest that the character of the diarrhoea would be particularly helpful in differential diagnosis. Suffice it to say that a very watery diarrhoea or one with much blood or mucous is unusual in regional enteritis unless the large bowel is involved.

The toxic aspects such as fever and joint pains may simulate malaria, rheumatic fever, subacute endocarditis, undulant fever, acute pulmonary tuberculosis and many other acute diseases.

Treatment

Unfortunately, the results of operation are frequently unsatisfactory and hence medical treatment is continued until the disease becomes inactive, or complications make surgery essential. Sometimes symptoms make life so intolerable that operation is undertaken. There is no specific medical treatment, but sulphasalazine in a dosage of 4 to 8 g daily sometimes gives benefit.

If the condition is acute, bed rest will be necessary, and a diet that is high in protein content and low in roughage should be given. Electrolyte disturbance should be controlled and the infusion of salt-free albumin may be valuable. The giving of multivitamin preparations is particularly relevant to treatment of the disease in the tropics, and vitamin K deficiency may also require attention. If the type of anaemia cannot be elucidated with certainty, it is reasonable to give ferrous sulphate (200 mg t.i.d.) and folic acid (15 mg daily) by mouth together with 1000 μg of hydroxocobalamin or cyanocobalamin intramuscularly weekly at first and monthly thereafter. If there is marked debility, blood transfusion will be helpful. Symptomatic treatment may include the use of codeine, kaolin, propantheline or sedatives.

Prednisone or another corticosteroid may sometimes cause improvement by improving well-being and reducing fever, but the patient is exposed to all the side effects of this form of treatment, perhaps without benefit. However, if an inflamed mass is felt, this may become smaller and less tender if a suitable dose of prednisone (60 mg daily) is given. The danger of perforation, haemorrhage and of exacerbation of symptoms on discontinuing the drug must be borne in mind.

Surgical treatment

This should be staved off as long as possible, since results of surgery are certainly no better than those obtained from medical treatment. If laparotomy is done and the disease found to be present, the abdomen should be closed unless there is obvious need to do something further. Obstruction may necessitate operation as may the formation of an abscess mass after local perforation. Fortunately, acute perforation is unlikely. If a perianal or perirectal fistula develops, local correction is unlikely to succeed, and removal of the primary lesion will be necessary.

If possible, the patient should be prepared for operation by correction of nutritional deficiencies and of electrolyte imbalance. Many surgeons prefer to give antibacterial treatment with a sulphonamide, possibly supplemented by neomycin prior to operation.

Resection of the bowel 12 to 18 inches (30–45 cm) proximal and distal to the limits of the lesion is advisable, but in most instances right hemicolectomy with removal of the requisite area of terminal ileum should be carried out. End-to-end ileocolic anastomosis is ideal, but more difficult to carry out than end-to-side anastomosis. An alternative operation that is possibly less satisfactory is ileotransverse colostomy with exclusion, the closed distal end of the ileum being retained to the abdomen. Such an operation acts by diverting faeces from the affected area. Ileostomy alone is advised only in advanced cases with extensive spread.

Prognosis

The outlook is better in older patients and some times remission occurs or the disease becomes quiéscent, but in the majority of patients it progresses. Medical treatment usually has to give way in time to surgery, and repeated recurrences may necessitate several operations. Fortunately, however, the results of surgery are not always unsatisfactory, and cure may occur.

WHIPPLE'S DISEASE

Definition

This rare condition of unknown aetiology tends to occur in middle or later life. It is a systemic disease which affects particularly the small intestine and its mesentery.

Pathology

The wall of the small intestine is thickened and there are irregular white patches on the serous surface which otherwise is bluish-red. The white patches are dilated lymph vessels laden with fat. The mesentery is thickened and indurated, but differs from that of regional enteritis in that its fat does not embrace the antimesenteric aspect of the serous coat. There are large firm lymph glands in the mesentery and they are porous when cut.

The intestinal villi are distended and if the mucosa is looked at with a magnifying lens they may be seen to be enlarged and club-shaped. In histological sections of the intestinal mucosa obtained at laparotomy or from biopsy by the oral route, there are clear areas of dilated lacteals in the lamina propria. The villi are distorted and distended by these and by so-called 'sickleform particle containing' (SPC) cells. Such cells are possibly derived from primitive reticulum cells and they elaborate an abnormal protein-carbohydrate complex. They have a 'frothy' appearance and occur not only as sickle-form particles, but also in amorphous clumps. They stain a purple-pink with periodic acid Schiff stain.

The SPC cells are found not only in the intestinal wall and mesenteric glands but also in many tissues of the body, including the stomach, large bowel, brain, spleen, heart, adrenal, kidney, peripheral lymph glands and bone marrow.

Clinical features

Because of its varied features the condition may not be diagnosed until it has progressed considerably. The first manifestation is usually pain in large and small joints, with little evidence of swelling or inflammation and this is followed months or years later by vague abdominal symptoms such as nausea, vomiting and cramp-like pains. Diarrhoea is common, but gross steatorrhoea is infrequent. Fever, dyspnoea and cough may occur.

The patient is wasted and may have pigmentation of the skin like that of Addison's disease. Palpable enlargement of peripheral lymph glands, dullness at the base of the lungs from pleural effusion, petechial haemorrhages and cardiac murmurs may be found. The abdomen is distended and doughy, and ill-defined masses may be felt, particularly in the upper abdomen. There may be hypertension.

Diagnosis

This is frequently made only at laparotomy, but jejunal biopsy or biopsy or a peripheral lymph gland may give the diagnosis. If there is X-ray evidence of malabsorption, enlargement of mediastinal glands may give a pointer to the diagnosis.

Treatment

No treatment is known to be of value, but there have been unconfirmed reports of benefit from corticosteroids.

EOSINOPHILIC GRANULOMA

Eosinophilia is common in the tropics and therefore the rare condition of eosinophilic gastroenteritis would be difficult to diagnose. There are believed to be two categories of eosinophilic granuloma.

The first is diffuse eosinophilic gastroenteritis, and it may cause constriction of the antrum or pylorus and segmental narrowing and dilatation of the small intestine. There is eosinophilia and commonly but not invariably a history of allergy particularly of bronchial asthma. Benefit may occur from treatment with adrenocortical steroids.

The second condition is circumscribed eosinophilic-infiltrated granuloma. Here there are demarcated lesions 1 to 12 cm in diameter occurring anywhere in the alimentary tract. The lesions are granulomata involving particularly the submucosa, but sometimes spreading beyond this. There is no evidence of eosinophilia in the peripheral blood and the radiographic appearances suggest a malignant tumour. Diagnosis prior to laparotomy is unlikely, and removal of the area is not usually followed by recurrence. Sometimes the granuloma is polypoid in character.

TUMOURS OF SMALL INTESTINE

Small intestinal tumours may be benign or malignant, and they may occur in the jejunum or ileum.

Benign tumours include adenomas, papillomas, lipomas, fibromas, myomas, fibromyomas, neurogenic tumours, haemangiomas and lymphangiomas. They frequently give rise to no symptoms, but may lead to partial or complete obstruction, cause melaena or initiate an intussusception. The growth may be seen on barium examination of the small bowel.

The condition of gastrointestinal polyposis with mucocutaneous pigmentation is known as the Peutz-Jeghers syndrome, and it is familial, occurring in both sexes. The areas of pigmentation occur particularly on the lips and buccal mucosa, and in dark-skinned races they consist of clearly demarcated small macules. The polyps occur in crops in various areas of the small intestine, and are usually benign. This is one form of hamartoma, the name being derived from a Greek word meaning 'to go wrong'.

Malignant tumours of the small intestine are uncommon and may have clinical features suggesting sprue. They are being reported increasingly as having developed in patients with gluten enteropathy and hence the question of whether this is potentially a premalignant disease requires consideration. There has, however, been no suggestion that tropical sprue may give rise to malignant disease.

The conditions that may develop in the small bowel include carcinoma, lymphosarcoma, reticulum cell sarcoma, lymphadenoma and leiomyosarcoma. There may be wasting, abdominal pain, diarrhoea, steatorrhoea, features of intestinal obstruction, intussusception, malabsorption of vitamins, minerals or other nutrients, megaloblastic or iron deficiency anaemia, melaena or frank bleeding, and sometimes the development of fistulae between loops of bowel. Treatment is unsatisfactory, but palliative surgery may be necessary.

CARCINOID OR ARGENTAFFIN TUMOURS

Argentaffin cells occur throughout the gastrointestinal tract, particularly in the crypts of Lieberkühn and the basilar portions of the gastric glands. Carcinoid tumours, which may arise from the argentaffin cells, are malignant in that metastases occur in regional lymph glands, liver, brain and elsewhere, but they grow very slowly.

Pathology

The majority of the tumours occur in the terminal ileum or appendix. The primary lesions and metastases have a bright yellow colour when cut. It is possible that some carcinoid tumours are benign.

Clinical features

The tumour and its secondary deposits are capable of liberating serotonin (5-hydroxytryptamine), and this leads to attacks of flushing, palpitations, diarrhoea and dyspnoea. Sometimes there are wheezing attacks as in bronchial asthma. Severe shock may occur suddenly, with considerable fall in blood pressure, and death may occur. It is to be noted that these dangerous attacks may occur when a tumour is squeezed on physical examination or during operation.

Pellagrinous features may develop because tryptophan, the precursor of nicotinic acid, is converted excessively to 5-hydroxyindolates.

If there are hepatic metastases, there may be thickening of the cusps of the tricuspid and pulmonary valves and this may lead to pulmonary stenosis and tricuspid stenosis or incompetence. The left side of the heart is seldom affected.

Carcinoid of the small intestine may lead to intussusception, but rarely causes true obstruction or bleeding.

Diagnosis

The bizarre nature of the symptoms should suggest the diagnosis. The urine contains an increased amount of 5-hydroxyindoleacetic acid.

Treatment

The tumour and metastases should be removed, but it must be remembered that there can be multiple primaries. Treatment with nicotinic acid may be required and operation for pulmonary stenosis is sometimes feasible in a suitably equipped centre.

Prognosis

The patient may live for 20 or more years, even if there are metastases.

DISACCHARIDASE DEFICIENCY

The final stages of digestion of sucrose, maltose, isomaltose and lactose are now believed to occur within the brush border of the cells of the small intestinal mucosa, and this requires the presence of the disaccharidases sucrase (invertase), maltase, isomaltase and lactase.

Juvenile forms

Two types of hereditary disaccharide intolerance have been clearly established as occurring in childhood. These may be described as hereditary sucrose intolerance, and hereditary lactose intolerance. The conditions are rare and their importance in tropical areas is uncertain. Even more complex combinations of deficiency states appear to exist.

Aetiology. In hereditary sucrose intolerance there is a deficiency or absence of sucrase activity in the jejunal mucosa, and at the same time, to a lesser extent, a deficiency of isomaltase. This can be shown directly by assaying the disaccharidase content in jejunal biopsy samples. Maltose does not occur in a free state in nature, but is split off from polysaccharides by amylase, and there are probably five different intestinal maltases. Accordingly, although there is intolerance to sucrose, the defect of starch breakdown is less serious.

Hereditary lactose intolerance is very rare, but this, too, can be shown by examination of biopsy samples.

Clinical features. Hereditary sucrose intolerance is inherited as a Mendelian recessive character, and hence there may be a family history. The child fails to thrive and has diarrhoea with acid, fluid stools.

In hereditary lactose intolerance, similar symptoms occur when milk is given.

Diagnosis. Apart from direct measurement of disaccharidases in jejunal biopsy samples, the abnormality may be shown by demonstrating that when the complex sugar (e.g. sucrose) is fed, no rise occurs in the blood glucose level, but if the two monosaccharides (e.g. glucose and fructose) are administered together, the rise does occur. If sucrose and starch are withdrawn from the diet of the child with sucrose intolerance or milk where there is suspected lactose intolerance, then improvement will occur. There is a form of lactose intolerance which is extremely rare and more severe than that referred to above in that lactosuria also occurs since lactose cannot be metabolised in the body.

Prognosis. There is a tendency for improvement with age. Although the inability to digest disaccharides continues, symptoms diminish.

Treatment. The offending sugar must be withheld from the diet, but after the first few years of life less rigid dietary restrictions may be possible. In lactase deficiency, feeding may be of a mixture of sucrose and a soya bean preparation.

Adult forms

The commonest deficiency state in the adult is of lactase, and this is not usually due to persistence of the childhood form. Instead it is an accompaniment of a variety of diseases, possibly because of damage of the jejunal mucosa, with greater depression of lactase than of other enzymes. Moreover, it has been shown that primary lactase deficiency occurs in apparently normal persons of certain races, such as the Baganda and certain other Bantu tribes.

The diseases associated with lactase deficiency in some patients include tropical sprue, kwashiorkor, regional enteritis, infective diarrhoea, gluten enteropathy and cystic fibrosis of the pancreas. It has also been reported after partial gastrectomy and from the use of contraceptive pills. The mechanism in these various conditions is far from being understood.

Clinical features. There may be none, or diarrhoea and abdominal distension may occur from the taking of milk.

Diagnosis. The enzyme deficiency state may be shown directly in biopsy samples, and it may be found that the expected increase in the blood glucose level does not occur when lactose is given. It should be remembered that some patients have milk intolerance without having lactase deficiency.

Treatment. Milk should be withdrawn from the diet, but after a few months the effects of reintroducing it should be tried.

MALABSORPTION FROM PARASITIC INFECTION

The extent to which parasites in the small intestine may cause steatorrhoea is uncertain, but giardiasis or hookworm infection may do this. It is also reported that infection with *Strongyloides stercoralis* may lead to duodenitis and jejunitis with steatorrhoea and wasting together with evidence of malabsorption of iron, xylose and other substances. The features to look for if malabsorption is suspected as being due to *Strongyloides* are persistent vomiting and X-ray changes in the duodenum consisting of mucosal oedema, dilatation and delay in the third part of the loop. Ulcerative duodenitis may also be seen in the radiograph.

MALABSORPTION FOLLOWING ADMINISTRATION
OF NEOMYCIN

When large doses of neomycin (e.g. 4 g t.i.d.) are taken for several days, the patient may develop steatorrhoea and malabsorption of glucose, xylose and vitamin B_{12}. There may be mild changes of partial villous atrophy in the jejunal mucosa.

BLIND OR STAGNANT LOOPS AND FISTULAE

Blind loops of small intestine are usually created by surgical operation, and stagnant areas may be formed in this way or by disease or adhesions. Reference to the formation of fistulae between loops of bowel as a result of disease has been made in various sections of this chapter. The small intestine is normally free of significant numbers of bacteria except in the lower part, but in stagnant areas coliforms and other organisms may proliferate. These do not appear to have toxic effects on the host, but they may lead to steatorrhoea, megaloblastic anaemia and perhaps some depletion of amino acids. The megaloblastic anaemia is due to vitamin B_{12} deficiency and it can be shown that the organisms are capable of removing vitamin B_{12} from a culture medium if they are grown in this under experiment conditions. The investigations that should be carried out include radiography of the small bowel, measurement of stool fats and a Schilling test of vitamin B_{12} absorption which is then repeated after a short course of tetracycline (page 447).

Treatment is by surgery if this is possible, but, if not, the anaemia should be treated by injections of hydroxocobalamin or cyanocobalamin (page 446). The giving of tetracycline or other antibiotics usually has only temporary benefit as the organisms soon develop resistance to this.

DUODENAL DIVERTICULA

The occurrence of diverticula in the duodenum is not very uncommon. These are found particularly on the inner border of the second part and they may be single or multiple. Frequently they are very small, but they may be large enough to contain as much as a litre of fluid. Such diverticula are seldom found in children and appear to develop by herniation of the mucosa and muscularis mucosae through the point of weakness where the biliary and pancreatic ducts enter, or where the blood vessels pass through the muscular coat to reach the submucosa. Duodenal ulceration is probably not a factor and the demonstration of both in the same patient is probably because the X-ray examination has been carried out for the symptoms of an ulcer.

Clinical features

Frequently there are no symptoms from a duodenal diverticulum, but there may be a fullness in the right hypochondrium, the epigastrium or around the umbilicus, made worse by eating a large meal. Sometimes the patient complains of true pain, and this may even be felt in the back. Relief may be obtained by alteration in posture. Occasionally there has been jaundice or pancreatitis, the latter being due to perforation of the diverticulum. Megaloblastic anaemia has been reported, the mechanism being similar to that with blind or stagnant loops.

Treatment

If pain is severe, there may be benefit from the use of propantheline bromide or from a diet as in duodenal ulceration. Postural drainage of the diverticulum may give relief, and guidance as to the best posture may be given by X-ray screening. Megaloblastic anaemia should be treated by giving hydroxocobalamin by injection in a dosage of 1000 μg every 6 weeks. Surgery should be avoided if at all possible, since this may lead to the formation of a duodenal fistula or to injury of the ampulla of Vater.

DIVERTICULA OF JEJUNUM OR ILEUM

These are less common than duodenal diverticula but may be associated with them. They are usually multiple and tend to be on the mesenteric border, appearing where the main blood vessels pierce the bowel wall. Their cause is uncertain, but irregular peristalsis has been said to be a factor. The solitary diverticulum, which may be on the antimesenteric border of the small intestine is believed to be congenital.

Clinical features

There may be vague abdominal discomfort and flatulence, and rarely there are complications such as haemorrhage, rupture, intestinal obstruction, intussusception, volvulus or diverticulitis. On the other hand, there may develop the combination of clinical features sometimes referred to as the 'blind loop syndrome', consisting of megaloblastic anaemia and steatorrhoea similar to what is sometimes found in association with other blind loops, stagnant areas and fistulae. As in such areas, the diverticula are colonised by coliforms and other organisms capable of assimilating vitamin B_{12}.

Treatment

There may be no need for treatment, but if megaloblastic anaemia develops, hydroxocobalamin should be given by injection as above. Sometimes it is possible to resect a large diverticulum or a short section of bowel containing multiple diverticula. If the terminal ileum is removed, this in itself will cause megaloblastic anaemia because the area for absorption of vitamin B_{12} has been eliminated.

MECKEL'S DIVERTICULUM

This is a vestige of the vitelline duct and it occurs on the antimesenteric border of the ileum, at about 15 to 35 inches (40–90 cm) from the ileocaecal junction. It has been said to occur in from 1 to 3 per cent of the population, but seldom gives rise to symptoms. It may contain heterotopic gastric or pancreatic tissue, and the complications that may arise from a Meckel's diverticulum include intestinal obstruction, intussusception, peptic ulceration of heterotopic tissue, the development of a carcinoid tumour, diverticulitis, haemorrhage, and the development of an umbilical fistula. The diverticulitis may simulate appendicitis, and may cause peritonitis. If the diverticulum is inflamed it is unlikely to be demonstrable on X-ray examination. Treatment is by excision.

INTUSSUSCEPTION

Definition

This is the prolapse of a part of the intestine into the lumen of another part distal to it. When this occurs the entering layers are gripped and passed onwards.

Aetiology

The condition occurs particularly in children, but in some areas of Africa it is more common in adults. In children no causative disease is usually found, but inflammatory swelling of collections of lymphoid tissue around the terminal ileum and ileocaecal valve or enlargement of Peyer's patches has been blamed. Alternatively, irregular peristaltic activity may lead to intussusception.

In the adult a localised cause such as a tumour or polyp may be the starting point, and the condition may occur in association with intestinal tuberculosis, inversion of a diverticulum or the presence of an amoeboma. It has been known to occur in the course of typhoid fever. Frequently in African adults no cause is found.

Pathology

The condition may be enteric with one portion of the small intestine passing into another; ileocaecal, with the ileocaecal valve pulling the ileum into the caecum; or ileocolic, with the ileum prolapsing through the ileocaecal valve into the colon. There is also a purely colic variety. The passage of one section of bowel into another may interfere with the blood supply. There may be considerable engorgement and oedema, with oozing of blood and mucus, followed by ulceration and even gangrene.

Clinical features

The condition may be acute or chronic, the acute form being common in children. In the latter variety there is sudden abdominal pain which is severe and colicky, occurring intermittently. Vomiting may occur, particularly at first and it is usually of bile-stained fluid. Diarrhoea is a feature rather than constipation, but the latter may develop later when obstruction becomes complete. At the onset there is frequently a loose motion containing red blood and mucus. Sometimes the intussusceptum passes onward sufficiently to be felt by the examining finger inserted in the rectum. A mass may be felt in the abdomen, but this is less likely in the enteric variety. The palpable tumour varies in size and shape, becoming more distinctly felt during attacks of pain.

In the adult, too, there may be similar symptoms, but sometimes there are long periods of days between attacks of pain. This may mean that the intussusception becomes spontaneously reduced and later recurs. In the tropics the symptoms may be so similar to those of amoebic dysentery that the correct diagnosis is not considered, and, of course, dysentery may coexist.

Diagnosis

The condition may be confused with amoebic or bacillary dysentery, enteric fever, appendicitis, abdominal tuberculosis, Henoch's purpura, mesenteric thrombosis or various causes of intestinal obstruction. In suspected enteric intussusception, Gastrografin may show the invagination, but in the other, commoner, forms, a barium enema will frequently suggest the diagnosis.

Treatment

If operation is carried out in a child, it should preferably be done within 12 hours, because young children do not tolerate intestinal resection well, and the mortality increases with the passage of time. The minimum operative procedure should be employed, reduction rather than resection being done if possible. This is also true in the adult, but if there is a tumour mass, it may be necessary to remove it.

Sometimes it is possible to reduce an intussusception without operation, provided this is attempted at an early stage. An anaesthetic should be given and the procedure carried out by the hydrostatic pressure of an enema combined with manipulation through the abdominal wall. Sometimes the reduction can be carried out successfully with a barium enema, but if there is any uncertainty about the completeness of reduction, this should be followed by operation.

MESENTERIC VASCULAR OCCLUSION

The occlusion of mesenteric arteries or veins leads to peritoneal irritation and small intestinal obstruction. When it occurs, it is usually in those over the age of 40 years, and it is possibly more commonly encountered in males.

Aetiology

Atheroma may lead to obstruction of an artery, or an embolus may cause this. Venous occlusion usually occurs from thrombosis or thrombophlebitis. It may follow pelvic or abdominal operations.

Pathology

It is usually the superior mesenteric vessels that are affected, and whether it is the artery or vein that is occluded, the bowel becomes congested and there is extravasation of blood. The bowel wall becomes engorged and obstruction occurs. Fluid passes into the peritoneal cavity and necrosis may occur in the bowel wall, with possible perforation.

Clinical features

Usually there is severe abdominal pain which may be constant or intermittent. Vomiting is sometimes of faecal character and bloody diarrhoea is likely to occur. The patient may be severely shocked and as peritonitis develops, he becomes very ill, with absent bowel sounds and a board-like abdominal wall.

Diagnosis

The condition has to be considered when acute abdominal pain occurs in those of middle age or older and differentiation is from the various causes of acute abdomen and intestinal obstruction. In sickle cell anaemia, intravascular sickling in the mesenteric vessels may cause pain, vomiting, absent bowel sounds, board-like rigidity and fever.

Treatment

Resection of the affected area is the only treatment likely to succeed, and the outlook is poor.

RESECTION OF SMALL INTESTINE

The small bowel varies considerably in length and it is important that the surgeon should remove as little as possible at operation in order to avoid troublesome after effects. There have been reports of a patient who lived for $3\frac{1}{2}$ years after losing all but 7 inches (18 cm) of his small bowel, and of survival after the duodenum had been anastomosed to the transverse colon, but diarrhoea, steatorrhoea and weight loss may be troublesome when much less heroic surgery is carried out. Moreover, the disease that necessitated resection and the type of operation are important, since the bowel must be healthy and free of blind loops or other abnormalities if it is to function properly. In massive resection, there may be malabsorption of protein, carbohydrate, fat and minerals, while resection or disease of the lower ileum will lead to vitamin B_{12} deficiency and megaloblastic anaemia.

PRIMARY ULCERATION OF SMALL INTESTINE

Ulceration of the small intestine may occur in association with a number of conditions including typhoid fever, tuberculosis, uraemia, parasitic infestation (e.g. *Strongyloides*), Meckel's diverticulum, tumours, gastroenterostomy or the giving of adrenocortical steroids. It is also found in the Zollinger-Ellison syndrome (page 461).

Sometimes, however, there is a primary ulcer of the small intestine unrelated to any such disease. It occurs very infrequently, but is found more often in males, and tends to be in the distal ileum or proximal jejunum. Ulceration of the small intestine may be caused by enteric-coated preparations of potassium chloride.

Clinical features

There may be cramp-like abdominal pain and vomiting, suggesting intermittent obstruction, or more persistent pain occurring after meals and possibly radiating to the back. Bleeding or perforation may occur.

Diagnosis

Occasionally an ulcer niche and distortion of the X-ray pattern may be seen on barium examination of the small bowel, or partial obstruction may occur and be found on barium examination.

In ulceration of the upper jejunum, it is most important to realise that this is likely to be associated with a non-beta cell islet tumour of the pancreas (Zollinger-Ellison syndrome).

Treatment

It is usually necessary to resect the affected segment.

ZOLLINGER-ELLISON SYNDROME

Definition

This is a syndrome of peptic ulceration of the jejunum associated with non-insulin producing islet cell tumours of the pancreas. The ulcers may be multiple, involving particularly the distal third of the duodenum and the proximal jejunum.

Pathology

There is hyperplasia of gastric glands with a marked increase in parietal cell mass, and these glands appear to secrete at their maximal rates even in the basal state. The normal volume of gastric juice is about 800 ml in 24 hours, but in this condition it may be from 4 to 18 litres. The acid concentration is greatly increased. The tumours of the pancreas may be malignant, with a tendency to spread locally or to distant organs. Gastrin-like activity has been demonstrated in extracts of the pancreatic tumours and of their metastases. In some instances there is evidence of multiple endocrine adenomas, the pituitary and parathyroids also being affected.

Clinical features

The patient may have symptoms of abdominal pain as in peptic ulceration, and there may be severe watery diarrhoea or steatorrhoea with or without symptoms suggesting peptic ulceration. In some cases the condition leads to recurrent ulceration, perforation or haemorrhage after an operation for a duodenal ulcer. In other instances it is noticed that a patient being investigated for a possible duodenal ulcer has marked evidence of gastric hypersecretion and acidity. Some patients have clinical evidence of hyperactivity in other endocrine glands such as the pituitary or parathyroids.

Diagnosis

The above features, particularly the gastric hypersecretion and acidity, should draw attention to this possible diagnosis. A barium meal examination may show coarse mucosal folds in the duodenum, and multiple ulcers may be seen. The diagnosis will only be made with certainty at laparotomy when the hyperplasia of pancreatic islet tissue or presence of non-beta cell tumours is demonstrated.

Treatment

Surgical treatment is essential but unsatisfactory. Total gastrectomy and hemipancreatectomy may be necessary.

Prognosis

The patient may die from the complications of ulceration or may have renal tubular degeneration secondary to the diarrhoea and potassium depletion. At operation all gastric tissue must be removed, and if the correct diagnosis is not made until pancreatic biopsy specimens have been examined after operation, it will be necessary for a second operation to be performed.

PROTEIN-LOSING GASTROENTEROPATHY

Albumin and other plasma proteins, except gamma globulin, are synthesised in the liver and eventually they are to a considerable extent secreted into the stomach or intestine. Digestion to amino acids occurs, and these are reabsorbed. If the rate of loss of albumin into the alimentary tract exceeds the ability of the liver to synthesise it, hypoalbuminaemia occurs.

It is obvious that in certain inflammatory conditions such as acute gastroenteritis, regional enteritis or ulcerative colitis there may be excessive protein loss into the gut, but modern techniques that have been developed to study the metabolism of albumin have revealed that in a number of diseases there is excessive loss into the gut. These pathological conditions include Menetrier's disease in which there is giant hypertrophy of the gastric mucosa and intestinal lymphangiectasia which is referred to below. Hypoalbuminaemia, because of increased protein loss into the gut, may also be found in some patients with idiopathic steatorrhoea or gluten enteropathy, in congestive heart failure, in Whipple's disease and in malignant disease of the stomach or small intestine.

Intestinal lymphangiectasia

This is a rare disease occurring in either sex and usually manifesting itself before the age of 30 years. The cause is unknown but it may be familial, indicating that at least in some instances there is a genetic fault. The main features are oedema and diarrhoea with low serum albumin and gamma globulin levels. If the latter is very low, there may be repeated infections. Steatorrhoea may occur.

The serosal lymphatic vessels are dilated and yellow nodules may be seen when the small intestine is examined. The villi are broadened and hence the mucosal surface may appear pebbly. If jejunal biopsy is carried out, the lymph vessels of the mucosa and submucosa are seen to be dilated and the dilated channels may contain foamy macrophages which differ from those of Whipple's disease in that they do not take up the periodic acid Schiff stain. A barium X-ray of the small intestine may show thickening and coarsening of the jejunal folds.

Demonstration of excessive protein loss into the small intestine involves such techniques as the intravenous administration of ^{131}Iodine-labelled polyvinylpyrrolidone with estimation of radioactivity in the faeces.

There is no satisfactory treatment for this condition.

PNEUMATOSIS CYSTOIDES INTESTINALIS

This is a very uncommon disorder in which there are multiple gas-filled cysts in the wall of the gastrointestinal tract. The cause is unknown in many cases, but the condition may occur in appendicitis, tuberculous enteritis, regional enteritis or ulcerative colitis, and possibly in amoebic or bacillary dysentery. There may be abdominal distension, pain, diarrhoea or features of partial intestinal obstruction. On X-ray examination of the abdomen there may be seen to be groups of radiotranslucent areas along the contours of the small and large intestine and the air may extend under the diaphragm and even into the mediastinum.

No treatment is available other than for any underlying disease, but the cysts may disappear spontaneously.

FURTHER READING

ADAMS, E. B. and HIFT, W. (1962) Pernicious anaemia among Africans and Indians in Durban. An investigation of 25 patients with megaloblastic anaemia and achlorhydria. *E. Afr. med. J.*, **39**, 172.

AQUINAS. M., ALLEN, W. G. L., HORSFALL, P. A. L., JENKINS, P. K., HUNG-YAN, W., GIRLING, D., TALL, R. and FOX, W. (1972) Adverse reactions to daily and intermittent rifampicin regimens for pulmonary tuberculosis in Hong Kong. *Brit. med. J.*, **1**, 765.

BAKER, S. J. (1972) Tropical sprue. *Brit. med. Bull.*, **28**, 87.

BAKER, S. J., MATHAN, V. I. and JOSEPH, I. (1962) *Amer. J. dig. Dis.*, **7**, 959.

BANWELL, J. G. and GORBACH, S. L. (1969) Tropical sprue. *Gut*, **10**, 328

BERRY, C. G. (1955) Anaemia of pregnancy in Africans of Lagos. *Brit. med. J.*, **2**, 819.

BJORN-RASMUSSEN, E., HALLBERG, L. and WALKER, R. B. (1972) Food iron absorption in man. 1. Isotopic exchange between food iron and inorganic iron salt added to food; studies on maize, wheat and eggs. *Amer. J. clin. Nutr.*, **25**, 312.

BOLEY, S. J., SCHWARTZ, S. S. and WILLIAMS, L. F. (1971) *Vascular Disorders of the Intestine*, 1st edn. London Butterworth.

BOTHWELL, T. H. (1964) Iron overload in the Bantu. In *Iron Metabolism*, p. 362. A Ciba Symposium, ed Gross, F., Naegeli, S. R. and Philips, H. D. Berlin: Springer.

BUSSEY, H. J. R. (1970) Progress report: gastrointestinal polyposis. *Gut*, **11**, 970.

CHATTERJEA, J. B. (1964) Some aspects of iron deficiency anaemia in India. In *Iron Metabolism*, p. 219. A Ciba Symposium, ed Gross, F., Naegeli, S. R. and Philips, H. D. Berlin: Springer.

DAWSON, A. M. (1971) *Intestinal absorption and its derangements*, 1st edn, published by *British Medical Journal*.

DAWSON, I. (1969) Hamartomas in the alimentary tract. *Gut*, **10**, 691.

DOIG, A. and GIRDWOOD, R. H. (1960) The absorption of folic acid and labelled cyanocobalamin in intestinal malabsorption. *Quart. J. Med.*, **29**, 333.

DUDRICK, S. J. and RUBERG, R. L. (1971) Principles and practice of parenteral nutrition. *Gastroenterology*, **61**, 901.

DUTZ, W, ASVADI, S., SADRI, S. and KOHOUT, E. (1971) intestinal lymphoma and sprue: a systemic approach. *Gut*, **12**, 804.

EVANS, N., FARROW, L. J., HARDING, A. and STEWART, J. S. (1970) New techniques for speeding small intestinal biopsy. *Gut*, **11**, 88.

FLEMING, A. F., ALLAN, N. C. and STENHOUSE, N. B. (1969) Folate activity, vitamin B_{12} concentration and megaloblastic erythropoiesis in anaemic pregnant Nigerians. *Amer. J. clin. Nutr.*, **22**, 755.

FRAZER, A. C. (1968) *Malabsorption Syndromes*. London: Heinemann.

FULLERTON, W. I. and TURNER, A. G. (1962) Exchange transfusion in treatment of severe anaemia in pregnancy. *Lancet*, **1**, 75

GIANNELLA, R. A., BROITMAN, S. A. and ZAMCHECK, N. (1972) Competition between bacteria and intrinsic factor for vitamin B_{12}: implications for vitamin B_{12} malabsorption in intestinal bacterial overgrowth. *Gastroenterology*, **62**, 255.

GILAT, T., KUHN, R., GELMAN, E. and MIZRAHY, O. (1970) Lactase deficiency in Jewish communities in Israel. *Amer. J. Dis.*, **15**, 895.

GIRDWOOD, R. H. (1948) Anaemia and marasmus in Indian troops on active service. *Trans. roy. Soc. trop. Med. Hyg.*, **42**, 65.

GIRDWOOD, R. H. (1956) The megaloblastic anaemias. *Quart. J. Med.*, **25**, 87.

GIRDWOOD, R. H. (1970) Some considerations of the sprue syndrome. In *Diseases of the Gastrointestinal Tract*, p. 65. Proceedings of a Boerhaave Course, ed Goslings, W. R. O. Leiden: Leiden University Press.

GIRDWOOD, R. H. (1972) Drug induced megaloblastic anaemia. In *Blood Disorders due to Drugs and Other Agents*, 1st edn. ed Girdwood, R. H. Amsterdam: Excerpta Medica.

GIRDWOOD, R. H. and SMITH, A. N. (eds) (1969) *Malabsorption*, University of Edinburgh Pfizer Medical Monographs, University of Edinburgh Press.

GRACEY, M. (1971) Intestinal absorption in the contaminated small bowel syndrome. *Gut*, **12**, 403.

GRAHAME-SMITH, D. G. (1970) Progress report: the carcinoid syndrome. *Gut*, **11**, 189.

GRAY, G. M. and COOPER, L. H. (1971) Protein digestion and absorption. *Gastroenterology*, **61**, 535.

GREGORY, R. A., TRACY, H. J., AGARWAL, K. L., and GROSSMAN, M. I. (1969) Aminoacid constitution of two gastrins isolated from Zollinger-Ellison tumour tissue. *Gut*, **10**, 603.

HALLBERG, L., HARWERTH, H. G. and VANOTTI, A. (eds) (1970) *Iron Deficiency—Pathogenesis, Clinical Aspects, Therapy*. 1st edn. London and New York: Academic Press.

HALSTED, C. H., SHEIR, S., SOURIAL, N. and PATWARDHAN, V. N. (1969) Small intestinal structure and absorption in Egypt: influence of parasitism and pellagra. *Amer. J. clin. Nutr.*, **22**, 744.

HARRISON, K. A. (1968) Anaemia in pregnancy: ethacrynic acid in blood transfusion; effects on plasma volume and urine in grossly anaemic women. *Brit. med. J.*, **4**, 84.

HOFFBRAND, A. V., TABAQCHALI, S., BOOTH, C. C. and MOLLIN, D. L. (1971) Small intestinal bacterial flora and folate status in gastrointestinal diseases. *Gut*, **12**, 27.

KLIPSTEIN, F. A. (ed) (1968) Symposium: Malabsorption and malnutrition in the tropics. Proceedings of a symposium held in Port-au-Prince. *Amer. J. clin. Nutr.*, **9**, 937.

KOTHARI, B. V. and BHENDE, Y. M. (1952) Nutritional megaloblastic anaemia of pregnancy. A study of 100 cases. *Indian J. med. Res.*, **40**, 387.

LOWENTHAL, M. N., O'RIORDAN, E. C. and HUTT, M. S. R. (1971) Tropical splenomegaly syndrome in Zambia: further observations and effects of cycloguanil and proguanil. *Brit. med. J.*, **1**, 429.

MARKS, J., and SHUSTER, S. (1971) Progress report: intestinal malabsorption and the skin. *Gut*, **12**, 938.

METZ, J., BRANDT, V. and STEVENS, K. (1962) Vitamin B_{12} and megaloblastic anaemia in South African Bantu. *Brit. med. J.*, **1**, 24.

MOUNTAIN, J. C. (1970) Cutaneous ulceration in Crohn's disease. *Gut*, **11**, 18.

OJO, O. A. (1965) The pattern of anaemia in Western Nigeria. *J. trop. Med. Hyg.*, **68**, 32.

OLINER, H. L. and HELLER, P. (1959) Megaloblastic erythropoiesis and acquired haemolysis in sickle cell anaemia. *New Engl. J. Med.*, **261**, 19.

PATWARDHAN, V. N., FARID, Z., DARBY, W. J., WOODRUFF, C. and FINCH, C. A. (1969) Symposium: Nutritional anaemias. *Amer. J. clin. Nutr.*, **22**, 495.

PEARSON, H. A. and COBB, W. T. (1964) Folic acid studies in sickle cell anaemia. *J. Lab. clin. Med.*, **64**, 913.

PETERS, T. J. (1970) Progress report: intestinal peptidases. *Gut*, **11**, 720.

RUSSELL, B. A. S. (1941) Macrocytic anaemia in pregnant women on the Gold Coast. *Lancet*, **2**, 792.

SAIDI, F. (1969) The high incidence of intestinal volvulus in Iran. *Gut*, **10**, 838.

SCHOFIELD, F. D. (1957) Aspects of nutritional anaemia in pregnancy in Gambia. *Trans. roy. Soc. trop. Med. Hyg.*, **51**, 221.

SHALDON, S. (1961) Megaloblastic erythropoiesis associated with sickle cell anaemia. *Brit. med. J.*, **1**, 640.

STEFANINI, M. (1948) Clinical features and pathogeneis of tropical sprue. *Medicine*, **27,** 379.

STEVENS, K., METZ, J., BRANDT, V. and VAN BROCKHUIZEN, L. (1962) Serum vitamin B_{12}, folic acid and urinary formiminoglutamic acid in megaloblastic anaemia in South African Bantu adults. *E. Afr. med. J.*, **39,** 222.

TANDON, B. N. SARAYA, A. K., RAMACHANDRAN, K. and SAMA, S. K. (1969) Relationship of anaemia and hypoproteinaemia to the functional and structural changes in the small bowel in hookworm disease. *Gut*, **10,** 360.

WATSON-WILLIAMS, E. J. (1965) The role of folic acid in the treatment of sickle cell disease. In *Abnormal Haemoglobins in Africa*, p. 435. A C.I.O.M.S. Symposium, ed Jon xs, J. H. P. Oxford and Edinburgh: Blackwell Scientific Publications.

WILLIAMS, P. O. (ed) (1971) *Tropical Sprue and Megaloblastic Anaemia.* (*Wellcome Trust Collaborative Study, 1961-1969*). Edinburgh and London: Churchill Livingstone.

WILSON, F. A. and DIETSCHY, J. M. (1971) Differential diagnostic approach to clinical problems of malabsorption. *Gastroenterology*, **61,** 911.

WOODRUFF, A. W. (1951) Anaemia of pregnancy among Africans in Nigeria. *Brit. med. J.*, **2,** 1415.

WOODRUFF, A. W. (1972) Recent work on anaemia in the tropics. *Brit. med. Bull.*, **28,** 92.

30
Haemoglobinopathies

Diseases caused by either a depression of haemoglobin formation (the thalassaemia syndromes) or the production of an abnormal haemoglobin molecule give rise to health problems of immense dimensions. About 1 per cent of children born in equatorial Africa will suffer from sickle cell anaemia and it has been calculated that the annual mortality from this disease in Africa alone is 80 000. The thalassaemias are probably responsible throughout the world for as many as 100 000 deaths in infancy or childhood per annum.

The massive problems involved are only just being realised. As public health programmes result in a steady diminution in childhood mortality from other causes, the enormous numbers of these deaths from the haemoglobinopathies and thalassaemia are becoming apparent. In England of 100 000 children born, 5 are expected to die of leukaemia in childhood. In Nigeria of 100 000 children born, 1000 will suffer from sickle cell anaemia and at present nearly all of them will be dead by adolescence.

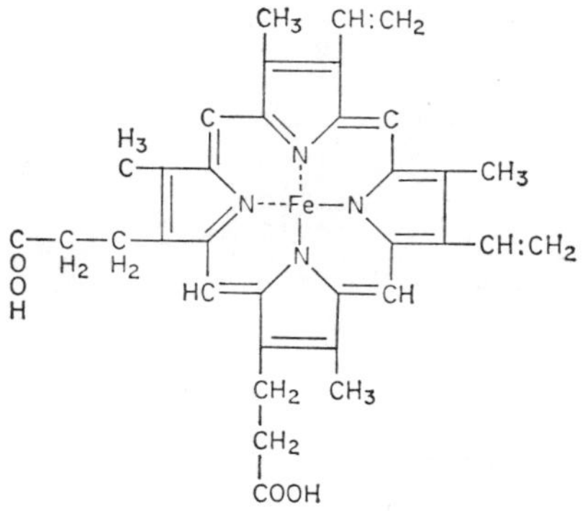

FIG. 30.1. *Haem is a metal-porphyrin complex. The exact nature of the atomic linkages between the iron atom, and its surrounding porphyrin ring and the globin is not clearly understood. The iron atom is attached to the globin by two histidine residues in such a way that molecular oxygen can be inserted between one of the histidine residues and the iron.*

Even the establishment of adequate diagnostic facilities will cause technical problems in the developing countries. However, these figures should demonstrate that the haemoglobinopathies must in the future become an increasingly important group of diseases.

STRUCTURE OF HAEMOGLOBIN

The haemoglobins are a group of related proteins (globins) to each of which the same prosthetic group, haem, is attached. The essential property of haemoglobin, which enables it to function as a respiratory pigment, is its ability to carry molecular oxygen.

Haem

The iron atom at the centre of the haem (Fig. 30.1) is normally in the ferrous state (Fe^{++}). When the oxygen pressure is high, an oxygen molecule becomes attached to this ferrous atom to form oxyhaemoglobin. This process is called *oxygenation*. The oxygen molecule is subsequently released when the pressure of oxygen falls. If at any time the iron atom becomes permanently *oxidised* to the ferric form (Fe^{+++}) the 'haem' becomes 'haematin' and the haemoglobin is converted to methaemoglobin. Methaemoglobin is unable to carry molecular oxygen and therefore cannot act as a respiratory pigment.

Previously it had been assumed that the iron atom of haemoglobin is present permanently in the ferrous form, even during oxygenation ($Fe^{++} + O_2 \rightarrow Fe^{++}O_2$). It is now thought, though not yet conclusively proved, that, in the absence of water, O_2 may in fact exchange an electron with the ferrous atom and thereby convert it temporarily into a ferric atom

$$(Fe^{++} + O_2 \rightarrow Fe^{++}O_2^-).$$

Before the now negatively charged oxygen can leave the haemoglobin molecule, it must return its electron to the iron atom and thereby leave it again in its ferrous state. It is reasonable to

This chapter first appeared in Woodruff, A. W. ed. (1970), *Alimentary and Haematological Aspects of Tropical Disease*, London: Edward Arnold Ltd., and is reproduced here by kind permission of the publishers.

465

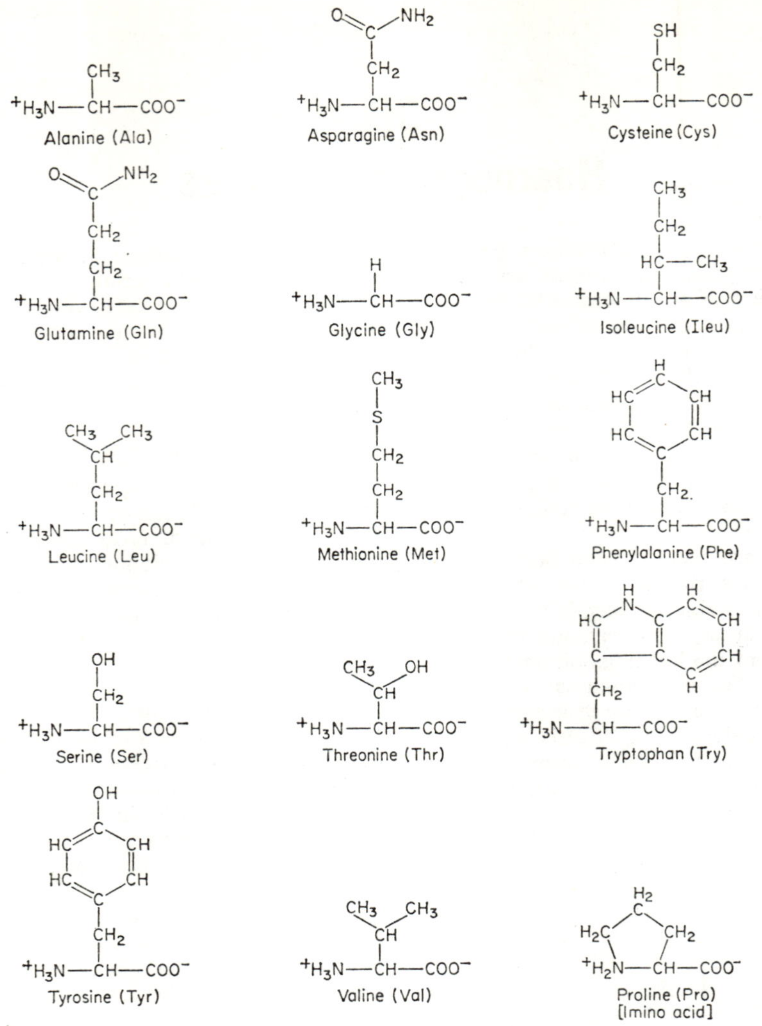

Alanine (Ala)

Asparagine (Asn)

Cysteine (Cys)

Glutamine (Gln)

Glycine (Gly)

Isoleucine (Ileu)

Leucine (Leu)

Methionine (Met)

Phenylalanine (Phe)

Serine (Ser)

Threonine (Thr)

Tryptophan (Try)

Tyrosine (Tyr)

Valine (Val)

Proline (Pro)
[Imino acid]

Fig. 30.2. *Amino acids with uncharged side chains.*

assume that it can only do this if water molecules are excluded from the region of the iron atom. The iron atom must therefore remain isolated from the watery environment of the haemoglobin molecule to prevent its permanent conversion to the ferric state. If this conversion were to occur methaemoglobin would be formed and no further oxygen molecules could be accepted by the iron atom.

Oxidation

Ferrous $\rightarrow$ Ferric
Fe^{++} $\rightarrow$ $Fe^{+++} + H_2O$
Haemoglobin $\rightarrow$ Methaemoglobin

Oxygenation

Ferrous $\rightarrow$ Ferric O_2
Fe^{++} $\rightarrow$ $Fe^{+++}O$
Haemoglobin $\rightarrow$ Oxyhaemoglobin

The manner in which water is normally excluded from the region of the iron atom and what happens when the mechanism for its exclusion breaks down are described on page 470.

Globin

Globin is a protein which is entirely composed of amino acids. The structure of any protein can conveniently be considered under the headings of *primary, secondary, tertiary* and *quaternary structures.*

Amino acids. All amino acids have the basic structure:

$$NH_2-CH-COOH \quad \text{or} \quad NH_3^--CH-COO-$$

They differ from each other only in their side chains (R). Proline is an exception because this particular 'amino acid' has a cyclical structure, and the peptide bond is formed with an NH_2^+ group (Fig. 30.2). Proline is therefore strictly an

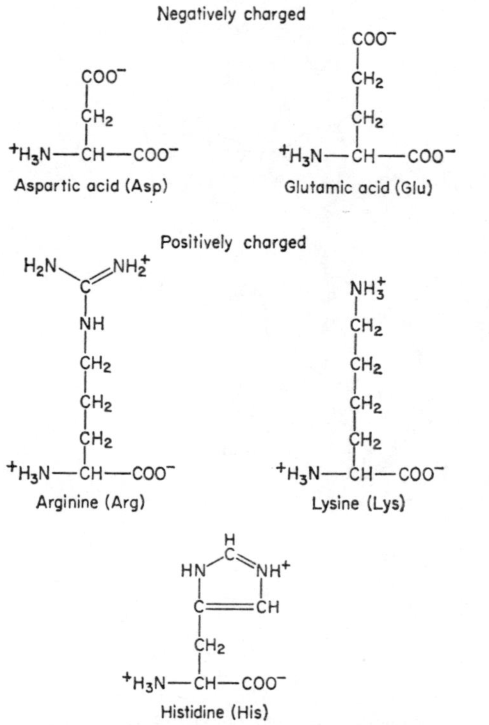

Negatively charged

Aspartic acid (Asp)

Glutamic acid (Glu)

Positively charged

Arginine (Arg)

Lysine (Lys)

Histidine (His)

FIG. 30.3. *Amino acids with charged side chains. These charged amino acids tend to point externally, thereby making the haemoglobin molecule soluble. A highly charged amino acid inserted into the centre of the haemoglobin molecule would result in a disturbance likely to disrupt the molecule. Such a mutation would be lethal. Note that histidine binds the iron to the globin.*

amino acid. The amino acids may be divided into those where the side chains are uncharged or poorly charged (Fig. 30.2) and those where the side chains are charged (Fig. 30.3).

Peptide link. The peptide link or bond is formed by the elimination of water between neighbouring

amino acids. When a polypeptide chain is formed there will be a free amino group at one end and a free carboxyl group at the other end of the chain (Fig. 30.4). The final charge carried by the polypeptide chain will depend upon the charges on the

Alanyl   Aspartyl   Valyl

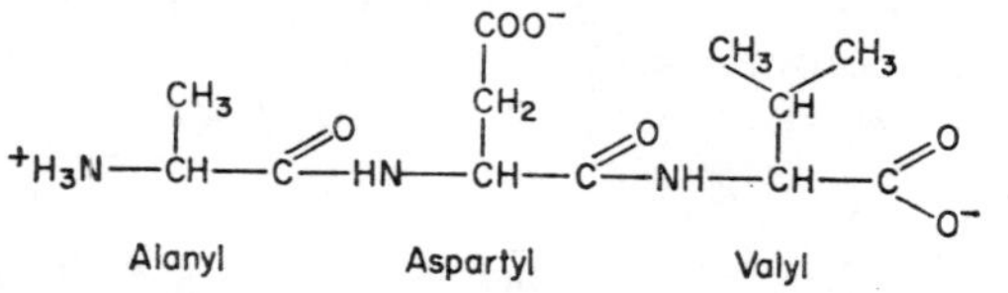

FIG. 30.4. *Peptide bond formation between three amino acids. Note the negative charge imparted to the peptide chain by the aspartyl side chain. The positive charge given by the NH_3^+ at the commencement of the peptide chain is cancelled by the negative charge given by the*

$$C \overset{O}{\underset{O^-}{\diagdown}} \quad \text{at its termination.}$$

side chains of the amino acids in Fig. 30.3. Once an amino acid has been incorporated into a peptide chain, it should strictly be referred to as an amino acid residue. It is convenient to name these by a form of shorthand, e.g. glutamyl for a glutamic acid residue or lysyl for a lysine residue or Glu or Lys (see Figs. 30.2 and 30.3).

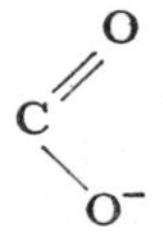

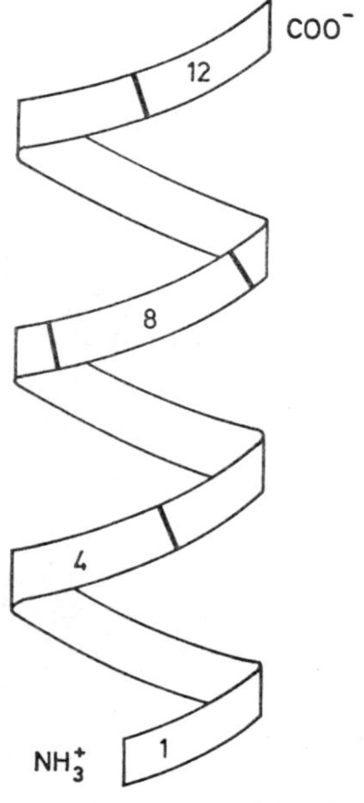

FIG. 30.5. *An α-helix. 3.7 amino acids complete each turn. Note the numbering of a polypeptide chain commences at the free amino end. The α-helix forms a rigid tube and gives the molecule a stable structure.*

Primary structure. If polypeptide chains were constructed from only one amino acid, the only variable factor would be their length. The variability of the side chains of the amino acids, together with the highly specific order in which they are introduced into a polypeptide chain, enables innumerable different protein molecules to be specifically constructed. A polypeptide chain may be likened to a paper chain constructed from

mutation of this gene may lead to an alteration of one amino acid in the total amino acid sequence. Such an amino acid substitution in the case of the polypeptide chains in haemoglobin gives rise to a haemoglobin variant.

Secondary structure. In order to gain molecular stability the amino acids are not just joined together in a straight line, but form a coil, shaped like a spring—the α-helix (Fig. 30.5). The turn of

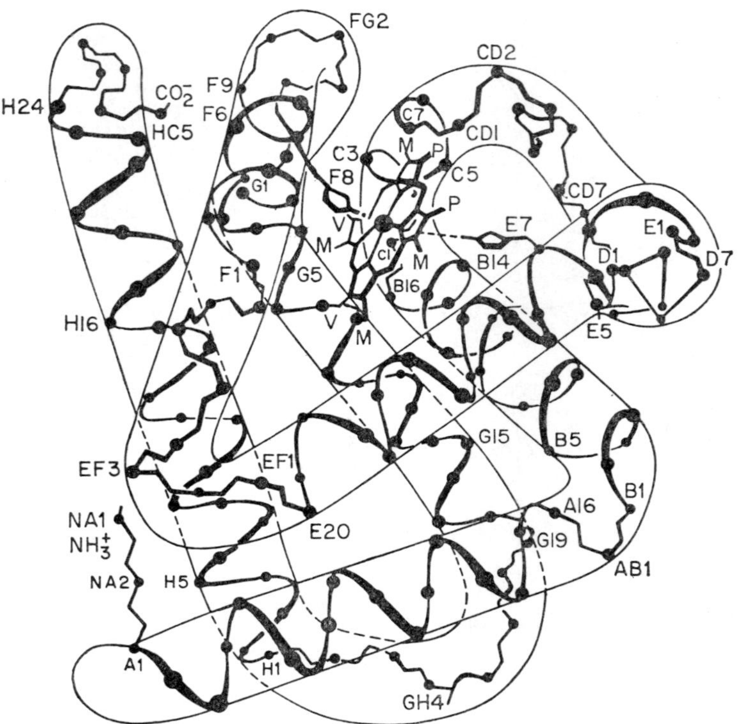

FIG. 30.6. *Figure to show that about 80 per cent of amino acids in myoglobin are in a helical structure. The helical parts are labelled with a letter. Non-helical parts are labelled with two letters, one the preceding and the other subsequent helical portion (e.g. A1→A16 = helical; EF1→EF8 = non-helical). Note the haem group between the two histidyls E7 and F8.* (From Dickerson, R. E., 1954. *The Proteins*, Vol. II, ed. Hans Neurath, p. 364. New York: Academic Press.)

gummed strips of about twenty different colours, each colour representing an amino acid. The probability of making two identical chains by random selection of colours would be infinitesimal.

The specific amino acid sequence of each individual polypeptide chain is called its primary structure. This amino acid sequence is controlled during manufacture by the gene responsible for producing that particular polypeptide chain. A

the helix may be right- or left-handed but the right-handed one appears to be the more stable and is found in many naturally occurring proteins.

In a protein not all of the amino acids are in the form of an α-helix; for instance, in myoglobin about 80 per cent of the amino acid residues in the polypeptide chain are arranged in helical segments. The remaining 20 per cent connect the helical segments together without themselves being coiled (Fig. 30.6).

Tertiary structure. The helix (the secondary structure of the protein) is a rigid, hollow, straight tube. Long, straight polypeptide chains occur in fibrous proteins, but in order to arrive at the

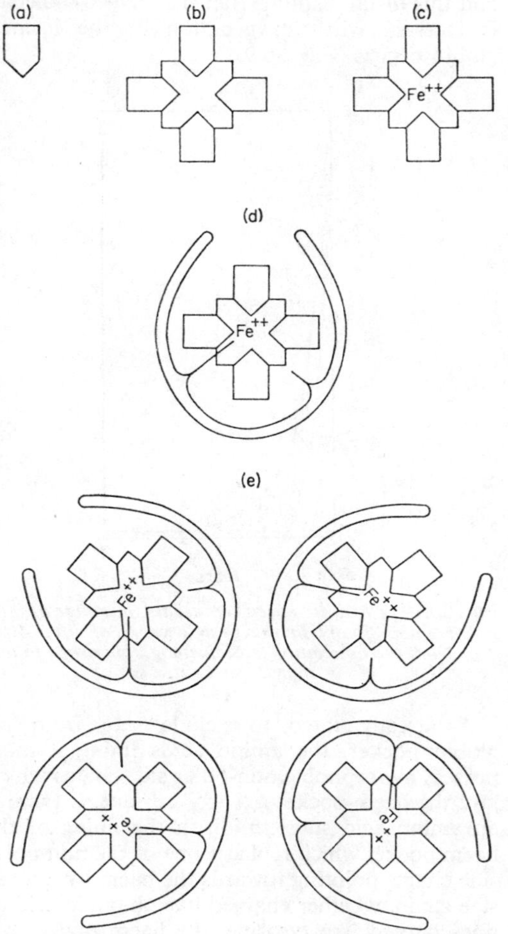

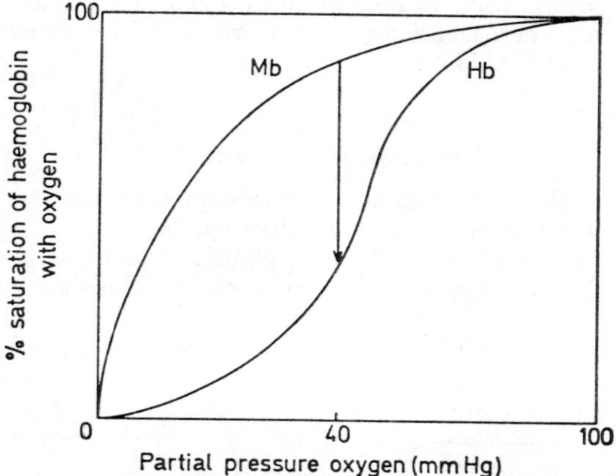

FIG. 30.8. *The oxygen dissociation curve of myoglobin (Mb) which is hyperbolic in shape and haemoglobin (Hb) which is sigmoid in shape. The length of the arrow represents the increased release of oxygen from haemoglobin when the oxygen pressure falls from 100 to 40 mm Hg.*

FIG. 30.7. *Steps in the development of haemoglobin. (a) Pyrrole unit; (b) porphyrin ring; (c) haem; (d) haem–globin complex (e.g. myoglobin); (e) four haem-globin units forming one complex molecule (e.g. haemoglobin). The units of haemoglobin are not in a fixed relationship to each other. On oxygenation, they move closer together and when the haemoglobin is reduced, they move farther apart. This has been likened by Perutz to paradoxical breathing. (In* Man's Haemoglobins, *North-Holland Publishing Company.)*

turns of the helix are a result of that specific amino acid sequence, the shape of the molecule being maintained by bonding of the side chains of amino acids lying in adjacent helices. If these bonds break down and the folding of the chain becomes distorted, the protein will become denatured. The presence of the haem gives the haem–globin unit stability, globin being easily denatured if the haem is allowed to escape. Some amino acid substitutions, particularly in the region of the haem group, result in an unstable haemoglobin molecule, which is easily denatured. These amino acid substitutions weaken the link between the globin and the porphyrin ring of the haem. After the haem has separated from the globin, the globin denatures.

Quaternary structure. Myoglobin exists as a single polypeptide chain in which one haem group is embedded (Fig. 30.6). The haemoglobin molecule consists of a combination of haem–polypeptide chain units of roughly similar shape (Fig. 30.7). The subunits do not form a fixed relationship with each other, because the molecule shrinks on oxygenation and expands on deoxygenation—a movement described as 'paradoxical breathing'.

This association of haem–polypeptide chain subunits to form one haemoglobin molecule favourably influences the oxygen dissociation curve. The oxygen dissociation curve of a single haem–polypeptide complex such as myoglobin is hyperbolic in shape (Fig. 30.8). With progressive

globular shape of myoglobin and haemoglobin, it is necessary for the helix to twist and turn in a complicated but fixed pattern (Fig. 30.6). Present evidence suggests that only the amino acid sequence is genetically determined and that the

2 H

oxygenation or deoxygenation the configuration of the haemoglobin molecule is continually altering. The sigmoid oxygen dissociation curve is an outward manifestation of the molecular changes made possible by the quaternary structure of haemoglobin.

In haemoglobin, when the polypeptide chains move apart on deoxygenation, amino acid residues which are not accessible in the oxygenated molecule are laid bare. These amino acid residues increase the buffering power of reduced haemoglobin. A small molecule (2 : 3 diphosphoglycerate) inserts itself in the centre of the deoxygenated tetramer. Deficiency of this compound increases oxygen affinity.

THE HAEM POCKET
ISOLATION OF THE IRON ATOM

Not many years ago it was thought that the haem groups were stuck like patches on to the surface of the underlying globin. If this was in fact so, there would be no possibility of isolating

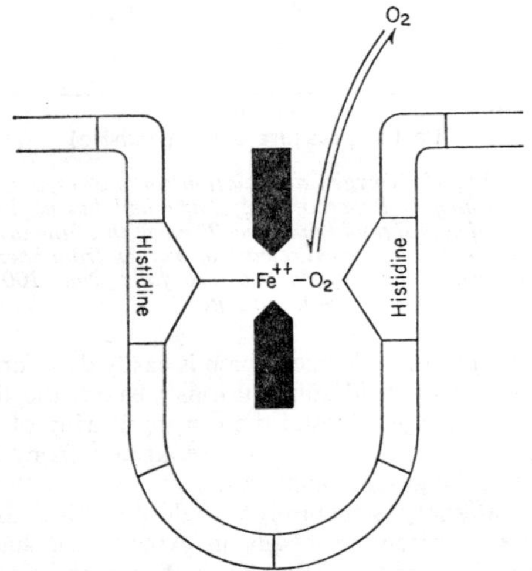

FIG. 30.9. *Diagrammatic representation of the haem group inserted in a fold of non-polar amino acid residues; only the histidines may become polar. Oxygenation and deoxygenation can only occur in one place, between the non-haem-linked histidine and the iron. (In* Man's Haemoglobins, *North-Holland Publishing Company.)*

the haem from the environment surrounding the molecule and as a result the ferrous atom would become oxidised to the ferric form.

X-ray crystallography has now visualised the position of the haem group and it is found to be embedded into the globin part of the molecule, surrounded by water repellent—hydrophobic—

amino acid residues. The iron atom is directly connected to the amino acid histidine on one side of the pocket (proximal histidine). There is another histidine on the other side of the pocket (distal histidine) and it is between the iron atom and this distal histidine that the oxygen molecule is inserted when oxygenation of the haemoglobin occurs (Fig. 30.9).

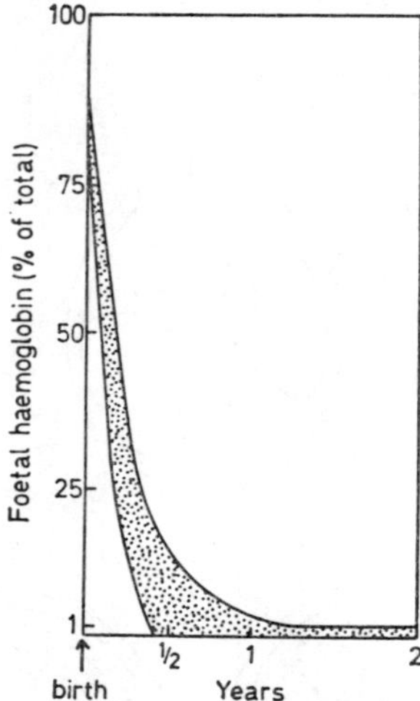

FIG. 30.10. *The dotted area represents the range of fetal haemoglobin found in the first 2 years of life. After 1–2 years the amount of fetal haemoglobin drops to less than 2 per cent.*

As already stated, to exclude water from this globin pocket, the amino acids lining it must possess hydrophobic non-polar side chains which give the haem pocket a 'waxy' surface. If there is an amino acid substitution in the lining of the haem pocket which replaces one of the non-polar side chains pointing towards the haem by a polar side chain, whether charged like glutamic acid or non-charged like tyrosine, the haem pocket becomes no longer water repellent and as a result the ferrous atom becomes oxidised to the ferric state.

The M haemoglobins (page 492) are a group of haemoglobin variants where, because of an amino acid substitution in the globin, the water-repellent nature of the globin pocket is disturbed. The resulting permanent oxidation of the ferrous atom to the ferric state converts the haem to haematin and therefore the haemoglobin to methaemoglobin. These interesting but unusual haemoglobin variants present not as a haemolytic anaemia but as cyanosis due to methaemoglobinaemia. On careful investigation some patients with haemoglobin M may show a haemolytic element.

NORMAL HAEMOGLOBINS

Man has at least four physiological haemoglobins.

Adult haemoglobin (haemoglobin A) comprises about 98 per cent of the haemoglobin of the adult.

Haemoglobin A_2 is a small fraction of the total circulating haemoglobin of the adult. The normal proportion of about 2 per cent may be raised or lowered in certain abnormalities of haemoglobin production which will be discussed later.

It is now realised that some of the γ chains in haemoglobin F are acetylated ($\alpha_2\gamma\gamma$ acetyl). In such a molecule, one γ chain would be normal and one acetylated. Similarly a proportion of the β chains form a bond with a sugar molecule. Although each individual has only one pair of β chain genes, there is evidence that there are two pairs of γ chain genes. The possible presence of two pairs of α chain genes is discussed on page 500.

Because all the above haemoglobins contain two α chains they are half alike; it is in the second half that they differ. The gradual change in the production pattern of these haemoglobins with the ageing of the fetus therefore depends

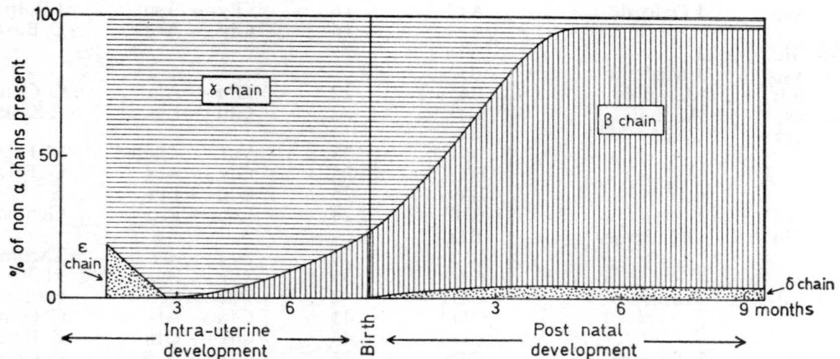

FIG. 30.11. *The changing pattern of production of non-α chains in man during the months preceding and following birth.*

Fetal haemoglobin (haemoglobin F), which forms up to about 80 per cent of the haemoglobin of the newborn, is produced in quantity only by the fetus and is rapidly replaced by adult haemoglobin during the first few months of extrauterine life (Fig. 30.10). Its persistence into adult life in a quantity above 2 per cent (the exact figure depending upon the method used for its detection) is abnormal.

Embryonic haemoglobin (haemoglobin Gower) is found only during the first 3 months of intra-uterine life. It has disappeared when the crown rump length of the embryo is about 8 cm.

The polypeptide chains of these haemoglobins have been named according to the Greek alphabet, alpha (α), beta (β), gamma (γ), delta (δ) and epsilon (ε). The composition of haemoglobins A, A_2, F and embryonic haemoglobins are as follows:

$$F = \alpha_2\beta_2$$
$$A_2 = \alpha_2\delta_2$$
$$F = \alpha_2\gamma_2$$
$$\text{Embryonic haemoglobin} = \alpha_2\varepsilon_2$$

on the differing output of the non-α chains. This is illustrated in Fig. 30.11.

VARIANT HAEMOGLOBINS AND HAEMOGLOBINS FOUND IN THALASSAEMIA

Amino acid substitutions in α, β, γ and δ chains

α, β, γ and δ chains which differ from those normally found in haemoglobins A, A_2 and F have been recognised (Table 30.1). Because of the difficulty in obtaining material, little is known of the structure of the ε chain and no variant embryonic haemoglobins have been described. Any change in the β chain ($\beta \rightarrow \beta^*$) can give rise to a variant of haemoglobin A ($\alpha_2\beta_2^*$) only. Haemoglobin A_2 ($\alpha_2\delta_2$) and F ($\alpha_2\gamma_2$) must be unaffected because haemoglobins A_2 and F contain no β chains. The common haemoglobin variants (S, C, D Punjab and E) differ from haemoglobin A in their β-polypeptide chains.

An amino acid substitution in the γ chain ($\gamma \rightarrow \gamma^*$) gives rise to a variant of haemoglobin F

TABLE 30.1. *List of known haemoglobin substitutions and deletions*

α chain variants			Helical	β chain variants		
No.		Name	No.	No.		Name
			NA2	2	His → Tyr	Tokuchi
5	Ala → Asp	J Toronto	A3	6	Glu → Val	S
			A3	6	Glu → Lys	C
			A3 or A4	6 or 7	Glu → deleted	Leiden
			A4	7	Glu → Gly	San José
			A4	7	Glu → Lys	Siriraj
			A6	9	Ser → Cys	Pôrto Alegre
12	Ala → Asp	J Paris	A10			
			A11	14	Leu → Arg	Sogn
15	Gly → Asp	J Oxford	A13	16	Gly → Asp	J Baltimore
			A13	16	Gly → Arg	D Bushman
16	Lys → Glu	I	A14			
22	Gly → Asp	J Medellin	B3			
23	Glu → Gln	Memphis	B4	22	Glu → Ala	G Coulshatta
23	Glu → Val	Audhali	B4	22	Glu → Lys	E Saskatoon
23	Glu → Lys	Chad	B4			
			B5	23	Val → deleted	M Freiburg
			B7	25	Gly → Arg	G Taiwan-Ami
			B8	26	Glu → Lys	E
			B10	28	Leu → Pro	Genova
30	Glu → Gln	G Chinese	B11			
			B12	30	Arg → Ser	Tacoma
			C1	35	Tyr → Phe	Philly
43	Phe → Val	Torino	CD1	42	Phe → Ser	Hammersmith
			CD2	43	Glu → Ala	G Galveston
			CD5	46	Gly → Glu	K Ibadan
47	Asp → Gly	L Ferrara	CD6	47	Asp → Asn	G Copenhagen
47	Asp → His	Hasharon	CD6			
50	His → Asp	Sardegna	CD8			
51	Gly → Arg	Russ	CD9			
			D7	56	Gly → Asp	J Bangkok
			E2	58	Pro → Arg	Dhofar
54	Gln → Arg	Shimonoseki	E3			
54	Gln → Glu	Mexico	E3			
			E5	61	Lys → Glu	N Seattle
			E5	61	Lys → Asn	Hikari
57	Gly → Asp	Norfolk	E6			
58	His → Tyr	M Boston	E7	63	His → Tyr	M Saskatoon
			E7	63	His → Arg	Zürich
			E11	67	Val → Glu	M Milwaukee
			E11	67	Val → Ala	Sydney
			E13	69	Gly → Asp	J Cambridge
68	Asn → Lys	G Philadelphia	E17	73	Asp → Asn	Korle Bu
68	Asn → Asp	Ube II	E17			
			A3	6	Glu → Val ⎱	C Harlem
			E17	73	Asp → Asn ⎰	
			E20	76	Ala → Glu	Seattle
			EF1	77	His → Asp	J Iran
			EF3	79	Asp → Asn	G Accra
78	Asn → Lys	Stanleyville II	EF7			
80	Leu → Arg	Ann Arbor	F1			
			F3	87	Thr → Lys	D Ibadan
			F4	88	Leu → Pro	Santa Ana
84	Ser → Arg	Etobicoke	F5			
85	Asp → Asn	G Norfolk	F6	90	Glu → Lys	Agenogi
			F7	91	Leu → Pro	Sabine
87	His → Tyr	M Iwate	F8	92	His → Tyr	M Hyde Park
			FG1	94	Asp → Asn	Oak Ridge

TABLE 30.1—*continued*

| α chain variants | | | Helical | β chain variants | | |
No.	Name		No.	No.		Name
90	Lys → Asn	Broussais	FG2	95	Lys → Glu	N
			F7–FG2	91–95		
			or	or	Leu, His	
			F8–FG3	92–96	Cys, Asp,	Gun Hill
			or	or	Lys	
			F9–FG4	93–97	deleted	
92	Arg → Gln	J Capetown	FG4			
92	Arg → Leu	Chesapeake	FG4			
			FG5	98	Val → Met	Köln
			FG6	99	Asp → His	Yakima
			FG6	99	Asp → Asn	Kempsey
			G4	102	Asn → Thr	M Kansas
102	Ser → Arg	Manitoba	G9			
			G15	113	Val → Glu	New York
112	His → Gln	Dakar	G19			
114	Pro → Arg	Chiapas	GH2			
115	Ala → Asp	J Tongariki	GH3	120	Lys → Glu	Hijiyama
116	Glu → Lys	O Indonesia	GH4	121	Glu → Lys	O Arab
			GH4	121	Glu → Gln	D Punjab
			H4	126	Val → Glu	Hofu
			H8	130	Tyr → Asp	Wien
			H10	132	Lys → Gln	K Woolwich
			H14	136	Gly → Asp	Hope
136	Leu → Pro	Bibba	H19			
			H21	143	His → Asp	Hiroshima
			HC2	145	Tyr → His	Rainier
141	Arg → Pro	Singapore	HC3			
141	Arg split off on haemolysis in plasma	Koellicker	HC3			

γ chain			
5	Glu → Lys	F Texas I	A2
6	Glu → Lys	F Texas II	A3
12	Thr → Lys	F Alexandra	A9
121	Glu → Lys	F Hull	GH4

δ chain			
2	His → Arg	A₂ Sphakia	HA2
12	Asn → Lys	A₂ N.Y.U.	A9
16	Gly → Arg	A₂ (or B₂)	A13
22	Ala → Glu	A₂ Flatbush	B4
136	Gly → Asp	A₂ Babinga	H14

($\alpha_2\gamma_2$*) only (Plate 33*a*) and one in the δ chain (δ→δ*) to a variant of haemoglobin A_2 ($\alpha_2\delta_2$*) (Plate 33*b*).

The consequences of an amino acid substitution in the α chain (α→α*) must give rise to three abnormal haemoglobins, an abnormal haemoglobin A (α_2*β_2), A_2 (α*δ_2) and F (α_2*γ_2). One would also expect an abnormal embryonic haemoglobin (α_2*ε_2).

The presence of a variant haemoglobin A may be caused by an amino acid substitution in the α(α_2*β_2) or β ($\alpha_2\beta_2$*) chain. If the substitution is in the α chain one would also expect to find a variant of haemoglobin A_2 (α_2*δ_2) present (Plate 33*c*). Such a finding of a double haemoglobin A_2 is sometimes of value in confirming that a variant of adult haemoglobin is due to a change in the α-polypeptide chains. A double haemoglobin A_2 may also be explained by the presence of a δ chain variant ($\alpha_2\delta_2$*) (Plate 33*b*) but in this case no variant of haemoglobin would be found.

The notation commonly employed in describing a variant haemoglobin gives information as to the polypeptide chain involved as well as the nature and the position of the amino acid substitution. $\alpha_2\beta_26$ Glu→Val, for instance, describes haemoglobin S. In haemoglobin S there is a substitution of a glutamic acid residue by a valine residue in the sixth position of both of the β-polypeptide chains.

DIMINISHED α AND β CHAIN FORMATION (α AND β THALASSAEMIA)

If there is decreased formation, either complete or partial, of the β chain it only depresses

there is a depression of α chain formation. When impairment of haemoglobin is due to α chain depression, there can be no compensatory increase in haemoglobins A₂ and F as they also contain α chains. Instead the lack of α chains results in the appearance of tetramers composed solely of β (β_4 or haemoglobin H) and γ chains (γ_4 or haemoglobin Bart's).

δ chain production can also be impaired and this condition, δ thalassaemia, is discussed on page 499.

The diagnosis of thalassaemia intermedia or thalassaemia minima is made purely on clinical severity. These terms tend only to confuse and

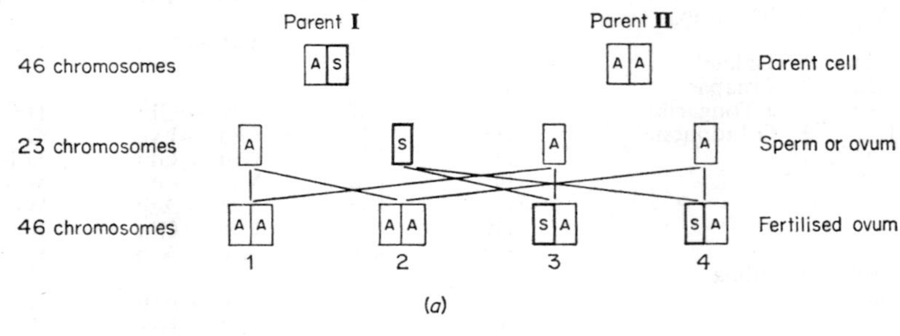

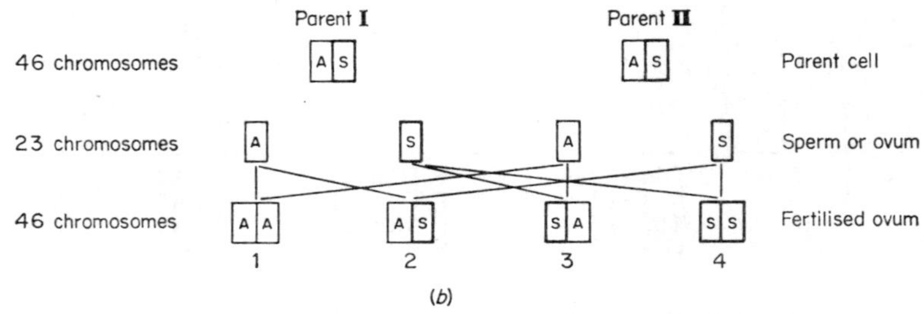

FIG. 30.12. (a) *If a sickle cell trait carrier (parent I) marries a normal individual (II) half the children would be normal (1 and 2) and half sickle cell trait carriers (3 and 4). (b) If two sickle cell trait carriers marry, on average one quarter of their children would be normal (1), one half would be sickle cell trait carriers (2 and 3) and one quarter would have sickle cell anaemia (4). The inheritance of thalassaemia is similar. A person with thalassaemia major must have parents who carry thalassaemia minor.*

the production of adult haemoglobin ($\alpha_2\beta_2$). Hence haemoglobin A₂ and/or haemoglobin F may, as a compensation, be raised in this situation. Because of the lack of β chains, traces of free α chains may be recognised in β chain deficiency.

Thalassaemia may exist in homozygous (major) or heterozygous (minor) form. Severe depression of β chain production is called β thalassaemia major, Mediterranean anaemia or Cooley's anaemia. In α thalassaemia and the form of α thalassaemia called haemoglobin H disease,

the diagnosis of β thalassaemia major or β thalassaemia minor should whenever possible be reached by means of a haematological and family study.

GENETICS

In genetics, human haemoglobin has come some way towards the position of eminence formerly occupied by the domestic pea. By now, about 100 variants of the haemoglobin molecule have been described, many of which have been chemically examined and found to possess a single amino acid substitution, which can be exactly identified. Every new variant of haemoglobin that is found is always of genetical interest as it permits the knowledge gained in great part from experimental work on viruses and bacteria to be tested in man.

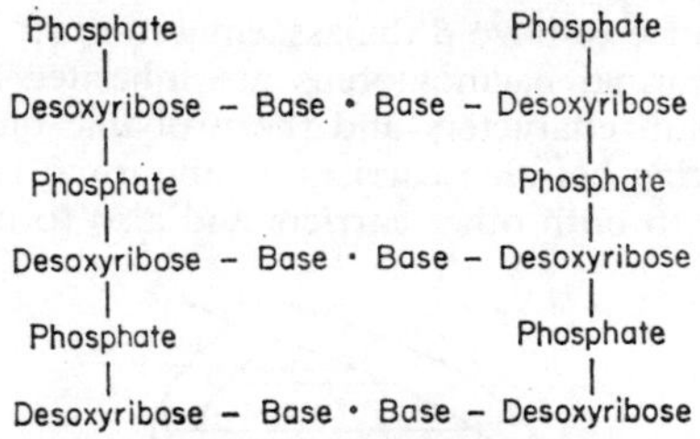

Phosphate   Phosphate
| |
Desoxyribose – Base · Base – Desoxyribose
| |
Phosphate   Phosphate
| |
Desoxyribose – Base · Base – Desoxyribose
| |
Phosphate   Phosphate
| |
Desoxyribose – Base · Base – Desoxyribose

FIG. 30.13. *A strand of desoxyribonucleic acid (DNA) consists of an alternating sugar (desoxyribose) molecule and phosphate. Ribonucleic acid which is a single stranded molecule has the sugar ribose substituted for desoxyribose. Specific bases are attached to the sugar molecules.*

A simple knowledge of classical Mendelian genetics is necessary in order that the clinician can advise on the possible outcome of a mating between individuals carrying haemoglobin variants or thalassaemia. In order, however, to appreciate the wider interest in haemoglobin variants, a

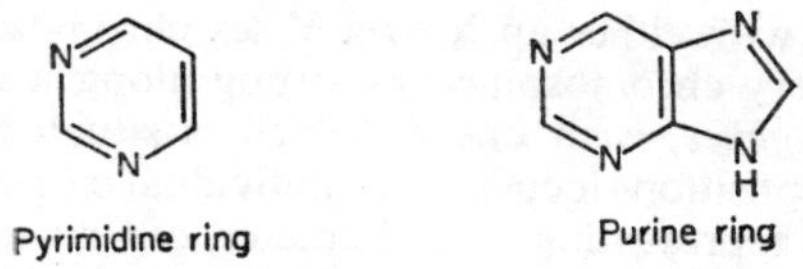

FIG. 30.14. *Of the four DNA bases, two (cytosine and thymine) have a pyrimidine ring and two (adenine and guanine) have a purine ring.*

knowledge of the chemical properties of genetic material and the mechanism of polypeptide chain formation is essential.

Chromosome

Man's genetic information is stored within the nucleus in the form of 46 thread-like chromosomes. With the exception of the two sex chromosomes (X and Y), the remainder are always present as pairs. The two chromosomes which constitute each pair are homologous, i.e. they are basically similar although not identical, because

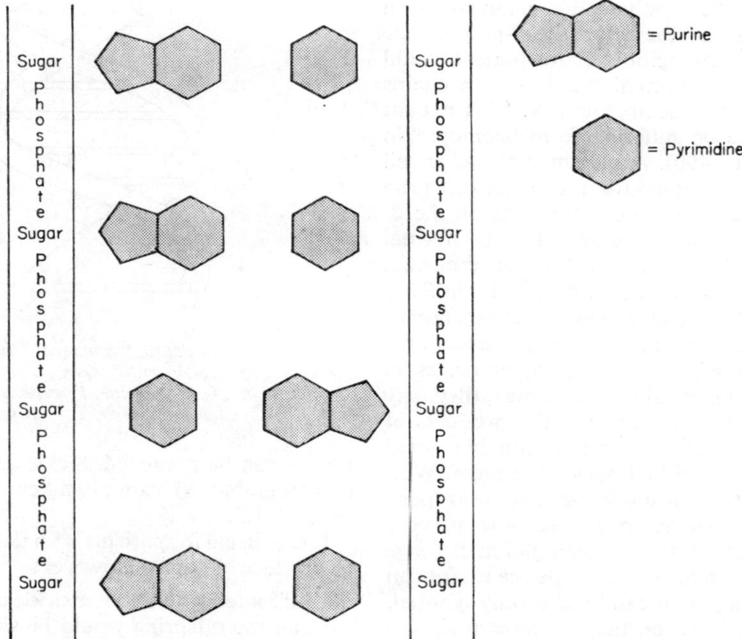

FIG. 30.15. *A short length of DNA to show the base pairing in the double-stranded structure. By pairing a purine with a pyramidine, the strands always remain the same distance apart.* (In *Man's Haemoglobins*, North-Holland Publishing Company.)

each one of the pair has been derived from a different parent. A mature cell contains 46 chromosomes, but an ovum or sperm contains only 23 chromosomes, one from each of the homologous pairs with either an X or a Y sex chromosome.

Every chromosome has strung along it about 3000 *genes*, each one of which is situated at a fixed position (locus). Each individual carries two genes representing each character, one on each of the paired chromosomes. If these paired genes are identical, the individual is *homozygous* for this character, and if they differ, the individual is *heterozygous*.

Different genes able to occupy the same locus on a chromosome are called *alleles*. For example, the genes responsible for the normal β-polypeptide chain and the abnormal β-polypeptide chains found in haemoglobins C, D, E and S are all alleles. Although different in detail, these genes are merely variations of one and the same β-polypeptide chain gene and these allelic genes therefore only occur on a chromosome at the specific locus which controls the manufacture of the β-polypeptide chain.

Because the chromosomes are paired, each specific polypeptide chain has two loci controlling its production. If, for example, one of these produces the β-polypeptide chain found in haemoglobin S and the other the β-polypeptide chain found in haemoglobin C, the patient would be unable to form normal β-polypeptide chains and therefore any haemoglobin A. This patient would therefore be suffering from haemoglobin SC disease (page 490). A patient with sickle cell anaemia is homozygous for the sickle cell gene and a patient with sickle cell trait has on the β-polypeptide chain loci one gene for the normal β-polypeptide chain and one for the abnormal β-polypeptide chain found in haemoglobin S.

When two allelic genes occupy a locus on homologous chromosomes, one of the characters may be *dominant* or *recessive* to the other or, as in inheritance of abnormal haemoglobins, they may be of equal dominance because the products of both genes are demonstrable in roughly equal amounts in the individual possessing them. With the exception of the unstable haemoglobins (page 495), haemoglobins M (page 492) and in very exceptional circumstances haemoglobin S (page 487), the possession of a single gene for an abnormal haemoglobin can be clinically ignored. Their presence, however, may become of significance if prospective partners seek marriage guidance in order to prevent the birth of a homozygous doubly abnormal offspring.

The presence of a single gene for β-thalassaemia

can on occasions give rise to clinical symptoms, but it must be remembered that, for instance, in parts of Italy over 20 per cent of the population have β-thalassaemia minor, and the very great majority without much disability. In a recent geriatric survey, a lady of 86, with every hope of going strong for another 20 years, was discovered by chance to have β thalassaemia minor.

Abnormal haemoglobins are inherited as co-dominant characters and the probable outcome of mating between carriers of abnormal haemoglobin to both other carriers and also to normal

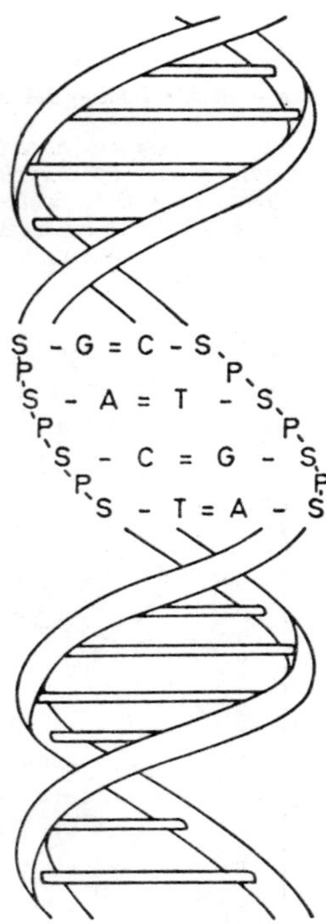

FIG. 30.16. *A model to demonstrate the double-stranded structure of DNA, with base pairing: A = adenine; C = cytosine; G = guanine; P = phosphate; S = sugar (desoxyribose); T = thymine.*

people can be predicted. Sickle cell haemoglobin (haemoglobin S) can be taken as an example (Fig. 30.12).

It is unusual for patients with sickle cell anaemia to produce children. However:

1. If mated with another sickle cell homozygote all the offspring would be sickle cell homozygotes.
2. If mated with a sickle cell trait carrier half the offspring will be sickle cell homozygotes and half will be sickle cell trait carriers.

3. If mated with a normal person all offspring will be sickle cell trait carriers (AS heterozygotes).

This can be easily checked by the construction of figures similar to Plate 33a and b.

Storage of genetic information

Desoxyribonucleic acid (DNA) is the sole carrier of genetic information except in a few viruses where ribonucleic acid (RNA) can be substituted for DNA. DNA is a long molecule consisting of alternating phosphate groups and desoxyribose molecules (Fig. 30.13). To each sugar (desoxyribose) is attached one of four bases. The selection of these four bases is the only variable factor in the DNA chain and genetic information is imparted solely by their sequence. Of the four DNA

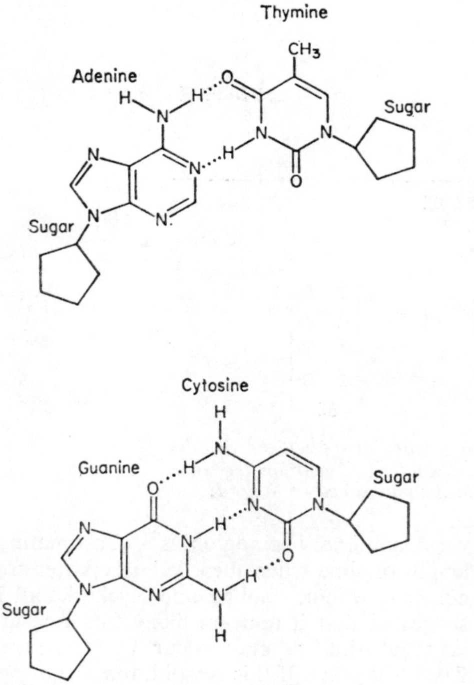

FIG. 30.17. *Specific base pairing is achieved by hydrogen bonding between guanine and cytosine and between adenine and thymine.*

bases, two (cytosine and thymine) have a pyrimidine ring and two (adenine and guanine) a purine ring structure (Fig. 30.14). The DNA strands within the resting cell are paired together in a manner reminiscent of a ladder with the uprights

consisting of desoxyribose molecules and phosphate groups and the rungs of purine and pyrimidine bases (Fig. 30.15). Although one can conceive of DNA as a ladder, in fact the strands are twisted together like an electric flex forming a double helix (Fig. 30.16). It is necessary, in order that the rungs remain the same width, that a purine base is always paired against a pyrimidine

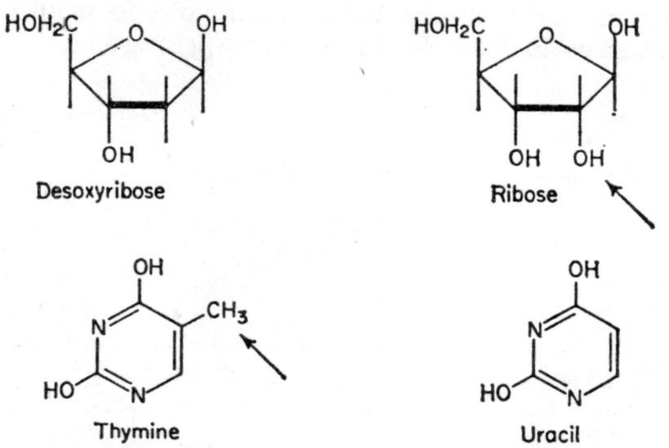

FIG. 30.18. *DNA and RNA have basically the same chemical constituents with two exceptions: desoxyribose in DNA is substituted by ribose in RNA; thymine in DNA is substituted by uracil in RNA.*

base. Because of hydrogen bonding, the base pairing is even more specific because cytosine will combine only with guanine and thymine will combine only with adenine (Fig. 30.17).

RNA differs from DNA in two particulars only. Firstly, in RNA the pyrimidine uracil takes the place of thymine in DNA. Secondly, in RNA the sugar ribose replaces desoxyribose in DNA (Fig. 30.18).

In order that each daughter cell possesses the same information as was contained in a single parent cell, reduplication of genetic material must occur at each cell division. This duplication of DNA is achieved by an unwinding of the two-stranded structure and forming two new strands of DNA, one alongside each of the single strands derived from the parent cell. Because of base pairing, each of the two new double helices finally formed are identical with the double helix in the parent cell (Fig. 30.19).

Genetic code

The genetic code is a triplet code, each of the twenty amino acids being represented on the DNA by three bases. Each unit of three bases is called a *codon* and represents a single acid (Fig. 30.20). Also, some triplet combinations represent the signal for terminating the construction of a polypeptide chain. The code is 'degenerate' which means that more than one triplet combination can represent the same amino acid. Other triplets also code for the commencement and termination of the polypeptide chain.

The genetic information in each cell of the human body has been likened to an encyclopaedia of 46 volumes, each chromosome representing a volume. If each triplet of three bases coding an amino acid is one word, each volume would average 20 000 pages! It is not surprising that the

It is probable that human haemoglobins originated from a single gene producing an α chain, and the β, γ and δ chains arose by a process of gene duplication. The number of amino acid differences between two polypeptide chains gives an indication of the length of time since gene duplication occurred, because from that moment in time a mutation of one gene would have no effect on the originally similar gene that had previously split away and become independent from it.

By examining the amino acid structure of

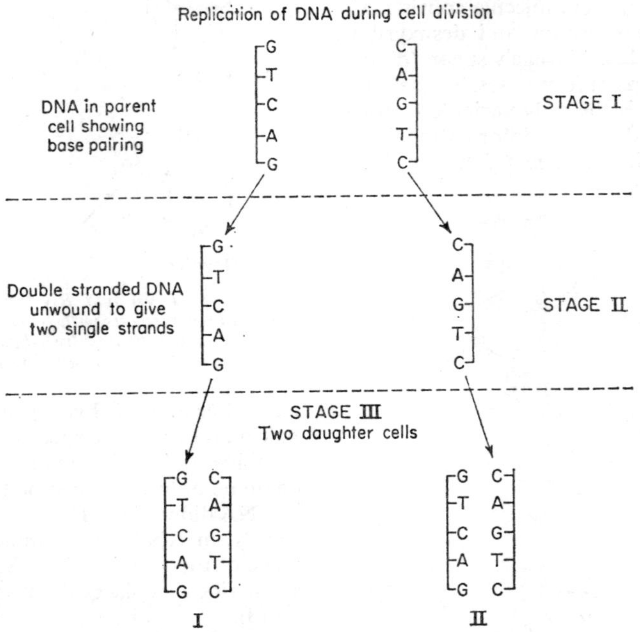

FIG. 30.19. *The newly formed strands I and II reform the double-stranded DNA and ensure that each daughter cell contains the same genetic information contained in the parent cell in Stage I.*

specification for a human body is complex. It is extraordinary that the structure of DNA permits the compression of such a mass of information into the compass of every cell nucleus. As there are 146 amino acids in the β chain of haemoglobin there will be 146 codons consisting of 438 bases representing these amino acids. A mutation resulting in an amino acid substitution is caused by an alteration of one of the DNA bases to another. It is apparent that in order to produce an abnormal haemoglobin with a single amino acid substitution, such as haemoglobins S, C, D and E, it requires only one base chain in the 438 bases representing the amino acids in that polypeptide chain.

various animal haemoglobins and estimating the length of time when these animals parted from a common origin, Pauling and Zuckerkandl have suggested that it appears likely that one amino acid substitution may occur by chance every 7 000 000 years. If this is valid, the β and δ genes separated 35 000 000 years ago and the β and γ 150 000 000 years ago. The α and β genes separated 380 000 000 years ago when the first amphibians were appearing. The multiple differences between the polypeptide chain in myoglobin and those that form haemoglobin suggests that these genes might have had a common origin 650 000 000 years ago, before the origin of the vertebrates!

By examining the amino acid structure of selected proteins of two species, one is able to hazard a guess as to when the species parted. This approach to a classification of species is in its infancy but appears of considerable potential.

Manufacture of polypeptide chain

Genetic information is stored in the nuclear DNA, but the polypeptide chain is manufactured by the ribosome in the cytoplasm. The coded information from the DNA is carried into the cytoplasm by a messenger ribonucleic acid (messenger RNA). This RNA has a base structure which is the consequence of base pairing upon a

Abnormal haemoglobins

All amino acid substitutions that have occurred in the abnormal haemoglobins have been proved to be compatible with a single base change in a DNA codon. It is this fact that has given striking confirmation that the DNA base triplets, which were postulated as a result of bacterial and virus work, are also true for man. An amino acid substitution caused by the mismatching of a single base is in any case an exceedingly rare occurrence. It would therefore be unsatisfactory to have to explain an amino acid substitution in a variant haemoglobin by requiring a simultaneous alteration of two bases in a codon.

Second letter

First letter	U	C	A	G	Third letter
U	UUU, UUC } Phe; UUA, UUG } Leu	UCU, UCC, UCA, UCG } Ser	UAU, UAC } Tyr; UAA ⊙; UAG ⊙	UGU, UGC } Cys; UGA ⊙; UGG Tryp	U C A G
C	CUU, CUC, CUA, CUG } Leu	CCU, CCC, CCA, CCG } Pro	CAU, CAC } His; CAA, CAG } GluN	CGU, CGC, CGA, CGG } Arg	U C A G
A	AUU, AUC, AUA } Ileu; *AUG Met	ACU, ACC, ACA, ACG } Thr	AAU, AAC } AspN; AAA, AAG } Lys	AGU, AGC } Ser; AGA, AGG } Arg	U C A G
G	GUU, GUC, GUA, *GUG } Val	GCU, GCC, GCA, GCG } Ala	GAU, GAC } Asp; GAA, GAG } Glu	GGU, GGC, GGA, GGG } Gly	U C A G

FIG. 30.20. *AUG and GUG, as well as coding for methionine and valine respectively, also indicate the commencement of the polypeptide chain. UAA, UAG and UGA do not code for the amino acid but signal the end of the polypeptide chain. Work on initiation and termination of polypeptide chains has so far been carried out exclusively on bacterial and virus ribosomes.

single parent DNA strand just as a new DNA strand manufactured during cell division is moulded on the DNA strand derived from the parent cell.

In order that amino acids should occupy their correct position in the polypeptide chain under construction they are themselves conjugated to a short coiled ribonucleic acid chain which contains under 100 bases which is called transfer RNA. The transfer RNA–amino acid complex appears to recognise its correct position in the polypeptide presumably because the transfer possesses a complementary base triplet which can lock into place on the messenger RNA triplet lying on the ribosome and waiting to receive it (Figs. 30.21 and 30.22).

The finding of a new rare haemoglobin variant yields information as to the relationship between amino acid structure of a protein molecule and its function. When the amino acid substitution is shown to be compatible with a single base change, it also provides further proof of the validity of the genetic code.

Once the genetic code was shown to be true for man, it was apparent that an amino acid substitution which involves a change of a positively charged amino acid (lysine or arginine) to a negatively charged amino acid (glutamic acid or aspartic acid) and vice versa, could only represent an interchange between glutamic acid and lysine. It is not possible for a mutation between lysine and aspartic acid to occur with only one base change, and similarly it is not possible for an interchange between arginine and aspartic acid or arginine and glutamic acid to involve only one base change in the specific codons responsible for these amino acids (Fig. 30.23).

haemoglobin S, there has been a substitution of valine for glutamic acid and in haemoglobin C a substitution of lysine for glutamic acid. For haemoglobin C to have arisen from haemoglobin S one must postulate the substitution of lysine

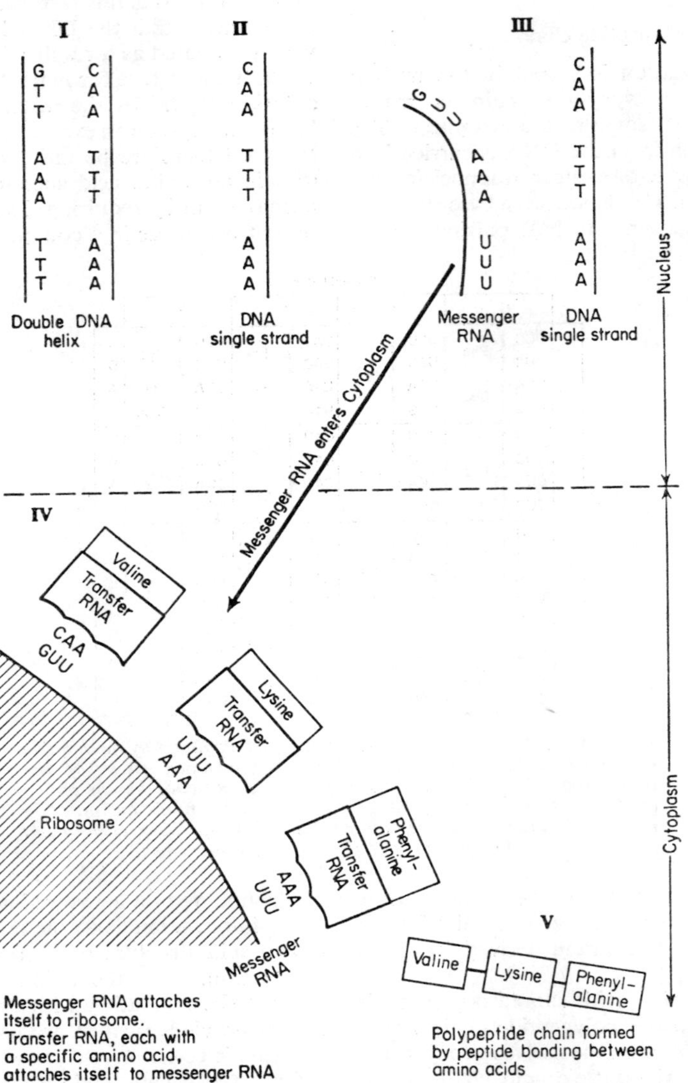

Fig. 30.21. *Formation of a polypeptide chain. C = cytosine; A = adenine; T = thymine; G = guanine; U = uracil.* (In *Man's Haemoglobins,* North-Holland Publishing Company.)

It has been suggested that haemoglobin C may have arisen from haemoglobin S, because haemoglobins S and C both have an amino acid substitution at the sixth position of the β chain. In

for valine. Such a substitution is not possible with one base change in the codon for these respective amino acids, whereas glutamic acid can change to both valine and lysine with only one base

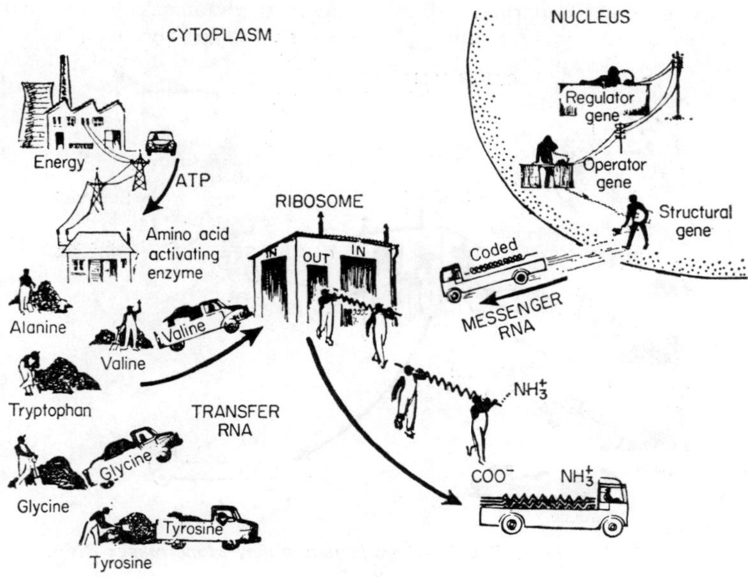

FIG. 30.22. *Formation of a polypeptide chain:*

(a)   *Normal haemoglobin synthesis.*

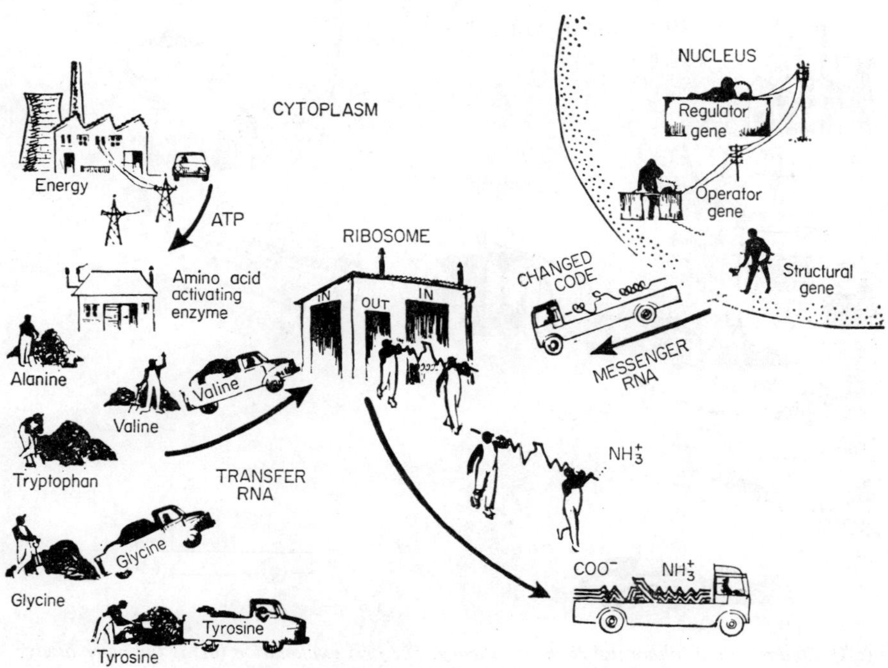

(b)   *Abnormal haemoglobin. The code is different from* (a).

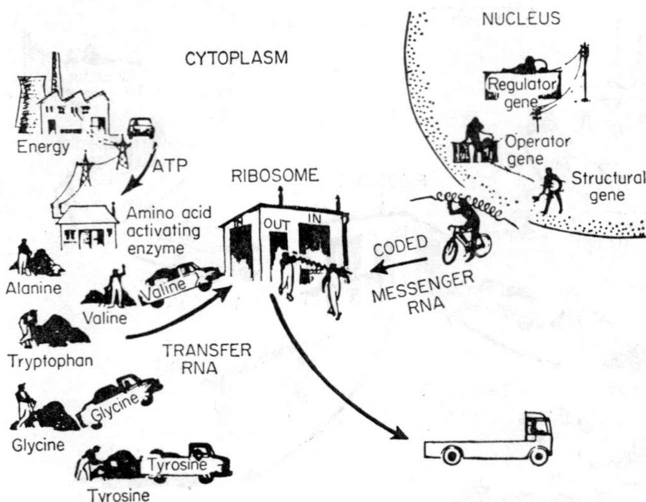

(cI) *Thalassaemia: diminished production of normal messenger RNA.*

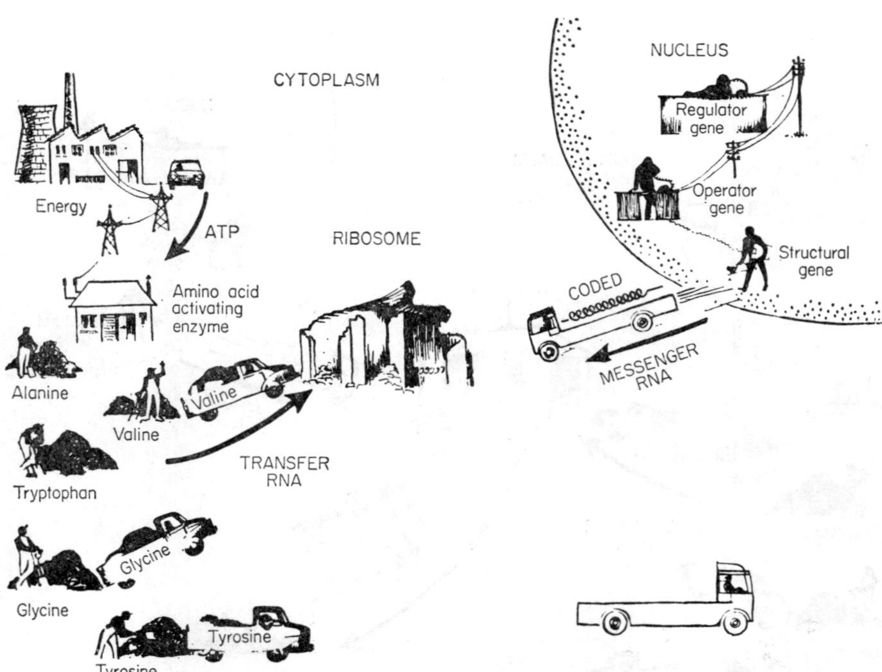

(cII) *Thalassaemia: abnormal ribosome theory. The first explanation* (cII) *is the more likely.*

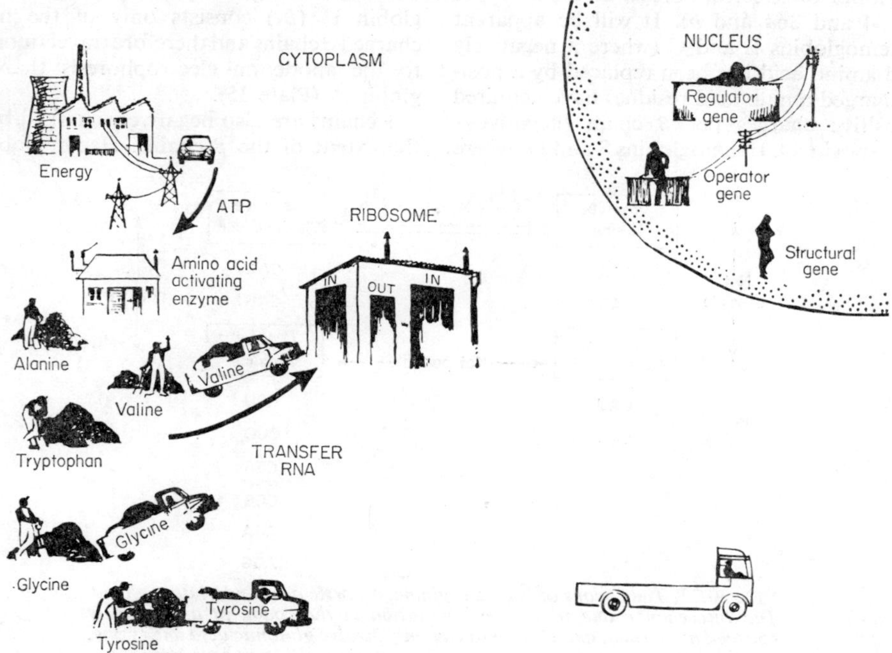

(d) *Persistence of high fetal haemoglobin. The structural gene for the β-polypeptide chain has not been 'turned on' or alternatively may be deleted.*

change (Fig. 30.24). In other words, haemoglobins S and C could both arise from haemoglobin A, but haemoglobin C could not have arisen from haemoglobin S. It therefore appears that haemoglobin C is an independent mutation from haemoglobin A despite the fact that it originated in an area where haemoglobin S occurs (see Fig. 30.25).

DETECTION OF ABNORMAL HAEMOGLOBINS BY ELECTROPHORESIS

Abnormal haemoglobins are usually identified by electrophoresis, although haemoglobin S may also be identified by sickling (Plate 38). Electrophoresis is a method which separates proteins of different overall charges by observing the mobility of the molecules in an electric field. A negatively charged molecule will move to the positive pole (anode) and a positively charged molecule will move to the negative pole (cathode).

If an amino acid substitution takes place in a polypeptide chain, and there is no resulting charge change (for instance, a neutral amino acid is replaced by another neutral amino acid), this amino acid substitution will not be detectable by

electrophoresis (see Figs. 30.2 and 30.3). It therefore follows that, when one relies upon electrophoresis as a method for the detection of amino acid substitutions, one can in fact only recognise a proportion of such substitutions, namely those that result in a charge change. The four common haemoglobin variants S, C, D, Punjab and E all have amino acid substitutions which result in the haemoglobin molecule receiving an increased positive charge.

Haemoglobin C. Substitution of glutamic acid by lysine in the sixth position of the β chain (negative amino acid→positive).

Haemoglobin D (Punjab). Substitution of glutamic acid by glutamine in the 121st position of the β chain (negative amino acid→neutral).

Haemoglobin E. Substitution of glutamic acid by lysine in the twenty-sixth position of the β chain (negative acid→positive).

Haemoglobin S. Substitution of glutamic acid by valine in the sixth position of the β chain (negative amino acid→neutral).

These four variants are all more positively charged than haemoglobin A and therefore move more slowly towards the anode than normal adult haemoglobin on electrophoresis at alkaline pH (Plates 34 and 36a and b). It will be apparent that haemoglobins E and C (where a negatively charged amino acid has been replaced by a positively charged amino acid residue) have acquired two positive charges per β chain (negative→neutral→positive). Haemoglobins S and D (where

α chains and negatively charged β chains. Haemoglobin H (β_4) consists only of the negatively charged β chains and therefore travels more rapidly to the anode on electrophoresis than haemoglobin A (Plate 35).

γ chains are also negatively charged but not to the extent of the β chains. Haemoglobin Bart's

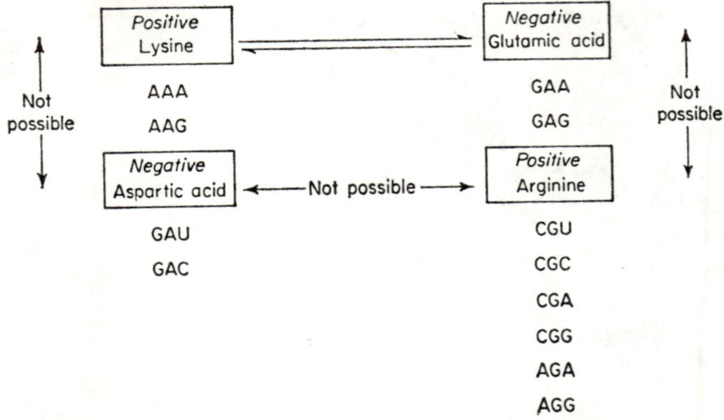

FIG. 30.23. *The codons of lysine, arginine, aspartic acid and glutamic acid. The interchange due to a single mutation in the codon of a negatively charged amino acid and vice versa can only involve glutamic acid and lysine. All other combinations will require a mutation with two base changes.*

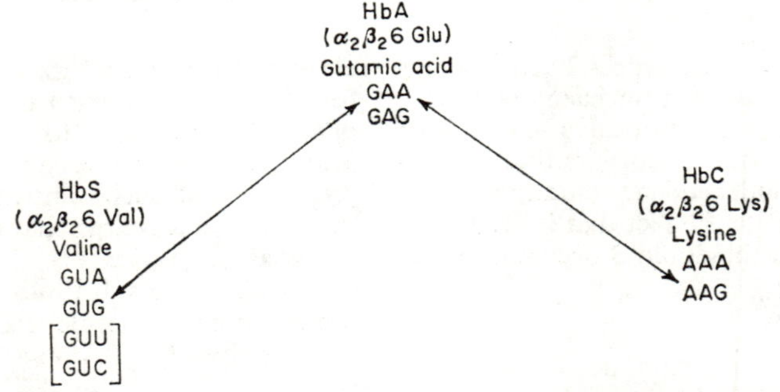

FIG. 30.24. *The codons for valine, glutamic acid and lysine. For haemoglobin C ($\alpha_2\beta_2$6 Lys) to arise from haemoglobin S ($\alpha_2\beta_2$6 Val) it is necessary to postulate two base changes. However, both haemoglobin C and S could arise as a mutation from haemoglobin A ($\alpha_2\beta_2$6 Glu), because both lysine and valine may arise from glutamic acid with only one base change.*

a negatively charged amino acid residue has been replaced by a neutral amino acid residue) have received only one positive charge per β-polypeptide chain (negative→neutral). It is thus logical to expect haemoglobins S and D to occupy a situation on electrophoresis between haemoglobin A and haemoglobins C and E.

The electrophoretic mobility of haemoglobin A at alkaline pH (TRIS buffer pH 8.9) is the outcome of a combination of positively charged

(γ_4) travels therefore slightly behind haemoglobin H (Plate 35).

δ chains are more positively charged than β chains and haemoglobin A_2 ($\alpha_2\delta_2$) moves in approximately the same position as haemoglobin E (Plate 35).

Fetal haemoglobin, on paper electrophoresis at alkaline pH, travels slightly behind haemoglobin A but fails to separate clearly. A haemolysate of fetal haemoglobin is commonly recognised by its

CHAPTER 30

PLATE 33

A   *Electrophoresis paper, barbiturate buffer pH 8·9, showing haemoglobin from baby carrying a γ chain variant (centre) with blood from parents on either side. One would not expect the parents to possess a visible chain variant as their fetal haemoglobin level is below 2 per cent.*
B   *Electrophoresis on cellulose acetate with benzidine staining. Right: Normal control. Left: δ chain variant. Note only an A_2 variant results from an amino acid substitution in the δ chain. This variant is found in about 1 per cent of American Negroes.*
C   *Electrophoresis on cellulose acetate with benzidine staining. Right: Normal control. Left: An α chain variant (α*) resulting in an abnormal haemoglobin $A(\alpha_2^*\beta_2)$ and an abnormal haemoglobin $A(\alpha_2^*\delta_2)$.*

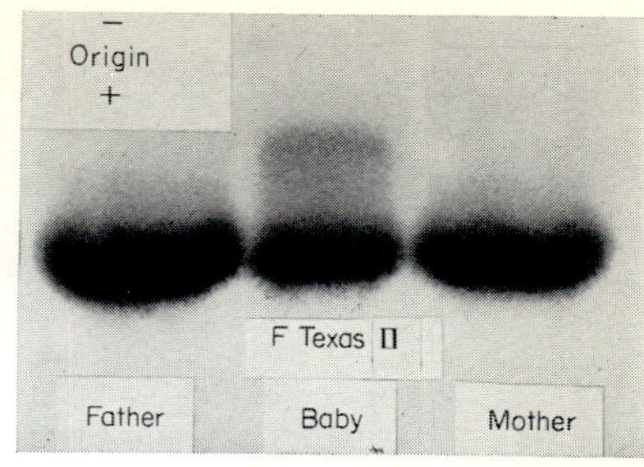

PLATE 33A

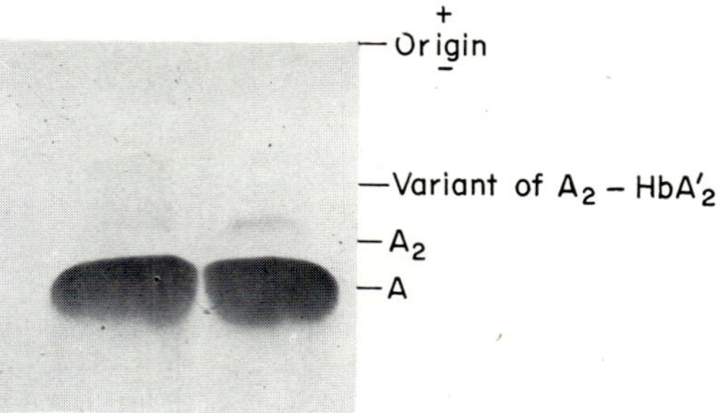

PLATE 33B

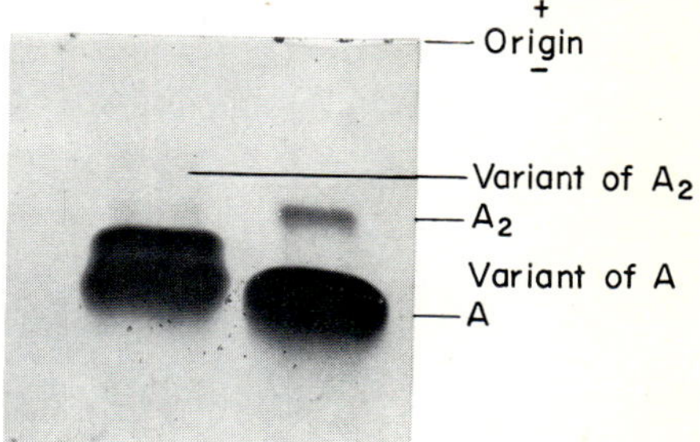

PLATE 33C

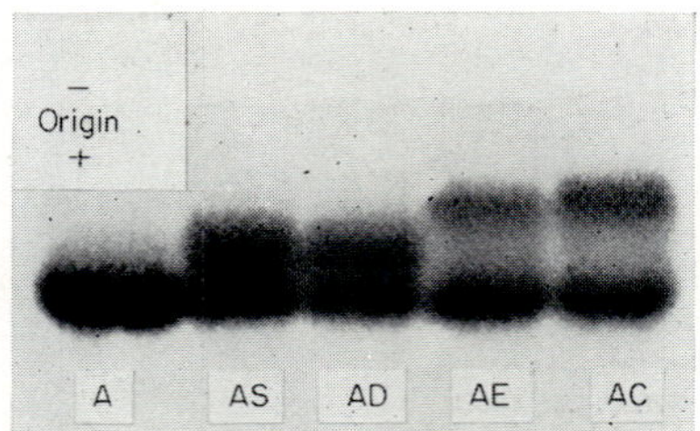

PLATE 34   *Electrophoresis of haemoglobins A, AS, AD, AE and AC on paper (barbiturate buffer pH 8·0). Haemoglobins S and D occupy identical positions. (See also Plate 36A and B.)*

PLATE 35   *Electrophoresis (TRIS buffer pH 8·9) to show the electrophoretic properties of haemoglobins A_1, A_2, Bart's (γ$_4$) and H (β$_4$).*

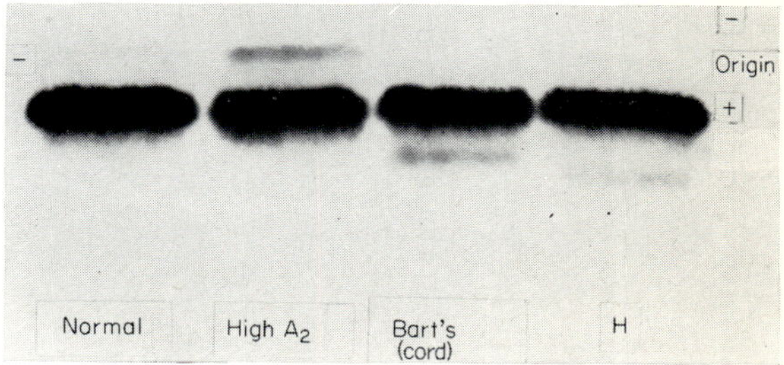

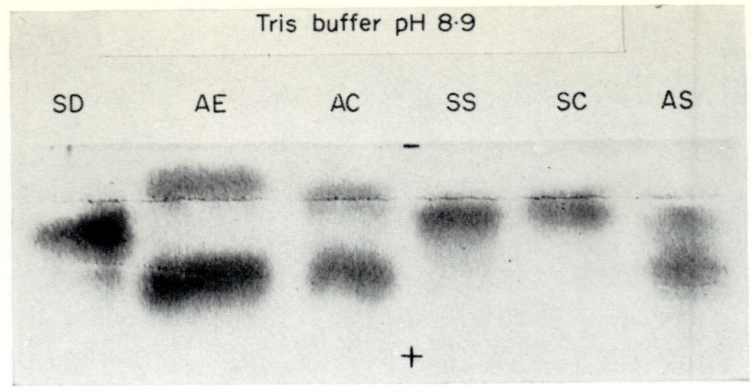

PLATE 36A

Paper electrophoresis: TRIS buffer system. Note SC and SS are identical in position. The blurring on the anodal side in the SS sample is due to fetal haemoglobin. When AC and AE are compared the C fraction is nearer the anode than the E fraction.

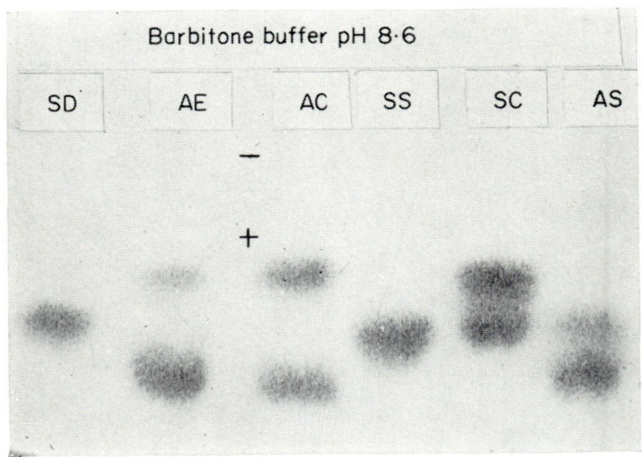

PLATE 36B

Paper electrophoresis barbitone buffer. Note SC and SS are easily distinguished. When AC and AE are compared the E fraction is nearer the anode than the C fraction. (See text.)

resistance to alkali denaturation. When in the intact red cell, adult haemoglobin may be eluted from the red cell by acid, leaving the fetal haemoglobin which is subsequently stained by eosin (Kleihauer staining).

CLINICAL AND LABORATORY RECOGNITION OF THE COMMON HAEMOGLOBINOPATHIES

Abnormal haemoglobins

The common haemoglobin variants (C, D, E and S) all result from amino acid substitutions in the β chain. Other uncommon variants with amino acid substitutions in the β chains have also been described (see Table 30.1). All the variants with substitutions in the α chain are uncommon and indeed many descriptions are limited to a single occurrence only.

It is therefore reasonable for a clinical haematologist to confine himself only to:

1. The recognition of the variants C, D, E and S.
2. The screening of an obscure haemolytic anaemia, in which Heinz bodies (denatured haemoglobin) are found in the red cells, for unstable haemoglobin (page 495).
3. Investigation of a methaemoglobinaemia for the presence of an amino acid substitution which permits the ferrous atom of the haem to become permanently oxidised to the ferric form (M haemoglobins, page 492).

Thalassaemia syndromes

It is now appreciated that the term 'thalassaemia' covers a number of disorders where there is impairment of the production of globin. Some of the rarer subdivisions of thalassaemia are of considerable theoretical interest but the clinician might well confine his interest to:

1. β thalassaemia major (Cooley's anaemia or Mediterranean anaemia), β thalassaemia minor, and the interaction of β thalassaemia with the variants C, D, E and S.
2. Haemoglobin H disease, a manifestation of α chain depression. (α thalassaemia major results in death *in utero* and α thalassaemia minor is symptomless.)
3. Haemoglobin Lepore and hereditary persistence of high fetal haemoglobin (high F gene) are both uncommon conditions worth brief consideration because they are liable to result in diagnostic errors.

2 I

Clinical severity of the haemoglobinopathies

In any description of the haemoglobinopathies an indication of the likely clinical state of the patient is usually valuable (Table 30.2). It must, however, be remembered that one of the characteristics of these haemolytic disorders is their variable severity. This variation can occur not only between individuals suffering from what is apparently the same disease but also in the same individual at different periods of time. For example, the clinical course of sickle cell anaemia is interspersed with crises which may be aplastic, haemolytic or infarctive in origin. Infections, (viral or bacterial), infestations (hookworms), dietary deficiency (folic acid) and pregnancy may all at times play a part in converting a symptomless or mild condition to a severe or lethal anaemia. It is found in practice that the patients who present in hospital may often be suffering from such complications as those mentioned above, while the patients found by survey would tend to be at the mild end of the clinical spectrum.

It must always be remembered that the patient with minimal symptoms usually found by survey has an erythropoietic system that is always under stress. If one of the complications outlined above has set in, for example an attack of virus pneumonia, that same patient may be found at a later date lying severely ill in hospital.

Value of a family study in diagnosis

The diagnosis of a clinically typical haemoglobinopathy may often be achieved with a reasonable degree of certainty without a family study. Family studies are always time-consuming and sometimes not possible. They are therefore best reserved for situations when laboratory tests will not permit a firm clinical opinion to be given. In the field of the haemoglobinopathies, a family study is most fruitful in differentiating the interaction of thalassaemia and an abnormal haemoglobin trait from the homozygous state of the abnormal haemoglobin. When no adult haemoglobin is detectable in the former, a family study then becomes essential for differentiation of the two conditions.

HAEMOGLOBINS

Haemoglobin S is relatively insoluble when it is in the reduced state. There is therefore a tendency for this haemoglobin to crystallise within the red cell, resulting in distortion of red cell shape. Some

TABLE 30.2. *A guide to the average clinical and haematological condition*

Disease or trait	Clinical				Haematological	
	Sickling crises	Degree of clinical disability	Spleen size	Anaemia (Hb g%)	Sickling test	Haemoglobins present [1]
Sickle cell anaemia	+++	Severe with, frequently, death in childhood. Good medical care increases life expectation	Usually impalpable [2]	6–10	+	S 90–95%: F 5–10%
Sickle cell trait	− [3]	Fit	Impalpable	Normal	+	S 20–40%: A 60–80%
Haemoglobin C disease	−	Mild to moderate disability	++	About 12	−	C 95%: F 0–5%
Haemoglobin C trait	−	Fit	Impalpable	Normal	−	C 40%: A 60%
Haemoglobin SC disease	++	Liability to defects of vision or postpartum maternal death	++	About 10	+	S 60%: C 40%: F 0–5%
Haemoglobin D trait	−	Fit	Impalpable	Normal	−	D 40%: A 60%
Haemoglobin SD disease	++	Less severe than sickle cell anaemia	+	About 10	+	S 60%: D 40%: F 5–10%
Haemoglobin E disease	−	Fit or mild disability	Sometimes just palpable	About 13	−	E 95%: F 0–5%
Haemoglobin E trait	−	Fit	Impalpable	Normal	−	E 40%: A 60%
β Thalassaemia major	−	Severe, almost always death in childhood. Good medical care can increase life expectation	+++	4–8	−	F 20–100%: A 0–80%. A_2 occasionally raised
β Thalassaemia minor	−	Mild or no disability	Sometimes palpable	11–14	−	A 90%: F 0–5%. A_2 usually raised
Haemoglobin H disease	−	Mild to moderate disability	+	8–10	−	A 90%: H 5–15%: Bart's 0–2%. F traces occasionally; A_2 low
Sickle cell thalassaemia	++	Not as severe as sickle cell anaemia	++	About 10	+	S 90%: F 10%. A sometimes demonstrable
Haemoglobin C thalassaemia	−	Mild to moderate disability	++	10–12	−	C 90–100%: F 0–7%. A_2 raised; A sometimes demonstrable
Haemoglobin E thalassaemia	−	Mild to moderate disability	++	10–12	−	E 75–85%: F 15–25%. A not usually demonstrable
Haemoglobin D thalassaemia	−	Mild to moderate disability	++	10–12	−	D 95%: F 5%. A not found; A_2 raised

[1] A_2 level normal unless otherwise stated. Children under 2 years may have a higher level of fetal haemoglobin.
[2] The spleen becomes impalpable after 5 years of age.
[3] Sickling only occurs under conditions of severe unphysiological anoxia. Haematuria may occur.

of the red cells adopt a characteristic sickle form, others appear like airships or bananas (see Plate 38).

Amino acid substitution

There is a substitution of valine for glutamic acid in the sixth position of the β-chain ($\alpha_2\beta_2$ 6 Glu→Val).

Geographical distribution (Fig. 30.25)

Haemoglobin S is distributed in Africa across a broad band bounded in the north by the Ethiopian highlands and Sahara Desert and in the south by

The severity of sickle cell anaemia appears to vary from one part of the world to another. Benign forms of the disease occur in the West Indies and North America, where it is not uncommon for a woman with sickle cell anaemia successfully to give birth to a child. In contrast, in parts of Africa where malaria is frequent it is uncommon for a patient with sickle cell anaemia to survive to the age of 4 years.

Clinical features. A patient with this condition tends to have a shorter trunk with comparatively long legs and an asthenic build. As well as the mucous membranes being pale, the patient may be noticed to be slightly jaundiced. Leg ulcers or scars of past ulcers may well be present, com-

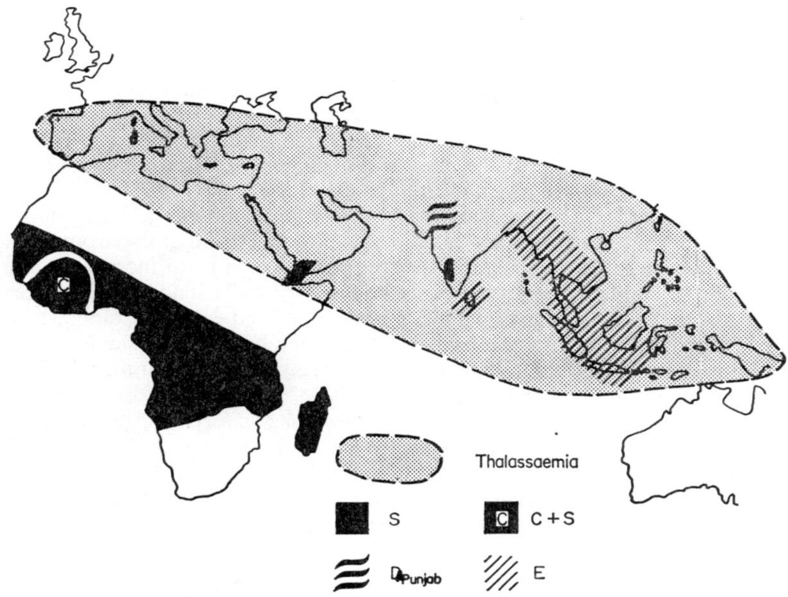

FIG. 30.25. *The source of the four major haemoglobin variants. The passage of Africans to the American continent has resulted in a further spread of haemoglobins S and C.*

the Rivers Zambesi in the east and the Kunene in the west. Haemoglobin S is also present in the Malagasi Republic and to a lesser extent in the Middle East, India and around the Mediterranean. The presence of sickle cell anaemia in both the West Indies and North America is a result of a direct spread from Africa.

Sickle cell anaemia

Sickle cell anaemia is the homozygous state for haemoglobin S and is the most severe form of sickle cell disease.

monly around the ankle. The liver is usually found to be somewhat enlarged, but the size of the spleen varies. Young children may show some splenomegaly, but from the age of 3 years splenomegaly becomes less common and eventually it is rare. Presence of an enlarged spleen in adults with sickle cell disease is always associated with an unusually bland form of the illness or indicates that, in fact, one is dealing not with sickle cell anaemia but with another form of sickle cell disease such as sickle cell haemoglobin C disease (page 490) or sickle cell thalassaemia (page 501).

Sickle cell anaemia is a haemolytic anaemia and like all haemolytic anaemias of any severity the course of the disease is interspersed with crises. These crises, although sometimes haemolytic in nature, are often aplastic crises. The hypertrophied bone marrow (Plate 40) becomes exhausted and blood formation stops. In a patient with a haemolytic process, any retardation of marrow output results in a catastrophic fall in the haemoglobin level. The cause of the marrow aplasia is usually a coincidental infection, which can be viral, bacterial or parasitic in nature. In West Africa there is a tendency for crises to be seasonal, occurring before the rainy seasons. Folic acid deficiency may also be responsible for an unexplained clinical deterioration.

OCCLUSIVE CRISES. In addition to the clinical manifestations of a haemolytic process common to all the haemoglobinopathies, sickle cell anaemia presents one severe additional complication due to the low solubility of the reduced sickle haemoglobin. The sickle cells that form when the haemoglobin crystallises within the red cell entwine one with the other in the small vessels and give rise to crises due to vascular occlusion. These occlusive crises may occur at any site in the body and account therefore for the multiple manifestations of sickle cell anaemia. In children, bones appear to be particularly affected and this may mimic osteomyelitis or rheumatism or, if vascular occlusion affects the femur, Perthes' disease (see Plate 40). At an early age dactylitis is particularly common, and when a child presents with swollen and painful fingers, this is highly suggestive of sickle cell disease. Patients with bony manifestations appear to be particularly liable to salmonella infections of bone.

Infarctions in the spleen may give rise to abdominal pain and it is because they are so frequent that the spleen will eventually become sufficiently scarred to shrink and clinically become no longer palpable. This is referred to as 'autosplenectomy'. Abdominal crises are common and if misdiagnosed can give rise to unnecessary surgical intervention. Like all haemolytic disorders, there is a liability to bilurubin stones, which creates an additional diagnostic difficulty.

Perhaps the most dramatic manifestations are those due to vascular occlusion affecting the nervous system. These may vary from sudden blindness to mental instability. Because of their bizarre nature there is always a danger of the diagnosis of hysteria.

A woman with sickle cell anaemia is at particular risk during and immediately after her pregnancy. A constant watch must be kept on the haemoglobin level and immediate transfusion should be available if the haemoglobin falls to a dangerous level. It is desirable to perform a Caesarean section at about the thirty-sixth week of pregnancy under carefully controlled anaesthetic.

As well as the variability in severity in each patient from time to time, certain patients, apparently suffering from typical sickle cell anaemia proved by family study, run a relatively bland course. These patients usually have an enlarged spleen and tend to have a higher level of fetal haemoglobin than is normally found in sickle cell anaemia (Table 30.2).

Other forms of sickle cell disease such as sickle cell haemoglobin C disease (page 490), sickle cell haemoglobin D disease (page 491) or sickle cell thalassaemia (page 501) also present as a sickle cell disease with splenomegaly and usually with milder clinical manifestations than sickle cell anaemia.

Routine haematology

Haemoglobin. Lies commonly between 6 and 10 g/100 ml.

Blood film. Shows a large number of target cells associated with polychromasia and nucleated red cells. There is an increase in the reticulocyte count. Red cells shaped rather like bananas can be seen in the peripheral blood. Numerous sickle forms may be seen in a sickle crisis when there is commonly also a granular leukocytosis (Plate 39).

Osmotic fragility. Shows an increased resistance to hypotonic saline.

Fetal haemoglobin. Increased, usually comprising 5–10 per cent of the total haemoglobin present. On rare occasions, larger amounts may be found and this is associated with a benign clinical course.

Sickle cell test. Positive.

Diagnosis is established by:
1. The combination of a severe haemolytic anaemia with sickling crises. The blood smear shows target cells with a variable number of sickle forms.
2. Splenomegaly is unusual in typical sickle cell anaemia after the age of 5 years. A massive spleen may be present in a sickle cell anaemia running an unusually mild course, but such patients warrant further investigation, including a family study.
3. Of the haemoglobin present 90–95 per cent is haemoglobin S and this may be confirmed by electrophoresis (Fig. 30.6) and a positive sickle cell test. (See haemoglobin SD disease (page 491).)

4. Racial origin of the patient.
5. Family study.

Haemoglobin S trait

This is the heterozygous or carrier state of haemoglobin S. The haemolysate of the blood of these individuals contains haemoglobins S and A, with haemoglobin S approximately 40 per cent of the total.

Clinical features. These patients are perfectly fit except for a slightly increased liability to haematuria, possibly of infarctive origin. Under severe conditions of deoxygenation sickling crises occur. Such conditions may arise in: (*a*) a badly administered anaesthetic, (*b*) severe pneumonia, (*c*) high altitude flying in unpressurised aircraft.

It therefore follows that the presence of the sickle cell trait does not explain the finding of an anaemia, and apart from the possible request for guidance on the choice of a partner in marriage (page 501) the finding of sickle cell trait can be totally ignored.

Routine haematology. This is normal except for a positive sickle cell test.

Diagnosis is established by:
1. The normal clinical and haematological findings.
2. Confirmation of the presence of haemoglobins S and A, haemoglobin S being approximately 40 per cent of the total (Plate 34). The presence of haemoglobin S, unlike haemoglobin D, will give a positive sickle cell test.
3. Racial origin of the patient.

Haemoglobin SC disease (see page 490)

Haemoglobin SD disease (see page 491)

Sickle cell thalassaemia (see page 501)

HAEMOGLOBIN C

Amino acid substitution

There is a substitution of lysine for glutamic acid in the sixth position of the β chain ($\alpha_2\beta_2$ 6 Glu$\rightarrow$Lys).

Geographical distribution (see Fig. 30.25).

Haemoglobin C was discovered in American Negroes and later found to occur in a remarkably circumscribed area in West Africa. In eastern Nigeria, across the River Niger, haemoglobin C

is virtually absent. Not only is haemoglobin C found in West Africa, it also will be present wherever people from this area have migrated, for instance in America and the West Indies.

On occasions haemoglobin C is found in North Africa, the Mediterranean area and even in northern Europe.

Any other haemoglobin variant which has an amino acid substitution of lysine for glutamic acid will have an electrophoretic mobility on paper and starch gel electrophoresis which may be very close to that of haemoglobin C. Haemoglobin E ($\alpha_2\beta_2$ 26 Glu$\rightarrow$Lys) and haemoglobin O Arab ($\alpha_2\beta_2$ 121 Glu$\rightarrow$Lys) are examples.

Because of their geographical distribution (Fig. 30.25) haemoglobins C and E may often be differentiated by a knowledge of the racial origin of the patient. However, in certain areas, particularly the West Indies and Central America, Asian and African populations have lived together for many years with consequent mixture of the racial groups and specific haemoglobin variants which these groups carry.

Some examples from Egypt reported as haemoglobin C and E may, in some cases, be examples of haemoglobin O Arab ($\alpha_2\beta_2$ 121 Gly$\rightarrow$Lys).

Haemoglobin C disease

This is the homozygous state for haemoglobin C.

Clinical features. In haemoglobin C disease the life span of the red cell is slightly shortened. Some patients with this condition are first seen because of their complaints, which include lassitude due to mild anaemia, slight jaundice and abdominal discomfort due to their splenomegaly. The majority of patients with haemoglobin C disease are relatively symptomless and are able to compensate for the mild haemolytic state. Such people are only discovered as a result of surveys. All patients with haemoglobin C disease may react badly to haematological stresses caused by pregnancy or infection in which circumstances the anaemia may become severe.

Routine haematology

Haemoglobin. Commonly between 10 and 13 g/100 ml.

Blood film. Shows a large number of target cells associated with some polychromasia and some increase in the reticulocyte count, due to the shortened red cell life.

Osmotic fragility. Shows an increased resistance to hypotonic saline.

Fetal haemoglobin. May be increased; up to 5 per cent may be present.

Diagnosis is established by:
1. Anaemia associated with target cells in blood smear.
2. Splenomegaly.
3. Presence of haemoglobin C with absence of haemoglobin A.
4. Racial origin of the patient.
5. Family study.

Haemoglobin C trait

This is the heterozygous or carrier state for haemoglobin C. The haemolysate of the blood of these individuals contains haemoglobins C and A, with haemoglobin C approximately 40 per cent of the total.

Clinical state. Normal.
Routine haematology. Normal.
Diagnosis is established by:
1. The normal clinical and haematological findings.
2. Confirmation of the presence of haemoglobins C and A in approximately equal proportions (see Plates 34 and 36).
3. Racial origin of the patient.

Haemoglobin SC disease

This is the double heterozygote state for haemoglobins S and C. Patients with this condition carry the genes for both the abnormal β chain producing haemoglobin S and the abnormal β chain producing haemoglobin C. The haemolysate of the blood of these individuals contains haemoglobins S and C with slightly more of haemoglobin S. A small quantity of fetal haemoglobin may be also present.

Clinical features. This condition manifests itself either as an anaemia arising in pregnancy or during an infection or as an infarctive incident. The latter may dramatically present as an impairment of vision due to occlusion of retinal vessels or as a liability to maternal death during the first few days following delivery. Apart from these two manifestations, patients with this condition are liable to attacks of abdominal pain. Splenomegaly is usual on clinical examination. Bone infarcts are commonly found on X-ray examination. Many patients with this condition are symptomless.

Routine haematology
Haemoglobin. Commonly about 10 g/100 ml.
Blood film. Shows some target cells together with occasional early sickle forms.
Osmotic fragility. Shows increased resistance to hypotonic saline.

Fetal haemoglobin. May be increased; up to 5 per cent may be present.
Sickle cell test. Positive.
Diagnosis is established by:
1. Sickling crises often result in impairment of vision of postpartum maternal death. Target cells with occasional early sickle forms are found in the blood smear.
2. Splenomegaly.
3. The presence on electrophoresis of haemoglobins S and C with an absence of haemoglobin A. Plate 36*a* and *b* show that using a TRIS paper electrophoresis system, haemoglobins S and C fail to separate. S and C are easily differentiated using paper electrophoresis and a barbiturate buffer system.
4. Racial origin of the patient.
5. Family study.

Haemoglobin C thalassaemia (see page 501)

HAEMOGLOBIN D PUNJAB

The name haemoglobin D was given to any haemoglobin variant (irrespective of the amino acid substitution) whose electrophoretic mobility on paper or starch gel was identical with haemoglobin S (see Plate 34). Unlike haemoglobin S, the haemoglobin D variants are normally soluble in the reduced state. The only common D variant is haemoglobin D Punjab, which will be discussed in this section.

Amino acid substitution

Haemoglobin D Punjab has an amino acid substitution of glutamine for glutamic acid in the 121st position of the β chain ($\alpha_2\beta_2$ 121 Glu→Gln).

Geographical distribution

Haemoglobin D was originally described in a Los Angeles family some years before the identical haemoglobin was discovered in the Punjab and strictly speaking this variant should be called D Los Angeles. In North-west India, particularly in the Punjab, 3 per cent of the people carry this variant (Fig. 30.25). The same haemoglobin is found at lower frequencies near by in Afghanistan and Iran and people who have migrated from the Punjab to Southern India. This pigment is occasionally found in Europe, especially among the Portuguese, French, British and Irish, and one possible explanation can be based on the close links between India and Europe. For example, there were probably about 400 intermarriages per annum between British soldiers and Anglo-Indian women in the early part of the nineteenth century.

Haemoglobin D disease

This is the homozygous state for haemoglobin D. Little is known about the clinical state or haematological findings of patients with haemoglobin D disease. In all probability they are symptomless and the cases reported previously are likely to have been examples of haemoglobin D thalassaemia (page 501).

Haemoglobin D trait

This is the heterozygous or carrier state of haemoglobin D. Haemolysates of the blood of these individuals contain haemoglobin A and D in approximately equal proportions.

Clinical features. Normal.
Routine haematology. Normal.
Diagnosis is established by:
1. The normal clinical condition and haematological findings.
2. Confirmation of the presence of haemoglobins A and D in approximately equal proportions (Plate 34). Although on starch gel and paper electrophoresis haemoglobin D and S travel identically, red cells containing haemoglobin D do not sickle.
3. Racial origin of the patient.

Haemoglobin SD disease

This is the double heterozygote state for haemoglobins S and D. Patients with this disease have slightly more haemoglobin S and D. Because haemoglobins S and D do not separate on paper and starch gel electrophoresis and because red cells from these patients will sickle, this condition is liable to be confused with sickle-cell anaemia.

Clinical features. These patients are not as severely affected as patients with sickle cell anaemia. The condition should therefore be suspected when a so-called sickle cell anaemia is found to have an enlarged spleen and to be running a relatively benign clinical course.

Routine haematology
Haemoglobin. Commonly about 10 g/100 ml.
Blood film. Shows a number of target cells and an occasional sickled cell.
Osmotic fragility. Shows an increased resistance to hypotonic saline.
Fetal haemoglobin. Increased; about 5–10 per cent of fetal haemoglobin may be present.

Sickle cell test. Positive.
Diagnosis is established by:
1. A clinical picture of a relatively benign sickle cell anaemia associated with splenomegaly. Target cells and occasional early sickle forms are found in the blood smear.
2. Presence of haemoglobins S and D. On paper and starch gel electrophoresis the haemolysates of patients with SD disease and sickle cell anaemia look identical (Plate 36). Haemoglobins S and D can, however, be distinguished by agar gel electrophoresis. The Itano solubility test measures the solubility of a reduced haemoglobin and by assessing the amount of precipitated haemoglobin gives an indication of the amount of haemoglobin S which is present in a haemolysate. The percentage of insoluble reduced haemoglobin (haemoglobin S) is lower in haemoglobin SD disease than in sickle cell anaemia.
3. Racial origin of the patient.
4. Family study.

Haemoglobin D thalassaemia (see page 501)

HAEMOGLOBIN E

Amino acid substitution

There is a substitution of lysine for glutamic acid in the twenty-sixth position of the β chain ($\alpha_2\beta_2$ 26 Glu→Lys).

Geographical distribution

Haemoglobin E is found in high frequency in Thailand, Burma and northern Malaya (see Fig. 30.25). In some areas of Thailand the frequency is over 30 per cent.

Haemoglobin E disease

This is the homozygous state for haemoglobin E.
Clinical features. Unless patients are under an additional haematological stress, it is likely that they suffer from no obvious disability. Often they are discovered because a routine examination has demonstrated a palpable spleen.
Routine haematology
Haemoglobin. Commonly between 12 and 14 g/100 ml.
Blood film. Shows a large number of target cells associated with some polychromasia and an

increase in the reticulocyte count due to the shortened red cell life span.

Osmotic fragility. There is an increased resistance to hypotonic saline.

Fetal haemoglobin. 0–5 per cent may be present.

Diagnosis is established by:

1. Mild anaemia associated with target cells in blood smear.
2. Splenomegaly.
3. Presence of haemoglobin E and absence of haemoglobin A.
4. Racial origin of the patient.
5. Family study.

Haemoglobin E trait

This is the heterozygous or carrier state for haemoglobin E. The haemolysate of the blood of these individuals contains haemoglobins E and A in approximately equal proportions.

Clinical state. Normal.

Routine haematology. Normal.

Diagnosis is established by:

1. The normal clinical and haematological findings.
2. Confirmation of the presence of haemoglobins E and A in approximately equal proportions (see Plates 34 and 36).
3. Racial origin of the patient.

Haemoglobin E thalassaemia (see page 501)

RARE HAEMOGLOBINS

A rare haemoglobin is suspected if either the physical characteristics of the haemoglobin variant or the racial origin of the carrier are other than those of the common variants C, D Punjab, E and S. Before it became possible to undertake an amino acid analysis of an abnormal haemoglobin, many variants were described and recognised by their electrophoretic properties alone. It is now realised that different amino acid substitutions may well give rise to identical changes in electrophoretic mobility. This is because the electrophoretic mobility of a variant is merely an indication of the overall charge change of the haemoglobin molecule resulting from an amino acid substitution. It gives no obvious clue to the position of the substitution in the polypeptide chain or, except in the case of a glutamic acid→ lysine or lysine→glutamic acid substitution (page 471), the amino acids involved.

Unless a rare haemoglobin variant has been described before in a particular part of the world, for example haemoglobin O β Arab in the northern Sudan, Egypt and Israeli Arabs, the identification of such variants ultimately depends upon the clinical analysis of the polypeptide chains. Because this is a lengthy procedure, it is necessary for the variant to be examined, either because its physical properties or geographical distribution is of unusual interest.

Two of the variants in Table 30.1, although considered under the heading of the rare haemoglobins, are nevertheless worthy of special mention. *Haemoglobin G Philadelphia*, which has been described under many names (α_2 68 Asn→Lys β_2), has been found many times in West Africans and American Negroes. On starch gel electrophoresis it travels in the same position as haemoglobins S and D, but on paper barbiturate electrophoresis it travels between haemoglobins A and S.

The second rare variant, *haemoglobin O Arab* ($\alpha_2\beta_2$ 121 Glu→Lys) travels in the same position as haemoglobin C and E but can be distinguished by electrophoresis using an agar gel. Examples of haemoglobin C and E from North Africa may in some cases be examples of haemoglobin O Arab (page 489).

The M haemoglobins (see below) and the unstable haemoglobins (page 495) are also rare. These haemoglobins are considered in some detail because of their theoretical interest and also because of their unusual clinical manifestations. Their clinical importance is obviously negligible when compared with sickle cell anaemia and β thalassaemia major.

M HAEMOGLOBINS

Causes of methaemoglobinaemia

In the normal individual there is a balance between the spontaneous process of methaemoglobin formation (1 per cent of the total circulating haemoglobin is spontaneously converted into methaemoglobin each day) and protective mechanisms dependent upon enzymes present in the intact red cell, which reconvert the pigment back again to haemoglobin. Methaemoglobinaemia may be caused in three ways.

NORMAL GLOBIN

1. Excessive formation of methaemoglobin often due to drugs or chemicals (*common*).

2. Diminished reconversion of methaemoglobin to haemoglobin due to a deficiency in the methaemoglobin reductase enzyme systems (*rare*).

ABNORMAL GLOBIN

3. An abnormality of the globin part of the haemoglobin molecule, which allows the haem

groups to exist only in the haematin (ferric) state. These globin abnormalities result collectively in the haemoglobins M (*rare*).

Molecular abnormality

When the structure of the haemoglobin molecule was considered (page 465), it was emphasised that the haem group was carefully protected from the external aqueous environment by being inserted into a globin pocket lined by hydrophobic side chains projecting from the neighbouring amino acid residues. The M haemoglobins result when the protective effect of the globin pocket proves to be inadequate. This can arise in a number of different ways.

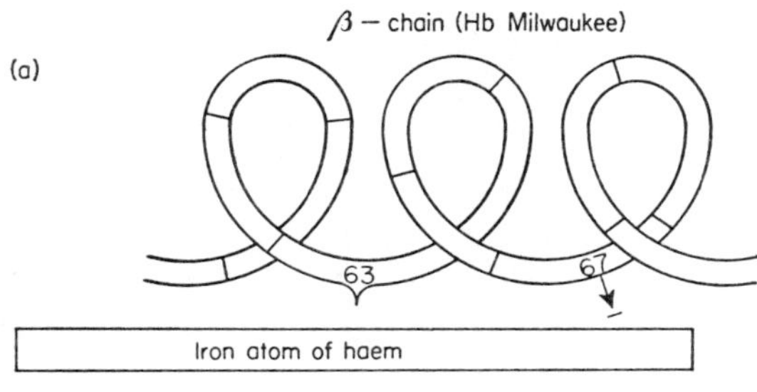

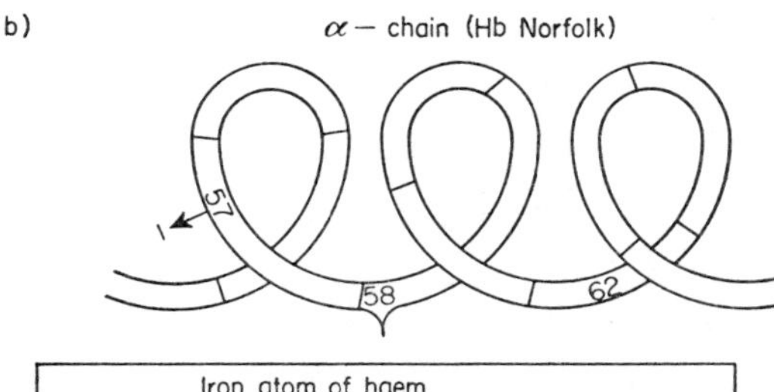

FIG. 30.26. *The influence upon the haem of the position of a mutation in the helical polypeptide chain. (a) A mutation of a neutral amino acid to a charged amino acid will point in the direction of the haem if it is four amino acid residues away from the distal histidyl (β63). A haemoglobin M results (M Milwaukee). (b) A similar type of mutation will point away from the haem pocket if it is alongside the distal histidyl (α58). Haemoglobin Norfolk is not an M haemoglobin. (In Man's Haemoglobins, North-Holland Publishing Company.)*

Substitution of the proximal or distal histidine residue

	α chain	β chain
Proximal	Iwate	M Hyde Park
histidyl	(α_2 87 His→Tyr β_2)	($\alpha_2\beta_2$ 92 His→Tyr)
Distal	M Boston	M Saskatoon
histidyl	(α_2 58 His→Tyr β_2)	($\alpha_2\beta_2$ 63 His→Tyr)

The replacement of distal histidine residue in the β chain by an arginine residue ($\alpha_2\beta_2$ 63 His→Arg) results not in an M haemoglobin but haemoglobin Zürich, an unstable haemoglobin (page 495).

Insertion of a charged group into the globin pocket. Because of the helical structure of the polypeptide chain, in the case of haemoglobin Milwaukee ($\alpha_2\beta_2$ 67 Val→Glu), an amino acid substitution four residues away from the distal histidyl will point in the direction of the iron atom.

In haemoglobin Norfolk a neutral glycyl in position 57 of the α chain has been replaced by a negatively charged aspartyl (α_2 57 Gly→Asp β_2). This mutation is next-door to the distal histidyl, which points into the pocket at position 58. Haemoglobin Norfolk is not a haemoglobin M, presumably because the charge on the aspartic acid residue, being only one position away, is at right angles to the previous amino acid and points away from the haem (Fig. 30.26).

Disturbance of the conformation of the haemoglobin molecule with a secondary effect on the haem pocket. Any amino acid substitution that results in an unstable haemoglobin molecule will also give rise to chemically detectable methaemoglobinaemia. The distortion of the haemoglobin molecule, even if not primarily within the haem pocket, appears to result in a secondary disturbance in the region of the haem.

Clinical features

The haemoglobins M occur sporadically in virtually every part of the world. Their rarity in deeply pigmented races appears due to the fact that cyanosis, the presenting feature, would be more difficult to recognise. Often there is no haemoglobin M present in the parents, which suggests that a mutation may have taken place at this generation. Indeed, it is possible that the incidence of haemoglobin M will be useful as an indication of human mutation rates.

The age of onset of cyanosis may give some indication as to whether the abnormality lies in the α or β chain of the haemoglobin molecule. If the abnormality lies in the α chain, because fetal haemoglobin ($\alpha_2\gamma_2$) is affected, cyanosis is present from birth. If the abnormality lies in the β chain, cyanosis does not appear until the formation of adult haemoglobin ($\alpha_2\beta_2$) becomes firmly established within a few months after birth. Because the haem group in any haemoglobin M cannot exist in the ferrous state, giving a reducing agent by mouth such as ascorbic acid or the in-

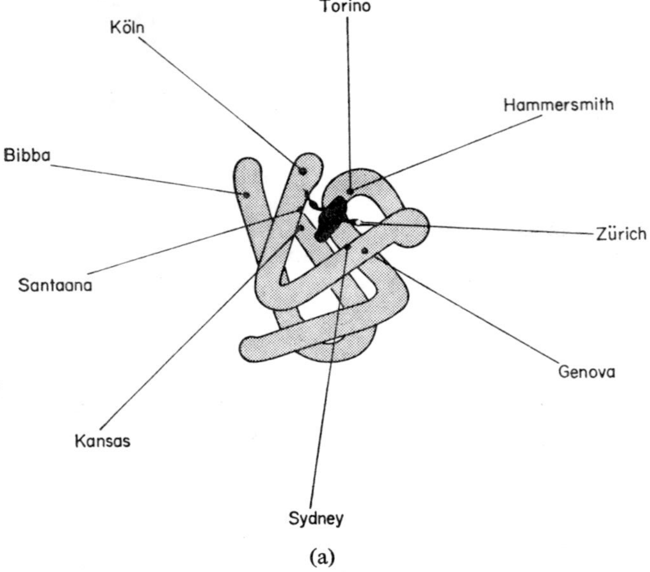

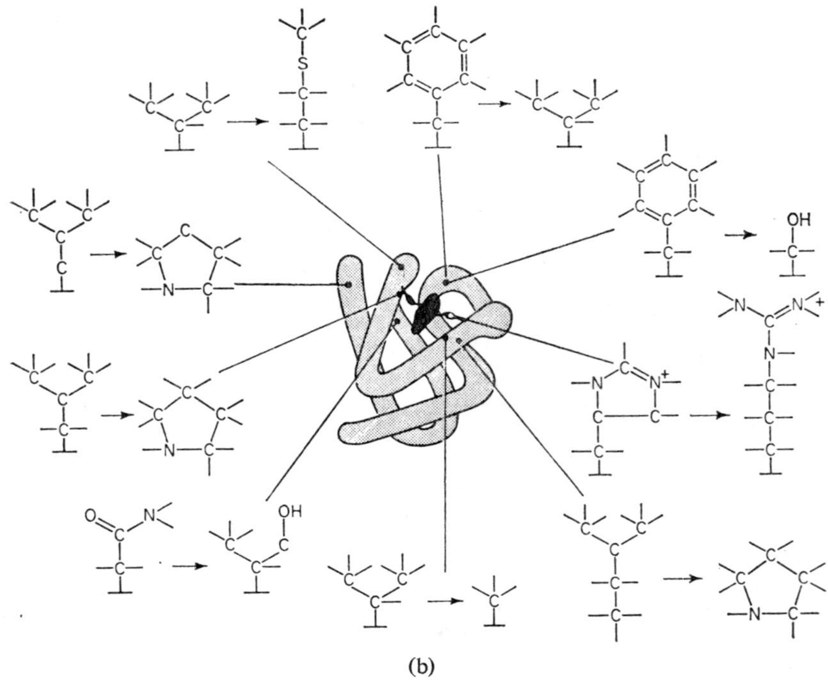

FIG. 30.27. *Unstable haemoglobins:* (a) *names;* (b) *amino acid substitutions.*

jection of methylene blue does not reduce the cyanosis if this is caused by an M haemoglobin. It must, however, be remembered that neither will these substances reduce the cyanosis if it is caused by sulphmethaemoglobin instead of methaemoglobin.

UNSTABLE HAEMOGLOBINS

The α- and β-polypeptide chains of the haemoglobin molecule and the single polypeptide chain of myoglobin are remarkably similar in shape although they differ considerably in their amino acid content. This strangely consistent shape, with the haem group embedded into the polypeptide chain, appears necessary for the function of the haem-globin complex, either as a single unit as in myoglobin or as a quaternary structure as in haemoglobin.

The conformation the polypeptide chain adopts depends basically upon amino acid constitution—for instance, proline is associated with a bend in the chain. The specific amino acid sequence must be compatible with the retention of the necessary contortions of the polypeptide chain. The helices are held in place by bonding between neighbouring amino acids and if an amino acid substitution so disrupts this bonding force that the natural shape (secondary and tertiary structure) of the polypeptide chain is disorganised, then the molecule will alter its form and become denatured.

It will be seen (Fig. 30.27a and b) that many of the variants have amino acid substitutions in the region of the haem. Such substitutions weaken the haemoglobin linkage. Haem appears to give mature globin stability—the globin easily denaturing if the haem is allowed to escape. Some amino acid substitutions such as the insertion of a charged amino acid into the centre of the molecule are probably totally incompatible with a functioning molecule and would not therefore be capable of existence. Others result in haemoglobin molecules which are somewhat unstable and permit the denaturation process to be easily triggered off. This denaturation is especially likely to occur when the haemoglobin molecule is already under some stress. Such situations arise when methaemoglobin-forming drugs are given or, in the laboratory, when the molecule is heated to 50°C in the heat denaturation test.

Even in the heterozygous state, patients carrying the trait for an unstable haemoglobin suffer from a haemolytic anaemia either continually or provoked by certain drugs. These drugs, or their metabolites, are likely to possess redox potential and would therefore be similar to those capable of causing haemolysis of glucose-6-phosphate-dehydrogenase-deficient cells. The denatured haemoglobin precipitates within the red cell as Heinz bodies and this precipitated material becomes markedly more noticeable after splenectomy, which is commonly carried out because of an associated splenomegaly.

The unstable haemoglobins may form only a small proportion of the total haemoglobin present and if one is screening to exclude an unstable haemoglobin as the cause of an obscure haemolytic anaemia, it is wise to rely on the heat denaturation test as a screening manoeuvre as well as an electrophoretic procedure. On page 466 it is explained that the ferrous atom of the haemoglobin molecule has to be protected from the external environment during the oxygenation and deoxygenation process. It is perhaps not surprising that, during the denaturation of the haemoglobin molecule, there is some disruption in the neighbourhood of the haem which permits the conversion of the ferrous atom to the ferric form. This explains why the patients with unstable haemoglobins have a chemically detectable increase in methaemoglobin.

As stated before, the stability of the haemoglobin molecule depends upon each polypeptide chain having a suitable amino acid constitution. As well as this, for the quaternary structure to be stable, the four polypeptide chains that compose it must form a satisfactory stable relationship with each other. Haemoglobin H (β_2) and to a lesser extent haemoglobin Bart's (γ_2) are both unstable, the former particularly giving rise to a positive heat denaturation test. It appears in these cases that the forming of a quaternary structure with solely β or γ chains results in an unstable molecule, although the β and γ chains are in every way identical to those found in haemoglobin A ($\alpha_2\beta_2$) and haemoglobin F ($\alpha_2\gamma_2$) respectively. The combination of the α and β chains in haemoglobin A, the α and γ chains in haemoglobin F, and the α and δ chains in haemoglobin A_2 must have a stabilising effect on the quaternary structure which is lacking when all four polypeptide chains are identical.

THALASSAEMIA

Since Cooley first described Mediterranean anaemia or thalassaemia in 1925 a number of different disorders have been included under this heading. All these conditions have in common a depression of synthesis of adult haemoglobin which, if sufficiently severe, results in a deficiency of haemoglobin in the red cells. The clinical severity of the conditions classified under thalassaemia is, however, highly variable. At one extreme thalassaemia causes death *in utero* and ranges from death in childhood through chronic anaemia to the other extreme when it is symptomless and virtually undiagnosable.

Now that the structure of the haemoglobin molecule is better understood, it has become possible to divide the great majority of the thalassaemias into those where there is an abnormality of β chain production (β thalassaemia) and those where there is an abnormality of α chain production (α thalassaemia and haemoglobin H disease). δ thalassaemia does not affect directly the production of adult haemoglobin ($\alpha_2\beta_2$) but primarily depresses the formation of haemoglobin $A_2(\alpha_2\delta_2)$. Hereditary persistence of high fetal haemoglobin (caused by the 'high F' gene) (page 499) and haemoglobin Lepore (page 496) although uncommon are worthy of consideration because they are liable to present difficulties of diagnosis.

In thalassaemia, there is a depression of production of normal haemoglobin A rather than its replacement by an abnormal haemoglobin. α and β thalassaemia may occur like the abnormal haemoglobins both in the heterozygous or homozygous state. The heterozygote suffers from thalassaemia minor and the homozygote from thalassaemia major. When a patient is a homozygote for an abnormal haemoglobin such as haemoglobin C, he is unable to produce any haemoglobin A. Both of his genes which should be capable of producing normal β chains are substituted by genes producing the abnormal β chains characteristic of haemoglobin C; in other words, β-polypeptide chains with a substitution of lysine for glutamic acid in the sixth position. In contrast, thalassaemia which is a depression of haemoglobin A production is quantitative rather than qualitative and some normal haemoglobin may yet be produced even in the homozygote state. This ability of a patient with thalassaemia to produce normal haemoglobin is of diagnostic importance when interaction between thalassaemia and an abnormal haemoglobin is considered (page 500).

β thalassaemia

Molecular abnormality. The genes responsible for the production of the β-polypeptide chains function abnormally. The cause of the impairment of β chain production may well be inadequate output of messenger RNA. The limitation of production is confined only to the β chains, therefore only the output of adult haemoglobin ($\alpha_2\beta_2$) is depressed. The production of haemoglobin F ($\alpha_2\gamma_2$) and haemoglobin A_2 ($\alpha_2\delta_2$) is not involved, and indeed, a compensatory increase in these two haemoglobins is at times a diagnostic feature of β thalassaemia.

Geographical distribution. By comparison with a survey for abnormal haemoglobins, where paper electrophoresis gives a clear-cut diagnosis, the recognition of thalassaemia is not as easy. One may well require a full blood examination with osmotic fragility and serum iron together with quantitation of haemoglobin A_2 and F. As a result, knowledge as to its distribution is not complete. β thalassaemia appears to be widely spread across the Mediterranean through the Middle East and into the Far East (Fig. 30.25). Very high incidences are seen notably in Greece and in Italy where, for instance, in the Po Valley about 20 per cent of the population have β thalassaemia minor, the heterozygous state of this condition. In Africa it is rare or absent in the East but frequent in some areas of the West.

β thalassaemia major

This is the homozygous state for β thalassaemia. As both genes responsible for β chain production are depressed very often little or no haemoglobin A ($\alpha_2\beta_2$) is found at all.

Clinical features. A person afflicted with β thalassaemia major can be expected to die in childhood or adolescence. The first symptoms are seen when haemoglobin A production becomes predominant at the age of about 4 months (Figs. 30.10 and 30.11). The child presents with anaemia of increasing severity, splenomegaly and usually hepatomegaly.

There is a compensatory hypertrophy of the bone marrow which is common to all severe congenital haemolytic anaemias. This hypertrophy is demonstrated on X-ray examination by the characteristic hair-on-end appearance in the skull, which is due to expansion of the diploe (Plate 40). Swelling of the marrow cavities within the zygoma bones results in a mongoloid facies. The child suffers from increasingly severe anaemia requiring repeated transfusions to retain the haemoglobin at a level compatible with life. Iron overloading is a danger and ultimately death may occur from cardiac failure due to severe anaemia or haemochromatosis of the cardiac muscle.

Routine haematology

Haemoglobin. Lies commonly between 4 and 8 g/100 ml.

Blood film. Shows hypochromic sometimes

fragmented red cells with target cells, nucleated red cells, polychromasia and basophilic stippling. There is an increase in the reticulocyte count.

Osmotic fragility. Shows increased resistance to hypotonic saline.

Fetal haemoglobin. Between 20 and 100 per cent of the total haemoglobin present is fetal haemoglobin.

Diagnosis is established by:

1. Presence of a severe anaemia in a child which is both dyshaemopoietic and haemolytic in nature. Despite the hypochromia, the serum iron level is raised and the iron stores in the marrow are found to be increased.
2. Massive splenomegaly with hepatomegaly.
3. Marked diminution of haemoglobin A. The majority of the haemoglobin present is usually haemoglobin F.
4. Racial origin of the patient.
5. Family study.

β thalassaemia minor

This is the heterozygous state for β thalassaemia.

Clinical features. The diagnosis of β thalassaemia minor is a common diagnostic problem that will frequently occupy the attention of the clinician and of the routine haematology department. The degree of anaemia in β thalassaemia minor is highly variable. Indeed, most people with this condition are able to live and work normally and may be discovered as a result of a survey. Like all chronic haemolytic anaemias, such people tend to react badly to haematological stresses and a severe anaemia may easily develop. They are often diagnosed because of an anaemia of pregnancy or alternatively as a severe anaemia precipitated by a complication such as a virus infection. Some patients present as a mild anaemia, which is found on blood film examination to be hypochromic in type.

After a course of iron therapy, the haemoglobin fails to rise and it is at this point that these patients, who are now labelled 'iron-resistant anaemia', are further investigated. The presence of hypochromia therefore makes the exclusion of iron deficiency the first requirement in the diagnosis and this is best achieved by a serum iron estimation. Thalassaemia complicated by iron deficiency is unusual and should become apparent when the iron deficiency is corrected. If the bone marrow is examined, the iron stores should always be assessed by a Prussian blue stain.

On clinical examination, the size of the spleen is highly variable but is usually palpable.

Routine haematology

Haemoglobin. Usually between 11 and 14 g/100 ml (unless complications arise, when the level will be lower).

Blood film. Shows hypochromia with occasional target cells, poikilocytes together with polychromasia and basophilic stippling. Blood film changes in some cases may show only minimal evidence of any abnormality.

Osmotic fragility. Shows an increased resistance to hypotonic saline. Red cells with hypochromia due to iron deficiency also show an increased resistance to hypotonic saline.

Fetal haemoglobin. Raised in about half the patients with β thalassaemia minor and does not commonly exceed 5 per cent of the total haemoglobin.

Diagnosis is established by:

1. Presence of anaemia. This anaemia is highly variable in severity and in many cases the haemoglobin is at the lower limit of the normal range. Although hypochromic in type, the anaemia fails to respond to iron and is associated with a normal or raised serum iron and iron stores unless the patient has iron deficiency as a complication.
2. Splenomegaly. The spleen may be palpable.
3. Haemoglobin A_2 is raised in the great majority of cases of β thalassaemia minor whereas only half the patients have a fetal haemoglobin above the normal level (see Plate 35). A small number of cases are found which, although in every way compatible with β thalassaemia minor, nevertheless have a normal or depressed haemoglobin A_2 level (see page 471).
4. Although the racial origin of the patient is of some value in reaching a diagnosis, β thalassaemia minor is present to a variable extent in virtually all populations.
5. Family study.

α thalassaemia

Molecular abnormality. The gene responsible for the production of the α polypeptide chains functions abnormally. The exact site of impairment of production is not certainly known but, as in β thalassaemia, may again be at the level of messenger RNA. Haemoglobins A ($\alpha_2\beta_2$), A_2 ($\alpha_2\delta_2$) and F ($\alpha_2\gamma_2$) all contain α chains and therefore a depression of α chain production must result in diminished production of all these three haemoglobins. No compensatory increase in haemoglobins F and A$_2$ is therefore possible as is the case in β thalassaemia and haemoglobin A$_2$ production may be depressed. There is, however, a tendency to produce haemoglobins which do not contain β chains. These haemoglobins are haemoglobin H (β_4) and haemoglobin Bart's (γ_4).

Haemoglobin H disease is another manifestation of impairment of α chain production. It is intermediate in severity between α thalassaemia major and minor and its mode of inheritance is not clear. However, it is possible to clarify the situation a little if one assumes that the α chain genes are duplicated on the chromosome, so that man has four α chain genes. The highly variable severity of α thalassaemia which contrasts with the sharp division between heterozygote and homozygote for β thalassaemia, could be due to four different types of α thalassaemia, depending on the number of the four α chain genes being affected.

Geographical distribution. It is very difficult to carry out a survey for α thalassaemia. One method of recognising the α thalassaemia gene is by detecting a raised haemoglobin Bart's (γ_4) in the cord blood. On this basis, α thalassaemia has been discovered in surveys carried out in Africa, the Mediterranean and in the Far East. We have examined 10 000 cord bloods in Britain and have yet to detect haemoglobin Bart's at a level above 2 per cent in a native British subject. It was, however, present above this level on many occasions in the cord blood of babies of immigrants from West Africa, West Indies, Hong Kong and the Mediterranean area.

Haemoglobin H disease is uncommon but present around the Mediterranean, in India and the Far East. It is occasionally reported from native British and Swedes. Although sometimes found in American Negroes, it appears remarkably rare in Africa. It is of interest that, although by estimating haemoglobin Bart's in the cord blood, α thalassaemia appears to be common in Africa, haemoglobin H disease is not frequent there. If the α thalassaemia gene is present in tropical Africa one would have expected to observe the occasional hydrops fetalis due to homozygosity for the α thalassaemia gene.

α thalassaemia presents clinically with three different conditions. These conditions are α thalassaemia major, α thalassaemia minor and haemoglobin H disease. Only haemoglobin H disease is likely to provide a diagnostic problem for the physician and α thalassaemia major and minor are therefore only briefly discussed.

α thalassaemia major

This is the homozygous state for α thalassaemia. In α thalassaemia major production resulting from all α chain genes are affected. As a result this condition is incompatible with life and results in stillbirth. Examination of the fetal blood shows mostly haemoglobin Bart's (γ_4), a small amount of haemoglobin F ($\alpha_2\gamma_2$) and traces of haemoglobin A ($\alpha_2\beta_2$) and haemoglobin H (β_4). Because the detection of α thalassaemia minor is so difficult, examination of parents may well prove to be negative.

α thalassaemia minor

This is the heterozygous state for α thalassaemia. When haemoglobin Bart's (γ_4) disappears a few months after birth, there may be no detectable abnormality of haemoglobin production. However, the red cells of adults may have a tendency to microcytosis and some increased resistance to hypotonic saline solution. The fact that carriers of the α thalassaemia trait are perfectly fit and have minimal or no abnormal haematological findings, makes the diagnosis of α thalassaemia minor difficult if not impossible.

Haemoglobin H disease

Haemoglobin H disease is a form of α thalassaemia, the mode of inheritance being uncertain. It is not uncommon that one parent can be diagnosed as having α thalassaemia minor, whereas the other is normal. It has been suggested that the normal parent carries a specific 'silent' α thalassaemia gene. Alternatively, assuming that there are four α chain genes, in the first parent two, and in the second one only may be affected.

Clinical features. The clinical severity of haemoglobin H disease tends to be somewhat more severe than that typically found in β thalassaemia minor. The spleen size also tends to be larger.

Routine haematology

Haemoglobin. Between 8 and 10 g/100 ml (it may rapidly fall in the presence of complications).

Blood film. Shows hypochromia with target cells, poikilocytoses and polychromasia with basophilic stippling.

Osmotic fragility. Shows an increased resistance to hypotonic saline.

Fetal haemoglobin. May occasionally be present in trace amounts only.

Diagnosis is established by:
1. Presence of anaemia which, as with β thalassaemia minor, may fluctuate greatly in

severity. This anaemia although hypochromic in type fails to respond to iron and is normally associated with a normal or raised serum iron and iron stores.

2. Splenomegaly.
3. Haemoglobin H is detectable both as finely distributed inclusion bodies (H bodies) within the red cell found after incubation with a vital dye (Plate 37) and as an abnormal haemoglobin band (5–15 per cent of the total pigment) which moves rapidly towards the anode on electrophoresis at alkaline pH (see Plate 35). Traces (0–2 per cent) of haemoglobin Bart's may also be seen. After splenectomy, inclusion bodies are particularly noticeable and some may be quite large, well over 1 μm in diameter. Haemoglobin H is unstable. Samples to be examined should be fresh and not be frozen, as under these conditions the haemoglobin H is precipitated out of solution.
4. Racial origin is not of help in making a diagnosis because haemoglobin H disease occurs sporadically across the Mediterranean, Middle and Far East as well as in many other populations.
5. Because of the difficulty in recognising α thalassaemia minor haemoglobin H disease is, like α thalassaemia major, one of the few haemoglobinopathies in which both parents may be found to be normal.
6. Haemoglobin H may not be found in iron deficiency and this condition must be excluded before absence of haemoglobin H disease is accepted.

δ thalassaemia

δ thalassaemia described mainly in Greece, is a condition where the primary lesion is a depression of the activity of the δ-polypeptide chain gene. The heterozygote shows reduced haemoglobin A_2 ($\alpha_2\delta_2$). The homozygous state is extremely rare. The heterozygous state may also include all cases of thalassaemia minor without raised haemoglobin A_2 but with a raised haemoglobin F (δ-β thalassaemia).

Associated conditions included in the thalassaemia syndromes

Hereditary persistance of high fetal haemoglobin and haemoglobin Lepore are discussed in conjunction with the thalassaemia syndromes. In both these conditions there is an impairment of normal β- and δ-chain production.

Hereditary persistence of high fetal haemoglobin (high F gene). If, after the age of about 2 years, one finds fetal haemoglobin above the normal level of 0–2 per cent, this nearly always indicates an anaemia which has been continually present since an early age. One of the exceptions to this statement is hereditary persistence of high fetal haemoglobin, an uncommon condition in which the pattern of haemoglobin production of the newborn is continued into adult life. The normal process of switching off the γ chain production and turning on the β and δ chain production has failed to occur.

The δ and β chain genes are close together on the same chromosome and they seem to be switched on together. When this switching-on mechanism fails, or the δ and β chain genes have been deleted, a high level of fetal haemoglobin production continues in the adult unassociated with anaemia. The heterozygotes for this condition (several dozen cases are now known) are found widely distributed across Africa, the Mediterranean and into India. On haematological examination, the majority of the haemoglobin is found to be haemoglobin A and, apart from the presence of 15–20 per cent of haemoglobin F, associated with a low A_2 level, they are normal. The homozygous conditions for the 'high F' gene is exceedingly rare, there being only three known cases. These people have a complete absence of adult haemoglobin and haemoglobin A_2 and possess 100 per cent fetal haemoglobin.

The fact that such individuals have no anaemia poses the question why evolution has resulted in the complex switching-over of one haemoglobin production line (fetal) to another (adult). Fetal red cells have a higher oxygen affinity than adult red cells, and this is of advantage to the embryo *in utero*. The carrier for the high F gene may be as fit as the normal person with haemoglobin A, and a mother with the high F gene might satisfactorily supply her offspring *in utero* with oxygen. The higher oxygen affinity of fetal red cells has nothing to do with their fetal haemoglobin but with a lower 2 : 3 diphosphoglycorate content.

There is now considerable interest in the mechanism of switching from fetal to adult haemoglobin production. If a patient with a β chain haemoglobinopathy was able to switch back to fetal haemoglobin production he would be cured of his illness.

A double heterozygote for the sickle cell gene and high F gene has haemoglobin S as the major component with haemoglobin F about 15–20 per cent. The haemolysate of the blood of these people may therefore be indistinguishable from the haemolysate from patients with sickle cell anaemia and yet clinically the condition is remarkably benign.

The two conditions can be distinguished haematologically by staining the red cells for fetal haemoglobin. In sickle cell anaemia the fetal haemoglobin present is distributed most unevenly in the red cells, some possess a lot, but the majority have no demonstrable fetal haemoglobin present. In contrast, the fetal haemoglobin in the double heterozygote state of hereditary persistence of high fetal haemoglobin and sickle cell trait shows that the fetal haemoglobin is more evenly distributed. It must be for this reason that the double heterozygote state is clinically a benign condition. Fetal haemoglobin protects the red cells against sickling and when the fetal haemoglobin is unevenly distributed, as in sickle cell anaemia, the majority of the red cells then have no protection against sickling.

Hereditary persistence of high fetal haemoglobin has also been found in association with haemoglobin C. When hereditary persistence of high fetal haemoglobin is found in association with β thalassaemia, it becomes possible, because of the high level of fetal haemoglobin, to confuse this condition with β thalassaemia major. A more benign clinical course combined with a family study will place the diagnosis beyond doubt.

Haemoglobin Lepore

Haemoglobin Lepore (two varieties have been described) is a haemoglobin molecule containing two normal α chains paired with two abnormal chains. Each of these abnormal chains consists of an initial segment of normal δ chain terminated by part of the normal β chain. Lepore haemoglobin may therefore be characterised as $\alpha_2 (\delta\beta)_2$. The Lepore haemoglobin found in American Negroes and the Mediterranean area (Lepore Washington) is different from the Lepore haemoglobin found in New Guinea natives (Lepore Hollandia). The two haemoglobins have differing points of fusion between the δ- and β-polypeptide chains.

The Lepore trait carrier is symptomless and there is demonstrable about 15–20 per cent Lepore haemoglobin in the haemolysate. Lepore haemoglobin does not separate from haemoglobin A on paper electrophoresis unless Tris buffer is used. It is easily demonstrable on a starch gel. Homozygotes for haemoglobin Lepore have been reported from New Guinea. Because

both δ and β chain loci are affected, no haemoglobin A and A$_2$ is present. The haemolysate consists of haemoglobin F and haemoglobin Lepore. A combination of haemoglobin Lepore with β thalassaemia trait results in severe disability which clinically and on routine haematological examination closely resembles β thalassaemia major. However, the haemolysate will show haemoglobin Lepore (5–10 per cent) with 20–95 per cent haemoglobin F. Haemoglobin A$_2$ is usually reduced. The amount of haemoglobin A present is highly variable but is usually less than 40 per cent of the total. Recently a patient with $\alpha_2(\beta\delta)_2$ haemoglobin has also been recognised.

Interaction between thalassaemia and haemoglobin variants

Thalassaemia can interfere with the formation of the α or the β chains of haemoglobin A ($\alpha_2\beta_2$). A rare type of thalassaemia decreasing the formation of the δ chains, and therefore the production of haemoglobin A$_2$ ($\alpha_2\delta_2$), has also been described.

A heterozygote for the common abnormal β chain variants (for example, haemoglobins S, C, D and E) will possess rather more of haemoglobin A than of the abnormal variant. These proportions are radically altered when such a heterozygote carries in the place of the normal β chain gene a β thalassaemia gene, i.e. is a double heterozygote for β thalassaemia and an abnormal β chain haemoglobin. Since these two genes are allelic, such people cannot possess a third normal gene for the production of β-polypeptide chains. Because the formation of the normal β chain is hindered by the β thalassaemia gene, the major proportion of haemoglobin present will be the abnormal variant. One therefore finds in, for example, sickle cell thalassaemia, that the sickle cell haemoglobin will be the prevalent haemoglobin, and little or no haemoglobin A will be formed. The term 'interaction' is used to describe this situation.

A double heterozygote for α thalassaemia and an abnormal β chain variant such as haemoglobin S will not show a preponderance of the abnormal variant. This is because the α thalassaemia gene will not depress the output of the normal β chains. As the normal and abnormal β chain haemoglobins contain the same normal α chains, α thalassaemia will not differentiate between the two. On the contrary when α chains are scarce, the concentration of the abnormal β chain haemoglobin may fall because its β chain may compete less successfully for the rare α chains.

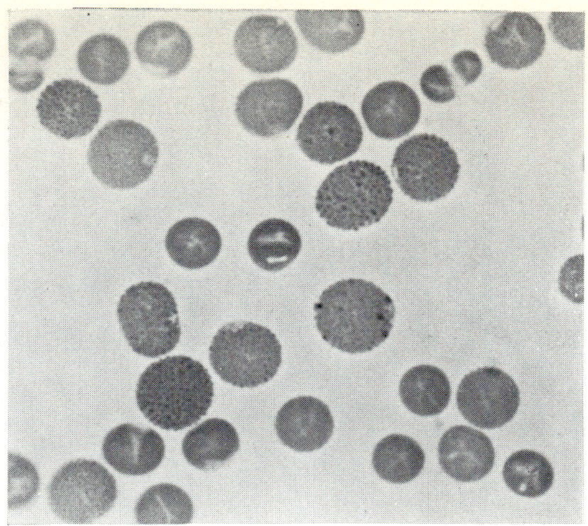

Plate 37 *Note the punctate appearance of the red cell due to 'H bodies'.*

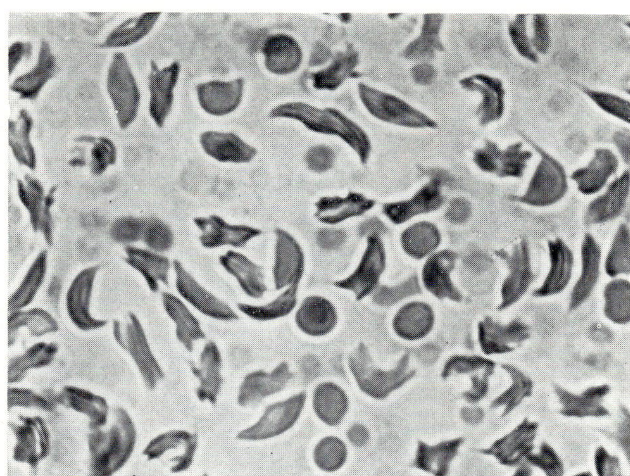

Plate 38 *Sickling test. It is common to find marked variation in the degree of sickling from cell to cell.*

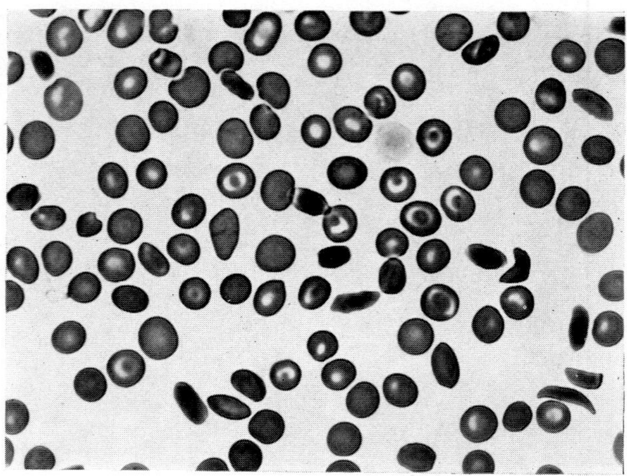

Plate 39 *Blood smear from a case of sickle cell anaemia. Note the target cells. The occasional sickle cells are mainly early forms. Note that in vivo sickle cells resemble bananas in shape rather than sickles.*

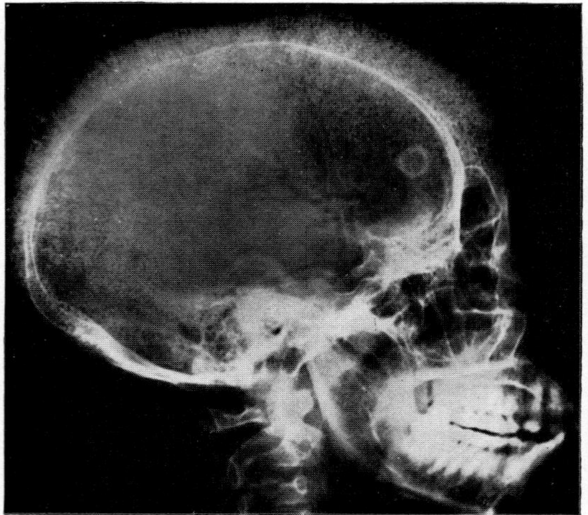

Plate 40 *The enlargement of the diploe gives the skull 'hair-on-end' appearance. Note the bony infarct, which can occur in sickle cell disease.*

These illustrations are from Woodruff, A. W. ed (1970), *Alimentary and Haematological Aspects of Tropical Disease*, London: Edward Arnold Ltd., and are reproduced by kind permission of the publishers.

However, α thalassaemia will interact with the uncommon α chain abnormal haemoglobins, whereas β thalassaemia would not.

Sickle cell thalassaemia

Because β thalassaemia is uncommon in most of tropical Africa, the main reservoir of the sickle cell gene, sickle cell thalassaemia occurs much less frequently than either β thalassaemia major or sickle cell anaemia. It is found sporadically in a widely scattered area, but principally in Liberia, Ghana, Southern Italy, Greece and North America, and areas where racial admixture has occurred.

Sickle cell thalassaemia presents as a condition which is clinically less severe than sickle cell anaemia. In contrast to sickle cell anaemia, the spleen is usually palpable and it is this combination of splenomegaly and a disability less severe than is usual in sickle cell anaemia, which alerts the physician to the possibility of this disorder. Haemoglobin SC disease (page 490) and SD disease where the blood also sickles (page 491) present in an exactly similar way.

On paper or starch gel electrophoresis, sickle cell anaemia and sickle cell thalassaemia may be indistinguishable, depending upon the amount of haemoglobin A present in the case of sickle cell thalassaemia. This haemoglobin A, if present, is best demonstrated by an agar gel electrophoresis.

The diagnosis is best achieved by a family study which should demonstrate β thalassaemia minor in one of the parents and the sickle cell gene in the other.

Haemoglobin C, D and E thalassaemia

Thalassaemia haemoglobin E disease is widely diagnosed in Thailand and Burma where it gives rise to mild or moderate disability, both the anaemia and splenomegaly being somewhat greater than that found in homozygous haemoglobin E disease.

Haemoglobin C thalassaemia and D thalassaemia, both uncommon conditions, are roughly similar in clinical severity to haemoglobin E thalassaemia. The patients present with a variable degree of anaemia and splenomegaly and, as with sickle cell thalassaemia, the diagnosis is best established by a family study.

TREATMENT OF THE HAEMOGLOBINOPATHIES

In assessing the treatment of the haemoglobinopathies two facts must always be borne in mind. Firstly, because many millions of people are likely to be involved, any suggested therapy should ideally be suitable for mass medication. Secondly, the great majority of people afflicted with the milder disorders may well require no treatment.

Because of the red cell hypochromia, iron therapy is often given. This may indeed be harmful because the usual danger is not iron deficiency but iron overload. A serum iron estimation should be undertaken to prove iron deficiency before iron therapy is commenced.

Most of the haemoglobinopathies are associated with a large spleen, which at times may reach massive proportions. Hypersplenism, which should be suspected if the anaemia becomes unusually severe, or the transfusion requirements increase, may at times develop. In such situations the value of a splenectomy should be assessed. Splenectomy is often of value in the rare anaemias due to the unstable haemoglobins.

Sickle cell trait

People with the sickle cell trait require no treatment. They should, however, avoid anoxia caused either by flying in unpressurised aircraft or from pneumonia or a badly administered anaesthetic. On occasions haematuria may occur and patients may be then submitted to an unnecessary operation.

In the future, marriage guidance may be requested.

Haemoglobin C, D and E trait

No treatment required.

Haemoglobin C and E disease, haemoglobin C, D and E thalassaemia

Treatment may not be practical, and indeed, apart from ensuring adequate nutrition, in many cases treatment may not be needed. However, these patients are liable to react to infection with severe anaemia, both haemolytic and aplastic in type. It is therefore wise to ensure that all infections are vigorously treated. As in all chronic haemolytic disorders, folic acid deficiency is liable to develop and prophylactic folic acid is particularly necessary in pregnancy.

Sickle cell disease

As with the other haemoglobinopathies adequate nutrition should be assured and infections

2 K

promptly treated. It is the sickle cell vascular crisis which differentiates the sickle cell diseases from the other haemoglobinopathies. The term 'sickle cell disease' includes sickle cell anaemia, sickle cell thalassaemia, haemoglobins SC and SD disease. Other sickling combinations such as haemoglobins S+E and S+O are rare.

Of the sickle cell diseases, sickle cell anaemia is the most severe, although even classical sickle cell anaemia at times may run a benign course. The therapy outlined below may well not prove necessary for sickle cell thalassaemia and for haemoglobin SD disease. A haemoglobinopathy may vary in severity from time to time (page 485) and therapy should therefore be adjusted according to the clinical disability and not according to the diagnosis.

Sickling crises may result in misdiagnoses and unnecessary surgery. When they occur they should be treated by combating shock and pain and vigorously treating any secondary infection present (often pulmonary) which may indeed have played a causative role in the crisis. Attempts should be made to prevent the further spread of thrombi and various therapeutic agents have been used. We favour the intravenous injection of magnesium sulphate (1–2 ml 50 per cent $MgSO_4$ given slowly every 4 hours). It acts as an anti-coagulant and causes vasodilatation. The number of sickle cell crises may be reduced by giving alkali (sodium bicarbonate) by mouth in sufficient quantity to keep the urine alkaline to litmus. This will counteract acidosis, which encourages intravascular sickling. Prophylactic antimalarial drugs and antibiotics have both played a part in reducing the incidence of sickling crises.

Sickle cell disease is a chronic haemolytic disease and, as in all such conditions, prophylactic folic acid is advisable. It is because the red cells in these patients have a shortened life span that any reduction in marrow activity, often caused by infection, results in a rapid and sometimes fatal fall in the haemoglobin level. This emergency, which is liable also to occur in pregnancy, must be met with by transfusion.

Leg ulcers may prove difficult to heal. Elastic stockings should be worn and the legs raised at night. In cold weather the limb should be kept warm.

Under normal circumstances sickle cell haemoglobin C disease may require no treatment. However, because up to 10 per cent of deliveries of women with haemoglobin SC disease may end in maternal death, it is perhaps wise prior to delivery to introduce the same management which is used for sickle cell crises. Sodium bicarbonate is given by mouth and 2 ml of 50 per cent magnesium sulphate is slowly given intravenously immediately the child has been delivered. This may be repeated every 4 hours if indicated clinically. Heparin has also been advocated whenever there was evidence prior to delivery of sickle cell crises, for example, attacks of bone pain.

β thalassaemia major

These patients require multiple transfusions in order to survive. There is therefore increasing danger of iron overload, which may ultimately prove fatal. The use of iron-chelating agents is now under trial, but the iron yield is not yet sufficient to make this therapy practical. Infections when they occur should be vigorously treated and folic acid routinely given. Disfiguration may be caused by expansion of the bone marrow in the facial bones. If this occurs, it may be reduced by keeping the haemoglobin within the normal range with frequent blood transfusions.

β thalassaemia minor

The clinical severity of β thalassaemia minor is variable and most of the millions of people with this condition remain undiagnosed. Infections should be vigorously treated and iron therapy avoided unless iron deficiency is proved. Folic acid should be given in pregnancy, although continuous mass prophylactic therapy is not practical. Improved diagnostic facilities may be needed to meet future demands for marriage guidance.

Haemoglobin H disease

This condition is somewhat more severe than β thalassaemia minor. Prophylactic folic acid is desirable and infections should be vigorously treated. The possibility of hypersplenism requiring splenectomy should be remembered. There is a theoretical objection to the administration of drugs capable of causing haemolytic anaemia (e.g. salicylates and sulphonamides). We have not been able to substantiate this danger in practice. It appears undesirable therefore that these valuable drugs should be withheld if they are the only ones available for therapy.

Unstable haemoglobins

These uncommon haemoglobin variants present with clinical symptoms in the carrier state. It is essential, particularly in the case of unstable haemoglobins, to be careful to avoid the ever-increasing number of drugs and chemicals capable of affecting the integrity of either the normal red cell or the glucose-6-phosphate-dehydrogenase-deficient red cell. Many of these drugs, or their metabolites, appear to have redox potential. Splenectomy may be helpful if the anaemia becomes disabling.

REFERENCES

BRAUNITZER, G., HILSE, K., RUDLOFF, V. and HILSCHMANN, N. (1964) *Advanc. Protein Chem.*, **19**, 1.

HUEHNS, E. R. and SHOOTER, E. M. (1965) *J. med. Genet.*, **2**, 48.

HUISMAN, T. H. J. (1963) *Advanc. clin. Chem.*, **6**, 231.

JONXIS, J. H. P. ed. (1965) *Abnormal Haemoglobins in Africa (Symposium Ibadan, 1963)*. Oxford: Blackwell Scientific Publications.

LEHMANN, H. and HUNTSMAN, R. G. (1966) *Man's Haemoglobins: including the haemoglobinopathies and their investigation*, p. 331. Amsterdam: North-Holland Publishing Co.

LEHMANN, H. HUNTSMAN, R. G. and AGER, J. A. M. (1966) In *Metabolic Basis of Inherited Disease*, 2nd edn. ed. Stanbury, J. B., Wyngaarden J. B. and Frederickson, D. S. New York and Maidenhead: McGraw-Hill.

LEHMANN, H. and CARRELL, R. W. (1969) *Brit. med. Bull.*, **25**, 14.

LIVINGSTONE, F. B. (1967) *Abnormal Haemoglobins in Human Populations*. Chicago: Aldine Publishing Co.

WEATHERALL, D. J. (1965) *The Thalassaemia Syndromes*, p. 262. Oxford: Blackwell Scientific Publications.

—— (1969) *Brit. med. Bull.* **25**, 24.

WORLD HEALTH ORGANIZATION (1966) *Wld Hlth Org. techn. Rep. Ser.* No. 338, Geneva.

31
Heat Disorders

The capacity of the human body to cope with the stresses of hot environments is a particularly well-developed characteristic of the human species. A large part of the world's population spends much of its active existence in tropical or equatorial regions. Many people carry out hard physical work in the continental summers of the northern hemisphere. So efficient is the heat regulatory system and ancillary to it the cardiovascular, osmotic, water regulatory and endocrine systems, that heat disorders must be reckoned uncommon conditions. This is not to say that even well-adapted people do not find their hot seasons oppressive and uncomfortable or that their working time may need to be curtailed. But these indigenous populations are sufficiently well acclimatised to make possible levels of activity and a tolerance to warm surroundings which newcomers certainly find very trying if not impossible.

Heat disorders, of all kinds, make their appearance only when individuals are exposed suddenly to heat loads at levels to which they are not acclimatised or at which adaptation is not possible. Heat disorders are therefore encountered in rather special and often artificial circumstances, as when temperate dwellers are transported to the tropics or find themselves in badly ventilated compartments of ships or motor cars and particularly in industrial conditions where high levels of air and radiant temperatures are generated. But tropical dwellers can also suffer heat disorders when they encounter abnormal heat waves or need to work in hot industries in their own countries.

The understanding of the aetiology and pathogenesis of heat illness rests to a large extent on an understanding of the normal physiology of heat adaptation and heat acclimatisation and of particular derangements of normal functioning which lead to the specific entities as described in some detail later. It is not necessary here to present an analysis of the physiology of adaptation to high temperatures. These are to be found in many accessible reviews. It is however necessary to make a comment on the measurement of heat stress.

A number of such indices are in use but in the account that follows reference is made only to the corrected effective temperature scale (C.E.T.).

Like many other indices the C.E.T. is a scale which measures the effect of a combination of the four environmental measurements necessary for specifying any hot environment. These are the air temperature, the wet bulb temperature, the black globe temperature as a measure of radiant heat and the air velocity. The C.E.T. is essentially a scale which is meant to assess the subject's responses to any combination of the four thermal environmental factors. The basic 'C.E.T. scale' refers to the responses of men stripped to the waist. It is read quite simply from a nomogram. The scale suffers from certain disadvantages, but for the levels of heat stress described below it is a sufficient guide.

General definition

Heat disorders, as encountered in the tropics, during abnormally hot weather or in hot industries, comprise a group of clinical conditions in which the heat regulatory and associated physiological systems are unable to adapt efficiently to the stresses imposed by life and work at high environmental temperatures.

Classification and nomenclature

That much confusion surrounds the recognition and naming of heat disorders is apparent from the nomenclature and coding as used in the *Manual of the International Statistical Classification of Diseases* (W.H.O., Geneva). Attempts have been made to improve this nomenclature by the removal of obsolete terms and synonyms, by repairing omissions and by putting the classification on a logical basis (Weiner and Horne, 1958). The present writer believes that an entirely satisfactory schedule of heat disorders can be drawn up based on recognisable clinical entities with reasonably well-established aetiology and pathogenesis. The terms suggested (Table 31.1) have been modified to avoid ambiguity, while still remaining close to those in general usage. In the table heat disorders are grouped into three subdivisions: (*a*) systemic disorders, (*b*) psychoneurotic disorders and (*c*) skin disorders.

Within the category of systemic disorders a clear distinction is made between the condition of heat stroke on the one hand and a group of four 'heat exhaustion' syndromes. It is justifiable to retain the term 'heat exhaustion' not merely because of long familiarity but because the presenting signs and symptoms of cardiovascular insufficiency is a common feature though brought about by different processes. The simple term 'heat exhaustion' is, however, too imprecise and it is essential to qualify it in the ways suggested so that the different clinical conditions can be clearly specified and recognised.

TABLE 31.1. *Heat disorders*

A. *Systemic disorders*
　　Heat stroke (hyperpyrexia)
　　Circulatory deficiency heat exhaustion (heat syncope)
　　Water deficiency heat exhaustion
　　Salt deficiency heat exhaustion (including heat cramps)
　　Anhidrotic heat exhaustion
B. *Psychoneurotic disorders*
　　Mild heat fatigue
　　Chronic heat fatigue (tropical fatigue)
C. *Skin disorders*
　　Prickly heat
　　Anhidrosis
　　Congenital sweat gland deficiency (anhidrotic ectodermal dysplasia)
　　Sunburn

The category of psychoneurotic conditions is not easy to characterise. The two conditions specified have been clearly recognised in the literature and the distinction between them is worth making on practical grounds.

The category of skin conditions comprises a miscellaneous group of which prickly heat is undoubtedly the most important. Sunburn is not due to high temperature; it is of course attributable to overexposure to ultraviolet rays, but it seems worth while retaining it here. Congenital defects of the sweat glands are extremely rare and are strictly not a condition peculiar to the tropics, but as the clinical effects are related to deficiency in heat regulation it seems reasonable to make mention of it in this category.

In the discussion of aetiology and pathogenesis of the various disorders presented below, the aim is to show that each entity rests on a distinctive aetiology and sequence of pathology. In addition to the clinical data, quite independent evidence is provided by the results of experiments on man and animals. In these experiments it has been possible to show that derangement of parti-cular physiological responses under high temperature conditions can lead to the appearance of recognisable syndromes. Of course, in clinical practice more than one of the entities may be present at the same time and indeed in some cases one syndrome may predispose to the appearance of another.

HEAT STROKE

SYNONYM. Heat hyperpyrexia

Definition

A serious condition characterised by derangement of the heat regulatory mechanisms with very high body temperatures and attended by profound disturbances of the central nervous system and other bodily functions.

Incidence and epidemiology

Statistics on the occurrence of the disorder are not readily available, partly because some returns do not make clear distinction between the different heat illnesses and partly because of the relative rarity and spasmodic appearance of cases. The most important factors governing the incidence are exposure to extreme heat conditions, in most cases combined with the performance of physical work. In populations at risk, the incidence appears to be of the order of 0.5–2.00 per 1000 persons per annum. The mortality rate has been reported as high as 80 per cent; in South African gold mining the mortality is 25 per cent (Wyndham, 1962).

In the South African gold mines at nearly saturated temperatures of wet bulb 90°F, the most probable risk of heat stroke is a rate of 0.30 per 1000 per annum, rising at wet bulb 94°F to 1.08 fatality rate per 1000 per annum and 4 per 1000 non-fatal cases. In line with these figures are the reports of heat stroke deaths during heat waves, e.g. 69 deaths in the course of a week or so in the St Louis, Missouri, area (1956) with temperatures reaching 105°F in many places.

The South African figures indicate that heat stroke may occur at wet bulb temperatures as low as 85°F. At temperatures of this level heavy physical efforts is an important factor in precipitating the condition as shown by an Israeli report (Gilat *et al*, 1963), though here solar radiation must also have contributed substantially to the heat load. A similar combination of factors was clearly responsible for inducing heat stroke among U.S. marines undergoing active field training. The dry bulb was 86°F, wet bulb 77.5°F with the globe temperature reading 104°F (Minard, Belding and Kingston, 1957).

Other factors predisposing to heat stroke, including obesity, lack of acclimatisation, alcoholism and water shortage, are discussed below.

Clinical features

Onset. In about 70 per cent the onset is quite sudden and dramatic with a rapid rise of body temperature to 105°F and over, the patient showing acute neurological effects, particularly disorientation, delirium, struggling or convulsions. In 20 per cent of cases prodromal symptoms may appear within a few hours of the attack, but in 10 per cent the onset is much more gradual and premonitory symptoms may be in evidence for several days. Prodromal features include restlessness, irritability, dizziness, headache, nausea, vomiting, polyuria and periods of mental confusion.

Acute attack. Outstanding features are (*a*) the hyperpyrexia, (*b*) neurological and mental disturbances and (*c*) the presence in many but not all cases of a hot dry skin.

Hyperpyrexia. The rectal temperature rises usually to between 105°F and 110°F, but values up to 114°F have been recorded. The higher temperatures are found in the rapidly developing cases.

Neurological and mental disturbances during the attack may involve only mild disturbances of consciousness, but usually these are pronounced, involving delirium and confusion, purposeless movements, maniacal struggling and convulsions. The pupillary light reflexes may be absent, especially as coma develops. The convulsions may take the form of tetanus-like seizures with involuntary spasms of the limb muscles; there may be incontinence of urine and faeces. The breathing is rapid and may be stertorous, and during coma it may be Cheyne-Stokes in character.

Cessation of sweating. Many reports testify to a stoppage of sweating immediately before the onset as well as during the acute attacks. Hearne (1932) could not evoke sweating in response to pilocarpine, but no systematic observations on the activity of the sweat glands to standardised doses of acetylcholine in the course of heat stroke and during recovery appears to have been made. Gilat *et al* (1963) cite instances from the literature and their own cases to show that failure of sweating is not an essential factor in precipitating heat stroke.

Course and complications. Without prompt removal of the patient from the hot surroundings and effective treatment by cooling, the outcome is certainly fatal. The persistence of the acute symptoms and the appearance of complications depend very largely on the duration and intensity of the hyperpyrexia.

If cooling is delayed, it will be more difficult to reduce the body temperature and stabilise it, to prevent serious neurological effects or to avoid a long period of coma. Complications, such as jaundice or oliguria, may ensue.

On admission pulse rates are high, mostly over 130 per minute, rising to 200 per minute in proportion to the pyrexia. In many patients (particularly in the age group of those in hot industries or in the services), the cardiovascular changes are usually not abnormal; the blood pressure is well maintained; there is no evidence in the ECG of damage to the myocardium or signs of heart failure. In elderly and obese patients however, where cardiovascular insufficiency may act as a predisposing cause, severe circulatory disturbances may be very noticeable. Low blood pressures have been recorded in a high proportion of some series. The pulse rate may be rapid and thready, lips and face are usually cyanotic; acute left ventricular failure has been reported, as have ECG changes indicative of myocardial damage. Haemorrhage into the skin and mucous membranes have been described in some series. The occurrence of such petechiae may be the result of delay in treatment. Jaundice is not often in evidence though liver damage with raised serum bilirubin has been found in about 15 or 20 per cent of individuals subjected to induced hyperpyrexia or fever therapy. Post-mortem pathological lesions in the liver, particularly centrilobular necrosis, have often been reported.

In a small number of cases acute renal failure supervenes with progressive uraemia and oliguria. The urine contains red cells, albumin, hyaline and granular casts. Though renal function tests appear not to have been done, post-mortem lesions such as acute tubular necrosis and multiple small haemorrhages along with congestion and softening of the kidney have been noted.

Of laboratory findings in heat stroke, the most interesting and fairly consistent are: thrombocytopenia, leucocytosis, increased bilirubin, raised blood urea and reduced plasma bicarbonate. How the raised body temperature brings about the thrombocytopenia is not clear, but this finding serves to explain the haemorrhagic tendency. The cause of the leucocytosis also remains unexplained. The raised urea is related to the acute tubular necrosis and the increased bilirubin to liver damage. The reduced plasma bicarbonate has been regarded as a consequence of hyperventilation, but in fact the urine is strongly acid in these patients. Increased blood lactate, both in man and animals, has been found. The reduced alkali reserve and increased lactate would plausibly be connected with the severe convulsions and muscle spasms. No definite changes occur on other blood constituents, e.g. the red blood cell number or in sodium or chloride, though hypokalaemia has been reported.

Duration. Of fatal cases the great majority are dead within 24 hours; the remainder die within the next 1 to 12 days, though occasionally after a much longer period. In these cases of long duration there may be either a continual deterioration and persistent coma or the course may be variable with early coma, some recovery of consciousness and terminal relapse.

Sequelae. The promptness and effectiveness of treatment influences the frequency and severity of sequelae. The high proportion of patients who recover have some disability, but in only a few are these really serious or permanent. Headache, dizziness, difficulties in concentration and sleeplessness are common complaints which almost always disappear within a matter of weeks or months. There may be some change of temperament, such as irritability, moodiness or childishness. Neurological disturbances include motor dysphasia early in the recovery period and occasionally signs of cerebellar dysfunction such as dysarthria, ataxia, motor incoordination, tremors and nystagmus. Ataxia is said to be the most persistent. Much less frequent are the residual effects of monoplegia, hemiplegia or epilepsy.

Diagnosis

The combination of hyperpyrexia, disturbance of the central nervous system and, in many cases, a hot dry burning skin in a patient known to have been subjected to heat stress are very striking presenting features. Nevertheless confusion is possible with other diseases characterised by hyperpyrexia or neurological signs in patients who happen also to be exposed to hot conditions. A differential diagnosis has to be made from malaria (malignant tertian), cerobrospinal fever, cerebral (pontine) haemorrhage, tetanus, typhus and typhoid fever. Patients found comatose from hypoglycaemia, alcoholism, drug excess or diabetes, under hot conditions, have to be excluded, but in these cases hyperpyrexia will not be present.

It may be very difficult with the ordinary mercury in glass rectal thermometers to obtain a rectal temperature (or even an axillary temperature) in a struggling patient, or one in convulsions. As Leithead (1964) advises, hospitals or clinics in places where heat stroke may occur should equip themselves with a clinical thermometer with a steel stem containing a thermosensitive bimetallic helix.

The response to cooling may also help materially in confirming the diagnosis of heat stroke.

Prognosis

The chances of recovery depend on the duration and extent of the hyperpyrexia. In the absence of treatment death is certain and it has been stated that if the temperature remains over 108°F for 2 hours, recovery is unlikely. If cooling is delayed, the outcome is uncertain and complications are to be expected. The outcome is also serious when hypotension and shock are present. The more rapid the response to cooling, the more favourable the prognosis and the fewer the sequelae. Rapid improvement in neurological disturbances is also a good prognostic sign.

Treatment

Heat stroke must be treated as an emergency requiring prompt attention. In localities where heat stroke is likely to occur, appropriate cooling equipment should be held in a state of readiness.

The immediate treatment is concerned primarily with reducing hyperpyrexia (and in so doing controlling the convulsions, restlessness or other violent activities) and, where it exists, treating the peripheral circulatory failure or shock condition. The aim in cooling the patient is to reduce the rectal temperature to 102°F within 1 hour; cooling should be discontinued at this level to avoid hypotension and shock. The temperature will continue to fall without further cooling by about 2°F to 100° or 99°F. Continual monitoring of the rectal temperature is obviously very important.

Rapid reduction of body temperature can be brought about by either evaporative cooling or by immersion in cold water. The relative merits of the procedures remain a matter of argument.

The simplest method is to wrap the patient in wet sheets or towels or to sponge him with cool water, while air is blown over him with one or more electric fans. Fanning by other methods may have to be improvised and must be contrived during transport to hospital. A more elaborate but more convenient procedure is to spray the patient with an ordinary hand-shower with cold water from a refrigerating unit and to combine this with a strong blast of dry air. This method requires the provision of cooling equipment in an air-conditioned room kept in a state of readiness: it has been used with success in the Kuwait Oil Company for many years (Guthrie and McCracken, 1960). Simultaneous with cooling the skin should be massaged (through the wet sheet if necessary) to promote circulation.

An alternative method of reducing the hyperpyrexia is by immersion of the patient in a bath of ice water. The rectal temperature must be continually followed as the temperature can easily fall to 102°F in under an hour. Again the body surface and limbs must be massaged to promote blood circulation. This method seems more drastic than evaporative cooling, but better results have been claimed for it particularly for patients who are admitted with extremely high hyperpyrexia (over 107°F).

The cooling must not be stopped except for the shortest period to clear the mouth and throat of vomitus.

Adjuvants to cooling: chlorpromazine. A number of favourable reports have appeared advocating the use of this drug for its thermolytic properties as an adjuvant to cooling and for its sedative and tranquillising properties to control restlessness and convulsions. Dosages of 20 or 50 mg have generally been used given intravenously. The claim that chlorpromazine should be used without cooling is not well supported at the present time; even as an adjunct the exact value and mode of action of the drug remains unclear.

Control of central nervous system disturbances: depressants. Valuable time may be lost if attempts are made to quieten a struggling or convulsant patient before cooling by the use of such drugs as chloral, phenobarbitone, paraldehyde or chlorpromazine. In fact, immediate and effective cooling will control the disturbances in most cases. Chlorpromazine should be given during the cooling treatment. Other depressants may be used if necessary after the hyperpyrexia has been reduced.

Control of shock. Treatment is aimed at correction of peripheral circulatory failure and prevention of cardiac failure, particularly in elderly patients. These measures must be undertaken immediately rapid cooling has been instituted. The basic measures are intravenous fluid therapy and administration of digitalis. Whether pressor agents (or corticosteroids) are really of benefit remains unproven.

Antimalarial treatment. If the locality is a malarious one, antimalarial treatment to combat possible cerebral malaria must be given. The conscious patient can be given chloroquine by mouth; if unconscious, intramuscular injection of nivaquine (1 ampoule) is necessary.

Prevention

Experience in the South African gold mines, U.S. military training programmes and from the Mecca pilgrimages have all shown that heat stroke can to a very large extent be prevented. Where individuals are moving deliberately into hot conditions as in industry or the armed services, or into a particularly hot region (as in the pilgrimage) and are therefore susceptible to some supervision, preventive measures can be applied with a high degree of success; at the same time when heat stroke does occur, fatalities can be greatly reduced. On the other hand, when severe heat waves afflict dense and widespread populations with little warning, prevention is much less easy, though even here medical officers of health could no doubt disseminate useful advice through public media.

Though the heat stroke incidence in situations of risk may be relatively small, preventive action is worth pursuing energetically. Firstly, the malady is extremely severe and even with good treatment the fatality rate may still be as high as 25 per cent. Secondly, in industry and the services, even a single case of heat stroke can have a serious effect on the morale of other personnel exposed to similar hot conditions. Thirdly, where heat stroke occurs, other heat disorders (while not so serious) will also be present. Measures taken to combat heat stroke will to a large extent be effective for dealing with most if not all other heat illnesses.

The aetiology and predisposing causes of the syndrome indicate that the lines on which prevention should be based comprise (a) management of the heat load, (b) ancillary measures concerning water supply, clothing, living conditions, (c) selection and screening, and (d) deliberate acclimatisation.

Only by attending to all these measures is it really possible to reduce heat stroke to negligible proportions. Thus Minard found that even when limits were placed on exposure to hard work in hot environments, five cases of heat stroke occurred because acclimatisation had not yet occurred and because four of these cases were obese.

One cannot with absolute assurance lay down 'safe' limits of temperature, but a reasonable guide to such limits is provided by the thermal conditions tolerable for moderately hard work, both by unacclimatised and acclimatised individuals. Thus in unacclimatised men a permissible upper limit for a work output averaging about

250 kilocalories per hour is a C.E.T. of 82°F, but the subjects must be fit and trained for the work. This limit would have to be reduced substantially, to about 78° C.E.T., for short bouts of extremely severe exertion. Acclimatised subjects can carry out sustained work at C.E.T. 86°F. One may conclude from available figures that 82° C.E.T. for acclimatised subjects carrying out fairly hard work are desirable upper limits if heat stroke is to be kept to a minimum. In these conditions dehydration must be avoided and a liberal supply of water must be available. Other factors to take into consideration are suitability of clothing and the avoidance of alcohol.

Where the risk of heat stroke is particularly pronounced, i.e. where conditions are unavoidably very near the upper desirable limits, some screening must be undertaken and even those who are selected must undergo some form of supervised graduated acclimatisation to heat. In selecting subjects, factors to take account of will include of course the medical history so as to eliminate those with cardiovascular disease, recent prickly heat, poor working capacity and obesity. More sophisticated selection requires a trial exposure of individuals to standardised heat tests for elimination of those that are heat intolerant.

Aetiology and pathogenesis

The characterisation of heat stroke as an identifiable entity rests on the recognition of its specific aetiology and of a pathogenetic sequence which explains the clinical signs and symptoms and causes of death as well as the features of the morbid anatomy. That the pathogenesis and concomitant clinical effects are the result of the hyperpyrexia is clear from experimental and clinical observation; but the cause of the hyperpyrexia remains a matter of uncertainty.

The uncontrollable rise of body temperature is obviously the consequence of the failure of the heat loss mechanisms to dissipate the combined environmental and metabolic heat load. With heat regulation out of physiological control there ensues the cumulative cycle of an increase in temperature stimulating an increase in metabolism and this in turn producing a further rise of body temperature and so on.

What is the nature of this failure in heat regulation? There are two possibilities: (*a*) a sudden failure of the sweating mechanism, centrally at the hypothalamus; (*b*) no absolute or total failure of the heat dissipating mechanism, but an incapacity of the sweating mechanism to meet the demands of the heat load.

Primary or total failure of sweating mechanism. In many clinical accounts of heat stroke there are reports of an arrest of sweating in apparently healthy men without any previous history of sweating difficulty. In the nature of the case, however, the sweating performance of heat stroke patients cannot be followed quantitatively and it is by no means certain that the appearance of the oft-reported hot dry skin had occurred as a primary event. It is quite likely that the cessation of sweating was at least in some instances a secondary result brought about by damage to the heat centre by the hyperpyrexia itself (Kuno, 1956). This is comparable to the way anoxia first stimulates, then 'wrecks', the respiratory centre.

Nevertheless, acute cessation of sweating is known to occur. Bannister (1959) reported this both in the field and in the experimental hot room, but whether this type of anhidrosis is long-lasting enough to cause heat imbalance and heat stroke is not certain. Arrest of sweating through a central action is certainly brought about by pyrogens. The pyrexia has been clearly shown to be accompanied by peripheral vasoconstriction and also by the arrest of sweating. Thus such conditions as malaria or encephalitis can certainly predispose to heat stroke in hot climates; and in these cases the failure of sweating could be attributed to a central action. However, many heat stroke cases occur of course outside known malarial areas. Failure of sweating through a pyrogen-like action can be true only of a minority of cases.

Insufficiency of sweating mechanism. Gilat *et al* (1963) have documented the evidence (including their own) to show that many cases of heat stroke occur without arrest of sweating. The continuance of sweating while control of body temperature is lost points to the failure of evaporative heat loss to balance the heat input. This failure may arise in two different ways, for both of which evidence is available. These are: (*a*) factors making for insufficiency of sweating, i.e. a reduction in sweat output; (*b*) overloading of the normal sweating capacity.

There are a number of factors which may reduce normal sweat output by interference with sweat secretion. The absence or reduction in the number of sweat glands as in ectodermal dysplasia would undoubtedly expose the sufferer to a high risk of heat stroke, but this very rare defect cannot account for the high incidence of heat stroke such as occurs in heat waves or in particular kinds of hot industry. In any case, heat stroke patients on recovery are known to regain their sweating ability. A second factor known to interfere with sweat secretion is the damage done to the skin by prickly heat. The anhidrosis so produced is part of the syndrome of anhidrotic heat exhaustion (see below); conceivably this could predispose to heat stroke. But the prior occurrence of prickly heat in heat stroke patients has rarely been described. The third factor is the occurrence of fatigue of the sweat glands. During prolonged sweating and particularly in hot humid conditions when the skin remains wet, a falling-off of sweating is noticeable and has been documented in numerous studies. It is conceivable that in some individuals this falling-off may be so marked that heat stroke is induced.

Disturbance in central nervous function can in favourable cases be reversed by cooling; any recrudescence of the hyperpyrexia will result in the reappearance of the central nervous effects. In experimental animals overheating leads to similar neurological disorders, particularly to convulsions, muscle spasm, struggling and coma with respiratory failure. Post-mortem examination reveals pathological changes in the central nervous system including degeneration of neurones, congestion, oedema and petechial haemorrhages. The degree of damage is related to the duration of hyperpyrexia. Damage by the hyperpyrexia to the heat centres as postulated by Kuno (1956) seems consistent with the pathological findings. Similarly, the respiratory centre, which is first stimulated by heat, would undergo damage by excess of heating, thus accounting for the respiratory failure commonly seen. Although overbreathing leading to alkalosis is known to accompany overheating, it appears that heat stroke patients are much more often in a state of acidosis, as evidenced by increased blood lactate, reduced alkali reserve, and a highly acid urine with increased lactate content. Presumably these are the results of the very severe muscular spasms and convulsions.

Outside the central nervous system it seems that the elevated temperature has a direct effect on other organs. In the liver centrilobular necrosis has been noted and this may underlie the appearance of jaundice in a small proportion of cases. Similarly, direct heating may account for acute tubular necrosis as the cause of the acute renal failure observed in some cases. Brauer *et al* (1963) have perfused the intact liver of the dog with blood at various temperatures. At high levels of temperature irreversible changes were noted, particularly a decline of bile secretion and depletion of liver glycogen.

The severe shock that occurs in a proportion of cases is not easy to explain. The fact that it occurs in a minority (about 20 per cent) may indicate that we are dealing with an additional syndrome. It is possible that the hypotension, cold clammy skin, cyanotic and congested appearance of the face, and thin thready pulse are all manifestations of a syncopal episode and that the patient has suffered a hyperpyrexial attack simultaneously with a circulatory collapse. Another possibility is that the shock is a manifestation of adrenal insufficiency or exhaustion.

CIRCULATORY DEFICIENCY HEAT EXHAUSTION

SYNONYM. Heat syncope

Definition

A condition characterised by disturbance of the vasomotor system with signs and symptoms of syncope.

Incidence and epidemiology

From the few available figures the incidence appears to be about 1 in 200 or 1 in 300 per year. In the hot humid conditions of Karachi, Horne (1954) recorded some 20–30 syncopal cases in 6000 men at risk in 1946. In a 3-year period Dreosti (1937) admitted from a population of about 9000 at risk, some 100 uncomplicated syncopal cases.

Heat syncope occurs over a wide range of hot conditions and not merely at extreme temperatures. This is because lack of acclimatisation, poor physical fitness and such variable factors as postural strain, individual susceptibility and coexistence of other illnesses all enter into the occurrence of the condition. It has been described amongst Indian and African gold miners, Egyptian agricultural labourers, Arab road-building labourers, American Army trainees and British servicemen.

Clinical features

Onset. The distinguishing features are the occurrence of a faint or near-collapse under hot conditions without the signs and symptoms of water or salt deficiency or of anhidrosis; the body temperature is usually not greatly raised. The syncopal signs may appear during or immediately after the heat exposure or after the subject has been standing for a while or working in the heat. The subject is pale, and in working individuals there may be a cyanotic hue; breathing is irregular or shallow with sighing and yawning; complaints of weakness, giddiness, nausea, 'cold' spells are common. If the patient does faint, the symptoms may be quite transitory and may pass off in a few minutes when he sits or lies down.

Immediately before and during the faint the blood pressure will be found to have fallen and in many, perhaps most, cases the faint is of the vasovagal type with slowing of the pulse rate; the pulse feels weak, the skin is moist and cold.

Course. A simple heat syncope is characterised by rapid recovery. Should the patient continue to complain of exhaustion or giddiness, or remain pale and hypotensive and to feel ill on standing up, one should suspect the coexistence of some infection or regard the faint as a sign of the more serious heat disturbances of salt deficiency, water deficiency or of anhidrosis. Fainting under hot conditions, therefore, should not be taken lightly.

Diagnosis

The combination of syncopal signs and symptoms in hot surroundings associated with postural changes during or after exercise or with prolonged standing followed by rapid recovery of consciousness, is highly characteristic. Other heat exhaustion disorders may occur with fainting as the presenting phenomenon, but the presence of salt in the urine will help to exclude salt deficiency and a copious urine output and low specific gravity will exclude water depletion, while the presence of a moist skin and moderate pyrexia will rule out anhidrotic heat exhaustion. Other causes of loss of consciousness must of course be considered, particularly epilepsy, anaemia and Adam-Stokes attacks. The possibility of infections such as influenza, acute tonsillitis, malaria, chickenpox etc. must be taken into account.

Prognosis

In a simple uncomplicated case recovery rapidly follows the head-down or recumbent posture.

Treatment

In a simple self-limiting case the patient needs only to be transported to cooler conditions, allowed to rest with the head down or kept recumbent with knees drawn up and with no special medication apart from simple beverages such as tea or plain drinks. The industrial worker needs reassurance that there will almost certainly be no recurrence of the disorder as he becomes accustomed to the working conditions.

Prevention

A medical examination of new entrants to eliminate those suffering from various maladies will help to reduce the incidence of heat casualties. A graduated introduction to the work and to the hot surroundings will also reduce the incidence.

Aetiology and pathogenesis

Vascular 'pooling' in skeletal muscles and skin, especially of the lower limbs, is the causal factor. Important predisposing causes are lack of heat acclimatisation and poor physical fitness for work, since these are associated with an insufficiency of adjustment of the circulatory system to activity and postural change in the heat.

The pathogenesis is quite straightforward. During exercise the blood flow through the working muscles may be fifty or more times greater than at rest in order to deliver the oxygen needed. When work stops, the blood flow through the muscles will remain high for some time and only gradually approach the resting level. The widely opened capillaries and vessels will be able to hold a large amount of blood; immediately after work, when the pumping action of the muscles has stopped, the legs may contain more than 25 per cent of the total blood volume. The effect is, therefore, to reduce the return of blood to the heart and consequently to reduce the cardiac output and with it the blood pressure.

In hot conditions the peripheral pooling is aggravated since the working subject has widely dilated skin vessels and arteriovenous anastomoses. This orthostatic syncope can be induced after work in the heat or even on prolonged standing in the heat. When this is done deliberately (Weiner, 1938) the effects are very similar to those noted clinically in heat syncope. If fainting does not occur, or for a time before it does occur, there is evidence of compensatory visceral and skin vasoconstriction to maintain the blood pressure and heart output. The diastolic pressure and systolic pressure will usually rise, the pulse accelerate and there will be pallor. But if the heart output remains reduced, the blood pressure rise may not be maintained and the pooling may be so great that the blood pressure falls precipitately. At the same time there is a slowing of the heart, thus presenting the features of a vasovagal faint due to the anoxia stimulating the vagus and therefore inducing bradycardia.

Definition

A condition characterised by dehydration and attributable to insufficient drinking water.

Incidence and epidemiology

This variety of heat exhaustion is encountered amongst workers in hot industry, in open air employment in the tropics (e.g. open-cast mining, road building, etc.); amongst servicemen during training or active service in hot climates; in individuals adrift in warm climates or stranded in desert conditions; in long-distance athletes running in the heat; in infants during exceptionally hot weather.

The rate of dehydration will depend on the rate of water loss from lungs, skin and kidney in relation to water intake; the rate of cutaneous loss in turn being dependent on environmental conditions, on activity of the subject and on his body size. In the circumstances of the castaway, no water for drinking may in fact be available and dehydration will naturally develop relatively fast. It is important to recognise that some degree of water deficiency may develop even when drinking water is readily available—so-called 'voluntary dehydration'.

The rate of dehydration on various levels of water replacement can be calculated from the sweat rate induced by the observed thermal conditions, the level of activity, amount of clothing, body size. The time it would take for a certain degree of water depletion (say 5 or 10 per cent of gross body weight) to develop can be estimated. Such 'survival' curves define the likelihood of water deficiency heat exhaustion under the specified conditions. For example (Adolph, 1947) on an intake of 1 quart (1.1 litres) daily at 80°F mean shade air temperature, 4 days, or at 90°F, 2 days would elapse before a 10 per cent body weight deficit develops (the limit of ability to work); a 20 per cent deficit (maximum endurance limit) would be reached in about 8 days at 80°F, or 6 days at 90°F.

Clinical features and course

The earlier stages of the syndrome with moderate degrees of dehydration, say up to 5–8 per cent body weight reduction, are attended by vague symptoms and by reduced working efficiency. Soldiers marching in the sun and carrying their packs, or workers in a hot industry—glass or metallurgical—may complain of lassitude and drowsiness, restlessness, irritability, thirst, at the end of a day's hard work. Compared with individuals well hydrated, their pulse rate and body temperature can be shown to be significantly increased, and oliguria is often noticeable.

The full syndrome (as presented by castaways) is characterised by thirst, dryness of the throat, hoarseness, great weariness and oliguria. There is a strong inclination to sit or lie down. There may be incoordination, inability to stand. In the later and irreversible stages, the tongue swells, swallowing becomes impeded, vision is dim, there is hysteria and delirium leading to death. In children excessive thirst is the presenting complaint, oliguria is often noticed by the parents, the urine being dark yellow; vomiting after feeding and anorexia is common; as in adults there is lethargy, restlessness, insomnia and the children cry excessively.

Diagnosis

The diagnosis is made from a combination of circumstances—the environmental conditions prevailing, the appearance of the patient, and complaints of intense thirst if conscious. In the comatose subject the temperature may be raised. Severe cases may be difficult to distinguish from heat stroke and in fact both hyperpyrexia and severe dehydration may exist together. The urine is reduced and of high specific gravity and the salt content is high. Exclusion of salt deficiency dehydration may sometimes be difficult, but the high salt content in the urine, the absence of heat cramp, a high level of sodium in the plasma and the presence of intense thirst are distinguishing features.

Treatment

This depends on whether the patient is able to take fluid by mouth or is unconscious and is difficult to manage. In all cases the patient must be kept at rest in a cool room. In the milder cases the patient is encouraged to drink water and flavoured drinks to ensure a large positive gain in the first few days. This can be monitored by watching the subject continually on the first day and regularly thereafter and keeping a continuous record of fluid intake, including some fluid food, and output. A net gain of about 2 to 3 litres is the first day and 0.5 to 1 litre a day in the following 2 or 3 days will restore deficiencies of about 7 per cent of body weight. Clinical recovery will be evident not only by the condition of the patient but by the establishment of a satisfactory urine output and an increase in body weight to a steady level.

In an unconscious patient intravenous 5 per cent glucose must be given, 4 litres in the first 24 hours, but the urine output must be carefully watched to make sure that the anuria is being overcome and there is no risk of water overload. After the first 24 hours the intravenous flow depends on the patient's condition and the urine output. If it is not clear whether the patient is suffering from water or salt depletion, isotonic saline should be given at the outset.

Prevention

Protection against the danger of water deprivation requires an assessment of water requirements, given a knowledge of the air and radiant temperatures and the amount of work and clothing. The upper value for sweat loss can be taken as 1 litre per hour, a value which applies strictly to well-acclimatised men working hard in severe heat. This rate is not sustained for a whole shift of 8 hours, but men working and living in a hot climate may lose as much as 10 litres over the 24 hours. It is clear, therefore, that for many situations an allowance of 12 pints (7 litres) of water a day is not excessive. The risks involved where only a limited amount of fluid is available can also be calculated (see Adolph).

Medical Officers may be called on to provide a list of rules for the use of military or industrial personnel working in hot climates. Such a code can be found in Leithead and Lind (1964, page 153).

Aetiology and pathogenesis

The aetiology of this syndrome, i.e. water deprivation, is not in doubt. The lack of water may simply be the outcome of a failure to provide sufficiently for the needs of individuals living or working in hot conditions, but dehydration may occur even when adequate water is available. This 'voluntary' dehydration is well known to occur in the desert, in the hot room or in hot industries when the men do not replace by drinking all the water lost by sweating and it is only during meals that the water deficit is made up. Thus some people consistently fail to correct this deficit and so build up a chronic water debt. Infants who cannot make their needs understood are at risk in hot climates: vomiting will exacerbate the water deficit as will diarrhoea.

Heat exhaustion water deficiency as a clear clinical entity is fully confirmed by experiments such as those of McCance (1936), who reproduced the main clinical and biochemical features of the condition by depriving a group of subjects of water but not of food. The food itself yielded about 600 ml of water a day, sufficient to cover the minimal urinary output, but water loss from skin and lungs reduced the body weight by about 1 kg/ day. When the body weight was reduced by about 5 per cent the clinical effects were quite obvious— the mouth and throat dry, the voice husky, swallowing difficult, face pinched, pale and slightly cyanotic, and the subject felt tired and irritable. As in the clinical syndrome, the water loss affected the extracellular volume primarily. There was a gradual decrease in blood volume, and since the excretion of salt was not sufficiently increased, the osmotic pressure of the extracellular fluid and later the intracellular compartment steadily rose. In the first stages of the syndrome the ill effects are attributable to the reduction of circulating blood volume, but in the later and irreversible stages the abnormal rise of osmotic pressure appears to be the responsible factor in bringing about cellular damage.

The effects of the shrinkage of the extracellular compartment and particularly of the blood volume have been followed in detail by Adolph and his colleagues in the desert, i.e. in conditions under which the syndrome actually develops. In the dehydrated subject it is found that the plasma gives up more than its share of water and there is also loss of volume by the red corpuscles. Reduction in the circulating blood volume accounts for the undue acceleration of pulse rate (compared with normal hydrated controls) in the lying or standing position or during work and also for the increased breathing since the blood supply to the head becomes inadequate. The pulse rate increment is closely related to the degree of water deficit. Adolph (1947) and others believe that in hot environments death is ultimately due to heat stroke because body temperature control is lost as a result of cellular damage. In cool environments dehydration results in coma and depression of central nervous activity.

SALT DEFICIENCY HEAT EXHAUSTION

SYNONYM. 'Heat cramps' is not an exact synonym since it refers to a variant of the syndrome.

Definition

A condition in which there has been excessive loss of chloride from the body by sweating without sufficient replacement to maintain normal chloride level; characterised by 'asthenic' symptoms—fatigue, dizziness, sleeplessness, vomiting and in the heat cramps variety by painful limb and abdominal spasms.

Incidence and epidemiology

The syndrome is encountered amongst workers in ships' boiler-rooms, iron foundries, travellers and service personnel in hot dry deserts and in mining. In the South African mining industry salt depletion heat exhaustion occurs with a frequency of about 2 per 1000 employees per annum. Caplan (1943) found a reduced plasma chloride in 70 per cent of all cases of 'exhaustion' in underground workers at the Kolar goldfields. The salt deficiency syndrome without cramps is the more common variety.

The syndrome occurs in conditions where the thermal load induces sustained sweating and consequently a sudden and greatly increased salt loss. The usual circumstances comprise a combination of hard physical work and thermal conditions above about 80–83°F effective temperature. Lack of acclimatisation is also a factor; salt deficiency heat casualties were induced within 48 hours in 15 out of 1500 servicemen transferred rapidly from cool conditions to hard training activities in the heat (Minard, 1957).

Clinical features

Unless muscle cramps are in evidence the presenting features, like those of water depletion heat exhaustion, may be vague. There may be complaints of fatigue, muscle weakness, headache, irritability and less frequently of nausea and vomiting. The appearance of a state of exhaustion in these patients may be quite striking, with dehydration evident in the sunken eyes and loss of skin elasticity. The patient may complain of dizziness on standing and in this posture the pulse rate may be found to be unduly high. Some cases of the syndrome are brought in after fainting. Cramps may vary from fasciculation of a few muscle groups to severe and agonising spasms. If cramps are complained of they may, if not present, be reinvoked by exercise of the foot or calf muscles. The body temperature is not raised and thirst is not complained of. Laboratory examinations are very important in revealing that the salt content of the urine is very low (below 10 mg/100 ml) whilst the specific gravity is not raised. Haemoconcentration is present,

the blood urea often raised (values rising to 80–100 mg/100 ml) and—highly significant—the blood chloride level reduced. Plasma volumes fall by about 10–15 per cent and extracellular volumes by as much as 30 per cent (Ladell *et al*, 1944). When there is continuous vomiting and, less often, diarrhoea the signs of salt and water depletion will be seriously aggravated.

Removal from the heat with the reduction in sweating and therefore of salt loss brings about some improvement in the patient's condition, but a minority who continue to vomit or suffer diarrhoea will present a progressive picture of salt depletion and dehydration. In rare cases a patient may be comatose and in a state of oligaemic shock.

The patient's condition on examination may present a less serious or dramatic picture than that complained of during the actual conditions of heat exposure when the patient may have suffered heat cramps and have fainted.

Diagnosis

Complaints of fainting may easily lead to confusion of this syndrome with the water depletion and the circulatory deficiency varieties of heat exhaustion. In the latter the syncope commonly appears on the first exposure and improves rapidly, whereas in salt depletion the subject may have been feeling unwell for quite a long time. The distinction from water depletion rests on the absence of thirst and on the laboratory finding of a low urine specific gravity and chloride as contrasted with the oligaemia and high salt content in water depletion. Where cramps are present, the diagnosis is quite straightforward when taken in conjunction with the history of exposure, though the possibility of tetany due to alkalosis following prolonged hyperventilation should not be overlooked. Other conditions that lead to fluid and electrolyte imbalance should be borne in mind—acute gastroenteritis, uraemia, Addison's disease and diabetic ketosis.

Prognosis

Heat cramps with or without nausea, vomiting or fainting are responsible for hospitalisation in most salt deficiency cases. In many cases the patients get better simply on removal from the hot conditions and by increasing salt intake in the diet. Serious cases recover rapidly on intravenous administration of saline. There are no sequelae and relapses are very rare.

Treatment

In mild cases the patient takes 4 to 500 ml of 0.8–1.0 per cent saline (2 level teaspoonfuls per pint) per hour until the drink is found too salty. Thereafter drinks of 0.1 per cent saline are given and extra salt added to the food. Severe cases are treated by replacement of salt and water by the intravenous route and this may necessitate the administration of as much as 5 litres of fluid and 25 g of salt, e.g. where 12 per cent of the body weight has been lost since each kg contains about 3.2 g of salt.

The procedure at the Ernest Oppenheimer Mine Hospital in the Orange Free State, South Africa, is to give 2 litres of normal saline (0.9 per cent NaCl) to correct the reduced osmolarity of the extracellular fluid and to relieve the cramps, followed by 3 litres of half-strength saline (0.45 per cent NaCl) in 5 per cent dextrose during the subsequent 24 hours. The first litre is given rapidly. The urine must be monitored for its volume, specific gravity and chloride content and if possible the patient should be weighed daily. Patients are not discharged until the sodium chloride of the urine exceeds 300 mg per cent. After recovery, patients should be advised to consume extra salt (say 3 g in a pint of water) and as additional intake at meals.

Aetiology and pathogenesis

The syndrome can be reproduced in its essentials in laboratory conditions by inducing salt loss through profuse sweating by unacclimatised subjects, while keeping them on a diet adequate in all constituents but low in salt. This makes it plain that the aetiology rests on salt depletion.

There is a demonstrable fall in osmolarity, and this leads to a movement of water into the intracellular compartment, thus affecting the muscle fibres, and a continuing loss of water by the kidney. There is a contraction of the extracellular compartment which may affect the plasma component disproportionately. Although the movement of water tends to maintain the plasma colloid osmotic pressure it does not prevent the reduction in blood and plasma chloride. The fall in chloride output from the kidney is a compensatory response. McCance (1936) showed further that in severe salt deficiency the kidney increases its reabsorption of urea leading to a rise in blood urea which is often also observed clinically. All these changes are reversed when salt is given in the diet. Both the experimental and clinical evidence suggest that the factor of individual suscepti-

bility is very important. Some individuals lose much more salt in the sweat and the compensating reduction from the kidney may be less in evidence.

SYNONYM. Other terms in use are 'tropical anhidrotic asthenia' and 'postmiliarial hypohidrosis'.

Definition

A condition characterised by some impairment of sweating resulting from damage or interference with the sweat glands over large skin areas, the anhidrosis being associated usually with past or present prickly heat. It is attended by symptoms of fatigue, circulatory distress and overheating whenever the patient attempts physical effort in the heat.

Incidence and epidemiology

No systematic records over a long period of time are available. Over a 3-year period Horne (1954) found very great variability. In hot humid conditions at Karachi with 5000–6000 men at work there were 58 cases in 1 year and very few (4 and 20) in the preceding and succeeding years. Ladell *et al* (1944) in Shaiba, Iraq, found cases about as frequently as salt deficiency heat exhaustion and at least twice as commonly as heat stroke.

The circumstances under which anhidrotic heat exhaustion occurs are not clear, but the frequent association of the syndrome with prickly heat was fairly close both in Iraq and Karachi.

Clinical features

The patient complains of a general feeling of exhaustion and overheating. Even on slight exertion these become particularly marked. The patient is usually aware of the reduction in sweating. A history of severe prickly heat is usual. Frequency of micturition and polyuria may also have been noticed.

On examination, even at rest, sweating on the face may be profuse in contrast to dryness elsewhere; and this becomes even more striking under heat stress. The rash resembles that of prickly heat; the skin feels rough and granular: there is usually no itching or irritation. If the patient performs a moderate step-climbing task his distress becomes noticeable; there is hyperpnoea and tachycardia, and collapse may ensue. Symptoms are rapidly relieved when the heat stress is removed, and returns when it is reapplied.

The anhidrosis may persist for many weeks, even when the patient has been moved to cooler climates. In due course the skin appears always to return to normal.

Diagnosis

The diagnosis depends on the demonstration of anhidrosis. For this either a starch-iodine or alizarin test should be used. Other diagnostic features are the profuse facial sweating and the association with past or present prickly heat. If the patient presents with syncopal features the history and particularly anhidrosis and the associated prickly heat will differentiate from simple circulatory deficiency heat exhaustion. The presence of chloride in the urine and the absence of cramps and the presence commonly of polyuria differentiates the condition from salt and water deficiency.

Prognosis

Symptoms are rapidly relieved when heat stress is removed; the anhidrosis may persist for many weeks but eventually returns to normal. Recovery does not ensure against a recurrence in a subsequent season.

Treatment

No special treatment is indicated apart from the provision of a cooler climate; there are no known measures for hastening the restoration of sweating.

Prevention

In so far as the anhidrosis is associated with skin changes associated with prickly heat, measures to avoid miliaria would reduce the incidence of the exhaustion syndrome.

Aetiology and pathogenesis

The underlying cause of the condition is believed to be a partial suppression of sweating over a large part of the body consequent on damage to and blocking of sweat gland ducts, brought about by miliaria rubra. Histological studies of biopsy material from actual cases have been interpreted by O'Brien (1960) and others as showing a mechanical obstruction of sweat ducts.

2L

Sweat glands can be blocked deliberately by a variety of agents, and these may act by occlusion of the ducts through swelling of surrounding cells of the stratum corneum or by actual plugging of the outlet or both. Injury to the skin induced by stripping of the superficial layers, by chemicals such as turpentine and formaldehyde has been shown by Shelley (1951) to bring about the appearance of miliarial-like skin lesions, and sweat suppression. Histological study has revealed the existence of actual blockages of the duct with retention of fluid producing the vesicles. Maceration of the skin by prolonged soaking has also been found to produce sweat suppression probably because of swelling of the stratum corneum. The whole syndrome has been reproduced on volunteers by Sulzberger and his colleagues (1969). By wrapping about one quarter of the skin surface in plastic film for 2 or 3 days they produced a substantial area of miliaria and vesicles and this was accompanied and followed not only by hypohidrosis but by signs and symptoms of heat exhaustion. As expected, the subjects are not able to maintain body temperatures when heat stress is applied. The skin is flushed and hot and circulatory and other signs of collapse are evident.

MILD HEAT FATIGUE

SYNONYM. Acute heat neurasthenia

Definition

A condition characterised by 'psychological' symptoms—tiredness, disinclination to work, and inefficiency in skilled work, due to acute or short-term heat exposure.

Incidence and epidemiology

Undoubtedly widespread in factories, offices, public transport, operating theatres and other places where ventilation is inadequate, and where environmental temperatures rise above the comfort zone and exposure of several hours is required. Probably the ill-effects of hot dry desert winds (sirocco, hamsin, etc.) may be included in this syndrome.

The symptoms of fatigue and inefficiency can be elicited on acute exposure to hot conditions; probably lack of acclimatisation plays a part since with continual exposure some degree of adjustment is apparent. Many studies have pointed to a relationship of increased environment temperature to reduced vigilance, error in skilled work.

Above an effective temperature of 82°F deterioration of performance and mild heat fatigue is to be expected. The more skilled the operator the more resistant will he be.

Clinical features

This is not strictly a 'clinical' condition calling for clinical treatment, but it is of real economic significance and its detection draws attention to the need for improvement in environmental conditions in the interest of working efficiency, output and safety. The symptoms are predominantly 'psychological' and shows itself in extreme tiredness, falling of work, errors in manipulation. The subject may complain of headache and fatigue, but physical signs are lacking. The exposure may only have been a matter of a few hours. The subject can probably withstand the conditions without undue distress if not required to work systematically or skilfully.

Diagnosis

This should be quite clear from the absence of physical symptoms, the shortness and acuteness of the exposure, the rapid improvement on removal of stress, the association of heat discomfort with inefficiency.

Prognosis

The subject's feelings of distress disappears at once when he leaves the hot conditions.

Treatment and prevention

This is a matter of reorganising and improving the working conditions so that comfortable conditions are obtained. The amount of clothing worn will affect the level of acceptable conditions.

CHRONIC HEAT FATIGUE

SYNONYM. Tropical fatigue, tropical neurasthenia.

Definition

A condition characterised by deterioration, principally of character and performance, associated with prolonged residence in a hot climate and affecting in particular white settlers in the tropics; physical signs are lacking.

Incidence and epidemiology

Exact figures are difficult to obtain, but there is no doubt that amongst service personnel during the Second World War psychoneurotic illness in the tropics made up a large proportion of cases invalided home. 'Tropical fatigue' affected all three services of the British military services as well as American and Australian troops. The syndrome has been noted also in civil servants invalided from East and West Africa and occurs amongst the more settled population of northern Australia. The syndrome of course figures dramatically in the fiction of civilian life in the tropics by such authors as Conrad, Maugham and Kipling. Native populations are not exempt from behaviour disorders or emotional or psychological upsets related to climate, but these are associated with poor working conditions, heat waves or with the arrival of hot winds. These short-term effects are probably better classified under 'mild heat fatigue'.

The condition is more particularly associated with hot humid areas and especially where monotony of climate prevails. But it seems clear that climate, while a necessary factor, is not the sole or sufficient factor. Social conditions are nearly always involved—isolation and boredom, excessive consumption of alcohol, discontent with conditions of service or employment, lack of recreational and other activities. A constitutional factor must also be involved. Macpherson found the incidence amongst military personnel greatest in those lacking 'courage and strength of mind'.

While the belief in tropical fatigue is or was widespread, Macpherson found from very careful checking that a high proportion did not consider that they had deteriorated. Thus even where social conditions may be irksome, tropical fatigue is by no means the inevitable lot of the newcomer.

Clinical features

The complaints make up a large and miscellaneous list—loss of energy, constant feeling of tiredness and general malaise, loss of output, dizziness on standing up, loss of appetite, of memory, of initiative, of concentration, increase in irritability, and sleeplessness. As Macpherson (1960) has shown in both his military and civilian studies, these complaints can be clearly seen in many subjects as a kind of protest against the living and working conditions. The patient is in fact motivated by a strong if thinly veiled desire to return home. While many cases may be regarded as minor functional disorders, in some the mental and behavioural deterioration may be serious enough to take the form of definite psychoneuroses —anxiety, hysteria or obsession (see Chapter 36).

On examination it is unusual to detect any overt changes indicative of circulatory, respiratory or digestive disorders. But the existence of skin trouble in many subjects has been often observed, most of these being quite mild. Skin rashes in the crural and axillary regions, prickly heat, otitis externa, which are in any case common, no doubt contribute to the sleeplessness and loss of efficiency which is commonly complained of.

Diagnosis

This rests on a recognition of the essentially subjective nature of the complaints and the absence of any tangible physical disturbance. The absence of raised body temperature, of fainting, or cramps, of deficient salt in the urine and of anhidrosis, makes the diagnosis from other heat disorders quite clear. The exact degree of 'functional' disability and the character of any manifest psychoneurosis require expert psychiatric examination, but such elements as anxiety or hysteria can usually be established without doubt. In cases presenting with psychiatric symptoms it is of course necessary to eliminate organic disease.

Prognosis

The natural history of 'psychological deterioration' in the tropics is by no means clear. It seems certain that the condition will persist or get worse unless ameliorative measures are carried out in particular as regards amenities, housing, etc. But the really serious cases will require removal to a cooler and easier climate or invalidation home if there is to be a good prospect of recovery.

Treatment

To correct the effect of tropical life, measures to combat the heat stress as well as the non-climatic stresses must be undertaken. This may range from simple measures such as attention to suitable clothing or change of work routine, to major improvements in the environment—housing ventilation, labour-saving equipment or air conditioning—and in social amenities—swimming pools, recreation facilities. Medical treatment as such would include attention to skin diseases, but in the absence of immediate environmental improvement, removal of the patient to cooler conditions with more of the social amenities will

be necessary. In extreme cases specialist psychotherapy will be necessary.

Aetiology

The aetiology of the syndrome of tropical deterioration is by no means clear. Understandably an environment which places a subject outside the 'comfort zone' for long periods will be very trying, leading to irritability and sleeplessness. But the body has good adaptive processes to heat load and there is evidence that with continued exposure to warmer conditions, some degree of wetness of the skin is tolerated. The 'comfort' zone is raised by reduction in clothing as well as by physiological acclimatisation. The factors which make for intolerance seem to be partly social as already indicated and partly constitutional. As Macpherson (1960) puts it: 'There is no place in the tropics for the poor in spirit.' It is possible that 'stress' effects affecting the endocrine system would be demonstrable but no studies appear to have been made.

PRICKLY HEAT

SYNONYM. Miliaria rubra

Definition

A skin condition characterised by a fine, superficial, papular eruption surrounded by vesicles and reddening of skin and usually accompanied by prickling.

Incidence and epidemiology

Prickly heat is an important cause of morbidity in service personnel in the tropics, in gold mines in South Africa and coal mines in Australia. It is known to occur in children and adults even amongst indigenous peoples.

In servicemen entering the tropics the time of onset is more likely to be within the first 10 weeks or so but the chance of contracting it increases with length of tropical service. In gold mines a primary transient attack may occur in the first 6 months of work; a more refractory miliaria may develop after years of freedom. The condition is independent of age, skin colour and physical type. Undoubtedly the condition occurs far more in hot humid areas than in hot arid conditions.

Clinical features

The patient complains of a rash accompanied by a tingling, burning or prickling feeling. The rash is usually described as symmetrical in distribution and is often characterised by reddening and itching. The skin condition may be associated with complaints of sleeplessness, interference with work and discomfort on sweating, depending on the site and extent of the rash. The patient may say that the rash is made worse by clothing, work, hot conditions or under stress.

On examination the lesion is seen as a papulovesicular rash with papules surrounded by erythematous areas and surmounted by vesicles and pustules. The rash affects usually the parts normally covered or subject to friction but is not necessarily confined to these.

Course and complications

The rash may last for a few days or up to several weeks. It is subject to remissions and exacerbations and it is aggravated by heat exposure and frequently becomes infected and eczematised. Secondary infections attributed to the miliaria include multiple boils, impetiginous rash, fungus infection and local adenitis.

Miliaria profunda is a more advanced stage arising from severe miliaria rubra and is characterised by non-inflammatory papules over the sweat pores; obstruction of the duct at the epidermodermal junction leads to anhidrosis. Miliaria profunda is thought to be the characteristic lesion in patients with anhydrotic heat exhaustion.

Diagnosis

This presents little difficulty as its distribution and appearance and the prickling when the patient sweats are all very characteristic.

Prognosis

It is difficult to make a very definite prognosis for the individual case. The rash may last for a few days or for several weeks and is subject to remissions and exacerbation. If the patient is successfully treated and regular prophylactic measures taken, the chances are in favour of continued freedom from the malady.

Treatment

The only reliable treatment is to transfer the patient to cool surroundings or to move him from the tropical to a temperate climate. A host of skin treatments designed to clear the skin of keratotic plugs or to counteract maceration have been advocated, but no reliable treatment has been forthcoming. The beneficial results claimed appear to have been merely episodes of natural remission. There is, however, a firm conviction that in many cases salt intake is excessive, and if this is so a reduction to moderate levels combined with an increased water intake may prove beneficial. To prevent secondary infection the patient should take cool showers regularly with thorough drying and the application of calamine lotion. If infection has occurred, the area should be washed with cetrimide solution and dibromopropamidine cream applied.

Prevention

Preventive measures are more hopeful. Exposure to humid heat should be limited; in particular, sleeping in cool quarters will do much to prevent the syndrome. Clothing should be loose fitting and well ventilated; the use of soap should be limited to once a day, hot water should be avoided and powders applied sparingly.

Aetiology and pathogenesis

In recent years clinical observers have favoured the view that the miliaria are caused by closure of the orifices of the sweat ducts. Histological evidence from biopsy material from actual cases to support this has been brought forward. A number of different agencies acting under hot and humid conditions might well be involved. The plugging could arise from a keratotic reaction in response to intense sunlight, degreasing of the skin by excessive washing, irritants such as excessive use of soaps and lotions, dermatitis from other causes, or from extensive hydration or waterlogging of the stratum corneum.

In general support of these ideas are experiments in which miliarial lesions have been produced deliberately. A variety of agents applied to the skin will produce visible as well as histological changes in the sweat gland very similar to the natural lesion. These agents include turpentine, soap, formaldehyde, wet dressings, adhesive tape and ultraviolet irradiation. Miliaria appears thus to be a non-specific response to local injury of the skin (Sargent, 1957). In hot, humid climates the accumulation of sweat in some parts of the skin, leading to maceration combined with friction, would represent a prime aetiological factor.

Miliaria rubra similar to the clinical entity has been provoked in volunteers exposed for at least 3 days for 24 hours a day to effective temperatures above 85°F. The incidence was greatly diminished by reducing the exposure to 7–12 hours a day.

Several careful observers believe that excess of

salt intake combined with low water intake is implicated in the aetiology. Patients have been improved by increasing the fluid intake and have been made to relapse by increasing the intake of table salt (Horne and Mole, 1949). Since artificial miliaria rubra has been produced quite readily with hypertonic salt compresses, it is possible that the secretion of sweat and high salt content following excessive salt ingestion could act as a dietary causal factor.

REFERENCES

ADOLPH, E. F. (1947) *Physiology of Man in the Desert*. New York: Interscience Publishers.
BANNISTER, R. G. (1959) *Lancet*, **2**, 313.
BRAUER, R. W., BALAM, R. W., BOND, H. E., CARROLL, H. W., GRISHAM, J. W. and PESSOTTI, R. L. (1963) *Fed. Proc.*, **22**, 724-1.
CAPLAN, A. (1943) *Trans. Inst. Mining Metall.*, **53**, 95.
DREOSTI, A. O. (1937) *S. Afr. med. J. Sci.*, **2**, 29.
GILAT, T. SHIBOLET, S. and SOHAR, E. (1963) *J. Trop. Med. and Hyg.*, **66**, 204-212.
GUTHRIE, J. and McCRACKEN, A. V. (1960) *Lancet*, **1**, 682.
HEARNE, K. G. (1932) *Med. J. Aust.*, **1**, 226.
HORNE, G. O. (1954) *Edin. med. J.*, **61**, 349.
HORNE, G. O. and MOLE, R. H. (1949) *Lancet*, **2**, 279.
KUNO, Y. (1956) *Human Perspiration*. Springfield, Illinois: Thomas.
LADELL, W. S. S., WATERLOW, J. C. and HUDSON, M. F. (1944) *Lancet*, **2**, 491, 527.
LEITHEAD, C. S. and LIND, A. R. (1964) *Heat Stress and Heat Disorders*. London: Cassell.
McCANCE, R. A. (1936) *Lancet*, **1**, 823.
MACPHERSON, R. K. (1960) *Spec. Rep. Ser. Med. Res. Council*, no. 298. London: H.M.S.O.
MINARD, D., BELDING, H. S. and KINGSTON, J. R. (1957) *J. Amer. med. Ass.*, **165**, 1813.
MINARD, D. (1961) *Milit. Med.*, **126**, 261.
O'BRIEN, J. P. (1960) *Trans. roy. Soc. trop. Med. Hyg.*, **54**, 235.
SARGENT, F. and SLUTSKY, H. L. (1957) *New Engl. J. Med.*, **256**, 401, 451.
SHELLEY, W. B. (1951) *J. invest. Derm.*, **16**, 53.
SULZBERGER, M. B. and GRIFFIN, T. B. (1969) *Arch. Derm.*, **99**, 145.
WEINER, J. S. (1938) *J. industr. Hyg.*, **20**, 389.
WEINER, J. S. and HORNE, G. O. (1958) *Brit. Med. J.*, **1**, 1533.
WYNDHAM, C. H. (1962) *Ergonomics*, **5**, 115.

32
Occupational Diseases

What is your occupation? This commonplace query in a patient's clinical history is becoming more important in the tropics. New materials and processes pose health risks in agriculture, mines, mills, factories, transport and construction work. Familiar communicable diseases have occupational aspects. Industrialisation can pose risks to individual workers, to the public and be accompanied by social changes which affect health. The recognition of occupational disease is important for diagnosis, treatment, and also for prevention. This chapter aims to describe general principles, illustrating these in relation to some of the more significant examples of occupational disease in the tropics, and to other aspects of the influence that working environments may have on health.

Occupational diseases may present with symptoms and signs simulating non-occupational disease, and may be easily missed if no enquiry is made about the patient's occupation and the materials he handles. Virtually any system of the body may be affected by exposure to a wide range of chemical, physical and biological agents which are increasingly used in tropical countries. A few examples will suffice to illustrate how some common occupational illnesses in the tropics may present.

Respiratory disease

Occupational respiratory diseases caused by exposure to *mineral dusts* such as quartz, coal or asbestos produce specific changes in chest radiographs and may be discovered at routine X-ray examination before the onset of symptoms.

By contrast the *organic dusts* such as cotton, flax and soft hemp which cause byssinosis do not produce specific X-ray changes, and the changes in bagassosis or farmer's lung caused by exposure to mouldy hay may be indistinct and not easily recognised (Gilson, 1960).

In the mineral dust pneumoconioses, the patient may present first with dyspnoea of insidious onset which may be accompanied by wheezing, cough and the production of sputum. Cyanosis and finger clubbing are often present in asbestosis but are rarely seen in the other pneumoconioses.

Byssinosis, which is discussed in more detail with other organic dust diseases on page 528, is characterised by chest tightness which is worse at the beginning of the working week. It is relatively easy to diagnose in workers routinely examined at their work place by medical staff aware of the hazard; but the disease is often missed in patients seen by doctors unfamiliar with the effects of exposure to such dusts; the patient may consult his doctor in the late stages of the disease when the characteristic symptoms are masked by irreversible and severe respiratory damage.

The more acute forms of occupational respiratory disease likely to be seen in the tropics are those associated with *inhalation of spores* from moulding crops of hay and bagasse (see page 529), and severe pulmonary oedema from *exposure to gases* such as oxides of nitrogen which accumulate in silage towers or storage bins (Gilson, 1969; Edson, 1969).

Pesticides

As many insecticides attack cell enzymes common to both insects and mammals, they are often toxic to man and particularly dangerous in countries with hot climates where it is necessary to destroy a variety of insect pests and where there are low precautionary standards. The early symptoms of poisoning by the *organophosphorus chemicals* include headache, nausea, anorexia and extreme fatigue (see page 529); their significance is easily missed and the same may be said of later symptoms such as nausea, abdominal cramps, vomiting, diarrhoea, convulsions and pulmonary oedema if the occupation of the patient is not ascertained.

The *organochlorine insecticides* such as DDT, Dieldrin and Aldrin are more persistent and less destructible than the organophosphorus chemicals and may be stored in the fatty tissues of the body. Although acute poisoning from these compounds is uncommon there is some doubt as to the long-term effects of this type of exposure; however, poisoning has occurred among those with long exposures, and presents as disordered personality, convulsions and changes in the central nervous system.

Health hazards may arise from the use of *rodenticides* such as fluoracetamide and zinc phosphide, *fumigants* such as methyl bromide, ethylene dibromide and HCN, all of which are toxic to both man and pests (Edson, 1969).

The main users of insecticides are agricultural workers and staff of public health departments who should be effectively supervised so that poisoning does not occur; nevertheless, poisoning amongst agricultural workers still occurs. Immediate diagnosis is important to ensure the right treatment is given and that action is taken to prevent further poisoning.

Other occupational diseases

The ways in which the metal poisonings may present are legion; some are briefly discussed on page 527. They usually occur as acute episodes which are quite easily related to recent occupational exposures. But in chronic diseases like occupational cancer and respiratory disease, which usually occur after prolonged exposure and frequently after the patient has changed his occupation, it is important to take a chronological occupational history in order to identify the aetiological agent; by asking whether other workmates have been similarly affected may provide a valuable clue to the identification of an occupational disease.

IDENTIFICATION AND CONTROL

Identification is not limited simply to the recognition of physical, chemical or biological risks, but includes the health characteristics of individuals exposed to these risks, and their interplay with job requirements. Apart from illness directly caused by work, occupational conditions may be aetiologically important in certain diseases although they do not directly cause them. Certain tropical diseases can limit work capacity: hookworm anaemia limits ability for heavy manual work; persons with the sickle cell trait are at special risk in occupations with definite anoxic risks. There are occupations in which the subject as a result of some illness or disability is a potential danger to his colleagues or the general public. The most important group in this category are drivers of public vehicles and other mechanically propelled vehicles. Thus medical responsibility extends from the identification of such risks to suitable job placement, treatment and control.

Clinical observation is often the starting point for identification of occupational diseases but they commonly require special investigations and the collaboration of other professions (such as engineering) for effective control. Problems may be approached systematically, as follows:

1. **Recognising the hazard**, by means of clinical observation, industrial sickness statistics, epidemiological surveys, and use of existing knowledge on the production process and its risks.

2. **Establishing criteria for diagnosis** and acceptable limits of risk which may be employed in biological monitoring and environmental monitoring. Diagnosis often depends on more than one type of evidence. For instance exposure to cotton dust and development of byssinosis is associated with *symptoms* of chest tightness related to occupational exposure, and with *changes in lung function*—but not with any changes in X-ray appearances. In mineral dust pneumoconioses there are characteristic *X-ray changes* which are graded according to an international classification (I.L.O., 1963). Some biologically inert dusts produce marked shadows but no disease at all; diagnosis thus depends not only on the X-ray appearance but on the occupational history, clinical findings and lung function tests.

   Environmental measurements are usually standardised, and for many toxic substances there are internationally accepted threshold limit values, which are periodically reviewed and revised (Department of Employment, 1972).

3. **Introducing preventive measures.** General principles are:
   —*substitution* of safe for unsafe substances or methods;
   —*enclosure* of dangerous processes;
   —safe *design and operation* of machinery, including guards over moving parts;
   —*removal at source* of dangerous dust or fumes by exhaust ventilation, or by suppression (e.g. wet drilling or grinding);
   —ensuring good *environmental hygiene*, tidiness and cleanliness, and suitable places for washing, eating and rest;
   —where other measures do not suffice in their own, the provision of individual *protective equipment*, safety gear or protective clothing.

It is wise to rely primarily on measures which operate constantly, independent of the whim of individuals. This principle is particularly applicable to developing countries where individual understanding, training and supervision may be defective. These points were well expressed by Sir Thomas Legge, the first Medical Inspector of Factories in Britain, who stated:

'Unless and until the employer has done everything—and everything means a good deal—the workman can do next to nothing to protect himself, although he is naturally willing enough to do his share. If you bring an influence to bear external to the workman (that is, one over which he can exercise no control) you will be successful. Influences which are not external but depend on the will or whim of the worker to use them (e.g. protective clothing) are useful up to a point but are not completely effective. All workmen should be told something of the danger of the material with which they come in contact and not be left to find it out for themselves.'

4. **Surveillance and follow-up.** Pre-placement periodic medical examinations are essential in hazardous occupations and of value in others. The examination can be limited to relevant diagnostic tests or screening procedures carried out by suitable medical auxiliary staff, and may not require the personal attention of the medical practitioner, apart from noting results in the medical records, and making appropriate recommendations. Work conditions may also require periodic inspection and testing by an occupational hygienist, engineer or safety officer.

5. **Education of management and workers.** Correct and accurate information on potential risks is essential to management; often it is a medical responsibility to provide this information and to recommend suitable measures for training and educating workers in safe practices. Here some general principles of health education in the tropics apply (Holmes, 1964); the motivation of both management and workers is not always easy but calculation of the costs to the individual and the enterprise of the existing hazard, and the ease and cheapness of prevention, is often available to reinforce other arguments.

Legge's axiom, quoted above, is an ideal which often cannot be achieved. In modern industry it is increasingly difficult to make work safe without the participation of the worker. In tropical countries the importance of careful training must be stressed. The worker must be shown his own responsibility in any health and safety programme. This needs patience, imagination and careful work on the part of management and the doctor, particularly with people in tropical countries who may be unfamiliar with modern industry. It is often the doctor's most important task to inspire both management and workers with enthusiasm for healthy working conditions. The employer can and must do a great deal, but total prevention may often be impossible without the cooperation of the worker (Lane, 1949).

6. **Role of authority: legislation and enforcement of minimum standards.** Authority—in the form of Government, usually a department of the Ministry of Health or Labour—has an important role in establishing standards of health and safety at workplaces and in seeing they are observed; in addition the authority plays an essential part in giving information and advice, particularly to newly developing enterprises. Legislation in most countries comprises principal laws (Acts) and subsidiary laws (Rules, Orders) on public health, employment of labour, factories, mines, workmen's compensation, social insurance and related matters. Doctors can play a useful part in seeing that employers and workers understand the *reasons* for such legislation on health, safety and welfare and do not view it as a meaningless requirement of authority. Some tropical countries do not yet have a fully developed legislation, or the means of enforcing it. In this respect the conventions, recommendations and Model Codes of the International Labour Office form helpful and reliable guides on many occupational risks.

Mechanical, thermal and electrical hazards

These are discussed in Model Codes and other publications of the I.L.O. (given in the bibliography) which are of particular assistance where local legislation and standards of safety are undeveloped. Occupational injuries are discussed in more detail in a later section of this chapter.

Heat: effects of climate and microclimate

Heat illnesses are discussed in detail in the previous chapter. In industry there are commonly two other types of problem concerning the thermal environment on which medical advice may be sought: (*a*) thermal comfort in offices and factories, which can affect working efficiency and safety, and (*b*) heat stress, or the limits of tolerance for manual work in hot environments. The investigation of these problems is well described by Leithead and Lind (1964), and an introduction to the principles of ventilation and air conditioning is given in Patty (1963).

Noise

Excessive noise in workplaces may be a hazard because of reduced intelligibility of speech, because of permanent hearing loss after months or years of intermittent exposures, and because it may cause temporary hearing loss after short exposures. The most significant variables to consider are the sound frequencies or pitch involved, and the sound pressure levels at each frequency; the effects of high sound pressure levels are different at each frequency.

High-pitched sound is more disturbing and damaging than low-pitched sound of the same intensity. Noise-induced hearing loss is preventable, and there is an obligation on employers in high-noise industries to promote hearing conservation programmes.

In extreme situations, the existence of a noise hazard is evident from its loudness, the occurrence of temporary hearing loss, with tinnitus, and muffling of sounds of speech and higher pitch (e.g. music). The technical assessment of noise exposure requires a sound level meter with octave band (or preferred frequency) analyser, and suitable microphone and sound level calibrator. The main methods of protection are reduction of noise by engineering control at source, or by suitable barriers to transmission, and by ear protection (plugs, muffs and acoustic helmets). Personal protection measures have limitations, and a recent welcome tendency is to consider engineering measures as prime methods of control. Modern sound level meters have what is called an 'A' weighting which mimics the response of the human ear, and the risk of noise-induced deafness from continuous, wide frequency sources is related to the 'A'-weighted level measured in decibels (dBA); levels of 90 dBA or more are hazardous in continuous 8-hour daily exposures. Non-continuous or narrow-frequency sources

must be assessed by measurement on a linear or 'C' weighting scale. The following levels (Matelsky, 1969) may be taken as guides to the values at which hearing conservation should be instituted; in any investigation it is of course necessary to consider the total durations of exposure which may occur.

Sound frequency band *Hz* (*cycles per second*)	*Sound pressure level* *dB* (*decibels, C weighting*)
75– 150	100
150– 300	90
300– 600	85
600–1200	85
1200–2400	80
2400–4800	80

Radiation

With the important exception of hospital radiography, problems in the control of ionising radiations are not common in the tropics. When they are encountered, however, adequate controls are essential. The essentials of safety in hospital radiography entail:

1. Adequate size and design of X-ray rooms and darkrooms, with the radiographer, his assistants, and neighbouring workers adequately screened (by thick walls, distance from machine during operation, and lead aprons).

2. Safe machine operation and maintenance (also methods to reduce unnecessary patient exposure, especially of gonads).

3. Monitoring—usually by film badge.

Industrial radiography may employ sealed radioactive sources, e.g. ^{60}Co to X-ray welded conduits in hydroelectric station construction, which may be carried out in remote areas. Radioactive sources are finding increasing use in many other industries. Uranium mining poses special problems due to atmospheric radon gas and its decay products. A reliable guide to control is the *I.L.O. Manual of Industrial Radiation Protection*, of which Part III (1963) is a general guide; Volume 1 of Patty (1963) may also be recommended. The problems of institutes using radioactive isotopes are best covered in the *U.K. Codes of Practice* (1963). Non-ionising radiations, ranging from ultraviolet, visible light, the infrared and radio frequencies, are finding increasing industrial applications in specialised fields; health aspects have been reviewed by Matelsky (1969).

CHEMICALS AND INDUSTRIAL MATERIALS

The recognition of these hazards depends on factors which are well described in standard works on occupational health or toxicology: the diverse industries involved, the chemical composition of the substance, its physical form and route of absorption, and the body systems in which clinical symptoms and signs become manifest. The sale and use of many chemicals and materials in the tropics has expanded in recent years much more than the simple growth of industry might indicate, and almost any major hazard may be encountered. In this section only a few representative examples can be mentioned.

Metals and their compounds

Inorganic lead and mercury are well-known heavy metal poisons; their effects are different from the corresponding organometal compounds. Thus, inorganic lead poisoning can cause anaemia, abdominal colic and muscle weakness, whilst organic alkyl lead compounds which are easily absorbed through intact skin cause encephalopathy. Inorganic mercury poisoning leads to tremor, gingivitis, erythism—timidity, irritability, depression or excitability—and albuminuria, whereas alkyl mercury compounds, once used extensively as fungicidal seed dressings, can lead to ataxia, visual field loss, with permanently impaired sight, hearing, mental capacity and personality.

Other metallic compounds used in industry have diverse effects, e.g. *arsenic* (gastroenteritis, dermatitis, peripheral neuritis), *cadmium* (emphysema, metal fume fever, anosmia, and other systemic effects), *chromium* and *chromates* (skin ulcer, perforation of nasal septum and bronchial carcinoma), *nickel* (dermatitis, haemorrhagic bronchopneumonia, nasal and bronchial carcinoma), *manganese* (extra pyramidal motor lesions, pneumonitis), *beryllium* (dermatitis, pneumonitis and pulmonary fibrosis), *vanadium* (eye irritation, bronchitis and pneumonitis).

Inorganic lead poisoning is taken as an example of the recognition and control of such hazards. Lead is used in numerous industries; it has been largely replaced in some common materials (e.g. paints, vitreous enamels) by less toxic compounds but may still be encountered in dismantling or refurbishing old structures. In the tropics, lead fume hazards are most likely to occur in small factory industries in which lead products are manufactured or renovated (e.g. lead battery manufacture).

Absorption of dust or fume is direct from the respiratory tract. Various degrees of absorption of lead occur, even in the normal population. Some increased absorption may occur and be detectable in blood or urinary lead levels, but may cause no symptoms. Higher degrees of absorption will cause mild or severe symptoms, dependent also on the duration of exposure. Some symptoms and signs are not specific to lead poisoning, and it is therefore important that a diagnosis of lead poisoning should be supported by laboratory evidence of excessive lead absorption.

Symptomatology. Mild symptoms of lead poisoning include lassitude, anorexia, constipation, irritability, sleep disturbance, abdominal discomfort or pain, sometimes nausea and diarrhoea; anaemia and a blue line in the gums may be seen. Severe symptoms and signs are abdominal colic, reduction of muscle power in commonly-used muscle groups (e.g. wrist drop), muscle tenderness, paraesthesia and in most severe cases, encephalopathy.

Diagnosis. Excessive lead absorption will concurrently give rise to levels of blood lead exceeding 80 μg/100 ml, urinary lead exceeding 150 μg/l, urinary coproporphyrin exceeding 500 μg/l, and urinary delta-amino laevulinic acid exceeding 2 mg/100 ml. A lowered haemoglobin concentration is also commonly found; punctate basophil counts are of less diagnostic value than the other tests, and are not now recommended. It should be noted that raised urinary coproporphyrins may also occur in subjects with an abnormal haemoglobin disease. Environmental measurements of inorganic lead in the atmosphere may provide strong evidence of a hazard, or of the efficiency of control.

Treatment of acute lead poisoning is by EDTA (versenate) orally or intravenously, and calcium by mouth, in order to displace lead from bone and other tissue stores and enable it to be excreted in harmless form.

Control of lead exposure entails engineering methods (isolation or enclosure of the process, local exhaust ventilation), clean handling of materials and maintenance of the workplace ('good housekeeping'), satisfactory toilets, washrooms, lunchrooms, education of the worker in the nature of the hazard, and periodic (monthly) examination of blood and/or urine for evidence of excessive lead absorption. The use of personal protective equipment (e.g. respirators) is *not* a suitable control measure, though such equipment may be available for use in some emergency or unusual occasion.

Dust diseases

Dust diseases may be considered together or separately, because their deposition and effects on various parts of the respiratory tract are related to particle size, and this characteristic also relates to their engineering control. However, in their chemical composition different dusts have very varying pathological effects, or none in the case of inert dusts such as chalk. Silica is taken as the most important example amongst inorganic dusts, though others have distinct effects, e.g. asbestos—asbestosis, bronchial carcinoma, mesothelioma (see Whipple, 1964); coal—pneumoconiosis; and cement—chronic bronchitis. Vegetable dusts produce distinct types of reaction, depending on the nature of the sensitisation, which is discussed later.

Silica dust can occur in a wide variety of occupations: the mining of ores or minerals in silica-bearing rock, sandstone, slate or flint quarrying and dressing, foundry workers (moulding, cleaning, grinding), and some trades where silica powders may be used (pottery glazing, abrasive soap or cleaning powder manufacture). Particles of size 1–10 μm are deposited in the alveoli, and get taken up by tissue macrophages in the lungs.

There have been many theories to account for the unique action of silica. A current explanation is that silica particles have the ability to break down the phagosome membrane within the macrophage, thus releasing hydrolytic enzymes into the cytoplasm and killing the cell, a process which can be repeated if the particle is taken up by a further macrophage. The dead cells produce a fibrotic reaction, and may also produce an auto-immune response, particularly in subjects predisposed to rheumatoid disease, in which the process of macrophage necrosis with concentric nodules of fibrosis is accentuated (Caplan's syndrome). Concurrent infection with tuberculosis may also accelerate this process. In some subjects the formation of discrete nodules of fibrosis progresses, leading to an irreversible progressive massive fibrosis (PMF) with extensive lung damage and disability, not altered by withdrawal from the dust exposure.

Diagnosis is provided by a history of occupational exposure, with characteristic changes on chest X-ray, which may be graded according to an international standard classification (U.I.C.C., 1970); concurrent changes in lung function (I.L.O., 1966) will be found in the later stages of the disease. Recognition of an occupational risk is confirmed by environmental measurements of the silica content of respirable (1–7 μm) dust; siliceous dusts are commonly of mixed composition, so that the method involves collection of the respirable fraction by a suitable sampler, weighing and/or particle counting and analysis of silica content. The present accepted threshold limit value is expressed in the formula

$$\frac{250}{\%SiO_2 + 5} \text{ million particles per ft}^3$$

$$(\text{or} \times 35.3 \text{ particles per cm}^3).$$

Control of the risk is by substitution (e.g. glass frits instead of silica powder for glazing), suppression at source (e.g. wet drilling methods in mining), enclosure or local exhaust ventilation (e.g. in foundries). Where any risk remains it is necessary to have a system of initial and periodic (usually annual) chest X-ray, and continued environmental measurements to ensure that the threshold limit value is not being exceeded.

Vegetable dust diseases may be classified for convenience into four main types, partly dependent on the site of deposition in the respiratory tract but also on the type of sensitivity response they involve.

ASTHMA involves an immediate reaction, dependent on a reaginic tissue sensitivity, but occupational sources are not common: some hardwood dusts, gum arabic and dust from castor or green coffee beans are recognised sensitisers.

BYSSINOSIS involves a delayed type of reaction to cotton, flax and soft hemp dust and may be encountered in most stages of cleaning and processing these fibres where dust concentrations exceed 1 mg/m^3. There is evidence that the reaction is caused by a histamine-releasing agent in the dust. The disease has a characteristic symptomatology, with chest tightness, dyspnoea and sometimes cough and intolerance to cigarettes, worse on return from holiday or weekend, and more pronounced towards the end of a shift. There is a characteristic diminution in forced expiratory volume (FEV$_{1\cdot0}$) following dust exposure, but no specific X-ray changes. In its late stages byssinosis presents a clinical picture of chronic bronchitis and emphysema. More detailed descriptions of the disease and international findings have been given by Schilling (1963, 1972a).

NON-BYSSINOGENIC. In the processing of other vegetable fibres like jute, St Helena hemp, manila and sisal, there is no specific hazard of byssinosis although these dusts may cause bronchial irritation, with persistent cough, expectoration, and a fall in FEV$_{1\cdot0}$ during the work shift. These effects are probably mechanical in origin and essentially a different response to that caused by byssinogenic dusts.

CONTAMINANT. The fourth type of response to vegetable dust is associated with the inhalation of dust contaminated by thermophilic actinomycetes, of which mouldy hay (causing '*farmer's lung*') is a common example, though similar contamination of other vegetable materials, e.g. sugar bagasse, palm kernels, can give a similar response, which is delayed in onset, several hours after exposure. The patient has a cough, malaise, dyspnoea and pyrexia and the chest X-ray shows miliary, nodular or diffuse shadowing. Lung function tests show diminished diffusion and compliance.

Control of byssinosis is directed towards dust extraction at source, with environmental monitoring to ensure that an acceptably low level is maintained (present TLV is 1 mg/m³ for total dust; this figure is likely to be revised). Entrants to the industry should have a medical examination including measurement of FEV_1, using a suitable spirometer (I.L.O., 1966), and periodic re-examination whilst exposed to dust is important in detecting susceptible workers and unhealthy occupations. In occupational asthma, engineering control of dust is a primary measure; individuals with extreme sensitivity may, however, have to be transferred to other work. In farmer's lung and similar diseases, risks arise during the handling of stored products; if the method of storage can be modified, e.g. by proprionic acid to prevent growth of the causative microorganism, this will resolve the problem; otherwise it will be necessary to devise an entirely mechanical enclosed process or use suitable respirators during handling of the material.

Pesticide poisoning

Toxic organic compounds are used in many industrial processes, and the literature on them is more extensive than on inorganic substances. In the tropics the commonest hazards from organic compounds are from pesticides, which are used in agriculture (food and fibre crops, and forests), industry (as fungicides for paint, leather, paper, wood and plastics), and in public health. The toxicology of pesticides is a wide subject, which has been well reviewed by Barnes and Edson (1960) and Edson (1969); here it is only possible to take one example, the organophosphorus insecticides which are in common use and generally favoured in agriculture because they do not have the persistence and cumulation of the earlier organochlorine compounds such as DDT,

HCH(BHC) or dieldrin. The organophosphorus compounds do however vary greatly in acute toxicity, from hazardous ones like parathion to relatively safe ones like malathion or diazinon.

Organophosphorous compounds inhibit the enzyme cholinesterase, and if absorbed (usually through intact skin), bind to this enzyme. This leads to an accumulation of acetylcholine in various organs, causing contraction of smooth muscle, glandular hypersecretion, bradycardia, muscle fasiculations and, in the central nervous system, disorientation, coma and depression of respiration. The inhibition of blood cholinesterase is, however, detectable much earlier than the first evidence of poisoning, and this is the basis for the biological monitoring of workers constantly exposed to these compounds; simple kits for estimating the enzyme are available.

Symptomatology. Where poisoning occurs, in individuals not subject to such surveillance, the first symptoms may occur an hour or two after exposure, and are commonly headache, nausea, vomiting and colic—easily confused with food poisoning if the possibility of exposure to organophosphate is not appreciated. Bradycardia, small pupils, excessive salivation, and muscle fasiculation are distinctive signs. Contaminated clothing and shoes should be removed, and the patient washed completely, to limit any further skin absorption. Atropine should be given intravenously (or intramuscularly) in high doses, in adults 2 mg every 10–20 minutes, and continued as long as necessary.

Treatment. Compounds which reverse the binding of organophosphate to enzyme, the so-called cholinesterase reactivators, such as pyridine-2-aldoxine methanesulphonate (P2S) or methiodide (P2AM) should also be given early in treatment to moderate or severe cases of poisoning; they are ineffective if administration is delayed about 24 hours after exposure. In adults these drugs may be given in an initial dose of 1 g, repeated if necessary after 3 hours. The main danger in organophosphorus poisoning is depression of respiration and anoxaemia. Artificial or controlled (positive pressure) respiration should be instituted immediately. In severe cases, excessive bronchial secretion, combined with bronchoconstriction, will tend to block the airway; it may then be necessary to pass an endotracheal tube or perform tracheostomy and bronchial aspiration, to ensure a clear airway.

Prevention of poisoning depends on safe procedures, especially in handling and mixing concentrates (preferably in an enclosed process), in personal protective clothing to obviate skin absorption, in personal hygiene (in regard to washing, food consumption and smoking), and in adequate labelling and safe disposal of containers to obviate accidents. Workers regularly using organophosphorus pesticides should have initial and periodic (monthly) blood cholinesterase estimations, and be withdrawn from such work if values fall below 30 per cent of the initial level (toxic symptoms do not occur until the level is below 10 per cent of normal). Many countries also adopt wider measures of control, particularly in the sale of these compounds, and in encouraging the use of less toxic compounds rather than the hazardous ones. W.H.O., I.L.O. and F.A.O. have collaborated in drafting Model Laws in pesticide control, which are due to be published shortly.

BIOLOGICAL HAZARDS

Rural workers in the tropics can be exposed to biological hazards to health to a greater extent than the general population, though exposure may not be exclusively occupational.

Agricultural, forestry, animal husbandry and some fishery workers become exposed to the risk of zoonoses, vector-borne disease, soil microorganisms, geohelminths and a variety of wild animals. Other tropical industries, e.g. mines, processing factories, hydroelectric stations, are often situated in rural areas where exposure to communicable disease may affect both production and safety, and offer a challenge to provide effective preventive as well as curative services. The *migrant* worker (and his family) may be at special risk from some disease to which they have not been exposed in their homeland, e.g. coming from a non-malarious to a malarious area, as in Africa. Conversely, the migrant coming from an endemic area (e.g. of schistosomiasis) can introduce a new disease where conditions for transmission are favourable; appropriate examination and treatment of new employees can obviate these risks. Migrant workers on engineering constructions (building railways, roads or dams) may live in temporary camps with inadequate water supplies, sanitation or vector control.

Occupational exposure can depend not only on the *place* but also on the *time* of working: whether, for instance, this corresponds with the peak of vector activity. Thus, the distinctive biting activity of different species of mosquito can create a greater hazard for night workers; this may include night workers in towns where *Culex fatigans* breeding is incompletely controlled. In forestry or agriculture an individual in the course of his work may enter a natural ecosystem in which he gets accidentally infected with a hazardous arbovirus; he brings back infection to a community and starts an epidemic if long years of apparent freedom from disease have bred complacency about vector control.

In some countries the rice-planting period coincides with seasonal breeding of malaria or schistosome vectors, and the erection of temporary dwellings in the fields (and associated changes in habit of the population) can produce *new conditions for transmission*. Communicable diseases such as malaria, hookworm and schistosomiasis merit the most vigorous control, which can be more easily financed, organised and applied in large-scale industrial or agricultural enterprises. Methods which do not have to rely on individual cooperation are more reliable, though careful explanation and education are required to obtain cooperation and support for mass treatment or chemoprophylaxis if these are necessary. Vaccination programmes to protect against smallpox, polio, tetanus, tuberculosis and other potential risks are also easily organised within industry.

Tuberculosis merits special mention as it is a major problem in most tropical countries and may be readily transmitted amongst overcrowded and perhaps undernourished periurban populations, and also at work where conditions may be crowded and ventilation poor. Special risks exist in relation to mining and other occupations with any silicosis hazard, in which tuberculosis can produce a serious complication (progressive massive fibrosis) and in relation to occupations where there are risks of spread to the community (or susceptible groups), as in food processing and handling, and schoolteaching. Medical, nursing and technical staff may be at risk in dispensaries and hospitals where close contact with infected patients is inevitable. Initial and periodic medical examination, including chest X-ray, tuberculin testing (and BCG vaccination of tuberculin negative subjects) are important control measures.

The possible occupational exposures to biological hazards are numerous, and can only be summarized here. The following text, giving diseases, causative agents, geographic distribution, animal reservoirs, transmission and control, is based on an annex to *Occupational Health Problems in Agriculture* (4th Report of the Joint I.L.O./W.H.O. Committee on Occupational Health, W.H.O., 1962), modified to incorporate later additions to knowledge. The authors are grateful to Dr Brian Southgate, Ross Institute of Tropical Hygiene, for assistance in revising this list.

In a number of infections of wild and domesticated animals, man is an occasional victim of a dead-end or accidental infection, but is not a normal host. Such infections, which may be a greater risk in certain agricultural or forestry occupations, are denoted by an asterisk.

Arboviruses

Group A arthropod-borne viruses are all mosquito-borne and most are natural infections in birds and rodents. Three, also harboured by horses, mules and donkeys, can cause encephalitis in man, although asymptomatic infections are common:

Eastern equine encephalitis (N.E., Central and S. America, Asia): transmitted by *Culiseta melanura*.

Western equine encephalitis (S. and N.W. America, Slovakia): *Culex tarsalis*.

Venezuelan equine encephalitis (S. America).

The following cause a fever and rash:

Chikungunya (Africa, S.E. Asia): *Aëdes* vector, monkey reservoir.

Sindbis (Africa, Asia): reservoir in birds.

Mayaro (S. America): monkey and rodent reservoir.

O'Nyong Nyong (Africa): *Anopheles* vector, natural reservoir unknown.

Group B arboviruses

Tick-borne encephalitis group includes:

Kyasanur forest disease (India): monkeys, rodents and cattle; tick vector *Haemaphysalis spinigera*; haemorrhagic fever with encephalitis.

Russian spring-summer encephalitis (Asia, E. Europe): birds and small mammals; tick vectors *Ixodes persulcatus, I. ricinus*.

Omsk haemorrhagic fever (Central Asian steppes): rodents; tick vectors *Dermacentor pictus, D. marginatus*.

Mosquito-borne infections include:

Dengue group (Asia, S. America, Australasia, S. Europe): *Aëdes* vectors; fever, rash, and with haemorrhagic complications in younger age groups.

Japanese B encephalitis (E. Asia and Pacific): bird reservoir, epidemic transmission to pigs, horses, other mammals; vector *Culex tritaeniorhynchus, C. gelidus*.

Murray valley encephalitis (New Guinea, Australia): from birds; vector *Culex annulirostris*.

St Louis encephalitis (Trinidad, Panama, S. United States): from birds; vector *Culex tarsalis*.

Spondweni and *Wesselsbron* viruses (Africa): monkey hosts; *Aëdes* vector; fever.

West Nile (Africa, Middle East, Asia): birds; *Aëdes* vector; fever and myocarditis.

Yellow fever, jungle type (Africa, subtropical Central and S. America): from monkeys, marmosets, marsupials; *Haemogogus* and *Aëdes* vectors.

Group C viruses are mosquito-borne infections of rodents in S. America, occasionally transmitted to man*.

Bunyamwera group

Bunyamwera (Africa): from monkeys, rodents, birds; *Aëdes* vectors; fever and rash.

Germiston, Ilesha viruses (Africa): fever without rash.

Guaroa (S. America): fever without rash.

Miscellaneous

Mosquito-borne:

Bwamba-Pongola group (Africa): monkeys, birds; *Aëdes* vector; fever.

California group (Asia, N. America): rodents, rabbits; *Culex* vector; fever, encephalitis.

Catu, Guama (S. America: rodents) and *Oropouche* (S. America: monkeys); fever.

Congo group (Africa, Pakistan): cattle, tick vectors; fever.

Rift valley fever (Africa): sheep, ungulates; vectors *Culex theileri, Aëdes caballus, Aë. circumluteolus*; fever, epistaxis.

Other vectors:

Nairobi sheep disease (Africa): sheep, rodents; tick vectors; fever.

Sandfly fever group (Africa, Asia, S. America, Europe): *Phlebotomus* vector; fever.

Vesicular stomatitis (N. and S. America): horses, ungulates; *Phlebotomus* vector; fever.

Tacaribe group (S. America): from rodents, possibly excreta or mites; fever, haemorrhage.

CONTROL OF ARBOVIRUS INFECTIONS. (*a*) use of insecticides varies according to the habits of the vector concerned; (*b*) barriers (mosquito-proofing; protective clothing against ticks); (*c*) insect repellents; (*d*) vaccination (yellow fever); (*e*) elimination of breeding sites of vectors or rodent reservoirs.

Other Viruses

Cowpox. Cattle, horses; world-wide, particularly where smallpox exists. Transmission by contact with lesions of animals. Fever and local skin lesions. Communicability: until lesions have healed.

CONTROL: (1) Vaccinate (for man) with smallpox vaccine. (2) Prohibit recently vaccinated persons whose vaccination lesions are unhealed, from milking and dairy work.

Lymphocytic choriomeningitis (LCM virus). Mice; world-wide. Transmission by (1) urine, (2) mechanical: arthropods. Communicability: considerable.

CONTROL: Rodent control in grain stores.

Newcastle disease (Myxovirus). Conjunctivitis in man, poultry; worldwide. Transmission by contact with infected poultry. Communicability: not transmissible man-to-man.

Orf. Contagious ecthyma of sheep; pustular dermatitis in sheep, goats; world-wide. Transmission by entrance through cuts and abrasions; by contact of hands and forearms with sheep and goats or their pelts; by transfer from hands to mouth. Communicability: as long as virus is present in lesions.

CONTROL: (1) Take hygienic precautions. (2) Keep contaminated pastures and premises out of use for long period of time. (3) Vaccinate lambs.

Bedsonia group. Viruses of the psittacosis LGV group; world-wide; reservoir parakeets, parrots, pigeons, finches, petrels, domestic fowl, turkeys and other birds, occasionally man. Transmission by contact with infected birds or their surroundings, particularly on duck and turkey-raising farms; man-to-man transmission rare. Communicability: during acute illness; birds shed virus while infected and for weeks thereafter if not treated.

CONTROL: (1) Keep farm flocks disease-free and isolate and treat or destroy infected birds. (2) Educate agricultural workers in dangers of exposure.

Rabies. World-wide except Australia, New Zealand, U.K., Scandinavia and some other countries and islands; from domestic and wild carnivores and other biting mammals, rarely from bats via ungulates to man. Transmission by bite of a rabid animal and rarely by deposition of saliva alone; man-to-man transmission not confirmed; saliva is infectious. Communicability: in animals, 3-5 days prior to frank clinical signs and during course of disease.

CONTROL: (1) Control stray dogs. (2) Apprehend and detain for observation animals known to have bitten a person. (3) Destroy or detain for 6 months unvaccinated dogs or cats bitten by known rabid animals. (4) Submit to a laboratory iced intact heads of animals dead of rabies; do not kill suspect animals that are well. (5) Wash with soap or detergent bite or scratch wounds by suspect animals; do not suture open wounds for 3-5 days. (6) Vaccinate persons bitten by a rabid animal (see Chapter 22).

Rickettsiae

Q fever (*Coxiella burneti*). Cattle, goats, sheep, wild animals. Transmission commonly by airborne dissemination of organisms near contaminated premises, establishments processing infected animals, or at autopsy. Communicability: transmission man-to-man uncommon.

CONTROL: (1) Use inactivated vaccine for those in hazardous occupations. (2) Vaccinate animals. (3) Boil milk or heat-treat at 65°C (150°F) for 30 minutes or 75°C (165°F) for 15 seconds. (4) Regulate movement of infected animals.

Rocky Mountain spotted fever (*Rickettsia rickettsi*). Rabbits, field mice, dogs in N. and S. America. Transmission by bite of infected tick; sick contaminated by crushed tissues or faeces of tick. Communicability not naturally transmissible man-to-man.

CONTROL: (1) Avoid tick-infested areas; remove ticks as soon as possible; use tick repellents. (2) Clear land, reducing wild animals, and use insecticides. (3) Use vaccines: killed *R. rickettsi* lessen chance of infection and lower mortality (annual doses necessary).

Scrub typhus (*R. tsutsugamushi*). Wild rodents in Asia, East Indies, Australia; reservoir mites, wild rodents. Transmission by bite of infected larval mites.

Communicability: not naturally transmissible man-to-man.

CONTROL: (1) Avoid contact with mites. (2) Impregnate clothes and blankets with mite-killing chemicals. (3) Clear camp sites of vegetation by bulldozer, burning and spraying. (4) Institute rodent-control measures.

African tick-borne fever, fievre boutonneuse (*R. conori*). Dogs, rodents in Africa, Europe; reservoir ticks, rodents. Transmission by bite of infected tick. Communicability: not transmissible man-to-man.

CONTROL: Avoid tick areas; use tick repellents.

Bacteria

Anthrax (*Bacillus anthracis*). Cattle, goats, sheep, horses, pigs; world-wide; reservoir tissues of animals that have died of the disease; contaminated hair, hides and wool; soil. Transmission by contamination of skin by contact with hair, hides, wool, bristles, bone-meal, infected tissues; inhalation of spores; ingestion of contaminated meat. Animals infected by eating contaminated bone meal, feeds or meat. Mechanical carrier: flies. Communicability: rarely transmitted man-to-man.

CONTROL: (1) Isolate sick animals and quarantine suspect animals. (2) Burn infected animal carcasses or bury deeply in quicklime; carcasses should not be eaten or their hides sold. (3) Certification of imported hides as free from contamination. (4) Vaccinate workers handling potentially contaminated material.

Brucellosis (*Brucella* spp. *melitensis, abortus, suis*). Goats, sheep, cattle, swine, hares; world-wide; reservoir tissues, blood urine, milk, placenta, vaginal discharges, aborted fetuses of animals involved. Transmission by contact with infected animals, tissues and secretions; ingestion of dairy products from infected animals. Communicability: rarely communicable man-to-man.

CONTROL: (1) Search for infection by serological test and segregate or slaughter infected animals. (2) Immunise calves, kids and lambs with vaccines. (3) Pasteurise milk and dairy products. (4) Handle with care and dispose of discharges and fetus from an aborted animal.

Erysipeloid (*Erysipelothrix rhusiopathiae*). Swine, fowl, fish; world-wide. Transmission by direct contact with infected animals or their products. Communicability: until lesions disappear.

CONTROL: (1) Eradicate disease in swine. (2) Care in handling infected animals.

Glanders (*Pfeifferella mallei*). Horses, mules, donkeys in Africa, Asia, S. America, E. Europe. Transmission by inoculation of skin by contact with diseased animals or tissues; to a lesser extent, indirect contact with soiled articles, hand-to-mouth; ingestion; rarely man-to-man. Communicability: until organisms disappear from discharges.

CONTROL in equine animals: (1) Abolish common feeding and watering troughs. (2) Mallein test.

Leptospirosis (*Leptospira* spp. *icterohaemorrhagiae, canicola, pomona, autumnalis*). Rodents, cattle, dogs, swine, other wild animals; world-wide. Transmission by contact with water contaminated with urine of infected animals, direct contact. Communicability: man-to-man transmission negligible.

CONTROL: (1) Avoid swimming or wading in suspect waters. (2) Protect with boots and gloves when exposed to hazard of infection. (3) Control rodents in rural habitations. (4) Prevent contamination of working areas by urine of infected animals. (5) Use vaccines —appreciable reduction of morbidity in exposed person.

Melioidosis (*Pseudomonas pseudomallei*) Whitmore, Haynes. Rodents, sheep, goats, equines, swine in Asia, W. Europe and United States; reservoir also mules, donkeys, man. Transmission by contact with diseased animals. Communicability: until organisms disappear from discharges.

CONTROL: same as for *Glanders* above.

Plague, sylvatic (*Pasteurella pestis*). Wild rodents; world-wide, particularly W. United States, S. America, Africa, E. Mediterranean, Central and S.E. Asia. Transmission by transfer of fleas from wild rodents to domestic rats where there is common contact. Communicability: not transmissible man-to-man except by terminal plague pneumonia.

CONTROL: (1) Suppress rats by trapping or poisoning. (2) Periodically inspect rodents and their ectoparasites. (3) Insecticides in epidemic.

Tetanus (*Clostridium tetani*). Horses and other domestic animals; world-wide. Transmission by spores entering body through wounds and burns. Communicability: not naturally transmissible man-to-man.

CONTROL: (1) Protect by active immunisation, especially workers in contact with soil or domestic animals. (2) Thoroughly clean and debride deep wounds; prophylactic pencillin. (3) Give booster dose of tetanus toxoid (plain) upon injury with danger of tetanus in previously inoculated workers. (4) In non-inoculated workers give tetanus antitoxin after testing for serum sensitivity upon injury with danger of tetanus; inoculation with tetanus toxoid should follow use of antitoxin within a few days.

Tuberculosis, bovine (*Mycobacterium tuberculosis*: var. *bovis*). Cattle, goats, swine, cats; world-wide. **Tuberculosis, human** (var. *hominis*). Dogs, swine, monkeys; world-wide. Transmission by inhalation of organisms, contact with lesions, drinking of raw milk. Communicability: as long as lesions contain viable organisms.

CONTROL: (1) Tuberculin-test all cattle. (2) Isolate and preferably destroy infected animals. (3) Pasteurise milk. (4) Use BCG when indicated.

Tularaemia (*Pasteurella tularensis*). Rabbits, hares, sheep, wild rodents in N. America, Europe, Asia; reservoir also wood ticks. Transmission by bite of infected flies or ticks; inoculation of skin or conjunctival sac through handling infected animals; drinking of contaminated water and ingestion of improperly cooked rabbit meat. Communicability: not naturally transmissible man-to-man.

CONTROL: (1) Use fly and tick repellents. (2) Thoroughly cook wild rabbit meat. (3) Avoid drinking raw water. (4) Attenuated vaccines may prove useful when indicated; killed vaccines of limited value.

Fungi

Actinomycosis (*Actinomyces israelii*, *A. bovis*). Cattle, swine, horses and other animals; sporadically world-wide; reservoir man, no external environmental source demonstrated. Transmission by fungus presumably passing by contact; transmission man-to-man not demonstrated. Communicability unknown.

CONTROL: none.

Blastomycosis, N. American (*Blastomyces dermatitidis*. Dogs, horses occasionally in Canada, United States, Central America; reservoir soil or spore-laden dust. Transmission by inhalation of spores or their introduction through abrasions or wounds. Communicability: unknown; not naturally transmissible from man or animals to man.

CONTROL: destroy diseased animals.

Blastomycosis, S. American (*Blastomyces brasiliensis*). No animals involved: distribution in S. America, particularly Brazil; reservoir wood, soil or vegetation. Transmission probably by contact with contaminated soil or vegetation. Communicability: not naturally transmissible man-to-man.

CONTROL: none.

Coccidioidomycosis (*Coccidiodies immitis*). Cattle, horses, burros, sheep, swine, dogs, wild rodents in W. United States, Argentina, Mexico, Russia; reservoir soil and spore-laden dust. Transmission by inhalation of spores in dust from soil and vegetation. Communicability: not directly transmissible from man or animals to man.

CONTROL: (1) Use dust-control measures. (2) Forbid recruitment of farm labour from non-endemic areas. (3) Destroy infected animals.

Farmer's lung (*Thermophilic actinomycetes*). Distribution probably world-wide; reservoir mouldy vegetable products, i.e. hay, bagasse, etc. Transmission by inhalation of spores, producing reaginic sensitivity to antigens from mould; usually after 2 or more months' exposure.

CONTROL: (1) Dry methods of storage to inhibit organism. (2) Withdraw workers from exposure. (3) Respirators (partial protection only).

Histoplasmosis (*Histoplasma capsulatum*). Rodents, dogs, cats, bats, chickens; nearly world-wide: Americas, Europe, Africa, Hawaii, Indonesia, Japan, Philippines; reservoir soil, dust. Transmission by inhalation of airborne saprophytic spores. Communicability: not directly transmissible man-to-man.

CONTROL: (1) Spray contaminated soil or dust with water or disinfectant. (2) If contact necessary, wear mask.

Trichophytosis. (*Microsporum* spp.). Dogs, cats; world-wide. (*Trichophyton*) Cattle, horses, rodents; world-wide. Transmission by direct contact with infected animals. Communicability: as long as infectious lesions are present.

CONTROL: (1) Effective control measures for animals difficult. (2) Examine suspect animals; early treatment. (3) Early recognition and treatment in man.

Protozoa

Leishmaniasis, cutaneous: New World, Chiclero's ulcer (*Leishmania mexicana*). Dogs, cats, jackals, gerbils in Mexico (endemic), most of Central S. America; reservoir man (exposed lesions with parasites), dogs, cats, jackals, gerbils. Transmission by bite of sandflies; possibly direct contact of abraded skin with lesion of infected person. Communicability: as long as parasites remain in lesions; untreated cases as long as 1 year.

CONTROL: (1) Apply residual insecticides, periodically spray possible breeding places—stone walls, rubbish heaps, duck and chicken pens, animal houses, damp area of dwellings, bed nets. (2) Insect repellents. (3) In infested areas locate dwelling 150 m from forest. (4) Educate population concerning transmission of the disease. (5) Rodent control.

Malaria (*Plasmodium* spp. *vivax, malariae, falciparum, ovale*). Usual transmission man-to-man by bite of infected anopheline mosquito. Communicability: as long as infective gametocytes circulate in the blood.

CONTROL: (1) Apply residual insecticides on inside walls of housing for entire community where vector is endophilic. (2) Eliminate breeding places by draining and filling. (3) Regular use of suppressive drugs. (4) Educate population in use of drugs for suppression and treatment, and in practical methods of prevention.

Metazoa

Ancylostomiasis (*Necator americanus, Ancylostoma duodenale*). No animals involved; reservoir soil. Transmission by third-stage larvae penetrating skin, usually around ankles. Communicability: as long as infected persons pollute soil; third-stage larvae remain alive for 3 weeks.

CONTROL: (1) Inculcate wearing of shoes. (2) Prevent soil pollution, especially by installation of sanitary privies in rural areas and by health education.

Creeping eruption (*Ancylostoma brasiliense, A. caninum*). Cats, dogs in S.E. United States; probably world-wide, especially tropics; reservoir soil. Transmission by larvae penetrating skin and causing dermatitis. Communicability: as long as soil pollution continues.

CONTROL: inculcate wearing of shoes.

Filariasis (*Wucheria bancrofti*). W. Indies, coastal Central America, N. and S. America, Saudi Arabia, Madagascar, Africa, India, Ceylon, S.E. Asia, China, Korea, Japan, N. Australia, most Pacific islands; reservoir man with microfilariae in blood. Transmission by bite of many spp. of mosquitoes: *Culex fatigans, Anopheles* (var. spp.), *Aëdes polynesiensis. Brugia malayi* (S.E. Asia, India, Central China, few islands of Indonesia; reservoir man with microfilariae in blood.) Transmission by *Mansonia* (several spp.), *Anopheles* (several spp.). Communicability: as long as microfilariae are present in blood of man; may be years; not naturally transmissible man-to-man.

CONTROL: (1) Determine local vectors. (2) Screen dwellings. (3) Eliminate larval breeding places or treat with larvicides. (4) Educate public concerning mode of transmission. (5) Mass treatment with diethylcarbamazine.

Hydatidosis, echinococcosis (*Echinococcus granulosus*). Dogs, foxes, sheep, swine, cattle, rodents; world-wide; reservoir carnivores. Transmission by hand-to-mouth transfer of eggs by objects soiled with dog faeces; dog licking face; ingestion of contaminated food and water. Communicability: not naturally transmissible man-to-man or from one intermediate host to another.

CONTROL: (1) Prevent access of dogs to scraps of uncooked meat and raw offal. (2) Antihelmintic treatment of dogs of some value but must be repeated at 4-month intervals. (3) Require licensing of dogs with resulting reduction in numbers in endemic areas. (4) Health education of public.

Onchocerciasis (*Onchocerca volvulus*). Africa; New World: Guatemala, S. Mexico, N.E. Venezuela; reservoir man, with skin microfilariae; vector *Simulium*. Transmission by *Simulium*. In Guatemala and Mexico: *S. ochraceum, S. callidum, S. metallicum*; in Africa: *S. damnosum, S. neavei*. Communicability: as long as living microfilariae persist in the skin.

CONTROL: (1) Eradicate vector larvae by insecticides in rivers. (2) Provide facilities and educate population in obtaining proper diagnosis and treatment. (3) Individual protection with clothing and insect repellents.

Schistosomiasis. (*Schistosoma haematobium*): Africa, E. Mediterranean, Portugal, India; reservoir man. (*Schistosoma mansoni*): Africa, Arabian peninsula, N.E. South America, Caribbean; reservoir man, primates, some rodent naturally infected, epidemiological significance doubtful. (*Schistosoma japonicum*): China, Japan, Philippines, Celebes; reservoir dogs, pigs, cattle, field mice, wild rats; also water buffalo, horses (not epidemiologically important). Transmission by free-swimming larvae emerging from infected snails penetrating skin of person in the water. Communicability: not communicable direct man-to-man; eggs discharged in faeces or urine of infected hosts produce infection in snail intermediate hosts.

CONTROL: (1) Provide safe domestic water supplies. (2) Treat snail breeding places with molluscicides, and use improved agricultural and irrigation practices. (3) Treat all infected cases; educate in need for treatment. (4) Dispose of faeces and urine where fresh water is not present. (5) Control animals infected with *S. japonicum.*

'Swimmer's itch'. From many known species of avian and mammalian schistosomes; many parts of the world, especially tropics. Transmission by free-swimming larvae penetrating the skin of the person in the water. Communicability: larvae do not migrate beyond skin in man; not communicable man-to-man.

CONTROL: safe areas for swimming.

Ectoparasites

Dermatitis (e.g. *Dermanyssus gallinae*). Birds, particularly domestic fowl, pigeons, starlings, sparrows, etc.; world-wide. Transmission by bite of mite, tick or louse. Communicability: not commonly transmitted man-to-man.

CONTROL: (1) Eradicate mites, ticks and lice in domestic fowl and their nesting places. (2) Use gloves in handling wild birds and their nests. (3) Use insect repellents on clothing while working with infected domestic fowl or wild birds and their nests.

Snake Bite

This hazard is dealt with in Chapter 33.

Injury from Wild Animals

This is mentioned for completeness. It may also include injury from farm animals, the preventive aspects of which merit more attention.

INDUSTRIAL INJURIES

Treatment of injuries forms a large part of clinical practice in the tropics: in areas of developing industry, mechanised agriculture and road transport many injuries are of occupational origin. Road accidents alone can absorb over half the surgical bedspace of an urban hospital in the tropics. The incidence of occupational injuries is often substantially greater than in developed countries, and there are several reasons why this may be so. Scarce capital can entail poor machinery, overloading, inadequate safeguards and maintenance, and defects in the working environment. On the human side, there may be poor management, poor supervision, difficulties in communication, poor training and technical understanding, and the effects of fatigue, to which endemic disease and climate can contribute.

A doctor concerned with a hazardous industry has to consider, amid the fascinating plethora of surgical cases, whether treatment and rehabilitation services are adequate, and what his contribution can be to the prevention of injury. Injuries often involve technically qualified and experienced people in industry as well as the unskilled, and a doctor called upon to organise services for a large industry or construction should not be too modest in his proposals.

Treatment and rehabilitation

The planning of medical and surgical facilities depends on the site, its distance from other hospitals, the population at risk and types of hazard, and several other factors. The probable volume of work will determine the need for different facilities: minor surgery, plaster work, anaesthesia, major surgery, blood transfusion, intensive care. Facilities for simple physiotherapy can speed recovery and reduce absence due to the effects of injury, and be linked to occupational therapy and vocational retraining for more seriously disabled.

In any industry first aid, rescue, resuscitation and transport need special consideration. The essentials of a successful first-aid organisation are: (*a*) adequate initial training and regular refresher training for supervisory and other first-aid staff, provided during the firm's time, (*b*) incentives to maintain qualifications and (*c*) careful supervision and periodic checking of first-aid equipment. Medical staff can encourage and assist first-aid organisations in industry; in most tropical countries there are branches of the Red Cross, Red Crescent or St John Societies which promote training adapted to local circumstances, and publish useful booklets and other aids. Thus, the St John publication *First Aid in Industry* gives details on equipment, sterile dressing procedures, and rescue and resuscitation. Rescue equipment for high-risk industries, such as mines, docks, oil refineries, is usually specified in legislation or codes of practice. Portable positive pressure oxygen sets should be provided in any industry with a gas or noxious fume hazard. All equipment must be inspected and tested regularly.

Rehabilitation of the injured begins right from the start of treatment, aiming at restoring maximum function and, if permanent disablement occurs, retraining for an alternative suitable occupation and placement. Enlightened employers in tropical countries are now providing sheltered occupations for the disabled, and this—together with early settlement of compensation—can engender an atmosphere of confidence and hope for those with severe disabilities.

Prevention

Industry, in which both the people and working environment are organised, with effective channels of authority, is particularly amenable to medical efforts in prevention. Time spent on prevention is usually fruitful.

An injury, whether it is due to mechanical, thermal or electrical sources, arises from a situation (the 'accident') which can usually be prevented. Two aspects need emphasis:

1. The causes of accidents are usually multiple,

and in rational investigation different environmental as well as human aspects must be considered. The investigation of accidents is usually imperfect, but the medical attendants are often in a position to ascertain some of the circumstances objectively, as they are not usually concerned with emotional or legal aspects of 'blame'. A succession of similar injuries from a workplace often indicates an unsafe work situation which can easily be investigated and remedied. *It is a medical responsibility to initiate the enquiry.*

2. Unsafe situations ('near misses') or accidents to equipment or plant are generally commoner than injuries, and efficient accident prevention is not limited to enquiry into the causes of current accidents but must include systems for *recognising and quickly eliminating defects or risks*, particularly those of any duration. This is the basic approach of Heinrich (1950); it is not a medical responsibility, though a doctor can do much to encourage friends in engineering or management to adopt this approach if they do not yet do so.

Most accidents, then, entail a combination of unsafe mechanical or physical conditions in the work environment with an unsafe act or other human failing. The relative importance of the *environment* is reflected in accident rates in different industries. Thus time-lost accidents in mining are usually at least 50 times more frequent than time-lost accidents in factories and may be 500 times more frequent than the rate in the safest factory. This is understandable from the combined effects in a mine of poor lighting, noise, rock falls, changing working areas, heavy tools and equipment, etc., compared with the well-lit, safe and static factory workplace.

The range of variation in accident frequency arising from *human factors* is of a lesser order of magnitude—roughly twofold for characteristics such as age, inexperience, fatigue, lack of sleep, neurosis, though somewhat more (about five to eightfold) for alcohol, narcotic effects, or serious social maladjustment (controlled studies quoted in Haddon *et al*, 1964). There are also effects from the size of the working group, for ease of communication and less personality conflict in small working groups are associated with lower injury rates (Revans, 1960). Acute illness or any defects in vision, hearing or musculoskeletal function also require investigation.

Simple enquiry into the circumstances of each injury can reveal bad work methods or lack of protection. Thus, hand or foot injuries may be common in men handling heavy materials where lifting equipment is inadequate and gloves or safety boots are not provided; lumbar back strain can be due to incorrect lifting methods. Particular attention should be paid to injuries occurring during maintenance work when protective devices may be dismantled.

Objective investigation of accident causation requires careful definition of the many possible factors involved, their inclusion in routine accident investigation so that significant causes are not missed, and comparability of the populations analysed. For those proposing a detailed study in this field, the review volume by Haddon, Suchman, and Klein (1964) can be recommended.

Statistical records of time lost from work due to various types of injury are easily kept and can provide convincing evidence to management on the savings which could accrue from specific safety measures. A number of methods of recording statistics on industrial injuries have been proposed (I.L.O., 1961, 1971). Injuries reportable under workmen's compensation or social insurance legislation are usually defined as causing several days' incapacity (e.g. 3 days or more); such a definition is rather too limiting for preventive purposes. That most widely used is the I.L.O. *international frequency rate*, in which the injury is defined as one causing loss of one complete shift (day's work) or more, e.g.

International frequency rate (IFR)

$$= \frac{\text{number of injuries} \times 1\ 000\ 000}{\text{total man-hours exposure}}$$

Example. An undertaking with 500 workers, working 50 weeks of 48 hours each, had 60 time-lost injuries during 1 year. Illness, injury and other reasons led to workers being absent 5 per cent of the aggregate working time, giving the real number of man-hours exposure as 1 140 000. This being so,

$$\text{IFR} = \frac{60 \times 1\ 000\ 000}{1\ 140\ 000} = 52.6 \text{ time-lost injuries}$$
per million man hours.

Safety organisations

Industrial safety is largely the responsibility of management and engineering staff, but medical staff obviously have an important contribution to make in detecting causes of accidents. They can also help by knowing how other organisations deal with safety, especially when managements seem in need of assistance. The expert services of Factories or Mines Inspectorates, in an advisory capacity, have already been mentioned; many in the tropics produce information bulletins and pamphlets particularly suited to local circumstances and problems. Voluntary organisations, such as the Royal Society for the Prevention of

Accidents (RoSPA) and the British Safety Council, are U.K.-based bodies which also offer corporate membership to overseas firms and provide useful material for safety education. Care has to be used, however, in selecting material for education in a different cultural context.

Trade associations and governments often assist with job training. Large industries such as mines, construction firms, railways, docks, large factories, often employ a safety officer, who should be responsible directly to the general manager to carry out spot checks on plant safety, equipment maintenance and work methods, to investigate the causes of accidents, recommend remedies, and check that decisions are fulfilled. Safety committees, representing supervisors and workers in each section, can also assist by discussing particular problems and their participation in the best methods to overcome them.

OCCUPATIONAL HEALTH SERVICES IN THE TROPICS

The general health services in tropical countries often suffer from shortages of skilled manpower, buildings, drugs and equipment. Such limitations do not necessarily apply to an industrial enterprise which organises its own medical service, for the resources of a large tropical industry are often adequate to maintain a first-class service, undertaking the total medical care of employees and their families.

Between these two extremes various other types of service can be organised, according to local conditions. For small industries or factories *group services* with a central base and mobile staff can be both economic and efficient; such a service, supplemented by a system of first-aid training for supervisors in each department, is also more reliable than employing a greater number of underemployed, less well supervised nurses or dressers in each firm.

The essential features of any service for industry have been described by I.L.O. (1959) and comprise emergency treatment together with preventive and promotive services. Their cost can be justified because they provide better and quicker access to medical care, the prevention of endemic diseases and occupational hazards, together with savings in sickness absence, morbidity and mortality.

The organisation of medical care in developing countries with limited resources is fully discussed by King (1966, 1969), whose work is a most helpful reference in the context of tropical industry. In underdoctored areas a medical service at the place of work usually relies on an occupational health nurse or medical auxiliary to undertake the primary 'sorting', treatment of minor ailments, disposal of more serious cases, and routine medical screening tests. In this way the doctor can give more adequate attention to individual cases and find time for preventive, promotive and educational work. The doctor is usually responsible for training as well as organising his auxiliary staff, who will seldom have grounding in occupational health. Regular weekly meetings of staff, to include those from outlying units, each devoted systematically to one or two aspects of diagnosis, treatment, prevention and control, illustrated by the example of some recent cases, are invaluable.

Industries, with their ordered and well-defined populations, allow the easy compilation of a reliable system of medical records from which case incidence and sickness absence statistics can be readily compiled. Usually there is a national system of monthly returns for hospitals and other medical units, based on the *International Classification of Diseases* (W.H.O., 1968), which can be used in industry. Such records and statistics are invaluable in identifying health problems, estimating their cost and measuring the success (or otherwise) in overcoming them. There is a tendency in most tropical industries to underestimate the savings which can accrue from provision of good medical facilities; the task of the doctor is made easier if proposals can be backed up by reliable figures as well as by reference to current expert opinion.

Government services

Governments have national responsibilities in the enactment and application of industrial health legislation, and in providing central information, advisory and investigational services on all types of occupational hazard. In Commonwealth countries such services are usually organised (for historical reasons) in the Ministries or Departments of Labour, whose medical consultants or advisers work in association with the Factories Inspectorate. The inspectors are usually qualified in some branch of engineering, chemistry or physics, with additional training in industrial safety and hygiene. These experts can be helpful in solving specific problems of the working environment. Some are equipped to investigate fume, dust, heat, noise, lighting and other environmental conditions. Sometimes advice can be obtained from occupational health units in universities or within industry, though in most developing countries expertise and equipment is usually concentrated in government units which have fuller access to, and influence upon, industry as a whole (W.H.O., 1967).

SOURCES OF INFORMATION

Asking *'what is your occupation?'* is not simply an enquiry of individual social interest but presupposes some appreciation of occupations and job environments and their effects on the health of individuals and groups. The purpose of obtaining knowledge of the patient's occupation is to answer three questions. Is the patient suffering from an occupational disease? Is his occupation likely to aggravate his illness or his disability? Does the patient's illness affect his ability to do his job?

A job in the tropics may imply very different conditions of work to those of the same occupation in a highly industrialised country, and a doctor is always assisted by first-hand knowledge of peoples' occupations in the area in which he practises. Nevertheless many problems are common to all countries, and reference to a standard text can help to solve them.

The most useful texts for general reference are the *Encyclopaedia of Occupational Health and Safety* (2 vols., I.L.O., Geneva, 1972); Schilling (1972*b*) *Occupational Health Practice*; and Donald Hunter (1969) *The Diseases of Occupations*, 4th edition, London: English Universities Press. The latter author's Pelican book, *Health in Industry* (Penguin Books, 1959) forms a stimulating introduction to the subject. Some further specialised texts are given in the bibliography to this chapter.

Amongst periodicals the *British Journal of Industrial Medicine* is notable for inclusion of papers pertaining to developing countries, and for a section entitled 'Current awareness' which gives references to recent key publications. Also useful is *Occupational Health* (monthly, Macmillan, London) intended particularly for industrial nurses and auxiliaries. A comprehensive abstracting service is run by the International Labour Office, Geneva (International Occupational Safety and Health Information Service, CIS), the card abstracts of which are usually taken by government centres (such as factories inspectorates) if not by medical libraries.

FURTHER READING

BARNES, J. M. and EDSON, E. F. (1960) Safety in the use of pesticides. In *Modern Trends in Occupational Health*, ed. Schilling, R. S. F., p. 97. London: Butterworth.

CREBER, F. L. (1967) *Safety for Industry: a manual for training and practice*. London: Royal Society for Prevention of Accidents.

EDSON, E. F. (1969) *Ann. occup. Hyg.*, **12**, 99.

GILSON, J. C. (1960) Industrial Pulmonary Disease. In *Modern Trends in Occupational Health*, ed. Schilling, R. S. F., p. 50. London: Butterworth.

—— (1969) *Ann. Occ. Hyg.*, **12**, 121.

GRANT, J. S., NORMAN, L. G. and HEGGIE, R. M. (1966) *Medical Services in Transport*. London: Butterworths.

HADDON, W., SUCHMAN, E. A. and KLEIN, D. (1964) *Accident Research, methods and approaches*. London and New York: Harper and Row.

HEINRICH, H. W. (1950) *Industrial Accident Prevention, a scientific approach*, 3rd edn., London: McGraw-Hill.

HOLMES, A. C. (1964) *Health Education in Developing Countries*. London: Nelson.

INTERNATIONAL LABOUR OFFICE:
 Model Code of Safety Regulations for Industrial Establishments, Geneva, I.L.O., 1949.
 Safety and Health in Dock Work, Code of Practice, 1958.
 Recommendation 112, on Occupational Health Services in Places of Employment, 1959.
 Accident Prevention, a workers education manual, 1961.
 Manual of Industrial Radiation Protection,
  Part I, Convention and Recommendation, 1963.
  Part II, Model Code of Safety Regulations (Ionising Radiations), 1959.
  Part III, General Guide on Protection Against Ionising Radiations, 1963.
  Part IV, Guide on Protection in Industrial Radiography and Fluoroscopy, 1964.
  Part V, Guide in the Application of Luminous Compounds, 1964.
 Man at Work, studies in the application of physiology to working conditions in a hot country. *Occup. Hlth and Safety Series*, No. 4, 1964.
 Report, International Symposium on Electrical Accidents, CIS, 1964.
 Safety and Health in Agricultural Work, 1965.

Respiratory Function Tests in Pneumoconioses. Occ. Hlth and Safety Series, No. 6, 1966.
Permissible levels of toxic substances in the working environment. *Occup. Hlth and Safety Series* No. 20, 1970.
Encyclopaedia of Occupational Health and Safety, 2 vols., 1972.
KING, M. (ed) (1966) *Medical Care in Developing Countries*. London and Nairobi: Oxf. Univ. Press.
—— (1969) *A Medical Laboratory in the Tropics*. London and Nairobi: Oxf. Univ. Press.
LEITHEAD, C. S. and LIND, A. R. (1964) *Heat Stress and Heat Disorders*. London: Cassell.
MATELSKY, I. (1969) The non-ionising radiations. In *Industrial Hygiene Highlights*, Vol. 1, ed. Cralley, Pittsburgh: Industrial Hygiene Foundation of America.
MINISTRY OF HEALTH (1963) *Code of Practice for Use of Radioactive Materials in Research and Teaching*. London: HMSO.
PATTY, F. A. (1963) *Industrial Hygiene and Toxicology*. Vol. 1, General Principles, Vol. 2, Toxicology, New York: Interscience.
REVANS, R. W. (1960) Morale and the size of the working group. In *Modern Trends in Occupational Health*, ed. Schilling, R. S. F., p. 196. London: Butterworth.
ROGAN, J. M. (ed.) (1972) *Medicine in the Mining Industry*. London: Heinemann.
SCHILLING, R. S. F. (1956) *Lancet*, **2**, 261, 319.
—— (1960) *Modern Trends in Occupational Health*. London: Butterworth.
—— (1963) International Surveys of Byssinosis. In *Epidemiology: Reports on Research and Training, 1962*. ed. Pemberton. London: Oxf. Univ. Press.
—— (1972a) In *Inhaled Particles in Clinical Practice*, ed. Muir, D. C. F. London: Heinemann.
—— (1972b) *Occupational Health Practice*. London: Butterworth.
U.I.C.C. COMMITTEE (1970) U.I.C.C./Cincinnati classification of the radiographic appearances of pneumoconiosis. *Chest*, **58**, 57.
WHIPPLE, H. E. (1964) Biological effects of asbestos. *Ann. N.Y. Acad. Sci.*, **132**, art. 1, 1-766.
WORLD HEALTH ORGANIZATION:
Joint I.L.O./W.H.O. Committee on Occupational Health, 3rd Report. *Wld Hlth Org. techn. Rep. Ser.*, **135**. Geneva, 1957.
—— 4th Report, Occupational Health Problems in Agriculture. *Wld Hlth Org. techn. Rep. Ser.*, **246**, 1962.
—— 5th Report. *Wld Hlth Org. techn. Rep. Ser.*, **345**, 1967.
International Classification of Diseases (1965 revision) Vol. 1, 1968; Vol. 2, 1969.

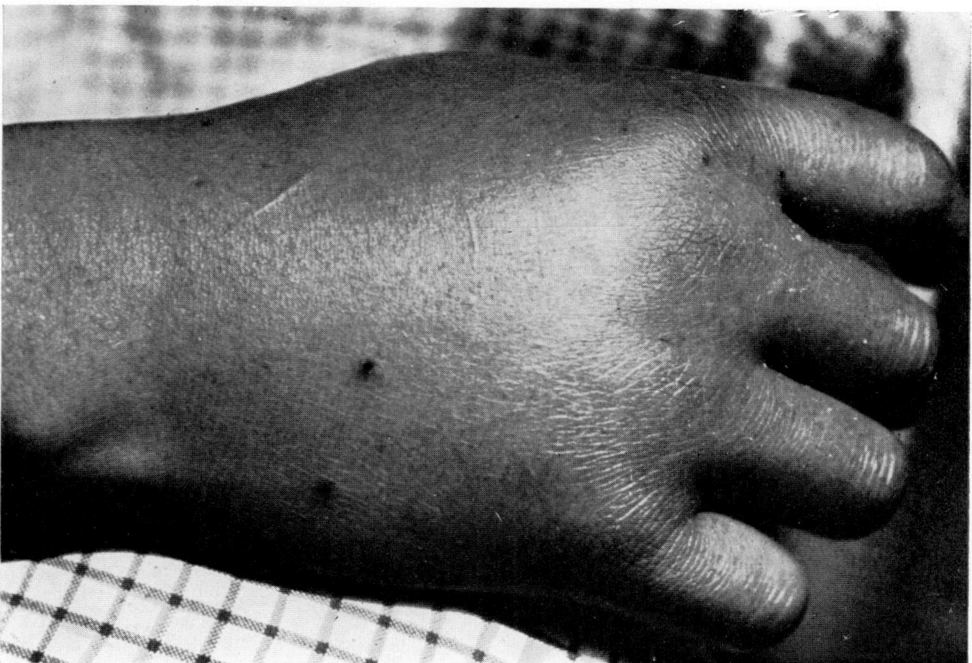

CHAPTER 33

Plate 41 *Twenty minutes after a viper bite; local swelling is a very valuable sign, confirming that venom has been injected.*

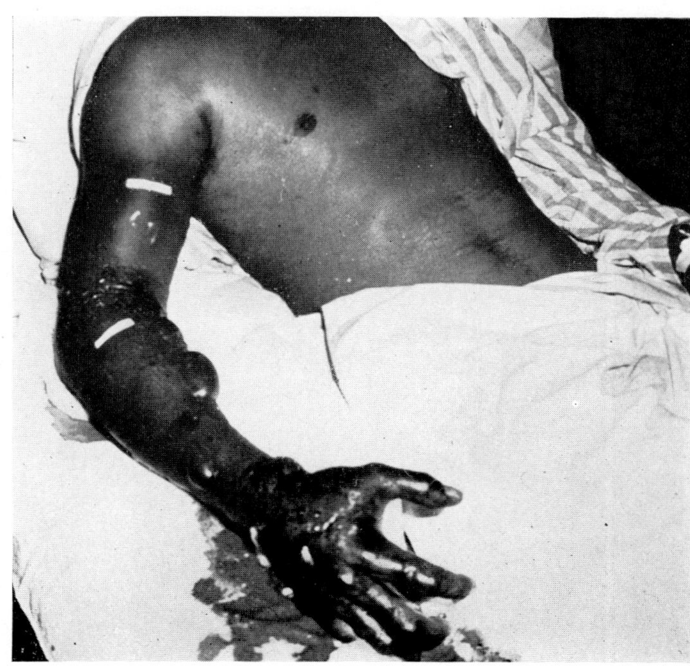

Plate 42 *Shock in severe systemic viper bite poisoning may be fatal. Blisters extending up the bitten limb also indicate a high venom dose. Specific antivenom can relieve the shock dramatically.*

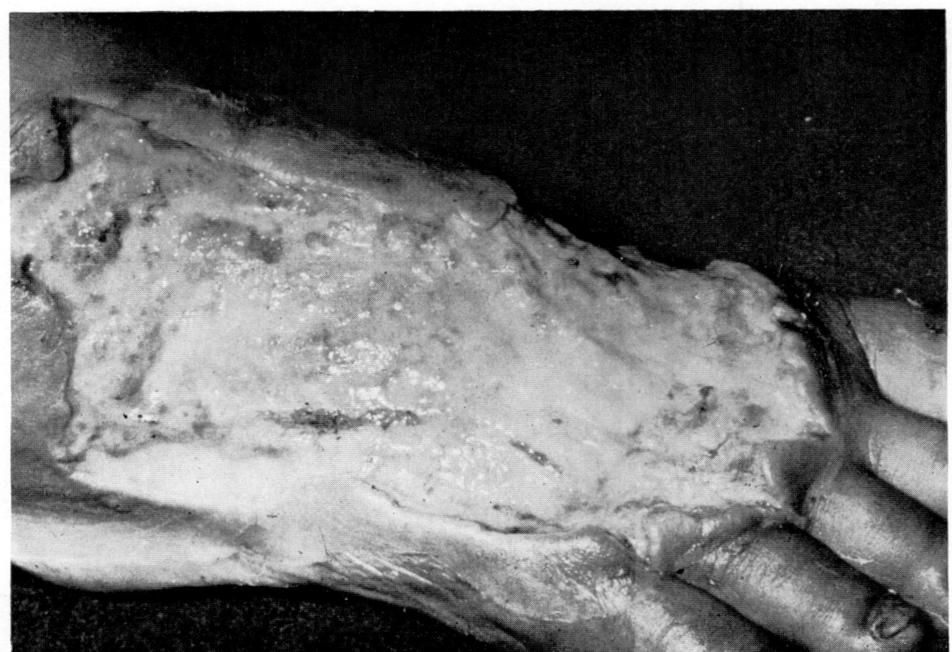

PLATE 43 *Local necrosis following the bite of a common cobra. No systemic poisoning developed and antivenom was therefore not indicated.*

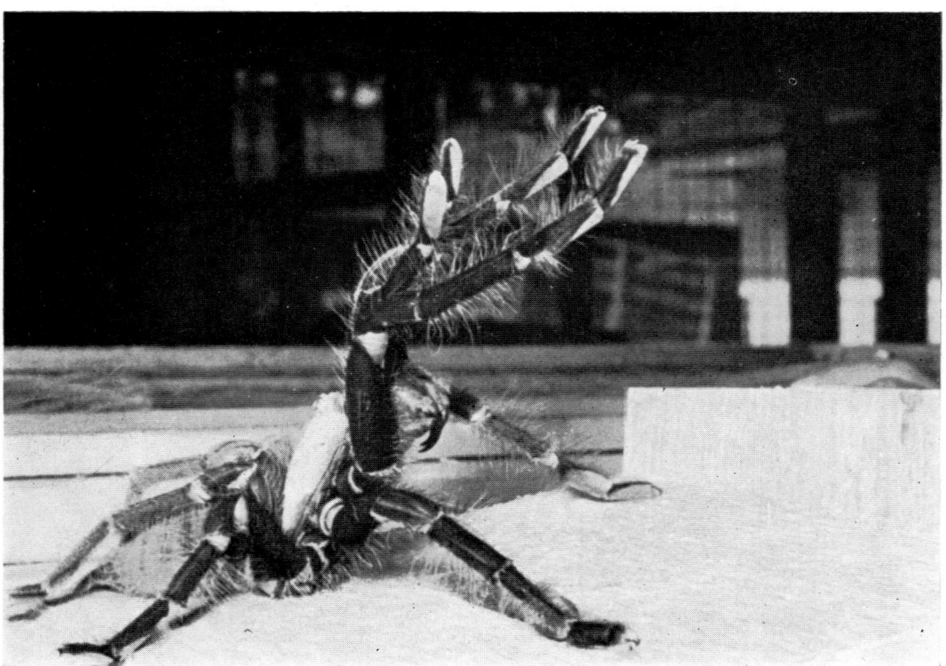

PLATE 44 *Spider 'fangs', or chelicerae.*

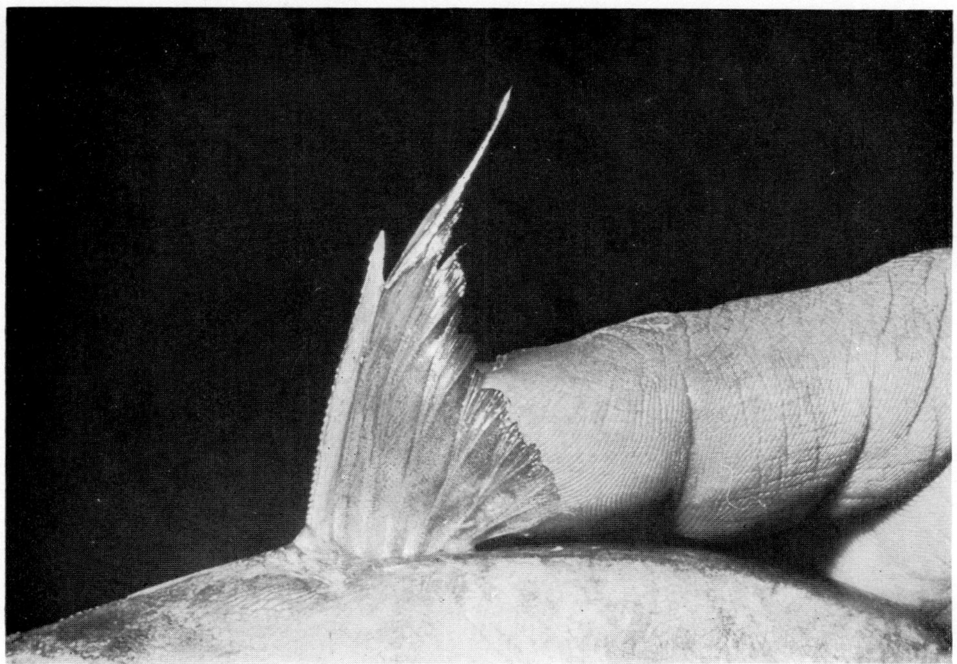

PLATE 45   *Dorsal sting of catfish.*

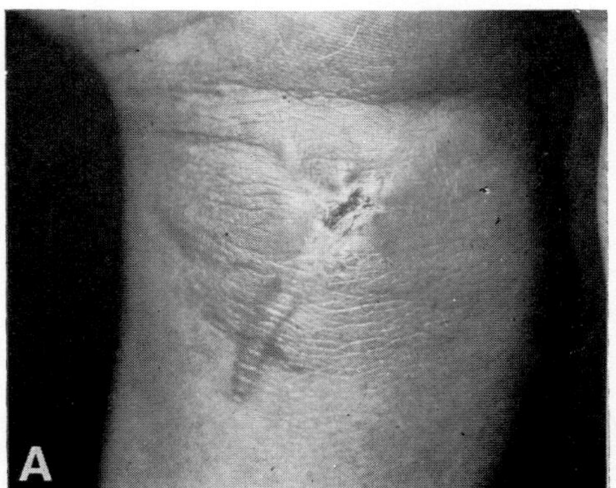
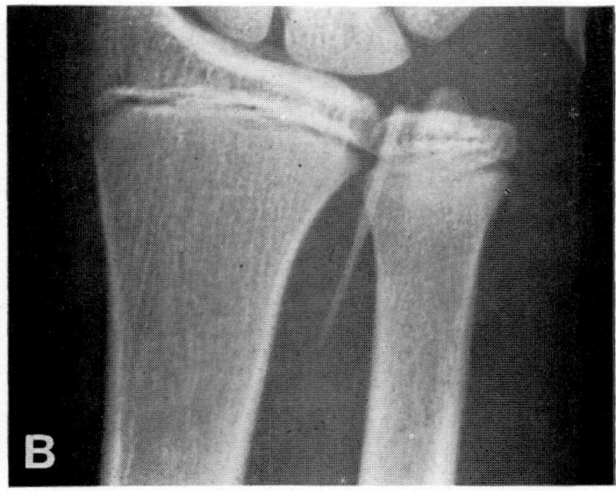

PLATE 46   *Sting of a stingray embedded in wrist of fisherman. The wound had been sutured on the day of the accident but it had continued to discharge for 3 months when the photograph (A) and radiograph (B) were taken.*

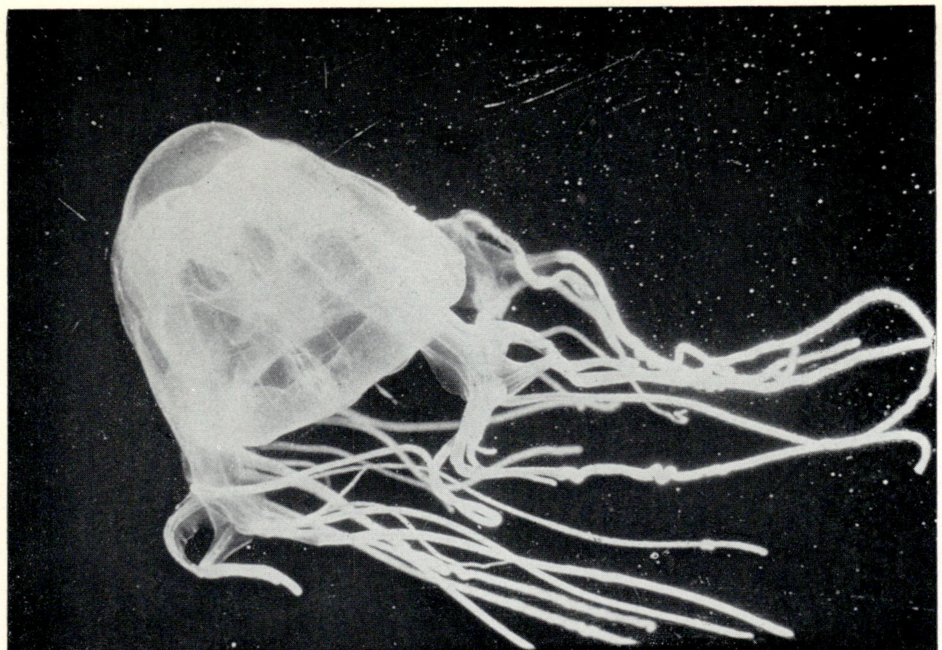

PLATE 47   *Wasp or box jellyfish*, Chironex fleckeri. *In its natural surroundings it is transparent and very difficult to see.* (Courtesy of K. Gillett.)

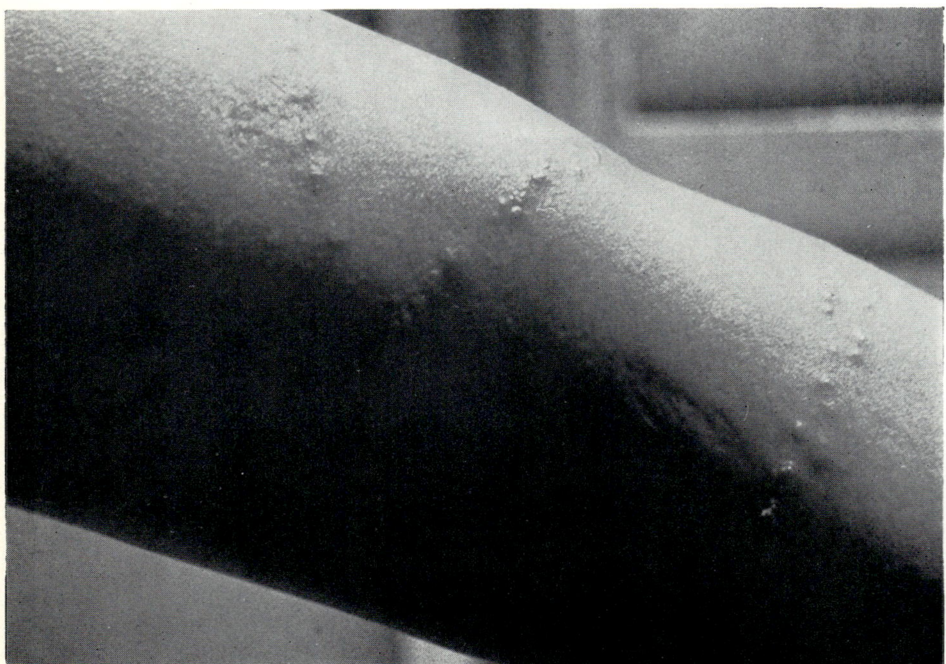

PLATE 48   *Jellyfish sting. Note the spaces between wheals, indicating the small proportion of nemato-cysts which have discharged venom.*

Copyright of Plates 41–48 is held by Dr H. A. Reid.

33
Venomous Bites and Stings

Bites and stings by venomous creatures such as snakes, scorpions, spiders and so on are quite common in the tropics, where they are mainly a rural and occupational hazard. Visitors to the tropics can be reassured that they are most unlikely to see, let alone be bitten or stung by, these creatures. The danger from venomous bites and stings has been greatly exaggerated. Thus it is commonly assumed that bites from venomous snakes are frequently fatal. This assumption is wrong. Although fatalities and serious poisoning undoubtedly *can* occur, careful observations of large series of patients coming to hospital following bites by reliably identified venomous and potentially lethal snakes have confirmed that more than one-half of the victims have minimal or no poisoning, and only about one-quarter will develop systemic poisoning. There are many reasons for this very important prognostic and therapeutic fact, but probably the most relevant is that bites or stings of human beings are defensive reactions which rarely result in the injection of much venom.

SNAKEBITE

Venomous snakes

Medically important snakes have fangs at the front of their mouths which enable them to inject venom. These are the 'poisonous' snakes of which there are three families—elapids (neurotoxic), seasnakes (myotoxic) and vipers (vasculotoxic). Elapids are landsnakes with short fixed fangs (covered by a gum-fold, the vagina dentis). Seasnakes have very short fixed fangs and characteristic flat tails; they are common only in Asian coastal waters. Vipers have long, erectile fangs, triangular heads and, usually, short fat bodies. Vipers are subdivided into crotaline or pit vipers, having a thermosensitive pit between eye and nose, and viperine vipers, without pits. The pit detects warm-blooded prey in the dark.

The 'non-poisonous' snakes are also of three types—small burrowing snakes often resembling worms, large constricting snakes such as pythons or boas, and the numerous family of colubrine snakes. Some colubrines have fangs at the back of the mouth, but, though technically venomous, their bits are harmless to man, with the rare exception of some back-fanged snakes in Africa such as the boomslang (*Dispholidus typus*).

Throughout the tropics viper bites are much more common than elapid bites, with the exception of the Pacific-Australian area in which vipers do not naturally occur. There are many different species of poisonous snakes but only a few are of medical importance. They include the tropical rattlesnake (*Crotalus durissus terrificus*), the fer-de-lance (*Bothrops atrox*) and the jararaca (*Bothrops jararaca*) in South America; the night adder (*Causus rhombectus*), the puff adder (*Bitis arietans*) and mambas (4 species of *Dendroaspis*) in Africa, and the saw-scaled viper (*Echis carinatus*) and cobras (mostly *Naja* species) which occur both in Africa and in Asia; Russell's viper (*Vipera russelli*), the Malayan pit viper (*Agkistrodon rhodostoma*) and the Indian krait (*Bungarus coeruleus*) are also important in parts of Asia; the tiger snake (*Notechis scutatus*), the death adder (*Acanthophis antarcticus*), the taipan (*Oxyuranus scutellatus*) and the Papuan black snake (*Pseudechis papuanus*) of the Pacific-Australian area. Medically important seasnakes include *Enhydrina schistosa*, *Hydrophis cyanocinctus* and *Lapemis hardwickii*.

The distinction of poisonous from non-poisonous snakes is often difficult, but is not usually important for the clinician; he should be able to diagnose whether or not a patient has poisoning, and, if so, of what type and severity.

Incidence of poisoning: fright

As already mentioned, the paramount fact about bites of man by poisonous snakes is that more than one-half of the victims will have minimal or no poisoning. Only about one-quarter will develop systemic poisoning. Hence poisonous snakebite is not synonymous with snakebite poisoning.

Fear in varying degrees is present in all victims bitten by snakes and often dominates the clinical picture. Emotional symptoms come on rapidly, within minutes of the bite, whereas symptoms of systemic poisoning rarely appear until a half to one hour after the bite. The frightened patient may appear semiconscious, with cold, clammy skin, feeble pulse and rapid shallow breathing. These symptoms resolve dramatically after a placebo injection.

Clinical features of poisoning

General. Snake venoms contain a complex mixture of many toxic factors, and it is uncertain which of the different factors discovered in laboratories are important either directly or indirectly (through autopharmacological substances) in poisoning symptoms displayed by human victims. But the clinical pattern can be divided conveniently, though arbitrarily, into local and systemic poisoning as in Table 33.1.

Early. Local swelling starts within a few minutes of a viper bite if venom is injected (Plate 41). It is a valuable clinical sign, because if swelling is absent and one knows the biting snake was a viper then poisoning can be immediately excluded. Local swelling is also a feature of poisoning by Asian cobra bites, though it may not appear for

TABLE 33.1. *Local and systemic effects of snake poisoning*

Snake family	Local effects	Systemic effects
Elapids		
1. Cobras	Swelling, later necrosis	Neurotoxic, cardiotoxic
2. Others	Nil	Neurotoxic
Seasnakes	Nil	Myotoxic
Vipers	Marked swelling; necrosis rare except in Africa	Vasculotoxic; often coagulation defect

1–2 hours (African cobra bites are not sufficiently documented to indicate whether local swelling is a reliable feature). Other elapids (such as mambas and kraits) and the seasnakes have no local effects.

Local pain almost invariably follows cobra and viper bites if venom is injected, and it may be severe for several days. But local pain may be minimal or absent in severe poisoning, and considerable in bites not involving poisoning; thus local pain is extremely variable and of no help in diagnosis.

The important early signs of systemic poisoning are as follows: *viper*—blood-stained spit, later non-clotting blood; *elapid*—ptosis, glossopharyngeal palsy; *seasnake*—general myalgia, 3–5 hours later myoglobinuria.

Non-clotting blood is best detected using a capillary tube with blood taken from a finger prick. The tube should be kept horizontal at room temperature for 20–30 minutes and then raised vertically. Non-clotting blood runs out of its own accord or can easily be blown out. Myoglobinuria shows as a brown or red colour of the urine (seasnake bite poisoning does not cause haemoglobinuria).

There are exceptions to the above generalisations. The tropical rattlesnake has neurotoxic, not haemorrhagic, effects although it is a pit viper. Some Australian elapid snakes have vasculotoxic and coagulation effects although they are principally neurotoxic. Some vipers (such as the puff adder and the gaboon viper in Africa) do not affect clotting in human victims.

Late. Blisters around the site of the bite are common in cobra and viper envenoming. Blisters extending up the limb in viper bites, African spitting cobra bites, *Naja nigricollis* (Plate 42) suggest a large dose of venom; they may be serous or sanguineous. Local necrosis is characteristic of poisoning from Asian cobra bites (Plate 43) and some viper bites (such as the African puff adder). Necrosis can be extensive but it is usually superficial; involvement of tendons, muscle and bones is exceptional. Bacterial infection follows necrosis and may spread to joints. But in the absence of necrosis or meddlesome local measures such as incision, application of dressings and so on, bacterial infection virtually never occurs.

Even without specific treatment the mortality in snakebite is low. Generally speaking, deaths are most rapid after elapid bites, especially cobra bites (average death time is about 5 hours after the bite), and most protracted after viper bites (average is 2–3 days after the bite). Death in seasnake bite (usually 12–24 hours after the bite) and in elapid bite is mainly due to respiratory failure; shock and haemorrhage into vital organs are the main causes of death in viper bites.

In the absence of necrosis, pain after viper bites rarely exceeds 2 weeks. Swelling usually resolves completely in 2–3 weeks, rarely in 2–3 months, and in exceptional cases the limb may remain permanently swollen. If blisters are left alone and no dressing is applied, they rupture spontaneously about 2 weeks after the bite and dry up in an additional 1–2 weeks. If dressings are applied, infection usually follows and greatly prolongs healing. Healing of local necrotic lesions varies according to the extent of the lesions and the treatment given, but requires at least a month, and may take 5–6 months or longer even with expert surgical attention. In patients who recover without receiving specific antivenom, systemic symptoms generally subside quickly. Neurotoxic features of elapid systemic poisoning resolve in 2–3 days as a rule, but exceptionally may persist as long as 2 weeks. However, the myotoxic effects of systemic poisoning from seasnake bite are prolonged and full recovery may take several months. The transaminases are a sensitive laboratory guide to the muscle damage. In systemic viper bite poisoning shock and haemorrhagic features generally resolve within a week, but in bites by some vipers coagulation changes may persist for 2–3 weeks or even longer if specific antivenom is not given.

Complications of systemic poisoning are extremely rare. Renal failure may occur with bites by all types of poisonous snake—vipers, elapids or seasnakes. Bilateral renal calcification after cortical necrosis, and blindness following retinal haemorrhage have been reported after viper bites. Neglected local necrosis can result in chronic osteomyelitis with sinuses discharging for years. Scarring may be extensive.

Clinical pathology

In cobra bites with severe poisoning, the white blood cell count is moderately raised during the first few days. Moderate haemolysis is shown by raised serum bilirubin and urine urobilinogen, followed by fall in the haemoglobin of 3 to 4 g/ 100 ml and increase of reticulocytes. The Schumm and direct Coombs tests are negative. Coagulation remain normal (Reid, 1964). In severe krait (*Bungarus candidus*) poisoning, no significant haematological abnormalities were observed. Most of the Australian elapid venoms are haemolytic and, with the exception of the death adder (Campbell, 1966, 1967) cause coagulation defects similar to those caused by viperine venoms. Clinically, these effects of elapid venoms on coagulation and haemolysis are of minor importance compared with the neurotoxic effects.

In systemic viper poisoning there is usually no abnormal haemolysis, but anaemia caused by loss of red cells into the bitten limb and haemorrhage may result in a fall in haemoglobin of over 8 g/ 100 ml (Reid *et al*, 1963a). Platelets are reduced during the first few days after the bite but bleeding time is usually normal. There is often a coagulation defect from defibrination (Reid *et al*, 1963b). Viper venoms have direct or indirect thrombin-like effects on fibrinogen and if the dose of venom is large, as, for example, when the viper attacks prey for food, massive intravascular clotting stops the circulation and causes extremely rapid death. But with smaller doses of venom, such as those injected into human victims, there is continual microcoagulation of fibrinogen with virtually simultaneous disposal of resulting fibrin. The venom thus eliminates fibrinogen as quickly as the liver provides it, and although viper venoms are basically 'coagulant', the paradoxical effect in human victims is non-clotting or poorly clotting blood because of absent or very low fibrinogen. Whole blood and plasma do not clot on addition of thrombin, and fibrinogen is low or absent as estimated by sodium sulphite precipitation or electrophoresis. The simplest procedure for assessing defibrination is the clot quality observation test (Reid *et al*, 1963b). After contraction of the clot is complete (1 hour at room temperature usually suffices), clot quality is graded according to the volume of extruded cell deposit and size of remaining clot.

Proteinuria lasting a few days is common in severe envenoming by any snake. Haematuria may occur in viper poisoning, haemoglobinuria may occur in poisoning by the tropical rattlesnake and by Australian elapids, and myoglobinuria is characteristic of seasnake bite poisoning. Exceptionally, acute renal failure develops, as shown by rising blood urea with fall in urinary output and specific gravity. In landsnake bite, bromsulphthalein retention tests, serum electrolytes, and serum transaminases are usually normal (Reid *et al*, 1963a; Reid, 1964). The latter emphasises that local necrosis affects skin and subcutaneous tissues but does not involve skeletal muscle, in contrast to the myotoxic seasnake envenomation, which is reflected by very high transaminase figures (Reid, 1962).

Diagnosis

The diagnostic importance of local swelling in viperine poisoning has already been stressed. The early signs of systemic poisoning have also been noted. Usually, the minority of victims who receive a venom dose large enough to cause systemic poisoning will already have signs of this by the time they see a doctor. In the rare cases seen soon after the bite, within the latent period between bite and possible onset of systemic symptoms (1–2 hours generally but up to 10 hours with some elapids), the patient should be given a placebo injection and then carefully observed every half-hour by the doctor for these early systemic signs.

Differentiation of viperine from elapid systemic poisoning is usually obvious from simple clinical evaluation. Identification of the snake (if available) is irrelevant. But in some parts of the tropics where different types of elapids or vipers are common, clinical distinction of individual types of systemic poisoning is difficult; reliable identification of the biting snake is then helpful and in most research projects it is essential.

Viperine poisoning is severe if within 1–2 hours of the bite swelling is above the knee or elbow, shock (Plate 42) is evident, or haemorrhagic signs besides haemoptysis develop (gum bleeding, ecchymoses, positive tourniquet test and so on, do not usually appear for 4–5 hours).

Elapid poisoning is severe if neurotoxic signs start within 1 hour or less of the bite and rapidly progress to respiratory failure. Mental confusion strongly suggests respiratory failure, though ptosis and glossopharyngeal palsy can make assessment of mental awareness difficult. Shock may also be a feature of severe elapid poisoning.

Severe seasnake poisoning is shown by myoglobinuria as early as 1–2 hours after the bite, and by the development within a few hours of respiratory failure.

In severe systemic poisoning following either elapid or viper bites, the electrocardiogram may show T-wave inversion and deviation of the ST-segment. In seasnake bites an electrocardiogram is specially valuable in detecting hyperkalaemia which can result from damage to muscle. Tall, peaked T-waves in chest leads may appear within 8 hours of the bite and give early warning of impending death or of acute renal failure.

Treatment

First-aid. First-aid comprises the measures taken by the victim or associates before receiving medical treatment. Recommendations (it will be rare indeed for the doctor to have to apply them personally) should be short, simple, practicable and more helpful than harmful. Reassurance is most important, as the danger of snakebite is greatly exaggerated. The site of the bite should be wiped and covered with a handkerchief or cloth; it should not be incised, as this frequently introduces infection, delays recovery and aggravates bleeding. A firm but not tight ligature should be applied just above the bite, using cloth, handkerchief or grass. The victim should then go to the nearest hospital. If available, aspirin or alcohol in moderation is helpful. If the snake has been killed it should be taken to hospital; otherwise it should be left alone, since attempts to find or kill it often result in further bites.

These recommendations are generally applicable to the tropics, but in special circumstances (for example, in the case of a sophisticated expedi-

tion) modifications may be appropriate. Thus if an expedition to remote areas includes a doctor or someone adequately trained in the administration of antivenom, adrenaline and so on, it might be advisable to take these drugs on the expedition. In areas of the tropics where it could take half a day or more to reach hospital, it might be desirable to teach a medical auxiliary when and how to give antivenom. Such a procedure, however, would be more accurately described as medical rather than first-aid treatment. But, generally speaking, antivenom should play no part in first-aid treatment.

General measures. Adequate reassurance is most important, so tetanus toxoid or a placebo injection should be promptly given unless systemic signs are already evident; in this event specific antivenom should be given. If a tourniquet has been applied it should be released. Unless one is confident that there is no possibility of significant poisoning ensuing, the patient should be carefully observed every half-hour for some hours. If tetanus toxoid has been given initially, a second dose should be injected about 6 weeks later.

After cleaning (if necessary), the site of the bite should be left alone. If the lower limb has been bitten it should be rested on the bed (the end of the bed being covered by rubber if there is oozing from the bite site; oozing soon stops after specific antivenom is given in effective dosage). If the upper limb has been bitten it should be rested in a sling. No coverings or dressings should be applied at this stage as they greatly increase the incidence of secondary bacterial infection. For the same reason, blisters should be left strictly alone; they will then break spontaneously and will quickly heal without infection provided there is no underlying necrosis. But as soon as local necrosis is obvious, sloughs should be excised. It may take several days for cobra bite necrosis to show, and over a week if steroids have been given. Necrosis is usually confined to subcutaneous tissues: tendons and muscles are rarely involved although muscles may appear necrotic. They should *not* be excised as they virtually always heal —and with surprisingly little permanent ill effect. Normal saline is the best local dressing to apply after excision of sloughs. At this stage systemic antibiotics may be helpful and skin grafting should be carried out early rather than late, even if infection is still evident. In neglected cases when the patient comes several days or weeks after the bite, secondary infection has often spread to the bones and joints; amputation may then be advisable. Tetanus antitoxin can be justified if necrosis develops—*after* necrosis is clinically evident.

Tetanus antiserum should not be given routinely in all snakebite cases. In the rare event that the patient has been actively immunised, then toxoid should be given instead of antitoxin.

Pain is rarely a problem once the patient has received an injection (placebo or antivenom). For the first night mild analgesics such as codeine or pethidine may be necessary but it is highly exceptional for morphine to be required.

Blood transfusion helps in viperine shock, especially if the victim was anaemic before the bite (but specific antivenom is usually dramatically successful in viperine shock if given in adequate dosage).

If respiratory failure develops in elapid or seasnake poisoning—shown by confusion, stupor, rapid shallow breathing, rise in pulse and blood pressure—a tracheostomy should be done (Campbell, 1964). Artificial respiration and intragastric drip feeds may also be needed.

Acute renal failure due to snakebite usually resolves with conservative treatment by limiting the intake of fluids and electrolytes, and avoiding drugs such as tetracycline which can aggravate renal failure (penicillins are safe). Otherwise peritoneal dialysis or haemodialysis would be needed.

Antivenom. In systemic snakebite poisoning, specific antivenom is the most important therapeutic agent available. If used correctly, it can be effective even though it is not given until hours or days after the bite. It is therefore not only safe but highly desirable to wait for clear clinical evidence of systemic poisoning before giving antivenom. It should not be given as a routine in all cases of suspected snakebite (particularly since less than one-quarter of the patients bitten by poisonous snakes experience systemic poisoning).

To be effective antivenom must, generally speaking, be specific. But recent work suggests that tiger snake antivenom (made in Australia) may constitute a 'broad spectrum' antivenom effective both against seasnake bite poisoning and against all commoner types of neurotoxic poisoning by Afro-Asian landsnakes, excepting mamba bite poisoning. Haemorrhagic signs indicate a viperine antivenom. Neurotoxic signs without local swelling indicate mamba antivenom in Africa and krait antivenom in Asia. Neurotoxic signs plus local swelling (not due to a ligature) indicate cobra antivenom. Clinical distinction of poisoning by the various Australian and Papuan elapid snakes is difficult. Non-clotting (defibrinated) blood is a feature of taipan poisoning, whereas coagulation is normal in death adder poisoning. Non-clotting blood is also a feature of systemic *Echis* poisoning and in Africa it is

very useful in differentiating from poisoning by other vipers such as the puff adder or night adder which do not affect clotting in man. *Echis* is the most deadly snake in the world to man. In some countries only polyvalent antivenom is available, so these distinctions are academic. The circumstances of the bite and generalised myalgia indicate the need for seasnake antivenom.

Serum sensitivity may be tested by injecting 0.2 ml antivenom subcutaneously; if severe reactions occur, desensitisation is needed before antivenom treatment. Adrenaline should be readily available for immediate antivenom reactions, which may occur despite negative sensitivity tests. Steroids are useful for delayed serum reactions, but controlled trials in human patients show that poisoning is not helped. Antivenom should always be given by intravenous drip. The intravenous route is much more effective than other parenteral routes, and if immediate serum reactions occur, administration can be slowed or stopped whereas there is little one can do about antivenom which has been injected intramuscularly or subcutaneously. At least 100 ml antivenom (usually contained in 10 ampoules) is needed, and this should be repeated, especially in neurotoxic poisoning, within 1 hour if there has been little significant improvement. The antivenom can be suitably diluted in two to three volumes of isotonic saline.

If antivenom is correctly used, the response in systemic poisoning is dramatic. Local effects of envenoming do not appear to benefit. If it were possible to inject antivenom locally at the site of the bite *within a few minutes of the bite* necrosis might well be prevented or minimised. But in practice this is virtually never possible, and therefore local injection of antivenom is not advocated.

The following is a list of some institutes making antivenom suitable for snakebite in the tropics—

1. *Algeria:* Institut Pasteur d'Algeria, Rue Docteur Laveran, Algiers.
2. *Australia:* Commonwealth Serum Laboratories, Parkville, Melbourne.
3. *Brazil:* Instituto Butantan, Caixa Postal 65, São Paulo.
4. *France:* Institut Pasteur, Service de Serotherapie, 36 Rue du Docteur Roux, Paris XV.
5. *Germany:* Behringwerke AG, Postachliessfach 167, 355 Marburg.
6. *India:* (*a*) Central Research Institute, Kasauli, R.I., Punjab. (*b*) Haffkine Institute, Parel, Bombay 12.
7. *Indonesia:* Perusahaan Negara Bio Farma, 9 Djalan Pasteur, Bandung.

8. *Iran:* Institut d'Etat des Serums et Vaccins Razi, Boite Postale 656, Teheran.
9. *Japan:* Institute for Infectious Diseases, University of Tokyo, Shiba Shirokane-daimachi, Minato-Ku, Tokyo.
10. *South Africa:* South African Institute for Medical Research, P.O. Box 1038, Johannesburg.
11. *Taiwan:* Taiwan Serum Vaccine Laboratory, 130 Fuh-lin Road, Shiling, Taipei.
12. *Thailand:* Queen Saovabha Memorial Institute, Bangkok.
13. *United States:* Wyeth Inc., Box 8299, Philadelphia, 1, Pa.

Scorpion antivenoms are made at institutes 1, 3 and 10; spider antivenoms at institutes 2, 3 and 10; jellyfish (sea-wasp) antivenom at 2.

Doctors who need supplies of antivenom for use in various geographical areas may find the following most useful—

Americas: polyvalent viper antivenom from 13; coral-snake antivenom from 3 or 13.
North Africa: viper antivenom from 1, 4 or 5.
Mid Africa: mamba antivenom from 10 (or 4); African cobra antivenom from 4, 5 or 10; viper antivenom from 4 (Bitis-Echis), 5 (Echis) or 10 (Echis).
South Africa: mamba, cobra, and viper antivenom from 10.
Middle East: viper-cobra antivenom from 4, 5 or 8.
Asia: (seasnake bite) seasnake antivenom from 2.
Burma, India, and Pakistan: cobra-krait-viper antivenom from 6(*a*) or 6 (*b*).
Cambodia, Laos, Malaysia, Vietnam, Thailand: viper and cobra antivenoms from 12.
Indonesia: cobra-krait-viper antivenom from 7.
Japan: viper antivenom from 9.
Philippines and Taiwan: cobra, krait and viper antivenoms from 11.

SPIDER BITES, SCORPION AND VENOMOUS FISH STINGS

Clinical features

Spiders have fangs similar to those of poisonous snakes (Plate 44). Some spiders, even large ones, are harmless; perhaps the most dangerous is *Latrodectus,* the black-widow spider. Scorpions have a poisonous sting at the end of their tail which is bent forward over the body to inject venom. They vary in length from less than an inch to about 8 inches, but some of the most dangerous scorpions never exceed 2–3 inches. The effects of scorpion stings and spider bites are very similar. If venom is injected, the main result is local pain which can be severe and may last some hours, even 1–2 days. Local necrosis may follow bites by spiders of the *Loxosceles* genus. General systemic symptoms are exceptional and include rapid breathing, salivation, sweating, vomiting, abdominal and generalised pains and, in very severe poisoning, falling blood pressure probably due to cardiotoxic effects. The latter can be fatal in children. Intravascular coagulation and abnormal haemolysis with haemoglobinuria can occur in severe spider bite poisoning by *Loxosceles,* and acute renal failure may ensue.

Venomous fish stings are common in the tropics. In coastal waters where the seabed is mud or sand, catfish occur—so called because they have whiskery mouthparts. They have serrated spines (Plate 45) in their fins which can inject venom. Stingrays have a flat triangular-shaped body varying in diameter from a few inches to 10 feet. When trodden on they whip forward their tail which has a serrated sting on it. In coral reefs, even more venomous fish are found such as stonefish and scorpion fish. They have multiple serrated venomous stings along their backs. The main effects of stings by these fish is an intense and often agonising local pain. Sometimes the sting becomes detached and remains embedded, leading to a chronic discharge (Plate 46).

Treatment

The most effective treatment for the local pain of venomous stings is hot water. The part stung is immersed in water as hot as the patient can bear (and only the patient can decide how hot this is). The pain is relieved within seconds and the part stung must be quickly removed from the water to avoid blistering. It should be reimmersed as pain recurs (within seconds at first, later within minutes). This procedure should be continued until the pain no longer recurs (usually about half an hour). It is important to explain details of this simple but highly effective treatment to the patient, who should be given a can of water recently brought to boiling point. This should be added to the immersing water to keep it as *constantly hot* as he can bear. If the water is not hot enough, the treatment is not effective; if the stung part is immersed too long in very hot water, blistering will result.

If the part stung is unsuitable for immersion in hot water (for example, the face or trunk), the area should be infiltrated through the puncture wound with 2–5 ml of 1 per cent lignocaine hydrochloride. Alternatively, intramuscular or intravenous pethidine should be given, 100 mg for an adult, 2 mg per kg for children.

For the general systemic symptoms of spider bites and scorpion stings, specific antivenom is available in a few parts of the tropics (see *Antivenoms* above). Otherwise adrenaline 0.5 ml should be injected subcutaneously (0.2 ml if aged under 2 years).

BEE AND WASP STINGS

Clinical features

Bees have a barbed sting which is left behind together with the venom sac. Wasp stings are not barbed and are therefore not left behind. The effects of stings are very similar to those following spider bites, including on rare occasions, general symptoms, haemoglobinuria or myoglobinuria and acute renal failure. In addition, victims may be allergic from previous bee or wasp stings; a subsequent sting, even a single one, can result in rapid collapse with death in 1–2 minutes. This rapid collapse is mainly caused by oedema of the throat and bronchospasm arresting respiration.

Treatment

The bee sting should be removed. It is a tiny black shaft with the white poison sac attached to its free end. It should not be grasped by forceps or fingers; this would express more venom from the sac. The sting should be scraped from the flesh with the finger or the blade of a knife. Local antiseptic is then applied. Pethidine may be needed for pain. Adrenaline is indicated for general symptoms by injection or inhalation of an aerosol; if these persist, an intravenous drip of hydrocortisone will be needed. People who are allergic to bee or wasp stings can be desensitised but this is usually temporary unless maintenance desensitising injections each month are continued indefinitely.

JELLYFISH STINGS

Clinical features

Jellyfish have myriads of microscopic stinging capsules called nematocysts on their tentacles. When touched, these capsules extrude a sting which can eject venom. However, only a small number of jellyfish have stings which can penetrate intact human skin. The most dangerous of all jellyfish, the cubomedusan or box jellyfish, sometimes called sea wasp, is confined to tropical waters. It has a cuboidal body or float, 1–3 inches in diameter, and a leash of several tentacles growing from each of the four body corners. It is translucent and difficult to see in the water (Plate 47).

Physalia or the Portuguese man-o'-war jellyfish has a coloured float from which numerous minor tentacles hang, together with a single main tentacle which can be over 10 feet long. Although it has an evil reputation, severe poisoning seldom follows the stings of the Portuguese man-o'-war; fatal stings are extremely rare. In contrast, several deaths following stings by the box jellyfish, *Chironex fleckeri*, have been recorded in Australian waters. Death is due to rapid collapse within a few minutes of the sting; these rapid deaths appear to be due more to heart failure than to respiratory failure. A smaller cubomedusan causes the Irukandji sting, so-named after an Australian aboriginal tribe. Local symptoms are minimal but after 10–20 minutes, violent generalised pains ensue, with restlessness and sweating. These symptoms may continue for 1–2 days. The Irukandji sting is never fatal.

Stings by most jellyfish other than box jellyfish cause only local wealing with tingling and discomfort, usually lasting a few hours. Only a small proportion (about 10–20 per cent) of the nematocysts discharge their stings and venom, and this has important implications for treatment (Plate 48). Local effects following box jellyfish stings can be more serious and necrosis of the skin may occur.

Treatment

Methylated spirits (or any other alcohol) should be applied to the stung parts to kill the undischarged nematocysts. If no alcohol is available, dry sand or any dry powder should be thrown on the sting and then the tentacles and slime should be scraped off. Dry sand is better than wet sand. The sting should *not* be rubbed with wet hands, cloth, and so on, as this will spread and aggravate the sting. After the spirits have dried, calamine lotion is a suitable local application. In severe cases with rapid collapse, the victim should be lain on his back, methylated spirits poured on the sting, and tourniquets put on affected limbs. If breathing stops, mouth-to-nose artificial respiration should be given; if the heart stops, closed-chest cardiac massage should be carried out.

A potent sea-wasp antivenom has recently been available from the Commonwealth Serum Laboratories, Australia. Administration has resulted in dramatic recovery from severe poisoning by *Chironex fleckeri* stings. A vaccine is now being developed for active immunisation of man.

REFERENCES AND FURTHER READING

General
Snakebite
CAMPBELL, C. H. (1964) *Trans. roy. Soc. trop. Med. Hyg.*, **58**, 263.
—— (1966) *Med. J. Aust.*, **2**, 922.
—— (1967) *Papua N. Guinea med. J.*, **10**, 117.
CHAPMAN, D. S. (1968) In *Venomous Animals and their Venoms*, Vol. I, Ch. 17, ed. Bucherl, W., Buckley, E. and Deulofeu, V. London: Academic Press.
CHRISTENSEN, P. A. (1968) In *Venomous Animals and their Venoms*, Vol. I, Ch. 16, ed. Bucherl, W., Buckley, E. and Deulofeu, V. London: Academic Press.
REID, H. A. (1961) *Lancet*, **2**, 399.
—— (1962) *Brit. med. J.*, **2**, 576.
—— (1964) *Brit. med. J.*, **2**, 540.
—— (1968) In *Venomous Animals and their Venoms*, Vol. I, Ch. 20, ed. Bucherl, W., Buckley, E., and Deulofeu, V. London: Academic Press.
—— (1970) *Clinical Toxicology*, **3**, 473.
REID, H. A., THEAN, P. C., CHAN, K. E. and BAHAROM, A. R. (1963a) *Lancet*, **1**, 617.
REID, H. A., CHAN, K. E. and THEAN, P. C. (1963b) *Lancet*, **1**, 621.
REID, H. A., THEAN, P. C. and MARTIN, W. J. (1963c) *Brit. med. J.*, **2**, 1378.
REID, H. A. (1972) In *Toxins of Animal and Plant Origin*, Vol. 3, p. 957, ed. de Vries, A. and Kochva, E. London: Gordon and Breach.

Scorpions
BARTHOLOMEW, C. (1970) *Brit. med. J.*, **1**, 666.
POON-KING, T. (1963) *Brit. med. J.*, **1**, 374.

Spiders
Annotation (1969) *Lancet*, **1**, 509.
VORSE, H., SECCARECCIO, P., WOODRUFF, K. and HUMPHREY, G. B. (1972) *J. Pediat.*, **80**, 1035.

Bees and Wasps
MARSHALL, T. K. (1957) *Practitioner*, **178**, 712.
ORDMAN, D. (1968) *S. Afr. med. J.*, **42**, 1194.
SHILKIN, K. B., CHEN, B. T. and KHOO, O. T. (1972) *Brit. med. J.*, **1**, 156.

Venomous Marine Animals
HALSTEAD, B. W. (1965) *Poisonous and Venomous Marine Animals of the World*, Vol. I, Invertebrates. Vol. II, Vertebrates, 1967. Vol. III, Vertebrates, 1970. Washington: U.S. Govt. Printing Office.
RUSSELL, F. E. (1965) In *Advances in Marine Biology*, Vol. 3, ed. Russell, F. S. London: Academic Press.

34
Hazards from Plants and Aquatic Organisms

In the main, diseases considered here are the result of the ingestion of toxins present in various plants although allergic reactions may occur on contact with a variety of species.

While many field fungi are poisonous, the most frequent offenders are those of the genus *Amanita*, especially *Amanita phalloides* which is often mistaken for a mushroom. In the United States 50 deaths occur per year following the ingestion of its polypeptide toxins for which there is no antidote. Ergot (*Claviceps purpurea*), a blackish mould growing on rye, has been responsible for epidemics of ergotism, one of the last being in France in 1951. These two types of fungal intoxication, namely with field fungi or as a result of consumption of various mouldy grains, have been briefly reviewed by Louria (1967). *Amanita muscarina*, a rather rare mushroom, is much prized in Siberia for the euphoria, hallucination and stupor it produces. Since muscarine is excreted unchanged in the urine, by drinking his own urine a subject can remain intoxicated on a single mushroom for days.

Recently there has been much interest in aflatoxin, one of the most potent carcinogens known, produced by *Aspergillus flavus* a frequent contaminant of groundnuts in the tropics. In repeated low doses it produces primary hepatoma in laboratory animals and it has been suggested that this may account for the high incidence of this tumour in man in Africa. However, to date no firm evidence has been produced to support this hypothesis.

PLANTS

The number of poisonous plants are legion and indeed most of the common garden plants in Britain have toxins which if ingested produce serious symptoms in man (North, 1967).

Many useful drugs are derived from plants (e.g. digitalis, ephedrine, reserpine). Most of our powerful narcotics are derived from the family *Papaveraceae*, and Taylor (1963) has reviewed these and other plant narcotics. The female Indian hemp (*Cannabis sativa*) provides marihuana, a fashionable drug among certain social groups at the present time. Nearly every large family of plants has its representatives producing powerful toxins, many of which have been identified. A classical example is *Atropa belladona* (deadly nightshade), the berries of which produce atropine intoxication, but there are many less well known and in the tropics a myriad of such toxic plants. A good example from the tropics is the crab's eye or rosary bean which is often made into necklaces and rosaries. It contains the phytoxin abrin and one bean is sufficient to kill an adult if the toxin is absorbed.

Many of the vetch and pea group produce important agents such as dicoumarol from spoiled sweet clover. *Lathyrus sativus* (Indian chickpea) is probably responsible for the spastic paraplegia encountered in some areas of India, and recently a similar condition has been produced in monkeys by the intrathecal injection of an amino acid extract of this legume (Rao *et al.*, 1967). *Argemone mexicana* (Mexican poppy) contaminating mustard oil has caused epidemic oedema among some Indian rice eaters using mustard oil for cooking.

Pyrrolizidine alkaloids occur in several groups of the compositae and are hepatoxic, producing thrombosis of the centrilobular veins and so-called venocclusive disease of the liver (Stuart and Bras, 1957). *Senecio jacobea*, the common ragwort, frequently causes liver disease in British livestock, but human disease has been reported from the West Indies, particularly Jamaica—where herbal medicines containing the toxic leaves are brewed as an infusion—Africa and India. The vomiting sickness of Jamaica was traced to the eating of unripe ackee fruit (*Blighia sapida*) which contains polypeptide hypoglycins producing a profound fall in blood sugar.

Plants are also important as irritants and five types of injury with examples can be classified as follows:

1. Mechanical injury—cactus spines, rose thorns.

2. Chemical injury—stinging nettles with the release of adrenaline and histamine.
3. Photosensitisation—*umbilliferae* (cow parsley) produces 5 methoxypsoralens.
4. Pseudophytodermatitis—due to chemicals and sprays on plants, e.g. mercurial fungicides.
5. True sensitisation—poison ivy, primulas.

Some fungi mentioned in the previous section may also produce allergic symptoms on inhalation (allergic alveolitis). Thus farmer's lung is thought to be due to thermophillic actinomycetes in mouldy hay and bird breeder's lung to *Aspergillus fumigatus*. An equivalent condition in the tropics has been described among those dwelling in huts with grass roofs in New Guinea (Blackburn, 1966).

Although the documentation of poisonous plants from certain parts of the world is good—for instance United States (Kingsbury, 1964), East and South Africa (Watt and Breyer Brandwijk, 1962)—it is obvious that much more information will become available in the future from tropical areas. The epidemic known as the Lusitu tragedy occurring in the Zambesi valley with the loss of 50 lives is a dramatic example of the sort of clinical problem where poisonous plants may be found to be playing a role (Gadd *et al*, 1962).

AQUATIC ORGANISMS

The effects of poisonous and venomous marine animals will be briefly discussed here. It must be remembered that many large freshwater rivers contain similar dangerous creatures. The Amazon, for instance, has not only piranha but freshwater sharks and rays, electric eels, and the little spiny candiru that is said to lodge in the urethra or vagina. However, documentation of such hazards is much less complete than those of the sea (Halstead, 1965).

Poisonous fish have toxic tissues (ichthyotoxism). Some are toxic at all times while in others the flesh is only toxic at certain seasons when the small fish feed on dinoflagellates and blue-green algae and are in turn ingested by larger fish. Common in the South Seas (Captain Cook was poisoned by fish) it is known there as ciguatera poisoning. Apart from the common gastrointestinal symptoms (diarrhoea and vomiting), anti-cholinesterase-like substances may block the neuromuscular junction with resultant ataxia and asphyxia. Paralytic shellfish poisoning from shellfish that have eaten the protistan dinoflagellates is similar. Fish commonly affected are barracuda (*Sphyraenidae*), sea bass (*Serranidae*), snappers (*Lutjanidae*) and parrot fish (*Scaridae*). The puffer fishes (*Tetraodontidae*) are good examples of the ability of fish to concentrate a potent toxin (tetrodotoxin, $C_{11}H_{17}O_8N_3$) in viscera such as ovaries, testes and liver. Twenty people a year die of this poisoning in Japan. The reader will recall that King Henry I of England died of a surfeit of lampreys and there are many examples of intoxication from over 500 species of fish.

Venomous fish have some apparatus for envenomating man. Seven hundred and fifty people a year are stung off the North American coast by stepping on sting rays (Russell, 1965). The venom can cause cardiac arrest. The weever fish caught by fisherman in nets in the North Sea has poisonous spines which produces tissue necrosis. In tropical waters scorpion fish and stone fish have similar poisonous spines and produce marked local pain and sometimes cardiovascular collapse or respiratory failure. Many species of shark may attack swimmers and inflict terrible injury.

Many invertebrates also constitute sea hazards, particularly the coelenterata (jelly fish, corals, etc). *Physalia* (the Portuguese man-of-war jellyfish) seldom kills but frequently causes local painful erythematous lesions which are slow to heal. In contrast the sea-wasp (*Chironex fleckeri*) has caused at least 50 deaths from cardio-respiratory failure off the east coast of Australia (Keen, 1970). Contact with the tentacles also results in acute local pain and inflammation often with permanent scarring. Among the mollusca, shellfish of the family *Conidae* (cone shells) inject a powerful venom into the unsuspecting through a modified tooth, and the bite of the little Australian blue-ringed octopus (*Hapalochlaena maculosa*) has proved fatal (Cleland and Southcott, 1965). Sea snakes are discussed elsewhere in this book, as is the pain following treading on sea urchin spines which will have been experienced by many who delight in holidaying on tropical beaches. Skin ulceration associated with coral implantation is another common problem. Diatoms and seaweeds have been responsible for outbreaks of dermatoses among fishermen (Beer *et al*, 1968).

REFERENCES

BEER, W. E., JONES, M. and EIFON JONES, W. (1968) Dermatoses in lobster fisherman. *Brit. med. J.*, **1**, 807–809.

BLACKBURN, C. R. B. (1966) *Lancet*, **2**, 1396.

CLELAND, J. B. and SOUTHCOTT, R. V. (1965) *Injuries to Man from Marine Invertebrates in the Australian Region.* National and Medical Research Council, Special report series No. 12, Canberra.

GADD, K. G. *et al.* (1962) The Lusitu tragedy. *Cent. Afr. J. Med.* Suppl, 8, 491–507.

HALSTEAD, B. W. (1965) *Poisonous and Venomous Marine Animals of the World.* 1: *Invertebrates.* United States Government Printing Office, Washington.

KEEN, T. E. B. (1970) Recent investigation on sea wasp stingings in Australia. *Med. J. Aust.*, **57** (6), 266–270.

KINGSBURY, J. M. (1964) *Poisonous Plants of U.S. and Canada.* New Jersey: Cornell Prentice Hall.

LOURIA, D. B. (1967) *New Engl. J. Med.*, **227**, 1128.

NORTH, P. (1967) *Poisonous Plants and Fungi.* London: Blandford Press.

RAO, S. L. N. *et al.* (1967) *Nature*, **214**, 610.

RUSSELL, F. E. (1965) Marine toxins and venomous and poisonous marine animals. In *Advances in Marine Biology*, 3, ed. Russell, F. S., pp. 255–384. New York: Academic Press.

STUART, K. L. and BRAS, G. (1957) *Quart. J. Med.*, **26**, 291.

TAYLOR, N. (1963) *Narcotics. Nature's Dangerous Gifts.* New York: Delta Books.

WATT, J. M. and BREYER BRANDWIJK, M. G. (1962) *Mediaeval and Poisonous Plants of Southern and Eastern Africa.* Edinburgh: Livingstone.

35
Cardiovascular Diseases

This chapter on cardiovascular disease in tropical countries will refer only to certain selected topics and it is in no way intended to be a comprehensive review of all cardiovascular disorders in these areas. Those cardiovascular diseases which appear to be predominantly problems of the tropical or subtropical environment are described in some detail, while those diseases which occur in both tropical and temperate situations are discussed only in as much as their presentation in the tropics requires special mention.

A lack of basic information is a major problem common to many tropical countries, and precise data on the population structure or the health and disease patterns in the community are rarely available. A considerably body of information on cardiovascular disease has accumulated from clinical and necropsy studies carried out in the major hospitals, and while this data is extremely valuable, it is limited by multiple factors of selection. Few epidemiological studies in cardiovascular function and disease have been carried out in the tropics, but basic information is beginning to become available on such measurements as height, weight, blood pressure levels, electrocardiographic patterns and radiological heart size. Necropsy studies are providing valuable information on heart weight in relation to body weight in different communities and there is increasing documentation of the changes in cardiovascular morphology seen with increasing age. There is still urgent need for further 'baseline' studies in cardiovascular function as well as in the biochemical and morphological fields relevant to cardiovascular disease.

A sense of professional isolation is a common phenomenon in those working with cardiovascular problems in the tropical and underdeveloped regions of the world. For this reason details are given of the major international organisations concerned with cardiovascular diseases. When advice, assistance or cooperation is required it is to these bodies that one should turn as their function is to provide precisely such services.

The World Health Organization established in 1959 a Cardiovascular Diseases Unit in Geneva, whose principal functions are: (*a*) to apply knowledge of cardiovascular diseases in order to strengthen public health services where this is needed and requested; (*b*) to promote, coordinate and assist research in cardiovascular diseases on an international or inter-regional scale.

The W.H.O. Cardiovascular Diseases Unit (Avenue Appia, 1211 Geneva, Switzerland) thus provides a focal point in an international sense for all those concerned with problems of cardiovascular disease and it is as much concerned with the disorders of the tropical environment as with those seen in the temperate and more well-developed regions. The World Health Organization also sponsors an Advanced Training Course in Cardiovascular Diseases for doctors from developing countries. This is held annually in Copenhagen under the auspices of the Danish Board of Technical Cooperation with developing countries and provides a sound training for those who already have a basis in internal medicine and some experience in cardiology.

The World Health Organization has recently published a handbook of methods for epidemiological studies of cardiovascular diseases (*Cardiovascular Population Studies: Methods*, by G. A. Rose and H. Blackburn, W.H.O. Monograph Series No. 56, 1968) and this valuable book outlines those principles which will provide a sound basis for obtaining comparable data. It is essential reading for any worker in the field of cardiovascular disease, perhaps more particularly in the tropical and rapidly developing areas of the world.

The International Society of Cardiology (22 rue de l'Athenee, 1206 Geneva, Switzerland) is the other major organisation with an international involvement in cardiovascular problems. The I.S.C. works very closely with the World Health Organization and with the national cardiac societies of all participating countries. It has a number of Scientific Councils dealing with such fields as atherosclerosis, rehabilitation, epidemiology, hypertension, cardiomyopathies, clinical science, paediatric cardiology and biophysics in cardiology and it is also the sponsoring body for the World Congress of Cardiology which is held every 4 years (London, 1970).

HYPERTENSION AND HYPERTENSIVE HEART
DISEASE

Hypertensive heart disease is one of the commonest of cardiovascular causes for admission to hospital in a tropical or subtropical environment. It may in some areas be the commonest single cause or it may rank just below rheumatic heart disease and/or idiopathic cardiomegaly.

Aetiology

Essential hypertension is the usual cause of hypertensive heart failure in subjects over 40 years of age, but a significant proportion of hypertensive heart disease in the tropics occurs in young adults with primary renal disease. They tend to present with both cardiac and renal failure and the manifestations of uraemia may overshadow those of the hypertensive heart disease. The cause is usually chronic renal disease and the precise proportion of this attributed to pyelonephritis or glomerulonephritis varies from one geographic region to another and, in any one geographic region, from one pathologist to another. One might even go further and add that any one pathologist's opinion concerning this problem will vary considerably from one time to another!

The role of urinary infections, urinary tract obstruction, schistosomiasis and the nephrotic syndrome are all much discussed but there have been few definite studies in this field. It has been suggested that a considerable number of cases of nephritis and nephrotic syndrome associated with quartan malaria progress to a chronic state (chronic glomerulonephritis) but the evidence for this is not available.

Epidemiology

In recent years there have been a large number of critical reviews dealing with the mass of information concerning the levels of blood pressure in different communities in various parts of the world. The patterns of blood pressure and the incidence of hypertension vary considerably from country to country and from group to group within each country. In most tropical communities there is a tendency for the blood pressure level to rise with age in a way similar to or identical with that observed in advanced societies in more temperate climates. There are groups of people however, usually little affected by the inroads of civilisation, in whom blood pressure levels tend to be low and who show little or no tendency for the blood pressure level to rise with increasing age. Among these groups, hypertension and hypertensive heart disease appear to be minimal or non-existent. It must be emphasised that these groups represent the exceptional rather than the usual finding in tropical and subtropical countries.

Clinical features

In the diagnosis and management of hypertension in tropical environments, reference must be made to those studies on hypertension carried out in the more highly developed temperate regions. There have been, quite understandably, virtually no studies carried out into the natural history of hypertension in tropical countries and this lack of information makes for extreme difficulty in the problems of prognosis and management. In most tropical communities individuals do not suffer from advanced or complicated arterial atheromatous lesions and the pattern of development of hypertensive disease, its clinical manifestations and its complications must be modified in some significant manner by this difference. There is an urgent need for such studies to be initiated for they will provide essential information concerning the natural history of hypertension uncomplicated by the presence of severe atherosclerosis.

RHEUMATIC FEVER AND RHEUMATIC
HEART DISEASE

It is difficult to form any clear view on the prevalence of rheumatic heart disease in the tropical and subtropical countries. Hospital inpatient studies and autopsy surveys, highly selective though they may be, make it evident that rheumatic heart disease is one of the commonest forms of heart disease in most tropical countries, comprising 10–20 per cent of cardiovascular disorders admitted or coming to necropsy.

Epidemiology

In some tropical countries there has been an apparent increase in the amount of chronic rheumatic heart disease as revealed by hospital and necropsy studies over the past decade. Chronic valvular lesions, e.g. mitral stenosis, may be seen in very young children, i.e. under 10 years of age, and this observation of a younger age of presentation with established valvular disease has been recorded in many tropical countries, e.g. Uganda, Nigeria, India, Indonesia, Philippines.

Despite the large numbers of patients with chronic rheumatic heart disease, many observers in tropical countries have commented on the relatively few cases of acute rheumatic fever seen. When young children present with acute rheumatic fever they not only have a severe carditis but also evidence of established valvular lesions. It is said that a history of polyarthritis is rarely obtained and that rheumatic nodules are exceptional. In the cooler parts of the tropics such as Ethiopia, the Kenya highlands and in South Africa, acute rheumatic fever and chorea are seen much more frequently than in the hotter, more humid regions.

It is clear that while impressions abound regarding rheumatic fever and its sequelae in the tropics, very little factual evidence is established regarding its prevalence or epidemiology.

Pathogenesis

Equally little is known about the streptococcus beyond that it is common and that streptococcal infections are even more inadequately treated than in the temperate and more advanced countries. It seems likely that streptococcal infection in impetigo, chronic leg ulcers and other skin lesions may be of importance in the pathogenesis of rheumatic disease in the poorer countries of the world, but very little attention has been paid to these problems.

In the field of pathology, remarkably little is known about the microscopic or histochemical features of rheumatic heart disease in the tropics and it is usually assumed by the pathologist that it is the same as in more developed countries. Available evidence suggests that the whole rheumatic process in the heart may be much more florid than is seen in Europe or America and that the fibrous tissue reaction may be excessive.

The natural history of rheumatic heart disease in tropical countries still requires to be established and it demands the combined efforts of clinicians, pathologists and epidemiologists.

PULMONARY HEART DISEASE

Whenever pulmonary heart disease in tropical or subtropical regions is discussed, the problem of schistosomal cor pulmonale is very much in mind. There is no doubt that in certain parts of the world where schistosomiasis is an endemic problem, this disorder is of some importance, e.g. in Egypt and Brazil. But even in these areas of high prevalence of schistosomiasis, its cardio-pulmonary aspects cannot be considered among its most important features from a public health point of view.

Epidemiology

Of subjects with schistosomiasis at autopsy approximately one third show involvement of the pulmonary vessels and only 1 per cent show cor pulmonale. Of all cardiac patients treated in general hospitals in Egypt, about 4 per cent are considered to have schistosomal cor pulmonale. In areas of schistosome endemicity other than Egypt and Brazil, cor pulmonale due to schistosomiasis does occur but seems to be very infrequent as a cause of pulmonary heart disease, e.g. East and West Africa, West Indies.

Studies in recent years indicate that cor pulmonale (unassociated with schistosomiasis) accounts for a significant proportion of cardiovascular disease in many tropical and subtropical countries. In many parts of India, particularly the northern provinces, some 20 per cent of all cardiac patients admitted to hospital are suffering from it. The majority are relatively young for this disorder; the maximum incidence is between 30 and 59 years and the underlying pulmonary disorder is chronic bronchitis and emphysema in at least two thirds, with bronchiectasis and bronchial asthma accounting for most of the remainder. Despite the high prevalence of pulmonary tuberculosis, only a small proportion were thought to be due to it.

Aetiology

Previously it has been assumed that chronic bronchitis and emphysema were associated with the big industrialised cities and were not problems of the underdeveloped countries. Workers in India attribute the lung disease there to untreated respiratory infections associated with squalid living conditions and a smoke-filled atmosphere. Cor pulmonale of this pattern is seen in other tropical countries, e.g. Kenya, Ghana, Nigeria, West Indies, Philippines.

In South Africa and Rhodesia, silicotic cor pulmonale occurs in mine workers and is often complicated by tuberculosis. This aetiological complex was found to be present in half of the cases of cor pulmonale seen in one study in Johannesburg.

In general, cor pulmonale is an underdiagnosed disorder even at autopsy examination and there should be an increased awareness not only of its existence in tropical environments but of the relative frequency of chronic bronchitis and emphysema in such communities.

ENDOMYOCARDIAL FIBROSIS

SYNONYMS. The term 'endomyocardial necrosis' was originally used by Davies in his MD thesis but later he labelled this 'endocardial fibrosis'. At present 'endomyocardial fibrosis' (EMF) is the more common synonym. In order to differentiate the tropical condition from those non-tropical cases in which there is fibrosis in the endocardium and myocardium, the term 'Davies disease' has also recently been used.

Definition

Endomyocardial fibrosis (EMF) is a form of heart disease endemic in several tropical countries and characterised in the established condition by endomyocardial fibrosis in the ventricular cavities, affecting in particular the apex and subvalvular regions. It is an active and possibly progressive disorder, not merely 'scarring in the heart'. Without any prejudice towards the various concepts of aetiology, it can be thought of in the same general pattern of behaviour as rheumatic heart disease.

Aetiology

The cause has not been established but it appears to be a disease of the wetter parts of the tropics and there is some suggestion of a seasonal variation.

1. *Malnutrition.* Although it is predominantly a disorder of the poorer socioeconomic groups in the areas in which it is endemic, its absence from many areas in which malnutrition is common and its occurrence in well-nourished Europeans who have lived in the endemic areas indicate that malnutrition cannot be a primary factor.

2. A *viral* aetiology has been postulated but without any evidence to support the suggestion.

3. *Filariasis* has been incriminated as a possible factor in Nigeria but not in Uganda, and argument still continues as to whether this infection may play a major or a contributory role in its pathogenesis or may merely be an ecologically associated phenomenon.

4. Much attention has been paid to the *serotonin* (5-hydroxytryptamine) content of the plantain (banana) diet of East and West African groups and an analogy is drawn between the fibrotic lesions of carcinoid heart disease and those of endomyocardial fibrosis. While the geographic distribution of the disease and the banana overlap considerably, there is little firm evidence to involve serotonin in the aetiology.

5. There is considerable evidence to indicate that endomyocardial fibrosis is a *hypersensitivity disorder* of cardiac connective tissue, similar in many ways to rheumatic heart disease. Recent detailed studies of the microscopic findings in endomyocardial fibrosis reveal mucinous swelling of the cardiac ground substance and vessels with excessive deposition of acid mucopolysaccharide and foci of collagen necrosis. These features strongly suggest that hypersensitivity may be the underlying mechanism.

One hypothesis is that the disease represents a response to haemolytic streptococcal infection modified by previous immunological experience, particularly by malaria. It has been demonstrated in Uganda that those groups most prone to develop endomyocardial fibrosis tend to differ in their immunological background from those less susceptible to it. This immunological difference is manifest as a syndrome which includes high levels of malarial antibody, immunoglobulin (IgM) and circulating autoantibodies to heart, thyroid and gastric parietal cell mucosa.

There is as yet no direct evidence to incriminate the streptococcus, but considerable evidence to suggest that the pattern of development of the disease is similar in many ways to that of rheumatic heart disease.

Epidemiology and distribution

Endomyocardial fibrosis was first described in West African troops serving in the Middle East and in indigenous African subjects in Uganda. The main areas of endemicity appear to be Uganda (Kampala) and western Nigeria (Ibadan) but the condition has been described from the Sudan, the Congo (Brazzaville), Kenya, Tanzania (Dar-es-Salaam), Ceylon, South India (Kerala), Malaya, Ghana, Gabon, Brazil and Colombia. There have also been convincing reports of endomyocardial fibrosis occurring in Europeans who have lived for long periods in certain of these endemic areas, in particular the Congo, Nigeria and the Cameroons. In Nigeria, an initial illness has been described which usually begins during the rainy season and relapses also tend to occur during this season. Some patients, whose disease was thought to be quiescent, suddenly became ill at this time and died with evidence of an acute carditis.

In Uganda, a peculiar epidemiological situation regarding endomyocardial fibrosis is that it appears to affect predominantly people of immigrant origins, coming from Ruanda, Burundi and the south-western districts of Uganda (Kigezi, Ankole). These migrants move from areas of low to high malarial endemicity. They also tend to form the lower socioeconomic group in the community and differ from the peoples indigenous to the Kampala region in a variety of social, educational and environmental factors.

Sporadic cases called 'endomyocardial fibrosis' have been reported in people who have never lived in the tropics and there are several possible approaches to these. One may accept that the term is purely descriptive, that the heart has a

ventricles; the lesions affect predominantly the endocardium and the inner portion of the myocardium. Pericardial effusion is present in more than one-third of cases (Fig. 35.1).

The fibrous tissue is frequently localised to the apex but may extend along the inflow tract to involve the papillary muscles and chordae tendinae. The fibrosed papillary muscles and chordae may lead to the atrioventricular valves being held rigidly, even though they are not abnormal. In the

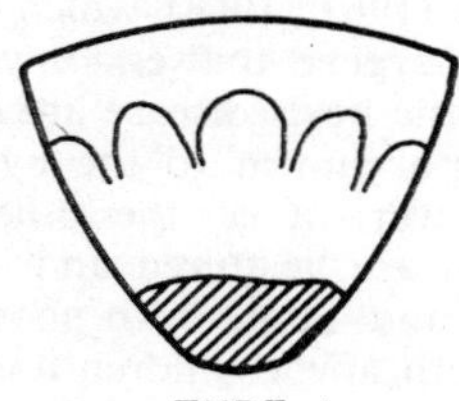

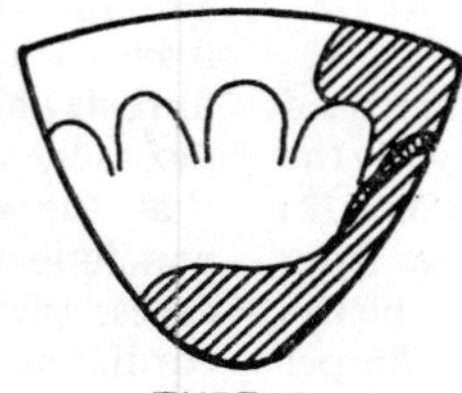

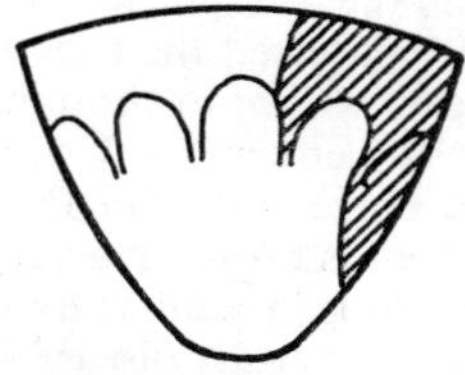

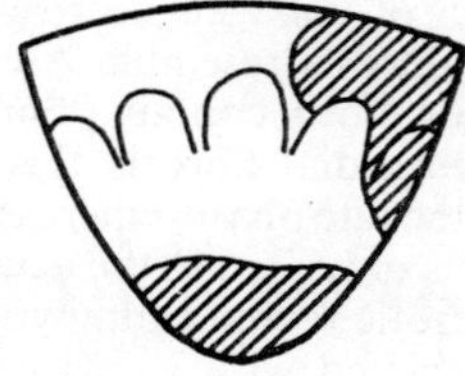

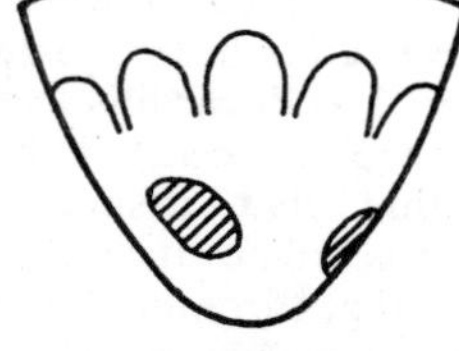

FIG. 35.1. *Diagram to show the distribution of endomyocardial fibrosis in the left or right ventricles.*

limited pattern of morphological response to injury and that these cases are due to aetiologic factors other than those usually responsible. On the other hand, they may represent the genuine tropical type of the disease occurring in subjects who have never been in the tropics, and in the ultimate analysis these sporadic non-tropical cases may be of considerable significance to the complete story. They should not be ignored.

Pathology

Macroscopic. Endomyocardial fibrosis is characterised in the established condition by fibrosis in the inflow tract and at the apex of one or both

left ventricle, a characteristic lesion affects the posterior mitral leaflet, the chordae attached to it and the adjacent endocardium of the outflow tract. In this form of the disease the anterior mitral cusp may show no evidence of thickening or scarring and its tethering structure may be normal. This posterior cusp lesion may be continuous with a lesion in the apex; alternatively it may occur on its own or both the areas may be affected but with a clear uninvolved area of endocardium between them.

In the more acute cases the endocardial lesions are covered with a soft, spongy, greyish-green layer of material; in more chronic cases the endocardial lesions are hard and white.

Pure right ventricular lesions occur in about 10 per cent of cases, almost always involving the apex and often extending to the tricuspid valve. Pure left ventricular lesions occur in about 40 per cent of cases, almost always affecting the apex and in half of those with apical fibrosis, the lesion extends continuously to involve the posterior mitral valve cusp. There are also many cases in which the posterior mitral cusp alone is affected.

Combined right and left ventricular lesions occur in about 50 per cent of cases, and in biventricular cases the left ventricle tends to be more predominantly affected than the right.

The heart weight in those affected is increased by about 40 per cent; in Uganda, hearts with the disease average 310 g in females and 380 g in males. There is however a very wide range, from 190 g to 680 g in adults. By comparison, hearts with rheumatic heart disease weigh about 66 per cent more than normal hearts and in idiopathic cardiomegaly the hearts tend to be even heavier.

Antemortem thrombi (atrial and ventricular) occur far more commonly in endomyocardial fibrosis (43 per cent) than in rheumatic heart disease (15 per cent). Ventricular thrombi show an even greater predilection for endomyocardial fibrosis (29 per cent) than rheumatic heart disease (2 per cent). However, embolic phenomena in the absence of bacterial endocarditis occur with the same frequency (15 per cent) in both heart disorders, suggesting that despite the frequent presence of intracardiac thrombi in endomyocardial fibrosis, the thrombi do not readily become dislodged, possibly because of their firm attachment to the underlying endocardial lesions. When they become detached, they may do so on a massive scale and aortic embolisation has been seen in seven such cases in Kampala but not in rheumatic heart disease over the same period.

Microscopic. In the endocardium, the connective tissues and underlying myocardial interstices contain excessive acid mucopolysaccharide (AMP). This is also increased in the mitral and tricuspid valve leaflets. In some areas, capillaries and fibroblasts penetrate from below, and within this organising zone, acid mucopolysaccharide is diminished and there are large numbers of Anitschkow myocytes (Aschoff cells) and a scattering of lymphocytes and other cells. In early lesions there are thin strands of hyalinised scar tissue between the overlying mucin and the myocardium. In older lesions, the entire endocardium is composed of hyalinised collagen.

The largest deposits of acid mucopolysaccharide are found in the areas of myocardium adjacent to the thickened endocardium; the middle and outer thirds of the myocardium are less severely involved, but random traces occur between individual myofibres throughout all portions of the myocardium. Peculiar foci of necrosis are seen in the endocardial collagen, situated in the scar tissue at the junction of the thickened endocardium and the underlying myocardium. In some hearts, similar foci of necrotic collagen are seen in the scars of the myocardial interstices.

In the detailed histological study by Connor and his colleagues (1967, 1968) which is summarised above it is argued that endomyocardial fibrosis and rheumatic heart disease are different diseases, a counter argument to the hypothesis that the one is a variant of the other. They conclude that both are 'acquired and in many cases, progressive and fatal. Both show endocardial scarring, both affect children and young adults and both are characterised by swelling of the cardiac ground-substance and by foci of collagen necrosis.'

However, they indicate differences considered to make for a clear distinction between the microscopic changes in the two:

1. The foci of collagen necrosis in endomyocardial fibrosis resemble Aschoff bodies in that they both contain 'fibrinoid', but in endomyocardial fibrosis this fibrinoid persists in the late phase, whereas in the Aschoff body it is only seen in the acute phase.
2. The necrotic foci in endomyocardial fibrosis are associated with a less pronounced cellular infiltrate than in Aschoff bodies.
3. The majority of necrotic foci in endomyocardial fibrosis are in the scar at the endomyocardial junction while Aschoff bodies are more widespread throughout the heart.

It would seem that the microscopic differences emphasised between the two conditions are in degree rather than being complete and indeed Connor and his colleagues conclude from their microscopic findings that hypersensitivity may be the underlying mechanism of endomyocardial fibrosis. The two disorders are thus at least similar histologically in that they are both disorders of cardiac connective tissue and in both the possible mechanism is hypersensitivity.

Symptomatology

The natural history has not been established, but in Nigeria an attempt has been made to define the early symptoms and signs. From nearly 100 patients in whom a clinical diagnosis had been made, 14 were selected because they described initial symptoms from which, in retrospect, their heart disease appeared to date.

The symptoms were non-specific with malaise, loss of appetite and commonly a fever which occasionally persisted for weeks. One child complained of joint pains. These general symptoms lasted from 1 week to 6 months and then merged imperceptibly into symptoms denoting pulmonary or systemic congestion, i.e. cough, breathlessness, swelling of the face and/or abdomen.

The majority of subjects with endomyocardial fibrosis present with established cardiac failure and the symptoms are in no way particular to the disease. With predominantly left ventricular lesions there is cough, chest pain, progressive effort dyspnoea and haemoptysis. With predominantly right ventricular lesions there is ascites, hepatomegaly and peripheral oedema. The onset is usually insidious and may progress over several weeks and end fatally in months, or the patient may live many years. Unexplained fevers may occur and loss of weight may be marked.

Diagnosis

A diagnosis is rarely established in the early stage and in the Nigerian study mentioned above, the 14 subjects presumed to be affected were unquestionably ill with fever, tachycardia, swelling of the face, abdomen or ankles and with a troublesome cough. The signs were those of a carditis plus an established heart lesion. It is clearly not possible to predict from this clinical picture that the individual will develop endomyocardial fibrosis.

Endomyocardial fibrosis is a disorder predominantly affecting children and young adults and in Fig. 35.2 the ages of subjects coming to necropsy with it are contrasted with those coming to necropsy with rheumatic heart disease. More than two-thirds of the subjects with endomyocardial fibrosis are below 35 years of age. The age range is wide, however, and in an individual problem the age will be of little help in its differential diagnosis for it has been encountered at autopsy at 3 years and at 73 years of age.

The clinical signs will depend on the pattern of lesions affecting the heart but there are three main clinical syndromes encountered.

1. Chronic pericardial effusion. The patient presents with ascites, hepatomegaly, slight peripheral oedema, raised jugular venous pressure, pulsus paradoxus and a quiet heart. There is no clinical evidence of either significant left or right ventricular hypertrophy. This syndrome is particularly

common in affected children but may occur in any age group. It appears to be more frequent in subjects with the right ventricular form.

2. Right ventricular endomyocardial fibrosis. The pure right ventricular form is relatively uncommon and yet until recently this has been the only group in the complex in which clinical diagnosis could be reasonably straightforward. The ventricular cavity is at first restricted and later diminished in size, resulting in a small stroke

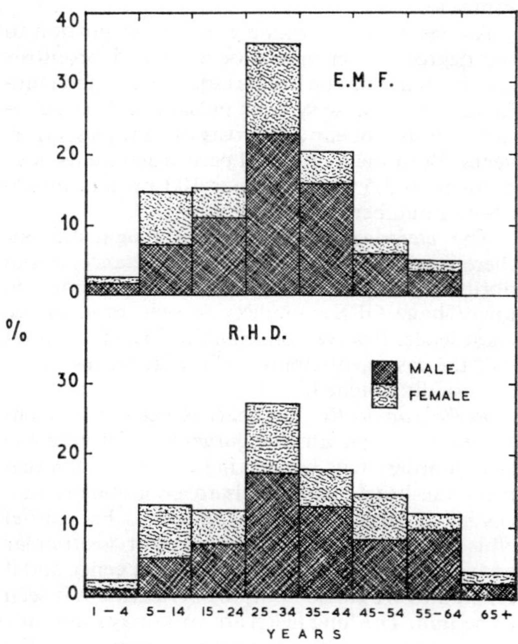

FIG. 35.2. *Age and sex distribution of endomyocardial fibrosis in subjects coming to autopsy in Kampala, Uganda, 1950–65.*

volume and cardiac output. The outflow tract dilates and hypertrophies. Tricuspid valve incompetence is almost always present. Invariably there is a high pressure in the right atrium and great veins, and the grossly enlarged right atrium may compress areas of the lung, affecting pulmonary perfusion.

Most cases present with tricuspid incompetence, but the murmur may not be audible, although it can more frequently be recorded on the phonocardiogram. The systemic venous pressure is always raised, sometimes very grossly and there is active systolic pulsation pathognomonic of tricuspid incompetence. The y descent is nearly always a prominent feature of the venous pulse.

The dilated outflow tract is responsible for producing pulsation in the second and third left intercostal spaces. There is no left parasternal heave and the apical impulse is usually between the mid-clavicular line and the anterior axillary line or beyond the anterior axillary line; it is sometimes impalpable. It is far more usual not to hear any significant murmurs (i.e. only soft short systolic murmurs than to hear murmurs of tricuspid and/or mitral incompetence. A third heart sound is usually present over the right ventricle.

Ascites may be strikingly out of proportion to the degree of dependent oedema and proptosis may be marked. The liver is large, tender and painful and may show systolic pulsation. This pulsation may disappear as fibrosis or cirrhosis supervenes. Both the ascitic and pericardial fluids have more than 3.5 g protein per 100 ml and an increased number of lymphocytes.

The *electrocardiogram* is not diagnostic but there is no right ventricular predominance. Atrial fibrillation or atrial ectopic beats are common and low-voltage QRS complex are seen even in the chest leads. P wave abnormalities occur in about half the cases with abnormally wide waves which are usually notched.

Radiographically, the heart is usually very enlarged and right atrial enlargement forming the right border may be striking. In gross enlargement the heart shape tends to be globular, suggesting a large pericardial effusion. Pericardial effusion is indeed common in right ventricular endomyocardial fibrosis (about 50 per cent), and if air studies are carried out, the pericardium is seen to be thin. The lung fields are strikingly oligaemic and pleural effusions are seen in about half the cases. In films with good penetration, calcification may occasionally be seen in the region of the apex. On fluoroscopy the movements of the heart are greatly diminished but sometimes expansile pulsation of the right atrium during systole can be detected.

On *angiographic examination*, the right ventricle is seen to have lost its trabeculations and the apex and inflow portions become partly obliterated while the outflow tract is usually dilated but may appear normal. There is tricuspid incompetence and a greatly enlarged right atrium and contrast medium may persist in the atrium for a considerable time (12–15 seconds).

Catheterisation studies of right ventricular endomyocardial fibrosis reflect the ventricular restriction, tricuspid incompetence and impairment of right ventricular myocardial function. Introduction of the catheter into the pulmonary artery or even into the right ventricle may be difficult. Pulmonary capillary and arterial pressures are normal. Because of the reduced right ventricular compliance, the end-diastolic pressure and right atrial pressures become raised and right ventricular systole may only raise the right ventricular pressure a few millimetres of mercury above the end-diastolic pressure. Tricuspid incompetence results in atrial and ventricular pressures being almost equal during ventricular systole. In advanced disease pressures in the right atrium, right ventricle and pulmonary artery may be similar. Intravenous digoxin is without effect on the raised right atrial pressure or the low cardiac output in subjects with normal rhythm.

3. Left ventricular endomyocardial fibrosis. In some areas, e.g. Ibadan, it is considered that pure left ventricular endomyocardial fibrosis is uncommon. This may be because in the biventricular form the clinical picture is often dominated by the right-sided disease and/or because the differential diagnosis between rheumatic mitral incompetence and left ventricular endomyocardial fibrosis may be difficult. A recent study of patients with left ventricular or biventricular endomyocardial fibrosis carried out in Uganda suggests that there is a clinical syndrome which is possibly diagnostic of the disease and it is hoped that this syndrome may lessen the diagnostic confusion with rheumatic mitral incompetence or functional mitral incompetence in idiopathic cardiomegaly.

Cardiac enlargement is unusual and the apical impulse is rarely prominent and never heaving. The presence of pulmonary hypertension in left ventricular endomyocardial fibrosis is determined by the *absence* of right ventricular disease. A palpable left parasternal heave associated with a narrow splitting of the second heart sound is thus only found in subjects with the advanced pure left ventricular form. Auscultation reveals an early, moderate to loud systolic murmur occupying not more than the early half of systole. There is a loud third heart sound, and in half the cases an audible and widely distributed opening snap. The systolic murmur often radiates, not only towards the axilla, but towards the base of the heart.

The *electrocardiogram* is rarely helpful and may show low voltage QRS complexes, T wave changes and P mitrale. Occasionally there is evidence of right, but not of left, ventricular hypertrophy.

Radiographically the heart may be normal; when enlarged, it frequently shows a 'mitral' configuration. There may be evidence of pulmonary hypertension with perihilar clouding, large main pulmonary vessels and relative oligaemia of the peripheral lung fields. Pleural effusions may be present. Very occasionally, calcification is visible in the left ventricle but this is unusual.

Angiography. Interpretation of left ventricular angiograms in endomyocardial fibrosis are at present controversial. Occasionally the presence of left ventricular scarring is unmistakeable with marked reduction in size of the left ventricle, but severe scarring may be present and not be fully reflected angiographically. Reflux into the atrium which is never grossly enlarged can usually be demonstrated.

On catheterisation the left ventricular pressure tracing shows a raised pressure at the end of diastole of the 'dip-and-plateau' type. There is pulmonary hypertension and the pulmonary vascular resistance is often raised. The cardiac output is low.

Combined right and left ventricular endomyocardial fibrosis. This is the largest group within the complex and the clinical picture tends to be dominated by the signs of right ventricular involvement. Cases classified after study as lone right ventricular disease are often found at autopsy also to have advanced disease of the left ventricle. Mitral incompetence is usual, but with associated right-sided disease the mitral incompetence may be clinically inapparent; pulmonary hypertension is absent and the right-sided features dominate together with tricuspid incompetence and systolic jugular venous pulsation. The low cardiac output of the affected right ventricle presumably protects the left ventricle from haemodynamic stress.

Evidence of left-sided endomyocardial fibrosis in the presence of the established disease in the right ventricle may thus be very difficult to demonstrate without angiography. Plain radiography usually shows the heart to be enlarged with a large right atrium and pulmonary veins but with no significant left atrial enlargement.

Differential diagnosis

Pericardial effusion. The differential diagnosis is from other causes of pericardial effusion such as tuberculosis and pyogenic infections.

Right ventricular endomyocardial fibrosis must be differentiated from constrictive pericarditis. The diagnosis is favoured by tricuspid incompetence and the presence of marked cardiac enlargement. Murmurs and systolic venous pulsation in the neck or hepatic pulsation are not found in constrictive pericarditis. The pattern of peri-

cardial calcification may be diagnostic but the occasional case of endomyocardial fibrosis with calcification in the visceral pericardium will produce a difficult diagnostic problem. In rheumatic tricuspid incompetence, right ventricular hypertrophy is usually present. Very rarely, the possibility of Ebstein's anomaly will be raised in the differential diagnosis of endomyocardial fibrosis. A much more common problem of differential diagnosis is from primary hepatic disease, in which the jugular venous pulse wave is normal.

Left ventricular endomyocardial fibrosis. The pure left ventricular form must be differentiated from other causes of pulmonary hypertension such as severe mitral stenosis or chronic lung disease. In rheumatic mitral incompetence the murmur is pansystolic and often louder than in endomyocardial fibrosis, and left ventricular hypertrophy occurs. In addition, there may be evidence of aortic valve disease, which is not seen in typical endomyocardial fibrosis. The differentiation from idiopathic cardiomegaly may be extremely difficult and may require angiography for a final assessment.

Treatment

There is little that is specific in the management of heart failure in endomyocardial fibrosis, and on the whole the results of treatment are disappointing. Particularly in the right ventricular form, digitalis appears not to be effective in reducing the raised venous pressure, although it may slow the cardiac rate when atrial fibrillation is associated with a fast ventricular rate. Ascites may be extremely resistant to diuretics and as abdominal paracentesis removes such a large amount of protein, many clinicians are reluctant to tap the ascites unless it is producing physical distress. Corticosteroids have no place in the treatment of the disease.

Prophylaxis and prevention

Until the aetiology of this condition is established there are no preventive measures possible.

Prognosis

The usual pattern of behaviour is one of continuing cardiac failure but patients have been known to survive for up to seven years from the time of first presentation in cardiac failure. There is some suggestion that the prognosis is better in those with right-sided endomyocardial fibrosis and is somewhat better in adults presenting in cardiac failure than in children. Signs which are regarded as of grave prognostic significance include cyanosis, finger clubbing and jaundice.

Bacterial endocarditis is a relatively uncommon complication, occurring in about 2 per cent of patients coming to autopsy compared with an incidence of bacterial endocarditis of 26 per cent in rheumatic heart disease coming to autopsy. However, when endomyocardial fibrosis and rheumatic heart disease are concurrently present, the incidence of bacterial endocarditis is similar to that seen in rheumatic heart disease.

Historical footnote

It is now over 20 years since Bedford and Konstam (1946) observed a form of heart failure in African troops serving in the Middle East. The soldiers were mostly from West Africa, were usually aged 20–30 years and presented in heart failure with gross cardiomegaly, a prominent pulmonary artery and often with a diastolic blood pressure of 100 mmHg or more. Seventeen of their 40 patients came to necropsy and in two cases there was old mitral endocarditis. In *some* cases there was an obvious and extensive subendocardial fibrosis, with fibrous areas resembling shallow infarcts in the ventricles, adherent to which was organised antemortem clots. Some sections showed extensive subendocardial necrosis and fibrosis without appreciable inflammatory reaction.

Bedford and Konstam considered that the clinical pathological findings corresponded to 'isolated myocarditis' or 'Fiedler's myocarditis'. Their material—in the light of present knowledge —probably included cases of endomyocardial fibrosis, idiopathic cardiomegaly, rheumatic heart disease and possibly non-specific myocarditis, and it fell to Davies in Uganda to produce shortly thereafter a more complete pathological description of the disorder and to Davies and his clinical colleagues to delineate the clinicopathological picture of what they termed endomyocardial fibrosis.

IDIOPATHIC CARDIOMEGALY (ICM)

SYNONYMS. Heart muscle disease, nutritional heart disease, cryptogenic heart disease, cardiovascular collagenosis with parietal thrombosis, primary myocardial disease, cardiomegaly of unknown origin, congestive cardiomyopathy, myocardosis, peripartal heart disease, alcoholic heart disease.

Definition

The basic definition is a large heavy heart in relation to body weight for which there is no apparent cause. It is extremely unlikely that all the conditions named above are manifestations of a common cause and pathogenesis, and it is now generally agreed that 'multiple factors result in a myocardial fault: all of these may present a similar clinical, roentgenological, electrocardiographic and pathologic picture'. In these many disorders, pericardial and endocardial involvement are infrequent and rarely of any significant degree.

Aetiology

The very attempt to discuss aetiology in a condition labelled as idiopathic indicates that some forms of idiopathic cardiomegaly may be less idiopathic than others! Wherever possible, an attempt should be made to relate the presence of a large heart to some factor or set of factors in the clinical history or the environmental situation of the patient, for it is in this way that we will eventually do away with the idiopathic title. Association is not causation and the clinical collector of large hearts should attempt to retain a critical attitude towards the factors apparently associated with the group of patients in his environmental situation.

1. Malnutrition. Because idiopathic cardiomegaly appears to be endemic in many poor tropical and subtropical countries, malnutrition is constantly brought forward as a primary aetiological factor. Gillanders (1951) focused attention on this by referring to the big hearts encountered in Johannesburg as 'nutritional heart disease'. A critical review of those observations reveals no convincing evidence that the problem encountered was primarily due to chronic malnutrition and later studies from the same hospital made it clear that alcohol may well have played a considerable role. 'Nutritional heart disease' has also been described from Ceylon, where alcohol was clearly not involved, but it must be emphasised that the association of a poor nutritional background, with clinical or biochemical evidence of malnutrition and an otherwise unexplained cardiomegaly is not adequate proof of a nutritional basis for the cardiac disorder.

There is also a postulate made that nutritional disturbances in childhood may lead to metabolic abnormalities in the myocardium which may not be completely reversible. In this view, childhood malnutrition, e.g. kwashiorkor, could conceivably result in the appearance of a cardiac disorder in childhood or perhaps in later life. There is no evidence that children who have been treated for severe kwashiorkor have in later life stigmata of cardiovascular disease. Cardiomyopathies (idiopathic cardiomegaly) in children have been reported from many tropical and subtropical countries and in none is there any suggestion that malnutrition has played a role.

While it is tempting to accept the supposition that severe and chronic malnutrition can permanently damage the myocardium or render it more susceptible to injury from other factors, there is at present no clear evidence that this happens in man. One should stress that people with big hearts in a poor environment may have suffered not only from malnutrition but from a wide variety of other insults associated with poverty and overcrowding.

2. Myocarditis. Myocarditis may be associated with almost every known bacterial, viral, rickettsial or parasitic disease and it may be the most common of all heart diseases. The prognosis in acute myocarditis associated with infectious diseases has always been regarded as favourable except in diphtheria and Chagas' disease. However, studies by Bengtsson and Lamberger (1966) have focused attention on the possible relationship between myocarditis and idiopathic cardiomegaly. They have shown that acute myocarditis may occur in as much as 1 per cent of patients admitted to hospital with acute infectious diseases, particularly streptococcal and Coxsackie B viral infections. Many of these patients have signs of impaired cardiac function during convalescence and a significant number have persisting symptoms and signs for many years afterwards. In a series of patients who had been healthy before the onset of their acute myocarditis, examination was carried out 5 years later. The resting electrocardiogram showed abnormalities in 19 per cent and the exercise ECG was abnormal in 30 per cent. The physical working capacity was abnormally low in 40 per cent and an abnormally large heart volume was present in 20 per cent.

Thus in a significant number of patients with a non-specific myocarditis there may ultimately develop an enlarged heart with no features to indicate the nature of the original injury to the heart. In tropical and subtropical countries, where the environmental situation is still one in which bacterial, viral, rickettsial and parasitic diseases are widespread and to a major degree uncontrolled, the significance of this work in Sweden is clear and very important. This may turn out to be a factor of major importance in the

development of idiopathic cardiomegaly as an endemic problem in certain areas. The possibility of a preceding myocarditis must be considered in all with idiopathic cardiomegaly and ways will eventually be found for the making of a retrospective diagnosis.

3. Alcohol. There is now general acceptance amongst those concerned with cardiac metabolism, if not amongst the general public, that alcohol can have a direct effect upon the myocardium. Experimental evidence has in recent years confirmed that alcohol, at mildly intoxicating levels, can affect the mitochondrial enzymes of the myocardium and that chronic alcohol ingestion can induce permanent alterations in the membrane permeability and metabolic pathways of the heart. It is surprising how often alcohol as a possible agent in idiopathic cardiomegaly in the tropics is either completely ignored or lightly dismissed. It seems reasonable to believe that in countries in which alcohol is as important a social phenomenon as it is in the more temperate parts of the world and where heavy drinking of an episodic or chronic nature is common, that the population is not immune to the myocardial effects of alcohol. It requires that careful and repeated attempts are made to obtain a true history of the pattern of alcohol ingestion and that the investigator should not be satisfied with the usual assurances of temperate habits.

4. Cirrhosis of the liver. There is a considerable literature on the haemodynamic changes and on alterations in myocardial metabolism in subjects with cirrhosis of the liver. Occasional cases of cardiac failure have been attributed to hepatic cirrhosis and in one autopsy survey of patients dying with alcoholic portal cirrhosis, cardiac enlargement was reported to be present in 11 per cent of subjects. In a study of 472 subjects with cirrhosis coming to autopsy in Kampala, the author could find no abnormally heavy heart for which there was not an adequate explanation. It is almost certain that obscure cardiomegaly in subjects with alcoholic cirrhosis is due to alcoholic heart disease and is not a result of the hepatic disorder.

5. Pregnancy and the puerperium. A form of idiopathic cardiomegaly, particularly in the early puerperium but which may occur in the last trimester of pregnancy, has been reported for many years. While some regard this as a 'vague, perhaps disappearing syndrome', there is convincing evidence from many tropical and subtropical countries of its existence as a recognisable entity.

The aetiology is as obscure as in most forms of idiopathic cardiomegaly, but the basic problem possibly lies in a complex metabolic situation affecting the myocardium. The condition occurs particularly in poorly nourished communities with a low socioeconomic status, although the patients themselves do not appear to be malnourished. There is considerable evidence, however, that repeated childbearing under adverse conditions, e.g. in Africa and Asia, is a considerable nutritional stress. Weight gain in pregnancy is considerably less than in more developed countries and the serum lipid increases normally encountered during pregnancy are minimal. Lactation makes even greater energy demands than pregnancy and those women who have been unable to store fat during pregnancy will be under even greater nutritional stress during subsequent lactation. It is not difficult to conceive that the physiologic changes in blood volume and cardiac output which normally occur during pregnancy may be radically altered by this nutritional situation, and that the metabolism of the myocardium may be affected, particularly in the lactating period.

If one accepts peripartal heart disease as an entity, it is possible that a small proportion of cases of idiopathic cardiomegaly in women in areas of inadequate nutrition may be the late result of repeated pregnancies and lactations. On the other hand, puerperal cardiomyopathy may merely represent the effects of myocarditis consequent upon infection in the early puerperium. It should perhaps be emphasised that it is yet to be established that the stress of a normal pregnancy alone may result in damage to a normal heart.

Epidemiology and distribution

Big hearts of unexplained aetiology are relatively common in many tropical and subtropical countries and there is an increasing number of reports of this from more temperate areas. The larger series come from South Africa, Nigeria, India, Brazil, Colombia, Venezuela and Jamaica, but even in the United States and Japan there is increasing recognition that many large heavy hearts cannot be explained in terms of the usual aetiological factors.

Surveys in rural Jamaica reveal an incidence of about 7 per cent of unexplained cardiomegaly in subjects aged 35–64 years. In chest X-ray population surveys conducted by the World Health Organization in Gambia, Liberia, Sierra Leone and East Africa the prevalence of a greatly increased heart shadow varied from 0.3 to 2.2 per cent. In Singapore, 7.6 per cent of subjects found to have heart disease during a tuberculosis survey had cardiomegaly of unknown cause. In Ethiopia,

again in subjects referred from chest X-ray screening because of cardiac enlargement, 16.6 per cent had idiopathic cardiomegaly. Idiopathic cardiomegaly comprised 3.5 per cent of cases with a diseased heart at autopsy in Kampala, while in Jamaica the figure was 4.1 per cent and in Colombia 5.6 per cent. These randomly selected figures from the data available on idiopathic cardiomegaly are merely intended to indicate the existence of a significant proportion of big hearts in population, hospital and autopsy studies which are at present unexplained aetiologically.

Pathology

The usual criterion for heaviness is a heart greater than 400 g in the male and 350 g in the female. Studies in Jamaica and Uganda suggest that these levels might be reduced to 350 g and 300 g if early cases of idiopathic cardiomegaly are not to be missed. It is essential, however, to emphasise that the normal heart weight is related to body weight and that this relationship should be determined for each sex in the area in which studies are being carried out.

Macroscopic. The endocardium of the ventricular cavities usually shows a lacework pattern due to stretching of the trabeculae carnae, and there may be thinning of the left ventricular apex. Patchy superficial white endocardial scars are irregularly distributed over the inflow or outflow tracts. Thrombi are frequent but their incidence seems to vary in different geographic areas.

Enlargement is usually due to dilatation and hypertrophy of both ventricles, but sometimes one ventricle may be predominantly affected. In typical cases there is an increase in the measurement of the tricuspid and mitral valves and functional mitral and tricuspid incompetence are common sequelae of the stretched valve rings. The greatest transverse diameter of the left ventricle is increased, but because of the dilatation, the ventricular walls may or may not be thick and rarely measure more than 12 mm (cf in hypertension $\pm$ 20 mm).

Microscopic. There is hypertrophy of muscle fibres and a variable increase in connective tissue. Focal scarring is nearly always found and may be extensive; it may follow obvious foci of myocytolysis or represent replacement of atrophy of fibres. Marked diffuse or focal collections of chronic inflammatory cells are usually classified as myocarditis, but scattered lymphocytes may be present in idiopathic cardiomegaly.

Pathological diagnosis. Given such a large heart at autopsy, the following conditions must be excluded before making a diagnosis of idiopathic cardiomegaly:

1. 'Significant' hypertension.
2. Organic valvular disease.
3. Coronary artery disease.
4. Intra- or extra-cardiac shunt.
5. Hypertrophic obstructive cardiomyopathy.
6. Histological evidence of myocarditis, amyloidosis, haemochromatosis.
7. Cor pulmonale.
8. Severe anaemia.

Clearly, the nature of 'significant' hypertension is difficult to define and for a final and definitive diagnosis of idiopathic cardiomegaly it is necessary to have a full and accurate clinical record as well as a detailed macroscopic and microscopic work-up. 'Significant' hypertension could perhaps be defined as clear-cut evidence of advanced hypertensive vascular disease, persistent albuminuria, grade III retinopathy or signs of renal failure.

Symptomatology

Most reports concern adults aged 30–60 years and males are more frequently affected than females. The course is variable and may be acute, subacute or chronic. The acutely ill patients may recover completely or go rapidly downhill and die within months with recurrent or constant heart failure and thrombotic/embolic episodes. The commonest form, however, is chronic, with frequent relapses over several years and eventually a fatal outcome.

Symptoms point characteristically to biventricular failure and their duration is often brief relative to the physical signs on presentation. Dyspnoea on effort, orthopnoea, nocturnal dyspnoea, ill-defined chest pain which is not anginal and sometimes cough and hepatic pain occur in more than 50 per cent of subjects in all series reported.

Swelling of the legs and/or abdomen tends to occur much later than breathlessness in most subjects with this disorder and tiredness and loss of energy are frequent.

Diagnosis

The characteristic presentation is in biventricular heart failure with a hypokinetic circulation. The hands are cold and the circulation time prolonged. Signs of right-sided failure are often more disturbing and impressive than those of left-sided failure and may persist longer. There is usually marked generalised oedema often out of

proportion to the degree of heart failure present, with ascites, tender hepatomegaly, raised jugular venous pressure with systolic pulsation and sometimes proptosis and/or chemosis. The pulse is of small volume, rapid and usually in sinus rhythm, ectopic beats are frequent but atrial fibrillation is rarely found.

The diastolic blood pressure is often elevated on admission and this 'hypertension of failure' appears to be a more common and more pronounced phenomenon with idiopathic cardiomegaly than with any other form of heart disease. Readings of 130–150/100–120 mmHg are common; even 160/130 mmHg. All such pressures return to normal within 1–3 days of bed rest and digitalis therapy. Pulmonary oedema is rarely seen.

The heart is enlarged in all cases, often markedly so but the cardiac impulse is variable. It is usually heaving over the left or right ventricles but may be feeble or impalpable. This may represent the difference between a hypertrophied heart and one with hypertrophy and considerable dilatation. A third heart sound is almost invariably present and a fourth sound may be heard.

About half of the cases have an apical pansystolic murmur sometimes accompanied by a thrill and short systolic murmurs in the aortic or pulmonary areas. When the myocardial failure is severe, the murmur of tricuspid incompetence may be present. On rare occasions the murmurs are so harsh as to simulate organic valvular disease. It is characteristic of this group that the murmurs diminish promptly during treatment for heart failure and may disappear. Pericardial effusion is not a feature of this condition. Embolic phenomena (pulmonary and arterial) are frequent and commoner in this cardiomyopathy than in any other.

Straight radiological examination shows generalised globular cardiac enlargement often suggesting predominant involvement of the left ventricle. Screening reveals reduced movements, especially of the left border. Generalised pulmonary oedema is rare and congestive changes are predominantly hilar with perihilar clouding, enlarged pulmonary veins and small pleural effusions.

There is no pathognomonic *electrocardiographic pattern* and the ECG usually shows sinus rhythm with frequent ectopic beats. Incomplete left and occasionally right bundle branch block may be present. The majority show left axis deviation. Atrial fibrillation is rare. In idiopathic cardiomegaly (primary myocardial disease) in the United States of America, atrial fibrillation is recorded in as many as 30 per cent, equally

20

affecting left and right bundles. Large peaked P waves of bi-atrial enlargement are seen and non-specific QRS and ST-T wave changes. A normal ECG may be regarded as strong evidence against the diagnosis of clinically significant disease of heart muscle.

Left ventricular angiography reveals an often grossly enlarged left ventricle and there is no evidence of obstructive hypertrophy of the out-flow tract. Great reduction in the normal variation in the size and shape of the left ventricular chamber throughout the cardiac cycle is striking. In some, the impairment of myocardial contraction is so great that there is little difference between films taken in systole and diastole. In cases with clinical signs of mitral incompetence, reflux of contrast into the left atrium can be demonstrated. The left atrium is normal or moderately enlarged in size and shows no significant systolic expansion. In about half, thinning of the left ventricular apex can be seen.

Right ventricular angiography reveals similar enlargement of the ventricular chamber and reduction in the change in size and shape during the cardiac cycle.

Differential diagnosis

The diagnosis may only be reached after lengthy observation, particularly once the patient is no longer in severe heart failure. Careful recording of the cardiovascular findings at each examination is essential.

Hypertensive heart disease. In idiopathic cardiomegaly there is usually no evidence of hypertensive retinopathy and the fall of blood pressure to normal levels with recovery from heart failure is characteristic of it.

Rheumatic mitral incompetence. In idiopathic cardiomegaly the murmur of mitral incompetence usually diminishes or disappears as the patient recovers from cardiac failure. In rheumatic heart disease, the murmurs are often intensified with improvement in cardiac compensation. The differential diagnosis may however be difficult unless additional valvular lesions of rheumatic heart disease are present; fluoroscopic demonstration of aortic or mitral valve calcification is virtually diagnostic of it.

Endomyocardial fibrosis of the left ventricle. The features described by Fowler and Somers (1968) may be of value in differentiating this from idiopathic cardiomegaly but in some cases angiography may be the only certain method.

Ischaemic heart disease. This, due to coronary atherosclerosis and obstruction, is uncommon in most tropical and subtropical countries, where the majority of the population are relatively poor. It is mainly in Europe and North America that in middle-aged or elderly people it must be excluded before a diagnosis of idiopathic cardiomegaly can be made. Unless angina pectoris or evidence of a recent or healed myocardial infarction is present, the differential diagnosis may be extremely difficult and in some areas, e.g. Jamaica, the situation is even further complicated by the frequent presence of angina-like chest pains and pathological Q waves in rural subjects with idiopathic cardiomegaly.

Pericardial disease (i.e. constrictive pericarditis or pericardial effusion with tamponade). The considerable cardiac dilatation in idiopathic cardiomegaly may simulate pericardial disease. A feeble or impalpable apical impulse, a persistently raised jugular venous pressure despite intensive treatment for heart failure, distant heart sounds, a paradoxical arterial pulse or rise in jugular venous pressure with inspiration (Kussmaul's sign) may all suggest pericardial disease. The presence of murmurs and a gallop rhythm favour the diagnosis of myocardial disease.

Chagas' disease. See section on **Chagas' disease.**

Secondary myocardial disease. Once a diagnosis of myocardial disease has been made it must be decided whether a primary or a secondary form is present. The secondary forms are many and varied and most are extremely rare, e.g. amyloid disease, glycogen storage disease, various neuro-muscular and neurologic disorders (progressive muscular atrophy, Friedreich's ataxia) haemachromatosis. Specific myocarditis produced by Coxsackie B virus, influenza virus or poliomyelitis virus must, however, be kept in mind particularly if the illness begins with an influenzal-like syndrome, followed by cardiac enlargement. Serum neutralising antibodies for the virus and isolation of the virus from the stools, nasopharynx or myocardium may help confirm the diagnosis. Persistent fever in a patient with myocardial disease always suggests the possibility of myocarditis.

Treatment

This is never satisfactory and in the advanced stages the results are disappointing.

Bed rest. Strict bed rest has often been beneficial in treatment and restriction to bed for months or even years has been recommended. The social and financial problems which this involves are often insurmountable and it is important that an individual evaluation be made to determine the degree of activity to be allowed. Bed rest can lead to marked reduction in heart size and improvement in signs and symptoms and should be regarded as fundamental.

Digitalisation. Digitalis is indicated when congestive heart failure is present. Numerous warnings are given concerning the unusual degree of digitalis sensitivity or myocardial irritability in all forms of primary myocardial disease, but most observers agree that these patients need digitalis and are able to tolerate it without undue difficulty. It is, however, essential to establish the electrocardiographic and electrolyte pattern in each patient before and during treatment if digitalis toxicity is to be avoided. The vigorous use of diuretics may produce haemoconcentration, dehydration and electrolyte imbalance and this may render the patient more susceptible to digitalis toxicity. Digitalis toxicity contributes to the high incidence of arrythmias in patients with idiopathic cardiomegaly.

Sodium restriction and diuretics. Salt restriction is essential and there is now a very wide choice of oral and intravenous diuretics available. Potassium supplements may be required as thiazide diuretics, frusemide and ethacrynic acid are likely to lead to potassium deficiency.

Steroids. There is no specific indication for steroids.

Anticoagulants. Embolic phenomena are common and systemic emboli are twice as common as pulmonary emboli. Although many authorities are firm about the need for anticoagulants, they are vague about indications. Presumably anticoagulants are indicated during phases of congestive cardiac failure when cardiac dilatation is greatest and cardiac output at its lowest and all patients in whom embolic episodes have already occurred should be placed on anticoagulants.

Cardioversion. Atrial flutter may require the use of low-voltage D-C countershock therapy. In atrial fibrillation, both the use of quinidine and electric cardioversion are accompanied by considerable risk and reversion to normal sinus rhythm may be extremely difficult.

Long-term therapy consists mainly in finding a suitable level of physical activity which can be tolerated without symptoms or with minimal symptoms, maintenance digitalisation and the judicious use of diuretics and sodium restriction.

Prognosis

Initial response to therapy with regression of symptoms is common and in many cases the heart returns to normal size on radiological examination. In the majority of cases some degree of cardiomegaly persists, the ECG remains abnormal and heart failure is recurrent. While it is not possible to generalise about a problem which clearly includes many causes, long survival is the exception rather than the rule. Some survive 5 or more years following a first heart failure; others die on their first admission.

Idiopathic cardiomegaly in children

From South Africa, Nigeria and the Middle East there have been reports of 'cardiomyopathy' in children aged 6 months to 8 years. The clinical and radiological picture is similar to that in adults with idiopathic cardiomegaly. Its causation in children in the tropics is unknown, but studies suggest that an antecedent myocarditis may frequently be responsible.

PERIPARTAL CARDIOMYOPATHY

This usually presents within the first 10 weeks of the puerperium and occasionally in the last trimester. Lactation has usually occurred in the puerperium and some consider this an important factor. An ill-defined 'toxaemia' during pregnancy has been reported in some series. The condition occurs more frequently in multipara (over five births), in women over 25 years of age and in twin pregnancies.

Symptomatology

The onset is usually gradual with weakness, fatigue, breathlessness on exertion, ankle swelling and eventually nocturnal dyspnoea. Occasionally it is acute with sudden pulmonary oedema. Recurrent praecordial or substernal discomfort is common and nausea, vomiting and colicky abdominal pain are described. Left heart failure may be rapidly progressive and followed by right heart failure. Embolic phenomena are frequent and may be the presenting feature.

Diagnosis

Examination usually reveals cardiac failure although cardiac enlargement may merely be found on routine examination. The cardiac failure is of the low-output variety and there may be a considerable rise in diastolic pressure. This labile and transient diastolic hypertension is not usually associated with a systolic hypertension. The heart is enlarged and a left ventricular heave is frequent. There is usually a pansystolic praecordial murmur and sometimes a tricuspid systolic murmur, but these may be inconspicuous and disappear with recovery. An apical diastolic gallop rhythm is constantly present.

The condition occurs particularly in poorly nourished communities with a low socioeconomic status but the patients do not appear to be malnourished.

Radiologically the heart shows generalised enlargement and on screening pulsation may be diminished. The electrocardiogram is usually abnormal with non-specific ST-segment and T-wave changes and these may progress to complete left bundle branch block. It has been suggested that the presence of left ventricular hypertrophy changes on ECG indicate a worse prognosis and that their absence indicates the likelihood of complete recovery.

Management and prognosis

The management of this condition is the same as that described for other forms of idiopathic cardiomegaly with emphasis on bed rest, suppression of lactation and consideration of sterilisation.

The prognosis varies widely. Cardiomegaly may persist with a fatal outcome after further pregnancies or even after an apparently satisfactory response. There may be prolonged survival but a marked tendency to relapse persists. There may be a reversion to normal heart size but there still remains a marked tendency to the insidious development of cardiomegaly and heart failure later, usually precipitated by further pregnancies. There is doubt whether the myocardium ever returns to normal despite the normal heart size sometimes achieved radiologically.

ALCOHOLIC HEART DISEASE

Clinical studies in recent years have resulted in a better understanding of the range of manifestations of cardiovascular disease associated with alcoholism. There appear to be two main types of clinical problems:

1. *Thiamine* (*vitamin B₁*) *deficiency* causing beriberi heart disease.
2. *Direct injury to cardiac muscle* (alcoholic cardiomyopathy), often occurring in well-nourished alcoholics.

Sometimes these clinical syndromes appear together but usually they are separate. It has frequently been suggested that beriberi heart disease and alcoholic cardiomyopathy are phases of the same underlying disease resulting from alcoholism with or without malnutrition, and there is some evidence that the high cardiac output of beriberi heart disease can progress to persistent cardiomegaly and low cardiac output. Further haemodynamic studies in individual patients are needed to confirm this and to demonstrate its frequency in alcoholic heart disease.

Cardiac beriberi (thiamine-responsive disease)

This occurs least frequently in series of subjects with alcoholic heart disease and is the least serious disorder. There is usually a good response to alcohol withdrawal and to thiamine therapy.

The patient is almost always a male, is often obese and usually has ready access to beer and wines. He complains of palpitations, dyspnoea on exertion and paroxysmal nocturnal dyspnoea, and ankle swelling may be a presenting feature. Excessive sweating and paraesthesiae of the limbs are occasional complaints.

The *physical signs* are those of a hyperkinetic state with a high cardiac output and cardiac failure. The extremities are warm and moist, the pulse regular, rapid and bounding and the blood pressure variable; the systolic level may be raised. The jugular venous pressure is raised, a third heart sound frequent and a systolic murmur common. With considerable cardiac enlargement, murmurs of mitral and/or tricuspid incompetence may be present. Pulmonary crepitations are heard at the bases and there may be pleural effusions, hepatic enlargement, ascites and ankle swelling.

The *clinical criteria* for the diagnosis of beriberi heart disease as listed by Blankenhorn (1955) include a history of a thiamine-deficient diet for 3 months or more, exclusion of other forms of heart disease, raised jugular venous pressure, oedema, cardiomegaly, minor electrocardiographic changes, evidence of peripheral neuritis or pellagra and a response to thiamine with a decrease in heart size.

Haemodynamic studies. In beriberi heart disease there is a high cardiac output and an abnormally low peripheral resistance. Recent studies suggest that there are peripheral vascular and myocardial lesions, resulting in vasodilatation or loss of peripheral vascular tone, associated with high cardiac output and biventricular failure. Although the peripheral lesion may respond rapidly to treatment with thiamine the response of the myocardial lesion may be delayed and thus a state of low output failure may appear (Akbarian *et al*, 1966).

A normal or nearly normal electrocardiogram in heart failure of unknown origin is strongly suggestive of beriberi. Changes seen are variable and transient and mainly concern inversion of T waves over the right ventricle.

Radiological examination shows generalised cardiac enlargement, prominence of the right atrium, right ventricle and pulmonary conus and artery; pulmonary congestion is uncommon.

Treatment consists primarily of withdrawal of alcohol and the institution of a normal diet. Thiamine hydrochloride 100 mg intravenously is administered daily for 5 days and thereafter 50 mg daily (subcutaneously) is given until alcohol restriction and a normal diet have ensured an adequate supply of thiamine.

Bed rest is important, as a tendency to sudden death has been recorded. Digitalis appears to have little effect but sodium restriction and diuretics are of value.

Prognosis. Very little is known regarding the long-term sequelae of severe thiamine-deficient heart disease and if the patient survives, the condition is regarded as being completely reversible.

Alcoholic cardiomyopathy

This is probably the most common way in which alcohol injures the heart and it is also a fairly common form of heart injury. Most subjects are men aged 40–70 years who have been alcoholics for at least 10 years and whose nutritional status is good at the time of onset of symptoms. A striking finding is the difficulty in obtaining a reliable history of the extent of the alcoholic habit; evasion and indifferent cooperation are hallmarks of these patients.

The *cardiac symptoms* are non-specific, with dyspnoea on exertion and palpitations. Tachycardia and irregularities due to ectopic beats are common and atrial fibrillation occurs frequently. A high diastolic blood pressure is sometimes found during periods of severe congestive heart failure and the pressure returns to normal following a good response to therapy. The heart size and the degree of pulmonary congestion are variable. With each successive episode of heart failure there is a diminishing response to treatment and thiamine is without effect. These subjects appear to have a very high tolerance to alcohol and frequent drunkenness is not associated with the development of the cardiomyopathy.

Haemodynamic changes consist of a low stroke volume with failure to respond normally to exercise and an increase in peripheral resistance.

Pressures recorded from the right side of the heart may be elevated and a further rise occurs with exercise.

In contrast with beriberi, reports of the electrocardiogram in alcoholic cardiomyopathy emphasise the frequency and importance of electrocardiographic alterations. Sinus tachycardia and multifocal ventricular ectopic beats are common and atrial fibrillation or flutter is often present. Left bundle branch block is more often present than right and occasionally pathological Q waves are seen in subjects who at autopsy have no significant coronary artery disease. T-wave changes of all descriptions are reported but their specificity is difficult to assess.

Treatment. The general treatment is no different from that outlined for idiopathic cardiomegaly; that is, alcohol restriction, bed rest, adequate diet, digitalis and diuretics, and, when indicated, anticoagulants. Steroids are without value.

CHAGAS' HEART DISEASE

SYNONYMS. Chronic chagasic myocarditis, cardiomegalia Chagasica, miocarditis obscura, miocarditis tropica, cardiopathia parasympathicopriva, etc.

Definition

Chagas' heart disease is an acute, subacute or chronic condition resulting from infection with *Trypanosoma cruzi*.

Aetiology

T. cruzi is transmitted by reduvid bugs of the Triatomid family, by blood transfusion or transplacentally. The trypanosome form circulates but never multiplies in the blood. It invades the cells of certain organs in man and animals and becomes a leishmanial form which divides to form a pseudocystic agglomeration of leishmania in the invaded cell. The cyst ruptures, the leishmanial forms are liberated and develop into trypanosome forms in the blood. Infected blood containing trypanosomes is taken up by the blood-sucking Triatomid bugs, and the trypanosomes change to a crithidial form which multiplies in the posterior gut. When the bug is taking its large blood meal, it evacuates faecal material containing trypanosomes and this may be inoculated into the skin or mucous membranes by scratching.

The disease may be transmitted by the vector from man to man or from other vertebrate reservoirs to man. The cat and dog are known domestic reservoirs and the armadillo is a much-mentioned wild reservoir which does not really appear to be as important as has previously been thought. Poor socioeconomic conditions with thatched mud-walled houses are the essential ecological conditions for the development of human infection on an endemic pattern.

Epidemiology and distribution

The disorder is found in almost all the countries of South and Central America, e.g. Brazil, Argentine, Uruguay, Panama, Venezuela. It is predominantly a problem of the rural areas and is closely linked to poverty and poor housing conditions. In some rural areas the prevalence of *T. cruzi* infections as judged by positive complement fixation tests is as high as 40–50 per cent and in such areas the prevalence of chronic Chagas' heart disease may be as high as 15 per cent. The condition is twice as frequent in males and the highest incidence is in the 25–45 year age group.

There is little doubt that in these tropical and subtropical regions of South and Central America, Chagas' heart disease is responsible for an enormous amount of morbidity and mortality and that it constitutes a major public health problem.

Pathology

Many possibilities have been put forward:
Toxic or *mechanical effects* of the parasite upon the tissues
Vascular lesions
Immunological mechanisms
Inflammatory processes
Nervous origin
There is considerable evidence to support destruction of the autonomic ganglion cells of the heart as the cause, with secondary or associated lesions of the myocardium.

Acute. This is manifest as a severe myocarditis. There is no cell reaction to the presence of the parasite in the myofibre before it ruptures, but once it has done so, there is a polymorphonuclear infiltration with considerable numbers of eosinophils. As more pseudocysts rupture, an eosinophilic granulomatous reaction develops with the presence of lymphocytes, monocytes and an occasional giant cell. Fibrous tissue develops around these lesions.

Leishmania are also found in cells in many other parts of the body, e.g. skeletal and smooth muscle fibres, bronchial epithelial cells, spleen, adrenal, thyroid and in ganglion cells of the peripheral nervous system.

In animal experiments (mice) intense infection of the ganglion cells in Meissner's and Auerbach's plexuses in the gut wall is seen, with large numbers of leishmania in the cytoplasm of the ganglion cells. When the cell ruptures, there is an intense inflammatory response with granuloma formation, first the nuclei of the ganglion cells and then the cells themselves disappear. These lesions can be produced by parasites derived directly from human cases. An analogous situation in humans is seen following death from acute Chagas' disease consequent upon blood transfusion. A severe myocarditis is present with a similar invasion and response around ganglion cells in the oesophagus, stomach and intestine.

It appears that in acute Chagas' disease the main damage is in the myocardium and in the ganglion cells of the peripheral nervous system and it would be anticipated that the lesions seen in the chronic stage would reflect this damage. There is also evidence that the major part of the destruction of ganglion cells takes place in the acute phase, and that up to 80 per cent of the ganglion cells in the heart may then be irreversibly damaged.

Chronic. There is marked hypertrophy and dilatation of the heart, often affecting the pulmonary conus which may appear aneurysmal. The heart may be globular in shape but there is usually separation of the left and right ventricular apices producing 'cor bifidum'. Heart weights average 500–600 g but may reach 1000 g.

Dilatation affects all chambers, mainly on the right side and most markedly affecting the right atrium. There is a characteristic thinning of the apex of the left ventricle and in some 50 per cent of cases coming to autopsy there is an 'aneurysm' in this situation. The wall of this aneurysm consists of endocardium and epicardium and may appear translucent. Less frequently, this aneurysm affects the right ventricular apex. These aneurysms virtually never rupture and appear to be almost unique to Chagas' heart disease. The anatomical basis for the apical aneurysm appears to be a slackening of certain muscle bundles which leads to an unwinding of the vortex region of the apex. A similar phenomenon is seen in the aneurysmal dilatation of the pulmonary conus. Thrombosis is common in these aneurysms and thrombosis is also commonly seen in the ventricle and greatly enlarged right atrium. Frequent embolic phenomena (about 30 per cent) occur in both pulmonary and/or systemic circulations.

Fibrotic areas of varying degree may be found in the wall of the left ventricle, the anterior part of the interventricular septum and left papillary muscles. Similar lesions occur in the right ventricle but are less marked. Endocardial thickening in the ventricles and right atrium is frequent but is not marked. There is sometimes evidence of a preceding pericarditis and the pericardium may be thickened. The coronary arteries show no gross pathology.

Microscopy of the myocardium reveals hypertrophy and atrophy of muscle fibres with discrete interstitial fibrosis. There is a varying degree of interstitial cellular fibrosis with a predominance of mononuclear cells and large areas of myocytolysis. Parasites are rarely seen. In Brazil, in addition to the above features, all cases of Chagas' heart disease have shown a marked decrease in the number of parasympathetic ganglion cells in the heart and other organs but with great individual variation, and this denervation is considered to be the essential lesion. In Venezuela, by contrast, this striking reduction in ganglion cells has not been observed.

Other pathology. In parts of central Brazil, megaoesophagus is extremely common and the condition has a significant association with positive complement fixation reactions for *T. cruzi*. There seems to be no reason to doubt on clinical and epidemiological grounds that megaoesophagus is due to Chagas' disease. The main lesion is a severe deprivation of ganglion cells and at least in the acute cases, this loss is due to invasion of the ganglion cells by leishmania with subsequent rupture and destruction of the ganglion cells.

Symptomatology and diagnosis

The natural history of Chagas' heart disease is only partly known, but there appears to be an acute stage, a long latent period and a chronic phase (Chagas' cardiomyopathy).

Acute. The acute stage of Chagas' disease is usually seen in infants and children. Local signs are usually present such as Romañas sign and the chagoma of inoculation together with more general signs and a varying degree of carditis.

Romañas sign is a non-painful unilateral oedema of the eyelids, often accompanied by a purple discoloration of the skin, conjunctivitis and enlargement of the preauricular and cervical lymph nodes. The sign may remain present for several weeks and is seen in perhaps half of the acute infections.

Chagoma of inoculation appears on the face, arms or legs as a hard, hot, purplish swelling of the skin which may ulcerate and leave a scar. It is seen in less than one quarter of the acute cases.

General signs include an irregular fever which may persist for several weeks, with sweating, anorexia, vomiting and diarrhoea. There may be a generalised oedema of varying degree, slight to moderate hepatomegaly and splenomegaly and a generalised lymphadenopathy.

Carditis. The myocardial involvement is manifest by varying degrees of tachycardia, arterial hypotension, gallop rhythm, cardiac enlargement, cardiac failure and electrocardiographic changes which are usually transient and variable. There may be prolongation of the P-R and Q-T intervals, disturbances of T wave and of ST segments and occasionally low QRS voltage. Conduction defects and rhythm disorders are exceptional at this stage. The majority of subjects with acute infection and associated cardiac involvement apparently recover.

Diagnosis in the acute stage
1. Parasitaemia is the fundamental finding, either directly in the peripheral blood film or on culture.
2. Xenodiagnosis, i.e. the patient is bitten by non-infected reduviid bugs (usually 5–12) bred in the laboratory and after 6–9 weeks the intestinal contents of the bugs are examined for *T. cruzi*.
3. Complement fixation test (Machado-Geurreiro reaction) begins to become positive from 2–4 weeks after infection.
4. A lymphocytosis is a frequent finding in the acute stage.

Latent period. The period between the acute and chronic phases of Chagas' disease may be as long as 10–20 years. The complement fixation test is positive and about 20 per cent of such asymptomatic patients will show a positive reaction to a single 5-bug xenodiagnosis test feed. In 10–30 per cent of people with positive complement fixation tests there will be some evidence of cardiac abnormality.

Chronic (Chagas' cardiomyopathy). The heart disease in chronic Chagas' disease usually appears in subjects between 15 and 50 years of age and there need be no history of an acute phase. The complement fixation test is almost always positive and the xenodiagnosis test is positive in about one third of patients.

In the initial stages there may be no symptoms in spite of the presence of objective evidence of heart disease, but symptoms appear as the disease progresses. Sudden death may occur at any stage.

The earliest symptoms tend to be related to rhythm disorders, viz. palpitations, faintness and syncope. Ectopic beats may be present but there may be no cardiac enlargement or cardiac failure. The electrocardiogram will however show definite signs of myocardial involvement, e.g. multifocal ventricular extrasystoles and complete right bundle branch block.

The clinical manifestations persist or increase, cardiac enlargement becomes apparent and the electrocardiographic changes become progressive with increasing evidence of myocardial damage. Cardiac failure now develops and thromboembolic phenomena are common. Signs of functional mitral and tricuspid incompetence are usually present. There are severe and complex arrhythmias and Adams-Stokes syndrome with complete atrioventricular block may occur and produce sudden death.

Radiologically there is generalised cardiac enlargement but the lung fields are usually clear. Cardiac pulsation on fluoroscopy may be so diminished as to resemble pericardial effusion. The electrocardiogram shows atrioventricular or intraventricular block, multifocal ventricular extrasystoles and sometimes abnormal Q waves. Death in cardiac failure usually occurs within 1–3 years if sudden death has not supervened.

In most large series in which a diagnosis of Chagas' cardiomyopathy has been made (and confirmed by autopsy) the complement fixation test is positive in about 80 per cent of cases only. The test is positive in about 10 per cent of other forms of heart disease and in about 10 per cent of those without heart disease. It has been suggested that it underestimates the true frequency of infection by 15–20 per cent.

Differential diagnosis

In endemic areas, the very high incidence of positive reactions to serological tests for Chagas' disease may make the recognition of other cardiomyopathies very difficult.

Endomyocardial fibrosis. Pulmonary hypertension is not a feature of Chagas' heart disease unless it is complicated by chronic pulmonary thromboembolism. Excessive ascites is not seen and pericardial effusion is uncommon in Chagas' disease. The electrocardiographic features of Chagas' heart disease, viz. right bundle branch block and abnormal Q waves are not usual in endomyocardial fibrosis. Idiopathic cardiomegaly (ICM) may be a major problem to diagnose in an endemic area of Chagas' cardiomyopathy. The 'hypertension of failure' so commonly seen in idiopathic cardiomegaly is not a feature of Chagas' disease and the presence of atrioventricular block, right-bundle branch block and abnormal Q waves,

while more frequently reported in Chagas' disease, are being recorded with increasing frequency in some varieties of idiopathic cardiomegaly, e.g. in Jamaica.

Ischaemic heart disease. Angina pectoris is not a feature of Chagas' heart disease and the Q waves seen on ECG tend to develop gradually and in the absence of a clinical story suggestive of angina or myocardial infarction. Arrhythmias and severe conduction defects are more common in Chagas' heart disease.

Treatment

There is at present no drug that will kill the parasite in the host and thus there is no specific treatment for this disorder.

Prevention

Prevention of new infections may be achieved by insecticidal control.

Prognosis

In subjects with a positive complement fixation test a normal ECG generally indicates a good prognosis. Electrocardiographic changes such as multiple extrasystoles, bundle branch block, total atrioventricular block or paroxysmal ventricular tachycardia all indicate a much worse prognosis than do less marked alterations such as those of the T wave or a low-voltage QRS complex. Sudden death occurs in about half the subjects affected.

CARDIAC DISEASE IN AFRICAN TRYPANOSOMIASIS

Trypanosoma rhodesiense

Some 40 years ago, attention was drawn to the occurrence of myocarditis in monkeys infected with virulent strains of *T. rhodesiense*. In humans, fibrotic lesions and cellular infiltration in the myocardium and endocardium were described in two subjects treated for *T. gambiense* infection (Lavier and Leroux, 1939) and a generalised cardiac involvement with predominant myocarditis was reported in two subjects with *T. rhodesiense* infection (Hawking and Greenfield, 1941). Two patients presenting with cardiac failure and responding rapidly to treatment for their trypanosomiasis have been described from Kenya (Manson-Bahr and Charters, 1963).

More recently, the clinical and pathological features in six necropsied cases of *T. rhodesiense* infection in Kenya have been presented (de Raadt and Koten, 1968). In all cases the epicardium was thickened and showed varying degrees of cellular exudate, predominantly mononuclear. The myocardium showed a diffuse interstitial infiltration of chronic inflammatory cells with focal collections, often in the vicinity of blood vessels. Collections of Anitschkow cells of the type seen in rheumatic myocarditis were present. All the hearts showed interstitial oedema, focal haemorrhages and shrinkage of the muscle fibres with loss of cross-striation.

Trypanosomiasis in Africa can clearly be associated with a myocarditis. Whether this is ever responsible for cardiac disease in later life in those who recover from this disease is not known but it is probably not a problem of major endemic importance.

Trypanosoma gambiense

The literature on cardiovascular disease in subjects with *T. gambiense* is similar to that concerning *T. rhodesiense*. Bertrand *et al* (1965) in Abidjan observed a patient with sleeping sickness who had gross cardiac enlargement radiologically and a low voltage ECG with a prolonged P-R interval. These cardiac signs cleared after treatment. They then studied the ECG in untreated and in other subjects following treatment with melarsoprol. Electro-cardiographic abnormalities were more frequent in the untreated (47 per cent) than in the treated patients (26 per cent); the changes were mainly flattening or inversion of the T waves, but four showed conduction defects and two showed ischaemic changes. The same group later reported on a somewhat larger series of untreated and treated patients. Chest radiographs suggested cardiac enlargement in 35 per cent and ECG abnormalities were present in about one third. Again, the ECG changes were mainly T-wave abnormalities, but atrioventricular block was occasionally seen. The incidence of abnormal findings was not higher in the group who had received arsenical therapy. Five subjects were examined at necropsy and all had small pericardial effusions. Histological examination in three cases revealed aggregates of lymphocytes, histiocytes and plasma cells, sometimes forming granulomas in the myocardium and pericardium.

Cardiovascular symptoms and signs appear to occur very infrequently in patients with *T. gambiense* infections, but the histological findings from Abidjan and in a further series from Dakar (Collomb *et al*, 1967) suggest that a myocarditis does occur.

OBLITERATIVE ARTERITIS

In recent years there have been a number of reports from tropical and subtropical countries of an arteritis of unknown aetiology, affecting particularly the aorta and its larger branches. It has been described in Nigeria, South Africa, Rhodesia, Malaya and India and while its relationship to Takayasu's syndrome (pulseless disease) is uncertain, it bears strong resemblance clinically and pathologically to this disorder or its variants described from Japan and other temperate countries. Females are affected somewhat more frequently than males and the age group under 20 years seems particularly susceptible.

Pathology

Pathologically the lesion is an arteritis with mononuclear and small round cell infiltration of the adventitia and media, particularly around the vasa vasorum, and a marked proliferation of the intima which ultimately produces stenosis or obstruction. The elastic tissue of the artery is replaced by fibrous tissue and the affected artery may show saccular dilatations. Thrombus formation on the intimal lesion may lead to a sudden clinical deterioration.

Symptomatology

The site of the lesion may vary considerably and the clinical symptoms and signs will be related to the site of vascular obstruction.

1. Lesions at the origin of the brachiocephalic branches of the aortic arch, as seen in the classical Takayasu syndrome, produce *eye signs* and *neurological symptoms*, occasionally with convulsions.
2. Lesions in the thoracic and upper abdominal aorta, from the origin of the left subclavian artery to the coeliac axis, result in *hypertension in the upper limbs* and *absent or diminished femoral pulsation* and a *systolic murmur* may be heard in the lower thoracic or upper abdominal regions ('atypical coarctation').
3. Lesions around the coeliac axis, mesenteric and renal vessels of the abdominal aorta will produce *abdominal symptoms* or *severe hypertension*. This latter presentation is among those more usually encountered in this disorder and in some areas the disorder is suspected 'in any child presenting with hypertension and a radiologically dilated or tortuous aorta'.

Diagnosis

While there may be few signs or symptoms initially, and a dilated aorta on routine radiological examination may be the only cause for suspicion, the vast majority of diagnosed cases present with severe (even malignant) hypertension and cardiac failure. Aortic incompetence, palpable aneurysms and impalpable pulses are less frequently observed. On investigation chest radiography may be of value but aortography is required to define the site and extent of the lesions. Intravenous pyelography may reveal a shrunken kidney if a renal artery is stenosed.

Treatment

No medical treatment has been shown to be of value. Unilateral nephrectomy has been performed with success in several cases with renal artery stenosis and surgical repair or replacement of damaged arteries has been advocated and employed with varying degrees of success. The natural history of the disorder is obscure but once diagnosed, the prognosis is limited unless surgery is attempted.

ANNULAR SUBVALVULAR LEFT VENTRICULAR
ANEURYSMS

Aneurysms of the left ventricle, unless they are secondary to disease of the coronary arteries, are extremely unusual. In Nigeria, however, this is a not uncommon cardiac lesion and it has been recognised in South Africa and in Uganda.

SYNONYMS. Cardiac aneurysm of unknown cause.

Definition

An aneurysm occurring just below the aortic and/or the mitral valve and with no established aetiology.

Aetiology

In most reports the aneurysm is believed to be due to a congenital defect in the ventricular wall in the region of the atrioventricular groove. Tuberculosis and rheumatic heart disease have also been incriminated as causal factors and several cases have occurred in association with endomyocardial fibrosis.

The most recent attempt to ascribe some aetiology other than that of congenital weakness to this unusual phenomenon arises from a detailed study of a young Congolese boy with a diffuse panaortitis, focal aneurysms of the aorta and right subclavian artery and a focal granulomatous myocarditis and pericarditis. One area of granulomatous myocarditis corresponded to the location of the aneurysm described in Nigeria and elsewhere, with invagination of the endocardium surrounded by inflammation and the authors regard the myocarditis as a possible cause of endemic ventricular aneurysms (Roberts and Wibin, 1966).

Epidemiology and distribution

The disorder has been described from Nigeria, South Africa, Uganda and the Congo.

Pathology

These aneurysms occur just below the aortic and the mitral valves and the aneurysmal cavities extend in the substance of the fibrous ring to which the valves are attached. The aneurysms are usually single and the margins of the opening are surrounded by dense fibrous tissue which is sometime calcified. A large aneurysm will stretch and narrow the circumflex branch of the left coronary artery and lead to myocardial ischaemia. For some reason (possibly previous myocarditis), the heart itself is usually large even in the presence of a very small aneurysm, and dense adhesions may be present between the aneurysm and the overlying pericardium. Histologically the appearances suggest a herniation of the endocardium into the wall of the heart with the subsequent deposition of fibrous tissue in the region.

Symptomatology

Most of the cases described have presented in cardiac failure, some few are found on routine radiographic examination and in the remainder the aneurysm is an autopsy finding following the sudden onset of severe left-sided cardiac failure and death. The subjects are usually males aged 20–40 years.

Diagnosis

The condition of *submitral aneurysm* should be suspected in an indigenous inhabitant of a tropical region, with mitral incompetence, cardiomegaly and a localised bulge on the left cardiac border on radiological examination. There may be a double impulse over the left ventricle produced by the aneurysm filling in ventricular systole. The diagnosis should particularly be considered if the electrocardiogram shows evidence of myocardial ischaemia. The bulge on the left cardiac border may show calcification. Systolic pulsation on fluoroscopy and opacification on ventriculography will confirm the diagnosis.

The diagnosis of *subaortic aneurysm* is virtually impossible to make in life. The presence in a young indigenous African subject of aortic incompetence associated with electrocardiographic evidence of myocardial ischaemia or infarction in the absence of syphilitic aortitis or bacterial endocarditis could perhaps raise the possibility of this diagnosis.

Treatment

There is no effective medical therapy and the few cases treated surgically have not done well. If we keep in mind the fact that the heart is almost always considerably enlarged even with small aneurysms, we are confronted with the likelihood that this is probably not a congenital lesion capable of repair but a more generalised cardiac disorder in which repair of the aneurysm may not improve the overall prognosis.

Prognosis

This is poor with a steady downhill course.

ABNORMAL ELECTROCARDIOGRAM IN
HEALTHY SUBJECTS

Littman (1946) was the first to draw attention to the fact that diphasic or inverted T waves in the praecordial leads occurred more frequently in the adult American Negro than in adult American white subjects. This finding was more common in Negro women, 4 per cent of whom had an inverted T wave in V4 while 1 per cent of the Negro males and no white subjects showed this change. Littman regarded this phenomenon as a persistence of the 'juvenile pattern', for most children have acquired upright T waves in the chest leads by the middle teens. He observed that these changes were variable over time but could suggest no adequate reason for the persistence of this juvenile pattern.

Since Littman's original observations, a number of reports have come from Africa describing the electrocardiographic patterns in African subjects and while none of these reports

have ever suggested that the peculiarities indicate organic diseases of the heart, a number of investigators concerned with the study of cardiomyopathies in African subjects, have tried to compare and relate these patterns to those found in various cardiac disorders in Africa.

The patterns of abnormality encountered fall into two main groups:

Pattern A. Inverted T waves in the praecordial leads, these being deeply inverted and occurring mainly in the right ventricular surface leads. This change is commonly seen in V1 and V2 and occurs in V3 and V4 in less than 5 per cent of African

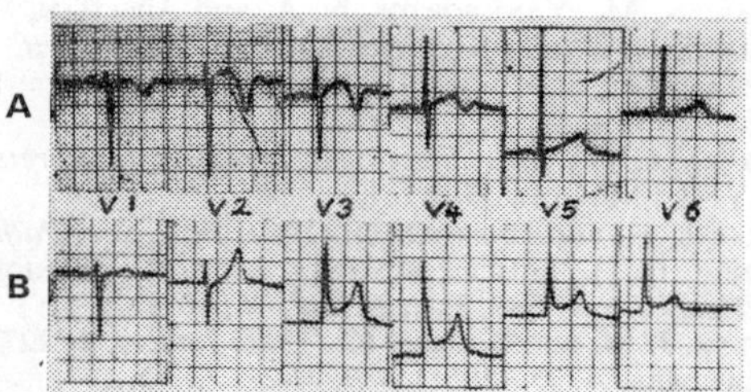

FIG. 35.3. *Abnormal electrocardiograms in healthy subjects.* (*From* Powell, S. J., *Brit Heart J.,* 1959, vol. 21, p. 263—*reproduced by permission.*)

subjects. It seems that females are more affected than males, as in Littman's original observations.

Pattern B. S-T segment elevation and tall T waves in the praecordial leads mainly affecting left ventricular surface leads and occurring far more frequently in males than in females.

Both these patterns show a striking day-to-day spontaneous variability and respond markedly to exercise, respiration, various drugs and to physical interference, strongly suggesting that they are functional in nature. The fact that these changes are also seen in some white subjects, and that when encountered in them, they respond to various stimuli in the same manner as they do in Negro subjects, suggests that this 'persistence of the juvenile pattern' is not a racial phenomenon and that it may be related to some environmentally induced factors.

In Mexico, the juvenile T-wave pattern is commonly seen until the age of 40 or 50 years and again more frequently in the female (Cabrera, 1963). In a study of the electrocardiogram in some North Indian population groups it is reported that 'Grusin's anomaly' was present in about 1 per cent of subjects, but they do not define their findings (Padmavati and Sandhu, 1964). In a study in South India, ST and T wave changes were even more frequent, occurring in some 10 per cent of subjects, but again no details are available (Srikantia *et al*, 1964).

It is important that those studying cardiovascular problems in underdeveloped or tropical countries be aware of these peculiarities and in particular, aware of their variability over a period of time. While their nature remains obscure, and one would hesitate to suggest that they may be nutritional in origin, there seems no evidence to link them with any of the tropical cardiomyopathies.

REFERENCES

AKBARIAN, M., YANKPORTOS, N. A. and ABELMAN, W. H. (1966) *Amer. J. Med.*, **41**, 197.

BEDFORD, D. E. and KONSTAM, G. L. S. (1946) *Brit. Heart J.*, **8**, 236.

BERTRAND, E., SENTILHES, L., DUCASSE, B., VACHER, P. and BAUDIN, L. (1965) *Med. trop. (Marseilles)*, **25**, 603.

BLANKENHORN, M. A. (1955) *Circulation*, **11**, 288.

CABRERA, E. (1963) In *Electrocardiographic Interpretation*, ed. Hurst, J. W. and Wenger, N. K., p. 70. New York: McGraw-Hill.

COLLOMB, H. and BARTOLI, D. (1967) *Bull. Soc. Path. exot.*, **60**, 142.

CONNOR, D. H., SOMERS, K. HUTT, M. S. R., MANION, W. C. and D'ARBELA, P. G. (1967, 1968) Part 1. *Amer. Heart J.*, 74, 687; Part II *ibid*, 75, 107.

FOWLER, J. M. and SOMERS, K. (1968) *Lancet*, **1**, 227.

GILLANDERS, A. D. (1951) *Brit. Heart J.*, **13**, 177.

HAWKING, F. and GREENFIELD, J. G. (1941) *Trans. roy. Soc. trop. Med. Hyg.*, **35**, 155.

LAVIER, G. and LEROUX, R. (1939) *Bull. Soc. Path. exot.*, **32**, 927.

LITTMAN, D. (1946) *Amer. Heart J.*, **32**, 370.

MANSON-BAHR, P. E. C. and CHARTERS, A. D. (1963) *Trans. roy. Soc. Trop. Med. Hyg.*, **57**, 119.

PADMAVATI, S. and SANDHU, I. (1964) *Proc. 3rd Asian Congr. Cardiol.*, **1**, 26.

RAADT, P. DE and KOTEN, J. W. (1968).

ROBERTS, W. C. and WIBIN, E. A. (1966) *Amer. J. Med.*, **41**, 453.

SRIKANTIA, S. G., PADMAVATI, S. and GOPELAN, C. (1964) *Circulation*, **29**, 118.

FURTHER READING

General

SHAPER, A. G. (1967) On the nature of some tropical cardiomyopathies. *Trans. roy. Soc. trop. Med. Hyg.*, **61**, 458.

SHAPER, A. G. ed. (1968) *Introduction to the Cardiomyopathies*. Basel: Karger. (*Cardiologia*, Vol. 52, No. 1-2, 1968.)

SHAPER, A. G. (1972) Cardiovascular disease in the tropics. *Brit. med. J.*, **3**, 683-686, 743-746, 805-807.

STAMLER, J. (1967) *Lectures on Preventive Cardiology*. New York: Grune and Stratton, Inc.

WORLD HEALTH ORGANIZATION (1965) Cardiomyopathies. Report of a W.H.O. meeting, Kampala 1965. *Bull. Wld Hlth Org.*, **33**, 257.

—— (1967) The Cardiomyopathies. Report of a W.H.O. meeting, New Delhi 1966. *W.H.O. Chronicle*, **21**, 407.

—— (1968) Idiopathic cardiomegaly. Report of a W.H.O. meeting, Jamaica 1967. *Bull. Wld Hlth Org.*, **38**, 979.

Hypertension and hypertensive heart disease

AKINKUGBE, O. O. (1972) *High Blood Pressure in the African*. London: Churchill Livingstone.

SHAPER, A. G. ed. (1969) Symposium on blood pressure and hypertension in Africa. *E. Afr. Med. J.*, **46**, 5.

STAMLER, J., STAMLER, R. and PULLMAN, T. N. (1967) *The Epidemiology of Hypertension*. New York: Grune and Stratton.

Pulmonary heart disease

CAVALCANTI, I. DE L., TOMPSON, G., DE SOUZA, N. and BARBOSA, F. S. (1962) Pulmonary hypertension in schistosomiasis. *Brit. Heart J.*, **24**, 363.

EL MOFTY, A. (1962) Clinical aspects of bilharziasis. *Bilharziasis: Ciba Foundation Symposium*, ed. Wolstenholme, G. E. W. and O'Connor, M., pp. 174-195. London: Churchill.

PADMAVATI, S. S. and PATHAK, S. N. (1959) Chronic cor pulmonale in Delhi. *Circulation*, **20**, 343.

Endomyocardial fibrosis

PARRY, E. H. O. and ABRAHAMS, D. G. (1965) The natural history of endomyocardial fibrosis. *Quart. J. Med.*, **34**, 383.

SOMERS, K., BRENTON, D. P., D'ARBELA, P. G., FOWLER, J. M., KANYEREZI, B. R. and SOOD, N. K. (1968) Haemodynamic features of severe endomyocardial fibrosis of the right ventricle including a comparison with constrictive pericarditis. *Brit. Heart J.*, **30**, 322.

SOMERS, K., BRENTON, D. P. and SOOD, N. K. (1968) Clinical features of endomyocardial fibrosis of the right ventricle. *Brit. Heart J.*, **30**, 309.

SOMERS, K., D'ARBELA, P. G. and PATEL, A. K. (1972) Endomyocardial fibrosis. *Medicine in a Tropical Environment*, ed. Shaper, A. G., Kibukamusoke, J. W. and Hutt, M. S. R., p. 348. London: British Medical Association.

Idiopathic cardiomegaly

BENGTSSON, E. and LAMBERGER, B. (1966) Acute myocarditis. Five-year follow-up study of cases. *Amer. Heart J.*, **72**, 751.

BURCH, G. E. and DePASQUALE, N. P. (1968) *Heart Muscle Disease. Disease-a-Month*, May 1968. Chicago: Year Book Medical Publishers.

DYE, C. L., ROSENBAUM, D., LOWE, J. C., BEHRIKE, R. H. and GENOVESE, P. D. (1963) Primary myocardial disease. *Ann. intern. Med.*, **58**, 426, 442.

EDINGTON, G. M. and JACKSON, J. G. (1963) The pathology of heart muscle disease and endomyocardial fibrosis in Nigeria. *J. Path. Bact.*, **86**, 333.

FODOR, J., MIALL, W. E., STANDARD, K. L., FEJFAR, Z. and STUART, K. L. (1964) Myocardial disease in a rural population in Jamaica. *Bull. Wld Hlth Org.*, **31**, 321.

HIGGINSON, J., ISAACSON, C. and SIMSON, I. (1960) The pathology of cryptogenic heart disease. *Arch. Path.*, **70**, 497.

MASSUMI, R. A., RIOS, J. C., GOOCH, A. S., NUTTER, D., DE VITA, V. T. and DATLOW, D. W. (1965) Primary myocardial disease. *Circulation*, **31**, 19.

SHAPER, A. G. (1968) Cardiomegaly of unknown origin in South Africa. *Trop. geog. Med.*, **20**, 291.

STEIN, H., SHNIER, M. H., WAYBURNE, S. and ISAACSON, C. (1964) Cardiomyopathy in African children. *Arch. Dis. Child.*, **39**, 610.

STUART, K. L. and HAYES, J. A. (1963) A cardiac disorder of unknown aetiology in Jamaica. *Quart. J. Med.*, **32**, 99.

Peripartal cardiomyopathy

BROCKINGTON, I. F. (1971) Postpartum hypertensive heart failure. *Amer. J. Cardiol.*, **27**, 650.

MEADOWS, W. R. (1960) Postpartum heart disease. *Amer. J. Cardiol.*, **6**, 788.

REID, J. V. O. (1961) Post-partal cardiomyopathy. *S. Afr. med. J.*, **35**, 165.

SEFTEL, H. and SUSSER, M. (1961) Maternity and myocardial failure in African women. *Brit. Heart J.*, **23**, 43.

STUART, K. L. (1968) Cardiomyopathy of pregnancy and the puerperium. *Quart. J. Med.*, **37**, 463.

WALSH, J. J., BURCH, G. E., BLACK, W. C., FERRANS, V. J., and HIBBS, R. G. (1965) Idiopathic myocardiopathy of the puerperium (post-partal heart disease). *Circulation*, **32**, 19.

Alcoholic heart disease

ALEXANDER, C. S. (1966) Idiopathic heart disease. An analysis of 100 cases with special reference to chronic alcoholism. *Amer. J. Med.*, **41**, 213.

EVANS, W. (1966) Alcohol and the heart. *Practitioner*, **196**, 238.

FERRANS, V. J. (1966) Alcoholic cardiomyopathy. *Amer. J. med. Sci.*, **252**, 89.

PRIEST, R. G., BINNS, J. K. and KITCHIN, A. H. (1966) Electrocardiogram in alcoholism and accompanying physical disease. *Brit. med. J.*, **1**, 1453.

Trypanosomal heart diseases

KÖBERLE, F. (1963) Enteromegaly and cardiomegaly in Chagas' disease. *Gut*, **4**, 399.

LARANJA, F. S., DIAS, E., NOBREGA, G. B. and MIRANDA, A. (1965) Chagas' disease. A clinical, epidemiologic and pathologic study. *Circulation*, **14**, 1035.

MOTT, K. E. and HAGSTROM, J. W. C. (1965) The pathologic lesions of the cardiac autonomic nervous system in chronic Chagas' myocarditis. *Circulation*, **2**, 175.

PUIGBO, J. J., NAVA-RHODE, J. R., GARCIA BARRIOS, H., SUAREZ, J. A. and GIL YEPEZ, C. (1966) Clinical and epidemiological study of Chagas' chronic involvement. *Bull. Wld Hlth Org.*, **34**, 655.

ROSENBAUM, M. B. (1964) Chagasic myocardiomyopathy. *Prog. cardiovasc. Dis.*, **7**, 199.

WORLD HEALTH ORGANISATION (1960) Study group on Chagas' disease. *Techn. Rep. Ser.*, 202.

—— (1965) Chagas' Disease in Brazil (prepared by Davies, J. N. P. and Fejfar, Z.). RES 4/10 Pan-American Health Organisation/W.H.O., Washington D.C.

Obliterative arteritis

ABRAHAMS, D. G. and PARRY, E. H. O. (1962) Hypertension due to renal artery stenosis caused by abdominal aortic aneurysm. *Circulation*, **26**, 104.

DANARAJ, T. T., WONG, H. O. and THOMAS, M. A. (1965) Primary arteritis of aorta causing renal artery stenosis and hypertension. *Brit. Heart J.*, **25**, 155.

HUDSON, R. E. B. (1965) Other arterial diseases. *Cardiovascular Pathology*, p. 531. London: Edward Arnold.

ISAACSON, C. (1961) An idiopathic arteritis in young Africans. *J. Path. Bact.*, **81**, 69.

PATON, B. C., CHARTIKAVARIJ, K., BURI, P., PRACHUABMOH, K. and JUMBULA, M. R. B. (1965) Obliterative aortic disease in children in the tropics. *Circulation*, **31**, Supp. I, 197.

SEN, P. K., KINARE, S. G., ENGINEER, S. D. and PARULKAR, G. B. (1963) The middle aortic syndrome. *Brit. Heart J.*, **25**, 610.

Ventricular aneurysms

ABRAHAMS, D. G., BARTON, C. J., COCKSHOTT, W. P., EDINGTON, G. M. and WEAVER, E. J. M. (1962) Annular subvalvular left ventricular aneurysms. *Quart. J. Med.*, **31**, 345.

CHESLER, E., JOFFE, N., SCHAMROTH, L. and MEYERS, A. (1965) Annular subvalvular left ventricular aneurysms in the South African Bantu. *Circulation*, **32**, 43.

COCKSHOTT, W. P., ANTIA, A., IKEME, A. and UZODIKE, V. O. (1967) Annular subvalvular LV aneurysms. *Brit. J. Radiol.*, **40**, 425.

ROBERTS, W. C. and WIBIN, E. A. (1966) Idiopathic panaortitis, supra-aortic arteritis, granulomatous myocarditis and pericarditis. *Amer. J. Med.*, **41**, 453.

ROBERTSON, J. H. and JACKSON, J. G. (1960) Cardiac aneurysms in Nigeria. *J. Path. Bact.*, **80**, 101.

SCHRIRE, V. and BARNARD, C. N. (1963) The surgical cure of a cardiac aneurysm of unknown cause. *J. cardiovasc. Surg.*, **4**, 5.

Electrocardiographic abnormalities

BRINK, A. J. (1956) The normal electrocardiogram in the adult South African Bantu. *S. Afr. J. lab. clin. Med.*, **2**, 97.

GRUSIN, H. (1954) Peculiarities of the African's electrocardiogram and the changes observed in serial studies. *Circulation*, **9**, 860.

POWELL, S. J. (1959) Unexplained electrocardiograms in the African. *Brit. Heart J.*, **21**, 263.

SERIKI, O. and SMITH, A. J. (1966) The electrocardiogram of young Nigerians. *Amer. Heart J.*, **72**, 153.

SOMERS, K. and RANKIN, A. M. (1962) The electrocardiogram in healthy East African (Bantu and Nilotic men). *Brit. Heart J.*, **24**, 542.

SWANEPOEL, A., SMYTHE, P. M. and CAMPBELL, J. A. H. (1964) The heart in kwashiorkor. *Amer. Heart J.*, **67**, 1.

TURNER, P. P. (1959) The electrocardiogram in fifty normal young adult Kikuyu males. *E. Afr. med. J.*, **36**, 555.

36
Psychiatry in the Tropics

INTRODUCTION

It has been known for years that psychiatric illness of all sorts forms a substantial part of medical practice in the tropics. The main emphasis used to be on the problem of the European expatriate living and working abroad, but more recently the psychiatric illnesses of the local inhabitants of tropical areas have received more attention. Since 1960 an increasing amount of work has been done on psychiatric illnesses in urbanised and rural tropical populations, and it is now possible to give some sort of picture of these and how they differ from the manifestations of psychiatric illness in Europeans.

EPIDEMIOLOGY

In attempting to find out the true psychiatric morbidity in any group of people, many problems are encountered, the main one being that of diagnosis, for each practitioner uses marginally different criteria for any illness. A psychiatrist, for instance, will more readily diagnose psychiatric illness than will a physician, who tends to be preoccupied with organic illness. Shepherd *et al* (1960), in a study of psychiatric morbidity in outpatients attending at a London hospital, showed that 3·4 per cent of all patients seen were referred for a psychiatric opinion, but when a full-time psychiatrist was available the number diagnosed as being psychiatrically disturbed rose to between 38 and 51 per cent. These diagnostic discrepancies are also apparent in other studies, and many different figures have been obtained. Pearson and Pennell (1938) found 16 per cent of new admissions to a general hospital to be psychiatrically ill, and Pemberton in 1951, studying a similar population, found 11 per cent. Helsborg (1958), a psychiatrist, gives a figure of 22 per cent of a consecutive series of 500 admissions to hospital as psychiatrically ill. Rowland Hill (1943) found 10 per cent of neurotic illness in expatriates seen at a tropical unit.

Obviously, more standardised criteria for diagnosis are needed before really reliable figures for any populations are reached. One recent advance in this direction has been by Goldberg (1970), who has produced a simple questionnaire which measures the degree of 'illness' present in any patient, the results of which can be checked against the findings of a clinical psychiatrist.

Certain points are, however, generally known about the incidence of psychiatric illness in the tropics:

1. Neurotic illness seems to be far more prevalent among those people who are in an alien cultural environment.
2. There are no real differences in total incidence of psychiatric disease between endemic populations all over the world.
3. The type of psychiatric symptomatology seen differs widely between the different races and cultures.

CLASSIFICATION

There is widespread controversy over the classification of psychiatric illness at present, ranging from those who see definite, separate disease entities into which all manifestations can be fitted to those who see no such rigid demarcation and consider it would be better simply to make a distinction between those who are ill and those who are not. A similar argument is present over the aetiology of psychiatric illness. One extreme school considers that all illness is organically based, and that organic or biochemical reasons for it will come to light given enough painstaking research, while others put more emphasis on social, environmental and constitutional factors, and tend to deny or overlook the organic factors. A simple classification is what is needed here, and the most useful one would be to divide psychiatric illness into two main groups.

1. **Organic disease**, where an organic cause for the disturbance exists and can be demonstrated.
2. **Functional disease.** No such cause is discernible. Functional disease may be subdivided into two further categories:

(*a*) *Psychotic illness* where a cause for an acutely disturbed pattern of behaviour is not to be found in the patient's background, and it is generally accepted that he is not in touch with reality—two main examples are schizophrenia and manic depressive psychosis.

(*b*) *Neurotic illness*, which can be seen as an abnormal extension of what is a normal defence mechanism and as such, of course, has its roots in the patient's personality. Examples of these conditions are anxiety states, reactive depression, obsessional and hysterical illnesses.

In the light of this simple classification, the various syndromes as they are seen in different populations in the tropics, and some predisposing causes will now be considered.

council estate dwellers who showed one or more major psychiatric symptoms (Martin *et al*, 1957), or Shepherd's (1960) study of medical outpatients, 38 per cent of whom were judged to be disturbed there are no major differences in total morbidity.

German and Arya (1969) studied various student populations at Makerere University College, East Africa, 1966–67. His results were compared with similar figures from Edinburgh and Belfast Universities (Kidd and Caldbeck-Meenan, 1966), and the overall illness rate is similar in all (Table 36.1).

The slight preponderance of psychotic illness amongst the Africans should be noted. Otherwise, however, there seem to be few differences. Short-lived psychotic reactions seem more prevalent among Africans, who more often react to stress in a psychotic way than do Caucasian groups.

TABLE 36.1. *Comparison of student populations*

	Total morbidity	Psychoses	Neuroses	Personality disorders
Makerere University	10.8%	6.7%	85.9%	7.4%
Edinburgh University	11.6%	4.6%	90.2%	5.2%
Belfast University	10.2%	2.0%	91.0%	7.0%

PSYCHIATRIC DISORDERS IN AFRICANS

Many believe that psychiatric illness is rare in rural tribalised Africans, and is only seen in urban populations where the traditional patterns of communal and religious life have been disrupted and where there are the new stresses of developed countries, poor relationships, lack of communication and intense competition. In fact, recent work in East and West Africa suggests that this is not so, and that psychiatric illness is at least as prevalent in rural Africa as it is in Western Europe. Geil and Van Luijk (1969), working in Ethiopia in a rural health centre, give a psychiatric morbidity figure of 19.5 per cent of patients seen being psychiatrically disturbed. Annual consultation rate was 14.8 per cent. This compares with Shepherd's figure of 13.9 per cent for a group of practices in London (Shepherd *et al*, 1966). Lambo, who has made extensive studies of psychiatric illness among the Yoruba of Nigeria (Leighton, Lambo *et al*, 1963), states that 42 per cent of the general population show at least one major psychiatric symptom. When compared with Martin's figure of 35 per cent of English

German also noted that most Ugandans presented with somatic complaints. This is also confirmed by Wilson (1973) in studies on Africans at the Hospital for Tropical Diseases, London. Common symptoms being chest pains, headaches and general aches and pains—some very bizarre.

In studying the effects of urbanisation on Africans various factors common to all developed urban communities must be noted. Firstly, towns containing hospitals attract psychiatrically disturbed patients seeking treatment. Secondly, disturbed people naturally seem to gravitate to towns and therefore towns seem to have more sick people. Thirdly, in urban society, people who do not conform are more likely to be ostracised and pushed into a 'sick' category, thus reaching the doctor, whereas in a rural community they might merely be considered eccentric.

SYMPTOMATOLOGY IN AFRICANS

Organic disease

This is extremely common in Africa. Lamont and Bignault (1953) report that 40 per cent of admissions to a South African mental hospital were suffering from organic states; 10.7 per cent of the admissions were from mental subnormality. German and Arya (1969) state that in Uganda in 1967 46 per cent of patients were in this category. Furthermore, 75 per cent of these were below 40 years old. In Europe, of course, exactly the reverse is true, the majority of organic states being in the over-60 age group, and being caused mainly by degenerative conditions. The acute and chronic brain syndromes seen in Africans are similar to those in any other racial group but often acutely disturbed behaviour is sparked off by seemingly trivial systemic disturbances. Altered consciousness is often seen in these episodes. Whether this is a response to stress or a true organic state is unclear, as the reason is seldom found. Most acute organic states are found in association with alcoholism in Africans, and these are very much more common than they are with Europeans. The whole cultural background of alcoholism differs. Africans tend to regard alcohol as a potent strengthener and aphrodisiac, and brew up very strong and lethal potions for this and also as a specific remedy against various tropical diseases. Furthermore, there is little moral censorship over drunkenness, and the toxic and long-term side-effects of alcohol are not understood. Children, too, tend to indulge in heavy drinking from an early age. Hypoglycaemia is also a factor which occurs with alcoholism in Africans and this increases brain damage. Europeans tend more to drink to allay clinical anxiety or increase social contact, and alcohol is not considered in the same magical therapeutic light. Delirium tremens is very common in Africans. Other common causes of organic states include viral and bacterial meningitis, malaria, syphilis and typhoid. Fifty-seven per cent of a sample of typhoid patients from University College Hospital, Ibadan, Nigeria, 1972 presented with a typical acute toxic confusional state (Osunokun *et al*, 1972). Chronic brain syndromes occur, but are far commoner in Europeans. The most common cause in Africans would appear to be syphilitic. This was the state of affairs in nineteenth-century Britain.

Functional diseases

PSYCHOSES. Schizophrenia in Africans has been extensively studied by Lambo (1968) and is common. There does not seem to be any marked difference in symptomatology between schizophrenia in Africa and in developed countries and it occurs at all levels in the community. However,

schizophreniform psychoses are also common. These are psychotic illnesses of sudden onset, characterised by florid hallucinations and delusions and extreme behavioural disturbances. Hallucinations are often visual (this is unusual for schizophrenia) and concern wild animals chasing the patient. There are often delusions with religious or magical content. The condition usually subsides quickly and there is no residual personality defect as is found in true schizophrenia. The prognosis is good. Schizophreniform psychoses are often seen among West Africans and West Indians in British psychiatric units. It is generally thought to be 'crisis behaviour' caused by changes in cultural patterns. Lambo (1968) points out that it is commoner in illiterate people, and my own observations confirm this. Rarely, a schizophreniform psychosis without obvious organic elements such as a disturbance of consciousness can occur in Africans as a result of a relatively minor infection with typhoid fever. In the above-mentioned study of 959 cases (Osunokun *et al*, 1972) of typhoid fever, seven presented with schizophrenic symptoms.

Manic depressive illness is also common in Africans. Contrary to the patterns seen in Europe, it is mania that occurs most frequently. Most authors report that mania is three times as common as depression in African patients. It may well be that this pattern of behaviour is far more 'mad' than the withdrawal of the depressive phase, which therefore goes unnoticed. Suicidal attempts among Africans are rare. German (1972) reports that in outpatient work just as much depression is seen as in Europe, and this usually masquerades as physical illness. There is no marked difference between the symptomatology of manic depressive psychosis in Europeans and Africans. Depression is far more often complained of amongst urbanised Africans than in the illiterate rural population, but the physical concomitants of apathy, anorexia and sleep disturbances seem to be common to all. Paranoid delusions, and those of guilt seem to be rare in Africans, and again only occur in those with a literate, urban background.

NEUROSES. *Anxiety states*. These are common at all levels in Africans, and anxiety is usually found to be fixed to a certain area of the body, depending on the nature of the complaint. For instance, a man worried about his fertility is likely to present with a pain in the penis or perineum; his anxiety will be fixed to this and he will worry that something dreadful has happened to it. Africans seldom present with non-fixed, i.e. free-floating, anxiety.

2P

Hysterical states (which will be more fully discussed with reference to Europeans) also occur frequently and are found to be more common among the unsophisticated African. African students studying in Europe are especially prone to neurotic illness, and their particular problems should be mentioned here. Several excellent papers have been written on this aspect of African psychiatry, notably by Hertzberg (1964), who stresses the importance of understanding the African's attitude to European life. He arrives to study and is often disillusioned. There are firstly the problems of learning. Often having been considered clever in their own countries, some students find they are not equal to the standard of work required to gain their qualifications. In addition to this, there are the problems of communication and language, accommodation, loneliness and racial prejudice. Most Africans are used to group living and the isolation common in European cities is a great problem to them. To return home without the qualification would be extremely difficult as it means a good job in the parent country and often the hopes of the family are at stake. Furthermore, the student is one of a greatly favoured minority chosen by, and financed by, the government and is expected to succeed. He presents to the doctor with a physical complaint, thus avoiding the need to take the dreaded examination and possibly failing it. Although this pattern of symptom presentation is hysterical, there is often a strong depressive element in it which can be treated, and if support and understanding are forthcoming the student will more often than not succeed in his quest. Hertzberg (1964) stresses that the essential difference between Africans and Europeans in the handling of stress is that the European intellectualises it and can say to himself 'I am depressed', whereas the African tends to internalise the concept which is then dealt with as a somatic feeling, so he says 'I have a pain in the chest' rather than 'I'm so depressed my heart aches'!

Case history No. 1

Patient Aged 24. Origin—West Africa. Time of residence in Britain—6 months.

This young man was admitted complaining of severe abdominal pain for four years. For 6 months prior to admission he also complained of dyspnoea, dizziness, extreme tiredness and alternating constipation and diarrhoea. He had an uneventful early life, worked hard at school, managed to pass his 'A' levels and won a government scholarship to study surveying in Britain.

His abdominal pain first started when he was working for his 'A' levels but worsened after his arrival in Britain. This is when his other symptoms began. He had eight brothers at home and he was the youngest. On further questioning it transpired that he could not concentrate, sleep was affected, he was always tired and had lost his appetite. Since starting his course six months previously he had spent most of the time attending various hospitals for investigation. He explained that it was only his abdominal pain which prevented him from concentrating and from succeeding in his work. His tutor at the technical college, who was in contact with the hospital, stated that in his view the patient was not really up to the course.

Like so many West Africans, this man was unable to conceptualise his problems and expressed them as physical symptoms. It was too much for him to face the fact that he might not succeed at his work. Clearly to return to West Africa without his qualification would mean considerable 'loss of face' for him and his family, and so he sheltered behind his physical symptoms which prevented him from working and also from possible failure in his final exams. Most of his symptoms were depressive in origin, and examination of his mental state showed him to be depressed although he could not admit this.

He was treated with a course of tricyclic antidepressants which improved the depressive symptoms considerably but left him with shortness of breath and mild abdominal pain. He was, however, able to return to work in spite of the symptoms, and succeeded finally in obtaining his qualification.

PSYCHIATRIC ILLNESS IN ASIANS

The migration of peoples from India and Pakistan to Western Europe has gathered momentum in recent years, so it is as well to add something on their problems here. As is the case with Africans, these Asians tend to show a similar incidence of psychotic and neurotic illness. They are largely urbanised when living either in Africa and Europe, and most illness is contained within the very strict family circle, which is all embracing. Organic illness, especially due to alcoholism, is far less common than in Africans, but hysterical illness is even more prevalent, and especially the crude acting out with florid hysterical symptoms. Language and communication problems are even more acute than with Africans. Depression is common, but as with Africans, usually hides behind a physical symptomatology. Complaints such as faintness, dizziness, sweating attacks, nausea and abdominal pain are seen and are, it seems, commoner in women than in men. Asian customs seem to clash far more with those of the west than do African customs, and much illness is caused by this, especially in young people who fall between the two cultural patterns. Arranged marriages are still the rule in India and it is common for a girl of 18 to be sent to Europe to marry a man she has never seen. Breakdown under these conditions is frequent.

Case history No. 2

Miss M. Aged 21. Country of origin—India. Time of residence in Britain—14 months.

This girl was admitted to the Hospital for Tropical Diseases, London, for the investigation of roundworms. She was from a low-caste Indian family and was sent to Britain from India 14 months before admission to marry her first cousin whom she had not seen since she was 13 years old. She married him within a month of her arrival and became pregnant soon afterwards. At the time of admission her baby was 9 weeks old. Her first symptoms appeared in August 1970 and consisted of muteness, stiffness of the arms and legs, hyperventilation attacks, and many hours of lying on her bed with her eyes flickering and arms twitching.

This worried her family considerably. She went out very seldom but when her husband did take her out she fainted. The symptoms cleared up spontaneously after 2 months but recurred 3 months later and continued up to and after admission.

She and her husband lived with 12 other members of the family in an east London tenement where they had one room. Her in-laws looked after the house. Her husband was indifferent to her, and her only interest in life was the baby. She spoke no English and had made no attempt to learn it, consequently she was quite isolated.

A diagnosis of hysterical acting out was made and the course of the illness in hospital was similar to that seen at home. She showed no emotion and no anxiety about her symptoms but she got considerable primary and secondary gain from them. Unfortunately all communications with her took place through an interpreter but she would say nothing about her problems except, 'If God wills it I am happy'. This was in fact a typical Indian woman's reaction to circumstances like this. She would never betray her family or her husband by showing her feelings and would obey him at all times.

She was put in the hands of an Indian social worker who did a good deal of work with the family and eventually persuaded her husband to take her and the baby back home to India, at least for a little while. On her discharge from hospital there were no further symptoms.

PSYCHIATRIC ILLNESS IN EUROPEANS IN THE TROPICS

As early as 1940 Manson-Bahr's textbook of tropical diseases stated that 'as a cause of invaliding home from the tropics, neurasthenia now exceeds tropical illness'. Certainly Europeans in the tropics are especially at risk. In the old days, a condition called 'tropical neurasthenia' was diagnosed. There are all sorts of descriptions of this. Rowland Hill (1943) and Cook (1945) give a depressive picture with the emphasis on bad dreams, withdrawal from society and anxiety, whereas Cilento (1933) felt that it was mainly a manic depressive illness. Cameron (1949), writing about Royal Navy personnel in the tropics, described a paranoid type of neurotic illness. Clearly the topic needs clarification.

The manifestation of psychiatric illness in the tropics depends greatly on the personalities of the people who go and serve there, and of course on the ability of those people to adapt to the particular stresses of the tropics. It is certainly true that stress factors in the tropics are vastly greater than those found in temperate regions and are especially telling on those people who are not equipped to deal with life in the environment, which requires adaptation on both emotional and physical levels.

Obviously not all people who go abroad suffer from psychiatric illnesses. It is the people who show obsessional personality traits who tend to be the most prone to psychiatric disorders. In a study carried out in 1971 at the Hospital for Tropical Diseases, London, those patients referred for psychiatric opinion and treatment were markedly more obsessional than those who were not (Wilson, 1973). They also tended to show more anxiety, more depression, and have more difficulties with authority figures than a normal population. The study also showed an overall morbidity of 45 per cent in a sample of 208 consecutive admissions to the hospital.

Obsessional patterns of behaviour are recognised psychoanalytically to be a defence against anxiety, and anxiety itself can similarly be said to arise from a conflict over the handling of aggression, which cannot be tolerated in consciousness and is repressed, only to appear as anxiety.

It seems that one of the ways of attempting to escape from oneself is to move frequently. Hence the flight to overseas jobs lasting to 2–5 years of many disturbed people who see the tropics as an escape from themselves. It may also be an escape from restrictive authority for those whose aggressive problems make it difficult for them to work in a more structured environment. The tropics offers them a chance to 'do their own thing'. Alas, they are very much more prone to break down when things go against them (see Case History No. 3).

A third group are those in missionary work, who seek to protect themselves from their own feelings by throwing themselves into helping others. They may break down for many reasons, especially isolation and overwork, and tend to be rigid and unyielding. It should be added that those workers in the missionary and V.S.O. fields who have learned about themselves before taking up this work are probably the most stable group of Europeans abroad.

The final group, and one which increases in size yearly, are those sent overseas by their companies or who go abroad because they are unlikely to gain promotion at home. Furthermore, tropical service has financial advantages. They are frequently unable to express their feelings about being 'trapped' abroad. To return home for them would be to risk unemployment, as they have lost their niche in the career structure at home. Often, people who are awkward at home tend to be offered overseas posts to get them away from head office.

Many of the patients who break down under tropical conditions have a past history of symptoms under stress. Of 151 patients referred for psychiatric opinion over 18 months at the Hospital for Tropical Diseases, 47.5 per cent had a previous history of psychiatric symptoms (Wilson, 1973). The majority of them were married and had been more than 5 years continuously in the tropics.

Case history No. 3

Mr C. Aged 32. British. Abroad 5 years—in Tanzania and Burma.

This man was admitted to the Hospital for Tropical Diseases for investigation of diarrhoea which had been severe for 3 years. No organic cause was found. After admission, however, he was found to be a heavy drinker, but he would not admit this despite drinking approximately one bottle of whisky a day.

He was one of five children from a working-class family. He did very well, reaching grammar school and university. For a short time he worked as a university lecturer in English, and then specialised in the teaching of English abroad. He did a 2-year tour in Tanzania before going to the Far East, where he held a position of great responsibility.

On examination he was extremely intense, never blinking and smiling only occasionally.

It was clear that he was ambitious, ruthless, very intolerant and drove himself continuously. His difficulties with authority figures were obvious and he said that he could only function when he was in charge. He consistently denied that he had any emotional troubles, even though his tension and anxiety were obvious. He was especially worried that the physicians at the hospital would prevent him from going abroad again. He only mentioned his wife at the second interview. He had married four years previously and said that the marriage was perfect. It was not surprising to hear that his wife was invalided home from the Far East with fainting, night sweats, headaches and vomiting attacks, which were found to be functional.

This patient was suffering from a severe anxiety state which had only become apparent in the previous 6 months and was connected with his excessive drinking (which he denied). Before this he had suffered from severe diarrhoea for 3 years which followed a genuine attack of dysentery. Clearly this was the way his emotions were able to show themselves as an admission of failure would be unthinkable for him. He was treated with valium 15 mg t.d.s. and was advised to go overseas again as soon as possible, the danger being that if he stayed in this country he would sooner or later become intensely depressed or his aggression would show itself openly despite his attempts to control it with alcohol.

STRESS FACTORS IN THE TROPICS

These have been adequately described in several papers, notably by Rowland Hill (1943) and McPherson (Lee and McPherson, 1948). They are of great importance in understanding the aetiology of psychiatric illness in European expatriates.

Heat and humidity. Studies carried out by Pepler (1964) show that efficiency is marginally affected at temperatures up to 21°C and severely impaired at temperatures over 26.7°C. The effect of heat is profound: it produces a sense of lassitude and apathy and pronounced memory loss which may be disturbing; sleep is difficult, and sexual activity low. Appetite is reduced. Humidity produces a sense of claustrophobia until 'acclimatisation' takes place. Clearly the loss of efficiency will be a serious blow to someone whose standards are inflexible. Mild depression is common among people who have been in the tropics for over 5 years.

Other climatic factors. These include the monotony of perpetually unchanging weather conditions. Lack of twilight, as the sun rises and sets quickly in the tropics, local insects which may terrify the newcomer, and the constant fear of tropical infection. It is safer to think before doing anything.

Work conditions. These are frequently full of problems, not only because of the effects of heat and humidity, but because of the vast number of petty frustrations of working with people of a different culture. There may be language difficulties and the worry of making a serious *faux pas*. Often local workers require constant supervision if the job is to be done to European standards. Frequently, excessive demands are made on the man on the spot by his superiors back home who do not understand the true difficulties of the situation. Isolation at work is another extremely stressful factor

Social factors. Tropical countries have different cultural norms from Europe, and boredom is a factor. Often, small groups of Europeans are huddled together and intrigue is common. So is drinking, although surprisingly alcoholism is less prevalent than is often imagined. Married women are the most at-risk group. They seldom choose to go abroad, but do so to avoid separation from their husbands. Work is not encouraged, even in one's own house, where it is accepted that servants do everything. There is lack of privacy, and also lack of communication, as the wife feels she cannot bother her husband with her own petty worries. If children are taken to the tropics, then the fear of disease becomes much more acute, but sending them home for schooling brings damaging separation. Libido is greatly decreased in humid conditions and this further adds to a wife's emotional stresses. One more factor often mentioned is the monotony of diet which has a predominance of starch.

Returning home. There is finally the problem, frequently financial, of eventual return to Europe. There is often the risk of unemployment, and this is getting worse with the contraction of European interests in the tropics.

Case history No. 4

Mrs W. Aged 28. British. Abroad $5\frac{1}{2}$ years—in Nigeria.

This lady was admitted to the Hospital for Tropical Diseases having been rushed to Britain from Nigeria with severe fainting attacks, numbness of both arms and continuous headaches for the previous 2 weeks, which she claimed were driving her insane. The history was as follows. She had been married for $5\frac{1}{2}$ years to an engineer. All that time she had been abroad. She came from a sheltered, middle-class, suburban background and had never been away from home before her marriage. She was very close to her family. When she went to Nigeria she made a reasonable

adaptation to life there but began to suffer from migraine which worsened during her stay. At the time of her return to Britain she had totally rejected the possibility of returning to Nigeria. She said that the people were false and two-faced and she had no friends. She complained that she could not talk to anyone and did not want to bother her husband with her petty worries. This had simmered for about a year before she finally went to the Company doctor, who was unsympathetic but gave her tryptizol. She did not take the tablets and began to be aggressive towards her baby girl, aged 3. She finally confessed to her husband that she felt suicidal, whereupon she was brought home to England.

In hospital her symptoms cleared fairly rapidly. Her husband showed enormous concern about her and revealed that he had decided to leave his career in Nigeria with some regret but felt that his wife was more important.

Mrs W. was taken on for limited supportive psychotherapy, during which many of the problems which had brought her home were discussed. She eventually decided that she would try to persuade her husband to return to Nigeria and would go with him herself but only for limited periods at a time. So she succeeded in making something of a compromise, and the symptoms did not return. This case illustrates fairly well the history of a girl of previously sound personality who succumbed to the strain of an isolated existence in an alien cultural environment.

SYMPTOMATOLOGY

Because of some degree of prior selection, people suffering from organic disease or from psychoses are rare. When psychosis occurs, it is typical of manic depressive psychosis or schizophrenia. Depression is a far commoner manifestation than mania. However, the incidence of neurotic behaviour patterns is extremely high. Three main syndromes are seen in Europeans:

Depression. This is a typical reactive depression and arises as a result of the patient's inflexible character and his relative intolerance to an extremely stressful situation and presents as follows:

Acute anxiety
Insomnia, frequently with difficulty in getting off to sleep and early morning waking
Appetite disturbance
Lassitude
Apathy
Forgetfulness
There may also be constipation, loss of weight and loss of libido.

Very often depression itself is not complained of but is covered up by a physical presentation: tiredness for no reason, which needs investigation; symptoms of abdominal pain and diarrhoea; very often sexual and gynaecological problems tend to be those presented to the doctor.

It is only later that the depression itself comes to light. In a recent study by the author (Wilson, 1973), 33.1 per cent of a sample of patients referred for psychiatric opinion were depressed and 55 per cent of those showed on personality testing severe obsessional personality traits such as ritual checking, intolerance of authority, resistance to change, etc. Depressive illness is far commoner among married men than any other group. In the same study it was noted that sexual problems are much commoner among single women.

Anxiety states. These are common among Europeans in the tropics: 14.6 per cent of patients referred for psychiatric opinion at the Hospital for Tropical Diseases in 1970–71 had anxiety states. This is usually the initial presentation of a much later depressive illness and the anxiety may be very intense. The typical picture is one of tension, preoccupation, forgetfulness, irritability, inability to concentrate, and various autonomic signs such as sweating, frequency of micturition and diarrhoea. Headaches are often found among women, but on the whole there seems to be no sexual difference in the symptoms. Usually in Europeans the anxiety is free-floating, but it is not unusual for it to become fixed to a particular part of the body which is then a source of extreme obsessional anxiety. This gives a hypochondriacal picture. The belief in the existence of a much feared tropical illness is very difficult to shake. Later on a true depressive picture usually becomes apparent. In obsessional people, the anxiety may be further complicated by florid obsessional symptoms frequently concerned with bowel habits, and imaginary alimentary companions! Rowland Hill in his 1943 study gives a 19 per cent incidence of hypochondriasis, but in the author's experience it is less common.

Hysterical manifestations. This term is so often misused that it really needs explanation. There are three types of hysterical manifestation which are all complicated unconscious defences for dealing with anxiety. In each case anxiety is denied by the patient and falls on the shoulders of friends, family, nurses or doctors, who then feel the emotion denied by the patient. This accounts for the extreme reactions seen when this type of illness is encountered by the medical profession. In all cases there is some sort of short-term gain to be had from hysterical behaviour: the so-called 'primary gain', which simply means that the patient has succeeded in dealing with the anxiety through his illness, and 'secondary gain', which is the advantage gained through the illness; firstly removing the patient from the source of stress, and secondly aiming to ensure continuance of love and support from friends and employers. To say that one wishes to give up one's job because one is not equal to it causes consternation, but to be 'ill' is quite acceptable, especially in a tropical setting.

1. *Conversion* is the commonest hysterical manifestation whereby conflicts are converted into physical symptoms. Symptoms are often symbolic of the problem to be solved but more often an actual physical illness is seized upon and the symptoms of that illness persist long after the original cause is removed, to the consternation of everyone.

2. *Dissociation*—much rarer but also seen. Here the patient removes himself from anxiety by cutting off the conscious element of his mind. This may be seen as a *partial dissociation*, such as amnesia, where the memory loss concerns only certain aspects of the patient's life; or *complete dissociation*, as in an hysterical fugue state where the patient appears stuporose for no reason. This also causes consternation among doctors.

3. *Acting out*—a much cruder and more child-like defence mechanism containing more obviously manipulative elements, but still unconscious, though it is often difficult to detect whether conscious exaggeration (malingering) has also occurred. In its extreme form it may be epileptiform in type or simply discoordinated and destructive. There is often amnesia for the event. Because of the embarrassment, an onlooker usually experiences extreme hostility or fear; some patients, by contrast, are anxiety-free. Others, however, do retain their anxiety. Contrary to popular belief, people suffering from the hysterical mechanisms of conversion and dissociation often tend to appear mature and capable. They are the typical stiff-upper-lip types who show little emotional reaction to stress until their breaking point comes, and this is usually sudden and unexpected. In tropical practice the nature of the symptomatology gives ample scope for hysterical manifestations. They are the second commonest presentation seen after depression and are usually based on an original bona fide infection. This clears up but the symptoms persist. In a series of psychiatric referrals at the Hospital for Tropical Diseases (Wilson, 1973) 27.8 per cent of the patients were

suffering from hysterical conversion symptoms. In contrast, only 1.3 per cent showed hysterical acting-out. Often it is difficult to distinguish between hysterical conversion symptoms and psychosomatic illness but in the latter an actual organic lesion is present though it may have a psychological basis.

Diarrhoea and abdominal pain are easily the commonest physical symptoms seen. They are invariably persistent and defy organic diagnosis. The patients are usually invalided home for investigation for medical, not psychiatric reasons; thus, there is considerable secondary gain. Removal from the source of stress, the tropics, and the avoidance of loss of face. Headaches (especially among married women), nausea and vomiting, faintness, dizziness and night sweating attacks (which are usually blamed on some non-specific tropical infection) are common. Parasthesiae are also commonly seen, and vary with the patient's cultural background. Among Europeans backache is frequent as are various symptoms of numbness, joint pains, tingling in the body, arms and legs, diplopia, feelings of extreme heat and extreme thirst, pains in the tongue, pains in the genitalia and also in the bladder.

Hysterical manifestations seem to be equally common among European men and women, but what at first appears hysterical may in fact be a depressive symptom. This is often the case with diarrhoea but examination of the patient's mental state and especially his attitude to his illness will provide the answer.

Neurotic manifestations of the depressive and hysterical type are easily the commonest psychiatric disease patterns seen in tropical practice, but of course other syndromes occur.

Case history No. 5

Mr G. Age 53. British. Abroad for 18 months in India in 1943 and not since.

This man was admitted to the Hospital for Tropical Diseases with a 28 year history of frequent episodes of thirst, generalised aches and pains, dizziness and malaise. These occurred about five times a year, lasting a week and causing him to take to his bed. Full investigations were carried out with negative results.

He was the son of a country parson and was one of four boys. He had a strict upbringing with no love from his parents. He was allowed to see his mother for an hour every evening and was sent away to preparatory school at the age of 7 and to public school after that. He had just qualified at Oxford when the Second World War broke out. He was commissioned in the Royal Air Force and sent to India as an instructor. He hated it and

was invalided home with amoebic dysentery after 18 months. After the war he qualified as a solicitor and did well. He was married at the age of 25 for 6 months after which his wife left him. Then at the age of 47 he married again. During the intervening time he had no girl friends and had always been painfully shy with the opposite sex. The patient was a quiet, charming person. He showed no emotion when talking and was always perfectly under control. He thought before he said anything. He was a markedly obsessional character, showing ritual patterns of behaviour including checking and tidying. His wife was a dominant, neurotic and aggressive woman who tended to control him. His mother was similar. It was interesting that it was he rather than his wife who nursed his mother during her last illness. His wife was most anxious that an organic diagnosis of his troubles should be made whereas he himself was not worried about this. He derived considerable gain from the symptoms in that he could take to his bed and escape from his work during the attacks. His wife also looked after him when he was ill. He himself showed no anxiety about his illness. His conversation consisted mainly of his obsessional ideas of discipline and control.

After the initial interview he urgently demanded another. He said he had carefully weighed up the interpretation of his illness in which it had been suggested that perhaps he was expressing some of his conflicts in a physical way. He strongly disagreed with this and launched into a long and angry legal tirade about the term 'obsessional' which had been mentioned. Although he tried to control himself he was very agitated. It transpired that his wife was a great deal more agitated about it than he was. Shortly after this he discharged himself.

This man's hysterical conversion symptoms which had started with an attack of amoebic dysentery which probably gave him similar symptoms had adequately succeeded in maintaining his defence mechanisms for a long time and it was only his wife's anger at being forced into looking after him that brought him to hospital.

Psychosomatic illness. This is generally accepted to mean physical illness, the course of which is profoundly influenced by psychological factors. It, too, is common in tropical practice. Of 151 patients referred to the author at the Hospital for Tropical Diseases in 1970–71 13.4 per cent had various forms of psychosomatic disease. People having difficulties in coming to terms with their feelings abound in the tropics. One of the ways of showing aggression subconsciously is through the body. Various skin conditions, asthma, peptic ulceration, and spastic colon are common examples. They are not more prevalent than they would be in the general population. It is often difficult to find the border-line between hysterical and psychosomatic illness.

Alcoholism. This is comparatively rare in comparison to its incidence amongst the endemic African population, but it occurs in about 5 per cent of referrals. Alcoholism is usually seen as a thinly disguised attempt to treat anxiety in a socially acceptable way. European community life in the tropics greatly favours heavy drinking and it is surprising that alcoholism is not more common.

A new problem has shown itself in the last 3 or 4 years: that of the young pilgrims who visit the Indian subcontinent in search of the 'truth', which is often sought through drugs. This is fortunately usually a temporary state of affairs and, like the wandering, is a phase in a personality crisis, which may need psychiatric help to resolve itself.

DIAGNOSIS

The diagnosis of psychiatric illness depends on two factors: (1) A good history, with exploration of possible stress factors: (2) assessment of the patient's mental state.

If these are used properly no psychiatric condition will be missed. It is very important to be sure the patient is not suffering from an undiagnosed organic illness, and if this is suspected it should be thoroughly investigated. There is considerable danger that once a patient has been labelled as suffering from psychiatric illness the diagnosis sticks and any other symptoms seen tend thereafter to be attributed to it. The importance of the history cannot be overestimated and good history-taking only comes with practice. Special care should be taken to ask about the patients' life style, his reactions to stress, his job, home and relationships, especially with wife or parents, and also about past illnesses. While doing this the doctor should be assessing the patient's mental state, his mood (is he depressed, flat, anxious?) and his speech, memory and orientation. If there is any suggestion of clouding of consciousness or of memory loss, especially for recent events, an organic state should be suspected which must be investigated.

The diagnosis of the various psychotic states is more difficult to make. There are many diagnostic criteria for the schizophrenic states which are adequately discussed in the psychiatric textbooks and it is unnecessary to repeat them here. However, the treatment of acutely psychotic behaviour does not necessarily need to wait for a firm diagnosis.

Depression may not present as such but may be covered by other symptoms and strenuously denied, especially in Asians and Africans and to some extent among upper-class Europeans. Nevertheless, the patient will always appear depressed or anxious and direct questioning will usually uncover the typical depressive symptomatology. Anxiety is frequently the first symptom and alcohol may be used to remove it.

Psychotic depression which cannot be attributed to stress factors or the patient's personality is very rare in Europeans in the tropics but may develop from a longstanding untreated reactive depression.

A sizeable number of depressed patients present with feelings of tiredness, apathy and general malaise sometimes complicated by more obviously physical symptoms such as headaches, pains or dizzy spells. Examination of the patient's mental state will show the depressive aetiology.

Hysterical manifestations. These are much more difficult to diagnose, and patients are often exhaustively and wastefully investigated because of the patient's insistence that he has a physical illness; all the same, thorough investigation is vital and physical illness should be suspected if hysterical symptoms appear in someone over 40 (Slater, 1965) with a previously good personality. Stress situations in the patient's past life may well have produced symptoms. Enquiries should also be made about the natural history of the symptoms and whether they were in any way connected with an initial infection or whether they first appeared at a time of stress. The mental state here will give the answer. The patient is usually not anxious or not anxious enough about persistent and serious symptoms. The patient is frequently supported by an over-anxious spouse who usually worries the doctor by persisting in asking for more to be done for the sick relative; often one finds that it is not the sufferer himself who looks for help but he has been persuaded to come by well-meaning friends. It is as well to look for primary and secondary gain from the illness and to observe the reactions of the patient and those around him.

The differential diagnosis of hysterical illness involves almost every type of disease but the symbolic nature of the hysterical symptoms should be noted. If neurological in type, they never show the true neurological distribution which one would expect. The symptomatology frequently changes and is seldom constant. Treatment of any type may temporarily relieve the symptoms which then return in a different form. A patient may also be very angry if his illness is not supported by the doctor, and he will frequently manipulate the situation by spreading stories and trying to split the loyalties of those who surround him, especially other patients in hospital.

TREATMENT

General principles

The same general rules apply when treating people of all races. The two main approaches to treatment in psychiatry are the physical approach using drugs, or physically oriented procedures like electroconvulsive therapy or surgery, and the psychotherapeutic approach which aims to give support, alleviate adverse social factors, and where possible increase the amount of insight of the patient into the reasons for and nature of the illness. Clearly, use of the latter approach may be seriously limited by language and cultural barriers. In practice the two are usually combined.

Organic states

The investigation and treatment of the underlying physical cause is of the first importance. This cannot be overstressed. If this is not done, the patient's chances of survival will be minimal. The physical results of an acute confusional state must be treated. Dehydration is the most important result especially in a tropical setting. Food may also be refused, and nursing difficulties be severe. Intravenous fluids are indicated and vitamins given through a drip. Avitaminosis is often a potent factor, especially in the alcoholic confusional states so common in Africans. Retention of urine may also worsen the confusional state, and this should be corrected. If possible the patient should be nursed in a side room and relatives should be actively encouraged to stay with him. There is a temptation to over-sedate confused patients because of the trouble they cause, but this should be resisted. Chlorpromazine 50–250 mg daily should be sufficient. In older people promazine (Sparine) 50–100 mg or valium 10 mg may be preferable. Barbiturates should always be avoided.

Acute psychotic states

Schizophrenia and the schizophreniform psychoses are best treated by admission to hospital followed by regular drug treatment which may have to be maintained for a considerable time to prevent relapse. The phenothiazine group of drugs are especially useful in controlling symptoms. Those most commonly prescribed are chlorpromazine (Largactil) 50–250 mg q.d.s., trifluoperazine (Stelazine) 2–10 mg t.d.s., thioridazine (Melleril) 25–200 mg t.d.s. All these drugs are complicated by parkinsonian side effects and should be combined with antiparkinsonian drugs such as Artane (4 mg t.d.s.) or Disipal (50 mg t.d.s.) if used for long periods. Hypotension and jaundice of an obstructive type may appear. The jaundice clears when drug therapy is stopped. Alternatively, haloperidol 1.5–4.5 mg t.d.s. may be used.

Acute mania is usually controlled by large doses of phenothiazines; doses in the region of 500 mg of Largactil t.d.s. are realistic. Subsequently lithium carbonate in a dose of 250–500 mg t.d.s. may reduce relapses. Care should be taken to avoid overdosage, which produces renal damage. The first signs are usually tremor, pallor and abdominal pain. To avoid these problems lithium carbonate should never be given without regular blood lithium levels being taken. These should not exceed 1.3 mEq/litre. The dangers of dehydration in tropical conditions should not be overlooked.

Neuroses

Depression. The condition most commonly encountered by the practitioner in the tropics is depression in its various forms and it requires urgent treatment. It may present in any of the ways already mentioned and very occasionally may be serious enough for suicide to be a risk. In practice, suicide attempts are very rare in the tropics and the depressive illnesses most commonly seen are reactions to environmental stress rather than any psychotic process in action.

Many authorities do not accept the separate aetiologies of the various types of depression, viz. psychotic or reactive, but consider that depression represents a continuous scale and the differences are only a matter of degree. When the diagnosis is made, treatment should be instituted at once on the following guide-lines:

1. Simple psychotherapy. The patient may well find the symptoms intolerable and re-assurance from the doctor is vital. Too often patients are told to 'pull their socks up'. Of course they would if they could.
2. Social factors. Although the action of choice is to keep the patient in his environment, it may be necessary to remove him from the source of stress if the depression is bad, and this may involve sending him

back to his home country for a period of rest, or admitting him locally to hospital if this is feasible.

3. Symptomatic drugs to correct sleep and relieve anxiety.
4. Antidepressant drugs for the specific treatment of depression.

There are two main groups of antidepressant drugs: the tricyclic group and monoamine-oxidase inhibitors (MAOIs).

1. TRICYCLIC GROUP

Imipramine (Tofranil). Dosage 25 mg t.d.s. up to a maximum of 225 mg in 24 hours. It is usually thought best to increase the dose gradually. There is little antidepressant effect for the first 14–21 days but the sedative effects are noticed immediately. Doses of up to 50 mg at night may be given to help sleep, and if the patient is a poor tablet-taker it is probably better to give him the whole daily dose when he goes to bed. Many side effects have been reported and it is wise to warn the patient about these—dryness of the mouth, sweating, dizziness due to postural hypotension, skin rashes and urinary retention, and, rarely, cardiac arrythmias, parkinsonian symptoms and confusion in some elderly patients; agranulocytosis has occasionally been reported.

Amitriptyline (Tryptizol). Dosage 25 mg t.d.s. up to 75 mg t.d.s. Has more of a sedative effect but few side effects.

Trimipramine (Surmontil). Dosage 50 mg b.d. also has a marked sedative effect and can be given at night.

Nortriptyline (Aventyl). Dosage 10–50 mg t.d.s. This drug, together with protriptyline (Concordin) dosage 5–20 mg t.d.s., tends to have much less sedative effects but has an antidepressant effect in 10–15 days.

2. MONOAMINE OXIDASE INHIBITORS (MAOIS)

Common ones include *phenelzine* (*Nardil*) dosage 15 mg t.d.s., *isocarboxazid* (*Marplan*) dosage 10 mg t.d.s., and *tranylcypromine* (*Parnate*) dosage 10 mg t.d.s. All take on average 10–14 days to act but Parnate, which has the most side effects, acts more quickly.

Foods containing tyramine should be avoided by patients on MAOIs (beef extract, cheese, beer, bananas, and some rich meats).

It is unwise to give opiates to patients on MAOIs, and it used to be thought risky to mix tricyclic antidepressants with MAOIs but encouraging results have lately been reported in severe anxiety states especially of the phobic variety and obsessional illnesses when small doses of the two drugs are mixed. The MAOI is given in the day and the tricyclic antidepressant at night. This should only be done when adequate medical supervision is available (Sargant and Dally, 1962; Kelly, 1970; Winston, 1971).

Side effects of MAOIs include hypertensive crises with severe headaches and possible subarachnoid haemorrhages which are always precipitated by the eating of tyramine-containing substances. It is worth pointing out that these side effects are rare and only occur in 1 in 100 patients even if diet is not strictly adhered to. Tricyclic antidepressants do not, however, carry these risks and are in practice easier to use.

Because of the reactive nature of most depressive illness in the tropics, the importance of support and communication cannot be overstressed. A chance of discussion and a feeling that somebody understands is the mainstay of treatment, and the lift given by antidepressants will help considerably. If anxiety is the main problem then MAOIs are very effective and if necessary can be combined with sedative drugs such as chlordiazepoxide (Librium) dosage 10–20 mg t.d.s. or diazepam (Valium) dosage 5–15 mg t.d.s. The patient's progress should be carefully watched and frequent visits to the doctor are indicated. Relatives and employers can also help by their understanding of the stress factors which led to the illness.

Hysterical illness. As most of these patients present in tropical practice with persistent symptoms requiring investigation, the onus of treatment and management falls on the investigating hospital rather than on the doctor in the field. Having established the nature of the illness one has to decide whether it is treatable. Generally speaking, the younger the patient the more amenable to treatment. Older people, especially women, who may have many years' history of incurable symptoms are very resistant to treatment and it is unlikely that they will be able to face the true nature of their illness (see Case History No. 5). In older people hysterical symptoms are very often complicated by depression which should be treated since treatment may do something to alleviate some of the symptoms. The principles of treatment of all races with hysterical illness are the same, but in practice Africans and Asians prove more resistant to treatment than do Europeans.

The only real treatment of hysterical defence mechanisms is psychotherapy. The aim is not only to remove the symptoms, which almost always occurs if the patient wishes to cooperate, but also to bring about changes in the way the patient solves his problems. The first step is to try to understand the symptoms in the light of the patient's relationships with others and the stress of his life style. This is extremely important and relevant in a tropical setting. The next stage is to set about giving him insight into his behaviour and especially the meaning of his symptoms. There will be considerable anger with the therapist followed by a great deal of dependence on the therapist and attempts to manipulate him. These too must be resisted gently, understood and interpreted. The patient may see that anger itself is not as destructive as his efforts to avoid it. If the treatment goes well the patient will be cured of his original symptoms and one hopes to enable him to deal with his problems in a more mature way. The average time of treatment varies considerably, from a few weeks to several years, and relapses are common. Usually psychotherapy can only be carried out in a very superficial form by a doctor practising in the tropics and is really the province of the psychotherapist. Unfortunately it is frequently difficult for expatriates to stay long enough in their home country for treatment to be effective but it has been found that minimal treatment of the supportive variety, say 10 sessions, frequently helps to alleviate the symptoms and enables some sort of adaptation to take place.

In treating Africans, many more difficulties are encountered. Hysterical acting out is of course far more acceptable in simple, rural society and is adequately dealt with by magical remedies. However, in the towns, or in other alien cultural environments, this type of behaviour is unacceptable and is rapidly referred to the doctor. Psychotherapy, as we understand it, is extremely difficult, and suggestion, sedative drugs and rehabilitation are the only answers. In African students studying in the West, conversion symptoms are far commoner. These are frequently complicated by depression which responds very readily to tricyclic antidepressants. The physical symptoms, however, are defence mechanisms to deal with an impossible situation. Often the patient is under pressure from home to pass his examinations but cannot face the fact that he may fail. The only escape is through illness, and he will not lightly give up his symptoms. Supportive psychotherapy which aims to alter marginally the social situation by arranging special tuition or deferring examinations offers the best hope of success. A compromise situation is usually reached where the symptoms persist in

an attenuated form, so that the student is able to return to work in spite of the illness, and honour is satisfied (see Case History No. 1). Loneliness is another factor which can be dealt with. Because of the African method of dealing with emotion by internalising it, interpretative psychotherapy is usually valueless even in highly educated Africans. Drugs, when used, should be given with full authority and the strongest suggestion that they will work. African cultures all place great stress on the supernatural, even when overlaid with Western ideals. This can often be exploited to medical advantage.

Similar rules apply to Asians, who, in fact, are less at risk because of their strong family ties, especially when in the West. Language difficulties are often an even bigger problem, and when physical symptoms occur they are more florid and more intractable than in Africans. Often the answer here lies in an alteration of the social situation. Women from India and Pakistan seem to show many more gross hysterical symptoms than do Negro women, and are almost always caught in an impossible social situation. Indian women are most reluctant to discuss emotional problems for fear of bringing dishonour on the husband and family. Amongst Arabs, especially of the professional classes, phobic or fixed anxiety and hypochondriacal symptom patterns are common. Good results may be obtained with MAOIs. Again, absolute faith in the doctor is necessary for the best results.

PROPHYLAXIS

This is a very important and urgent aspect of psychiatry in the tropics.

Europeans in the tropics

All authorities agree that the breakdown rate among Europeans in the tropics is very high. In fact, recognised psychological illness accounts for only a minority of causes of invaliding home. Most people are sent home with physical symptoms which need investigation. These are usually found to have psychological causes, and often, a past history of psychiatric disturbance is found. In Wilson's (1973) study at the Hospital for Tropical Diseases, of a total of 208 consecutive admissions for all reasons, 31.8 per cent had a recognisable psychiatric illness. In addition, 13.4 per cent had psychosomatic conditions; a further 17.8 per cent had personality traits serious enough for future breakdown to be likely; 37 per cent were psychiatrically normal. This does not represent a cross-section of British people sent abroad, of course, only a minority who are investigated for medical conditions. More women are referred for psychiatric treatment than men. This is in line with the findings of psychiatric morbidity in Europe, where 66 per cent of psychiatric patients are women. Young married women are the most illness-prone group, followed by older married men. There is a high incidence of obsessional personality traits among those who break down. Some method of identification of these people is clearly needed. The Middlesex Hospital questionnaire (Crown and Crisp, 1966) is especially valuable in this respect. It gives a reliable measure of obsessional traits and also of depression and anxiety, which can be checked by clinical examination. Perhaps routine use of a questionnaire of this type in screening men and women for service abroad would help to identify those most likely to break down under tropical conditions. These people could then be prepared for life in the tropics and warned about the physical and psychological pitfalls, especially those of non-communication at home and at work. Psychiatric illness of all sorts can be minimised if treated early by the doctor on the spot. Doctors working in the tropics should have a good working knowledge of the common psychiatric illnesses seen in ex-patriates. Simple supportive measures given early may avoid the need for sending the patient home later.

Any steps which help to increase community life and cut down isolation are of primary importance. Women especially should be encouraged to work, where this is possible. Leave should be frequent.

Asians and Africans in Europe

Similar problems of isolation and cultural differences exist amongst Africans and Asians in an alien environment, but more important here is a proper preparation for them before they reach the West, and a thorough understanding of their problems once they arrive. Among these two racial groups more highly trained doctors and social workers are required. With them communication would be less of a barrier and they would be fully conversant with cultural patterns. Perhaps a more thorough understanding of the European language required for their studies would be a help to students. Young Asian married women, who tend to be the most disturbed group of all, could be greatly helped by the setting up of proper community centres, some by trained social workers.

REFERENCES

CAMERON, J. (1949) *J. ment. Sci.*, **95**, 133.

CILENTO, R. W. (1933) *Aust. med. J.*, 421.

COOK, SIR ALBERT (1945) See *Stitt's Tropical Diseases*, 7th edn, p. 1706. London: H. K. Lewis.

CROWN, S. and CRISP, A. H. (1966) *Br. J. Psychiat.*, **112**, 917.

GEIL, R. and VAN LUIJK, J. N. (1969) *Br. J. Psychiat.*, **115**, 149.

GERMAN, G. A. (1972) In *Medicine in a Tropical Environment*, ed. Shaper, A. G., Kibukamusoke, J. W. and Hutt, M. S. R. London: British Medical Assoc.

GERMAN, G. A. and ARYA, O. P. (1969) *Br. J. Psychiat.*, **115**, 1323.

GOLDBERG, D. P., EASTWOOD, M. R., KEDWARD, H. B. and SHEPHERD, M. (1970) *Br. J. prev. soc. Med.*, **24**, 18.

HELSBORG, H. C. (1958) *Acta psychiat. neurol. scand.*, **33**, 303.

HERTZBERG, I. M. (1964) *African Students in English Universities*. First International Congress of Social Psychiatry.

HILL, T. R. (1934) *Lancet*, **1**, 332.

KELLY, D. (1970) *Br. J. Psychiat.*, **116**, 387.

KIDD, C. B. and CALDBECK-MEENAN, J. (1966) *Br. J. Psychiat.*, **112**, 57.

LAMBO, T. A. (1968) In *Deuxième Colloque Africain de Psychiatrie, Association Universitaire pour le Développement de l'Enseignement et de la Culture en Afrique et à Madagascar*. Paris.

LAMONT, A. and BLIGNAULT, W. J. (1953) *S. Afr. med. J.*, **27**, 637.

LEE, D. H. K. and McPHERSON, R. K. (1948) *J. appl. Physiol.*, **1**, 60.

LEIGHTON, A. M., LAMBO, T. A., HUGHES, C. C., LEIGHTON, D.C., MURPHY, J. M. and MACKLIN, D. B. (1963) *Psychiatric Disorder Among the Yoruba*. Ithaca, N.Y.: Cornell Univ. Press.

MANSON-BAHR, SIR PHILIP (1940) *A Textbook of Tropical Diseases*. London: Cassell.

MARTIN, F., BROTHERSTON, J. H. and CHAVE, S. P. (1957) *Br. J. prev. soc. Med.*, **11**, 196.

OSUNOKUN, B. O., BADEMOSI, O., OGUNREMI, K. and WRIGHT, S. G. (1972). *Archs Neurol. Psychiat., Chicago*, **27**, 7.

PEARSON, K. and PENNELL, E. H. (1938) *Hospitals*, **12**, 42.

PEMBERTON, J. (1951) *Lancet*, **1**, 224.

PEPLER, R. D. (1964) In *Heat Stress and Heat Disorders*, ed. Leithhead, C. S. and Lind, A. R. London: Cassell.

SARGANT, W. and DAVEY, P. (1962) *Br. med. J.*, **1**, 6.

SHEPHERD, M., COOPER, B., BROWN, A. C. and KALTON, G. W. (1966) *Psychiatric Illness in General Practice.* Oxford Univ. Press.

SHEPHERD, M., DAVIES, B. and CULPAN, R. (1960) *Acta psychiat. neurol. scand.*, **35**, 518.

SLATER, E. (1965) *Br. med. J.*, **1**, 1395.

WILSON, C. R. M. (1973) *A Study of Psychiatric Morbidity in the Hospital for Tropical Diseases, London.* Unpublished.

WINSTON, F. (1971) *Br. J. Psychiat.*, **118**, 301.

Index

2R

Tetracycline
 in balantidiasis, 132
 in brucellosis, 298
 in cholera, 265, 266
 in intestinal amoebiasis, 120, 121
 in tropical sprue, 450
Tetramisole in ascariasis, 160
Thalassaemia, 495–498
 β 474, 496
 β major, 496
 β minor, 497
 α 474, 497
 α major, 498
 α minor, 498
 δ 499
 treatment, all forms, 502
 associated conditions, 499–500
 genetics, 474–483
  chromosome, 475–477
  code, 477–479
  storage of information, 477
 haemoglobins, 471–474
 and haemoglobin variants, interaction, 500–501
 haemoglobin C, 501
  treatment, 501
 haemoglobin D, 501
  treatment, 501
 haemoglobin E, 501
  treatment, 501
 sickle-cell, 486, 501
 syndromes, 485–503
Thiabendazole
 in ancylostomiasis, 168
 in capillariasis, 171
 in creeping eruption, 168
 in strongyloidiasis, 163
 in toxocariasis, 165
 in trichinosis, 170
 in trichuriasis, 170
Thiacetazone
 in abdominal tuberculosis, 452
 in leprosy, 308
Thiambutosine in leprosy, 308
Thiamine deficiency, 426–429
 in alcoholic heart disease, 568
 causing peripheral neuropathy, 435
 see also Beri-beri
Thiourea compounds in leprosy, 308
Tick-borne fever, African, 532
Tinea corporis, 374
 differential diagnosis from leprosy, 307
Tinea cruris, 374
Tinea favosa, 375
Tinea imbricata, 374–375
Tinea pedis, 373–374
Tinea versicolor, 374
Tixanthone in schistosomiasis, 209
Tofranil as antidepressant, 590
Torulosis, 378
Toxocara canis, 163
 characteristics and life cycle, 163–164
Toxocara cati, 163

characteristics and life cycle, 163–164
Toxocariasis, 163–165
 aetiology, 163–164
 clinical features, 164
 definition, 163
 diagnosis, 164–165
 epidemiology, 164
 pathology, 164
 prognosis, 165
 treatment, 165
Toxoplasma gondii
 characteristics, 125
 development cycles in different hosts, 126
 distribution, 125–126
 transmission, 126–127
Toxoplasmosis, 125–129
 acquired infection, 127
 congenital, 127–128
 diagnosis, 128–129
  Sabin-Feldman dye test, 128
  serology, 128–129
 disease in man, 127
 distribution, 125–126
 ocular, 127
 in pregnancy, management, 128
 Siim's disease, 127
 transmission, 126–127
 treatment, 128
Trachoma
 and inclusion conjunctivitis, 348–349
  clinical features, 349
  treatment, 349
Tranylcypromine as antidepressant, 590
Tremor, in African human trypanosomiasis, 83
Treponema cerateum, 355
Treponema pallidum, 356 *et seq.*
Treponema pertenne, 355 *et seq.*
Triacetoleandomycin in granuloma inguinale, 388
Triatoma rubrofasciata, 91
Triatominae, vectors of South American trypanoso-
 miasis, 93
Trichinella spiralis, characteristics, 169
Trichinosis, 169–170
 diagnosis, 170
 symptoms, 169–170
 treatment, 170
Trichomycosis axillaris, 375
Trichophyton spp., 374, 376
Trichophytosis, 533
Trichostrongyliasis, 168
Trichostrongylus, 168
Trichuriasis, 170
Trichuris trichuria, 170
Trichomonas hominis, 131
Trichomonas tenax, 131
Tricuspid incompetence in endomyocardial fibrosis,
 560
Trimelarsan, in African human trypanosomiasis, 88
Trimelarsan, in onchocerciasis, 240
Trimipramine as antidepressant, 590
Tropical sprue, 448–451
 aetiology, 448

Printed in Great Britain by T. & A. CONSTABLE LTD., Edinburgh